Review of ORTHOPAEDICS

Review of ORTHOPAEDICS

FIFTH EDITION

Mark D. Miller, MD
Professor, Department of Orthopaedic Surgery
Head, Division of Sports Medicine
University of Virginia
Charlottesville, Virginia
Team Physician
James Madison University
Harrisonburg, Virginia

Associate Editor-in-Chief
Jennifer A. Hart, MPAS, PA-C
Physician Assistant, Department of Orthopaedic Surgery
University of Virginia
Charlottesville, Virginia

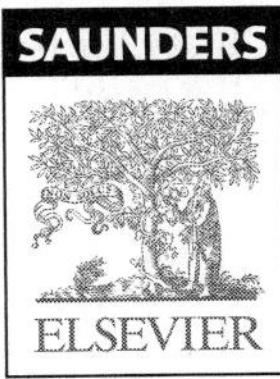

SAUNDERS
ELSEVIER

1600 John F. Kennedy Blvd.
Ste 1800
Philadelphia, PA 19103-2899

REVIEW OF ORTHOPAEDICS, 5th Edition ISBN: 978-1-4160-4093-4

Notice

Knowledge and best practice in this field are constantly changing. As new research and experience broaden our knowledge, changes in practice, treatment, and drug therapy may become necessary or appropriate. Readers are advised to check the most current information provided (i) on procedures featured or (ii) by the manufacturer of each product to be administered to verify the recommended dose or formula, the method and duration of administration, and contraindications. It is the responsibility of the practitioner, relying on their own experience and knowledge of the patient, to make diagnoses, to determine dosages and the best treatment for each individual patient, and to take all appropriate safety precautions. To the fullest extent of the law, neither the Publisher nor the Editors assume any liability for any injury and/or damage to persons or property arising out of or related to any use of the material contained in this book.

The Publisher

Library of Congress Cataloging-in-Publication Data

Review of orthopaedics / [edited by] Mark D. Miller.—5th ed.
p. ; cm.
Includes bibliographical references and index.
ISBN: 978-1-4160-4093-4
1. Orthopedics—Outlines, syllabi, etc. I. Miller, Mark D.
[DNLM: 1. Bone Diseases—Outlines. 2. Joint Diseases—Outlines. 3. Orthopedic Procedures—Outlines. WE 18.2 R454 2008]
RD731.R44 2008
616.7—dc22 2007026512

Publishing Director: Kimberly Murphy
Developmental Editor: Adrianne Brigido
Publishing Services Manager: Tina Rebane
Project Manager: Amy Norwitz
Design Direction: Louis Forgione

Printed in the United States of America

Last digit is the print number: 9 8 7 6 5 4 3 2 1

To my supportive and loving family—Thank you for allowing me to pursue my passion.
To all of the residents that I have had the pleasure of teaching—Continue to learn, prepare, and care!
To all of the patients that I have had the honor of caring for, either directly or indirectly—Thank you!
To the Great Physician—I remain your humble servant.

Contributors

Joshua A. Baumfeld, MD
Assistant Professor, Department of Orthopaedic Surgery
Lahey Clinic
Boston University
Peabody, Massachusetts
Sports Medicine

Judith Baumhauer, MD
Associate Chair of Academic Affairs
Department of Orthopaedic Surgery
Professor, Division of Foot and Ankle Surgery
Strong Foot and Ankle Institute
University of Rochester Medical School
Rochester, New York
Disorders of the Foot and Ankle

Mark R. Brinker, MD
Director, Acute and Reconstructive Trauma
Fondren Orthopedic Group
Texas Orthopedic Hospital
Houston, Texas
Clinical Professor, Department of Orthopaedic Surgery
Tulane University School of Medicine
New Orleans, Louisiana
Clinical Professor, Department of Orthopaedic Surgery
Baylor College of Medicine
Houston, Texas
Basic Sciences

Lance M. Brunton, MD
Chief Resident, Department of Orthopaedic Surgery
University of Virginia Health System
Charlottesville, Virginia
Hand, Upper Extremity, and Microvascular Surgery

A. Bobby Chhabra, MD
Associate Professor, Department of Orthopaedic Surgery
Division Head, Hand and Upper Extremity Surgery
University of Virginia Health System
Charlottesville, Virginia
Hand, Upper Extremity, and Microvascular Surgery

Luke S. Choi, MD
Resident, Department of Orthopaedic Surgery
University of Virginia
Charlottesville, Virginia
Tables 3–10, 9–6, 9–7, 9–8, 9–9, 9–10

Matthew R. Craig, MD
Instructor, Department of Orthopaedic Surgery
University of Minnesota
Minneapolis, Minnesota
Trauma Fellow, Regions Hospital
St. Paul, Minnesota
Trauma

Marc M. DeHart, MD
Clinical Assistant Professor, Department of Orthopaedics
University of Texas Health Sciences Center at San Antonio
San Antonio, Texas
Texas Orthopedics
Austin, Texas
Principles of Practice and Statistics

Deborah A. Frassica, MD
Associate Professor, Department of Radiation Oncology and Molecular Radiation Sciences
The Johns Hopkins University
Baltimore, Maryland
Orthopaedic Pathology

Frank J. Frassica, MD
Robert A. Robinson Professor of Orthopaedic Surgery and Oncology
Chair, Department of Orthopaedic Surgery
The Johns Hopkins University
Baltimore, Maryland
Orthopaedic Pathology

Brian D. Giordano, MD
Resident, Department of Orthopaedic Surgery
University of Rochester
Rochester, New York
Disorders of the Foot and Ankle

S. Raymond Golish, MD, PhD
Resident, Department of Orthopaedic Surgery
University of Virginia
Charlottesville, Virginia
Principles of Practice and Statistics

Frank A. Gottschalk, MD
Professor, Department of Orthopaedic Surgery
University of Texas Southwestern Medical Center at Dallas
Dallas, Texas
Rehabilitation: Gait, Amputations, Prostheses, Orthoses, and Neurologic Injury

Bradley P. Graw, MD
Chief Resident, Department of Orthopaedic Surgery
Georgetown University Hospital
Washington, DC
Spine

Jennifer A. Hart, MPAS, PA-C
Physician Assistant, Department of Orthopaedic Surgery
University of Virginia
Charlottesville, Virginia
Sports Medicine

William C. Lauerman, MD
Professor, Department of Orthopaedic Surgery
Georgetown University Hospital
Washington, DC
Spine

Edward F. McCarthy, MD
Professor, Departments of Pathology and Orthopaedic Surgery
The Johns Hopkins University
Baltimore, Maryland
Orthopaedic Pathology

Edward J. McPherson, MD, FACS
Director, Department of Orthopedic Surgery
California Hospital Medical Center
Los Angeles, California
Director and Founder
L.A. Orthopedic Institute
Los Angeles, California
Adult Reconstruction

Todd A. Milbrandt, MD
Assistant Professor, Department of Orthopaedic Surgery
Shriners Hospital for Children and the University of Kentucky
Lexington, Kentucky
Pediatric Orthopaedics
Trauma

Mark D. Miller, MD
Professor, Department of Orthopaedic Surgery
Head, Division of Sports Medicine
University of Virginia
Charlottesville, Virginia
Team Physician
James Madison University
Harrisonburg, Virginia
Sports Medicine

Daniel P. O'Connor, MD
Director, Joe W. King Orthopedic Institute
Houston, Texas
Basic Sciences

William M. Ricci, MD
Associate Professor
Chief, Orthopedic Trauma
Director, Clinical Operations
Washington University Orthopedics
Washington University School of Medicine
St. Louis, Missouri
Trauma

E. Greer Richardson, MD
Professor, Department of Orthopaedic Surgery
University of Tennessee-Campbell Clinic
Co-Director, Campbell Clinic Foot and Ankle Surgery Fellowship
Memphis, Tennessee
Disorders of the Foot and Ankle

Gregory J. Roehrig, MD
Chief Resident, Department of Orthopaedic Surgery
University of Rochester
Rochester, New York
Disorders of the Foot and Ankle

Franklin D. Shuler, MD, PhD
Director, Orthopaedic Research
Director, Molecular Orthopaedics Laboratory
Assistant Professor, Division of Orthopaedic Trauma
Department of Orthopaedics
West Virginia University
Morgantown, West Virginia
Anatomy

James P. Stannard, MD
Professor, Department of Surgery
Associate Director, Orthopaedic Surgery
Chief, Orthopaedic Trauma
Orthopaedic Trauma Fellowship Director
University of Alabama at Birmingham
Birmingham, Alabama
Trauma

Daniel J. Sucato, MD
Associate Professor, Department of Orthopaedic Surgery
Texas Scottish Rite Hospital for Children and University of Texas Southwest Medical Center
Dallas, Texas
Pediatric Orthopaedics
Trauma

David A. Volgas, MD
Associate Professor, Department of Orthopaedic Surgery
Orthopaedic Residency Director
University of Alabama at Birmingham
Birmingham, Alabama
Trauma

Preface

Vigorous writing is concise. A sentence should contain no unnecessary words, a paragraph no unnecessary sentences, for the same reason that a drawing should have no unnecessary lines and a machine no unnecessary parts. This requires not that the writer make all his sentences short, or that he avoid all detail and treat his subjects only in outline, but that every word tell.

William Strunk Jr., *Elements of Style*, 1919

Fifth edition—wow! When I was a resident, I thought that any orthopaedic textbook that was in its fifth edition meant that the original author had long since retired, and was likely pushing up daisies. Well, I'm happy to report that I am neither, and I hope to publish five more editions of this popular book before I retire.

So. . .what's new for *Review 5?* Is it just a rehash of previous editions? The answer is a resounding **NO!** Several chapters have had extensive revisions—all for the better. These include the Sports Medicine, Hand, Trauma, and Principles of Practice chapters. The Sports Medicine chapter (Chapter 4) benefited from the comprehensive review of the literature that we did to help prepare for the Subspecialty Examination in Sports Medicine that was offered for the first time in November 2007. The inclusion of color arthroscopic photos in the book enhances this topic. The Hand chapter (Chapter 7) was extensively revised by my partner and close friend, Dr. Bobby Chhabra, who worked with an aspiring hand surgeon/chief resident, Dr. Lance Brunton, to put together what may well be the best chapter ever written in the *Review* series! The Trauma chapter (Chapter 11) was updated extensively as well, and the trauma tables have been restored in this edition. In addition, both adult and pediatric trauma tables are included in a perforated Appendix that the user can remove and place in a binder. The Principles of Practice chapter (Chapter 12) benefited hugely from two very energetic authors with extensive experience and research interests in these difficult topic areas.

All of the chapters have been thoroughly updated and revised, with an emphasis on getting to *the bottom line*. Additionally, Elsevier has developed a companion website with full-text search capability and link-through to full text articles in PubMed and Cross Ref for all of the references in each chapter.

I would be remiss if I did not recognize the exhaustive efforts of my Associate Editor-in-Chief, Jennifer A. Hart, PAC-C, who did an amazing job in helping put this fifth edition of *Review of Orthopaedics* together.

I have been truly blessed that the *Review* text, and my *Review* Course, have been hugely successful. It is in part because of our fervent passion to be vigorous and concise, but it is also in large part because of the wonderful associates that I have had the honor and pleasure to work with. Orthopaedic education really is a lifelong process—let us help you continue in that process!

Mark Miller

Contents

Color Plates

Knee Arthroscopy

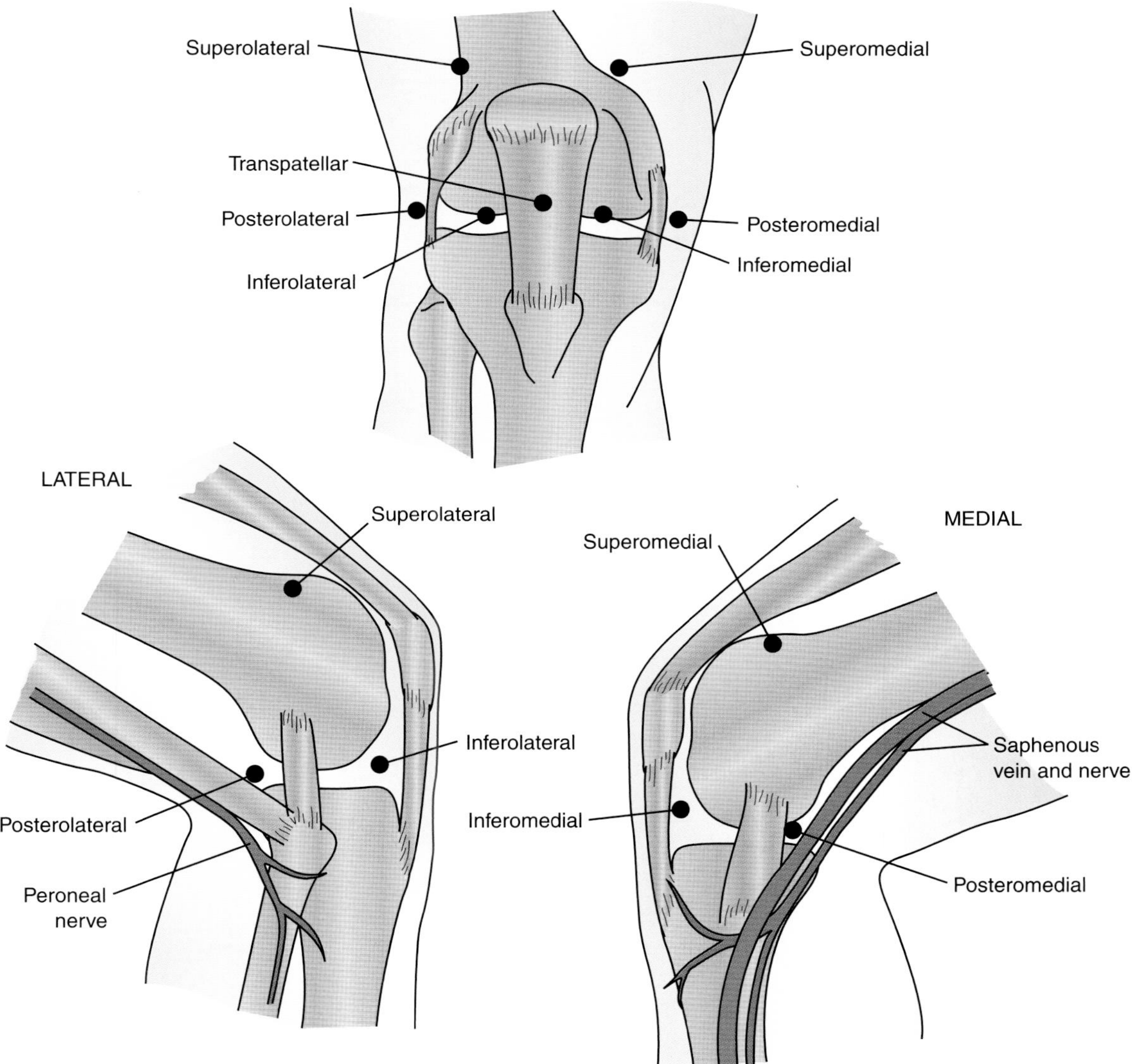

Knee arthroscopy portals*

*From Miller MD, Chhabra AB, Hurwitz SR, Mihalko WM, Shen FH: Orthopaedic Surgical Approaches. Philadelphia, WB Saunders, 2008.

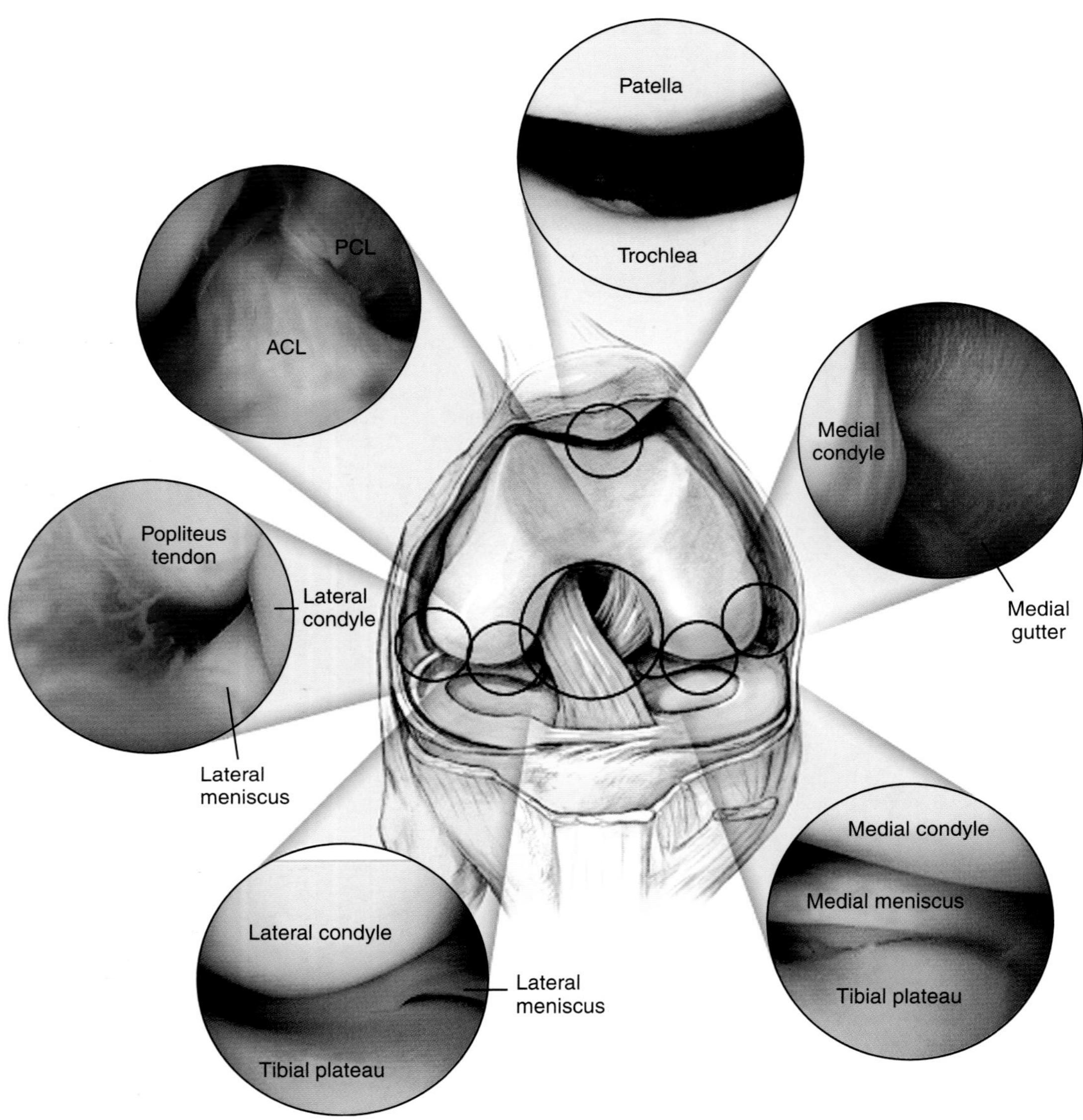

Knee arthroscopy overview*

ACL, anterior cruciate ligament; PCL, posterior cruciate ligament

*From Miller MD, Chhabra AB, Hurwitz SR, Mihalko WM, Shen FH: Orthopaedic Surgical Approaches. Philadelphia, WB Saunders, 2008.

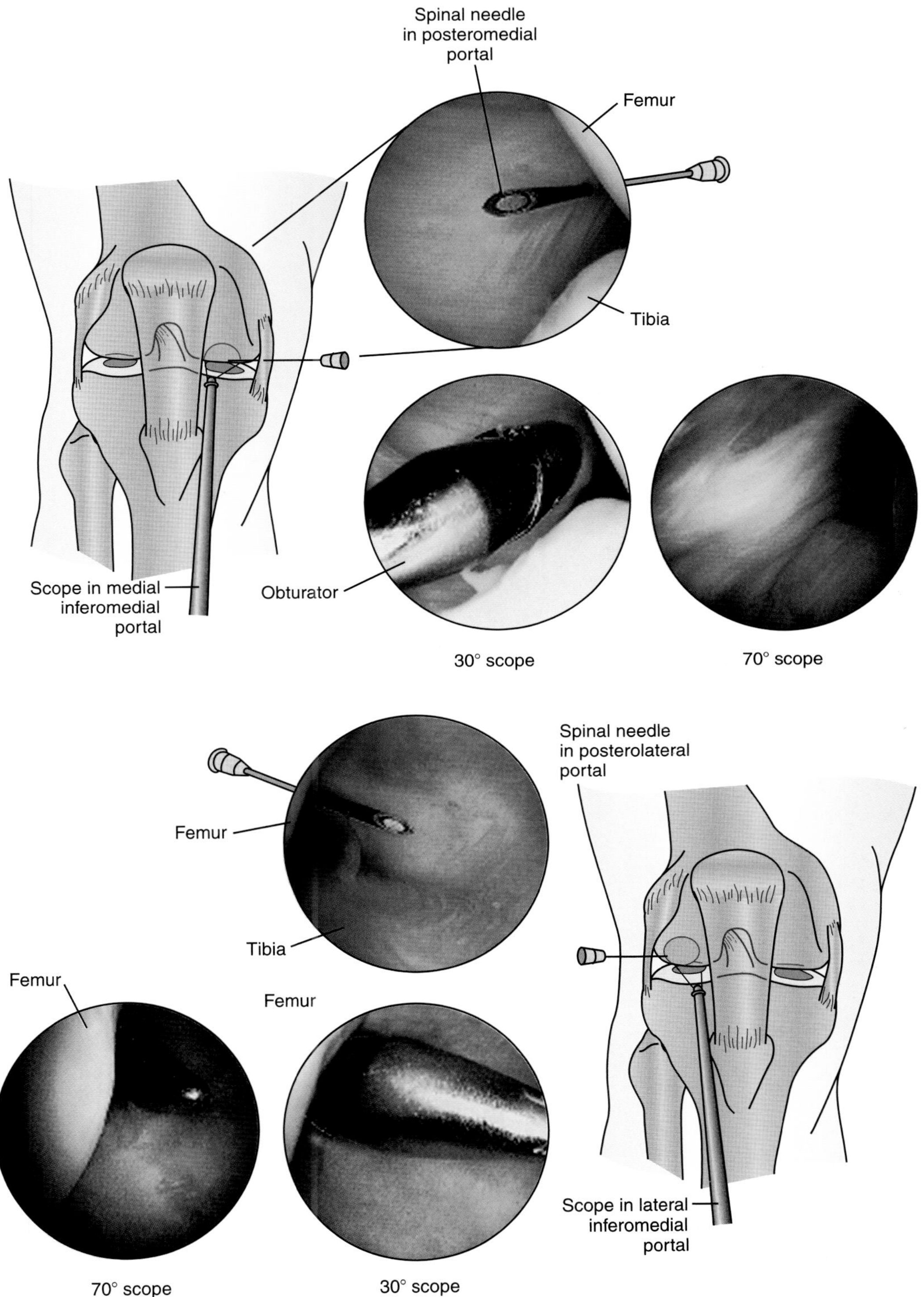

Knee arthroscopy posterior portals*

ACL, anterior cruciate ligament; PCL, posterior cruciate ligament

*From Miller MD, Chhabra AB, Hurwitz SR, Mihalko WM, Shen FH: Orthopaedic Surgical Approaches. Philadelphia, WB Saunders, 2008.

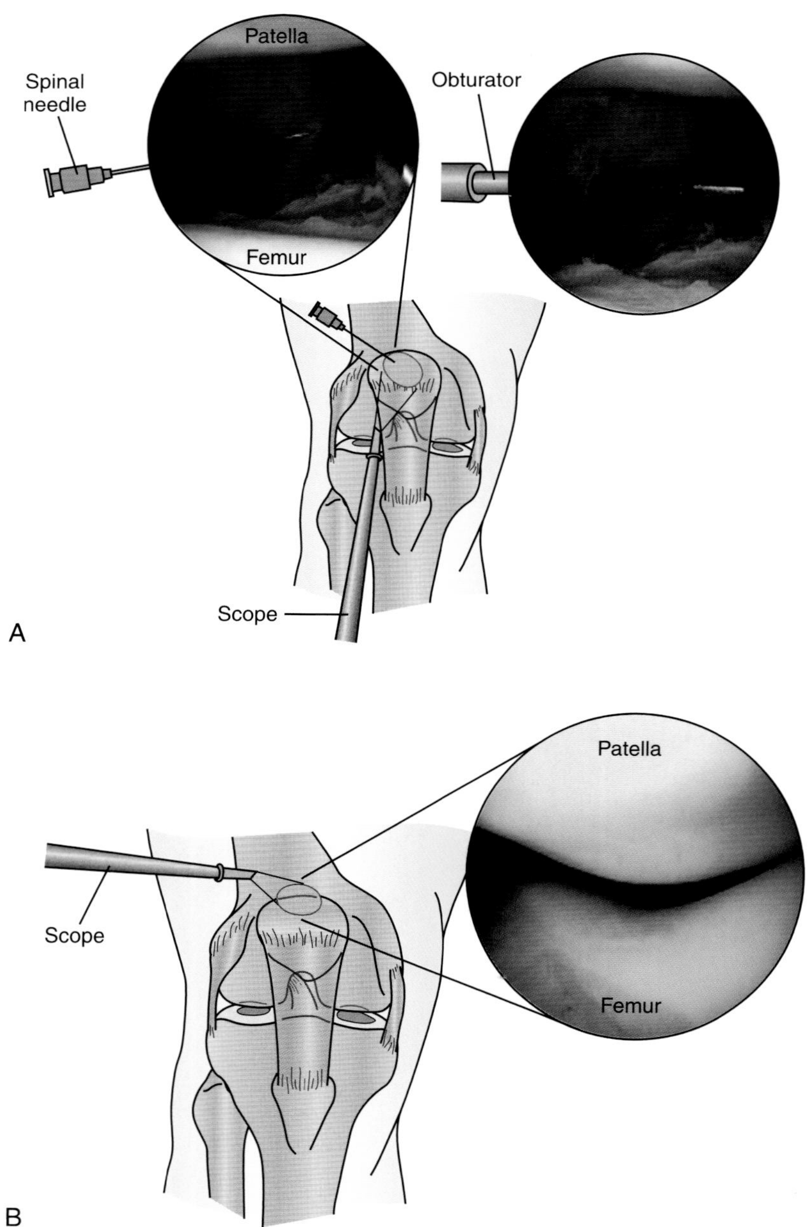

Knee arthroscopy, superolateral view*
A, Portal placement. B, View from superolateral portal.

*From Miller MD, Chhabra AB, Hurwitz SR, Mihalko WM, Shen FH: Orthopaedic Surgical Approaches. Philadelphia, WB Saunders, 2008.

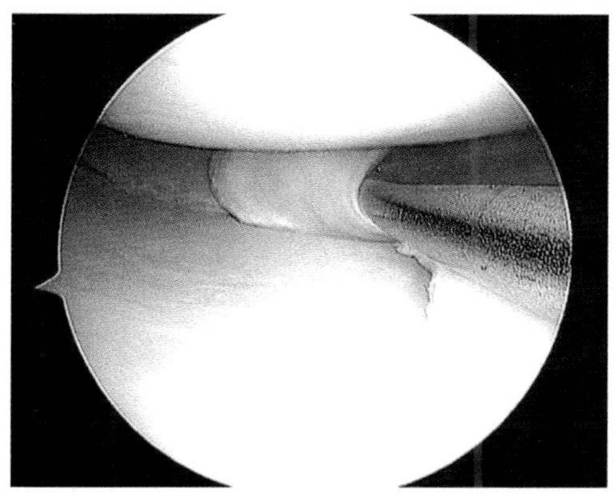

Displaced meniscal flap tear

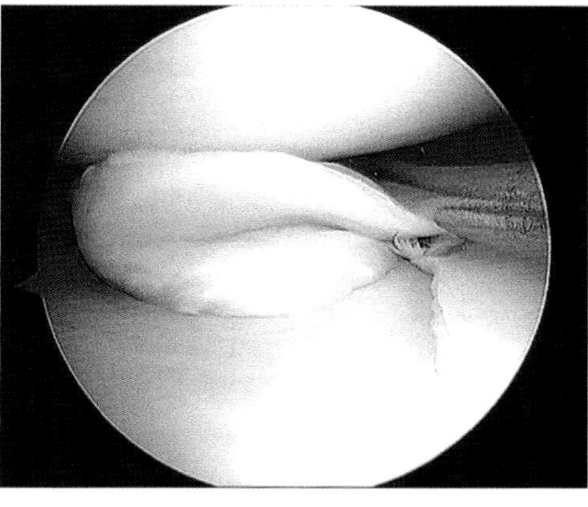

Displaced meniscal flap tear after probing

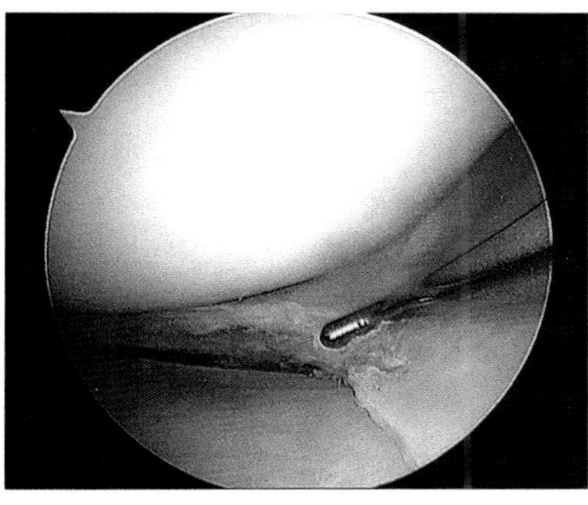

Displaced meniscal flap tear: partial medial meniscectomy

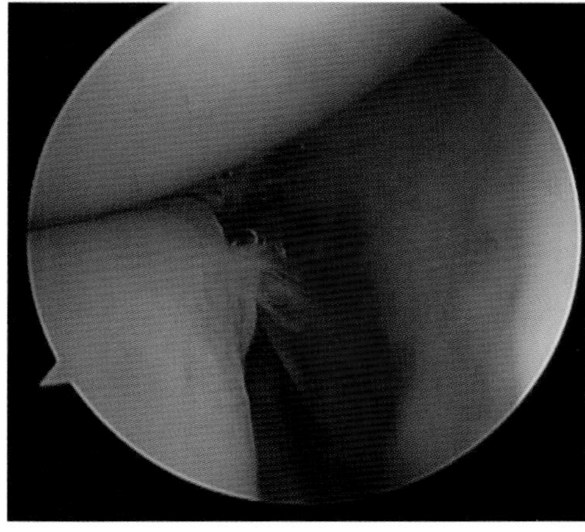

Peripheral longitudinal medial meniscal tear

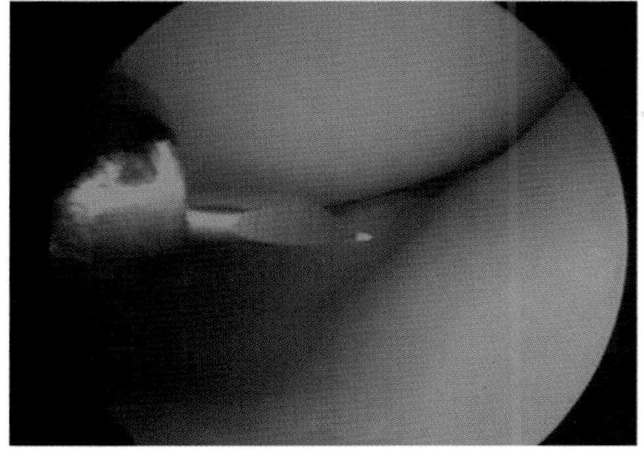

Inside-out meniscal repair

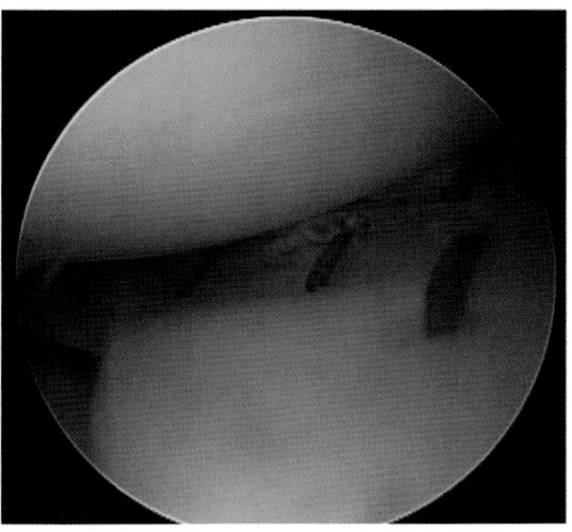

Tear after meniscal repair

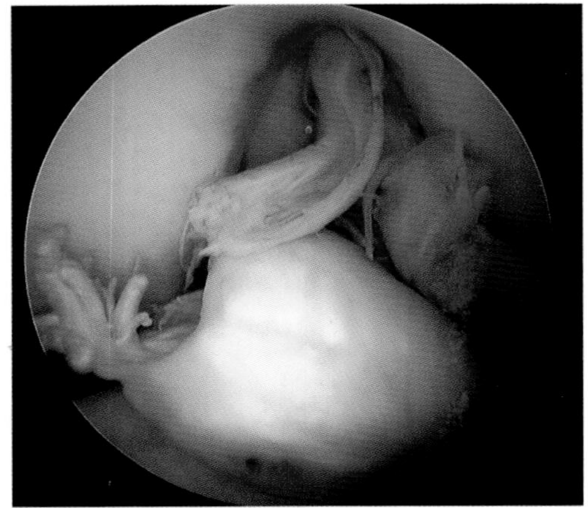

ACL tear

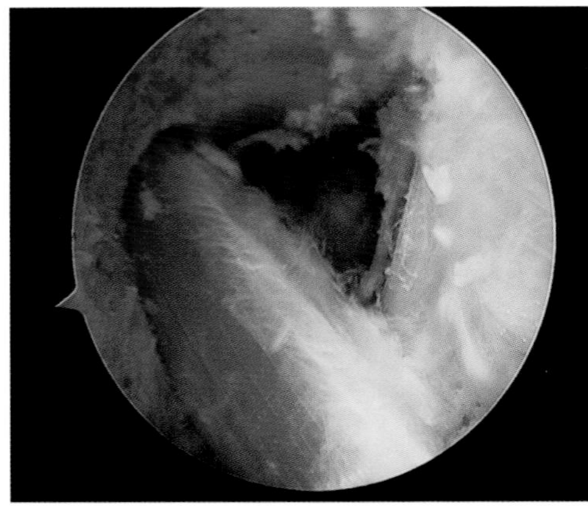

ACL reconstruction with hamstring graft

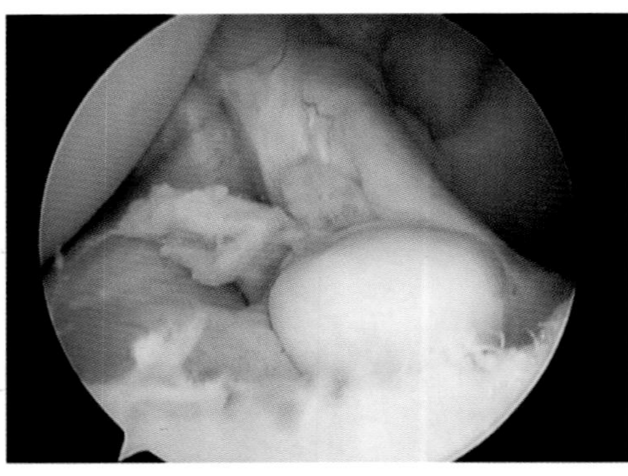

Single-bundle ACL tear

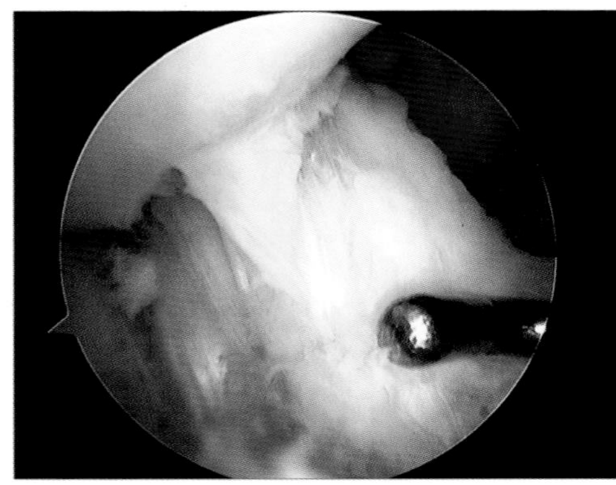

Single-bundle ACL reconstruction

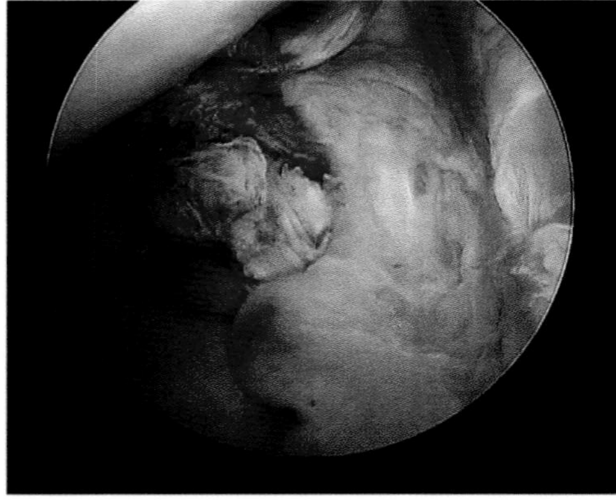

PCL tear (view from posteromedial portal)

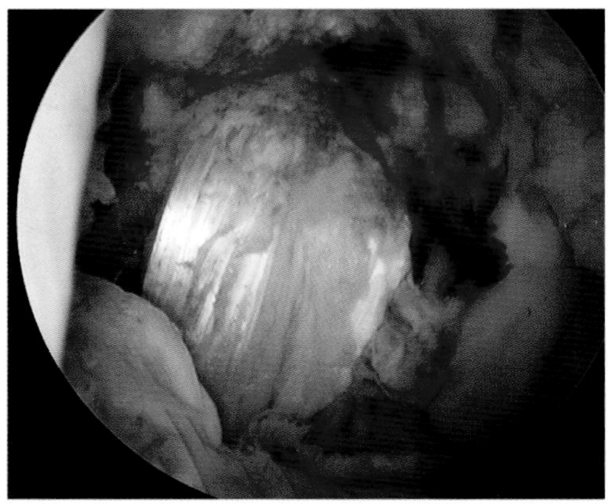

PCL reconstruction

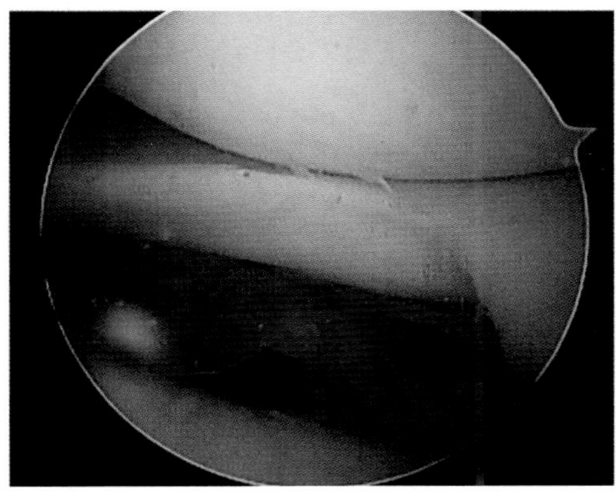

Posterolateral corner injury with "drive-through" sign

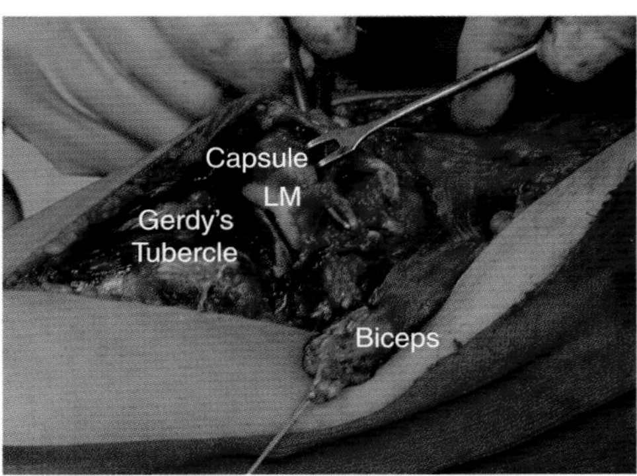

Open posterolateral corner repair

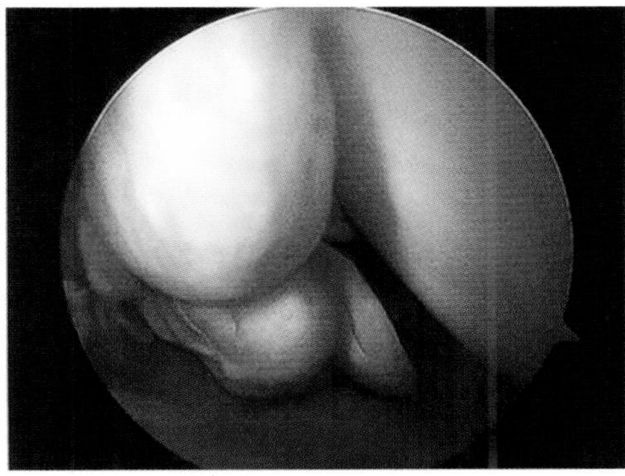

Pigmented villonodular synovitis débridement

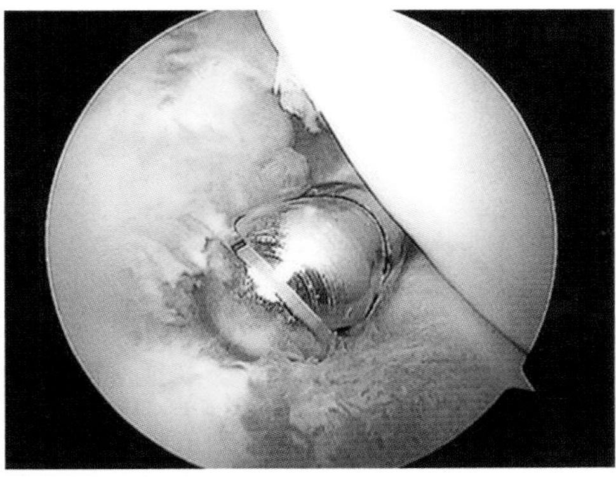

Pigmented villonodular synovitis débridement

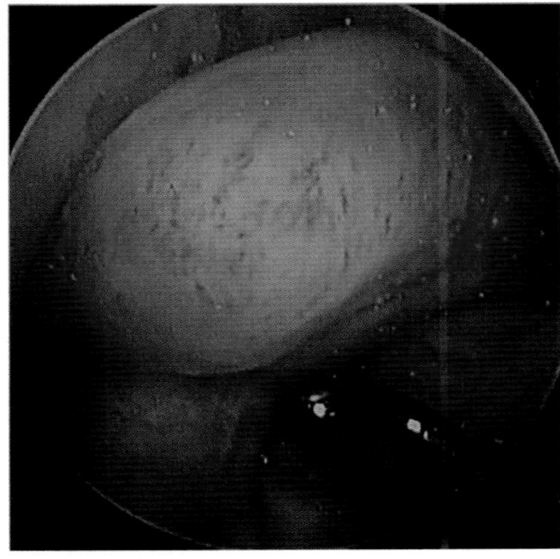

Cyclops lesion

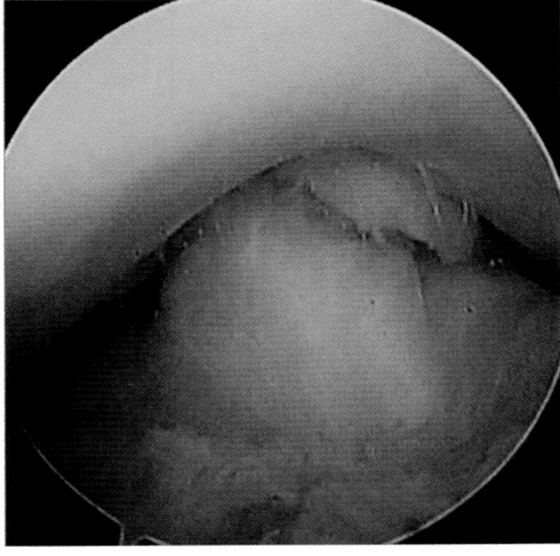

Cyclops lesion following débridement

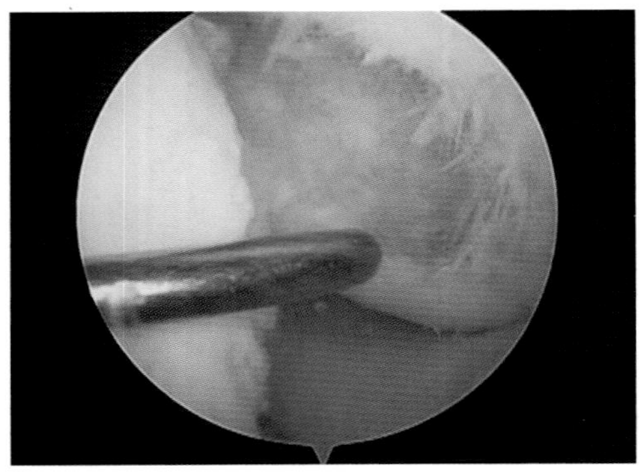

Medial femoral condyle chondral flap tear

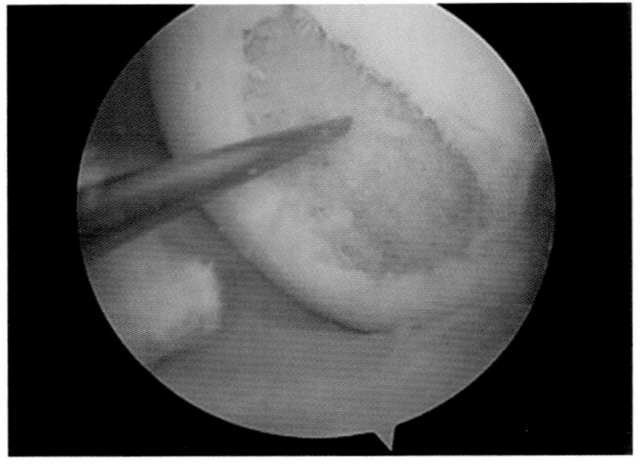

Cartilage débridement

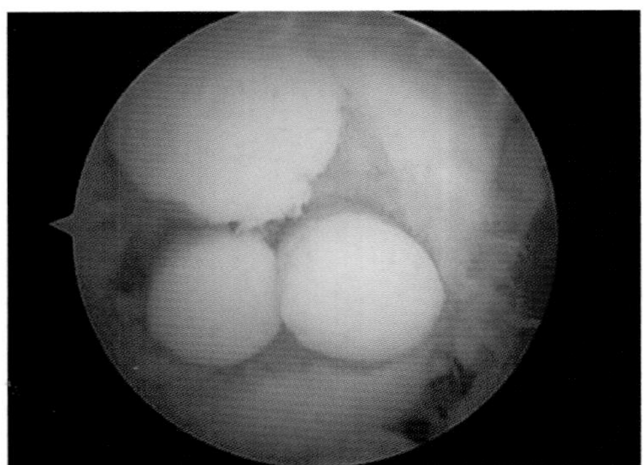

Osteochondral plug transfer

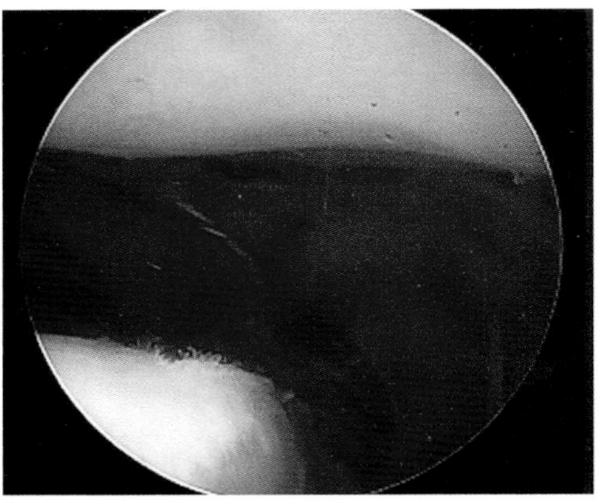

Patellar instability
(view from proximal lateral portal)

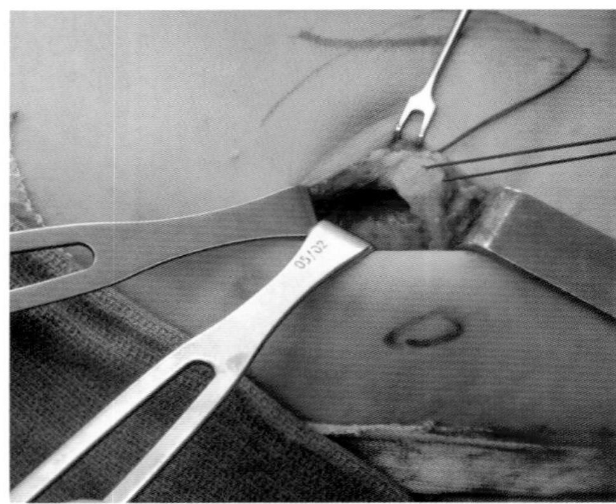

MPFL repair

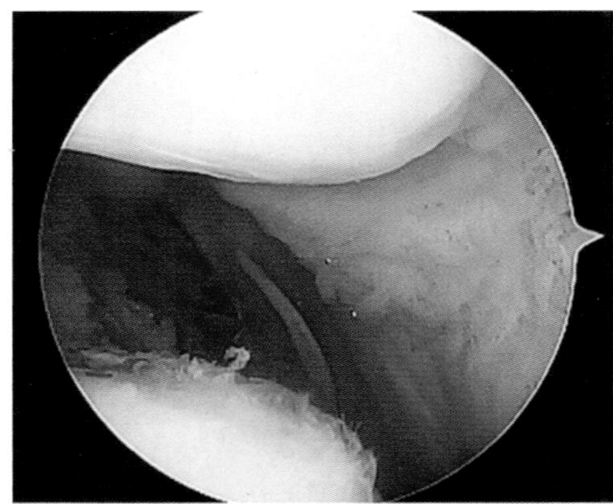

After MPFL repair
(view from superolateral portal)

Hip Arthroscopy*

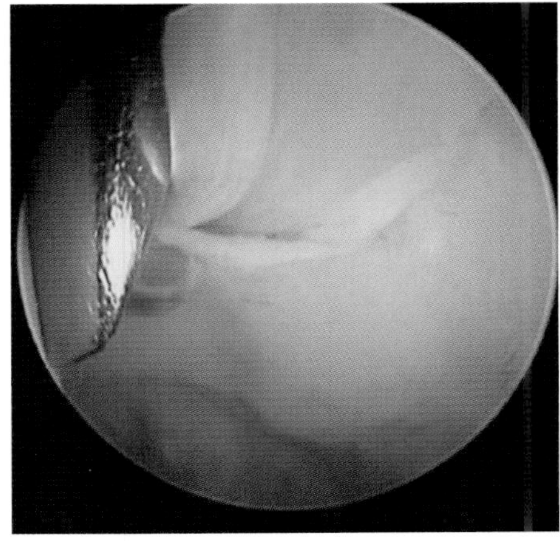

Anterior labral tear
(view from anterolateral portal)

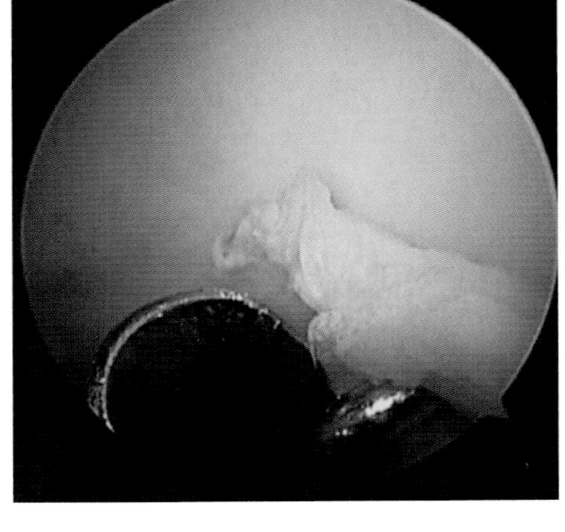

Anterior labral tear
(view from anterior portal)

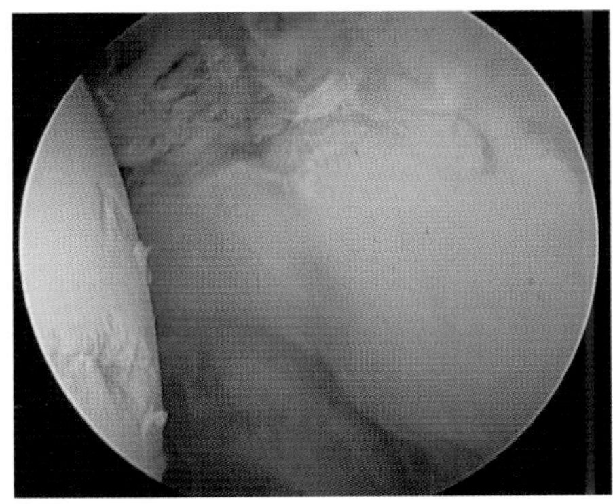

Labral tear after débridement

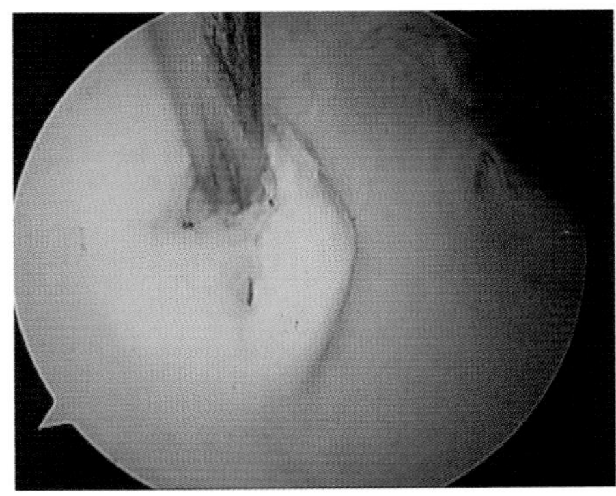

Acetabular chondral injury

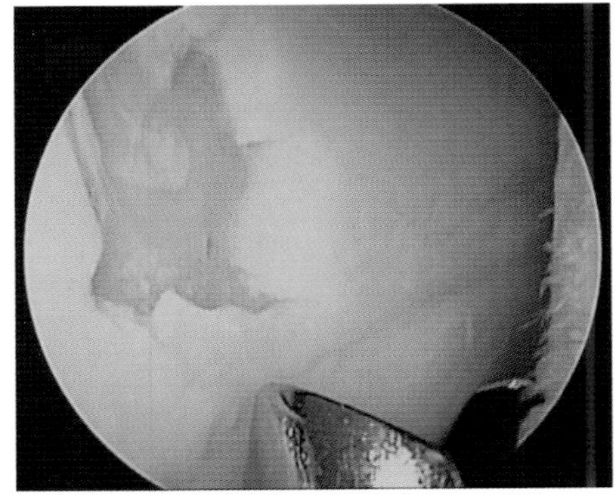

Chondral injury after débridement

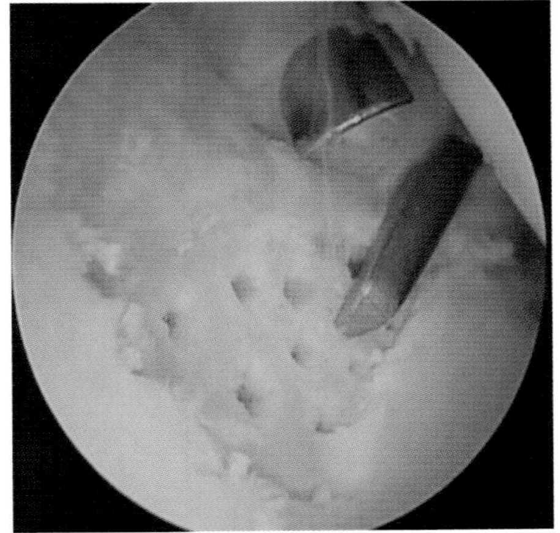

Chondral injury after microfracture

*Images courtesy of Marc Safon, MD.

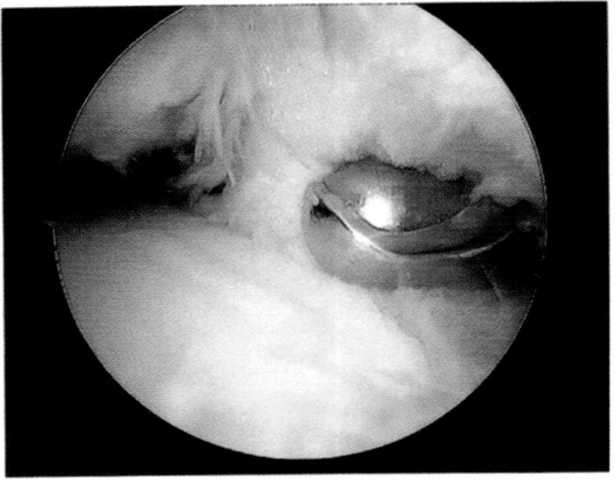

Ankle arthroscopy: initial débridement

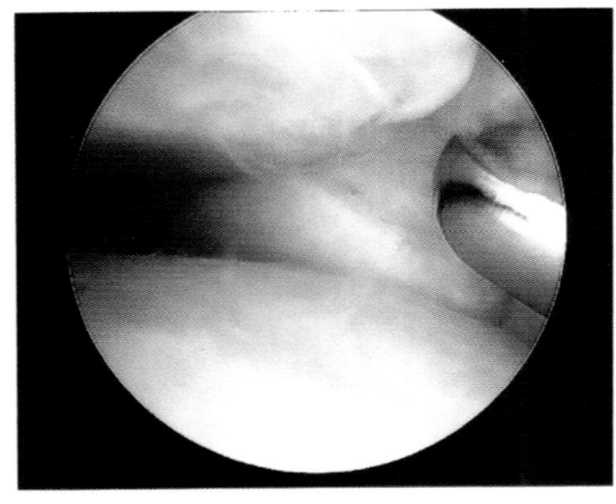

Ankle arthroscopy: after débridement

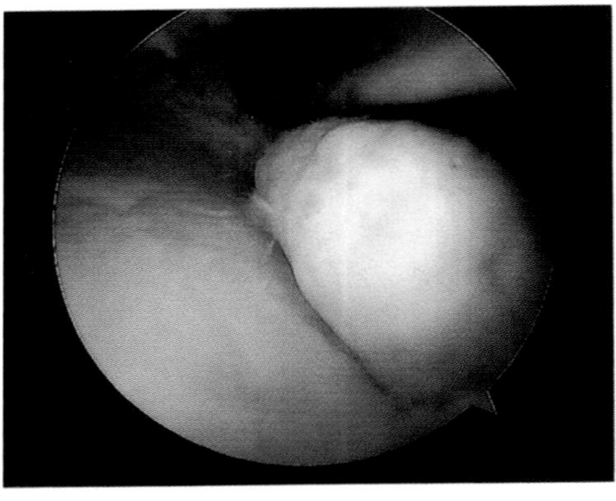

Ankle arthroscopy: loose body removal

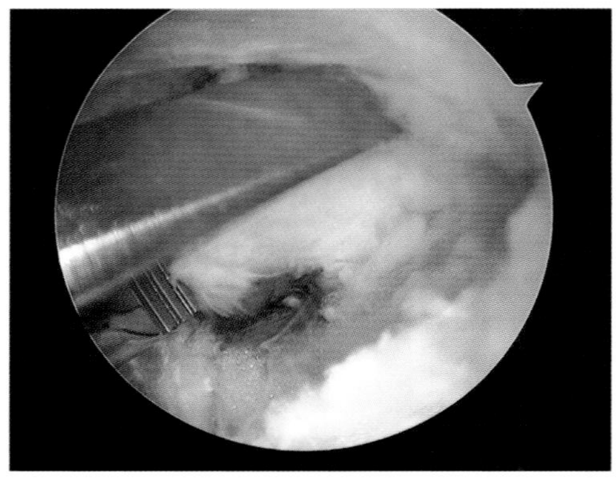

Posterior ankle arthroscopy: removal of os trigonum

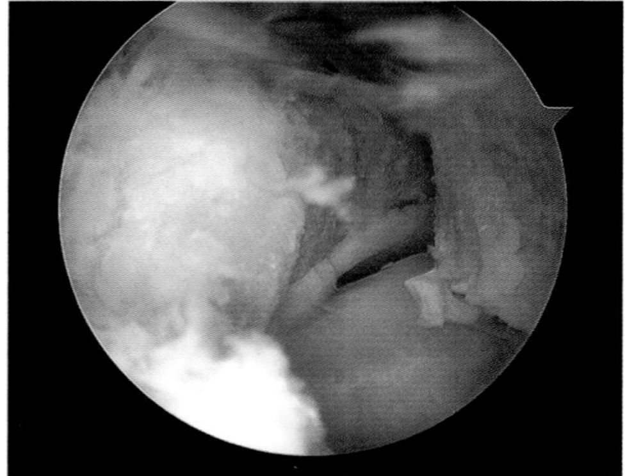

Posterior ankle arthroscopy: removal of os trigonum

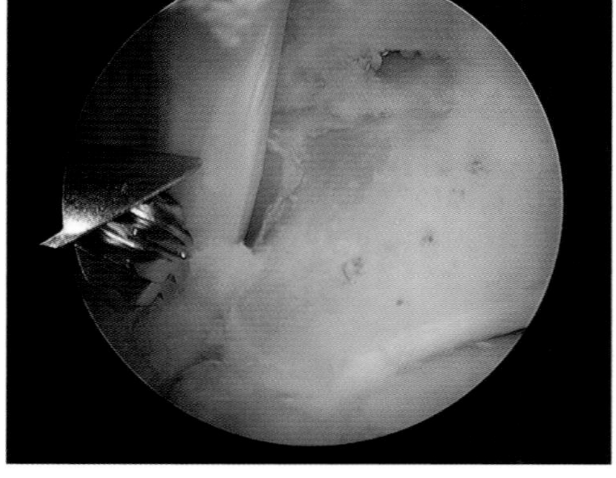

Posterior ankle arthroscopy: removal of os trigonum

Shoulder Arthroscopy

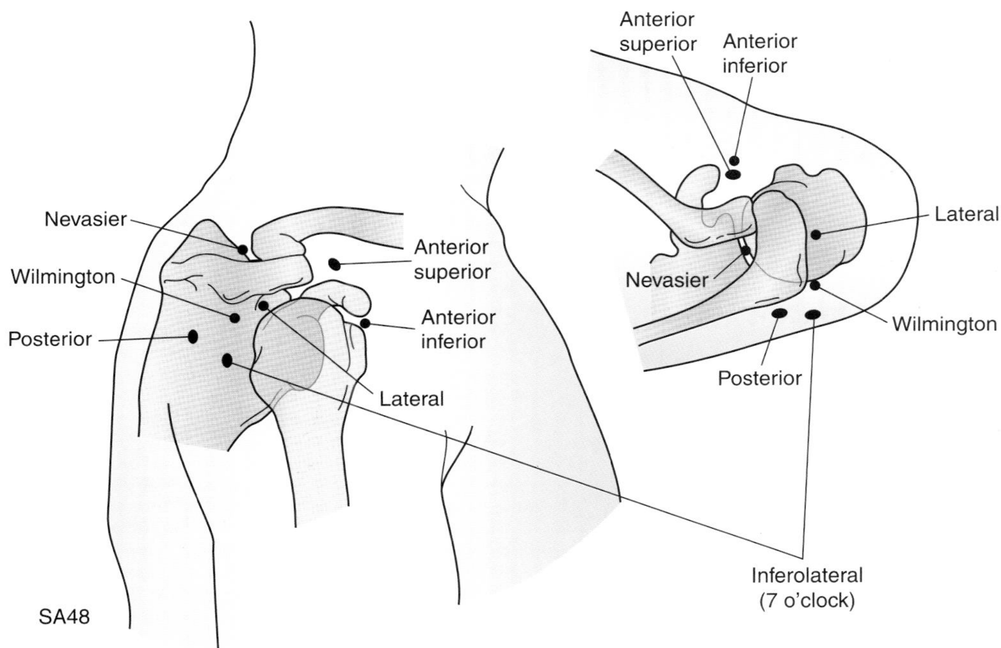

Shoulder arthroscopy portals*

*From Miller MD, Chhabra AB, Hurwitz SR, Mihalko WM, Shen FH: Orthopaedic Surgical Approaches. Philadelphia, WB Saunders, 2008.

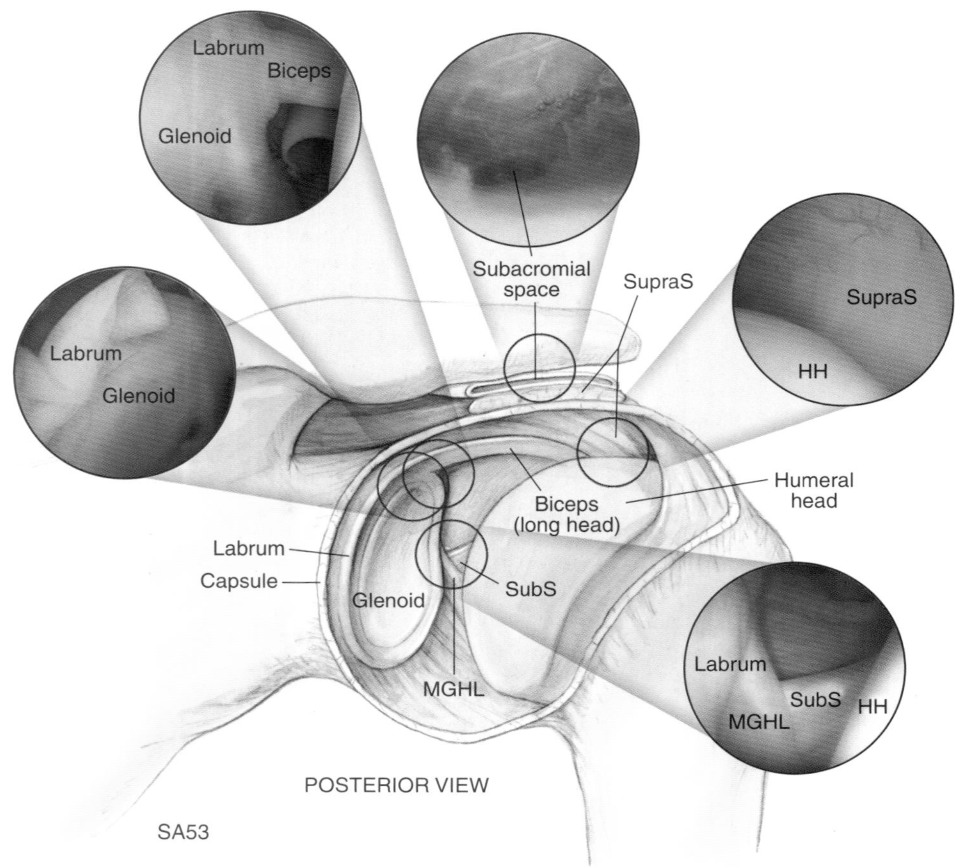

Shoulder arthroscopy overview*

HH, humeral head; MGHL, middle glenohumeral ligament; SupraS, supraspinatus; SubS, subscapularis

*From Miller MD, Chhabra AB, Hurwitz SR, Mihalko WM, Shen FH: Orthopaedic Surgical Approaches. Philadelphia, WB Saunders, 2008.

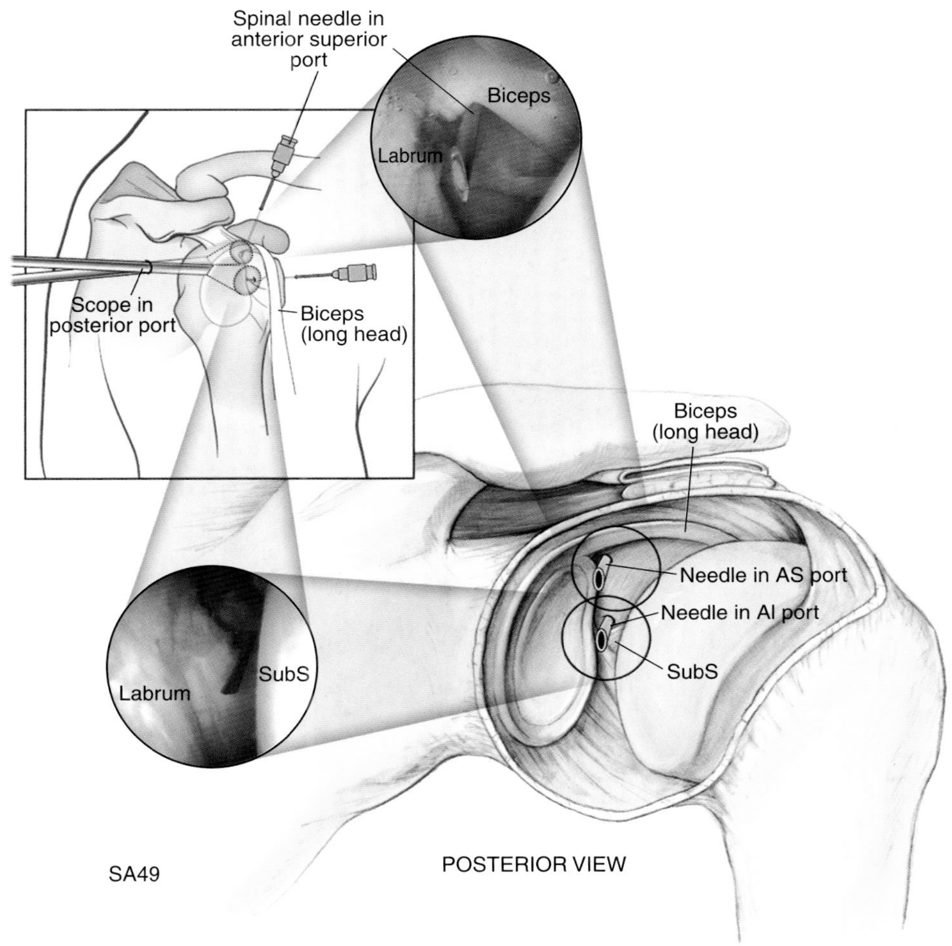

Shoulder arthroscopy: anterior portal placement*

AI, anterior inferior; AS, anterior superior; SubS, subscapularis

*From Miller MD, Chhabra AB, Hurwitz SR, Mihalko WM, Shen FH: Orthopaedic Surgical Approaches. Philadelphia, WB Saunders, 2008.

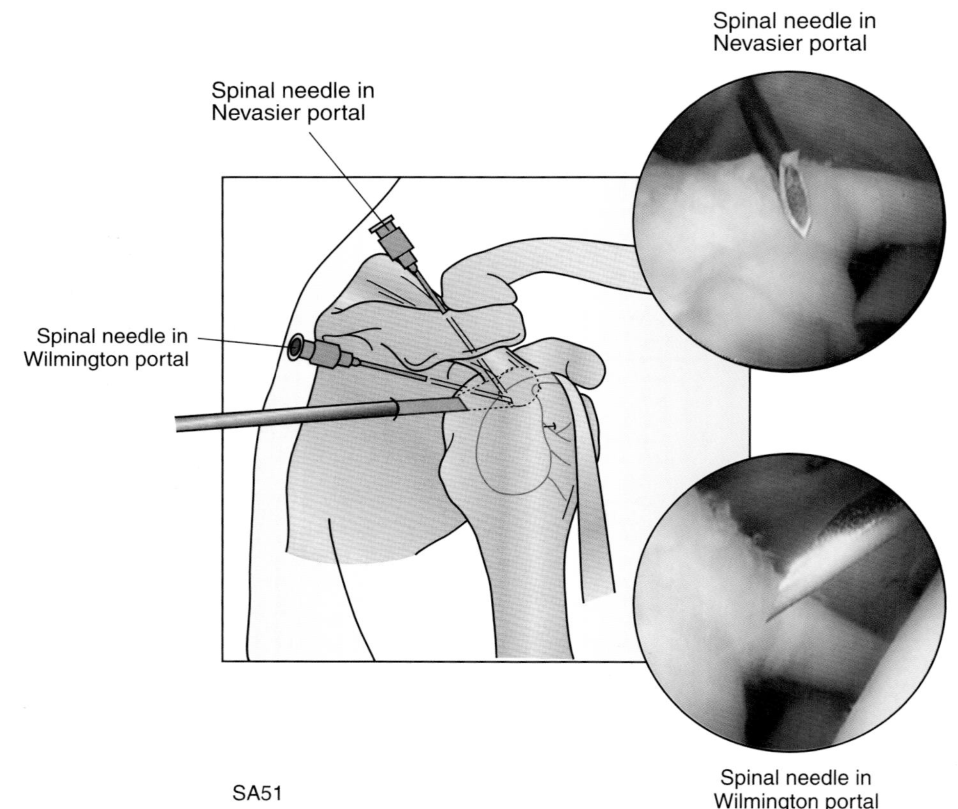

Shoulder arthroscopy: supplemental portal placement*

*From Miller MD, Chhabra AB, Hurwitz SR, Mihalko WM, Shen FH: Orthopaedic Surgical Approaches. Philadelphia, WB Saunders, 2008.

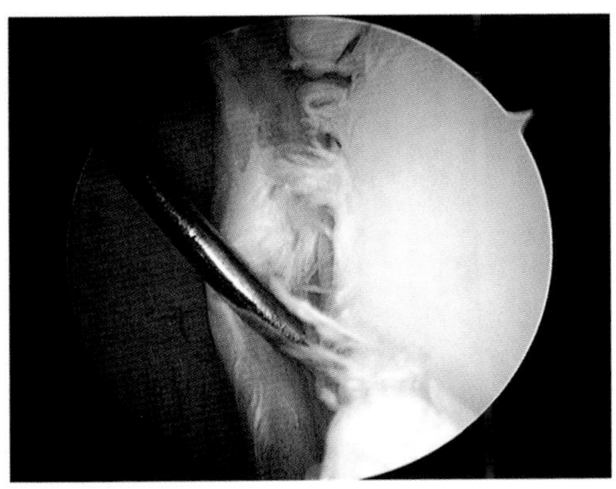

Bankart tear

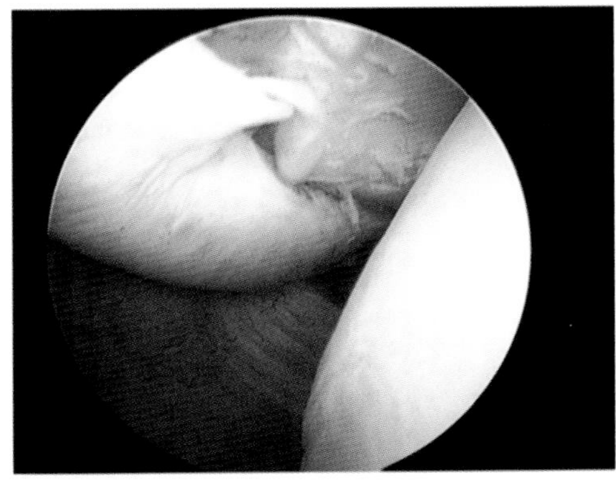

Bankart tear
(view from anterosuperior portal)

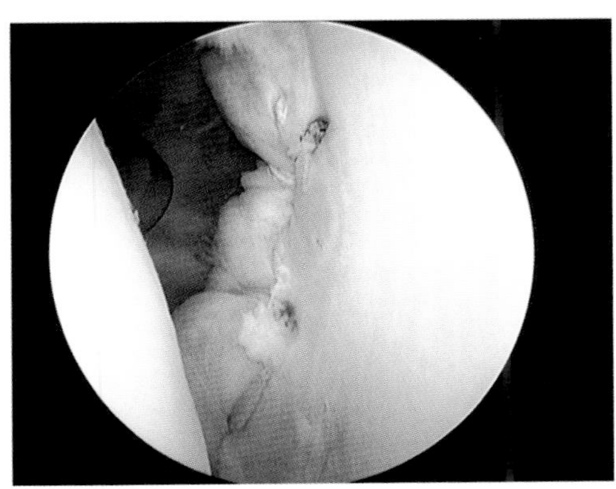

Bankart tear after repair

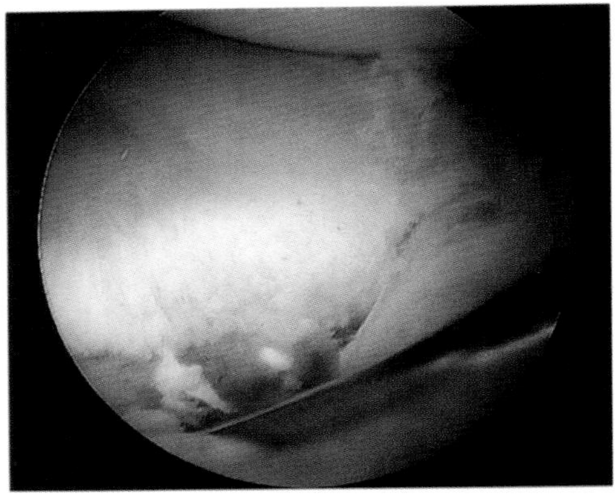

Posterior Bankart tear

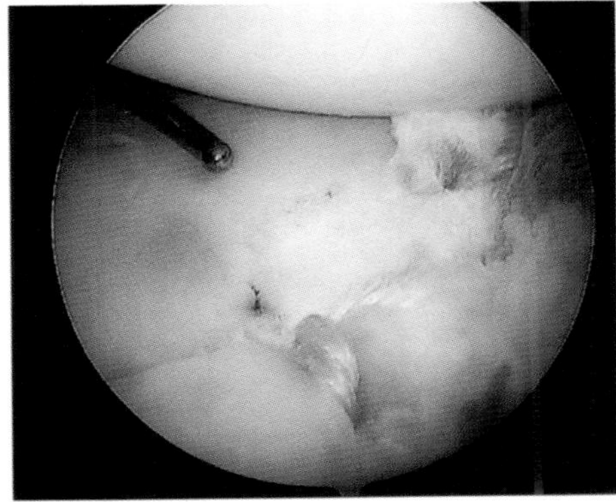

Posterior Bankart repair
(view from posterior portal)

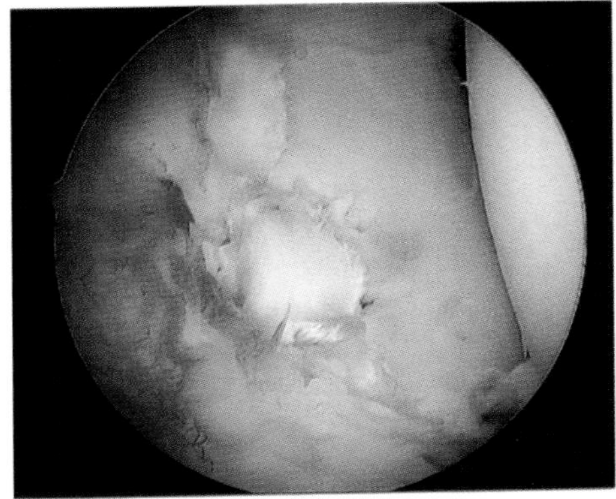

Posterior Bankart repair
(view from superior portal)

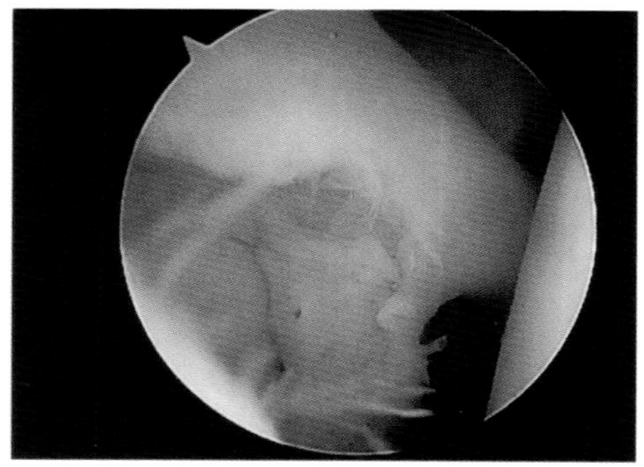

SLAP tear

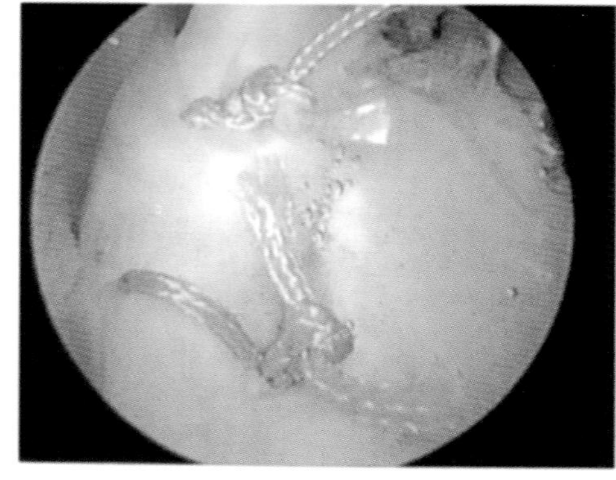

SLAP repair

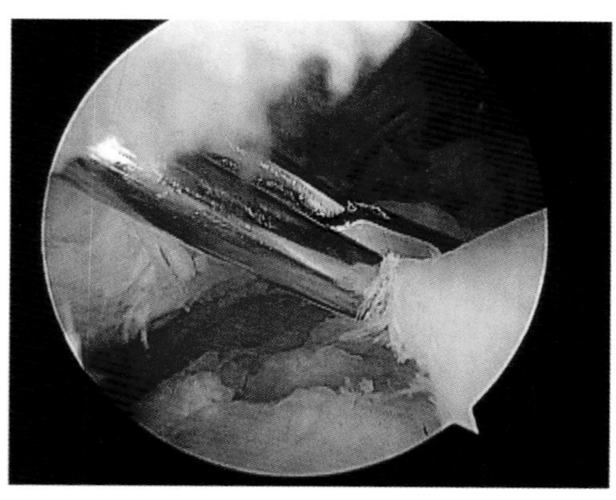

Rotator cuff tear

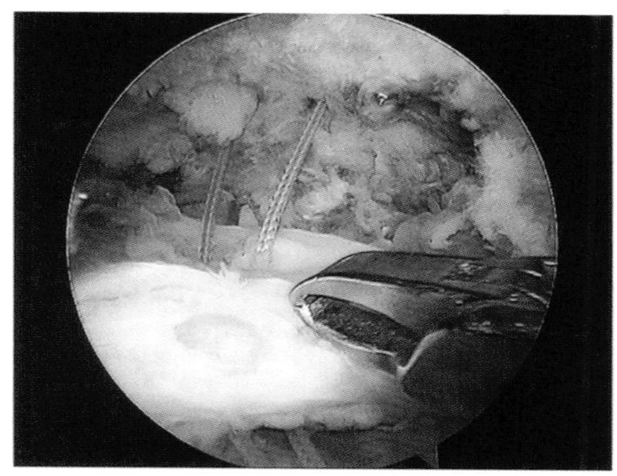

Rotator cuff suture passage

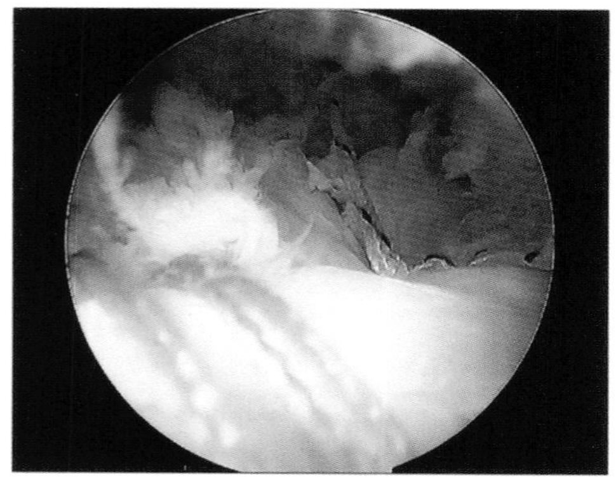

Rotator cuff repair

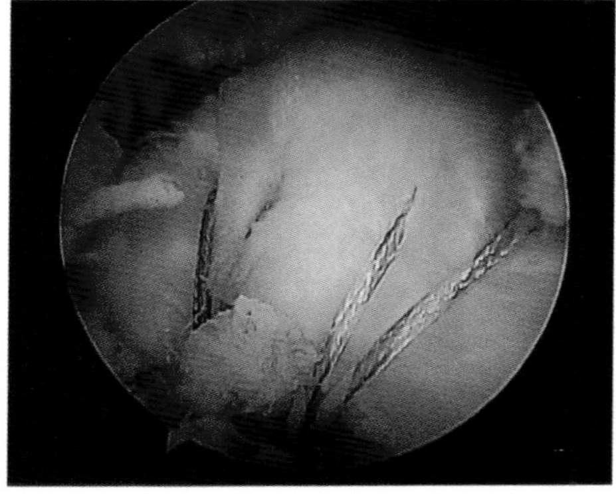

Rotator cuff repair

Elbow Arthroscopy*

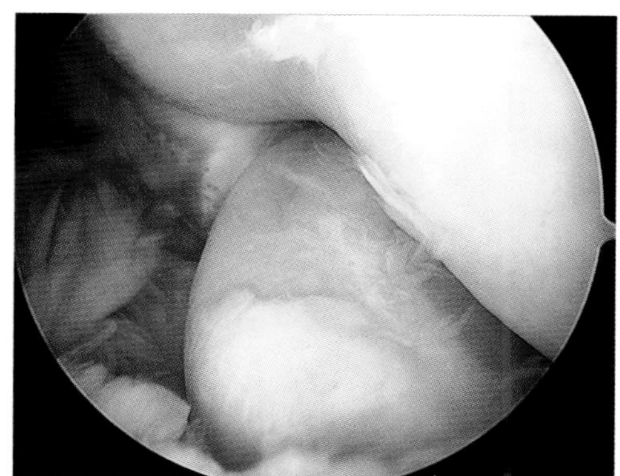

Synovitis

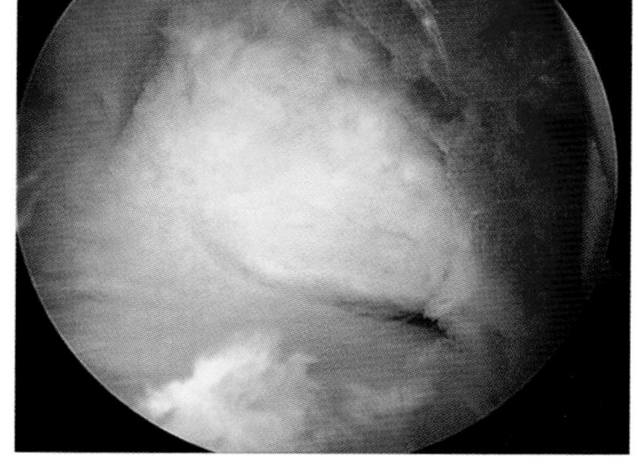

Olecranon fossa

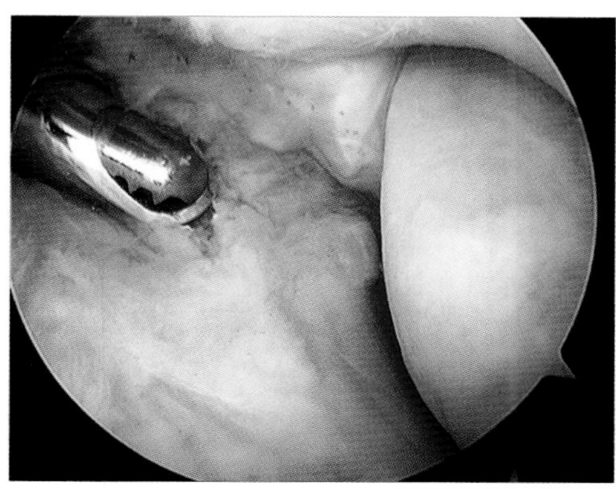

Synovectomy

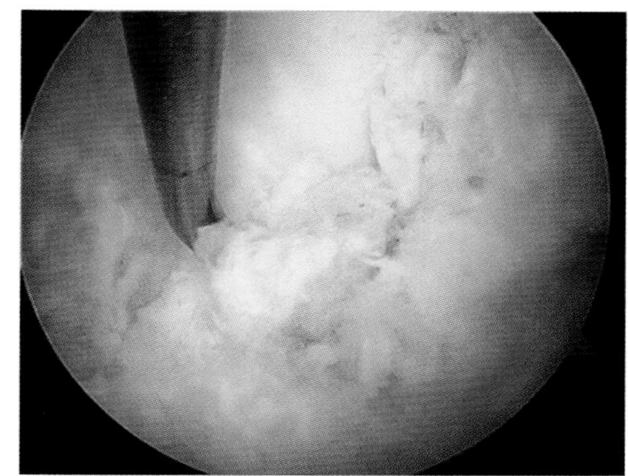

Olecranon osteophyte

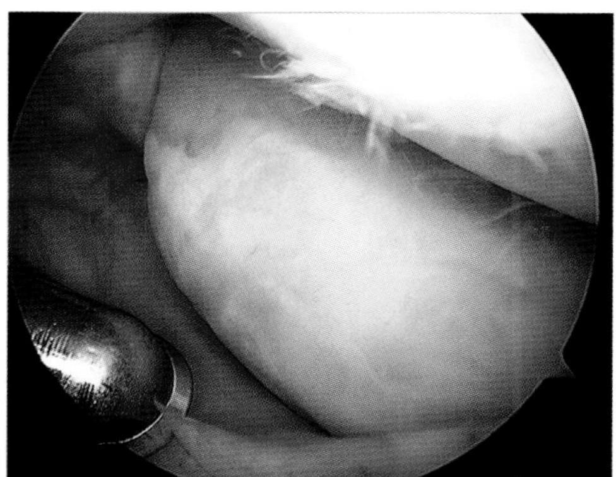

Radiocapitellar joint

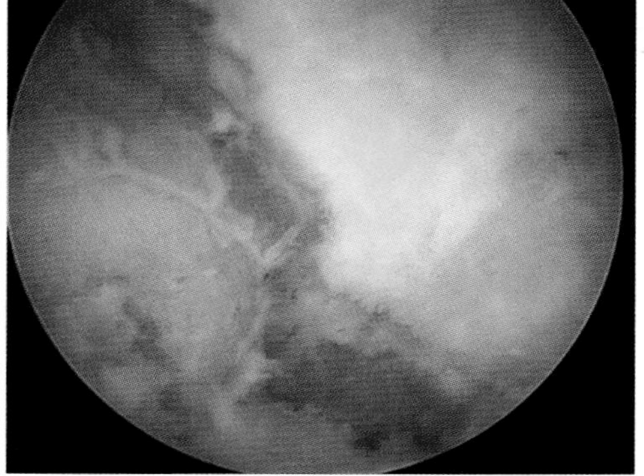

Olecranon fossa after osteophyte removal/débridement

*Images courtesy of A. Bobby Chhabra, MD.

Wrist Arthroscopy*

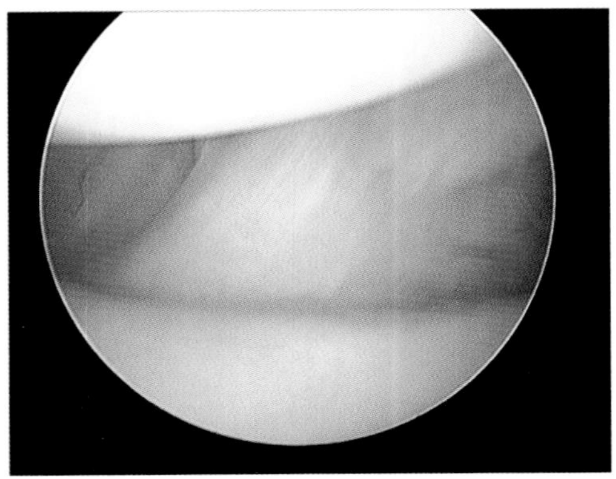

Radioscaphocapitate ligament

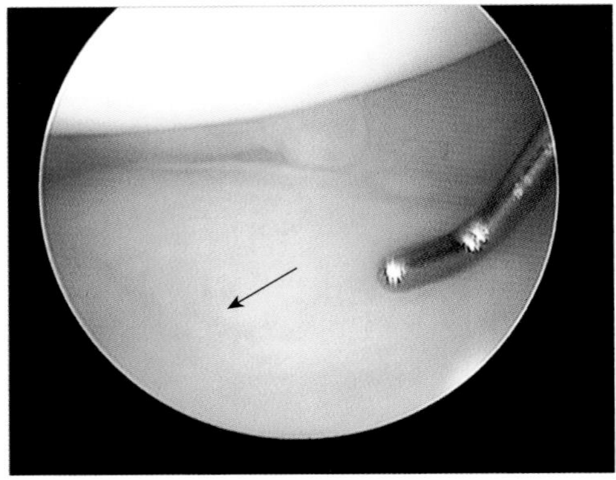

TFCC tear

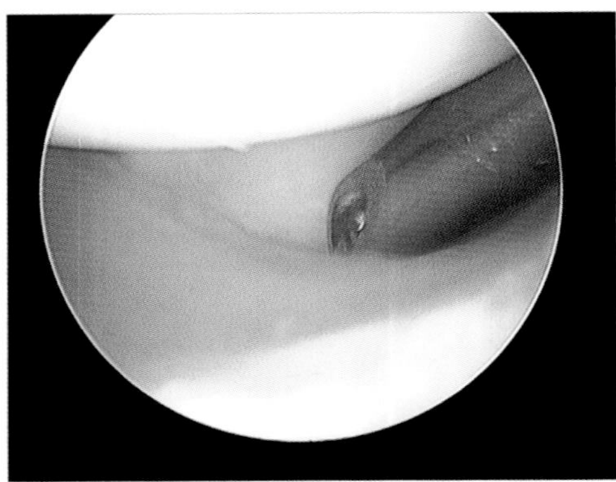

TFCC débridement

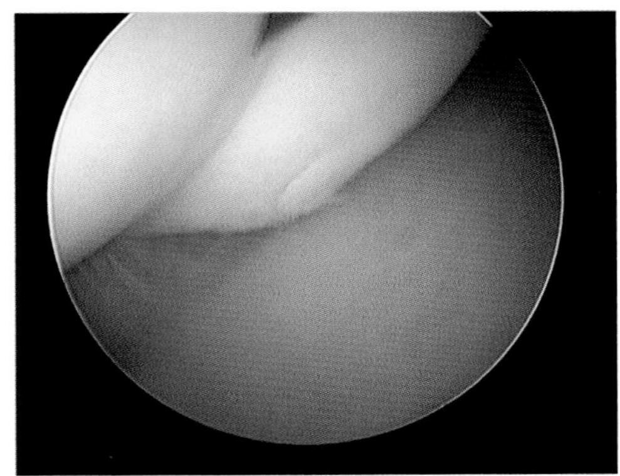

Mid-carpal joint: capitohamate

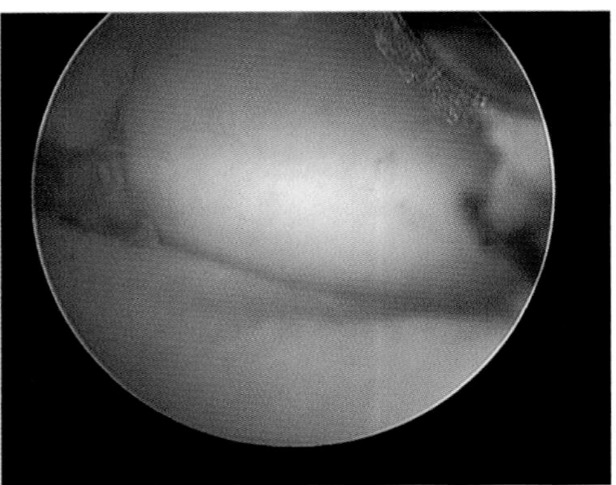

Lunotriquetral joint

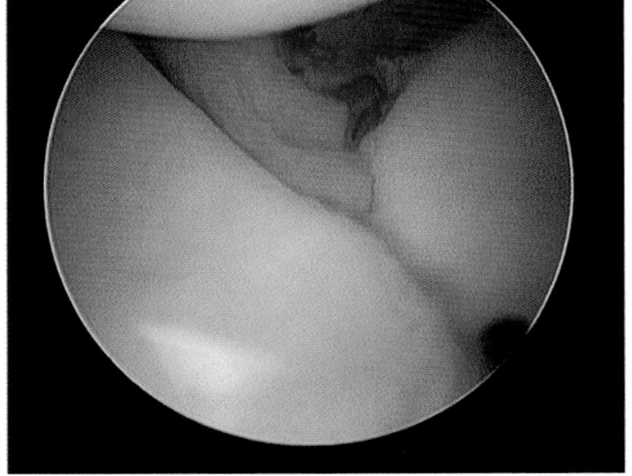

Scapholunate interval

*Images courtesy of A. Bobby Chhabra, MD.

CHAPTER 1

Basic Sciences

Mark R. Brinker AND Daniel P. O'Connor

CONTENTS

SECTION 1 Bone

I. Histology of Bone

A. Types (Fig. 1–1) (Table 1–1)—Normal bone is lamellar and can be cortical or cancellous. Immature and pathologic bone is woven, is more random with more osteocytes than lamellar bone, has increased turnover, and is weaker and more flexible than lamellar bone. Lamellar bone is stress oriented; woven bone is not stress oriented.

1. Cortical bone (compact bone)—Makes up 80% of the skeleton; composed of tightly packed osteons or haversian systems connected by haversian (or Volkmann's) canals containing arterioles, venules, capillaries, nerves, and possibly lymphatic channels. Interstitial lamellae lie between the osteons. Fibrils frequently connect lamellae but do not cross cement lines (where bone resorption has stopped and new bone formation has begun). Cement lines define the outer border of an osteon. Intraosseous circulation (canals and canaliculi [cell processes of osteocytes]) provides nutrition. Cortical bone has a slow turnover rate, a relatively high Young modulus (*E*), and a higher resistance to torsion and bending than cancellous bone.

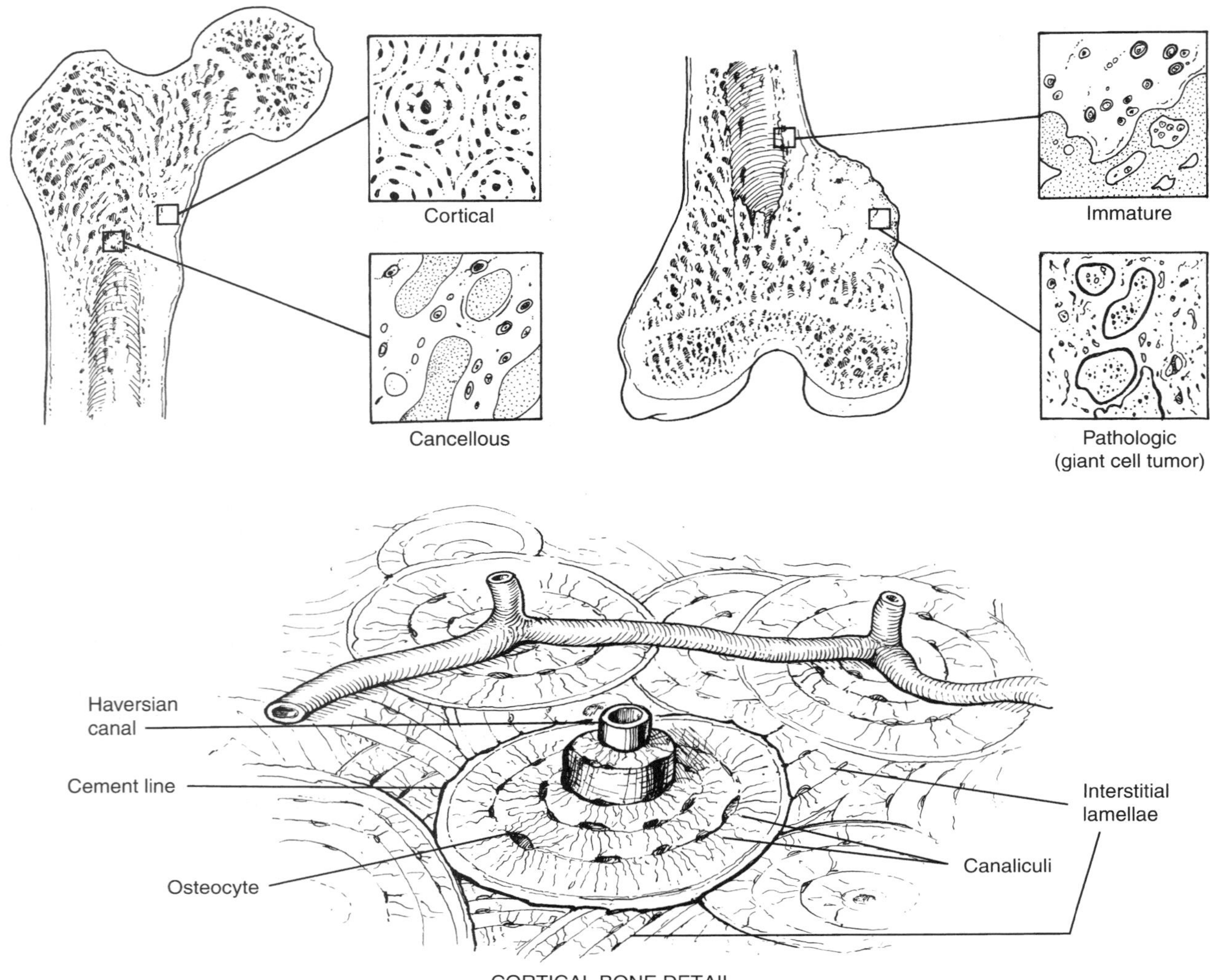

FIGURE 1–1 Types of bone. *Cortical* bone consists of tightly packed osteons. *Cancellous* bone consists of a meshwork of trabeculae. In *immature* bone, there is unmineralized osteoid lining the immature trabeculae. In *pathologic* bone, atypical osteoblasts and architectural disorganization are seen. (From Brinker MR, Miller MD: Fundamentals of Orthopaedics. Philadelphia, WB Saunders, 1999, p 2.)

2. Cancellous bone (spongy or trabecular bone) (see Fig. 1–1)—Less dense and undergoes more remodeling according to lines of stress (Wolff's law). It has a higher turnover rate, has a smaller Young modulus, and is more elastic than cortical bone.

B. Cellular biology
  1. Osteoblasts—Form bone by generating the organic, nonmineralized matrix. Derived from undifferentiated mesenchymal stem cells. These cells have more endoplasmic reticulum, Golgi apparatus,

TABLE 1-1 TYPES OF BONES

Microscopic Appearance	Subtypes	Characteristics	Examples
Lamellar	Cortical	Structure is oriented along lines of stress. Strong	Femoral shaft
	Cancellous	More elastic than cortical bone	Distal femoral metaphysis
Woven	Immature	Not stress oriented	Embryonic skeleton Fracture callus
	Pathologic	Random organization Increased turnover Weak Flexible	Osteogenic sarcoma Fibrous dysplasia

Modified from Brinker MR, Miller MD: Fundamentals of Orthopaedics, p 1. Philadelphia, WB Saunders, 1999.

and mitochondria than other cells (for synthesis and secretion of matrix). More differentiated, metabolically active cells line bone surfaces, and less active cells in "resting regions" or entrapped cells maintain the ionic milieu of bone. Disruption of the active-lining cell layer activates the entrapped cells. Osteoblast differentiation in vivo is effected by the interleukins, platelet-derived growth factor (PDGF), and insulin-derived growth factor (IDGF). **Osteoblasts respond to parathyroid hormone (PTH)** and produce alkaline phosphatase, type I collagen, osteocalcin (stimulated by 1,25-dihydroxyvitamin D), and **bone sialoprotein.** Osteoblasts have receptor-effector interactions for (1) PTH; (2) 1,25-dihydroxyvitamin D; (3) glucocorticoids; (4) prostaglandins; and (5) estrogen (Table 1–2). Certain antiseptic agents are toxic to cultured osteoblasts (including hydrogen peroxide and povidone-iodine [Betadine] solution and scrub); bacitracin is believed to be less toxic.

2. Osteocytes (see Fig. 1–1)—Maintain bone. Make up 90% of the cells in the mature skeleton; are former osteoblasts that are surrounded by a newly formed matrix (which they help preserve). Osteocytes have a high nucleus/cytoplasm ratio, with long interconnecting cytoplasmic processes projecting through the canaliculi. Not as active in matrix production as osteoblasts. Important for control of extracellular calcium and phosphorus concentration. Directly stimulated by calcitonin and inhibited by PTH.
3. Osteoclasts—Resorb bone. Multinucleated, irregularly shaped giant cells originate from hematopoietic cells in the macrophage lineage (**monocyte progenitors** form giant cells by fusion). Possess a ruffled ("brush") border (plasma membrane enfoldings that increase surface area; important in bone resorption) and a surrounding clear zone. Bone resorption occurs in depressions (Howship's lacunae); bone formation and resorption are linked ("coupled"), but resorption occurs more rapidly. **Osteoblasts (and tumor cells) express the receptor activator of NF-kβ ligand (RANKL), which is a molecule that binds to receptors on osteoclasts, stimulating differentiation into mature osteoclasts and thus increasing bone resorption;** this mechanism is inhibited by osteoprotegrin binding to RANKL and prevents interaction with osteoclasts. **Osteoclasts synthesize tartrate-resistant acid phosphate.** Osteoclasts bind to bone surfaces via cell attachment (anchoring) proteins (**integrins, specifically the $\alpha_v\beta_3$ or vibronectin receptor**), which effectively seal the space below the osteoclast. Osteoclasts produce hydrogen ions (via carbonic anhydrase), which lower the pH and increase the solubility of hydroxyapatite crystals, and the organic matrix is then removed by proteolytic digestion. Patients deficient in carbonic anhydrase cannot resorb bone by this mechanism. **Osteoclasts have specific receptors for calcitonin** to allow them to regulate bone resorption directly (see Table 1–2). **Osteoclasts are responsible for the bone resorption seen in multiple myeloma and metastatic bone disease. Interleukin-1 (IL-1) is a potent stimulator of osteoclastic bone resorption and has been found in the membranes surrounding loose total joint implants. By contrast, IL-10 suppresses osteoclast formation. Bisphosphonates inhibit osteoclast resorption of bone (by preventing the osteoclast from forming the ruffled border necessary for expression of acid hydrolases) and reduce the incidence of skeletal events in patients with multiple myeloma.**
4. Osteoprogenitor cells—Originate from mesenchymal stem cells and become osteoblasts (under low strain and increased oxygen tension), cartilage (under intermediate strain and low oxygen tension), or fibrous tissue (under high strain). Line haversian canals, endosteum, and periosteum, awaiting the stimulus to differentiate.
5. Lining cells—Narrow, flattened, "resting" osteoblasts that form an "envelope around bone."

C. Matrix—Composed of organic components (40%) and inorganic components (60%) (Table 1–3).
   1. Organic components—40% of the dry weight of bone.
      a. Collagen—Primarily type I collagen ("bone" contains the word "one"; remember that bone is primarily type I collagen). **Hole zones** (gaps) exist within the collagen fibril between the **ends** of molecules. **Pores** exist between the **sides** of parallel molecules. Mineral deposition

TABLE 1-2 BONE CELL TYPES, RECEPTOR TYPES, AND EFFECTS

Cell Type	Receptor	Effect
Osteoblast	PTH	Releases a secondary messenger (exact mechanism unknown) to stimulate osteoclastic activity Activates adenylyl cyclase
	1,25 vitamin D_3	Stimulates matrix and alkaline phosphatase synthesis and production of bone-specific proteins (such as osteocalcin)
	Glucocorticoids	Inhibits the synthesis of DNA, production of collagen, and synthesis of osteoblastic proteins
	Prostaglandins	Activates adenylyl cyclase and stimulates resorption of bone
	Estrogen	Anabolic (bone production) and anticatabolic (prevents bone resorption) effects on bone Increases the levels of mRNA for alkaline phosphatase and inhibits the activation of adenylyl cyclase
Osteoclast	Calcitonin	Inhibits the function of osteoclasts (inhibits bone resorption)

mRNA, messenger RNA; PTH, parathyroid hormone.

TABLE 1-3 COMPONENTS OF BONE MATRIX

Type of Matrix	Function	Composition	Types	Notes
Organic Matrix				
Collagen	Provides tensile strength	Primarily type I collagen		90% of organic matrix Structure: triple helix of one α_2 and two α_1 chains, quarter-staggered to produce a fibril
Proteoglycans	Partly responsible for compressive strength	Glycosaminoglycan (GAG)-protein complexes (see Section 2: Joints)		Inhibit mineralization
Matrix proteins (noncollagenous)	Promote mineralization and bone formation		Osteocalcin (bone γ-carboxyglutamic acid–containing protein [bone Gla protein])	Attracts osteoclasts; direct regulation of bone density; most abundant noncollagenous matrix protein (10-20% of total)
			Osteonectin (SPARC)	Secreted by platelets and osteoblasts; postulated to have a role in regulating Ca or organizing mineral in matrix
			Osteopontin	Cell-binding protein, similar to an integrin
Growth factors and cytokines	Aid in bone cell differentiation, activation, growth, and turnover		Transforming growth factor-β (TGF-β) Insulin-like growth factor (IGF) Interleukins (IL-1, IL-6) Bone morphogenetic proteins (BMPs 1-6)	Present in small amounts in bone matrix (for more information, see Table 1–9)
Inorganic Matrix				
Calcium hydroxyapatite [$Ca_{10}(PO_4)_6(OH)_2$]	Provides compressive strength			Makes up most of the inorganic matrix; primary mineralization in collagen gaps (holes and pores), secondary mineralization on periphery
Osteocalcium phosphate (brushite)				Makes up the remaining inorganic matrix

SPARC, secreted protein, acidic, rich in cysteine.

(calcification) occurs within the hole zones and pores (Fig. 1–2). Cross-linking decreases collagen solubility and increases its tensile strength.

b. Proteoglycans

c. Matrix proteins (noncollagenous)—**Osteocalcin, the most abundant noncollagenous protein in bone,** is inhibited by PTH and stimulated by 1,25-dihydroxyvitamin D. **Osteocalcin levels can be measured in the serum or urine as a marker of bone turnover;** elevated in Paget's disease, renal osteodystrophy, and hyperparathyroidism.

d. Growth factors and cytokines

2. Inorganic (mineral) components—60% of the dry weight of bone.
   a. Calcium hydroxyapatite [$Ca_{10}(PO_4)_6(OH)_2$]
   b. Calcium phosphate (brushite)

D. Bone remodeling
   1. General
      a. **Wolff's law**—Bone remodels in response to mechanical stress (Wolff's law). Increasing mechanical stress leads to significant bone gain. Removing external mechanical stress can lead to significant bone loss, which is reversible (to varying degrees) on remobilization.

Progressively increasing mineral mass due to:
1. Increased number of new mineral phase particles (nucleation)
   a. Heterogeneous nucleation by matrix in collagen holes (? pores)
   b. 2° crystal-induced nucleation in holes and pores
2. Initial growth of particles to ~ 400Å × 15–30Å × 50–75Å

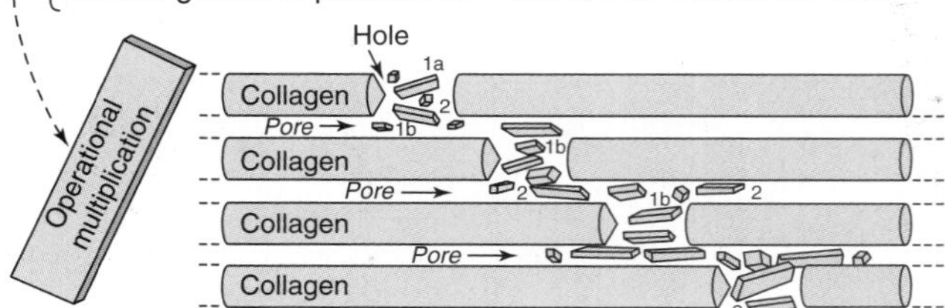

FIGURE 1–2 Biological considerations of mineral accretion: heterogeneity within a collagen fibril. (From Simon SR, ed: Orthopaedic Basic Science, p 139. Rosemont, IL, American Academy of Orthopaedic Surgeons, 1994.)

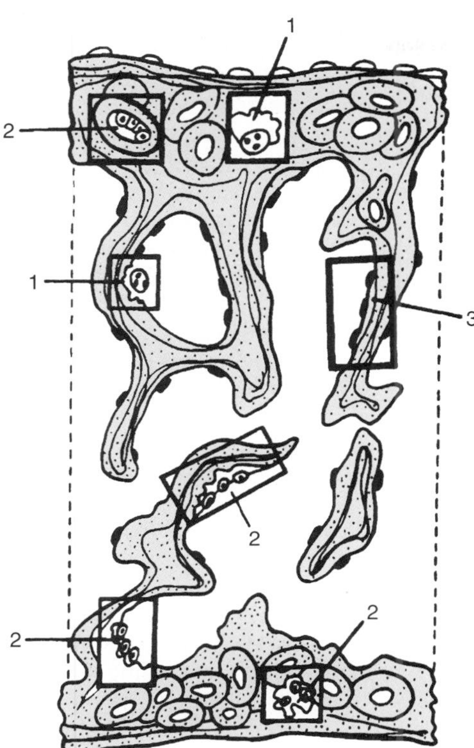

FIGURE 1–3 Bone remodeling 1, Bone resorbed by osteoclastic activity in the cortex and trabeculae. 2, Osteoblasts form new bone at the site of prior bone resorption. 3, Osteoblasts become incorporated into bone as osteocytes. (From Simon SR, ed: Orthopaedic Basic Science, p 141. Rosemont, IL, American Academy of Orthopaedic Surgeons, 1994.)

b. Piezoelectric charges—Bone remodels in response to electrical charges. The compression side of bone is electronegative, stimulating osteoblasts (formation); the tension side of bone is electropositive, stimulating osteoclasts (resorption). Cortical and cancellous bone is continuously remodeled throughout life by osteoclastic and osteoblastic activity (Fig. 1–3).

c. **Hueter-Volkmann law**—Remodeling occurs in small packets of cells known as **basic multicellular units (BMUs),** modulated by systemic hormones and local cytokines. The Hueter-Volkmann law suggests that mechanical factors can influence longitudinal growth, bone remodeling, and fracture repair; compressive forces inhibit growth and tensile forces stimulate growth, which may play a role in the progression of scoliosis and Blount's disease.

2. Cortical bone—Remodels by osteoclastic tunneling (cutting cones) (Fig. 1–4) followed by layering of osteoblasts and successive deposition of layers of lamellae (after the cement line has been laid down) until the tunnel size has narrowed to the diameter of the osteonal central canal. The head of the cutting cone is made up of osteoclasts, which bore holes through hard cortical bone. Behind the osteoclast front are capillaries, followed by osteoblasts that lay down osteoid to fill the resorption cavity.

3. Cancellous bone—Remodels by osteoclastic resorption followed by osteoblasts laying down new bone.

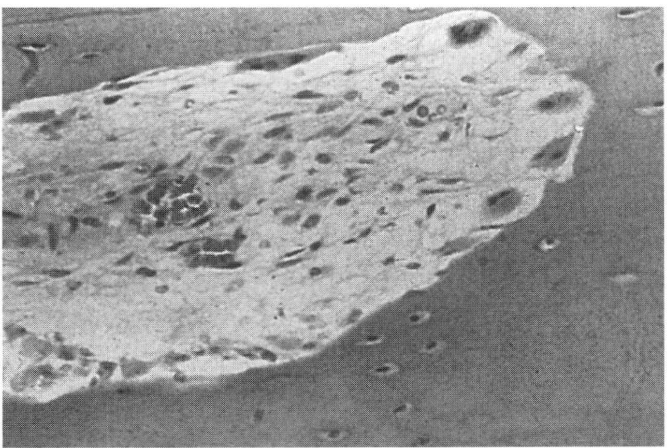

FIGURE 1–4 Mechanism of cortical bone remodeling via cutting cones. (From Simon SR, ed: Orthopaedic Basic Science, p 142. Rosemont, IL, American Academy of Orthopaedic Surgeons, 1994.)

E. Bone circulation

1. Anatomy—As an organ, bone receives 5-10% of the cardiac output. Long bones receive blood from three sources (systems): (1) nutrient artery; (2) metaphyseal-epiphyseal; and (3) periosteal. Bones with a tenuous blood supply include the scaphoid, talus, femoral head, and odontoid.

a. Nutrient artery system—Nutrient arteries branch from the major systemic arteries, enter the diaphyseal cortex (outer and inner tables) through the nutrient foramen, and then enter the medullary canal, branching into ascending and descending small arteries (Fig. 1–5). These branch into arterioles in the endosteal cortex and supply at least the inner two thirds of the mature diaphyseal cortex via vessels in the haversian system (Figs. 1–6 and 1–7). The nutrient artery system is **high pressure.**

b. Metaphyseal-epiphyseal system—Arises from the periarticular vascular plexus (e.g., geniculate arteries).

c. Periosteal system—Composed primarily of capillaries that supply the outer one third (at most) of the mature diaphyseal cortex. The periosteal system is **low pressure.**

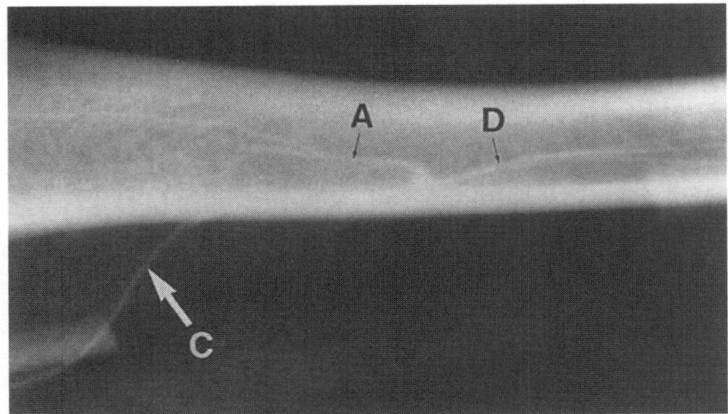

FIGURE 1–5 Intraoperative arteriogram (canine tibia) demonstrating ascending (A) and descending (D) branches of the nutrient artery. C, Cannula (From Brinker MR, Lipton HL, Cook SD, Hyman AL: Pharmacological regulation of the circulation of bone. J Bone Joint Surg [Am] 72:964-975, 1990.)

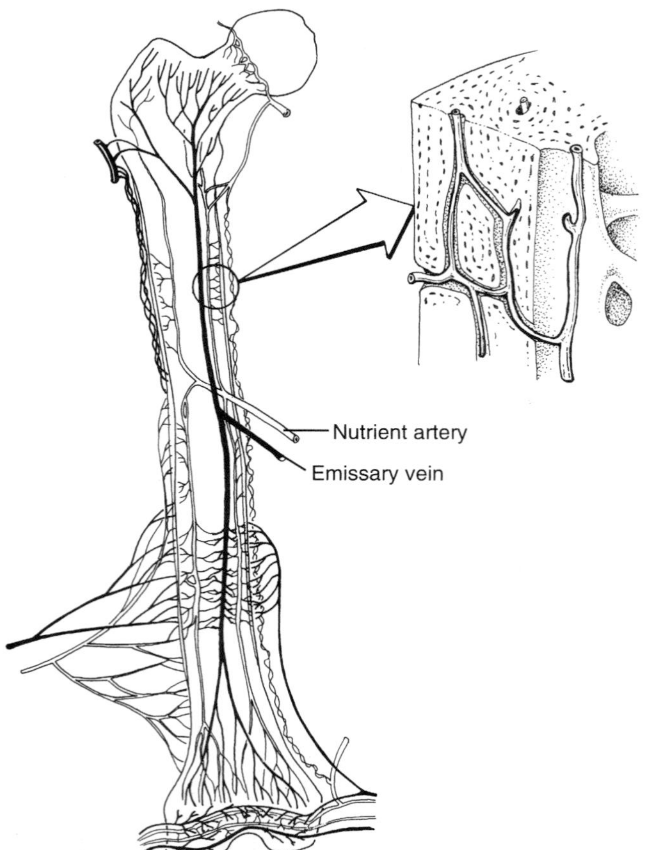

FIGURE 1–6 Blood supply to bone. (From Brinker MR, Miller MD: Fundamentals of Orthopaedics, p 4. Philadelphia, WB Saunders, 1999.)

2. Physiology
   a. Direction of flow (Fig. 1–8)—Arterial flow in mature bone is centrifugal (inside to outside), a result of the net effect of the high-pressure nutrient artery system (endosteal system) and the low-pressure periosteal system. In a completely displaced fracture with disruption of the endosteal (nutrient) system, the pressure gradient reverses, the periosteal system pressure predominates, and blood flow is centripetal (outside to inside). Arterial flow in immature, developing bone is centripetal because the periosteum is highly vascularized and is the predominant component of bone blood flow. Venous flow in mature bone is centripetal; cortical capillaries drain to venous sinusoids, which in turn drain to the emissary venous system.
   b. Fluid compartments of bone

Extravascular	65%
Haversian	6%
Lacunar	6%
Red blood cells (RBCs)	3%
Other	20%

   c. The effect of physiologic states on bone blood flow—Hypoxia, hypercapnia, and sympathectomy all increase flow.
3. Fracture healing—**Bone blood flow is the major determinant of fracture healing.** Bone blood flow delivers nutrients to the site of bony injury. The **initial response** is **decreased bone blood flow** after vascular disruption at the fracture site. **Within hours to days, bone blood flow increases** (as part of the **regional acceleratory phenomenon), peaks at approximately 2 weeks, and returns to normal in 3 to 5 months.** The major advantage of unreamed intramedullary (IM) nails is preservation of the endosteal blood supply. Loose-fitting nails spare cortical perfusion and allow more rapid reperfusion than canal-filling nails. Reaming devascularizes the inner 50-80% of the cortex; this is associated with the greatest delay in revascularization of the endosteal blood supply.
4. Regulation—Bone blood flow is under the control of metabolic, humoral, and autonomic inputs.

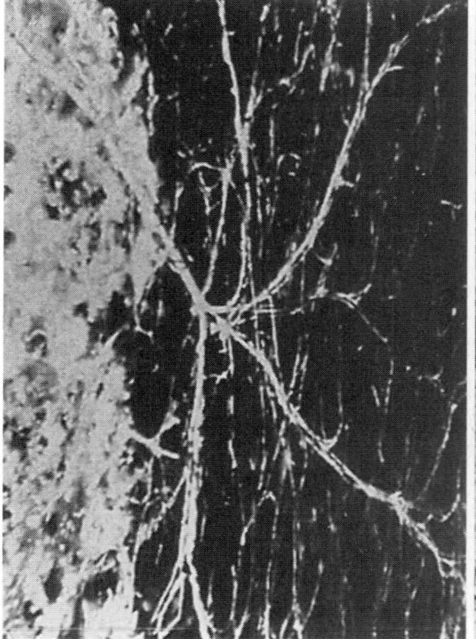
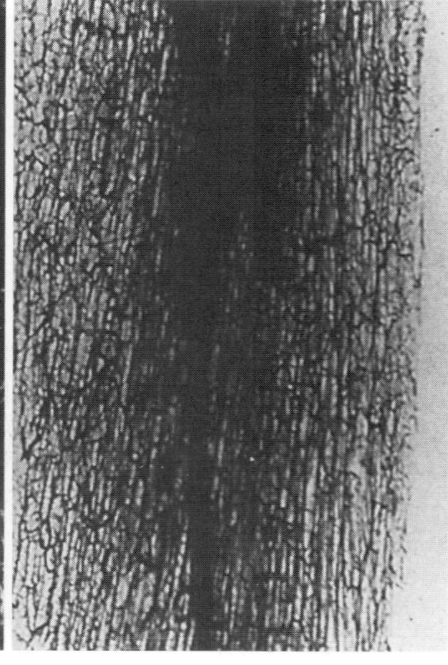

FIGURE 1–7 Vasculature of cortical bone. (From Simon SR, ed: Orthopaedic Basic Science, p 131. Rosemont, IL, American Academy of Orthopaedic Surgeons, 1994.)

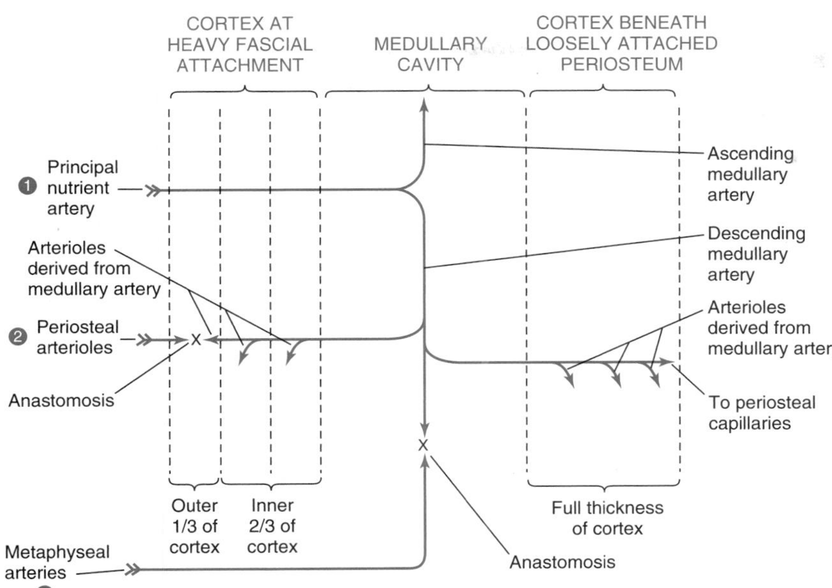

FIGURE 1–8 Major components of the afferent vascular system of long bone. Components 1, 2, and 3 constitute the total nutrient supply to the diaphysis. *Arrows* indicate the direction of blood flow. (From Rhinelander FW: Circulation in bone. In Bourne G, ed: The Biochemistry and Physiology of Bone, 2nd ed, vol 2, pp 1-77. Orlando, FL, Academic Press, 1972.)

The arterial system of bone has great potential for vasoconstriction (from the resting state) and much less potential for vasodilation. The vessels within bone possess a variety of vasoactive receptors (β-adrenergic, muscarinic, thromboxane/prostaglandin) that may be useful in the future for pharmacologic treatment of bone diseases related to aberrant circulation (e.g., osteonecrosis, fracture nonunions).

F. Tissues surrounding bone
   1. Periosteum—Connective tissue membrane that covers bone. It is more highly developed in children because of its role in the deposition of cortical bone, which is responsible for growth in bone diameter. The inner layer of the periosteum, or cambium, is loose, is more vascular, and contains cells that are capable of becoming osteoblasts (to form bone); these cells are responsible for enlarging the diameter of bone during growth and forming periosteal callus during fracture healing. The outer (fibrous) layer is less cellular and is contiguous with joint capsules.
   2. Bone marrow—Source of progenitor cells; controls the inner diameter of bone.
      a. Red marrow—Hematopoietic (40% water, 40% fat, 20% protein). Red marrow slowly changes to yellow marrow with age, beginning in the appendicular skeleton and later the axial skeleton.
      b. Yellow marrow—Inactive (15% water, 80% fat, 5% protein).

G. Types of bone formation (Table 1–4)
   1. Enchondral bone formation/mineralization
      a. General comments—Undifferentiated cells secrete the cartilaginous matrix and differentiate into chondrocytes. The matrix mineralizes and is invaded by vascular buds that bring osteoprogenitor cells. Osteoclasts resorb calcified cartilage, and osteoblasts form bone.

TABLE 1-4 TYPES OF BONE FORMATION

Type of Ossification	Mechanism	Examples of Normal Mechanisms	Examples of Diseases with Abnormal Ossification
Enchondral	Bone replaces a cartilage model	1) Embryonic long-bone formation 2) Longitudinal growth (physis) 3) Fracture callus 4) The type of bone formed with the use of demineralized bone matrix	Achondroplasia
Intramembranous	Aggregates of undifferentiated mesenchymal cells differentiate into osteoblasts, which form bone	1) Embryonic flat bone formation 2) Bone formation during distraction osteogenesis 3) Blastema bone	Cleidocranial dysostosis
Appositional	Osteoblasts lay down new bone on existing bone	1) Periosteal bone enlargement (width) 2) The bone formation phase of bone remodeling	Paget's disease Infantile hyperostosis (Caffey's disease) Melorheostosis

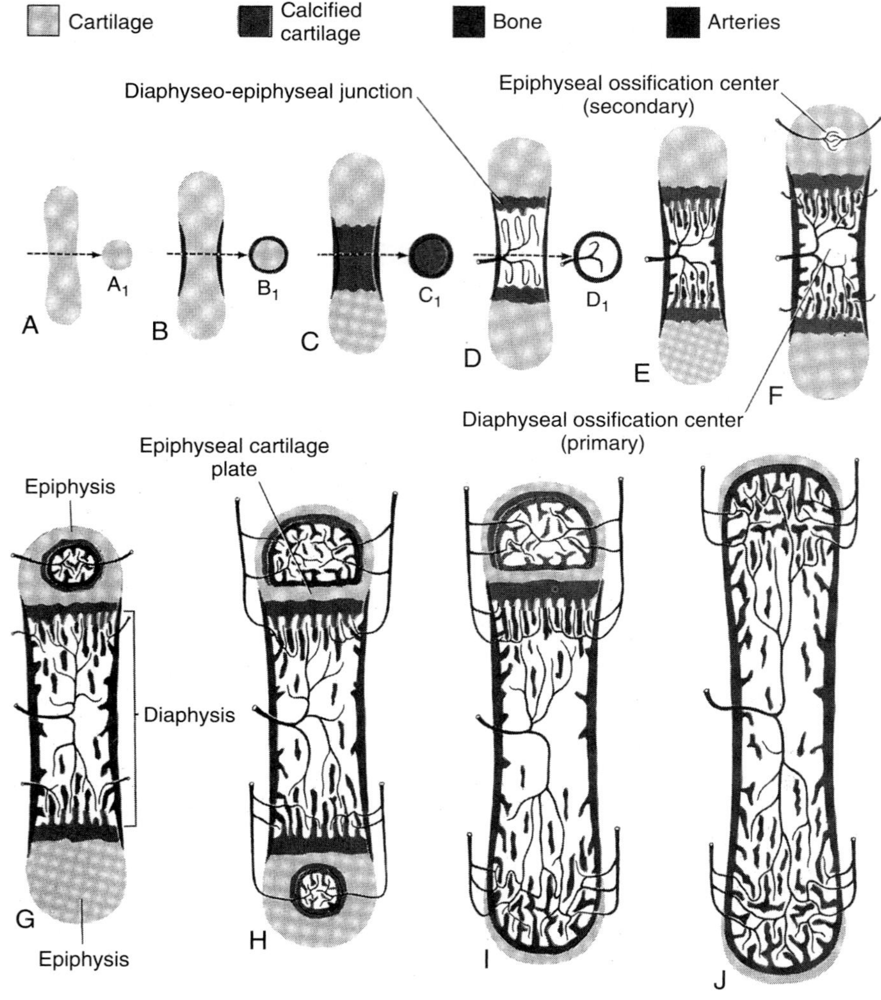

FIGURE 1–9 Enchondral ossification of long bones. Note that phases F through J often occur after birth. (From Moore KL: The Developing Human, p 346. Philadelphia, WB Saunders, 1982.)

Remember that bone replaces the cartilage model; cartilage is not converted to bone. Examples of enchondral bone formation include (1) embryonic long-bone formation, (2) longitudinal growth (physis), (3) fracture callus, and (4) the bone formed with the use of the demineralized bone matrix.

b. Embryonic long-bone formation (Figs. 1–9 and 1–10)—Formed from the mesenchymal anlage, usually at 6 weeks in utero. Enchondral bone formation is responsible for the development of embryonic long bones. Vascular buds invade the mesenchymal model, bringing in osteoprogenitor cells that differentiate into osteoblasts and form the primary centers of ossification at approximately 8 weeks. The cartilage model increases in size through appositional (width) and interstitial (length) growth. The marrow is formed by resorption of the central portion of the cartilage anlage by invasion of myeloid precursor cells brought in by the capillary buds. Secondary centers of ossification develop at the bone ends, forming epiphyseal centers of ossification (growth plates), which are responsible for longitudinal growth of immature bones. During this developmental stage, there is a rich arterial supply composed of an epiphyseal artery (which terminates in the proliferative zone), metaphyseal arteries, nutrient arteries, and perichondrial arteries (Fig. 1–11).

c. Physis—Two growth plates exist in immature long bones: (1) **horizontal** (the physis) and (2) **spherical** (allows growth of the epiphysis). The spherical growth plate has the same arrangement as the physis but is less organized. **The perichondrial artery is the major source of nutrition for the physis.** Acromegaly and spondyloepiphyseal dysplasia affect the physis; multiple epiphyseal dysplasia affects the epiphysis. Physeal cartilage zones are based on growth (see Fig. 1–11) and function (Figs. 1–12 and 1–13).

(1) Reserve zone—Cells store lipids, glycogen, and proteoglycan aggregates for later growth and matrix production. Decreased oxygen tension occurs in this zone. **Lysosomal storage diseases (Gaucher's)** and other disorders can affect this zone.

(2) Proliferative zone—Longitudinal growth occurs, with stacking of chondrocytes (the

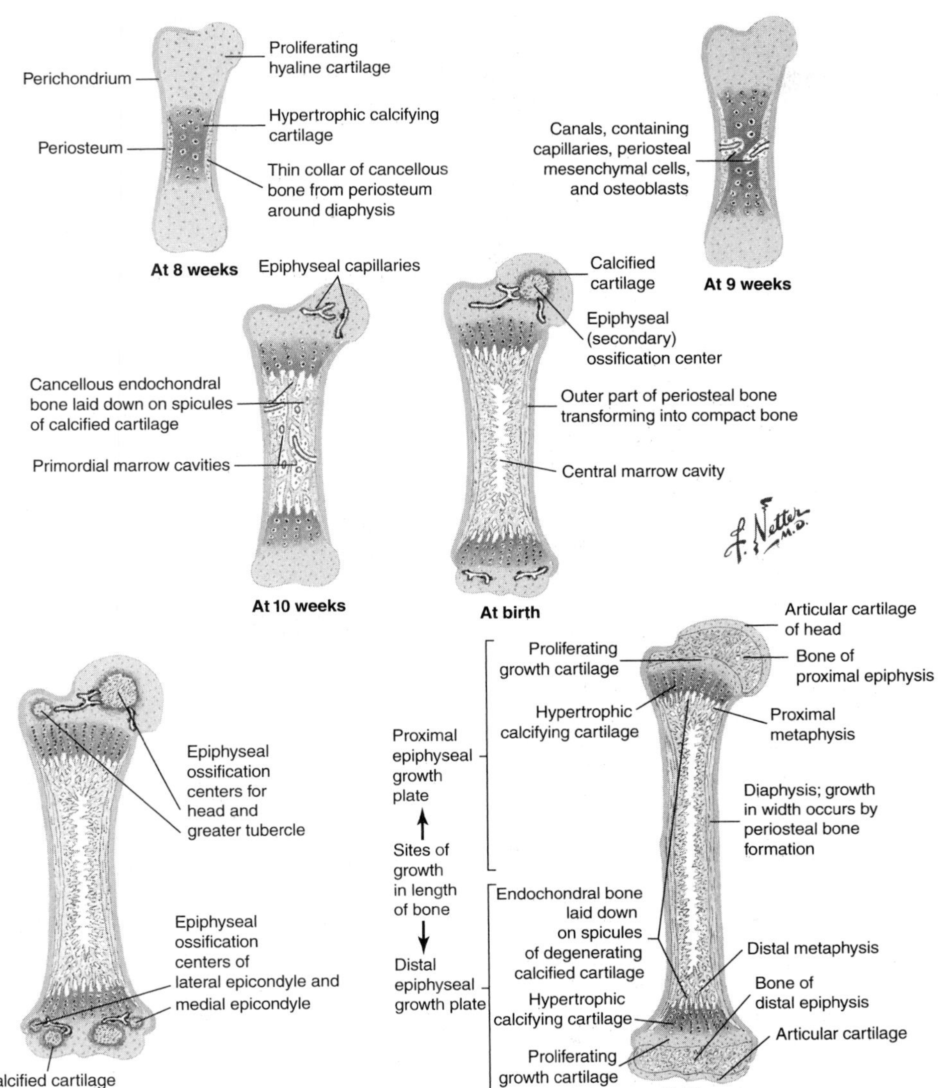

FIGURE 1–10 Development of a typical long bone: formation of the growth plate and secondary centers of ossification. (From The Ciba Collection of Medical Illustrations, vol 8, part I, p 136, 1987. Illustrated by Frank H. Netter. Reprinted by permission.)

top cell is the dividing "mother" cell). There are increased oxygen tension and increased proteoglycans in the surrounding matrix, which inhibit calcification. This zone functions in cellular proliferation and matrix production. Defects in this zone (chondrocyte proliferation and column formation) are seen in **achondroplasia** (see Fig. 1–13) (does not affect intramembranous bone [width]).

(3) Hypertrophic zone—Sometimes subdivided into three zones: **maturation, degeneration,** and **provisional calcification.** Normal mineralization of the matrix occurs in the lower hypertrophic zone where chondrocytes increase five times in size, accumulate calcium in their mitochondria, and then die (releasing calcium from matrix vesicles). **The rate of chondrocyte maturation is regulated by systemic hormones and local growth factors (parathyroid-related peptide inhibits chondrocyte maturation; Indian hedgehog is produced by growth plate chondrocytes and regulates the expression of parathyroid-related peptide).** Osteoblasts migrate from sinusoidal vessels and use cartilage as a scaffolding for bone formation. Low oxygen tension and decreased proteoglycan aggregates aid this process. **This zone widens in rickets** (see Fig 1–13), where little or no provisional calcification occurs. **Enchondromas** also originate in this zone. **Mucopolysaccharide diseases** (see Fig. 1–13) also affect this zone, leading to chondrocyte degeneration (swollen, abnormal chondrocytes). Physeal fractures were classically believed to occur through the provisional calcification zone (within the hypertrophic zone) but probably

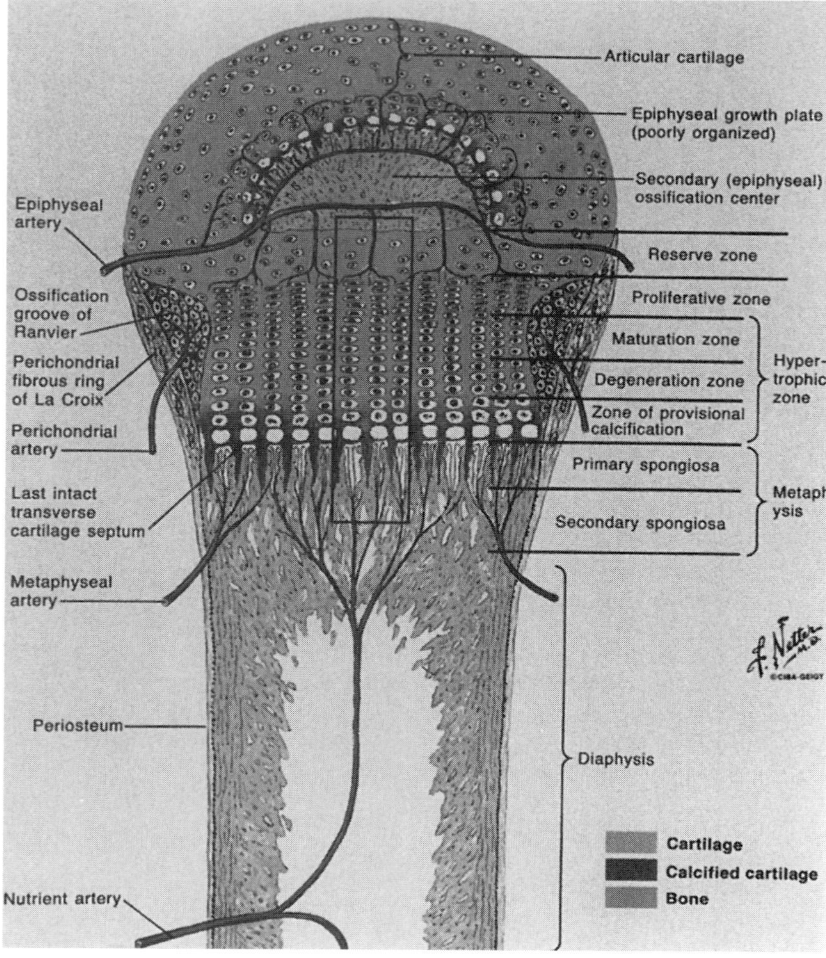

FIGURE 1–11 Structure and blood supply of a typical growth plate. (From The Ciba Collection of Medical Illustrations, vol 8, part I, p 166, 1987. Illustrated by Frank H. Netter. Reprinted by permission.)

traverse several zones, depending on the type of loading (Fig. 1–14). **The hypertrophic zone is believed to be involved in slipped capital femoral epiphysis (SCFE), except SCFE associated with renal failure, in which the slippage occurs through the metaphyseal spongiosa.**

d. Metaphysis—Adjacent to the physis, the metaphysis expands with skeletal growth. Osteoblasts from osteoprogenitor cells align on cartilage bars produced by physeal expansion. Primary spongiosa (calcified cartilage bars) mineralizes to form woven bone and remodels to form secondary spongiosa and a "cutback zone" at the metaphysis. Cortical bone is made by remodeling of physeal (enchondral) and intramembranous bone in response to stress along the periphery of the growing long bones.
e. Periphery of the physis—Composed of two elements:
   (1) Groove of Ranvier—Supplies chondrocytes to the periphery of the growth plate for lateral growth (width).
   (2) Perichondrial ring of LaCroix—Dense fibrous tissue that is the primary limiting membrane anchoring and supporting the periphery of the physis.
f. Mineralization—Consists of seeding of collagen hole zones with calcium hydroxyapatite crystals through branching and accretion (crystal growth).
g. Effect of hormones and growth factors on the growth plate—Several hormones and growth factors have both direct and indirect effects on the developing growth plate. Some factors are produced and act within the growth plate (paracrine or autocrine), and others are produced at a site distant from the growth plate (endocrine). Hormones and growth factors act via their effects on chondrocytes and matrix mineralization (summarized in Fig. 1–15 and Table 1–5).

2. **Intramembranous ossification**—Occurs without a cartilage model. Undifferentiated mesenchymal cells aggregate into layers (or membranes). These cells differentiate into osteoblasts and deposit an organic matrix that mineralizes to form bone. **Examples of intramembranous bone formation include (1) embryonic flat bone formation (pelvis, clavicle, vault of skull), (2) bone formation during distraction osteogenesis, and (3) blastema bone (occurs in young children with amputations).**

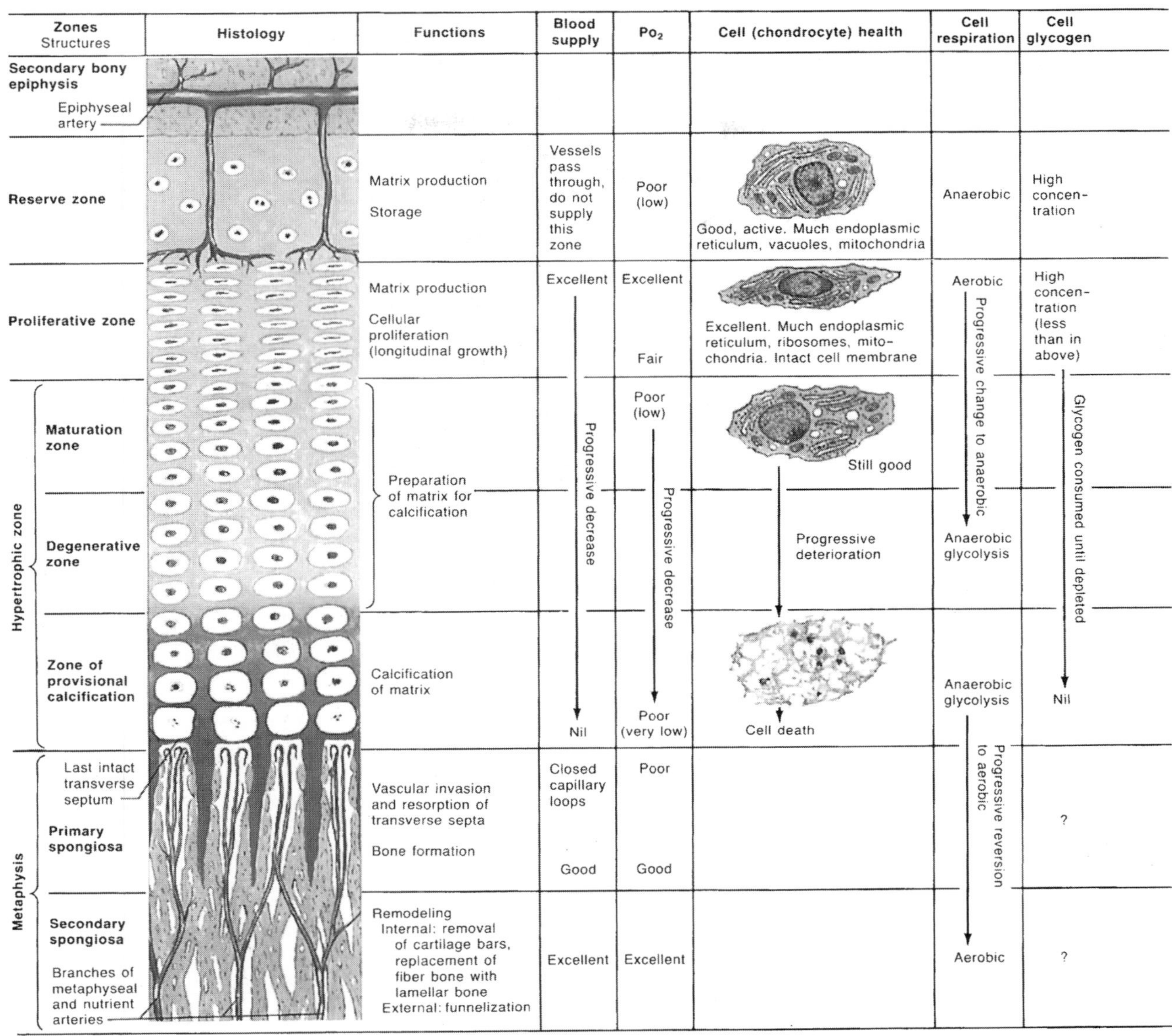

FIGURE 1–12 Zone structure, function, and physiology of the growth plate. (From The Ciba Collection of Medical Illustrations, vol 8, part I, p 164, 1987. Illustrated by Frank H. Netter. Reprinted by permission.)

3. **Appositional ossification**—Osteoblasts align themselves on the existing bone surface and lay down new bone. **Examples of appositional ossification include (1) periosteal bone enlargement (width) and (2) the bone formation phase of bone remodeling.**

II. Bone Injury and Repair

A. **Fracture repair**—A continuum proceeding from **inflammation** through **repair** (soft callus followed by hard callus) and ending in **remodeling.** Fracture healing may be influenced by a variety of biologic and mechanical factors (Table 1–6). **The most important factor in fracture healing is blood supply (bone blood flow).** Head injury can increase the osteogenic response to fracture. Nicotine from smoking increases the time to fracture healing, increases the risk of nonunion (particularly in the tibia), and decreases the strength fracture callus. Smoking also increases the risk of pseudarthrosis after lumbar fusion by up to 500%. Nonsteroidal anti-inflammatory drugs (NSAIDs) have an adverse effect on fracture healing and healing of lumbar spinal fusions.

1. Stages of fracture repair
   a. Inflammation—Bleeding from the fracture site and surrounding soft tissues creates a hematoma, which provides a source of hematopoietic cells capable of secreting growth factors. Subsequently, fibroblasts, mesenchymal cells, and osteoprogenitor cells are present at the fracture site, and granulation tissue forms around the fracture ends. Osteoblasts from surrounding osteogenic precursor cells, fibroblasts, or both proliferate.
   b. Repair—Primary callus response occurs within 2 weeks. If the bone ends are not in continuity, **bridging (soft) callus** occurs.

Zones Structures	Histology	Functions	Exemplary diseases	Defect (if known)
Secondary bony epiphysis; Epiphyseal artery	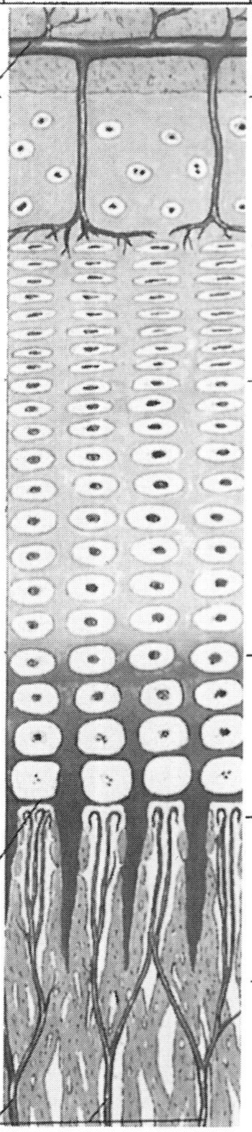			
Reserve zone		Matrix production Storage	Diastrophic dwarfism (also, defects in other zones)	Defective type II collagen synthesis
			Pseudoachondroplasia (also, defects in other zones)	Defective processing and transport of proteoglycans
			Kneist syndrome (also, defects in other zones)	Defective processing of proteoglycans
Proliferative zone		Matrix production Cellular proliferation (longitudinal growth)	Gigantism	Increased cell proliferation (growth hormone increased)
			Achondroplasia	Deficiency of cell proliferation
			Hypochondroplasia	Less severe deficiency of cell proliferation
			Malnutrition, irradiation injury, glucocorticoid excess	Decreased cell proliferation and/or matrix synthesis
Hypertrophic zone: Maturation zone; Degenerative zone		Preparation of matrix for calcification	Mucopolysaccharidosis (Morquio's syndrome, Hurler's syndrome)	Deficiencies of specific lysosomal acid hydrolases, with lysosomal storage of mucopolysaccharides
Hypertrophic zone: Zone of provisional calcification		Calcification of matrix	Rickets, osteomalacia (also, defects in metaphysis)	Insufficiency of Ca^{++} and/or P for normal calcification of matrix
Metaphysis: Last intact transverse septum; Primary spongiosa		Vascular invasion and resorption of transverse septa Bone formation	Metaphyseal chondro-dysplasia (Jansen and Schmid types)	Extension of hypertrophic cells into metaphysis
			Acute hematogenous osteomyelitis	Flourishing of bacteria due to sluggish circulation, low PO_2, reticuloendothelial deficiency
Metaphysis: Secondary spongiosa; Branches of metaphyseal and nutrient arteries		Remodeling Internal: removal of cartilage bars, replacement of fiber bone with lamellar bone External: funnelization	Osteopetrosis	Abnormality of osteoclasts (internal remodeling)
			Osteogenesis imperfecta	Abnormality of osteoblasts and collagen synthesis
			Scurvy	Inadequate collagen formation
			Metaphyseal dysplasia (Pyle disease)	Abnormality of funnelization (external remodeling)

FIGURE 1–13 Zone structure and pathologic defects of cellular metabolism. (From The Ciba Collection of Medical Illustrations, vol 8, part I, p 165, 1987. Illustrated by Frank H. Netter. Reprinted by permission.)

The soft callus is later replaced, via the process of enchondral ossification, by **woven bone (hard callus).** Another type of callus, **medullary callus,** supplements the bridging callus, although it forms more slowly and occurs later (Fig. 1–16). During callus formation in an unstable fracture, type II collagen is expressed early, followed by type I collagen. Fracture healing varies with the method of treatment (Table 1–7). The amount of callus formation is inversely proportional to the extent of immobilization of the fracture. **Differentiation of the progenitor cells depends on local oxygen tension and strain conditions. High strain promotes fibrous tissue; low strain and high oxygen tension promote woven bone; and intermediate strain and low oxygen tension promote cartilage.** Primary cortical (direct osteonal) healing via intramembranous ossification without visible callus, which resembles normal (haversian) remodeling, occurs with rigid immobilization (compression plate) and anatomic (or near-anatomic) reduction. With closed treatment, enchondral ossification with periosteal bridging callus occurs. The initial histologic change observed in hypertrophic nonunions treated with plate stabilization is fibrocartilage mineralization.

c. Remodeling—This process begins during the middle of the repair phase and continues long after the fracture has clinically healed (up to 7 years). Remodeling allows the bone to assume its normal configuration and shape based on the stress to which it is exposed (Wolff's law). Throughout the process, woven bone formed during the repair phase is replaced with lamellar bone. Fracture healing is complete when there is repopulation of the marrow space.

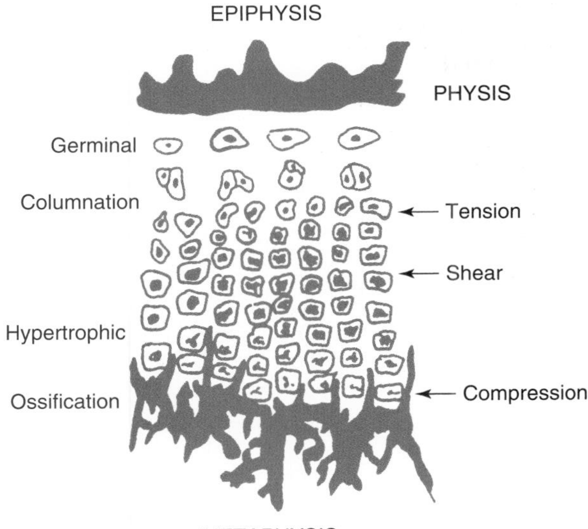

FIGURE 1–14 Histologic zone of failure varies with the type of loading applied to a specimen. (From Moen CT, Pelker RR: Biomechanical and histological correlations in growth plate failure. J Pediatr Orthop 4:180–184, 1984.)

2. Biochemistry of fracture healing—Four biochemical steps of fracture healing have been described (Table 1–8).
3. Growth factors of bone (Table 1–9)
4. Endocrine effects on fracture healing (Table 1–10)
5. Ultrasound and fracture healing—Clinical studies show that low-intensity pulsed ultrasound accelerates fracture healing and increases the mechanical strength of callus, including torque and stiffness. The postulated mechanism of action is that the cells responsible for fracture healing respond favorably to the mechanical energy transmitted by the ultrasound signal.
6. Effect of radiation on bone—High-dose irradiation causes long-term changes within the haversian system and also decreases cellularity. Immediate postoperative irradiation adversely affects the incorporation of anterior spinal interbody strut grafts (delaying radiation for 3 weeks eliminates these effects). High-dose irradiation (90 kGy, the dose needed for viral inactivation) of allograft bone significantly reduces its structural integrity.
7. Electricity and fracture healing
   a. Definitions
      (1) Stress-generated potentials—Serve as signals that modulate cellular activity. Piezoelectric effect and streaming potentials are examples of stress-generated potentials.
      (2) Piezoelectric effect—Charges in tissues are displaced secondary to mechanical forces.
      (3) Streaming potentials—Occur when electrically charged fluid is forced over a tissue (cell membrane) with a fixed charge.
      (4) Transmembrane potentials—Generated by cellular metabolism.
   b. Fracture healing—Electrical properties of cartilage and bone depend on their charged molecules. Devices intended to stimulate fracture repair by altering a variety of cellular activities have been introduced.
   c. Types of electrical stimulation
      (1) Direct current (DC)—Stimulates an inflammatory-like response (stage I).

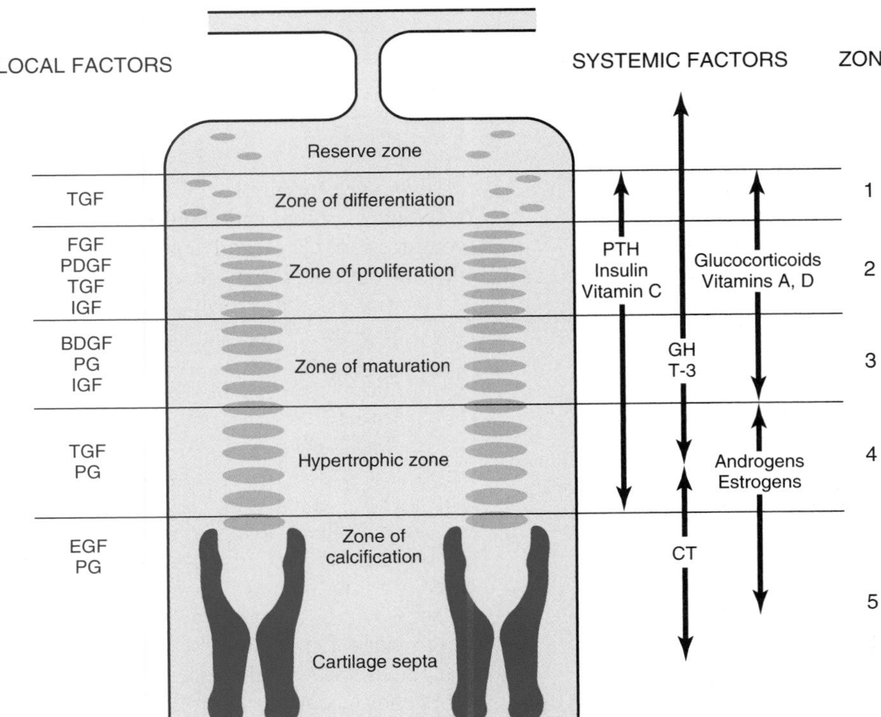

FIGURE 1–15 Growth plate demonstrating the proposed sites of action of hormones, growth factors, and vitamins. (From Simon SR, ed: Orthopaedic Basic Science, p 197. Rosemont, IL, American Academy of Orthopaedic Surgeons, 1994.)

TABLE 1-5 EFFECTS OF HORMONES AND GROWTH FACTORS ON THE GROWTH PLATE

Biologic Effect of Hormone/Factor	Systemic/Local Derivation	Proliferation	Macromolecule Biosynthesis	Maturation Degradation	Matrix Calcification	Zone Primarily Affected
Thyroxine	Systemic (thyroid)	+ (T3 with IGF-I)	0	+ (T3 alone)	0	Proliferative zone and upper hypertrophic zone
Parathyroid	Systemic (parathyroid)	+	++ (Proteoglycan)	0	0	Entire growth plate
Calcitonin	Systemic (thyroid)	0	0	+	+	Hypertrophic zone and metaphysis
Excess corticosteroids	Systemic (adrenals)	–	–	–	0	Entire growth plate
Growth hormone	Systemic (pituitary)	+ (through IGF-I locally)	+ (Slight)	0	0	Proliferative zone
Somatomedins	Systemic local paracrine (liver, chondrocytes)	+	+ (Slight)	0	0	Proliferative zone
Insulin	Systemic (pancreas)	+ (through IGF-I receptor)	0	0	0	Proliferative zone
1,25-$(OH)_2D_3$	Systemic (liver, kidney)	0	0	+ (Indirect effect serum [Ca] × [PO])		Hypertrophic zone
24,25-$(OH)_2D_3$	Systemic (liver, kidney)	+	+ (Collagen II)	0	0	Proliferative zone and hypertrophic zone
Vitamin A	Systemic (diet)	0	0	–	0	Hypertrophic zone
Vitamin C	Systemic (diet)	0	+ (Collagen)	0	+ (Matrix vesicles)	Proliferative zone and hypertrophic zone
EGF	Local paracrine (endothelial cells)	+	– (Collagen)	0	0	Metaphysis
FGF	Local paracrine (endothelial cells)	+	0	0	0	Proliferative zone
PDGF	Local paracrine (platelets)	+	+ (Noncollagenous proteins)	0	0	Proliferative zone
TGF-β	Local paracrine (platelets, chondrocytes)	±	±	0	0	Proliferative zone and hypertrophic zone
BDGF	Local paracrine (bone matrix)	0	+ (Collagen)	0	0	Upper hypertrophic zone
IL-I	Local paracrine (inflammatory cells, synoviocytes)	0	–	++ (Activates tissue metalloproteinases)	0	Entire growth plate
Prostaglandin	Local autocrine	±	+ (Proteoglycan) – (Collagen and alkaline phosphatase)	0	Bone resorption with osteoclasts	Hypertrophic zone and metaphysis

+, Increase stimulation; 0, no known effect; –, inhibitory; ±, depending on the local hormonal milieu.

EGF, epidermal growth factor; FGF, fibroblast growth factor; PDGF, platelet-derived growth factor; TGF-β, transforming growth factor-β; BDGF, bone-derived growth factor; IL-1, interleukin-1; IGF-I, insulin-like growth factor I.

From Simon SR: Orthopaedic Basic Science, 2nd ed, p 196. Rosemont, IL, American Academy of Orthopaedic Surgeons, 1994; reprinted by permission.

TABLE 1-6 BIOLOGIC AND MECHANICAL FACTORS INFLUENCING FRACTURE HEALING

Biologic Factors	Mechanical Factors
Patient age	Soft tissue attachments to bone
Comorbid medical conditions	Stability (extent of immobilization)
Functional level	Anatomic location
Nutritional status	Level of energy imparted
Nerve function	Extent of bone loss
Vascular injury	
Hormones	
Growth factors	
Health of the soft tissue envelope	
Sterility (in open fractures)	
Cigarette smoke	
Local pathologic conditions	
Level of energy imparted	
Type of bone affected	
Extent of bone loss	

(2) Alternating current (AC)—"Capacity coupled generators." Affects cyclic adenosine monophosphate (cAMP), collagen synthesis, and calcification during the repair stage.

(3) Pulsed electromagnetic fields (PEMFs)—Initiate calcification of fibrocartilage (cannot induce calcification of fibrous tissue).

8. Pathologic fracture—Occurs through areas of weakened bone from tumor, infection, or metabolic bone disease. The factors most predictive of the risk of pathologic fracture are pain, anatomic location, and the pattern of bony destruction (scoring system of Mirels). **The anatomic site with the highest risk of pathologic fracture is the subtrochanteric femur.**

B. Bone grafting—Bone grafts have four important properties (Table 1–11).
   1. Graft properties
      a. Osteoconductive matrix—Acts as a scaffold or framework into which bone growth occurs.
      b. Osteoinductive factors—Growth factors such as bone morphogenetic protein (BMP) and transforming growth factor-β (TGF-β that signal local factors to stimulate bone formation.
      c. Osteogenic cells—Include primitive mesenchymal cells, osteoblasts, and osteocytes.
      d. Structural integrity
   2. Overview of bone grafts—Commonly autografts (from same person) or allografts (from another person). Cancellous bone is commonly used for grafting nonunions or cavitary defects because it is quickly remodeled and incorporated (via creeping substitution). Cortical bone is slower to turn over than cancellous bone and is used for structural defects.
      a. Osteoarticular (osteochondral) allograft use is increasing in frequency for tumor surgery; they are immunogenic (cartilage is vulnerable to inflammatory mediators of immune response [cytotoxicity from antibodies and lymphocytes]); articular cartilage is preserved with glycerol or dimethyl sulfoxide (DMSO); and **cryogenically preserved grafts leave few viable chondrocytes.** Tissue-matched (syngeneic) osteochondral grafts produce minimal immunogenic effects and incorporate well.
      b. Vascularized bone grafts, though technically difficult, allow more rapid union and cell preservation; best for irradiated tissues or large tissue defects (may be donor site morbidity [i.e., fibula]).
      c. Nonvascular bone grafts are more common than vascularized grafts.
      d. Allograft bone
         (1) Types—(a) fresh—increased immunogenicity; (b) fresh-frozen—less immunogenic than fresh BMP preserved; (c) freeze-dried (lyophilized)—loses structural integrity and depletes BMP, **least immunogenic, purely osteoconductive, and lowest likelihood of viral transmission,** commonly known as "croutons." **Compaction is faster with freeze-dried allograft than with fresh-frozen allograft, so they may be more efficient to use in surgical situations.** (d) bone matrix gelatin (BMG, a digested source of BMP)—**demineralized bone matrix (Grafton) is osteoconductive and osteoinductive.**
         (2) Antigenicity—Bone allografts are composite materials and therefore possess a spectrum of potential antigens, **primarily from cell surface glycoproteins.** The primary mechanism of rejection is cellular, as opposed to humoral. Bone marrow cells of allograft incite the greatest immunogenic response. Classes I and II cellular antigens contained within allograft are recognized by T lymphocytes in the host. Cellular components that contribute to antigenicity include those of marrow origin, the endothelium, and retinacular activating cells. Both the cellular components and

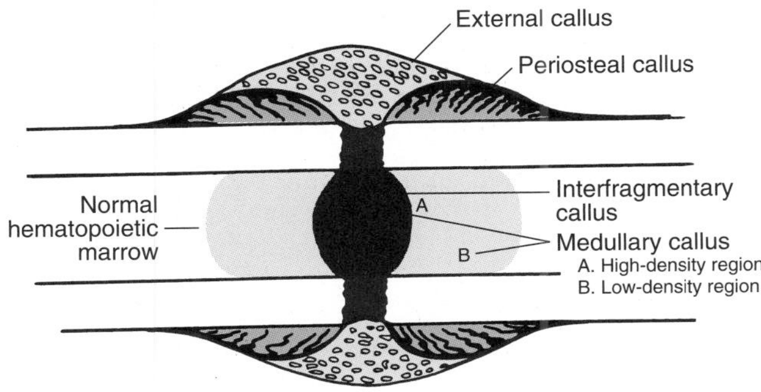

FIGURE 1–16 Histology of typical fracture healing. (From Brighton CT, Hunt RM: Early histological and ultrastructural changes in medullary fracture callus. J Bone Joint Surg [Am] 73:832-847, 1991.)

TABLE 1-7 TYPE OF FRACTURE HEALING BASED ON TYPE OF STABILIZATION

Type of Stabilization	Predominant Type of Healing
Cast (closed treatment)	Periosteal bridging callus and interfragmentary enchondral ossification
Compression plate	Primary cortical healing (cutting cone–type or haversian remodeling)
Intramedullary nail	Early: periosteal bridging callus; enchondral ossification Late: medullary callus and intramembranous ossification
External fixator	Dependent on extent of rigidity: Less rigid: periosteal bridging callus; enchondral ossification More rigid: primary cortical healing; intramembranous ossification
Inadequate immobilization with adequate blood supply	Hypertrophic nonunion (failed enchondral ossification); type II collagen predominates
Inadequate immobilization without adequate blood supply	Atrophic nonunion
Inadequate reduction with displacement at the fracture site	Oligotrophic nonunion

TABLE 1-8 BIOCHEMICAL STEPS OF FRACTURE HEALING

Step	Collagen Type
Mesenchymal	I, II (III, V)
Chondroid	II, IX
Chondroid-osteoid	I, II, X
Osteogenic	I

the extracellular matrix elicit an antigenic response, with the former eliciting a relatively greater response. Type I collagen (organic matrix) stimulates both cell-mediated and humoral responses. The noncollagenous portion of the matrix (proteoglycans, osteopontin, osteocalcin, and other glycoproteins) also stimulates an immunogenic response. **Hydroxyapatite has not been shown to elicit an immune response. Allograft incorporation is related to cellularity and major histocompatibility complex (MHC) incompatibility between host tissue and allogenic tissue.**

e. Five stages of graft healing (Urist) (Table 1–12)

3. **Specific bone graft types**
   a. Cortical bone grafts—Slower incorporation through remodeling of existing haversian systems via resorption (weakens the graft) followed by deposition of new bone (restores strength). Resorption confined to osteon borders; interstitial lamellae are preserved. Used for structural defects.
   b. Cancellous grafts—Revascularize and incorporate quickly; osteoblasts lay down new bone on old trabeculae, which are later remodeled ("creeping substitution"). Allografts must be harvested with a sterile technique, and donors must be screened for potential transmissible diseases. The major factors influencing bone graft incorporation are shown in Figure 1–17.
   c. Synthetic bone grafts—Composed of calcium, silicon, or aluminum.
      (1) Silicate-based grafts—Incorporate the element silicon (Si) as silicate (silicon dioxide): bioactive glasses and glass-ionomer cement.
      (2) Calcium phosphate–based grafts—Capable of osseoconduction and osseointegration. **These materials biodegrade at a very slow rate.** Many are prepared as

TABLE 1-9 GROWTH FACTORS OF BONE

Growth Factor	Action	Notes
Bone morphogenetic protein (BMP)	Osteoinductive; stimulates bone formation Induces metaplasia of mesenchymal cells into osteoblasts	Target cells of BMP are the undifferentiated perivascular mesenchymal cells; signal through serine/threonine kinase receptors. Intracellular molecules called SMADs serve as signaling mediators for BMPs.
Transforming growth factor-β (TGF-β)	Induces mesenchymal cells to produce type II collagen and proteoglycans Induces osteoblasts to synthesize collagen	Found in fracture hematomas; believed to **regulate cartilage and bone formation in fracture callus;** signal through serine/threonine kinase receptors Coating porous implants with TGF-β enhances bone ingrowth.
Insulin-like growth factor II (IGF-II)	Stimulates type I collagen, cellular proliferation, cartilage matrix synthesis, and bone formation	Signal through tyrosine kinase receptors
Platelet-derived growth factor (PDGF)	Attracts inflammatory cells to the fracture site (chemotactic)	Released from platelets; signal through tyrosine kinase receptors

TABLE 1-10 ENDOCRINE EFFECTS ON FRACTURE HEALING

Hormone	Effect	Mechanism
Cortisone	–	Decreased callus proliferation
Calcitonin	+?	Unknown
TH/PTH	+	Bone remodeling
Growth hormone	+	Increased callus volume

TH/PTH, thyroid hormone/parathyroid hormone.

ceramics (heated apatite crystals fuse into crystals [sintered]).
(a) Tricalcium phosphate
(b) Hydroxyapatite (e.g., Collagraft Bone Graft Matrix [Zimmer, Inc, Warsaw, IN]); purified bovine dermal fibrillar collagen plus ceramic hydroxyapatite granules and tricalcium phosphate granules.
(3) Calcium sulfate—Osteoconductive (e.g., OsteoSet [Wright Medical Technology Inc., Arlington, TN]).
(4) Calcium carbonate (chemically unaltered marine coral)—Is resorbed and replaced by bone (osteoconductive) (e.g., Biocora [Inoteb, France]).
(5) Coralline hydroxyapatite—Calcium carbonate skeleton is converted to calcium phosphate via a thermoexchange process (e.g., Interpore 200 and 500 [Interpore Orthopaedics, Irvine, CA]).
(6) Other materials
(a) Aluminum oxide—Alumina ceramic bonds to bone in response to stress and strain between implant and bone.
(b) Hard tissue—Replacement polymer

C. Distraction osteogenesis (Fig. 1–18)
1. Definition—The use of distraction to stimulate formation of bone.
2. Clinical applications
a. Limb lengthening
b. Hypertrophic nonunions
c. Deformity correction (via differential lengthening)
d. Segmental bone loss (via bone transport)
3. Biology
a. Under optimally stable conditions, bone forms via intramembranous ossification.
b. In an unstable environment, bone forms via enchondral ossification; in an extremely unstable environment, pseudarthrosis may occur.
c. Histologic phases
(1) Latency phase (5-7 days)
(2) Distraction phase (1 mm per day [approximately 1 inch per month])
(3) Consolidation phase (typically twice as long as the distraction phase)
4. Conditions that promote optimal bone formation during distraction osteogenesis
a. Low-energy corticotomy/osteotomy
b. Minimal soft tissue stripping at the corticotomy site (preserves blood supply)
c. Stable external fixation to eliminate torsion, shear, and bending moments
d. Latency period (no lengthening) of 5-7 days
e. Distraction at 0.25 mm 3-4 times per day (0.75-1.0 mm per day)
f. Neutral fixation interval (no distraction) during consolidation
g. Normal physiologic use of the extremity, including weight bearing.

D. Heterotopic ossification (HO)—Ectopic bone forms in the soft tissues, most commonly in response to an injury or a surgical dissection.
1. Myositis ossificans (MO) is a specific form of HO when the ossification occurs in muscle.
2. Patients with traumatic brain injuries are particularly prone to HO; recurrence after resection is likely if neurologic compromise is severe. **The timing of surgery for HO after traumatic brain injury depends on the time since injury (usually 3 to 6 months is adequate; there is usually no need to wait longer than 6 months) and evidence of bone maturation on plain radiographs (sharp demarcation and a trabecular pattern).**

TABLE 1-11 TYPES OF BONE GRAFTS AND BONE GRAFT PROPERTIES

Graft	Properties				
	Osteoconduction	*Osteoinduction*	*Osteogenic Cells*	*Structural Integrity*	*Other Properties*
Autograft					
Cancellous	Excellent	Good	Excellent	Poor	Rapid incorporation
Cortical	Fair	Fair	Fair	Excellent	Slow incorporation
Allograft	Fair	Fair	None	Good	Fresh has the highest immunogenicity Freeze-dried is the least immunogenic but has the least structural integrity (weakest) Fresh-frozen preserves BMP
Ceramics	Fair	None	None	Fair	
Demineralized bone matrix	Fair	Good	None	Poor	
Bone marrow	Poor	Poor	Good	Poor	

BMP, bone morphogenic protein.
Modified from Brinker MR, Miller MD: Fundamentals of Orthopaedics, p 7. Philadelphia, WB Saunders, 1999.

TABLE 1-12 STAGES OF GRAFT HEALING

Stage	Activity
1—Inflammation	Chemotaxis stimulated by necrotic debris
2—Osteoblast differentiation	From precursors
3—Osteoinduction	Osteoblast and osteoclast function
4—Osteoconduction	New bone forming over scaffold
5—Remodeling	Process continues for years

3. When resecting HO after total hip arthroplasty (THA) (should be delayed for ≥6 months after THA), adjuvant radiation therapy is useful to prevent HO recurrence; **irradiation (optimal therapy is a single postoperative dose of 600-700 rad) prevents proliferation and differentiation of primordial mesenchymal cells into osteoprogenitor cells that can form osteoblastic tissue.**
4. **Preoperative radiation helps to prevent the formation of HO following THA in patients who are at high risk.** The incidence of HO after THA in patients with Paget's disease is high (approximately 50%).
5. Oral diphosphonate inhibits mineralization of osteoid but does not prevent the formation of osteoid matrix; when oral diphosphonate therapy is discontinued, mineralization with formation of HO may occur.

III. Conditions of Bone Mineralization, Bone Mineral Density, and Bone Viability

A. Normal bone metabolism

1. Calcium—Bone serves as a reservoir for more than 99% of the body's calcium. Calcium is also important in muscle and nerve function, clotting mechanisms, and many other areas. Plasma calcium (<1% of total body calcium) is about equally free and bound (usually to albumin). It is absorbed in the duodenum by active transport (requiring adenosine triphosphate (ATP) and calcium-binding protein and regulated by 1,25-$(OH)_2$ vitamin D_3) and by passive diffusion in the jejunum. The kidney reabsorbs 98% of calcium (60% in the proximal tubule). **The primary homeostatic regulators of serum calcium are PTH and 1,25-$(OH)_2$ vitamin D.** The dietary requirement of **elemental calcium** is approximately 600 mg/day for children, about 1300 mg/day for adolescents and young adults (growth spurt [ages 10-25 years]), and 750 mg/day for adult men and women (age 25-65 years). Pregnant women require 1500 mg/day, and **lactating women require 2000 mg/day. Postmenopausal women and patients with a healing long-bone fracture require 1500 mg/day.** Most people have a positive calcium balance during their first 3 decades of life and a negative balance after the fourth decade. About 400 mg of calcium is released from bone daily. Calcium may be excreted in stool.
2. Phosphate—In addition to being a key component of bone mineral, phosphate is important in enzyme systems and molecular interactions (metabolite and buffer). Approximately 85% of the body's phosphate stores are in bone. Plasma phosphate is mostly unbound and is reabsorbed by the kidney (proximal tubule). Dietary intake of phosphate is usually adequate (requirement is 1000-1500 mg/day). Phosphate may be excreted in urine
3. PTH—An 84–amino acid peptide synthesized in and secreted from the chief cells of the (four) parathyroid glands PTH helps regulate plasma calcium. It directly activates osteoblasts and modulates renal phosphate filtration. Decreased calcium levels in the extracellular fluid stimulate β_2 receptors to release PTH, which acts at the intestine, kidney, and bone (Table 1–13). PTH may affect bone loss in the elderly. **PTH-related protein and its receptor have been implicated in metaphyseal dysplasia.**
4. Vitamin D—Naturally occurring steroid activated by ultraviolet irradiation from sunlight or utilized from dietary intake (Fig. 1–19). It is hydroxylated to 25-(OH) vitamin D_3 in the liver and is hydroxylated a second time in the kidney. Conversion to the 1,25-$(OH)_2$ vitamin D_3 form activates the hormone, whereas conversion to the 24,25-$(OH)_2$ vitamin D form

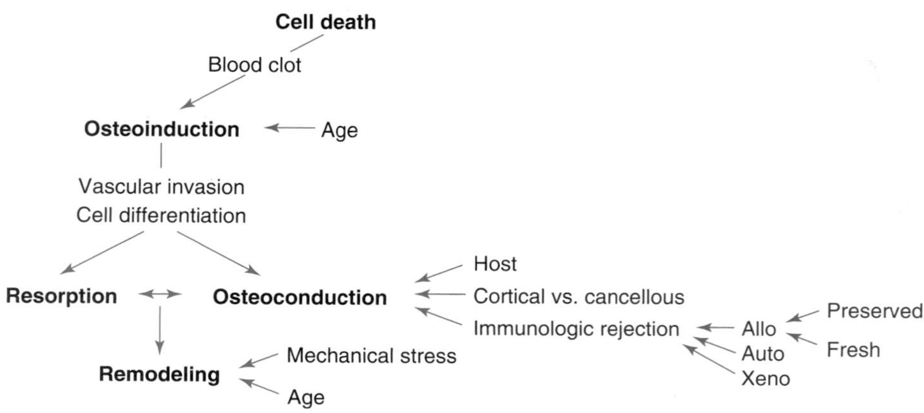

FIGURE 1–17 Major factors influencing bone graft incorporation. (From Simon SR, ed: Orthopaedic Basic Science, p 284. Rosemont, IL, American Academy of Orthopaedic Surgeons, 1994.)

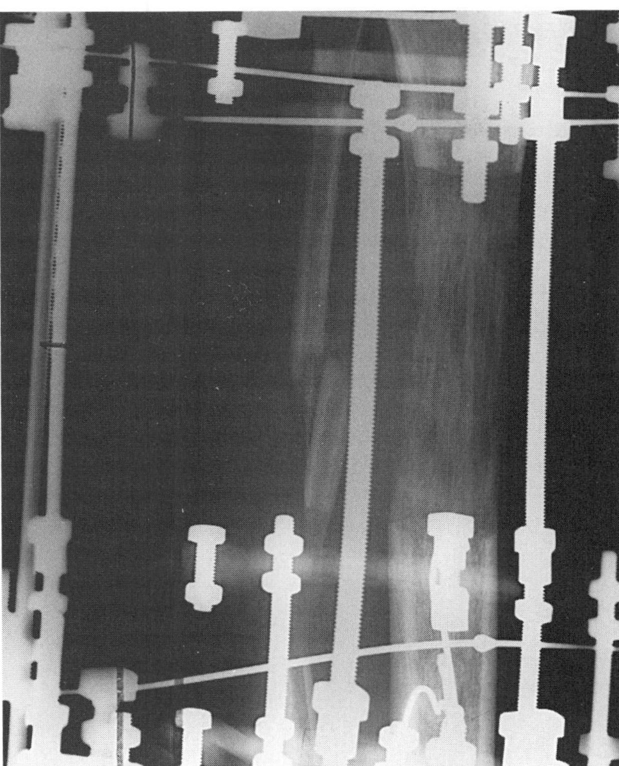

FIGURE 1–18 Radiograph of a patient who has undergone bone transport for a large distal tibial segmental defect. This anteroposterior radiograph of the proximal tibia shows early regeneration of distraction osteogenesis; bone formation is via intramembranous ossification.

inactivates it (Fig. 1–20). The active form works at the intestine, kidney, and bone (see Table 1–13). Phenytoin (Dilantin) causes impaired metabolism of vitamin D.

5. Calcitonin—A 32–amino acid peptide hormone produced by the clear cells in the parafollicles of the **thyroid gland;** has a limited role in calcium regulation (see Table 1–13). Increased extracellular calcium levels cause secretion of calcitonin, which is controlled by a β_2 receptor. **Calcitonin inhibits osteoclastic bone resorption (osteoclasts have calcitonin receptors; decreases osteoclast number and activity) and decreases serum calcium.** May also have a role in fracture healing and reducing vertebral compression fractures in high-turnover osteoporosis.
6. Other hormones affecting bone metabolism
   a. Estrogen—**Prevents bone loss by inhibiting bone resorption** (a decrease in urinary pyridinoline cross-links is observed). **However, because bone formation and resorption are coupled, estrogen therapy also decreases bone formation (see section on Bone Loss, below).** Supplementation is helpful in postmenopausal women only if started within 5-10 years after onset of menopause; the risk of endometrial cancer for patients taking estrogen is reduced when combined with cyclic progestin therapy. **Recent studies suggest a higher risk of heart disease and breast cancer with**

TABLE 1–13 REGULATION OF CALCIUM AND PHOSPHATE METABOLISM

Parameter	Parathyroid Hormone (Peptide)	1,25-(OH)$_2$ D (Steroid)	Calcitonin (Peptide)
Origin	Chief cells of parathyroid glands	Proximal tubule of kidney	Parafollicular cells of thyroid gland
Factors stimulating production	Decreased serum Ca^{2+}	Elevated PTH Decreased serum Ca^{2+} Decreased serum Pi	Elevated serum Ca^{2+}
Factors inhibiting production	Elevated serum Ca^{2+} Elevated 1,25-$(OH)_2$D	Decreased PT Elevated serum Ca^{2+} Elevated serum Pi	Decreased serum Ca^{2+}
Effect on end-organs for hormone action			
Intestine	No direct effect Acts indirectly on bowel by stimulating production of 1,25-$(OH)_2$D in kidney	Strongly stimulates intestinal absorption of Ca^{2+} and Pi	?
Kidney	Stimulates 25-(OH)D-1α-OHase in mitochondria of proximal tubular cells to convert 25-(OH)D to 1,25-$(OH)_2$D Increases fractional resorption of filtered Ca^{2+} Promotes urinary excretion of Pi	?	?
Bone	Stimulates osteoclastic resorption of bone Stimulates recruitment of preosteoclasts	Strongly stimulates osteoclastic resorption of bone	Inhibits osteoclastic resorption of bone ? Role in normal human physiology
Net effect on Ca^{2+} and Pi concentrations in extracellular fluid and serum	Increased serum Ca^{2+} Decreased serum Pi	Increased serum Ca^{2+} Increased serum Pi	Decreased serum Ca^{2+} (transient)

1,25-$(OH)_2$D, 1,25-dihydroxyvitamin D; PTH, parathyroid hormone; 25-(OH) D, 25-hydroxyvitamin D.
Adapted from an original figure by Frank H. Netter. From The Ciba Collection of Medical Illustrations, vol 8, part I, p 179. Copyright by Ciba-Geigy Corporation.

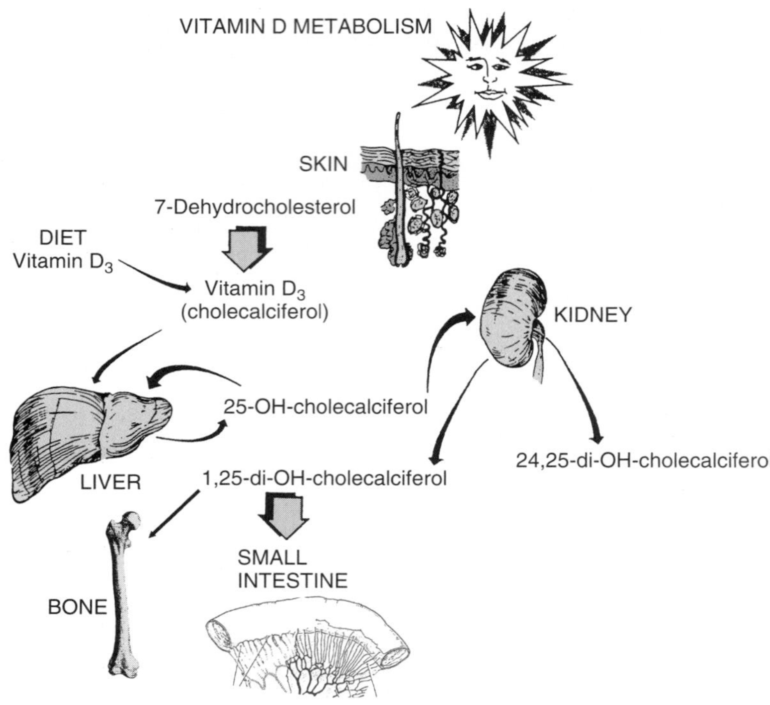

FIGURE 1–19 Vitamin D metabolism. (Modified from Orthopaedic Science Syllabus, p 11. Park Ridge, IL, American Academy of Orthopaedic Surgeons, 1986.)

certain regimens of hormone replacement therapy; therefore, other postmenopausal pharmacologic interventions (alendronate, raloxifene) should be strongly considered to slow bone loss in patients at lower risk.

b. Corticosteroids—Increase bone loss (decrease gut absorption of calcium by decreasing binding proteins; decrease bone formation [cancellous more affected than cortical bone] by inhibiting collagen synthesis and osteoblast productivity; they do not affect mineralization). Alternate-day therapy may reduce the effects.
c. Thyroid hormones—Affect bone resorption more than bone formation, leading to osteoporosis (large [thyroid-suppressive] doses of thyroxine can lead to osteoporosis). Regulates skeletal growth at the physis by stimulating chondrocyte growth, type X collagen synthesis, and alkaline phosphatase activity.
d. Growth hormone—Causes positive calcium balance by increasing gut absorption of calcium more than it increases urinary excretion. Insulin and somatomedins participate in this effect.
e. Growth factors—TGF-β, PDGF, and mono-/lymphokines have roles in bone and cartilage repair (discussed elsewhere in this chapter).

7. Interaction—Calcium and phosphate metabolism is affected by an elaborate interplay of hormones and even the levels of the metabolites themselves. Feedback mechanisms play an important role in the regulation of plasma levels of calcium and phosphate. Peak bone mass is believed to occur between 16 and 25 years of age and is greater in men and African Americans. After this peak, bone loss occurs at a rate of 0.3-0.5% per year (2-3% per year for untreated women during the sixth through tenth years after menopause).
8. Bone loss—Occurs at the onset of menopause, when there is both accelerated bone formation and resorption; a net negative change in calcium balance also occurs because menopause decreases intestinal absorption and increases urinary excretion of calcium. **Markers of bone resorption include urinary hydroxyproline and pyridinoline cross-links (when there is**

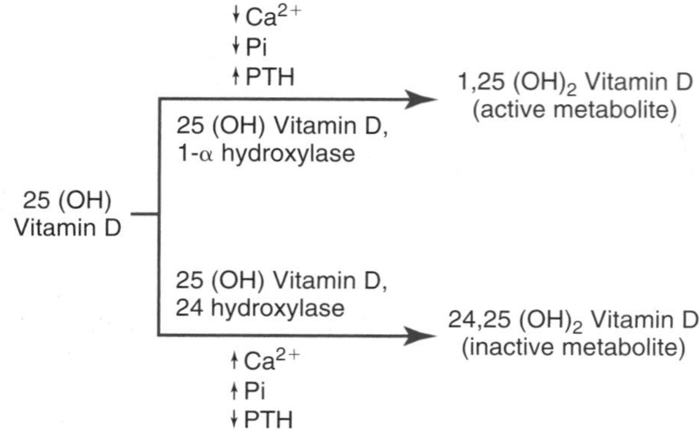

FIGURE 1–20 Vitamin D metabolism in the renal tubular cell. (From Simon SR, ed: Orthopaedic Basic Science, p 165. Rosemont, IL, American Academy of Orthopaedic Surgeons, 1994.)

TABLE 1-14 OVERVIEW OF CLINICAL AND RADIOGRAPHIC ASPECTS OF METABOLIC BONE DISEASES

Disease	Etiology	Clinical Findings	Radiographic Findings
Hypercalcemia			
Hyperparathyroidism	PTH overproduction—adenoma	Kidney stone, hyperreflexia	Osteopenia, osteitis fibrosa cystica
Familial syndromes	PTH overproduction—MEN/renal	Endocrine/renal abnormalities	Osteopenia
Hypocalcemia			
Hypoparathyroidism	PTH underproduction—idiopathic	Neuromuscular irritability, eye	Calcified basal ganglia
PHP/Albright's syndrome	PTH receptor abnormality	Short MC/MT, obesity	Brachydactyly, exostosis
Renal osteodystrophy	CRF—↓ phosphate excretion	Renal abnormalities	"Rugger jersey" spine
Rickets (osteomalacia)			
Vitamin D–deficiency rickets	↓ Vitamin D diet; malabsorption	Bone deformities, hypotonia	"Rachitic rosary," wide growth plates, fractures
Vitamin D–dependent (types I and II) rickets	See Table 1–15	Total baldness	Poor mineralization
Vitamin D–resistant (hypophosphatemic) rickets	↓ Renal tubular phosphate resorption	Bone deformities, hypotonia	Poor mineralization
Hypophosphatasia	↓ Alkaline phosphatase	Bone deformities, hypotonia	Poor mineralization
Osteopenia			
Osteoporosis	↓ Estrogen—↓ bone mass	Kyphosis, fractures	Compression vertebral fractures, hip fractures
Scurvy	Vitamin C deficiency—defective collagen	Fatigue, bleeding, effusions	Thin cortices, corner sign
Osteodense			
Paget's disease	Osteoclastic abnormality—↑ bone turnover	Deformities, pain, CHF, fractures	Coarse trabeculae, "picture frame" vertebrae
Osteopetrosis	Osteoclastic abnormality—unclear	Hepatosplenomegaly, anemia	Bone within bone

↓, Decreased; ↑, increased; CHF, congestive heart failure; CRF, chronic renal failure; MC, metacarpal; MEN, multiple endocrine neoplasia, MT, metatarsal; PHP, pseudohypoparathyroidism; PTH, parathyroid hormone.

bone resorption, both of them are elevated). Serum alkaline phosphatase is a marker of bone formation (elevated when bone formation is increased). Estrogen therapy for osteoporosis in high-risk patients results in a decrease in urinary pyridoline (decreased bone resorption) and a decrease in serum alkaline phosphatase (decreased bone formation); estrogen also increases bone density of the femoral neck, thereby reducing the rate of hip fracture.

B. Conditions of bone mineralization—Include hypercalcemic disorders, hypocalcemic disorders, and hypophosphatasia (Tables 1–14 through 1–16).

1. Hypercalcemia—Can present as polyuria, **polydipsia,** kidney stones, excessive bony resorption with or without fibrotic tissue replacement (osteitis fibrosa cystica), central nervous system (CNS) effects (confusion, stupor, weakness), and gastrointestinal (GI) effects (constipation). Can also cause **anorexia, nausea, vomiting, dehydration, and muscle weakness.**

a. Primary hyperparathyroidism—Caused by overproduction of PTH, usually as a result of a parathyroid adenoma (which generally affects only one parathyroid gland). Excessive PTH causes a net **increase in plasma calcium** and a **decrease in plasma phosphate** (due to enhanced urinary excretion). It results in **increased osteoclastic resorption** and failure of repair attempts (poor mineralization due to low phosphate). Diagnosis is based on signs and symptoms of hypercalcemia (described earlier) and characteristic laboratory results (increased serum calcium, PTH, urinary phosphate; decreased serum phosphate). Bony changes include osteopenia, osteitis fibrosa cystica (fibrous replacement of marrow), **"brown tumors"** (Fig. 1–21) (increased giant cells, extravasation of red blood cells (RBCs), hemosiderin staining, fibrous tissue hemosiderin), and chondrocalcinosis. Radiographs may demonstrate deformed, osteopenic bones; fractures; "shaggy" trabeculae; areas of radiolucency (phalanges, distal clavicle, skull); **destructive metaphyseal lesions;** and calcification of the soft tissues. Histologic changes include osteoblasts and osteoclasts active on both sides of the trabeculae (as seen in Paget's disease), areas of destruction, and wide osteoid seams. Surgical parathyroidectomy is curative.

b. Other causes of hypercalcemia—Familial syndromes. Hypercalcemia can result from pituitary adenomas associated with multiple endocrine neoplasia (MEN) types I and II and from familial hypocalciuric hypercalcemia (which is caused by poor renal clearance of calcium).

c. Other causes of hypercalcemia—Malignancy (most common), PTH-related protein secretion (lung carcinoma), lytic bone metastases and lesions (such as multiple myeloma), hyperthyroidism, vitamin D intoxication, prolonged immobilization, Addison's disease, steroid administration, peptic ulcer

TABLE 1-15 LABORATORY FINDINGS AND CLINICAL DATA REGARDING PATIENTS WITH THE VARIOUS METABOLIC BONE DISEASES

Disorder	Serum Ca	Serum Phos	Alk Phos	PTH	25-(OH) Vit D	1,25-(OH)$_2$ Vit D	Urinary Calcium	Other Findings/Possible Findings	Treatment	Comments
Primary hyperparathyroidism	↑	N or ↓	N or ↑	↑	N	N or ↑	↑	Active turnover seen on bone biopsy with peritrabecular fibrosis Brown tumors	Surgical excision of parathyroid edema Treat hypercalcemia (see text)	Most commonly due to parathyroid adenoma Because PTH stimulates conversion of the inactive form to the active form [1,25-(OH)$_2$ vitamin D] in the kidney, ↑ production of PTH leads to ↑ levels of 1,25-(OH)$_2$ vitamin D
Malignancy with bony metastases	↑	N or ↑	N or ↑	N or ↓	N	N or ↓	↑	Destructive lesions in bone	Treat cancer and hypercalcemia (see text)	↑ Calcium levels may lead to ↓ PTH production via feedback mechanism ↓ 1,25-(OH)$_2$ vitamin D levels are due to ↓ PTH (which is responsible for conversion of the inactive to the active form of vit D in the kidney) Multiple myeloma will display abnormal urinary and serum protein electrophoresis
Hyperthyroidism	↑	N	N	N or ↓	N	N	↑	↑ Free thyroxin index ↓ Thyroid-stimulating hormone Tachycardia, tremors		↑ Calcium levels due to ↑ bone turnover (hypermetabolic state)
Vitamin D intoxication	↑	N or ↑	N or ↑	N or ↓	↑↑↑	N	↑			History of excessive vitamin D intake Dietary vitamin D is converted to 25-(OH) vitamin D in the liver. This results in very high concentrations of 25-(OH) vitamin D that cross-react with intestinal vitamin D receptors to ↑ resorption of calcium to cause hypercalcemia
Hypoparathyroidism	↓	↑	N	↓	N	↓	↓	Basal ganglia calcification Hypocalcemic findings		↓ PTH production most commonly follows surgical ablation of the thyroid (with the parathyroid) gland ↓ PTH leads to ↓ serum calcium and ↑ serum phosphate (due to ↓ urinary excretion of phosphate) Because PTH stimulates conversion from the inactive to the active form of Vit D (in the kidney), 1,25-(OH)$_2$ vitamin D is also ↓
Pseudohypo-parathyroidism	↓	↑	N	N or ↑	N	↓	↓	Hypocalcemic findings		PTH has no effect on the target cells (in the kidney, bone, and intestine) due to a PTH receptor abnormality. This leads to a ↓ in the active form of vitamin D. Therefore, serum calcium levels are ↓ due to 1) the lack of effect of PTH on bone and 2) ↓ levels of 1,25-(OH)$_2$ vitamin D
Renal osteodystrophy (high-turnover bone disease due to renal disease [secondary hyperparathyroidism])	↓ or N	↑↑↑	↑	↑↑↑	N	↓	—	Findings of secondary hyperparathyroidism "Rugger jersey" spine Osteitis fibrosa Amyloidosis	1) Correct underlying renal abnormality 2) Maintain normal serum phosphorous and calcium	↓ Renal phosphorous excretion leads to hyperphosphatemia Phosphorous retention leads to ↓ serum calcium and ↑↑↑ PTH (which can lead to secondary

									3) Dietary phosphate restriction 4) Phosphate-binding antacid (calcium carbonate) 5) Administration of the active form of vitamin D—1,25-(OH)$_2$ vitamin D (calcitriol)	hyperparathyroidism) Elevated BUN and creatinine Associated with long-term hemodialysis
Renal osteodystrophy (low-turnover bone disease due to renal disease [aluminum toxicity])	↑ or N	N or ↑	↑	N or mildly elevated	N	↓	—	"Rugger jersey" spine Osteitis fibrosa Amyloidosis Osteomalacia may be seen		PTH levels are ↓ because of 1) frequent episodes of hypercalcemia and 2) direct inhibitory effect of aluminum on PTH **No secondary hyperparathyroidism is present** Elevated BUN and creatinine Associated with long-term hemodialysis
Nutritional rickets—vitamin D deficiency	↓ or N	↓	↑	↑	↓	↓	↓	Osteomalacia, hypotonia Muscle weakness, tetany Bowing deformities of the long bones Rachitic rosary	Oral administration of vitamin D (1500-5000 IU/day)	With ↓ vitamin D intake, intestinal calcium and phosphate absorption is reduced, leading to hypocalcemia. ↓ Serum calcium stimulates ↑ PTH (secondary hyperparathyroidism), which leads to bone resorption and ↑ serum calcium (toward or to normal levels) Sources of vitamin D include 1) Sunlight 2) Fish-liver foods 3) Fortified milk
Nutritional rickets—calcium deficiency	↓ or N	↓	↑	↑	N	↑ or N	↓	Clinical findings similar to those for vitamin D deficiency	Oral administration of calcium (700 mg/day)	Hypocalcemia leads to secondary hyperparathyroidism. ↑ PTH leads to enhanced renal conversion of 25-(OH) vitamin D to 1,25-(OH)$_2$ vitamin D
Nutritional rickets—phosphate deficiency	N	↓	↑	N	N	↑↑↑	N	No changes of secondary hyperparathyroidism are seen.	Oral supplementation of phosphate	Neither secondary hyperparathyroidism nor vitamin D deficiency is present ↓ Serum phosphate leads to ↑ renal production of 1,25-(OH)$_2$ vitamin D
Hereditary vitamin D–dependent rickets type I ("pseudo-vitamin D deficiency")	↓	↓	↑	↑	N or ↑	↓↓↓	↓	Osteomalacia Clinical findings similar to (but more severe than) nutritional rickets—vitamin D deficiency	Oral administration of physiologic doses (1-2 μg/day) of 1,25-(OH)$_2$ vitamin D	There is a defect in renal 25-(OH) vitamin D 1α hydroxylase. This enzymatic defect inhibits conversion from the inactive form [25-(OH) vitamin D] to the active form [1,25-(OH)$_2$ vitamin D] of vitamin D in the kidney
Hereditary vitamin D–dependent rickets type II ["hereditary resistance to 1,25-(OH)$_2$ vitamin D"]	↓	↓	↑	↑	N or ↑	↑↑↑	↓	Osteomalacia Alopecia Clinical findings similar to (but more severe than) nutritional rickets—vitamin D deficiency	Long-term (3-6 months) daily administration of high-dose vitamin D analogue [1,25 (OH)2 vit D or 1α (OH) vit D] plus 3 g/day of elemental calcium	There is an intracellular receptor defect for 1,25-(OH)$_2$ vitamin D Patients with this disorder have the highest 1,25-(OH)$_2$ vitamin D levels observed in humans; this ↑↑↑ level of 1,25-(OH)$_2$ vitamin D distinguishes hereditary vitamin D–dependent rickets type II from type I (the level of 1,25-(OH)$_2$ vitamin D is ↓↓↓)

Continued

TABLE 1-15 LABORATORY FINDINGS AND CLINICAL DATA REGARDING PATIENTS WITH THE VARIOUS METABOLIC BONE DISEASES—cont'd

Disorder	Serum Ca	Serum Phos	Alk Phos	PTH	25-(OH) Vit D	1,25-$(OH)_2$ Vit D	Urinary Calcium	Other Findings/Possible Findings	Treatment	Comments
Hypophosphatemic rickets (vitamin D–resistant rickets) ("phosphate diabetes") (Albright's syndrome is an example of a hypophosphatemic syndrome)	N	↓↓↓	↑	N	N	N	N or ↑	Osteomalacia No changes of secondary hyperparathyroidism Classic triad: 1) Hypophosphatemia 2) Lower limb deformities 3) Stunted growth rate	Oral administration of elemental phosphate (1-3 g/day) plus high-dose vitamin D (20,000-70,000 IU/day). Vitamin D administration is needed to counterbalance the hypocalcemic effect of phosphate administration, which otherwise could lead to severe secondary hyperpara-thyroidism.	There is an inborn error in phosphate transport (probably located in the proximal nephron). This leads to failure of reabsorption of phosphate in the kidney and "spilling" of phosphate (phosphate diabetes) in the urine. While the absolute levels of 1,25-$(OH)_2$ vitamin D are normal, they are inappropriately low, considering the degree of phosphaturia [production of 1,25-$(OH)_2$ vitamin D is normally stimulated by ↓ serum phosphorous (see Table 1–13)]. **This is the most commonly encountered form of rickets.**
Hypophosphatasia	↑	↑	↓↓↓	N	N	N		Osteomalacia Early loss of teeth	There is no established medical therapy.	There is an inborn error in the tissue-nonspecific (kidney, bone, liver) isoenzyme of alkaline phosphatase. Elevated urinary phosphoethanolamine is diagnostic.

↓, decrease(d); ↑, increase(d); Alk, alkaline; BUN, blood urea nitrogen; N, no(ne); Phos, phosphatase; PTH, parathyroid hormone.

TABLE 1-16 DIFFERENTIAL DIAGNOSIS OF THE METABOLIC BONE DISEASES BASED ON BLOOD CHEMISTRIES

↑ Calcium	↓ Calcium	Normal Calcium	↑ Phosphorus	↓ Phosphorus	Normal Phosphorus
Primary hyperparathyroidism	Hypoparathyroidism	Osteoporosis	Malignancy with bony metastasis	Primary hyperparathyroidism	Osteoporosis
Hyperthyroidism	Pseudohypoparathyroidism	Pseudohypoparathyroidism	Multiple myeloma	Malignancy without bony metastasis	Primary hyperparathyroidism
Vitamin D intoxication	Renal osteodystrophy (high-turnover bone disease)	Nutritional rickets—vitamin D deficiency	Lymphoma	Nutritional rickets—vitamin D deficiency	Malignancy with bony metastasis
Malignancy without bony metastasis	Nutritional rickets—vitamin D deficiency	Nutritional rickets—calcium deficiency	Vitamin D intoxication	Nutritional rickets—calcium deficiency	Multiple myeloma
Malignancy with bony metastasis	Nutritional rickets—calcium deficiency	Nutritional rickets—phosphate deficiency	Hypoparathyroidism	Nutritional rickets—phosphate deficiency	Lymphoma
Multiple myeloma	Hereditary vitamin D–dependent rickets (types I and II)	Hypophosphatemic rickets	Pseudohypoparathyroidism	Hereditary vitamin D–dependent rickets (types I and II)	Hyperthyroidism
Lymphoma	Malignancy with bony metastasis	Osteoporosis	Renal osteodystrophy	Hypophosphatemic rickets	Vitamin D intoxication
Sarcoidosis	Malignancy without bony metastasis	Malignancy with bony metastasis	Hypophosphatasia	Malignancy with bony metastasis	Renal osteodystrophy (only low-turnover bone disease)
Milk-alkali syndrome	Multiple myeloma	Multiple myeloma	Sarcoidosis	Malignancy without bony metastasis	Sarcoidosis
Severe generalized immobilization	Lymphoma	Lymphoma	Milk-alkali syndrome	Multiple myeloma	Milk-alkali syndrome
Multiple endocrine neoplasias	Hyperthyroidism	Vitamin D intoxication	Severe generalized immobilization	Lymphoma	Severe generalized immobilization
Addison's disease	Vitamin D intoxication	Pseudohypoparathyroidism	Primary hyperparathyroidism	Hypoparathyroidism	Osteoporosis
Steroid administration	Hypoparathyroidism	Renal osteodystrophy (only low-turnover bone disease)	Nutritional rickets—calcium deficiency	Pesudohypoparathyroidism	Primary hyperparathyroidism
Peptic ulcer disease	Sarcoidosis	Nutritional rickets—phosphate deficiency	Nutritional rickets—phosphate deficiency	Renal osteodystrophy	Malignancy with bony metastasis
Hypophosphatasia	Milk-alkali syndrome	Hypophosphatemic rickets	Hereditary vitamin D–dependent rickets type II	Nutritional rickets—vitamin D deficiency	Multiple myeloma
Primary hyperparathyroidism	Severe generalized immobilization	Hypophosphatasia	Sarcoidosis	Hereditary vitamin D–dependent rickets type I	Lymphoma
Pseudohypoparathyroidism		Sarcoidosis			Hyperthyroidism
Renal osteodystrophy		Hyperthyroidism			Vitamin D intoxication
Nutritional rickets—vitamin D deficiency		Milk-alkali syndrome			Nutritional rickets—calcium deficiency
Nutritional rickets—calcium deficiency		Severe generalized immobilization			Hypophosphatemic rickets
Hereditary vitamin D–dependent rickets (types I and II)					Hypophosphatasia

FIGURE 1–21 Radiograph (**A**) and photomicrograph (**B**) showing delineation of brown tumor *(arrows)* of hyperparathyroidism. (From Resnick D, Kransdorf MJ, eds: Bone and Joint Imaging, 3rd ed, p 608. Philadelphia, WB Saunders, 2005.)

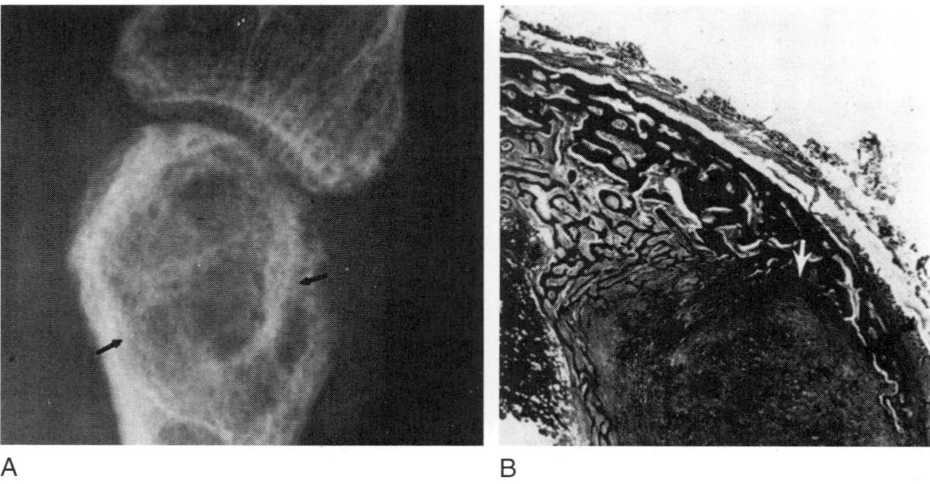

disease (milk-alkali syndrome), kidney disease, sarcoidosis, and hypophosphatasia. Hypercalcemia related to malignancy can be life threatening and is commonly associated with muscle weakness. Initial treatment should include hydration with normal saline (reverses dehydration). Hypercalcemia of malignancy can occur in the absence of extensive bone metastasis; hypercalcemia of malignancy most commonly results from the release of systemic growth factors and cytokines that stimulate osteoclastic bone resorption (at bony sites not involved in the tumor process).

d. Treatment of hypercalcemia
   (1) Hydration (saline diuresis)
   (2) Loop diuretics
   (3) Dialysis (for severe cases)
   (4) Mobilization (prevents further bone resorption)
   (5) Specific drug therapy (bisphosphonates, mithramycin, calcitonin, and gallium nitrate)

2. Hypocalcemia (Fig. 1–22)—Low plasma calcium can result from low PTH or vitamin D_3. Hypocalcemia leads to increased neuromuscular irritability (tetany, seizures, Chvostek's sign), cataracts, fungal infections of the nails, ECG changes (prolonged QT interval), and other signs and symptoms.
   a. Hypoparathyroidism—Decreased PTH decreases plasma calcium and increases plasma phosphate (urinary excretion not enhanced because of the lack of PTH). Common findings include fungal nail infections, hair loss, and blotchy skin (pigment loss; vitiligo). Skull radiographs may show basal ganglia calcification. **Iatrogenic hypoparathyroidism most commonly follows thyroidectomy.**
   b. Pseudohypoparathyroidism (PHP)—A rare genetic disorder caused by a lack of effect of PTH on the target cells. The PTH level is normal or even high, but PTH action at the cellular level is blocked by an abnormality at the receptor, by the cAMP system, or by a

FIGURE 1–22 Body's reaction to hypocalcemia, with the consequent resorption of bone. (From Favus MJ, ed: Primer on Metabolic Bone Diseases and Disorders of Mineral Metabolism, 3rd ed, p 302. Philadelphia, Lippincott-Raven, 1996.)

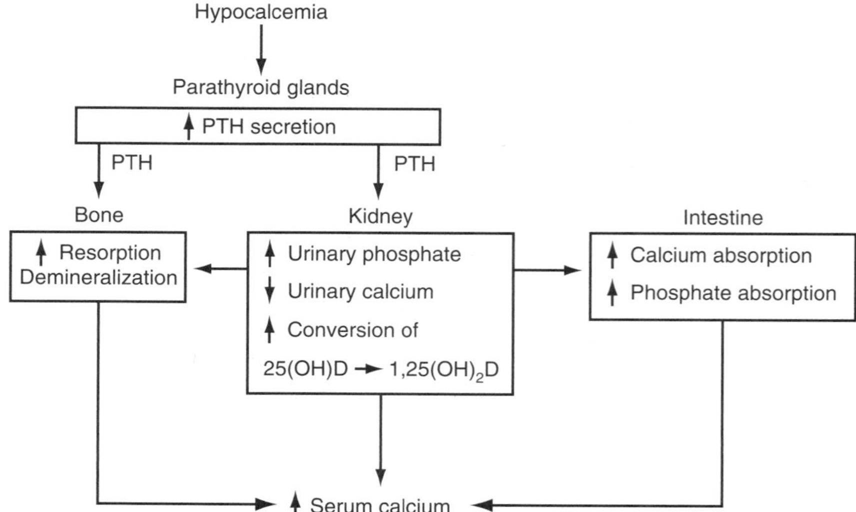

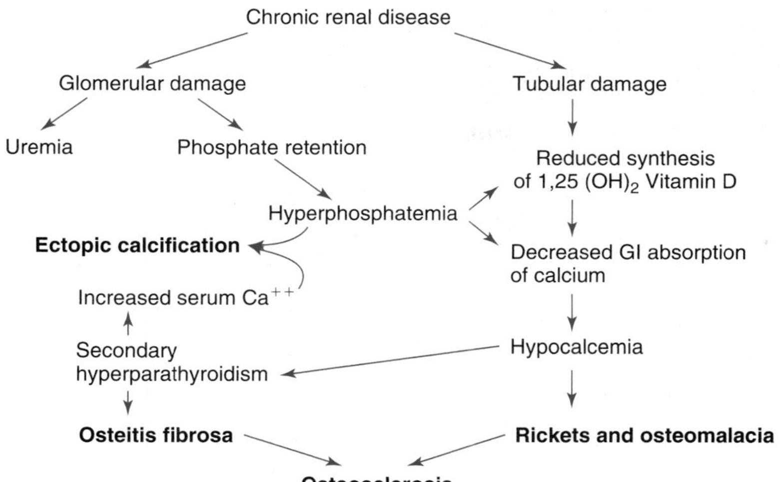

FIGURE 1–23 Pathogenesis of bony changes in renal osteodystrophy. (From Simon SR, ed: Orthopaedic Basic Science, p 171. Rosemont, IL, American Academy of Orthopaedic Surgeons, 1994.)

lack of required cofactors (e.g., Mg^{2+}). **Albright hereditary osteodystrophy,** a form of PHP, is associated with short first, fourth, and fifth metacarpals and metatarsals; brachydactyly; exostoses; obesity; and diminished intelligence. Pseudo-pseudohypoparathyroidism (pseudo-PHP) is a normocalcemic disorder that is phenotypically similar to PHP. However, in pseudo-PHP there is a normal response to PTH.

c. Renal osteodystrophy (Fig. 1–23)—A spectrum of disorders of bone mineral metabolism in patients with chronic renal disease. Renal disease impairs excretion of certain endogenous and exogenous substances and compromises mineral homeostasis, which leads to abnormalities of bone mineral metabolism. Renal bone diseases are subdivided into high-turnover and low-turnover diseases.

(1) High-turnover renal bone disease—Chronically elevated serum PTH leading to **secondary hyperparathyroidism** (hyperplasia of the chief cells of the parathyroid gland). Factors contributing to sustained, increased secretion of PTH and ultimately hyperplasia of the chief cells of the parathyroid gland (secondary hyperparathyroidism) include the following:

(a) Diminished renal phosphorous excretion—Chronic renal failure leads to an inability to excrete phosphate. Phosphorous retention promotes PTH secretion by three mechanisms: (1) hyperphosphatemia leads to lowered serum calcium directly, thereby stimulating PTH; (2) phosphorous impairs renal 1α-hydroxylase activity, thereby impairing production of 1,25-$(OH)_2$-vitamin D_3; and (3) phosphorous retention may directly increase the synthesis of PTH Increased secretion of PTH can lead to secondary hyperparathyroidism.

(b) Hypocalcemia

(c) Impaired renal calcitriol [1,25-$(OH)_2$-vitamin D_2]

(d) Alterations in the control of PTH gene transcription secretion

(e) Skeletal resistance to the actions of PTH

(2) Low-turnover renal bone disease (adynamic lesion of bone and osteomalacia)—**These patients do not have secondary hyperparathyroidism;** serum PTH is normal or mildly elevated. Bone formation and turnover are reduced. Excess deposition of aluminum into bone (aluminum toxicity) negatively affects bone mineral metabolism. It (a) impairs differentiation of precursor cells to osteoblasts; (b) impairs proliferation of osteoblasts; (c) impairs PTH release from the parathyroid gland; (d) disrupts the mineralization process; depending on the severity of involvement, the low-turnover lesion may represent an adynamic lesion or osteomalacia; (e) accounts for the majority of cases of low-turnover bone disease in patients with chronic renal failure (adynamic lesions); and (f) causes osteomalacia. In addition to slowed bone formation and turnover, there is a defect in the mineralization of newly formed bone. In renal osteodystrophy, radiographs may demonstrate a "rugger jersey" spine, like that in childhood osteopetrosis, and soft tissue calcification. **An additional complication of chronic dialysis is the accumulation of β_2-microglobulin, which leads to amyloidosis. Amyloidosis may be associated with carpal tunnel syndrome, arthropathy,**

and pathologic fractures. The material in amyloidosis stains pink with Congo red. Laboratory tests in renal osteodystrophy show an abnormal glomerular filtration rate (GFR); increased alkaline phosphatase, blood urea nitrogen (BUN), and creatinine; and decreased venous bicarbonate. Treatment should be directed at relieving the urologic obstruction or kidney disease.

d. Rickets (osteomalacia in adults)—**Failure of mineralization,** leading to changes in the physis in the zone of provisional calcification (increased width and disorientation) and bone (cortical thinning, bowing). The causes of rickets and osteomalacia are summarized in Box 1–1.
   (1) Nutritional rickets (see Table 1–15)
      (a) Vitamin D–deficiency rickets—Rare after addition of vitamin D to milk but still seen in Asian immigrants, patients with dietary peculiarities, premature infants, and those with malabsorption (sprue) or chronic parenteral nutrition. Decreased intestinal absorption of calcium and phosphate leads to secondary hyperparathyroidism (PTH continues to be produced because of low plasma calcium). **Laboratory studies** show **low-normal calcium** (maintained by high PTH), **low phosphate** (excreted because of the effect of PTH), **increased PTH, increased alkaline phosphatase** (a result of increased bone absorption from the increased PTH), and **low levels of vitamin D.** Enlargement of the costochondral junction (**"rachitic rosary"**), bony deformities (**bowing of the knees,** "codfish" vertebrae), retarded bone growth (a defect in the hypertrophic zone, with widened osteoid seams and physeal cupping), muscle hypotonia, dental disease, pathologic fractures (Looser's zones [pseudofracture on the compression side of bone]), **milkman's fracture** ([pseudofracture in adults] Fig. 1–24), a waddling gait, and other problems may result. Affected children are commonly below the fifth percentile for height. Treatment with vitamin D (5000 IU daily) resolves most deformities. Characteristic radiographic changes seen in rickets include physeal widening, physeal cupping, and coxa vara.
      (b) Calcium-deficiency rickets (Fig. 1–25)
      (c) Phosphate-deficiency rickets
   (2) Hereditary Vitamin D–dependent rickets, types I and II—Rare disorders with features similar to vitamin D deficiency (nutritional) rickets, except they **may be worse** and patients may have total baldness.
      (a) Vitamin D–dependent rickets, type I—**Defect in renal 25-(OH)-vitamin D 1α-hydroxylase,** inhibiting conversion of the inactive form of

Box 1–1 Causes of Rickets and Osteomalacia

NUTRITIONAL DEFICIENCY

Vitamin D deficiency
Dietary chelators (rare) of calcium
   Phytates
   Oxalates (spinach)
Phosphorus deficiency (unusual)
   Antacid (aluminium-containing) abuse leading to severe dietary phosphate binding

GASTROINTESTINAL ABSORPTION DEFECTS

Postgastrectomy (rare today)
Biliary disease (interference with absorption of fat-soluble vitamin D)
Enteric absorption defects
   Short-bowel syndrome
   Rapid-transit (gluten-sensitive enteropathy) syndromes
   Inflammatory bowel disease
      Crohn's disease
      Celiac disease

RENAL TUBULAR DEFECTS (RENAL PHOSPHATE LEAK)

X-linked dominant hypophosphatemic vitamin D-resistant rickets (VDRR) or osteomalacia
Classic Albright's syndrome or Fanconi's syndrome, type I
Fanconi's syndrome, type II
Phosphaturia and glycosuria
Fanconi's syndrome, type III
Phosphaturia, glycosuria, aminoaciduria
Vitamin D-dependent rickets (or osteomalacia), type I (a genetic or acquired deficiency of renal tubular 25-hydroxyvitamin D-1α hydroxylase enzyme that prevents conversion of 25-hydroxyvitamin D to the active polar metabolite 1,25-dihydroxyvitamin D)
Vitamin D-dependent rickets (or osteomalacia), type II (this entity represents enteric end-organ insensitivity to 1,25-dihydroxyvitamin D and is probably caused by an abnormality in the 1,25- dihydroxyvitamin D nuclear receptor)
Renal tubular acidosis
   Acquired–associated with many systemic diseases
   Genetic
      Debre-De Toni-Fanconi syndrome
      Lignac-Fanconi syndrome (cystinosis)
      Lowe's syndrome

RENAL OSTEODYSTROPHY–MISCELLANEOUS CAUSES

Soft tissue tumors secreting putative factors
   Fibrous dysplasia
   Neurofibromatosis
   Other soft tissue and vascular mesenchymal tumors
Anticonvulsant medication (induction of the hepatic P450 microsomal enzyme system by some anticonvulsants–e.g., phenytoin, phenobarbital, and Mysoline–causes increased degradation of vitamin D metabolites)
Heavy metal intoxication
Hypophosphatasia
High-dose diphosphonates
Sodium fluoride

Adapted from Simon SR: Orthopaedic Basic Science, 2nd ed, p 169. Rosemont, IL, American Academy of Orthopaedic Surgeons, 1994.

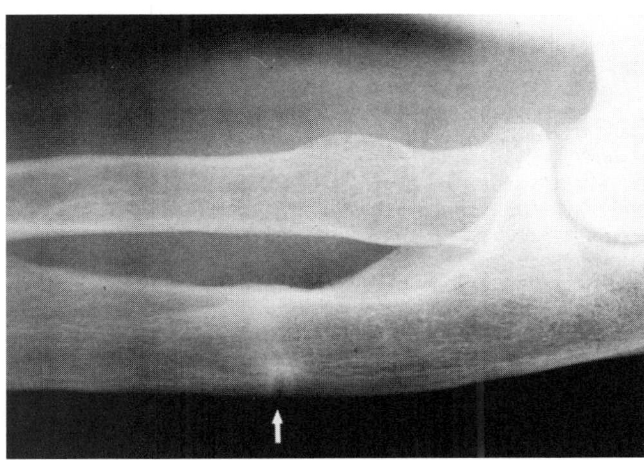

FIGURE 1–24 Pseudofracture *(arrow)* in an adult patient with X-linked hypophosphatemic osteomalacia occurring in characteristic location in the proximal ulna. Note bowing of the ulna. (From Pitt MJ, et al: Current concepts of vitamin D metabolism: Correlation with clinical syndromes. Crit Rev Radiol Sci 10:145, 1977.)

vitamin D to its active form. The inheritance pattern is autosomal recessive. The gene responsible is on chromosome 12q14.

(b) Vitamin D–dependent rickets, type II—**Defect in an intracellular receptor for 1,25-$(OH)_2$-vitamin D.**

(3) Familial hypophosphatemic rickets (Vitamin D–resistant rickets [“phosphate diabetes”])—**The most commonly encountered form of rickets. X-linked dominant disorder that is a result of impaired renal tubular reabsorption of phosphate.** Affected patients have a normal GFR and an impaired vitamin D_3 response. Phosphate replacement (1-3 g daily) with high-dose vitamin D_3 can correct the effects of the disorder, which are similar to those of the other forms of rickets.

3. Hypophosphatasia (Fig. 1–26)—Autosomal recessive disorder caused by an inborn error in the tissue-nonspecific isoenzyme of alkaline phosphatase that leads to **low levels of alkaline phosphatase,** which is required for the synthesis of inorganic phosphate and important in bone matrix formation. **Features are similar to those of rickets,** and treatment may include phosphate therapy. **Increased urinary phosphoethanolamine is diagnostic.**

C. Conditions of bone mineral density—Bone mass is regulated by the relative rates of deposition and withdrawal (Fig. 1–27).

1. Osteopenia

a. Osteoporosis—Age-related **decrease in bone mass** usually associated with loss of estrogen in postmenopausal women (Fig. 1–28). **The World Health Organization defines osteoporosis as a lumbar (L2-4) density level at least 25 standard deviations (SDs) below the peak bone mass of a 25-year-old individual; osteopenia is defined as a bone density level 10 to 25 SDs below the peak bone mass of a 25-year-old individual.** Osteoporosis is responsible for more

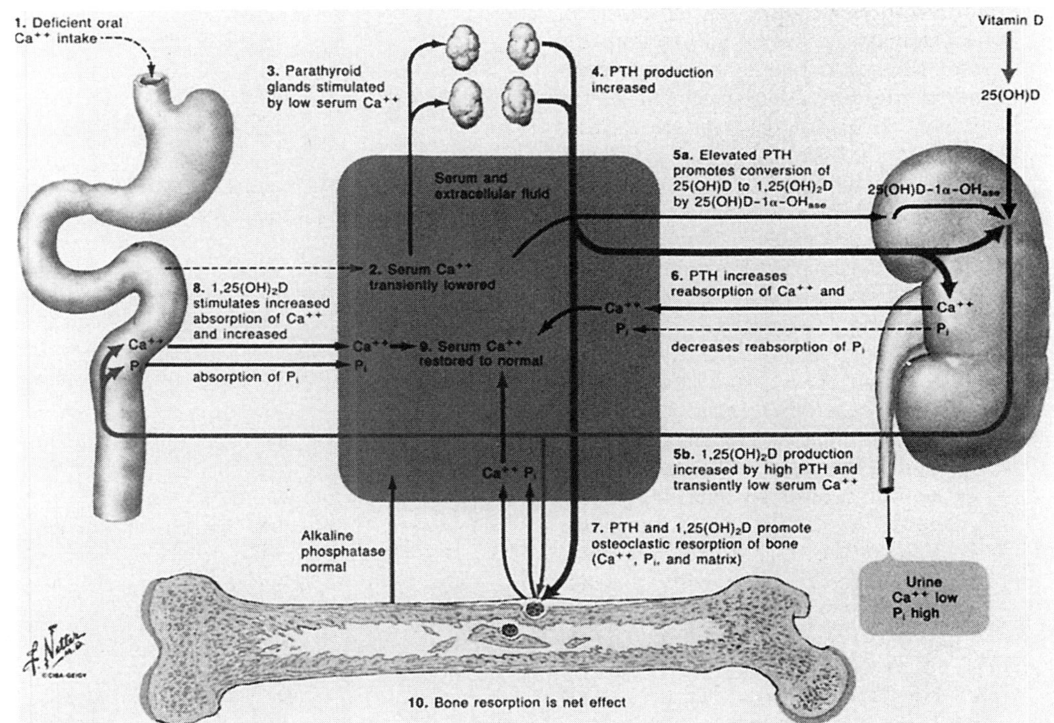

FIGURE 1–25 Nutritional calcium deficiency. (From The Ciba Collection of Medical Illustrations, vol 8, part I, p 184, 1987. Illustrated by Frank H. Netter. Reprinted by permission.)

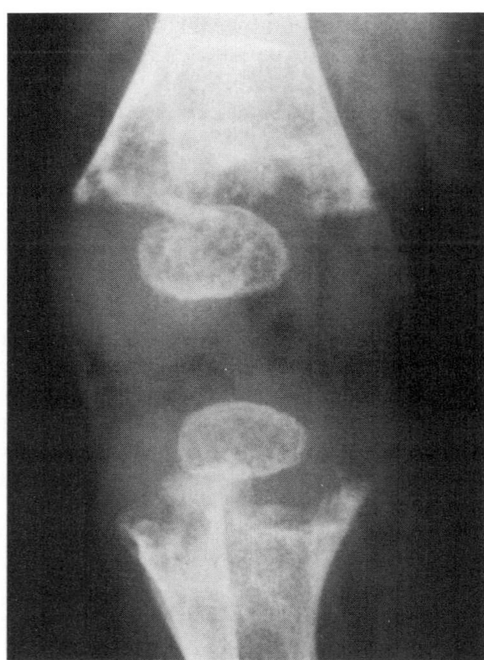

FIGURE 1–26 Hypophosphatasia. Deossification is present adjacent to the growth plates. Characteristic radiolucent areas extend from the growth plates into the metaphysis. (From Resnick D, Kransdorf MJ, ed: Bone and Joint Imaging, 3rd ed, p 574. Philadelphia, WB Saunders, 2005.)

than 1 million fractures per year (vertebral body most common). The lifetime risk of fracture in white women after 50 years of age is approximately 75%; the risk of hip fracture is 15-20%. **Osteoporosis is a quantitative, not qualitative, defect in bone; mineralization of bone remains normal.** Sedentary, thin **Caucasian women of northern European descent** (fair skin and hair), particularly smokers, heavy drinkers, and patients on **phenytoin (impairs vitamin D metabolism),** with diets low in calcium and vitamin D who **breast-fed their infants,** are at the greatest risk. **A history of two osteoporotic vertebral compression fractures is the strongest predictor of subsequent vertebral fracture in postmenopausal women; positive family history and premature menopause also increase the risk. Cancellous bone is the most markedly affected.** Clinical features include kyphosis and vertebral fractures (compression fractures of T11-L1 [creating an anterior wedge-shaped defect or resulting in a centrally depressed "codfish" vertebrae]), hip fractures, and distal radius fractures. Two types of osteoporosis have been characterized: type I (postmenopausal) and type II (age-related).

(1) Type I osteoporosis (postmenopausal)—Primarily affects trabecular bone; vertebral and distal radius fractures are common.

(2) Type II osteoporosis (age-related)—Seen in patients older than 75 years; affects both trabecular and cortical bone; is related to poor calcium absorption. Hip and pelvic fractures are common. Laboratory studies, including urinary calcium and hydroxyproline and serum alkaline phosphatase, are helpful for evaluating osteopenic conditions; **these studies are usually unremarkable in osteoporosis,** but hyperthyroidism (reversible osteoporosis), hyperparathyroidism, Cushing's syndrome, hematologic disorders, and malignancy should be ruled out. **Plain radiographs are usually not helpful unless bone loss is >30%.** Special studies used for the workup of osteoporosis include single-photon (appendicular) and double-photon (axial) absorptiometry, quantitative computed tomography (CT), and dual-energy x-ray absorptiometry (DEXA). **DEXA is most accurate with less radiation.** Biopsy (after tetracycline labeling) may be used to evaluate the severity of osteoporosis and to identify osteomalacia. Histologic changes: thinning trabeculae, decreased osteon size, and enlarged haversian and marrow spaces. Physical activity, calcium supplements (more effective in type II [age-related] osteoporosis), **estrogen-progesterone therapy (in type I [postmenopausal] osteoporosis; works best when initiated within 6 years of menopause),** and fluoride (inhibits bone resorption, but bone is more brittle) have a role in the treatment of osteoporosis. Bisphosphonates bind to bone resorption surfaces and inhibit osteoclastic membrane ruffling without destroying the cells. Other drugs, such as intramuscular calcitonin, may also be helpful but are expensive and may cause hypersensitivity reactions. The future of bone augmentation with PTH, growth factors, prostaglandin inhibitors, and other therapies remains to be determined. **An overview of recommended treatments for osteoporosis is shown in Figure 1–29.** The best prophylaxis for at-risk patients comprises (1) a diet with adequate calcium intake, (2) a weight-bearing exercise program, and (3) estrogen therapy evaluation at menopause.

(3) Idiopathic transient osteoporosis of the hip—Uncommon; diagnosis of exclusion; most common during the third trimester of pregnancy in women but can also occur in men. Presents with groin pain, limited range of motion (ROM), and localized osteopenia (without a

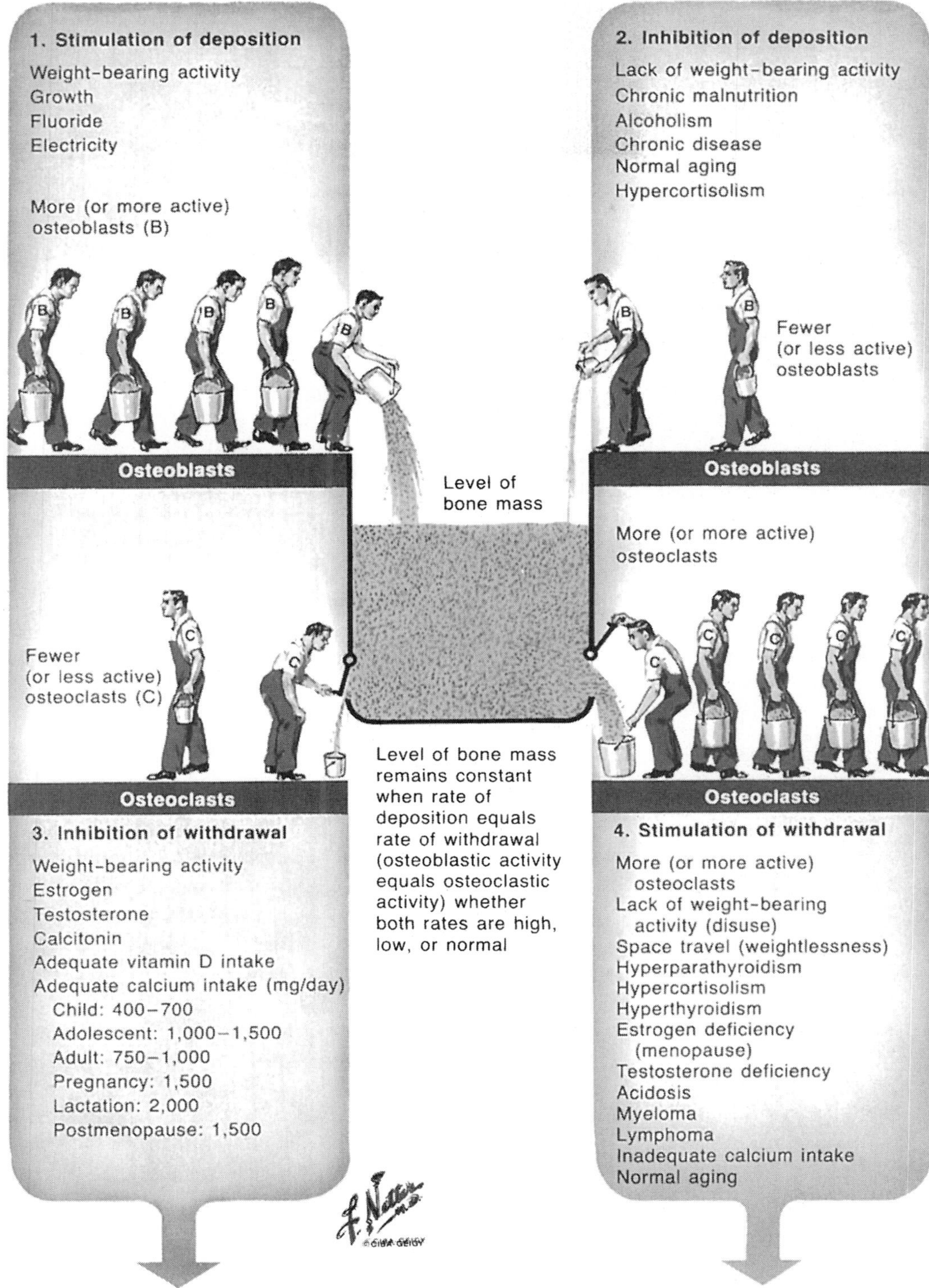

FIGURE 1–27 Four mechanisms of bone mass regulation. (From The Ciba Collection of Medical Illustrations, vol 8, part I, p 181, 1987. Illustrated by Frank H. Netter. Reprinted by permission.)

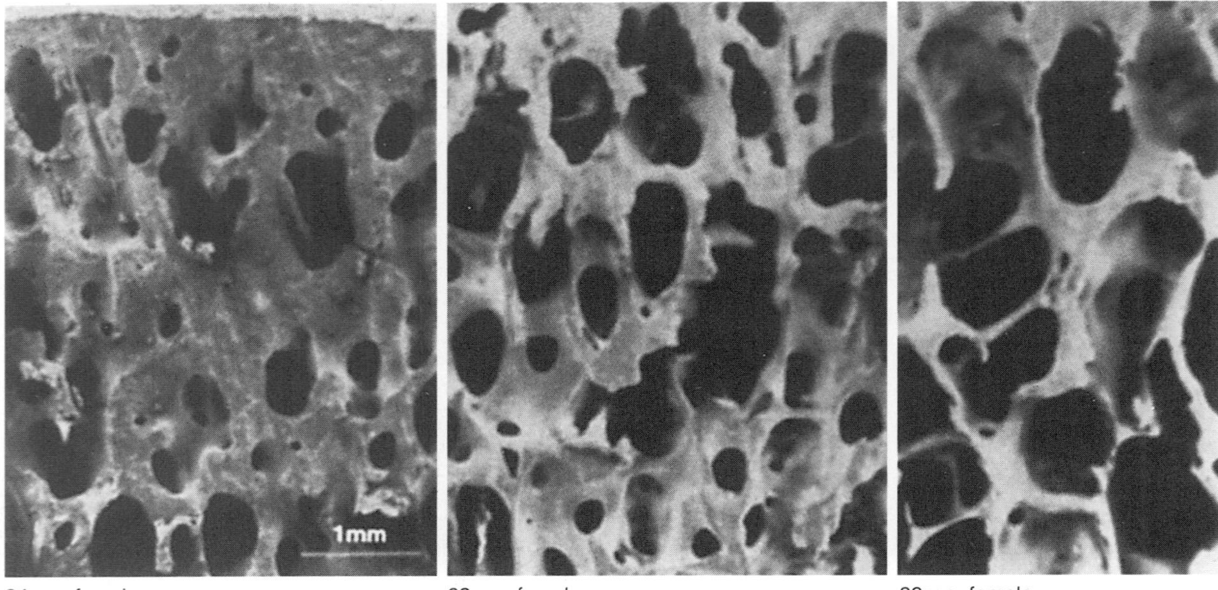

FIGURE 1–28 Age-related changes in density and architecture of human trabecular bone from the lumbar spine. (Reprinted from Keaveney TM, Hayes WC: Mechanical properties of cortical and trabecular bone. Bone 7:285-344, 1993, with permission from Elsevier Science.)

history of trauma). Treatment includes limited weight bearing and analgesics. The disease is generally self-limiting and tends to resolve spontaneously after 6-8 months (distinguishes it from ON, in which the symptoms are progressive and do not resolve spontaneously). Stress fractures may occur.

(4) Bone loss related to spinal cord injury—With paraplegia and quadriplegia, bone mineral loss occurs throughout the skeleton (except the skull) for approximately 16 months and levels off at two thirds of the original bone mass (high risk of fracture). Bone loss occurs to the greatest extent in the lower extremities.

b. Osteopenia—Discussed in conjunction with rickets. A **defect in mineralization** results in a large amount of **unmineralized osteoid (qualitative defect).** Osteomalacia is caused by vitamin D–deficient diets, GI disorders, renal osteodystrophy, and certain drugs (aluminum-containing phosphate-binding antacids [aluminum deposition in bone prevents mineralization] and phenytoin [Dilantin]). **Like osteoporosis, osteomalacia is also associated with chronic alcoholism.** It is commonly associated with Looser's zones (microscopic stress fractures), other fractures, biconcave vertebral bodies, and a trefoil pelvis seen on plain radiographs. Biopsy (transiliac) is required for diagnosis (widened osteoid seams are seen histologically). Femoral neck fractures are common in patients with osteomalacia. Treatment usually includes large doses of vitamin D. Osteoporosis and osteomalacia are compared in Figure 1–30.

c. Scurvy—**Vitamin C (ascorbic acid) deficiency produces a decrease in chondroitin sulfate synthesis, which leads to defective collagen growth and repair and impaired intracellular hydroxylation of collagen**

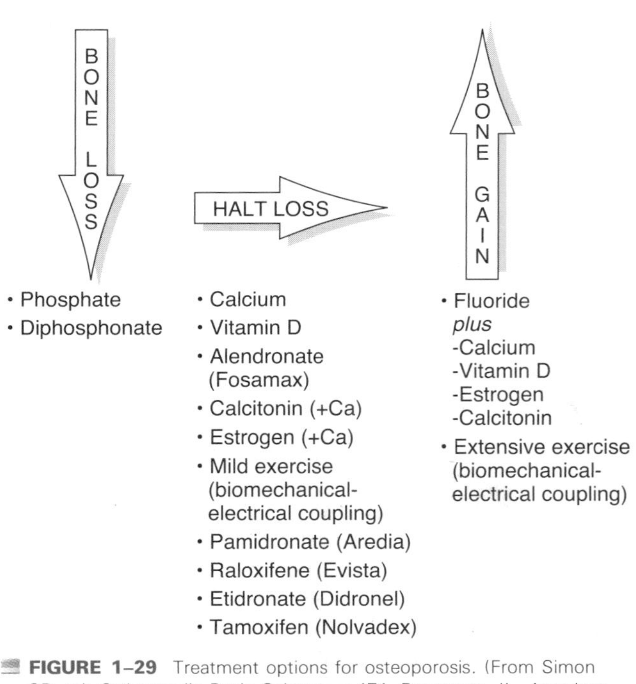

FIGURE 1–29 Treatment options for osteoporosis. (From Simon SR, ed: Orthopaedic Basic Science, p 174. Rosemont, IL, American Academy of Orthopaedic Surgeons, 1994.)

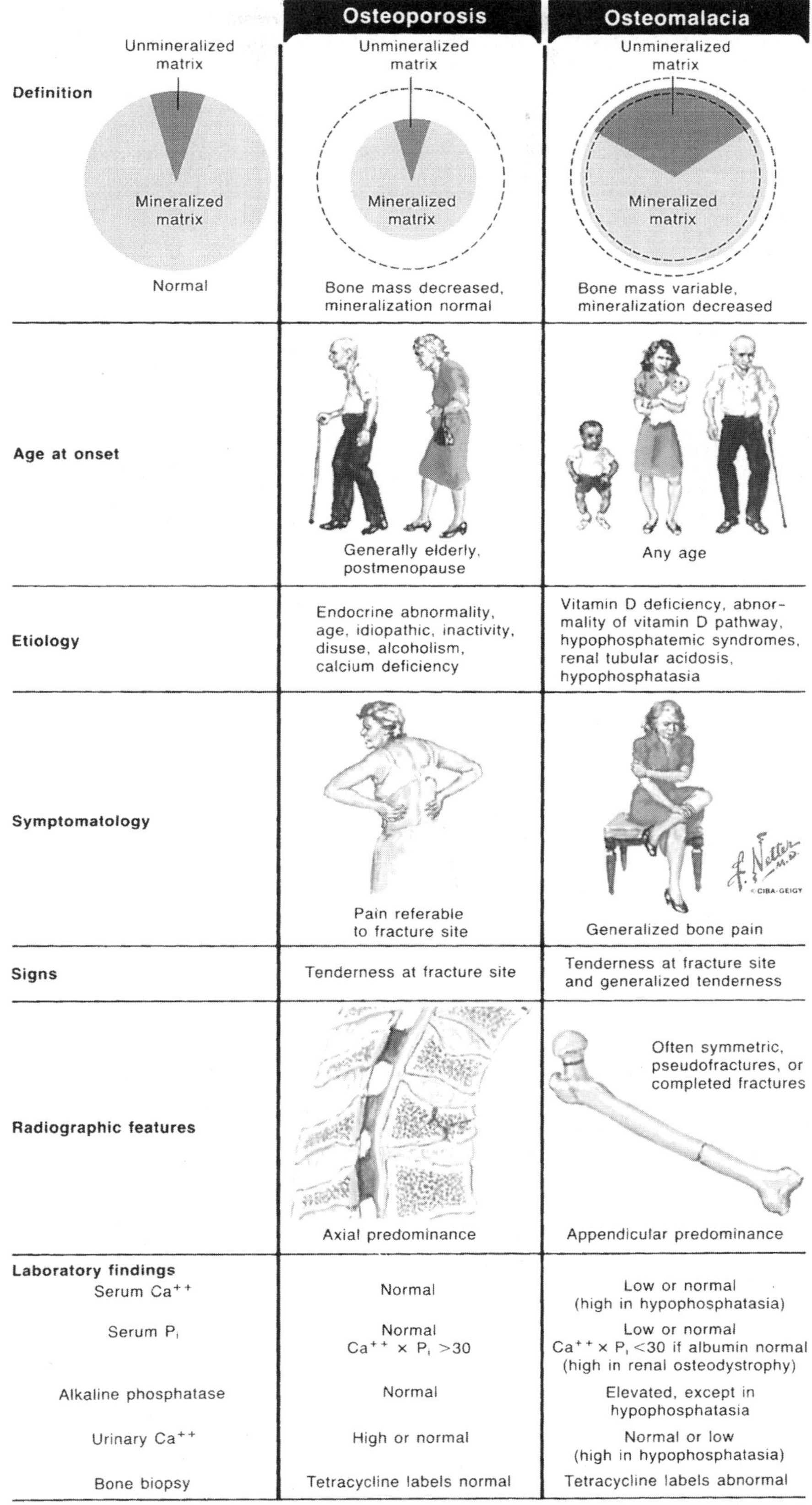

	Osteoporosis	Osteomalacia
Definition (Normal: Unmineralized matrix / Mineralized matrix)	Unmineralized matrix / Mineralized matrix Bone mass decreased, mineralization normal	Unmineralized matrix / Mineralized matrix Bone mass variable, mineralization decreased
Age at onset	Generally elderly, postmenopause	Any age
Etiology	Endocrine abnormality, age, idiopathic, inactivity, disuse, alcoholism, calcium deficiency	Vitamin D deficiency, abnormality of vitamin D pathway, hypophosphatemic syndromes, renal tubular acidosis, hypophosphatasia
Symptomatology	Pain referable to fracture site	Generalized bone pain
Signs	Tenderness at fracture site	Tenderness at fracture site and generalized tenderness
Radiographic features	Axial predominance	Often symmetric, pseudofractures, or completed fractures Appendicular predominance
Laboratory findings		
Serum Ca^{++}	Normal	Low or normal (high in hypophosphatasia)
Serum P_i	Normal $Ca^{++} \times P_i > 30$	Low or normal $Ca^{++} \times P_i < 30$ if albumin normal (high in renal osteodystrophy)
Alkaline phosphatase	Normal	Elevated, except in hypophosphatasia
Urinary Ca^{++}	High or normal	Normal or low (high in hypophosphatasia)
Bone biopsy	Tetracycline labels normal	Tetracycline labels abnormal

FIGURE 1–30 Comparison of osteoporosis and osteomalacia. (From The Ciba Collection of Medical Illustrations, vol 8, part I, p 228, 1987. Illustrated by Frank H. Netter. Reprinted by permission.)

peptides. Clinical features include fatigue, gum bleeding, ecchymosis, joint effusions, and iron deficiency. Radiographic changes may include thin cortices and trabeculae and metaphyseal clefts (corner sign). Laboratory studies are normal. Histologic changes include replacement of primary trabeculae with granulation tissue, areas of hemorrhage, and widening of the zone of provisional calcification in the physis. **The greatest effect on bone formation occurs in the metaphysis.**

d. Marrow packing disorders—Myeloma, leukemia, and other disorders can cause osteopenia (see Chapter 9, Orthopaedic Pathology).
e. Osteogenesis imperfecta (see Chapter 3, Pediatric Orthopaedics)—**Caused by abnormal collagen synthesis (failure of normal collagen cross-linking). Abnormality is primarily due to a mutation in the genes that are responsible for the metabolism and synthesis of type I collagen.**

2. Increased osteodensity
   a. Osteopetrosis (marble bone disease)—A group of bone disorders that lead to increased sclerosis and obliteration of the medullary canal due to **decreased osteoclast (and chondroclast) function** (there is failure of bone resorption). The number of osteoclasts may be increased, decreased, or normal. The disorder may result from an abnormality of the immune system (thymic defect). Histologically, osteoclasts lack the normal ruffled border and clear zone. Marrow spaces fill with **necrotic calcified cartilage,** and the cartilage may be trapped within the osteoid. Empty lacunae and plugging of haversian canals are also seen. The most severe infantile autosomal recessive ("malignant") form leads to a "bone within a bone" appearance on radiographs, hepatosplenomegaly, and aplastic anemia and can lead to death during infancy. Bone marrow transplantation (e.g., osteoclast precursors) can be life saving during childhood. High doses of calcitriol with or without steroids may also be helpful. The autosomal dominant "tarda" (benign) form **(Albers-Schönberg disease)** demonstrates generalized osteosclerosis (including the typical **"rugger jersey" spine**), usually without other anomalies (Figs. 1–31 and 1–32). Pathologic fractures through abnormal (brittle) bone are common.
   b. Osteopoikilosis ("spotted bone disease")—Islands of deep cortical bone appear within the medullary cavity and the cancellous bone of the long bones (especially in the hands and feet). These areas are usually asymptomatic, and there is no known incidence of malignant degeneration.
3. Paget's disease—**Elevated serum alkaline phosphatase and urinary hydroxyproline;**

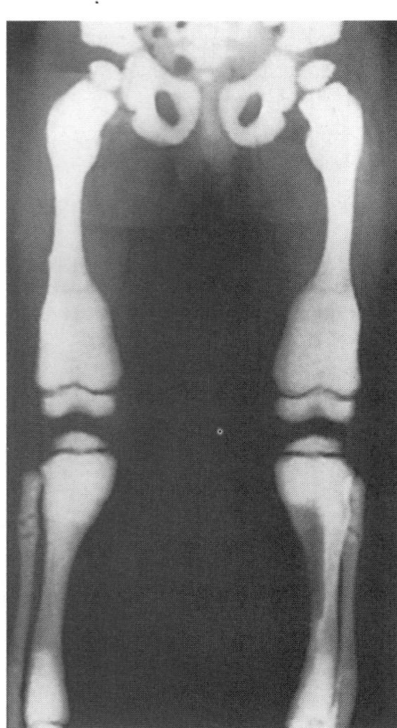

FIGURE 1–31 Typical "marble bone" appearance of osteopetrosis. (From Tachdjian MO: Pediatric Orthopaedics, 2nd ed, p 795. Philadelphia: WB Saunders, 1990.)

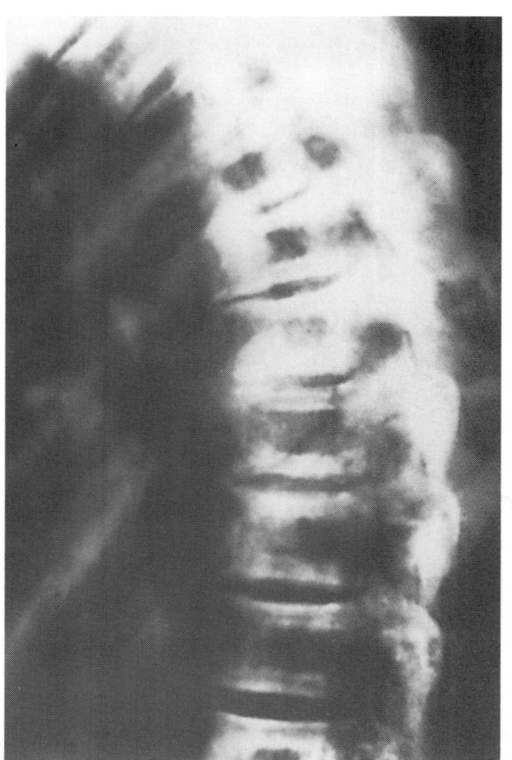

FIGURE 1–32 Typical "rugger jersey" spine seen in osteopetrosis. (From Tachdjian MO: Pediatric Orthopaedics, 2nd ed, p 797. Philadelphia, WB Saunders, 1990.)

virus-like inclusion bodies observed in osteoclasts. Can display both decreased and increased osteodensity (depending on the phase of the disease). Discussed in Chapter 9, Orthopaedic Pathology.

a. Active phase
   (1) Lytic phase—Intense osteoclastic bone resorption
   (2) Mixed phase
   (3) Sclerotic phase—Osteoblastic bone formation predominates

b. Inactive phase

D. Conditions of bone viability

1. ON—Death of bony tissue (usually adjacent to a joint surface) from causes other than infection. It is usually caused by loss of blood supply due to trauma or another etiology (e.g., after a slipped capital femoral epiphysis). **Recent studies suggest that idiopathic ON of the femoral head and Legg-Calvé-Perthes disease occur in patients with coagulation abnormalities** [deficiency of antithrombin factors protein C and protein S and increased levels of lipoprotein (a)]. ON commonly affects the hip joint, leading to eventual collapse and flattening of the femoral head, most frequently in the anterolateral region. The condition is associated with steroid and heavy alcohol use; it is also associated with blood dyscrasias (e.g., sickle cell disease), dysbarism (Caisson's disease), excessive radiation therapy, and Gaucher's disease.

   a. Etiology—Theories regarding the etiology of ON vary (Fig. 1–33), It may be related to enlargement of space-occupying marrow fat cells, which leads to ischemia of adjacent tissues. Vascular insults and other factors may also be significant. Idiopathic ON (Chandler's disease) is diagnosed when no other cause can be identified. Idiopathic, alcohol, and dysbaric ON are associated with multiple insults. ON may arise secondary to an underlying hemoglobinopathy (such as sickle cell disease) or a marrow disorder (such as hemochromatosis). Cyclosporine has reduced the incidence of ON of the femoral head in renal transplant patients.

   b. Pathologic changes—Grossly necrotic bone, fibrous tissue, and subchondral collapse may be seen (Figs. 1–34 and 1–35). Histology: (1) Early changes involve autolysis of osteocytes (14-21 days) and necrotic marrow, followed by (2) inflammation with invasion of buds of primitive mesenchymal tissue and capillaries; (3) later, **newly woven bone is laid down on top of dead trabecular bone;** and (4) this stage is followed by resorption of dead trabeculae and remodeling via **"creeping substitution."** The bone is weakest during resorption and remodeling, and **collapse (crescent sign, seen on radiographs)** and fragmentation can occur.

   c. Evaluation—A careful history (risk factors) and physical examination (e.g., decreased ROM, limp) should precede additional studies. Evaluation of other joints (especially the contralateral hip) is important in order to identify the disease process early. The process is bilateral in the hip in 50% of cases of idiopathic ON and up to 80% of steroid-induced ON. MRI **(earliest positive study; highest sensitivity and specificity)** and bone scanning are helpful for making an early diagnosis. Femoral head pressure

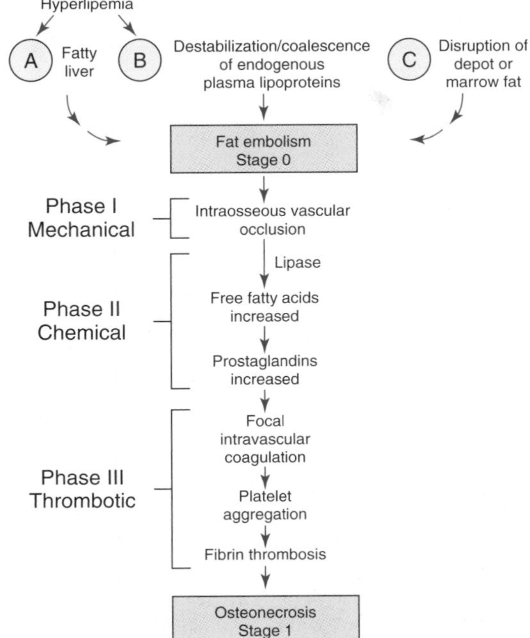

FIGURE 1–33 Possible mechanisms of intraosseous fat embolism leading to focal intravascular coagulation and osteonecrosis. (From Jones JP Jr: Fat embolism and osteonecrosis. Orthop Clin North Am 16:595-633, 1985.)

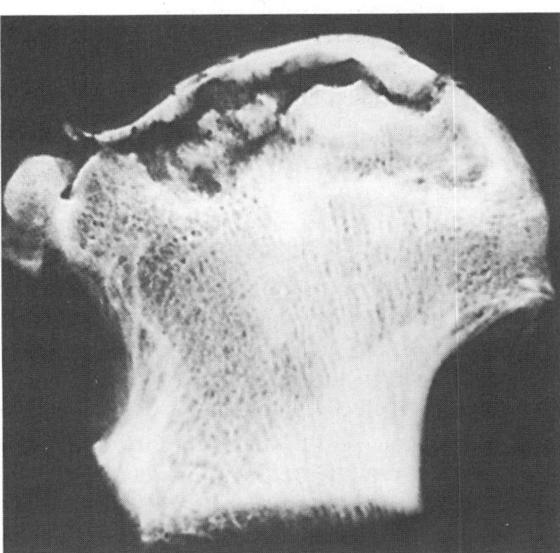

FIGURE 1–34 Fine-grain radiograph demonstrating space between the articular surface and subchondral bone: "crescent sign" of osteonecrosis. (From Steinberg ME: The Hip and Its Disorders, p 630. Philadelphia, WB Saunders, 1991.)

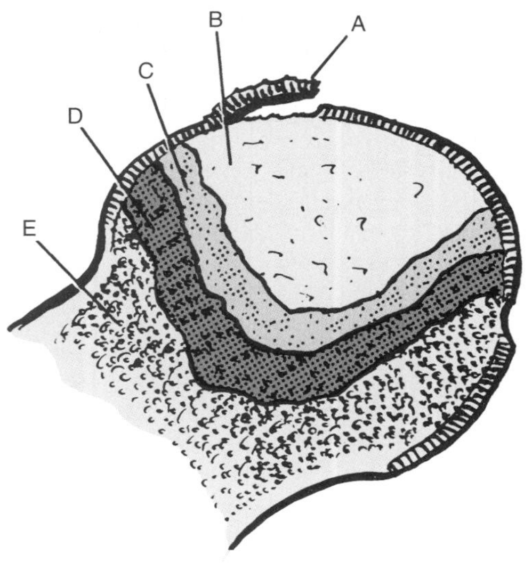

FIGURE 1–35 Pathology of avascular necrosis. A, Articular cartilage. B, Necrotic bone. C, Reactive fibrous tissue. D, Hypertrophic bone. E, Normal trabeculae. (From Steinberg ME: The Hip and Its Disorders, p 630. Philadelphia, WB Saunders, 1991.)

measurement is possible but invasive. Pressure >30 mm Hg or increased >10 mm Hg with injection of 5 mL of saline (stress test) is considered abnormal, but these values have varied widely from one investigation to another.

d. Treatment—Replacement arthroplasty of the hip is associated with increased loosening. Nontraumatic ON of the distal femoral condyle and proximal humerus may improve spontaneously without surgery. The precise role of core decompression remains unresolved, but results are best in early hip disease (Ficat stage I).

2. Osteochondroses—Can occur at traction apophyses in children and may or may not be associated with trauma, inflammation of the joint capsule, or vascular insult/secondary thrombosis. The pathology is similar to that described for ON in the adult. Table 1–17 shows the common osteochondroses. Most are discussed separately in the chapters covering the respective sites of disease.

TABLE 1-17 COMMON OSTEOCHONDROSES

Disorder	Site	Age (yr)
Van Neck's disease	Ischiopubic synchrondrosis	4-11
Legg-Calvé-Perthes disease	Femoral head	4-8
Osgood-Schlatter disease	Tibial tuberosity	11-15
Sinding-Larsen-Johansson syndrome	Inferior patella	10-14
Blount's disease (infant)	Proximal tibial epiphysis	1-3
Blount's disease (adolescent)	Proximal tibial epiphysis	8-15
Sever's disease	Calcaneus	9-11
Köhler's disease	Tarsal navicular	3-7
Freiberg's infarction	Metatarsal head	13-18
Scheuermann's disease	Diskovertebral junction	13-17
Panner's disease	Capitellum of humerus	5-10
Thiemann's disease	Phalanges of hand	11-19
Kienböck's disease	Carpal lunate	20-40

SECTION 2 Joints

I. Articular Tissues

A. Cartilage—Types: **growth plate (physeal) cartilage** (previously discussed); **fibrocartilage** at tendon and ligament insertion into bone (and healing articular cartilage); **elastic cartilage** in tissues such as the trachea; **fibroelastic cartilage,** which makes up menisci; and **articular cartilage,** the focus of this section, which is critical to joint function. Articular cartilage decreases friction and distributes loads and is classically described as avascular, aneural, and alymphatic;**as a result, chondrocyte metabolism appears to be modulated primarily via mechanical stimulation.** Chondrocytes receive nutrients and oxygen from synovial fluid via diffusion through the cartilage matrix. The pH of cartilage is 7.4; changes in pH can disrupt cartilage structure. **Unlike mature articular cartilage, immature articular cartilage has a stem cell population.** Animal models (rabbit knee) suggest that autologous osteochondral progenitor cells can be isolated from bone marrow and grown in vitro, apparently without losing their ability to differentiate into cartilage or bone. They therefore may be clinically useful for repairing articular cartilage defects (and subchondral bone). Animal models (rabbit) also suggest that TGF-β can induce chondrogenesis in periosteal explants cultured in agarose gel.

1. Articular cartilage composition
   a. Water (65-80% of wet weight)—Shifts in and out of cartilage to allow deformation of cartilage surface in response to stress. Water is not distributed homogeneously (65% in deep zone, 80% at surface). Water content increases (90%) in osteoarthritis (Table 1–18). Water is also responsible for nutrition and lubrication. Increased water content leads to increased permeability, decreased strength, and decreased Young's modulus *(E)*.
   b. Collagen (10-20% of wet weight; >50% of dry weight) (Fig 1–36)—Type II collagen accounts for approximately 95% of the total collagen content of articular cartilage and provides a cartilaginous framework and **tensile strength. Type II collagen is very stable, with a half-life of approximately 25 years.** Increased amounts of glycine, proline, hydroxyproline,

TABLE 1-18 BIOCHEMICAL CHANGES OF ARTICULAR CARTILAGE

Parameter	Effect of Aging	Effect of Osteoarthritis
Water content (hydration; permeability)	↓	↑
Collagen	Content remains relatively unchanged	Becomes disorderly (breakdown of matrix framework) Content ↓ in severe osteoarthritis Relative concentration ↑ (due to loss of proteoglycans)
Proteoglycan content (concentration)	↓ (also, the length of the protein core and glycosaminoglycan chains decreases)	↓
Proteoglycan synthesis		↑
Proteoglycan degradation	↓	↑↑↑
Chondroitin sulfate concentration (includes both chondroitin 4 and 6–sulfate)	↓	↑
Chondroitin 4–sulfate concentration	↓	↑
Keratin sulfate concentration	↑	↓
Chondrocyte size	↑	
Chondrocyte number	↓	
Modulus of elasticity	↑	↓

↓, decrease(d); ↑, increase(d).

and hydrogen bonding are responsible for its unique characteristics. Hydroxyproline is unique to collagen and can be measured in the urine to assess bone turnover. Small amounts of types V, VI, IX, X, and XI collagen are present in the matrix of articular cartilage. An overview of all collagen types is shown in Table 1–19. Collagen type VI is a minor component of normal articular cartilage, but its content increases significantly in early osteoarthritis. **Collagen type X is produced only by hypertrophic chondrocytes during enchondral ossification (growth plate, fracture callus, HO formation, calcifying cartilaginous tumors) and is associated with calcification of cartilage; a genetic defect in type X collagen is responsible for Schmid's metaphyseal chondrodysplasia (affects the hypertrophic physeal zone). Collagen type XI is an adhesive holding the collagen lattice together.**

c. Proteoglycans (10-15% of wet weight)—Protein polysaccharides provide **compressive strength.** Proteoglycans are produced by chondrocytes, are secreted into the extracellular matrix, and are composed of subunits known as

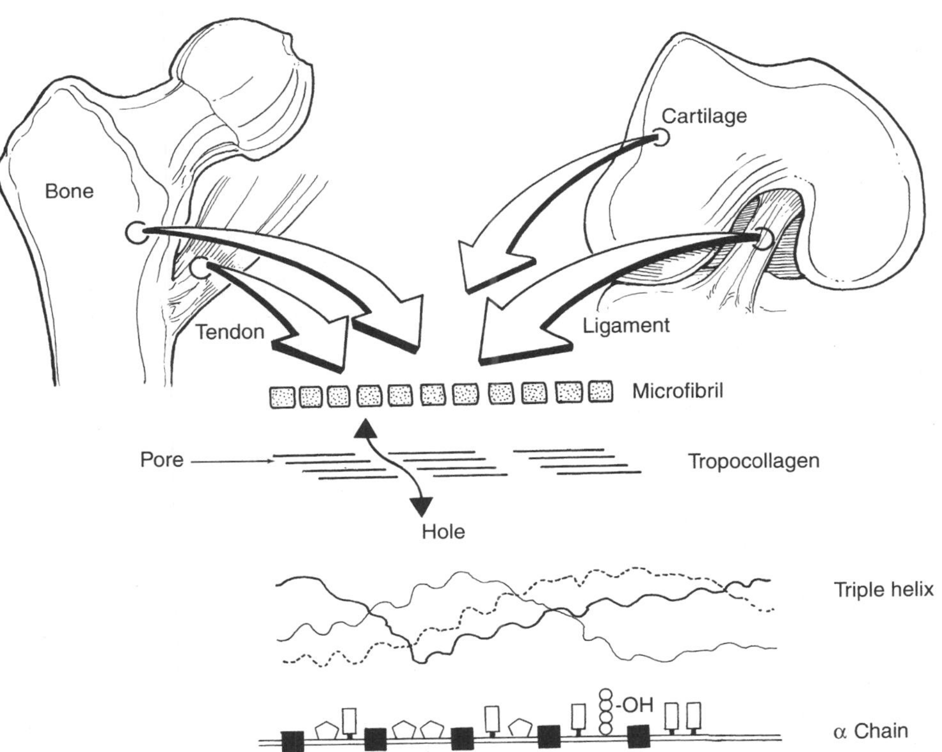

FIGURE 1–36 Microstructure of collagen. Collagen is composed of microfibrils that are quarter-staggered arrangements of tropocollagen. Note hole and pore regions for mineral deposition (for calcification). Tropocollagen in turn is made up of a triple helix of α chains of polypeptides. (From Brinker MR, Miller MD: Fundamentals of Orthopaedics. Philadelphia, WB Saunders, 1999, p 3.)

TABLE 1-19 TYPES OF COLLAGEN

Type	Location
I	Bone
	Tendon
	Meniscus
	Annulus of intervertebral disc
	Skin
II	Articular cartilage
	Nucleus pulposus of intervertebral disc
III	Skin
	Blood vessels
IV	Basement membrane (basal lamina)
V	Articular cartilage (in small amounts)
VI	Articular cartilage (in small amounts)
	Tethers the chondrocyte to its pericellular matrix
VII	Basement membrane (epithelial)
VIII	Basement membrane (epithelial)
IX	Articular cartilage (in small amounts)
X	Hypertrophic cartilage
	Associated with calcification of cartilage (matrix mineralization)
XI	Articular cartilage (in small amounts) (acts as an adhesive)
XII	Tendon
XIII	Endothelial cells

glycosaminoglycans (GAGs, disaccharide polymers). **These GAGs include two subtypes of chondroitin sulfate (the most prevalent GAG in cartilage) and keratin sulfate. The concentration of chondroitin-4-sulfate decreases with age, that of chondroitin-6-sulfate remains essentially constant, and that of keratin sulfate increases with age.** GAGs are bound to a protein core by **sugar bonds** to form a proteoglycan aggrecan molecule. **Link proteins** stabilize these aggrecan molecules to hyaluronic acid to form a proteoglycan aggregate. Proteoglycans have a half-life of 3 months, provide structural properties for the articular cartilage, provide elastic strength, produce cartilage's porous structure, and trap and hold water **(regulate and retain fluid in the matrix).** Figure 1–37 illustrates a proteoglycan aggregate and an aggrecan molecule.

d. Chondrocytes (5% of wet weight)—Active in protein synthesis, possess a double effusion barrier; produce collagen, proteoglycans, and some **enzymes for cartilage metabolism,** including the **metalloproteinases** (breakdown cartilage matrix) and **tissue inhibitor of metalloproteinases** (TIMPs; inhibit the metalloproteinases); least active in the calcified zone. Deeper cartilage zones have chondrocytes with a decreased rough endoplasmic reticulum (RER) and increased intraplasmic filaments (degenerative products). Chondroblasts, derived from undifferentiated mesenchymal cells (stimulated by motion), are later trapped in lacunae to become chondrocytes.
e. Other matrix components

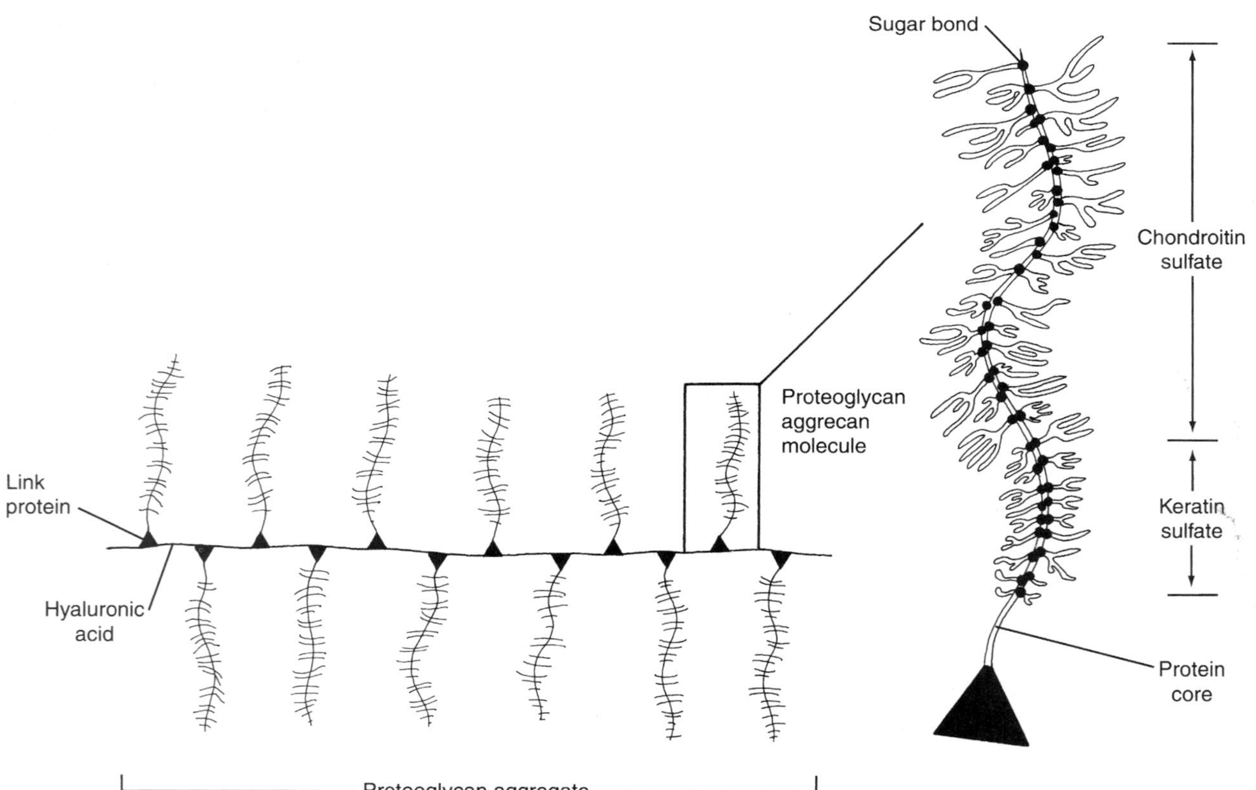

FIGURE 1–37 Proteoglycan aggregate and aggrecan molecule. (From Brinker MR, Miller MD: Fundamentals of Orthopaedics. Philadelphia, WB Saunders, 1999, p 9.)

TABLE 1-20 ARTICULAR CARTILAGE LAYERS

Layer	Width (μm)	Characteristic	Orientation	Function
Gliding zone (superficial)	40	↓ Metabolic activity	Tangential	vs. Shear
Transitional zone (middle)	500	↑ Metabolic activity	Oblique	vs. Compression
Radial zone (deep)	1000	↑ Collagen size	Vertical	vs. Compression
Tidemark	5	Undulating barrier	Tangential	vs. Shear
Calcified zone	300	Hydroxyapatite crystals		Anchor

↑, increased; ↓, decreased.

(1) Adhesives (noncollagenous proteins, such as fibronectin, chondronectin, and anchorin CII)—Involved in interactions between chondrocytes and fibrils. Fibronectin may be associated with osteoarthritis.

(2) Lipids—Unknown function

2. Articular cartilage layers—The various layers of articular cartilage are described in Table 1–20 and are illustrated in Figure 1–38. **The tangential zone has a high concentration of collagen fibers** arranged at right angles to each other (parallel to the articular surface). The calcified zone forms a transitional region of intermediate stiffness between articular cartilage and subchondral bone. The superficial zone has the greatest tensile stiffness. The deeper zones have increased chondrocyte volume; collagen fibers are oriented perpendicular to the joint surface.
3. Articular cartilage metabolism
   a. Collagen synthesis—Figure 1–39 shows the events and sites involved in collagen synthesis.
   b. Collagen catabolism—Little is known of the exact mechanism. Enzymatic processes have been proposed that involve metalloproteinase collagenase cleaving to the triple helix. Mechanical factors may also play a role.
   c. Proteoglycan synthesis (Fig. 1–40)—A series of molecular events beginning with proteoglycan gene expression and transcription of messenger RNA and concluding with proteoglycan aggregate formation in the extracellular matrix.
   d. Proteoglycan catabolism (Fig. 1–41)
4. Articular cartilage growth factors—Regulate cartilage synthesis; may have a role in osteoarthritis.
   a. PDGF—May affect healing of cartilage lacerations (and perhaps osteoarthritis).
   b. TGF-β—**Stimulates proteoglycan synthesis while suppressing synthesis of type II collagen.** Stimulates the formation of plasminogen activator inhibitor-1 and TIMP, which prevent the degradative action of plasmin and stromelysin.
   c. Fibroblast growth factor (basic) (b-FGF)—Stimulates DNA synthesis in adult articular chondrocytes; may affect cartilage repair.
   d. Insulin-like growth factor-I (IGF-I)—Previously known as somatomedin C. Stimulates DNA and cartilage matrix synthesis in adult articular

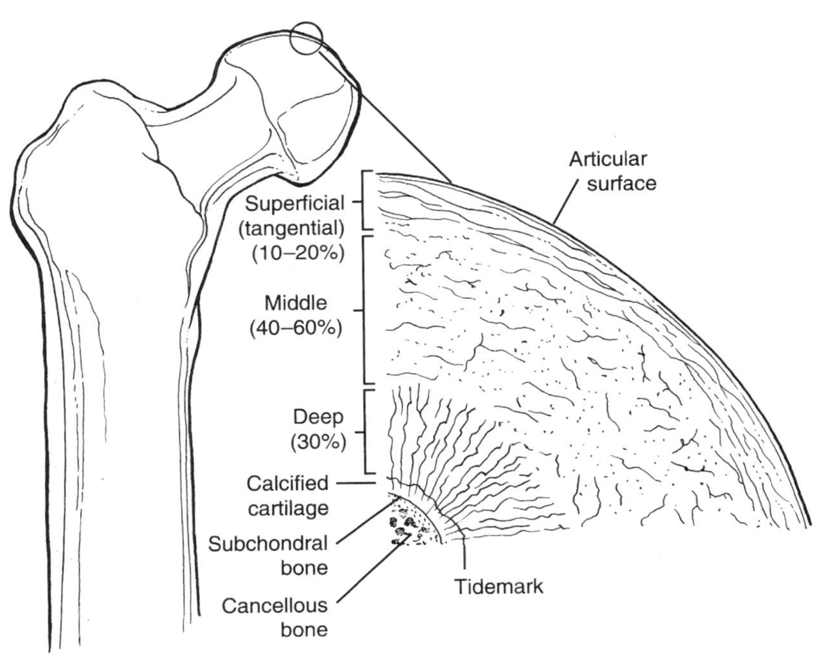

FIGURE 1–38 Articular cartilage layers. (From Brinker MR, Miller MD: Fundamentals of Orthopaedics. Philadelphia, WB Saunders, 1999, p 9.)

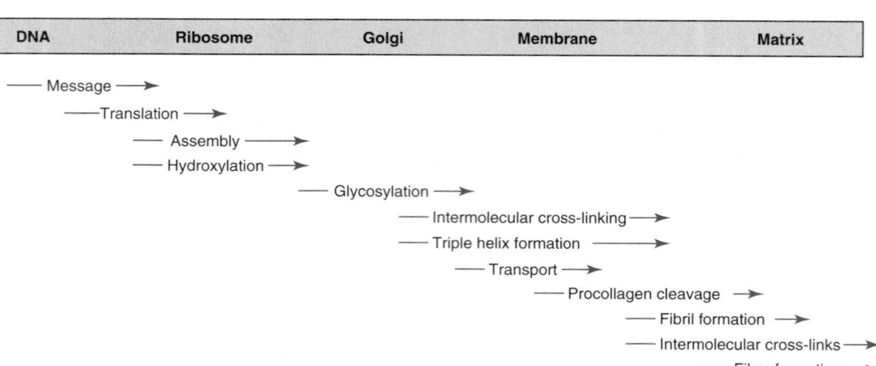

FIGURE 1–39 Collagen synthesis is accomplished at various intracellular sites. (From Mankin HJ, Brandt KD: Biochemistry and metabolism of articular cartilage in osteoarthritis. In Moskowitz RW, Howell DS, Goldberg VM, et al, eds: Osteoarthritis: Diagnosis and Medical/Surgical Management, 2nd ed, p 124. Philadelphia, WB Saunders, 1992.)

cartilage and immature cartilage of the growth plate.

5. Lubrication and wear mechanisms of articular cartilage (Figs. 1–42 through 1–44)
   a. General comments—The primary mechanism responsible for lubrication of articular cartilage (low coefficient of friction) during dynamic function is **elastohydrodynamic lubrication.** The coefficient of friction for human joints (such as the knee and hip) varies from 0.002 to 0.04. Factors decreasing the coefficient of friction of articular cartilage include fluid film formation, elastic deformation of articular cartilage, synovial fluid, and efflux of fluid from the cartilage An example of a factor that increases the coefficient of friction is fibrillation of articular cartilage. During ROM, almost all joints undergo both rolling and sliding (for more information, see the section on Biomechanics).
   b. Specific types of lubrication (see Figs. 1–42 and 1–43)
      (1) **Elastohydrodynamic lubrication—The predominant mechanism during dynamic joint function.** Elastic deformation of articular surfaces and thin films of joint lubricants separate the surfaces (the coefficient of friction is primarily a function of lubricant properties, not the surfaces). Coefficient of friction is generally low.
      (2) **Boundary lubrication** (slippery surfaces)—The bearing surface is largely nondeformable, and therefore the lubricant only partially separates the surfaces.

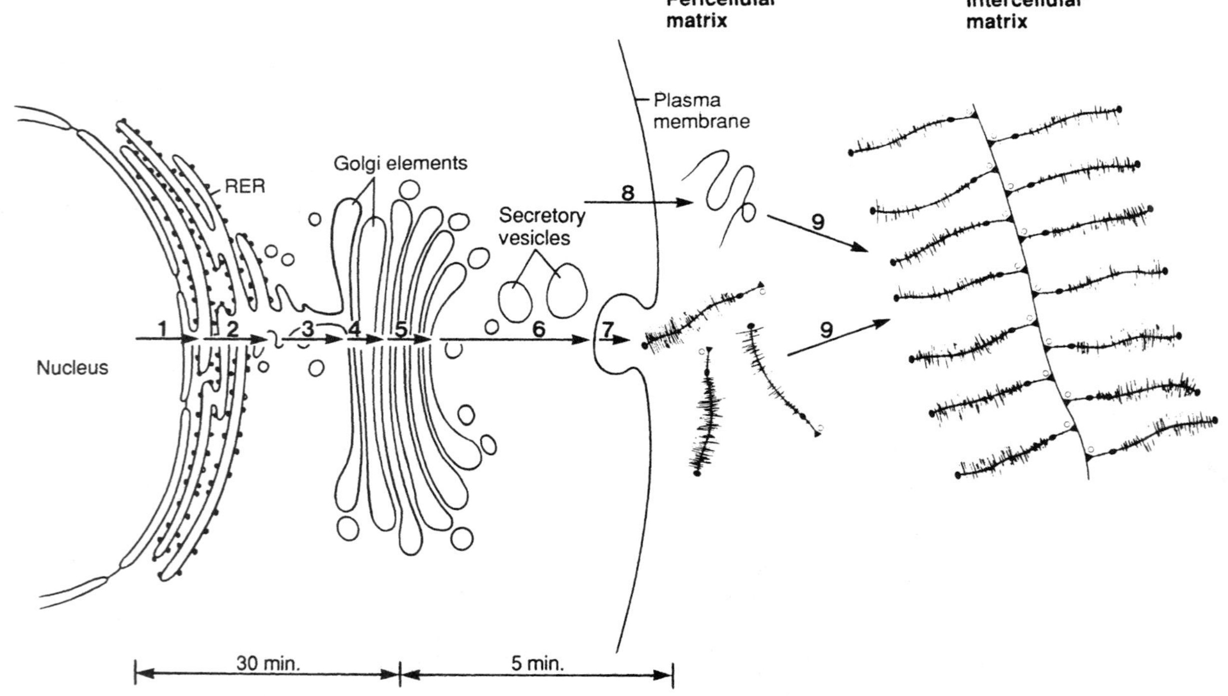

FIGURE 1–40 Synthesis and secretion of proteoglycan aggrecan molecules and link protein by a chondrocyte. 1, Transcription of aggrecan and link protein genes to mRNA. 2, Translation of mRNA to form protein core. 3, Transportation. 4, 5, cis- and medial trans Golgi compartments, respectively, where glycosaminoglycan chains are added to the protein core. 6, Transportation to the secretory vesicles. 7, Release into the extracellular matrix. 8, 9, Hyaluronate from the plasma membrane binds with the aggrecan and link proteins to form aggregates in the extracellular matrix. RER, rough endoplasmic reticulum. (From Simon SR, ed: Orthopaedic Basic Science, p 13. Rosemont, IL, American Academy of Orthopaedic Surgeons, 1994.)

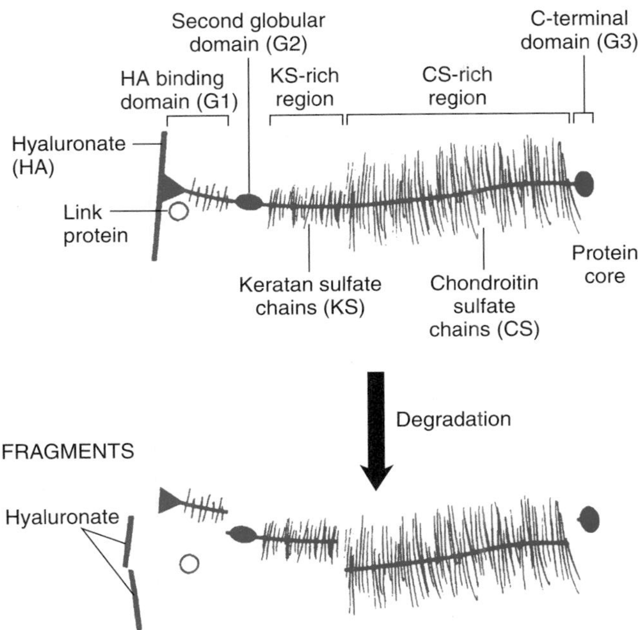

FIGURE 1–41 Proteoglycan degradation in articular cartilage. Cleavage of the G1 and G2 domains makes the fragments nonaggregating. (Modified from Simon SR, ed: Orthopaedic Basic Science, p 14. Rosemont, IL, American Academy of Orthopaedic Surgeons, 1994.)

Superficial zone protein appears to have a role in boundary lubrication.

(3) **Boosted lubrication** (fluid entrapment)—Describes the concentration of lubricating fluid in pools trapped by regions of bearing surfaces that are making contact. The coefficient of friction is generally higher for boosted than elastohydrodynamic lubrication.

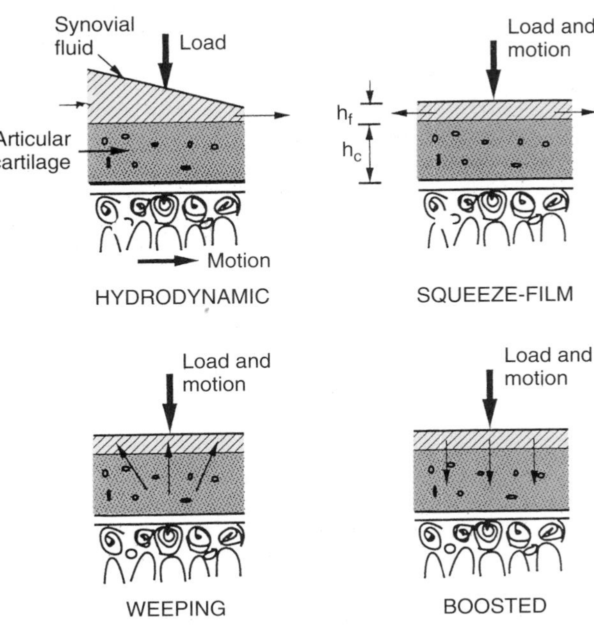

FIGURE 1–43 Fluid film lubrication models include Hydrodynamic, Squeeze-film, Weeping, and Boosted. (From Mow VC, Soslowsky LJ: Friction, lubrication, and wear of diarthrodial joints. In Mow VC, Hayes WC, eds: Basic Orthopaedic Biomechanics, pp 245-292. New York, Raven Press, 1991.)

(4) **Hydrodynamic lubrication**—Fluid separates the surfaces when one of the surfaces is sliding on the other.

(5) **Weeping lubrication**—Fluid shifts out of articular cartilage in response to load, separating the surfaces by hydrostatic pressure.

(6) Articular cartilage aging (and other special circumstances) (see Table 1–18)—With aging, chondrocytes become larger, acquire increased lysosomal enzymes, and no longer reproduce, so cartilage becomes relatively **hypocellular. Cartilage increases stiffness and decreases solubility with aging.** In addition, cartilage proteoglycans decrease in mass and size (decreased length

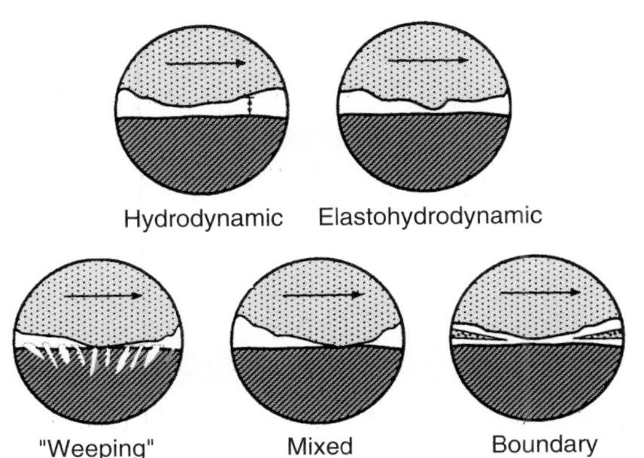

FIGURE 1–42 Types of lubrication. (From Simon SR, ed: Orthopaedic Basic Science, p 465. Rosemont, IL, American Academy of Orthopaedic Surgeons, 1994.)

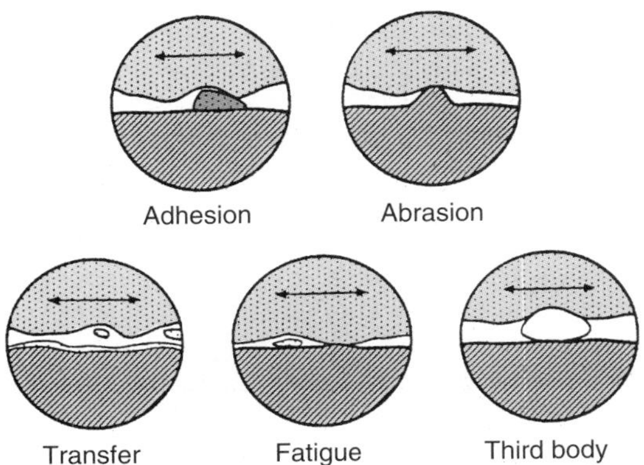

FIGURE 1–44 Wear mechanisms. (From Simon SR, ed: Orthopaedic Basic Science, p 466. Rosemont, IL, American Academy of Orthopaedic Surgeons, 1994.)

of the chondroitin sulfate chains) and change in proportion (decreased concentration of chondroitin sulfate and **increased concentration of keratin sulfate**). Protein content increases with aging, and **water content decreases;** these changes decrease cartilage elasticity. In a normal joint, **weight-bearing exercise increases proteoglycan content** and thickens the cartilage, but moderate joint impact (without a fracture) decreases proteoglycan concentration and increases tissue hydration.

6. Articular cartilage healing—Damage that is limited to the chondrocytes (type 1 injury) or articular cartilage surface (type 2 injury) do not cross the tidemark and have a poor potential for healing **because cartilage is avascular.** Lacerations extending below the tidemark that penetrate the underlying subchondral bone (type 3 injuries) cause an inflammatory response and may heal with fibrocartilage. **The fibrocartilage is produced by undifferentiated marrow mesenchymal stem cells** that differentiate into cells capable of producing fibrocartilage (this is the theory behind abrasion chondroplasty); an abundance of type I collagen is typical at 1 year after injury. Remember, fibrocartilage is not as durable as hyaline cartilage. Blunt trauma may induce changes in cartilage similar to those seen with osteoarthritis. Continuous passive motion is believed to benefit cartilage healing; joint immobilization leads to atrophy or cartilage degeneration. In animal models, 4 weeks of joint nonuse (knee immobilization) decreases the ratio of proteoglycan to collagen, which returns to normal after 8 weeks of joint mobilization. Joint instability (transection of the anterior cruciate ligament [ACL]) initially decreases the ratio of proteoglycan to collagen (at 4 weeks) but later (12 weeks) elevates the ratio of proteoglycan to collagen and increases hydration. Joint instability markedly decreases hyaluronan, whereas joint nonuse does not.

B. Synovium—The synovium mediates the nutrient exchange between blood and joint (synovial) fluid. Synovial tissue is composed of vascularized connective tissue that lacks a basement membrane.

1. Types—Two cell types are present: **type A,** important in **phagocytosis,** and **type B (fibroblast-like cells),** which produce synovial fluid (broth). Other undifferentiated cells have a reparative role. A third type of cell, type C, may exist as an intermediate cell type.
2. Components and function—**Synovial fluid** consists of hyaluronic acid, lubricin (a lubricating glycoprotein), proteinase, collagenases, and prostaglandins. Synovial fluid is an ultrafiltrate (dialysate) of blood plasma added to fluid produced by the synovial membrane; it contains no RBCs, clotting factors, or hemoglobin. It **lubricates articular cartilage and provides nourishment through diffusion. Synovial fluid exhibits non-Newtonian flow characteristics** (the viscosity coefficient μ is not a constant; the fluid is not linearly viscous); its **viscosity increases as the shear rate decreases. Lubricin** is the key lubricating component. **Hyaluronan molecules** in the knee become entangled and behave like an elastic solid during high-strain activities (running, jumping). Analysis of synovial fluid in disease processes is important and is discussed later in this section under Arthroses.
3. Histology—Chronic inflammation of the synovium causes an accumulation of lymphocytes and hyperplasia of the intimal lining, with an absence of neutrophils.

C. Meniscus—Deepens the articular surface of a variety of synovial joints (acromioclavicular, sternoclavicular, glenohumeral, hip, knee), broadening the contact area and distributing the load, such as that on the tibial plateau. The meniscus is more elastic and less permeable than articular cartilage. The meniscus of the knee is the focus of this section. **The meniscus transmits 50% of the force across the joint when the knee is extended and up to 90% in deep flexion. Three years after total meniscectomy of the knee, 20% of patients have significant arthritic lesions and 70% have x-ray changes; all experience arthrosis after 20 years. The severity of degenerative changes is proportional to the amount of meniscus excised.**

1. Anatomy (knee meniscus)—Triangular semilunar structure. Peripheral border is attached to the joint capsule. The medial meniscus is semicircular; the lateral meniscus is circular.
2. Histology—The meniscus is composed of **fibroelastic cartilage** (Fig. 1–45), with an interlacing network of collagen fibers (90% type I), proteoglycans, glycoproteins, and cellular elements (Box 1–2).
3. Innervation and blood supply (knee meniscus)—The peripheral two thirds is innervated by types I and II nerve endings (concentrated in the anterior and posterior horns; few fibers are found in the meniscal body); **the greatest concentration of mechanoreceptors is in the posterior horns. Blood supply is from the geniculate arteries.** Vessels branch circumferentially to form a plexus supplying the **peripheral 25% of the meniscus;** the remaining meniscus receives nutrition via diffusion. Peripheral meniscal tears in the vascularized

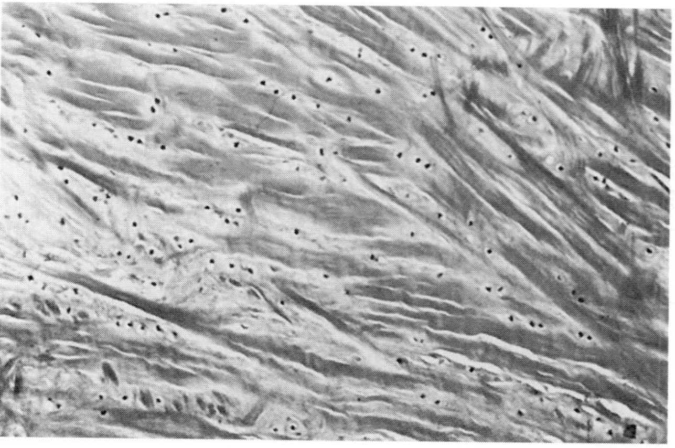

FIGURE 1–45 Histology of menisci.

Box 1–2 Histologic Features of Meniscus

EXTRACELLULAR MATRIX

Collagen
- Types
  - Primarily type I collagen (55-65% of dry weight)
  - Also types II, III, V, and VI (5-10% of dry weight)
- Layers
  - Superficial layer–meshlike fibers oriented primarily radially
  - Surface layer (deep to superficial layer)–irregularly aligned collagen bundles
  - Middle layer (deep)–parallel circumferential fibers

Elastin (0.6% of dry weight)

Proteoglycans, Glycoproteins } 1-3% of dry weight

Adhesive glycoproteins (fibronectin, thrombospondin)

CELLULAR COMPONENTS

Function
- Synthesize and maintain extracellular matrix
- Anaerobic metabolism (few mitochondria)

Components: chondrocytes and fibroblasts (fibrochondrocytes)
- Fusiform cells
  - Found in superficial layer
  - Resemble fibroblasts and chondrocytes
  - Found in lacunae
  - Contain abundant endoplasmic reticulum (ER) and Golgi
- Ovoid cells
  - Found in surface and middle layer
  - Contain abundant ER and Golgi

region ("red zone") can heal via fibrovascular scar formation, making surgical repair necessary; more central tears in the avascular region ("white zone") cannot. **The cell responsible for meniscal healing is the fibrochondrocyte. Peripheral acute meniscal tears with a rim width <4 mm have the best healing characteristics.**

II. Arthroses

A. Introduction—Arthroses may be classified into four basic groups based on their common characteristics (Table 1–21).

1. **Noninflammatory arthritides**—Include osteoarthritis, neuropathic arthropathy, acute rheumatic fever, and a variety of other entities (osteonecrosis, osteochondritis dissecans, osteochondromatosis).
2. **Inflammatory arthritides**—Include many rheumatologic disorders: rheumatoid arthritis (RA), systemic lupus erythematosus, the spondyloarthropathies, and crystalline arthropathies. These disorders may be associated with a human leukocyte antigen (HLA) complex region.
3. **Infectious arthritides**—Include pyogenic arthritis, tuberculous arthritis, fungal arthritis, and Lyme disease.
4. **Hemorrhagic arthritides**—Include hemophilic arthropathy, sickle cell joint destruction, and pigmented villonodular synovitis.

B. Joint fluid analysis (Table 1–22)

1. Noninflammatory arthritides—200 white blood cells (WBCs) with 25% polymorphonuclear neutrophils (PMNs); equal serum values of glucose and protein; normal viscosity (high), straw color, firm mucin clot.
2. Inflammatory arthritides—2000-75,000 WBCs with up to 50% PMNs; moderately decreased glucose (25 mg/dL lower than serum glucose); low viscosity, yellow-green, friable mucin clot. Synovial fluid complement is decreased in RA and normal in ankylosing spondylitis.
3. Infectious arthritides—More than 80,000 WBCs with more than 75% PMNs, a positive Gram stain (also positive cultures later), low glucose (25 mg/dL lower than serum glucose), opaque fluid, increased synovial lactate.

C. Noninflammatory arthritides

1. Osteoarthritis (degenerative joint disease) (see Table 1–21)—**Most common form** of arthritis, but little is known about this disease.
   a. Etiology—On a cellular level, osteoarthritis may be a result of a failed attempt of chondrocytes to repair damaged cartilage. Osteoarthritic cartilage is characterized by **increased water content** (in contrast with the decreased water content seen with aging) (see Table 1–18), **alterations in proteoglycans** (decrease in overall content, shorter chains, and increased chondroitin/keratin sulfate ratio), **collagen abnormalities** (disrupted by collagenase), and **binding of proteoglycans to hyaluronic acid** (caused by proteolytic enzymes from increased prostaglandin E [PGE] and decreased link proteins). Cathepsins B and D levels and **metalloproteinases** (collagenase, gelatinase, stromelysin) **increase in osteoarthritic cartilage** IL-1 enhances enzyme synthesis and may have a **catabolic effect** leading to cartilage degeneration; GAGs and polysulfuric acid may have a protective effect. **Biochemical changes seen in articular cartilage with aging and osteoarthritis are compared in Table 1–18**. Figure 1–46 shows the enzymatic cascade involved in articular cartilage degradation. Cartilage degeneration is encouraged by shear stress and is prevented by normal compressive forces. Excessive stress and inadequate chondrocyte response lead to degeneration. Genetic predisposition may be important in osteoarthritis. **Postmenopausal arthritis of the medial clavicle** seen on the side of the dominant extremity in elderly women is not associated with any systemic arthritis; treatment is with NSAIDs. **Rapidly destructive osteoarthritis** occurs most commonly in the hip and may mimic septic arthritis, RA, seronegative arthritis, neuropathic arthritis, or osteonecrosis. In the hip, the femoral head may be so flattened that it appears to have "sheared off."
   b. General characteristics—Osteoarthritis can be primary (intrinsic defect) or secondary (trauma, infection, congenital condition). Changes that occur in osteoarthritis begin

TABLE 1-21 COMPARISON OF COMMON ARTHRITIDES

Arthritis	Age	Sex	Symmetry	Joints	Physical Exam	Lab Tests	Radiography	Systemic	Treatment
Noninflammatory									
Osteoarthritis	Old	M > F	Asym	Hip, knee, CMC	↓ ROM, crepitus	Nonspecific	Asym. narrowing, eburnation, cysts, osteophytes	None	NSAID, arthrodesis, osteotomy, TJA
Neuropathic	Old	M > F	Asym	Foot, ankle, LE	Effusion, unstable	For underlying disease	Destruction/ heterotopic bone	None	Brace, TJA contraindicated
ARF	Child	M = F	Asym	Mig; lg joints	Red, tender joint; rash	ASO titer	Usually normal	Erythema marginatum nodules, carditis	Symptomatic
Ochronosis	Adult	M = F	Asym	Lg joints/spine	↓ ROM, locking	Urine homogentisic acid	Destruction, disc calcification	Spondylosis	Supportive
Inflammatory									
Rheumatoid	Young	F > M	Sym	Hands, feet	Ulnar dev, claw toes	ESR, CRP, RF	Sym. narrow, periart. resorp.	Pericardial and pulmonary disease	Pyramid Tx synovitis, reconstructive surgery
SLE	Young	F > M	Sym	PIP, MCP, knee	Red, swollen joint; rash	ANA	Less destruction	Cardiac, renal, pancytopenia	Drug therapy like RA
JRA	Child	F > M	Sym	Knee, multiple	Swollen joint, normal color	RF/ANA	Juxta-art. late, osteopenia	Iridocyclitis, rash	ASA; 75% remission
Relapsing polychondritis	Old	M = F	Sym	All joints	Eye, ear involved	ESR	Normal	Ear, cardiac	Supportive, dapsone?
Spondyloarthropathies									
AS	Young	M > F	Sym	SI, spine, hip	Rigid spine, "chin on chest"	ESR, alk phos, CPK, HLA-B27	SI arth., bamboo spine	Uveitis	PT, NSAID, osteotomy
Reiter's syndrome	Young	M > F	Asym	Wt-bearing	Urethral D/C, conjunctivitis	ESR, WBC, HLA-B27	MT head erosion, periostitis	Urethritis, conjunctivitis, ulcer	PT, NSAID, sulfa?
Psoriatic	Young	M = F	Asym	DIP, small joints	Rash, sausage digit, pitting	ESR, HLA-B27	DIP—pencil-in-cup	Rash, conjunctivitis	Drug therapy as for RA
Enteropathic	Young	M > F	Asym	Wt-bearing	Synovitis, GI manifestations	ESR, HLA-B27	Normal	Erythema nodosum, pyoderma	Tx bowel disease, symptomatic
Crystal Deposition Disease									
Gout	Young	M > F	Asym	Great toe, LE	Tophi, red, swollen	Uric acid: – Birefr. crystals; + Birefr. rod-shaped crystals	Soft tissue swelling, erosions	Tophi, renal stones	Colchicine, indomethacin
Chondrocalcinosis	Old	M = F	Asym	Knee, LE	Acute swelling		Articular fibrocartilage calcified	Ochronosis, hyperparathyroidism, hypothyroidism	Symptomatic, avoid surgery
Infectious									
Pyogenic	Any	M = F	Asym	Any joint	Red, hot, swollen	WBC, ESR, bacteria	Joint narrowing (late)	Fever, chills, infection	I&D, IV antibiotics
Tuberculous	Old	M > F	Asym	Spine, LE	Indolent, swelling	PPD, AFB, cultures	Both sides, cysts	Lung, multiorgan	Antibiotics ± I&D
Lyme disease	Young	M = F	Asym	Any joint	Acute effusion	Culture, ELISA	Usually normal	ECM rash, neuro., cardiac	Penicillin, tetracycline
Fungal	Any	M > F	Asym	Any joint	Indolent	Special studies/ cultures	Minimal changes	Immunocompromised	5-FU, amphotericin
Hemorrhagic									
Hemophilia	Young	M	Asym	Knee, UE (elbow, shoulder)	↓ ROM, swelling	PTT, factor VIII	Squared-off patella	Soft tissue bleeding	Support, synovectomy, TJA
Sickle cell	Young	M = F	Asym	Hip, any bone	Pain, ↓ ROM	Sickle prep.	Osteonecrosis	Infarcts, osteonecrosis	
PVNS	Young	M = F	Asym	Knee, LE	Pain, synovitis	Aspirate, biopsy	Juxtacortical erosion	None	Surgical excision

AFB, acid-fast bacilli; alk phos, alkaline phosphatase; ANA, antinuclear antibody; ARF, acute rheumatic fever; arth, arthritis; AS, ankylosing spondylitis; ASA, acetylsalicylic acid; ASO, antistreptolysin O; Asym, asymmetrical; Birefr., birefringent; CMC, carpometacarpal; CPK, creatine phosphokinase; CRP, C-reactive protein; D/C, discharge; DIP, distal interphalangeal; ECM, erythema chronicum migrans; ELISA, enzyme-linked immunosorbent assay; ESR, erythrocyte sedimentation rate; 5-FU, 5-flucytosine; GI,

TABLE 1-22 JOINT FLUID ANALYSIS

Types of Arthritis	White Blood Cells (/mm^3)	Polymorphonuclear Leukocytes (%)	Other Characteristics
Noninflammatory	200	25	Joint aspirate glucose and protein equal to serum values
Inflammatory	2000-75,000	50	↓ Joint aspirate glucose
Infectious	>80,000	>75	Thick, cloudy fluid + Gram stain + Cultures ↓ Joint aspirate glucose, ↑ joint aspirate protein

From Brinker MR, Miller MD: Fundamentals of Orthopaedics, p 26. Philadelphia, WB Saunders, 1999.

with deterioration and loss of the bearing surface, followed by osteophyte development and osteochondral junction breakdown. Later, cartilage disintegration and subchondral microfractures expose the bony surface. **Subchondral cysts** (which arise secondary to microfracture and may contain amorphous gelatinous material) and **osteophytes,** which are part of this process, along with **"joint space narrowing"** and eburnation of bone, are demonstrated on radiographs. Microscopic changes include loss of superficial chondrocytes, **chondrocyte cloning** (>1 chondrocyte per lacuna), replication and breakdown of the tidemark, fissuring, cartilage destruction with eburnation of subchondral "pagetoid" bone, and other changes (Figs. 1–47 and 1–48). Findings on physical examination include decreased ROM and crepitus. **The knee is the most common joint affected in osteoarthritis.**

c. Radiographic characteristics—Osteophytes, "joint space" narrowing, subchondral cysts (from microfractures/bone repair) on both sides of the joint, and subchondral sclerosis are typical. Tomograms or CT scans are best at showing these osteoarthritis-related changes.

   (1) Hand—Distal interphalangeal (DIP), proximal interphalangeal (PIP), and carpometacarpal (CMC) joints
   (2) Hip—Superolateral involvement
   (3) Knee—Asymmetrical involvement

d. Treatment— Treatment begins with supportive measures (e.g., activity modification, cane) and includes NSAIDs (misoprostol [Cytotec] may lower GI complications via a prostaglandin effect). Surgical procedures ranging from arthroscopic débridement to total joint arthroplasties (TJAs) may be useful in advanced cases that are resistant to nonoperative treatment.

2. Neuropathic arthropathy (Charcot joint disease) (see Table 1–21) (Fig. 1–49)—An extreme form of osteoarthritis caused by disturbed sensory innervation.
   a. Causes—Causes include diabetes (foot), tabes dorsalis (lower extremity), **syringomyelia (the most common cause of upper-extremity neuropathic arthropathy** [most common in the shoulder and elbow]), Hansen's disease (the second most common cause of upper extremity neuropathic arthropathy), myelomeningocele (ankle and foot), congenital insensitivity to pain (ankle and foot), and other

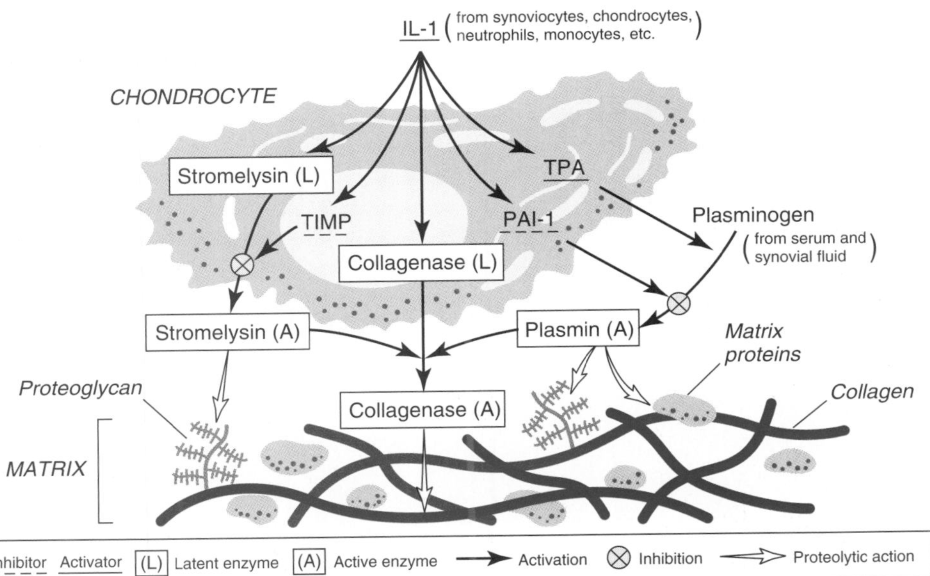

FIGURE 1–46 Enzyme cascade of interleukin-1-stimulated degradation of articular cartilage. (From Simon SR, ed: Orthopaedic Basic Science, p 40. Rosemont, IL, American Academy of Orthopaedic Surgeons, 1994.)

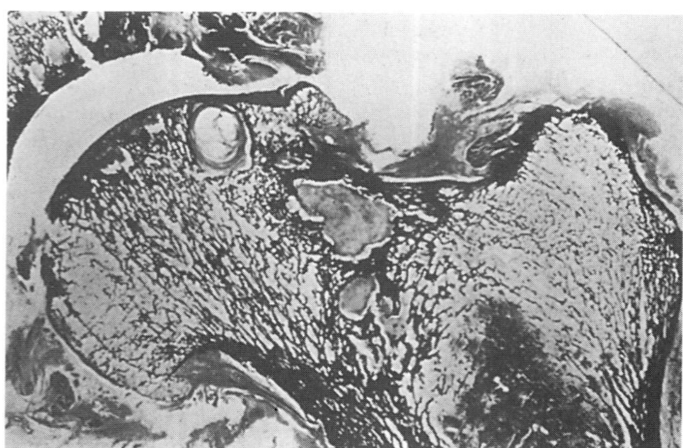

FIGURE 1–47 Macrosection of an osteoarthritic human femoral head demonstrating subarticular cysts, sclerotic bone formation, and an inferior femoral head osteophyte. (From Simon SR, ed: Orthopaedic Basic Science, p 35. Rosemont, IL, American Academy of Orthopaedic Surgeons, 1994.)

neurologic problems (such as spinal cord injury). A Charcot joint develops in 25% of patients with syringomyelia (80% involve the upper extremity).

b. Diagnosis—Typically seen in an older patient with an unstable, painless, swollen joint who may present with a hemarthrosis. Radiographs show advanced (severe) destructive changes on both sides of the joint, scattered "chunks" of bone embedded in fibrous tissue, joint distention by fluid, and heterotopic ossification. **It may be very difficult to differentiate Charcot's arthropathy and osteomyelitis based on physical examination and plain radiographs.** Symptoms common to the two conditions include swelling, warmth, erythema, minimal pain, and a variable WBC count and erythrocyte sedimentation rate (ESR); both are common in diabetic patients. A **technetium bone scan may look similar ("hot") for both osteomyelitis and Charcot's arthropathy; an indium leukocyte scan will be "hot" (positive) for osteomyelitis and "cold" (negative) for Charcot's arthropathy.**

c. Treatment—Treatment of Charcot's arthropathy is focused on limitation of activity and appropriate bracing or casting **(skin temperature of the involved side similar to that of the uninvolved side is the best indicator for discontinuing a total contact cast).** A Charcot joint is usually a contraindication for TJA and the use of other orthopaedic hardware.

3. Acute rheumatic fever (see Table 1–21) (sometimes included in the inflammatory group)—Formerly the most common cause of childhood arthritis, acute rheumatic fever has rarely been seen since the advent of antibiotics. Arthritis and arthralgias can follow **untreated group A β-hemolytic strep infections** and can present with acute onset of red, tender, extremely painful joint effusions. Systemic manifestations include carditis, erythema marginatum (painless macules with red margins usually on the abdomen but never on the face), subcutaneous nodules (extensor surfaces of the upper extremities), and chorea. The arthritis is **migratory** and typically involves **multiple large joints.** Diagnosis is based on the **Jones criteria** (preceding strep infection with two major criteria [carditis, polyarthritis, chorea, erythema marginatum, subcutaneous nodules] or one major and two minor criteria [fever, arthralgia, prior rheumatic fever, elevated ESR, prolonged PR interval on ECG]). **Antistreptolysin O titers are elevated in 80% of affected patients.** Treatment includes penicillin and salicylates.

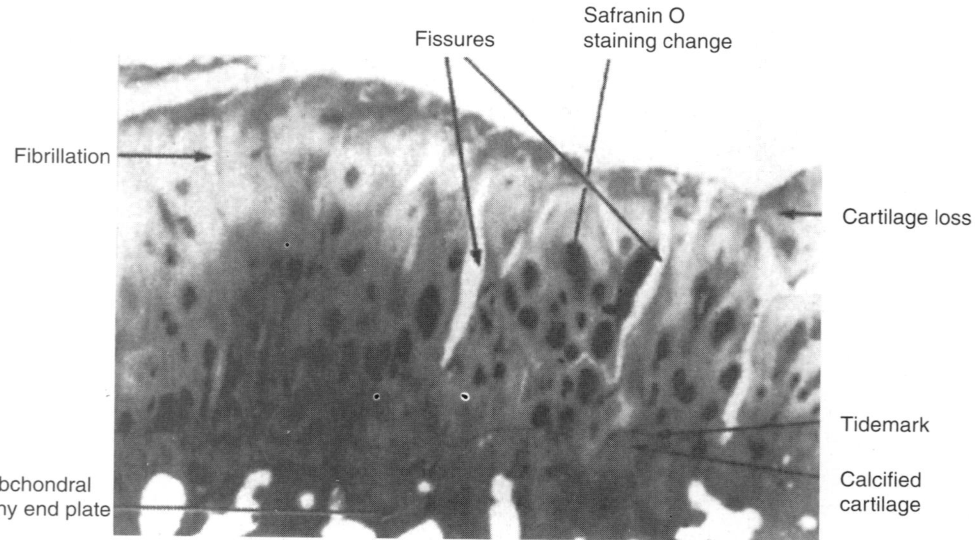

FIGURE 1–48 Low-power micrograph of osteoarthritis demonstrating fibrillation, fissures, and cartilage loss. (From Simon SR, ed: Orthopaedic Basic Science, p 34. Rosemont, IL, American Academy of Orthopaedic Surgeons, 1994.)

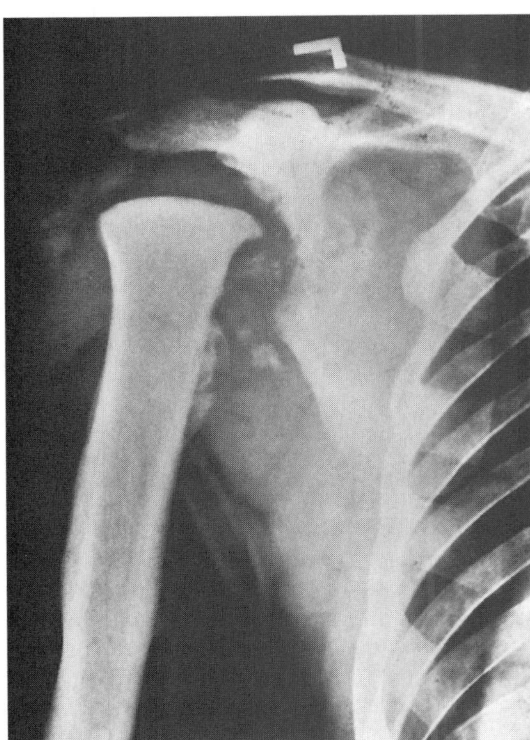

FIGURE 1–49 Anteroposterior radiograph of a shoulder showing severe destructive changes characteristic of neuropathic arthropathy. (From Weissman BNW, Sledge CB: Orthopedic Radiology. Philadelphia, WB Saunders, 1986, p 238.)

4. Ochronosis (see Table 1–21)—Degenerative arthritis resulting from **alkaptonuria,** a rare inborn defect of the **homogentisic acid oxidase enzyme system** (tyrosine and phenylalanine catabolism). **Excess homogentisic acid is deposited in the joints** and then polymerizes (turns black), leading to early degenerative changes (can also be deposited in other tissues, such as the heart valves). These patients may also present with **black urine. Ochronotic spondylitis** (Fig. 1–50), which usually occurs during the fourth decade of life, includes progressive degenerative changes and disc space narrowing and calcification (Table 1–23).
5. Secondary pulmonary hypertrophic osteoarthropathy—A clinical diagnosis. Involves a lung tumor mass, joint pain and stiffness, periostitis of the long bones, and clubbing of the fingers.

D. Inflammatory arthritides—Tables 1–24 and 1–25 show an overview of commonly confused laboratory findings in inflammatory arthritic conditions. Generally, inflammatory arthritides produce radiographic evidence of destruction on both sides of a joint.
   1. RA (see Table 1–21)—The most common form of inflammatory arthritis, RA affects 3% of women and 1% of men. Required diagnostic criteria, developed by the American Rheumatism Association, are morning stiffness, swelling, nodules, positive laboratory tests, and radiographic findings.
      a. Etiology—Unclear but probably related to a cell-mediated immune response (T cell) that incites an inflammatory response initially against soft tissues and later against cartilage (chondrolysis) and bone (periarticular bone resorption). **Mononuclear cells are the primary cellular mediators of tissue destruction in RA.** RA may be associated with an infectious etiology or an HLA locus **(HLA-DR4 and -DW4).** Lymphokines, cytokines

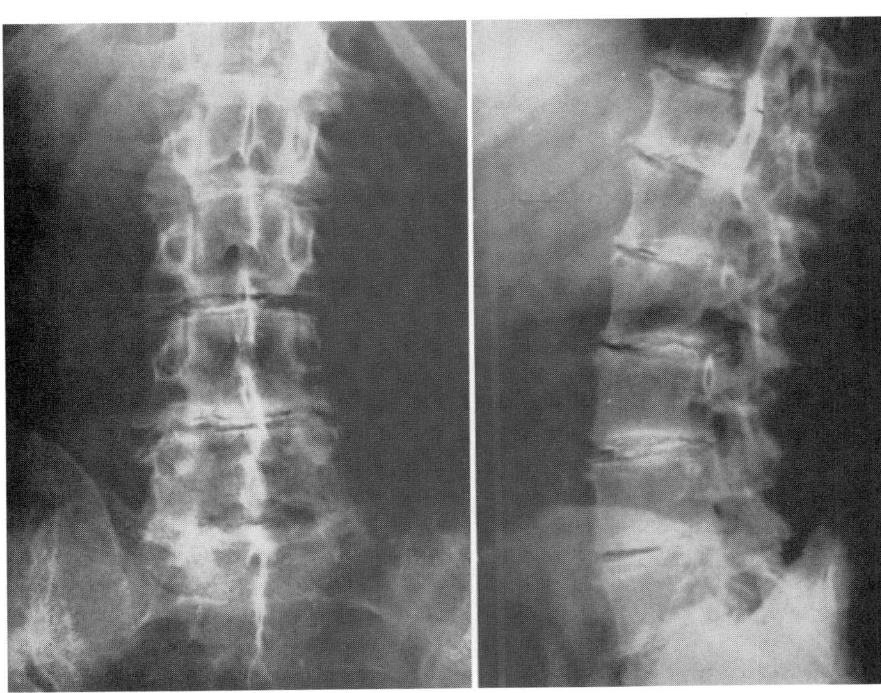

FIGURE 1–50 Ochronosis. Irregular calcification and narrowing of the intervertebral discs are present. Radiolucent streaks, evident anteriorly between the vertebral bodies, are not uncommon. There is only minimal slipping of the vertebral bodies. (Courtesy of Samuel Fisher, MD.)

TABLE 1-23 COMPARATIVE BONY CHANGES OF THE SPINE IN THE ARTHRITIDES

Disorder	Bony Change	Radiographic Appearance
Ochronosis	Syndesmophytes (ossification of the annulus fibrosis of the intervertebral disc)	Vertical syndesmophytes extending from the body of one vertebra to the adjacent vertebra
Ankylosing spondylitis	Syndesmophytes	Similar to above
Reiter's syndrome and psoriatic spondylitis	Ossification of the connective tissues adjacent to the spine	Area of ossification is separated from the margin of the vertebral body and/or the intervertebral disc
Disseminated idiopathic skeletal hyperostosis	Ossification of the connective tissues adjacent to the spine, the anterior longitudinal ligament, and the intervertebral disc	Undulating osseous extension along the anterior portion of the spine

(particularly IL-1 and tumor necrosis factor-α [TNF-α]), and other inflammatory mediators initiate a destructive cascade that leads to joint destruction; for example, **TNF-α increases chondrocyte secretion of matrix metalloproteinases, which degrades the cartilage extracellular matrix.** RA cartilage is sensitive to PMN degradation and IL-1 effects (phospholipase A_2, PGE_2, and plasminogen activators). **Class II molecules** are involved in antigen–T-lymphocyte interaction.

b. General characteristics—Usually an insidious onset of morning stiffness and polyarthritis. Most commonly the hands (ulnar deviation and subluxation of the metacarpophalangeal [MCP] joints) and the feet (metatarsophalangeal [MTP] joints, claw toes, and hallux valgus) are affected early, but also common in the knees, elbows, shoulders, ankles, and cervical spine. **Subcutaneous nodules,** which are strongly associated with positive serum rheumatoid factor (RF), are seen in 20% of RA patients during their lifetime. The synovium and soft tissues are affected first; only later are joints significantly involved. **Early in the disease process, the RA-inflamed synovium shows a proliferation of blood vessels.** Pannus ingrowth denudes articular cartilage and leads to chondrocyte death. **Laboratory findings** include **elevated ESR and C-reactive protein** and **a positive RF titer (immunoglobulin M [IgM])** in approximately 80% of patients. Joint fluid assays can also demonstrate RF, decreased complement levels, and other helpful findings. **Systemic manifestations** can include rheumatoid vasculitis, pericarditis, and pulmonary disease (pleurisy, nodules, fibrosis). Popliteal cysts in rheumatoid patients (confirmed by ultrasonography) can mimic thrombophlebitis. Felty's syndrome is RA with splenomegaly and leukopenia. Still's disease is acute-onset juvenile RA (JRA) with fever, rash, and splenomegaly. Sjögren's syndrome is an autoimmune exocrinopathy often associated with RA; symptoms include **decreased salivary and lacrimal gland secretion** (keratoconjunctivitis sicca complex) and lymphoid proliferation.

TABLE 1-24 COMMONLY CONFUSED LABORATORY FINDINGS IN INFLAMMATORY ARTHRITIC CONDITIONS

Finding	May Be Positive for	Usually Negative for
Rheumatoid factor (RF)	Rheumatoid arthritis Sjögren's syndrome Sarcoid Systemic lupus erythematosus	Ankylosing spondylitis Gout Psoriatic arthritis Reiter's syndrome
HLA-B27*	Ankylosing spondylitis Reiter's syndrome Psoriatic arthritis Enteropathic arthritis	
Antinuclear antibody (ANA)	Systemic lupus erythematosus Sjögren's syndrome Scleroderma	

Approximately 6% of all whites are HLA-B27 positive.
Modified from Brinker MR, Miller MD: Fundamentals of Orthopaedics, p 27. Philadelphia, WB Saunders, 1999.

c. Radiographic characteristics (Fig. 1–51)—Include **periarticular erosions** and **osteopenia.** The areas commonly affected are the hand (MCPs, PIPs, and carpal bones), wrist, and cervical spine. All three knee compartments may show osteoporosis and erosions. **Protrusio acetabuli** (medial displacement of the acetabulum beyond the radiographic teardrop with medial migration of the femoral head into the pelvis) is common in RA as well as ankylosing spondylitis, Paget's disease, metabolic bone diseases, Marfan's syndrome, Otto's pelvis, and other conditions.

d. Treatment—**RA treatment** goals: control synovitis and pain, maintain joint function, and prevent deformities. A multidisciplinary approach involving therapeutic drugs, physical therapy, and sometimes surgery is necessary. The "pyramid" approach to RA drug therapy begins with NSAIDs and then slowly progress to antimalarials, remittent agents (methotrexate, sulfasalazine, gold, and penicillamine), steroids, cytotoxic drugs, and finally experimental drugs. The pyramid approach

TABLE 1-25 ASSOCIATIONS BETWEEN HUMAN LEUKOCYTE ANTIGEN ALLELES AND SUSCEPTIBILITY TO SOME RHEUMATIC DISEASES

Disease	HLA Marker	Frequency (%) in Patients (Whites)	Frequency (%) in Controls (Whites)	Relative Risk
Ankylosing spondylitis	B27	90	9	87
Reiter's syndrome	B27	79	9	37
Psoriatic arthritis	B27	48	9	10
Inflammatory bowel disease with spondylitis	B27	52	9	10
Adult rheumatoid arthritis	DR4	70	30	6
Polyarticular juvenile rheumatoid arthritis	DR4	75	30	7
Pauciarticular juvenile rheumatoid arthritis	DR8	30	5	5
	DR5	50	20	4.5
	DR2.1	55	20	4
Systemic lupus erythematosus	DR2	46	22	3.5
	DR3	50	25	3
Sjögren's syndrome	DR3	70	25	6

From Nepom BS, Nepom GT: Immunogenetics and the rheumatic diseases. In McCarty DJ, Koopman WJ, eds: Arthritis and Allied Conditions: A Textbook of Rheumatology, 12th ed. Philadelphia, Lea & Febiger, 1993.

has been challenged recently in favor of a more aggressive approach with **disease-modifying antirheumatic drugs (DMARDs)** such as methotrexate, azathioprine, anakinra (an IL-1 inhibitor), and other TNF-α inhibitors, such as infliximab and etanercept. Surgery includes synovectomy (only if aggressive drug therapy fails), soft tissue realignments (usually not favored because the deformity progresses), and various reconstructive procedures (increased risk of infection after TJA). If done early, chemical and radiation synovectomy can be successful. **Operative synovectomy** (open or arthroscopic), especially in the knee, **decreases the pain and swelling associated with the synovitis but does not prevent radiographic progression or the future need for total knee arthroplasty (TKA), nor does it improve joint ROM.** After all forms of synovectomy, the synovium initially regenerates normally but degenerates to rheumatoid synovial tissue over time. Evaluation of the cervical spine with preoperative radiographs is important.

2. Systemic lupus erythematosus (SLE) (see Tables 1–23, 1–26, and 1–27)—Chronic inflammatory disease of unknown origin usually affecting women (especially African Americans). Probably related to the immune complex. Manifestations include **fever, butterfly malar rash,** pancytopenia, pericarditis, nephritis, and polyarthritis. **Joint involvement is the most common feature,** affecting more than 75% of SLE patients. Arthritis typically presents as acute, red, tender swelling of the PIPs, MCPs, carpus, knees, and other joints. **SLE is typically not as destructive**

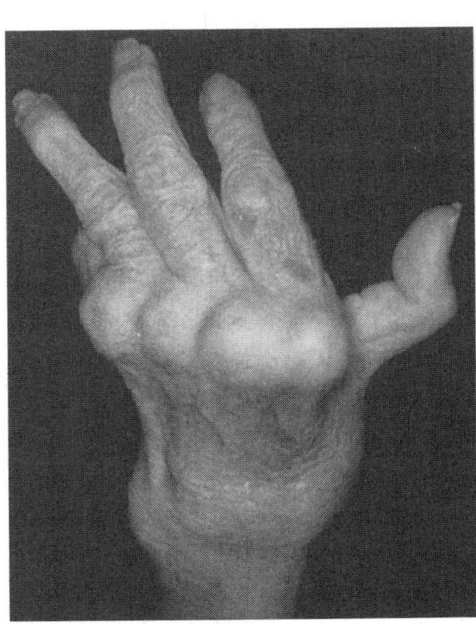
A

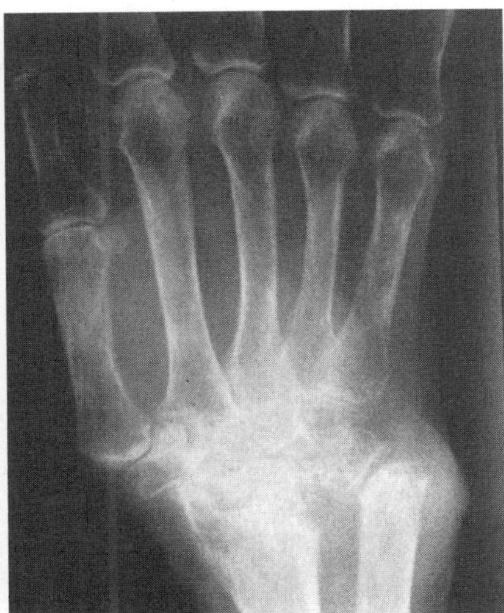
B

FIGURE 1–51 **A**, Clinical photograph of the hand of a patient with advanced rheumatoid arthritis. Note ulnar drift of the metacarpophalangeal (MCP) joints caused by the ulnar shift of the extensor tendons, dislocations of the MCP joints, and thumb deformities. **B**, Anteroposterior radiograph of the hand and wrist of a patient with rheumatoid arthritis. Note severe erosive destruction of the distal radioulnar joint and diffuse osteopenia. (From Bogumil GP: The hand. In Wiesel SW, Delahay JN: Essentials of Orthopaedic Surgery, 2nd ed, p 263. Philadelphia, WB Saunders, 1997.)

as RA. Treatment for SLE arthritis usually includes the same medications as those described for RA. Mortality in SLE is usually related to renal disease. The differential diagnosis of SLE includes polymyositis and dermatomyositis, which also present with symmetrical weakness with or without a characteristic "heliotropic" rash of the upper eyelids. SLE patients are typically positive for antinuclear antibody (ANA) and HLA-DR3 and may be positive for RF.

3. Polymyalgia rheumatica—Common among the elderly. Aching and stiffness of the shoulder and pelvic girdle, associated with malaise, headaches, and anorexia, are common symptoms. Physical examination is usually unremarkable. Laboratory studies show a **markedly elevated ESR,** anemia, increased alkaline phosphatase, and increased immune complexes. Usually treated symptomatically, with steroid use for refractory cases. **May be associated with temporal arteritis,** which requires a biopsy for definitive diagnosis and also requires timely treatment with high-dose steroids (if left untreated, may result in rapid total blindness).
4. JRA (see Tables 1–23 and 1–27)—Also discussed in Chapter 3, Pediatric Orthopaedics.
   a. Types—Three major types of JRA are recognized: systemic (20%), polyarticular (50%), and pauciarticular (30%). **Seronegative** denotes RF-negative, and **seropositive** denotes RF-positive; the incidence of seropositive JRA is estimated to be <15% and is associated with a higher incidence of chronic, active, and progressive disease. **Early-onset JRA** denotes onset of disease before the teens, **late-onset JRA** denotes onset of disease as a teenager or later.
      (1) Systemic
      (2) Polyarticular—**Polyarticular JRA** indicates that five or more joints are involved. **Seronegative polyarticular JRA** is characterized by involvement of more than five joints and is more frequent in girls. **Seropositive polyarticular JRA** also involves more than five joints, is more frequent in girls, exhibits a **positive RF** and **destructive degenerative joint disease (DJD),** and **frequently develops into adult RA.**
      (3) Pauciarticular—**Pauciarticular JRA** indicates that four or fewer joints are involved. **Early-onset pauciarticular JRA** involves four or fewer joints, is more frequent in girls, and is associated with **iridocyclitis** in 50% of cases (particularly those with a positive antinuclear antibody [ANA]). **Late-onset pauciarticular JRA** involves four or fewer joints and is **seen in boys more commonly than girls.** JRA may also be associated with an HLA locus (HLA-DR2, HLA-DR4, HLA-DR5, HLA-DR8, and HLA-B27 in boys).

   b. Treatment—Treatment of JRA includes high-dose aspirin, only occasionally gold or remittent agents (refractory polyarticular), and frequent ophthalmologic examinations (with a slit lamp) for asymptomatic ocular involvement. **The most common joint affected in JRA is the knee,** followed by the finger/wrist, ankle, hip, and cervical spine.
5. Relapsing polychondritis (see Table 1–21)—Rare disorder associated with episodic **inflammation; diffuse, self-limiting arthritis;** and progressive cartilage destruction with or without systemic vasculitis. The disorder typically involves the **ears (thickening of the auricle);** also seen are inflammatory eye disorders, tracheal involvement, hearing disorders, and sometimes cardiac involvement. It may be an autoimmune disorder (affected by type II collagen). Treatment is supportive, although dapsone may have a role in the future.
6. Spondyloarthropathies/enthesopathies (occur at ligament insertions into bone)—Characterized by a **positive HLA-B27** (sixth chromosome, D locus) and a **negative RF** titer.
   a. Ankylosing spondylitis (AS) (see Tables 1–21, 1–24, and 1–25)
      (1) Diagnosis—Bilateral sacroiliitis with or without acute anterior uveitis in an HLA-B27–positive man is diagnostic. There is insidious onset of back pain (with associated morning stiffness) and hip pain during the third to fourth decade of life. AS progresses for approximately 20 years **(progressive spinal flexion deformities).** Radiographic changes (Fig. 1–52; also see Table 1–23) in the spine include **squaring**

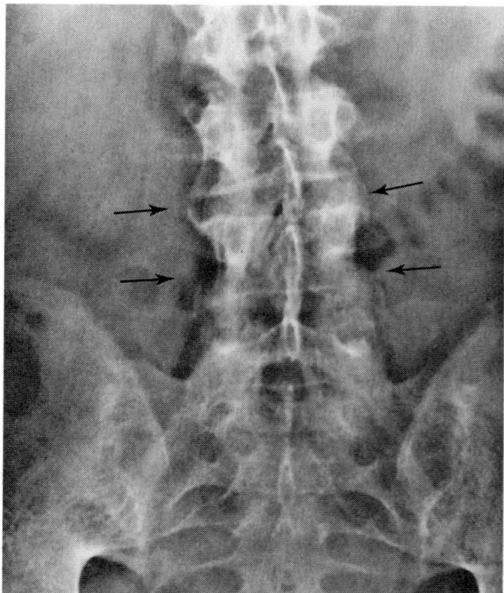

FIGURE 1–52 Anteroposterior radiograph of the lumbar spine and sacroiliac joints demonstrating marginal syndesmophytes *(arrows)* typical in ankylosing spondylitis. Note bilateral involvement of the sacroiliac joints. (From Bullough PG, Vigorita VJ: Atlas of Orthopaedic Pathology. Philadelphia, Gower Medical Publishing, 1984, p 811, by permission of Mosby.)

of the vertebrae, vertical syndesmophytes, obliteration of sacroiliac joints, and "whiskering" of the enthesis. Ascending ankylosis of the spine usually begins in the thoracolumbar spine, often causing the entire spine to become rigid. Spinal manifestations include the "chin on chest" deformity (which may require corrective osteotomy of the cervicothoracic junction), **difficult cervical spine fractures (associated with epidural hemorrhage [high mortality rate]) that are best diagnosed via a CT scan (75% rate of neurologic involvement),** and severe kyphotic deformities (corrected via a posterior closing wedge osteotomy). Spondylodiskitis may develop in the late stage. Other extraskeletal manifestations include iritis; aortitis, colitis, arachnoiditis, amyloidosis, and sarcoidosis. Pulmonary involvement (restriction of chest excursion [<2 cm]), hip involvement, and young age at onset are prognostic of poor outcomes.

(2) Treatment—Lower spinal deformities with hip flexion deformities and pain (plus **morning stiffness**) are often helped with bilateral total hip arthroplasty (THA). Associated protrusio acetabuli requires special THA techniques. The need for prophylaxis for heterotopic bone formation has been questioned in patients with AS undergoing routine primary, noncemented THA. Initial treatment with physical therapy (PT) and NSAIDs (phenylbutazone is best but can cause bone marrow depression) may be helpful. AS is often associated with heart disease and pulmonary fibrosis.

b. Reiter's syndrome (see Tables 1–21 and 1–23 through 1–25) (Fig. 1–53)—The classic presentation is a young man with the triad of **conjunctivitis, urethritis, and oligoarticular arthritis** ("can't see, pee, or bend the knee"). Painless **oral ulcers, penile lesions,** and **pustular lesions** on the extremities, **palms,** and **soles (keratoderma blennorrhagicum)** and plantar heel pain are common. The arthritis usually causes sudden asymmetrical swelling and pain in weight-bearing joints. Recurrence is common and can lead to metatarsal head erosion and calcaneal periostitis. Approximately **80-90% of patients with Reiter's syndrome are HLA-B27 positive,** and 60% with chronic disease have **sacroiliitis.** Treatment includes NSAIDs, PT, and possibly sulfa drugs.

c. Psoriatic arthropathy (see Tables 1–21 and 1–23 through 1–25)—Affects approximately 5-10% of patients with psoriasis. Many HLA loci may be involved, but HLA-B27 is found in 50% of patients with psoriatic arthritis. Many forms exist; most patients have the oligoarticular form, which asymmetrically affects the small joints of the hands and feet. **Nail pitting** (also fragmentation and discoloration), **"sausage" digits, and "pencil-in-cup" deformity (with DIP involvement)** are characteristic (Fig. 1–54). Treatment is similar to that for RA.

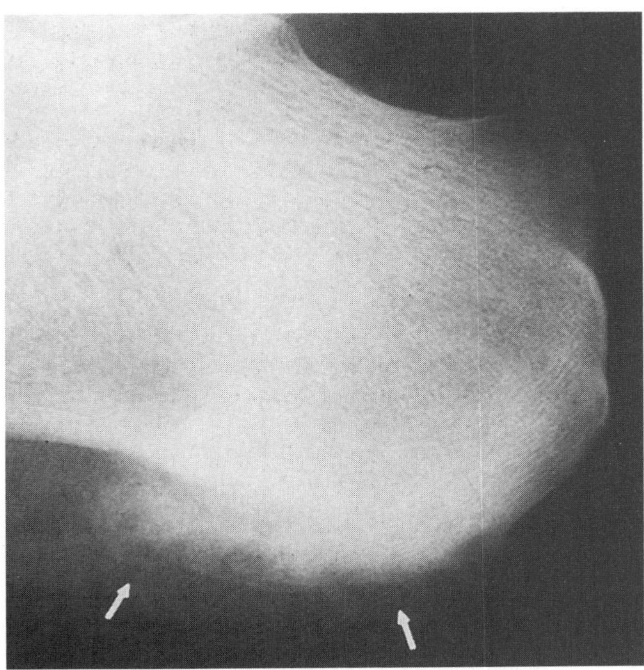

FIGURE 1–53 Lateral radiograph of the calcaneus of a patient with Reiter's syndrome shows fluffy periosteal calcifications *(arrows)*.

d. Enteropathic arthritis (see Tables 1–21, 1–24, and 1–25)—Approximately 10-20% of patients with Crohn's disease and ulcerative colitis experience peripheral joint arthritis, and 5% or more experience axial disease. This nondeforming arthritis occurs more commonly in large, weight-bearing joints. It usually presents as an acute monarticular synovitis that may precede any bowel symptoms. Enteropathic arthritis is HLA-B27 positive in approximately half of all affected persons and is associated with AS in 10-15% of cases.

7. Crystal deposition disease

a. Gout (see Table 1–21; Fig. 1–55) —Disorder of nucleic acid metabolism causing hyperuricemia, which leads to monosodium urate (MSU) crystal deposition in joints.

(1) Cause—Crystals activate inflammatory mediators (proteases, chemotactic factors, prostaglandins, leukotriene B_4, and free oxygen radicals). The inflammatory mediators are **inhibited by colchicine.** The crystals also activate platelets, IL-1, and the complement system. **Phagocytosis is inhibited by phenylbutazone and indomethacin (Indocin).** Local polypeptides may inhibit the crystal inflammatory response via a glycoprotein "coating."

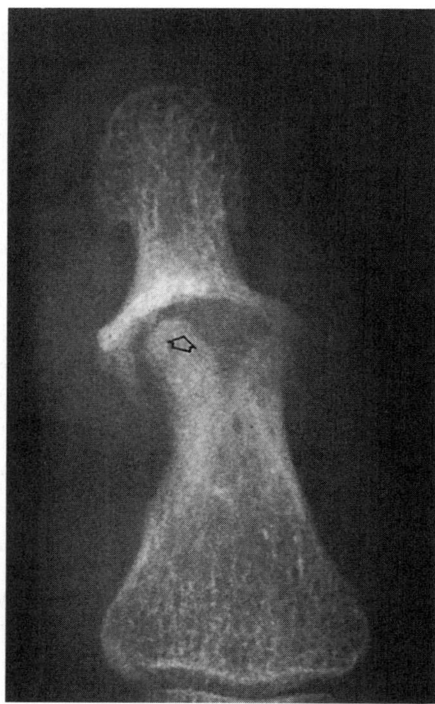

FIGURE 1–54 Anteroposterior radiograph of the distal interphalangeal joint of the foot in a patient with psoriatic arthritis shows the classic pencil-in-cup deformity.

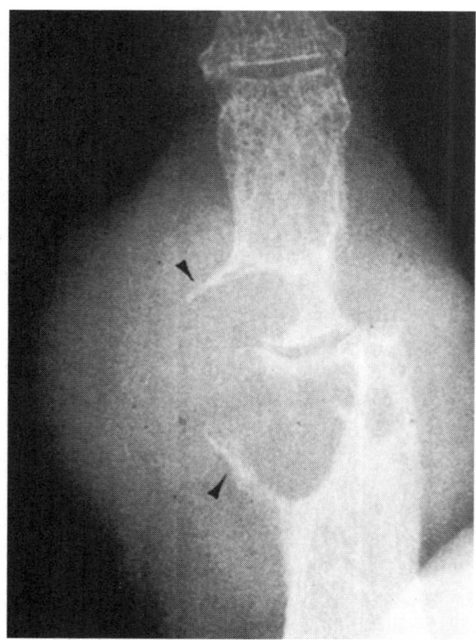

FIGURE 1–55 Anteroposterior radiograph of the proximal interphalangeal joint of a finger in a patient with gout. Note the soft tissue swelling, "punched out" periarticular erosions, and sclerotic overhangings bordering the joint *(arrowheads)*. (From Resnick D, Niwayama G: Diagnosis of Bone and Joint Disorders, p 1478. Philadelphia, WB Saunders, 1981.)

Gout may be precipitated by chemotherapy for myeloproliferative disorders.

(2) Diagnosis—Recurrent arthritis attacks, especially in men 40-60 years of age (usually in the lower extremity, **especially the great toe [podagra]**), crystal deposition as **tophi** (ear helix, eyelid, olecranon, Achilles; usually seen in the chronic form), and renal disease/stones (2% Ca^{2+} versus normal [02%]), are characteristic. The kidneys are the second most commonly affected organ. **Radiographs may show soft tissue changes and "punched-out" periarticular erosions with sclerotic overhanging borders** (see Fig. 1–55). Elevated serum uric acid level is not diagnostic of gout; MSU crystals, which are **thin, tapered intracellular crystals that are strongly negatively birefringent** (Fig. 1–56) in joint aspirate, are essential for diagnosis.

(3) Treatment—**Initial treatment with indomethacin** (50-75 mg tid) is indicated, followed by a rheumatology consultation (patients with GI symptoms or a history of peptic ulcer disease should receive intravenous colchicine for acute attacks). **Allopurinol** is used to lower the serum uric acid levels in hyperuricemic patients with chronic gout and is given prior to chemotherapy for myeloproliferative disorders. **Allopurinol is a xanthine oxidase inhibitor** (xanthine oxidase is needed for the conversion of hypoxanthine to xanthine and xanthine to uric acid). Colchicine can be used for **prophylaxis after recurrent attacks.**

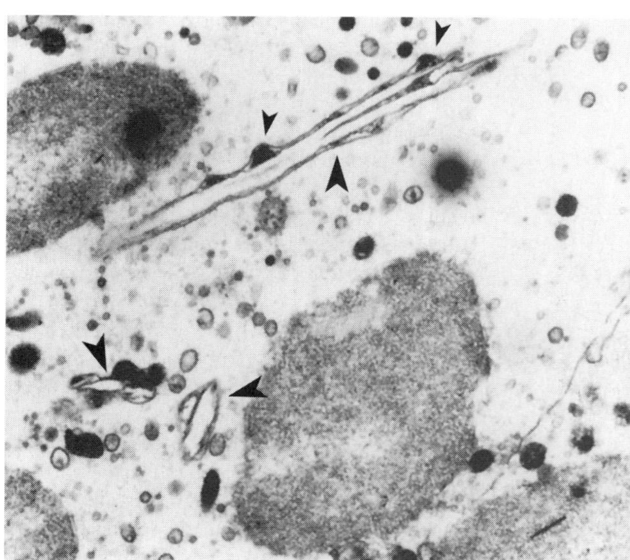

FIGURE 1–56 A neutrophil has phagocytosed a number of monosodium urate crystals *(large arrowheads)*. Although the crystals have almost completely dissolved, the outlines of the vacuoles remain, one still needle shaped. Lysosomes discharge their contents directly into the phagosomes *(small arrowheads)*. (Magnification, 22,000; original magnification, ×31,250.) (From Krey PR, Lazaro DM: Analysis of Synovial Fluid. Summit, NJ, Ciba-Geigy, 1992.)

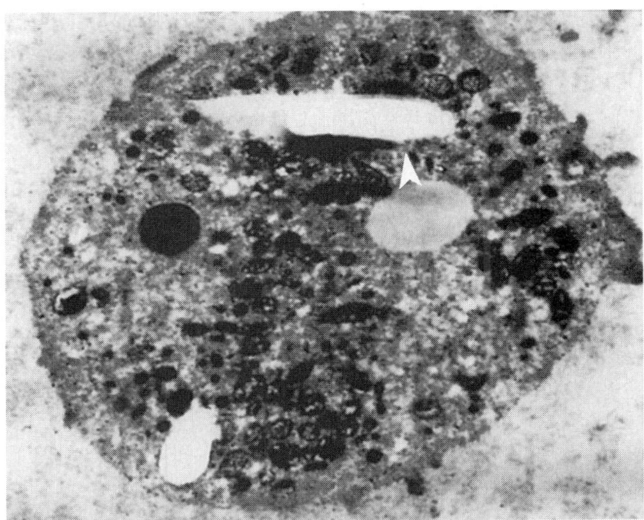

FIGURE 1–57 A synovial fluid leukocyte showing the outline of a phagocytosed calcium pyrophosphate dihydrate crystal that has dissolved *(arrowhead)*. (Magnification, ×14,000; original magnification, ×17,000.) (From Krey PR, Lazaro DM: Analysis of Synovial Fluid. Summit, NJ, Ciba-Geigy, 1992.)

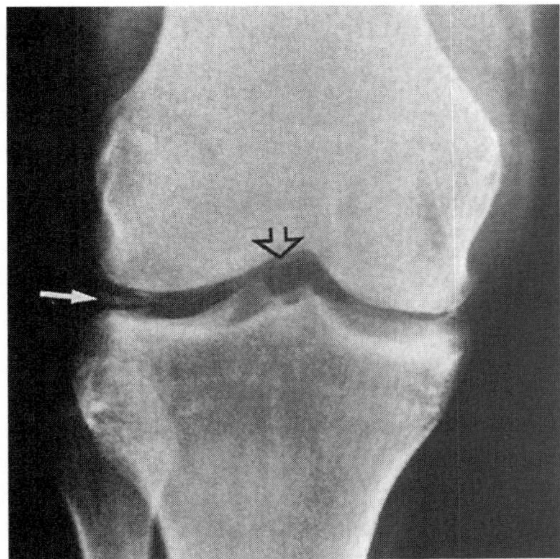

FIGURE 1–58 Anteroposterior radiograph demonstrating calcium pyrophosphate deposition disease (pseudogout) in the meniscus of the knee. Note calcification within the (fibrocartilage) meniscus *(closed arrow)* and articular involvement, with fine linear calcification of hyaline cartilage *(open arrow)*. (From Weissman BNW, Sledge CB: Orthopaedic Radiology, p 549. Philadelphia, WB Saunders, 1986.)

b. Chondrocalcinosis (see Table 1–21)—Caused by several disorders, including (1) **calcium pyrophosphate (dihydrate crystal) deposition disease (CPPD [pseudogout]),** (2) ochronosis, (3) hyperparathyroidism, (4) hypothyroidism, and (5) hemochromatosis. **CPPD** (a common cause of chondrocalcinosis) is a disorder of pyrophosphate metabolism that occurs in older patients and occasionally causes acute attacks (usually in the lower extremities, especially the **knee**), which can be mistaken for septic arthritis. **Short, blunt, rhomboid-shaped crystals that are weakly positively birefringent** (Fig. 1–57) are seen in neutrophilic leukocytes in knee aspirate. **Chondrocalcinosis of knee menisci is often related to a previous knee injury.** Radiographs show fine linear calcification in hyaline cartilage and more diffuse calcification of **menisci** (Fig. 1–58) **and other fibrocartilage (triangular fibrocartilage complex,** acetabular labrum). NSAIDs are often helpful. Intra-articular yttrium-90 injections have also been successful in chronic cases.

c. Calcium hydroxyapatite crystal deposition disease—Also associated with chondrocalcinosis and DJD. It is a **destructive arthropathy** commonly seen in the knee and shoulder. The "**Milwaukee shoulder**" is basic calcium phosphate deposition in the shoulder along with cuff tear arthropathy. Calcium hydroxyapatite crystals are too small to see with light microscopy; treatment is generally supportive.

d. Birefringence
   (1) Positive—Long axis of crystal parallel to the compensator (of the microscope): the crystal is blue.
   (2) Negative—Long axis of crystal parallel to the compensator: the crystal is yellow. (*Note:* when the crystal's long axis is perpendicular to the compensator, the color rules are reversed.)
   (3) Weak—Dull crystal
   (4) Strong—Bright, shiny crystal

E. Infectious arthritides

1. Pyogenic arthritis (see Table 1–21)—Results from hematogenous spread or by extension of osteomyelitis. Commonly occurs in children (see Chapter 3, Pediatric Orthopaedics). In adult patients, pyogenic arthritis occurs more commonly in persons who are at risk, including intravenous drug abusers (especially in the sternoclavicular and sacroiliac joints); sexually active young adults (*Neisseria gonorrhoeae* infection [intracellular diplococci], especially if seen with skin papules); diabetics (in the feet and lower extremities); and RA patients. It is also seen after trauma (fight bites, open injuries) or surgery (iatrogenic). Histology may demonstrate synovial hyperplasia, numerous PMNs, and cartilage destruction. Destruction of cartilage can be direct (proteolytic enzymes) or indirect (caused by pressure and lack of nutrition). Treatment includes incision and drainage (I&D) and up to several weeks of antibiotics.

2. Tuberculous arthritis (see Table 1–21)—Chronic granulomatous infection caused by *Mycobacterium tuberculosis* usually invades joints by **hematogenous spread.** The spine and lower extremities are most often involved, typically in Mexicans and Asians. Eighty percent of cases are monarticular. Radiographically, tuberculous arthritis causes changes on both sides of the joint. Diagnosis is helped with a **positive PPD,** demonstration of **acid-fast bacilli** and "**rice bodies**"

(fibrin globules) in the synovial fluid, positive cultures (may take several weeks), and characteristic radiographs (subchondral osteoporosis; cystic changes; notchlike, bony destruction at the joint edge; and joint space narrowing, with osteolytic changes on both sides of the joint). Histology may demonstrate **characteristic granulomas with Langhans giant cells** (peripheral nuclei). Treatment includes I&D and long-term antibiotics (isoniazid, rifampin, pyrazinamide, and pyridoxine).

3. Fungal arthritis (see Table 1–21)—More common in neonates, **AIDS patients,** and drug users. Pathogens include *Candida albicans.* Potassium hydroxide (KOH) preparations of synovial fluid are helpful because cultures require prolonged incubation. Arthritis can be treated with 5-flucytosine. Blastomycosis, coccal infections, and other fungal infections often require treatment with amphotericin (this treatment is sometimes administered intra-articularly, with fewer side effects).
4. Lyme disease (see Table 1–21)—Acute, self-limiting joint effusions (especially in the shoulder and knee) that recur frequently. Caused by the **spirochete *Borrelia burgdorferi*** (*Borrelia garinii* in Europe), which is transmitted by **tick bites** *(Ixodidae),* endemic in half of the United States. Transmission of *B. burgdorferi* occurs in approximately 10% of bites by infected ticks. Sometimes called the "great mimicker." Systemic signs may include a characteristic "bull's-eye" rash **(erythema chronicum migrans)** or neurologic (Bell's palsy is common) or cardiac symptoms. The disease occurs in three stages: I—rash, II—neurologic symptoms, III—arthritis. **Immune complexes and cryoglobulins accumulate in the synovial fluid** of affected persons. Diagnosis is confirmed by **enzyme-linked immunosorbent assay (ELISA) testing,** which should be sought in endemic areas after a Gram stain and joint cultures of an infectious aspirate show no organisms. **Treatment** is with doxycycline (most effective), amoxicillin, cefuroxime, erythromycin, or ceftriaxone (for carditis).

F. Hemorrhagic effusions

1. Hemophilic arthropathy (see Table 1–21)—**X-linked recessive disorder; factor VIII deficiency** (hemophilia A—classic) or factor IX deficiency (hemophilia B—Christmas disease) associated with repeated hemarthrosis due to minor trauma, leading to synovitis, cartilage destruction (enzymatic processes), and joint deformity. Disease severity related to the degree of factor deficiency (mild, 5-25% levels; moderate, 1-5% levels; severe, 0-1% levels), Repeated episodes of hemarthrosis lead to replacement of the normal joint capsule with dense scar tissue.
   a. Diagnosis—**The knee is most commonly involved,** followed by the elbow, ankle, shoulder, and spine. Joint swelling, decreased ROM, and pain are characteristic. **A joint aspirate should be obtained to rule out a concomitant infection.** Radiographs later in the disease process may demonstrate variable changes to the patella (**"squared off" patella is Jordan's sign** [also seen in JRA]), widening of the intercondylar notch, and enlarged femoral condyles that appear to "fall off" the tibia (Fig. 1–59). Ultrasonography can be used to diagnose and follow intramuscular bleeding episodes. **Iliacus hematomas can cause femoral nerve palsies.**
   b. Treatment—Management includes correction of factor levels, splints, compressive dressings, bracing, and analgesics. Occasionally, steroids are helpful. Surgical management includes synovectomy (for recurrent hemarthroses and synovial hypertrophy refractory to conservative treatment), TJA (for end-stage arthropathy), and arthrodesis (especially for the ankle). **Synovectomy** has been shown to reduce the incidence of recurrent hemarthroses (less pain and swelling). **Synoviorthesis** (destruction of synovial tissue by intra-articular injection of a radioactive agent) with colloidal ^{32}P chromic phosphate may be useful for the treatment of chronic hemophilic synovitis that is resistant to conventional treatment. **Factor levels** should be maintained near 100% during the first postoperative week and at 50-75% during the second week. There is a high incidence of HIV positivity in hemophiliacs (up to 90%). **The presence of an inhibitor that represents an IgG antibody to the clotting factor protein (causing the patient to have no response to factor replacement therapy) is a relative contraindication to any elective surgical procedure.** Inhibitor is present in 5-25% of patients and can develop at any time. New monoclonal recombinant factor VIII products are prone to induce inhibitors. When an inhibitor to factor VIII develops, other strategies to provide hemostasis must be used.
2. Sickle cell disease—Hemoglobin SS is found in 1% of North American blacks and leads to local infarction due to capillary stasis. Bony infarcts and ischemic necrosis may occur in multiple bones in sickle cell disease (thalassemia does not produce infarcts or ischemic necrosis). Dactylitis with metacarpal/metatarsal periosteal new bone formation may also be seen. Osteomyelitis is not uncommon in patients with sickle cell disease **(*Salmonella* is the most characteristic organism, and *Staphylococcus* is the most common);** *Salmonella* spread can come from a gallbladder infection. The ESR is usually falsely low. Osteonecrosis (especially of the femoral head, which leads to joint destruction and may require THA) is common in sickle cell patients. The results of TJA are poor due to ongoing negative bone remodeling.
3. Pigmented villonodular synovitis (PVNS) (see Table 1–21) (Fig. 1–60)—Synovial disease often

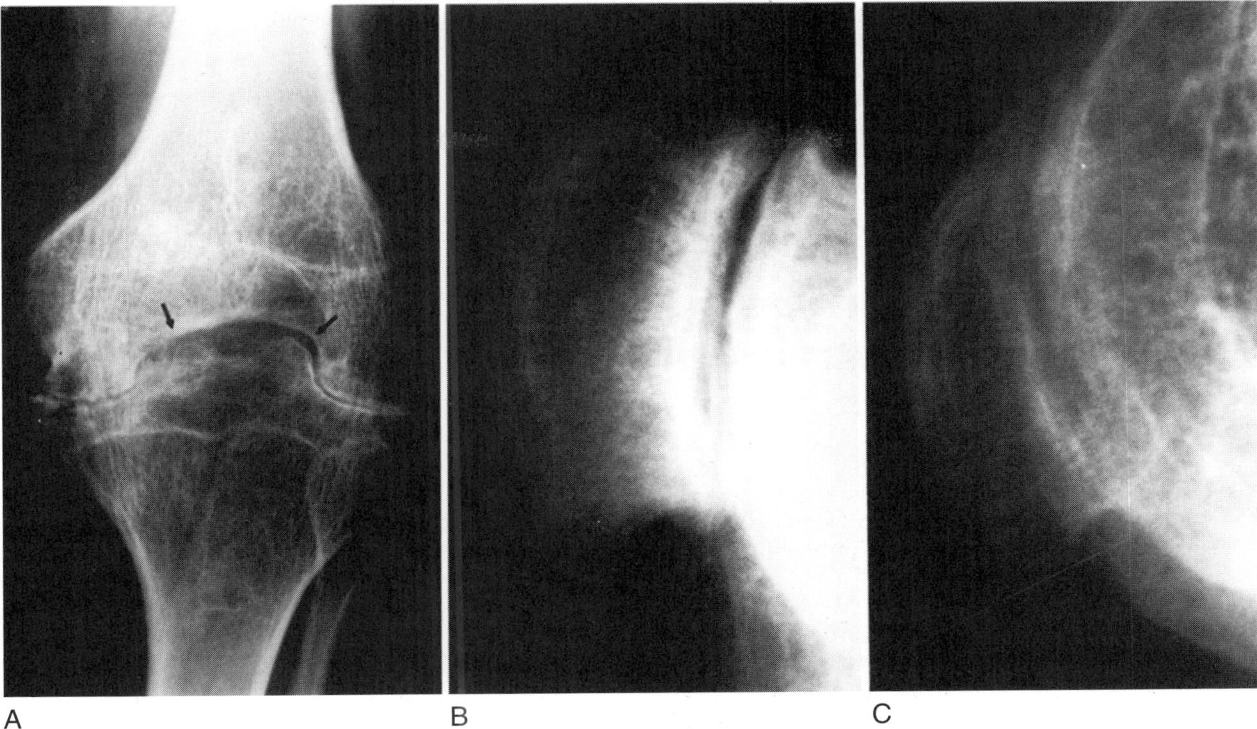

FIGURE 1–59 Radiographic changes of hemophilia. **A**, AP radiograph of the knee shows enlargement and ballooning of the distal femur, flattening of the distal femoral condyles, marked joint space narrowing, and severe widening of the intercondylar notch *(arrows)*. **B** and **C** show the variable radiographic changes that can occur in the patella, with **B** appearing "squared off" (Jordan's sign) and **C** appearing elongated and thinned. (From Resnick D, Niwayama G: Diagnosis of Bone and Joint Disorders, p 2025. Philadelphia, WB Saunders, 1981.)

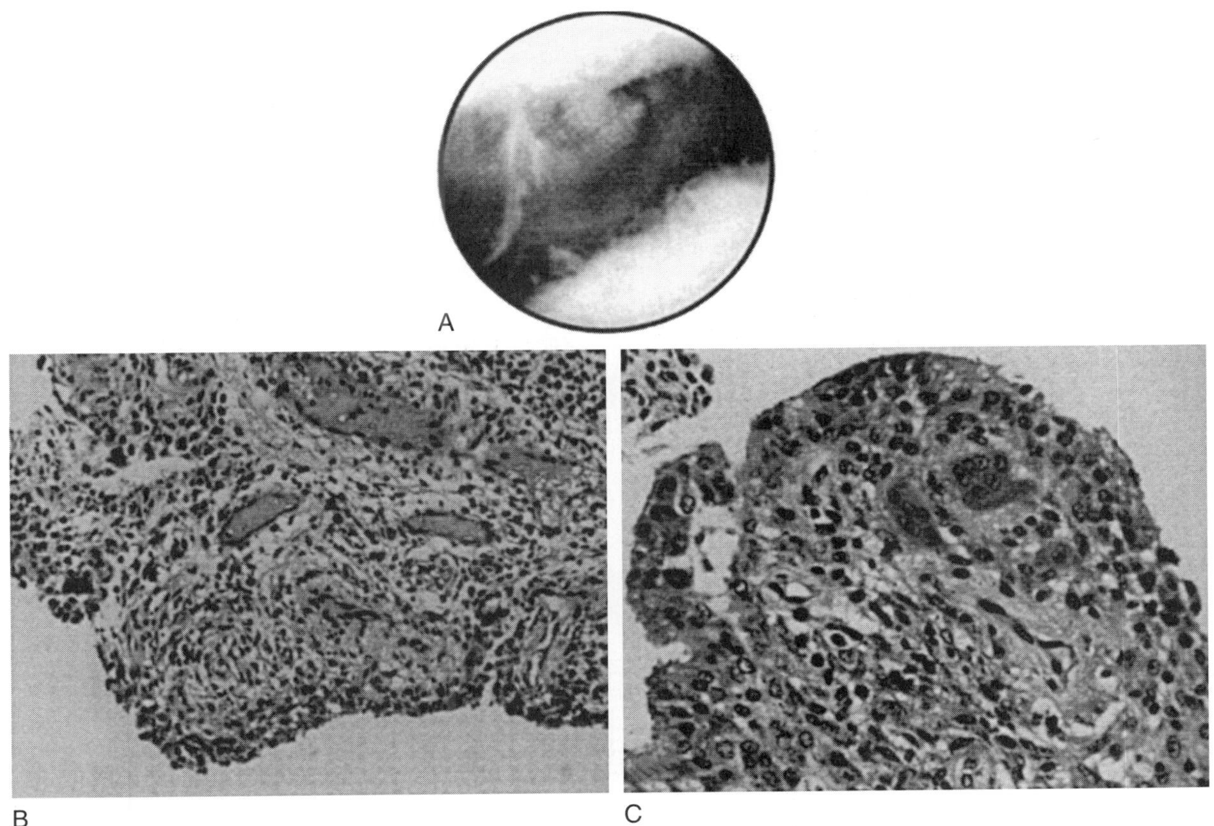

FIGURE 1–60 Localized pigmented villonodular synovitis. **A**, Arthroscopic view localized to the medial knee joint. **B**, Histologic picture shows vascular channels, giant cells, and blood pigments (hematoxylin and eosin stain, ×100). **C**, Giant cells in synovial villus (hematoxylin and eosin stain, ×400).

affecting young adults with **exuberant proliferation of villi and nodules.** The synovium is frequently rust colored or brown because of extensive **hemosiderin deposits.** Pain, swelling, synovitis, and a **rust-colored or bloody effusion** are common. **The knee is the most frequent site of PVNS,** with occasional involvement of the hip and ankle. Radiographs show well-defined juxtacortical erosions with sclerotic margins. Histologic features include pigmented synovial histiocytes, foam cells (lipid-laden histiocytes), and multinucleated giant cells. Treatment is by surgical excision **(total synovectomy)** of the affected synovium. Microscopic residual disease may be treated with intra-articular dysprosium (a radioisotope).

SECTION 3 Neuromuscular and Connective Tissues

I. Skeletal Muscle and Athletics

A. Noncontractile elements (Fig. 1–61)

1. Muscle body—**Epimysium** surrounds individual muscle bundles, **perimysium** surrounds muscle fascicles, and **endomysium** surrounds individual fibers.
2. Myotendinous junction—**The weak link in the muscle, often the site of tears,** especially with eccentric contractions. Sarcolemma filaments interdigitate with the basement membrane (type IV collagen) and tendon tissue (type I collagen). Involution of muscle cells in this region gives maximum surface area for attachment. Linking proteins and specialized membrane proteins are also present.
3. Sarcoplasmic reticulum—Stores calcium in intracellular membrane–bound channels, including

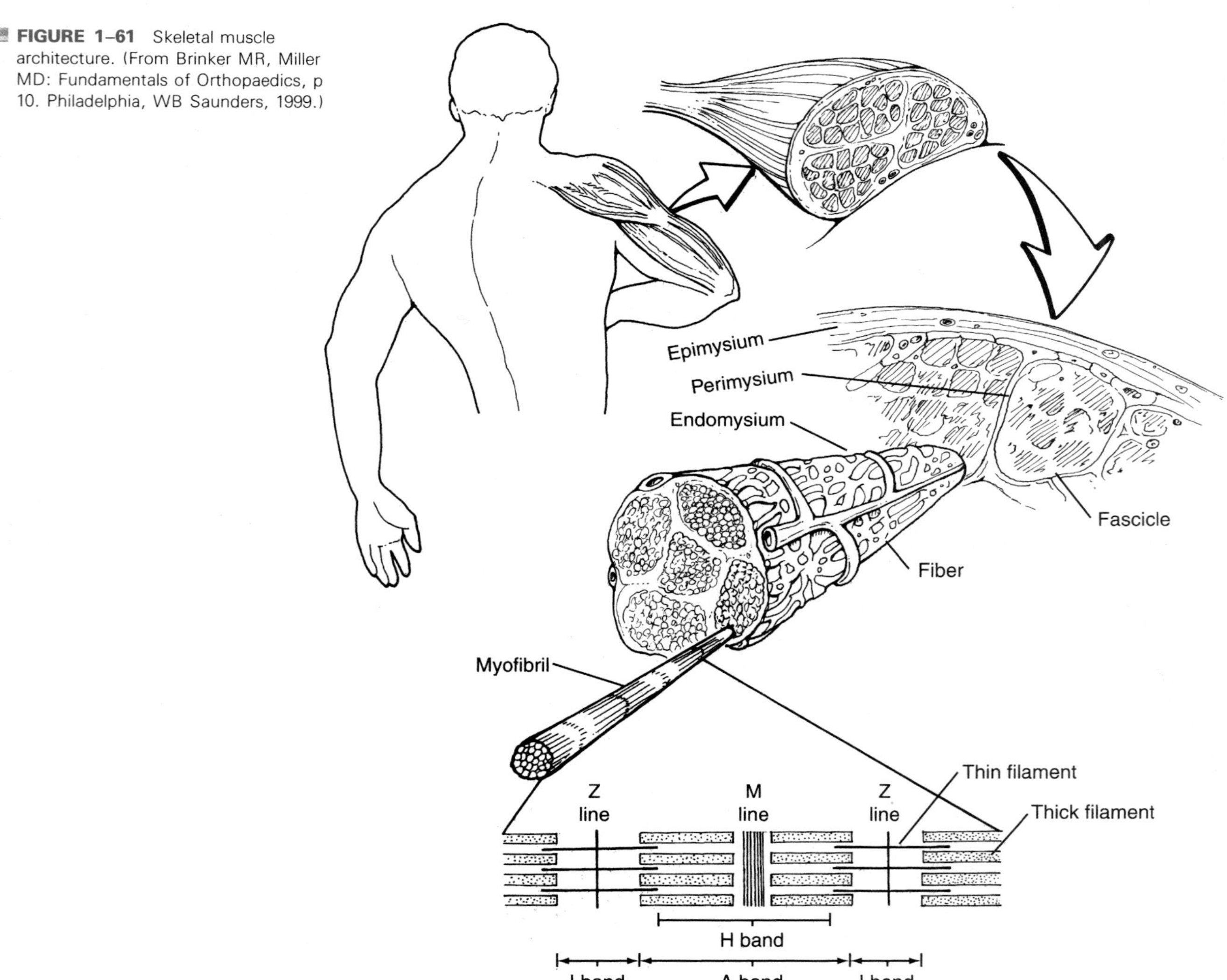

FIGURE 1–61 Skeletal muscle architecture. (From Brinker MR, Miller MD: Fundamentals of Orthopaedics, p 10. Philadelphia, WB Saunders, 1999.)

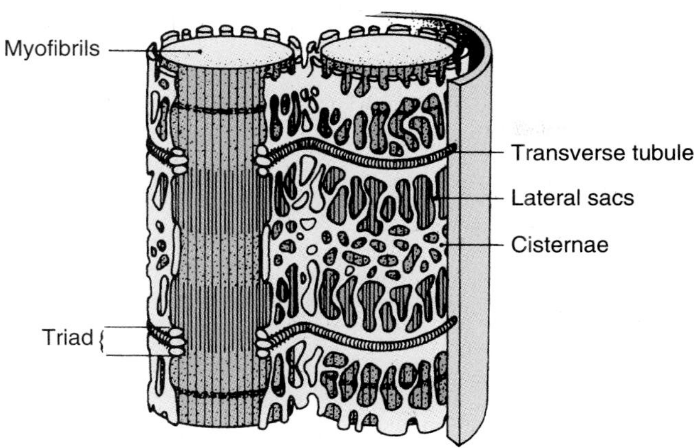

FIGURE 1–62 Sarcoplasmic reticulum. Action potentials travel down the transverse tubules, causing calcium release from the outer vesicles. (From Simon SR, ed: Orthopaedic Basic Science, p 94. Rosemont, IL, American Academy of Orthopaedic Surgeons, 1994.)

T-tubules (which go to each myofibril) and cisternae (small storage areas) (Fig. 1–62).

B. Contractile elements (see Fig. 1–61)—Derived from myoblasts. Each muscle is composed of several muscle **fascicles,** which in turn contain muscle **fibers** (the basic unit of contraction). Fibers are composed of **myofibrils** (1-3 μm in diameter and 1-2 cm long); a myofibril is a collection of **sarcomeres.** A muscle fiber is an elongated cell. Fibers are usually parallel but can run oblique to one another (e.g., bipennate muscle). Muscle fiber architecture is specific for the required function.

1. Sarcomere—Composed of thick **(myosin)** and thin **(actin)** filaments intricately arranged to allow the fibers to slide past each other. The sarcomere is arranged into bands and lines (see Fig. 1–61) (Table 1–26). The **H band** contains only thick (myosin) filaments, and the **I band is composed solely of thin (actin) filaments.** Thin filaments are attached to the **Z line,** extending across I bands and partially into the A band. Each sarcomere is bounded by two adjacent Z lines.

TABLE 1-26 SARCOMERE

Band	Description
A band	Contains actin and myosin
I band	Contains actin only
H band	Contains myosin only
M line	Interconnecting site of the thick filaments
Z line	Anchors the thin filaments

From Brinker MR, Miller MD: Fundamentals of Orthopaedics, p 11. Philadelphia, WB Saunders, 1999.

C. Action—Muscle tissue responds to electrochemical or mechanical stimuli by developing tension (contracting). The stimulus for a muscle contraction originates in the cell body of a nerve and is carried toward the neuromuscular junction via an electrical impulse that is propagated down the entire length of the axon (from the spinal cord to skeletal muscle). Once the impulse reaches the **motor end plate** (a specialized synapse formed between muscle and nerves) (Fig. 1–63), acetylcholine (stored in presynaptic vesicles) is released. Acetylcholine then diffuses across the **synaptic cleft** (50 nm) to bind a specific receptor on the muscle membrane (myasthenia gravis is a shortage of acetylcholine receptors; botulinum A injections reduce spasticity by blocking acetylcholine release at the end plate). Acetylcholine binding triggers depolarization of the sarcoplasmic reticulum, which releases calcium into the muscle cytoplasm. Calcium binds to troponin (on the thin filaments), causing them to change the position of tropomycin (also on the thin filaments) and exposing the actin filament. Actin-myosin cross-bridges form, and with the breakdown

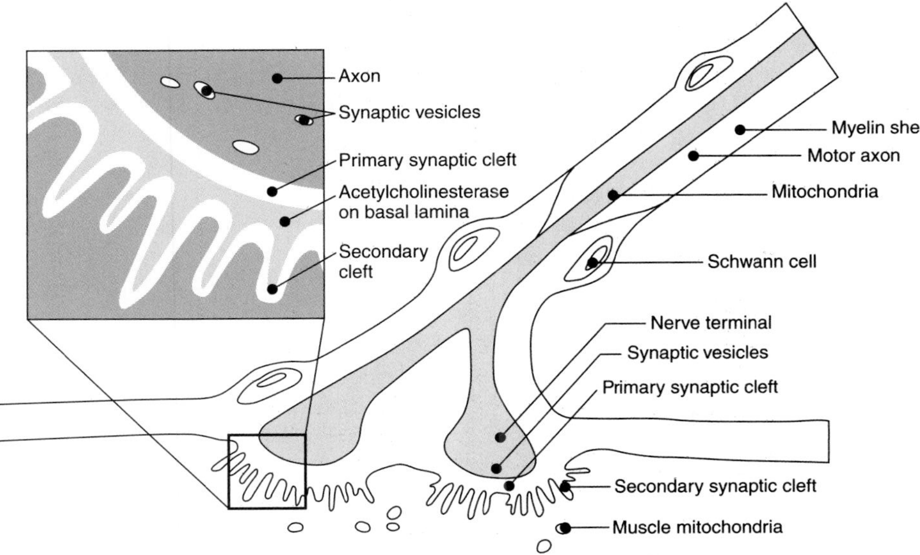

FIGURE 1–63 Motor end plate. (From Simon SR, ed: Orthopaedic Basic Science, p 93. Rosemont, IL, American Academy of Orthopaedic Surgeons, 1994.)

TABLE 1-27 AGENTS THAT AFFECT NEUROMUSCULAR IMPULSE TRANSMISSION

Agent	Site of Action	Mechanism	Effect
Nondepolarizing drugs (curare, pancuronium, vecuronium)	Neuromuscular junction	Competitively binds to acetylcholine receptor to block impulse transmission	Paralytic agent (long-term)
Depolarizing drugs (succinylcholine)	Neuromuscular junction	Binds to acetylcholine receptor to cause temporary depolarization of muscle membrane	Paralytic agent (short-term)
Anticholinesterases (neostigmine, edrophonium)	Autonomic ganglia	Prevents breakdown of acetylcholine to enhance its effect	Reverses effect of nondepolarizing drugs; muscarinic effects (bronchospasm, bronchorrhea, bradycardia)

of ATP, the thick and thin filaments slide past one another, contracting the muscle. Table 1–27 shows the effects of some commonly used agents that affect impulse transmission.

D. Types of muscle contractions (Table 1–28)

E. Types of muscle fibers—Include slow twitch (ST) (type I) and fast twitch (FT) (type II); fibers are part of a motor unit, which is a motoneuron and the muscle fibers it innervates. Table 1–29 shows the characteristics of types I and II muscle fibers.

1. ST (type i; oxidative [''red'']) fibers—**Aerobic** and therefore have **more mitochondria,** enzymes, and triglycerides (energy source) than type II fibers. They have low concentrations of glycogen and glycolytic enzymes (ATPase). Remember **''slow red ox''** (type I fibers are slower, more vascular [red], and undergo aerobic oxidation). Type I fibers perform **endurance activities** and are the first lost without rehabilitation.
2. FT (type ii; glycolytic [''white'']) fibers—Anaerobic; contract more quickly and have larger and stronger motor units (increased ATPase) than ST fibers but are for these reasons less efficient. Type II fibers develop a large amount of force per cross-sectional area, with high contraction speeds and quick relaxation times. Type II fibers are well suited for high-intensity, short-duration activities (sprinting) and fatigue rapidly. They have low intramuscular triglyceride stores. Types IIA and IIB fibers are associated with sprinting (ATP-creatine phosphate (CP) system); subtypes of type II fibers are based on myosin heavy chains.

TABLE 1-28 TYPES OF MUSCLE CONTRACTIONS

Type of Muscle Contraction	Definition	Example	Phases
Isotonic	**Muscle tension is constant through the range of motion**. Muscle length changes through the range of motion. This is a measure of dynamic strength.	Biceps curls using free weights	Concentric contraction—The muscle shortens during the contraction. Tension within the muscle is proportional to the externally applied load. An example of an isotonic concentric contraction is the ''curl'' (elbow moving toward increasing flexion) portion of a biceps curl. Eccentric contraction—The muscle lengthens during the contraction (internal force is less than external force). Eccentric contractions are the most efficient way to strengthen muscle but have the greatest potential for high muscle tension and muscle injury. An example of an isotonic eccentric contraction is ''the negative'' (elbow moving toward increasing extension) portion of a biceps curl.
Isometric	Muscle tension is generated, but the length of the muscle remains unchanged. This is a measure of static strength.	Pushing against an immovable object (such as a wall)	
Isokinetic	Muscle tension is generated as the muscle maximally contracts at a constant velocity over a full range of motion. Isokinetic exercises are best for maximizing strength and are a measure of dynamic strength.	Isokinetic exercises require special equipment, such as a Cybex machine.	Concentric contraction Eccentric contraction

TABLE 1-29 CHARACTERISTICS OF TYPES OF HUMAN SKELETAL MUSCLE FIBERS

Characteristic	Types		
	Type I	*Type IIA*	*Type IIB*
Other names	Red, slow twitch Slow oxidative	White, fast twitch Fast oxidative glycolytic	Fast glycolytic
Speed of contraction	Slow	Fast	Fast
Strength of contraction	Low	High	High
Fatigability	Fatigue-resistant	Fatigable	Most fatigable
Aerobic capacity	High	Medium	Low
Anaerobic capacity	Low	Medium	High
Motor unit size	Small	Larger	Largest
Capillary density	High	High	Low

From Simon SR: Orthopaedic Basic Science, p 100. Rosemont, IL, American Academy of Orthopaedic Surgeons, 1994.

F. Energetics—Three energy systems generate muscle activity, depending on the duration and intensity of the muscular activity required (Fig 1–64).

1. **ATP-CP system (phosphagen system).** Meets the metabolic requirements for intense muscle activities that last up to 20 seconds, such as **sprinting a 100- to 200-meter dash.** Converts stored carbohydrates from within the muscle fiber itself to energy. **Does not use oxygen and does not produce lactate.** Energy is derived from the high-energy phosphate bonds during hydrolysis:

ATP→adenosine diphosphate (ADP) + P + Energy

ADP→AMP + P + Energy

2. **Lactic anaerobic system (lactic acid metabolism)** (Fig. 1–65)—Meets the metabolic requirements for intense muscle activities that last for 20-120 seconds, such as a **400 meter sprint.** Involves hydrolysis of one glucose molecule to ultimately produce lactic acid plus energy, converting two molecules of ADP to two molecules of ATP.
3. **Aerobic system** (see Fig. 1–65; Fig. 1–66)—When oxygen is available, the aerobic system replenishes ATP through oxidative phosphorylation and the Krebs cycle; uses glucose or fatty acids to produce ATP. Meets the metabolic requirements for **episodes of longer duration and lower-intensity muscle activities.**

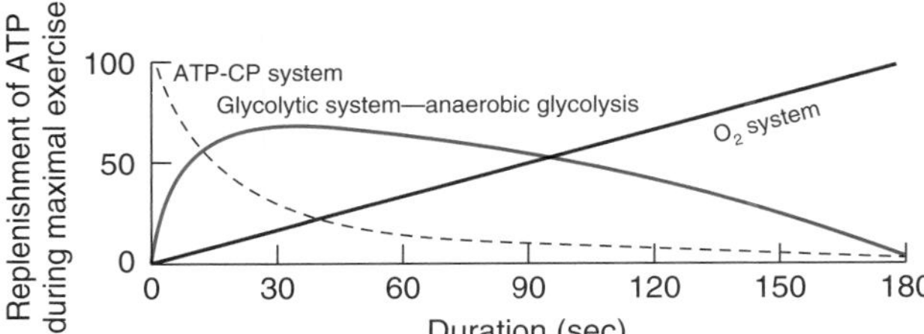

FIGURE 1–64 Energy sources for muscle activity. (From Simon SR, ed: Orthopaedic Basic Science, p 102. Rosemont, IL, American Academy of Orthopaedic Surgeons, 1994.)

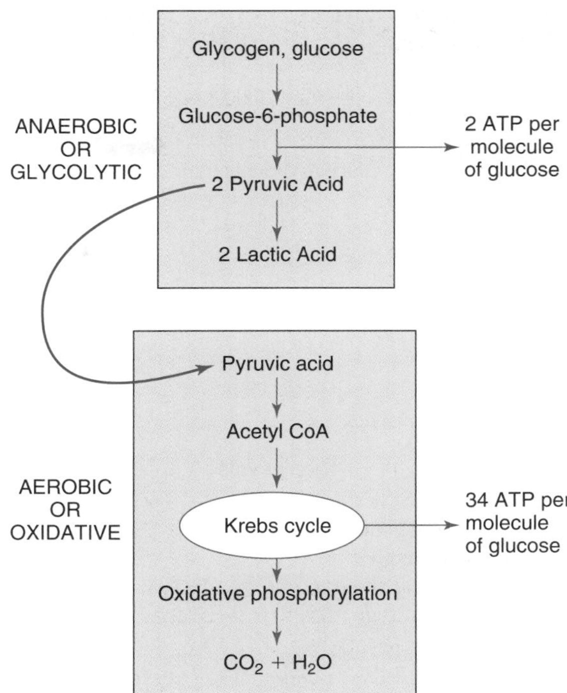

FIGURE 1–65 Adenosine triphosphate production via anaerobic and aerobic breakdown of carbohydrates: Glycolysis and anaerobic metabolism occur in the cytoplasm; oxidative phosphorylation occurs in the mitochondria. (From Simon SR, ed: Orthopaedic Basic Science, p 104. Rosemont, IL, American Academy of Orthopaedic Surgeons, 1994.)

G. Athletes and training—The distribution of FT versus ST fibers is genetically determined; however, specific training can selectively improve these fibers. **Endurance athletes typically have a higher percentage of ST fibers,** whereas athletes participating in "strength"-type sports (and sprinters) have more FT fibers.

1. Endurance training—**Training for endurance sports** consists of decreased tension and increased repetitions, which induces hypertrophy of the ST fibers and increases the number of mitochondria, capillary density, and oxidative capacity, resulting in increased resistance to fatigue. This type of training also improves blood lipid profiles.
2. Strength training—**Training for strength** consists of increased tension and decreased repetitions, which increases the number of myofibrils/fibers and induces **hypertrophy (increased cross-sectional area) of FT (type II) fibers;** a well-conditioned muscle may be able to fire over 90% of its fibers simultaneously. Both types of training slow the lactate response to exercise. The cross-sectional area of skeletal muscle reliably predicts the potential for contractile force. **Isokinetic exercises produce more strength gains than isometric exercises.** Isotonic exercises produce a uniform

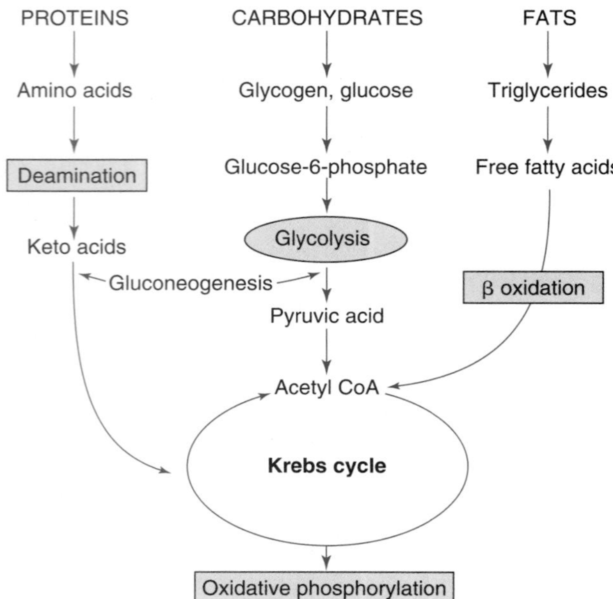

FIGURE 1–66 Aerobic system for adenosine triphosphate (energy) production of skeletal muscle. (From Simon SR, ed: Orthopaedic Basic Science, p 103. Rosemont, IL, American Academy of Orthopaedic Surgeons, 1994.)

strength increase throughout joint ROM. **Plyometric ("bounding") exercises** consist of a muscle stretch followed immediately by a rapid contraction. The stretch stores elastic energy, which increases the force of the concentric muscle contraction. **Plyometrics is the most efficient method of conditioning for improvement in power. Closed-chain exercise** refers to loading an extremity with the most distal segment stabilized or not moving; this allows muscular co-contraction around a joint, which minimizes joint shear (e.g., placing less stress on the ACL). Oxygen consumption (VO_2) is an important consideration when training athletes.

3. Aerobic training—**Aerobic conditioning (cardiorespiratory fitness)** in a healthy adult is recommended 3-5 days per week for 20-60 minutes per session (training at 60-90% of maximum heart rate). Long-distance runs increase aerobic capacity and endurance but decrease flexibility and optimum explosive strength. Aerobic conditioning has proved effective in lowering the incidence of back injury in workers and in helping the elderly to remain ambulatory. **In contrast to resistance exercise, aerobic exercise increases stroke volume, which increases cardiac output.** A significant decline in aerobic fitness ("detraining") occurs after just 2 weeks of no training.
4. Use of anabolic steroids and growth hormone—**Anabolic (androgenic) steroids** cause increased muscle strength (due to increased protein synthesis and an increase in aggressive behavior that promotes increased weight training), increased body weight, testicular atrophy, irreversible deepening of the female voice, reduction in testosterone and gonadotropic hormones, growth retardation, oligospermia, azoospermia, gynecomastia, hypertension, striae, cystic acne, alopecia (irreversible), liver tumors, increased low-density lipoprotein (LDL), decreased high-density lipoprotein (HDL), and abnormal liver isoenzyme lactate dehydrogenase (LDH). Anabolic steroids do not increase aerobic power or capacity for muscular exercise but have been shown to be more effective than corticosteroids for long-term muscle strength recovery after contusion injury. Athletes who use pure testosterone extract to enhance performance have both anabolic and androgenic effects. The anabolic effects include muscle development, increased muscle mass, and erythropoiesis. Drug testing for anabolic steroids is conducted by the International Olympic Committee through urine sampling. Abuse of the **growth hormone somatotropin** among adults causes selective hypertrophy of type I muscle fibers, which produces atrophy of type II fibers and leads to muscle hypertrophy, with weakness and fatigue.
5. Risk of sudden death and injury prevention—A syncopal episode in a young athlete suggests a serious underlying cardiac abnormality (and a risk of sudden death); a timely medical evaluation is mandatory prior to returning to athletics. The most common cause of **sudden death** in young athletes is hypertrophic obstructive cardiomyopathy. Abdominal injuries in athletes most commonly affect the kidney. Wraparound polycarbonate glasses should be worn to protect the eyes in racquet sports.
6. Nutrition—**Weight reduction** with fluid and food restriction (wrestlers, boxers, and jockeys trying to "make weight") is associated with reduced cardiac output, increased heart rate, smaller stroke volumes, lower oxygen consumption, decreased renal blood flow, and electrolyte loss. **Carbohydrate loading** involves increasing carbohydrates three days prior to an event (marathon) and decreasing physical activity. The best **fluid replacement** regimen for a competitive athlete is to consume enough water to maintain prepractice weight and maintain a normal diet. Fluid, carbohydrate, and electrolyte replacement is most effective when the osmolality of the replacement fluid is <10% (glucose polymers minimize osmolality); fluid absorption by the gut is enhanced by solutions of low osmolality. **Creatine supplements** are used by some athletes to attempt to enhance performance. The physiologic basis for this is that creatine is converted to phosphocreatine, which acts as an energy reservoir for ATP in muscle. Recent studies have shown that **creatine supplementation can increase the amount of work that is produced in the first few maximum-effort anaerobic trials but does not increase peak force production**. Treatment of **heat cramps** includes

passive stretching, cooling, and fluid/electrolyte replacement.

H. Female athletes—The "female athletic triad" is **amenorrhea, osteoporosis,** and **anorexia.** Amenorrhea results from a decrease in the percentage of body fat, increased training, hormonal changes, competitive running before menarche, and changes in the hypothalamic-pituitary axis. Exercise-induced secondary amenorrhea leads to premature bone demineralization. Female athletes presenting with stress fracture and a history of amenorrhea should undergo bone mineral density testing (dual-energy x-ray absorptiometry [DEXA]) to assess bone loss. Initial management includes increasing weight, decreasing exercise, and possibly administration of cyclic estrogens or progesterones.

I. Muscle injury
   1. Muscle strains—Most **muscle strains** (the most common sports injury) occur at the myotendinous junction in muscles crossing two joints (hamstring, gastrocnemius) that have increased type II fibers Initially there is inflammation and later fibrosis.
   2. Muscle tears—**Muscle tears occur most commonly at the myotendinous junction, often during a rapid (high-velocity) eccentric contraction; eccentric contractions develop the highest forces observed in skeletal muscle.** Muscle tears typically heal with dense scarring. Surgical repair of clean lacerations in the mid-belly of skeletal muscle usually results in minimal regeneration of muscle fibers distally, scar formation at the laceration, and recovery of about one-half of muscle strength. Muscle activation (via stretching) allows twice the energy absorption prior to failure; "bouncing" types of stretching are deleterious.
   3. Muscle soreness—**Delayed-onset muscle soreness (DOMS) occurs 24-72 hours after intense exercise** and may result from eccentric muscle contractions and be associated with changes in the I band of the sarcomere. **NSAIDs relieve DOMS in a dose-dependent fashion, and massage has varying effects; other modalities (ice, stretching, ultrasound, electrical stimulation) have not been shown to affect DOMS.**
   4. Denervation causes muscle atrophy and increased sensitivity to acetylcholine, causing spontaneous fibrillations at 2-4 weeks after damage to the motor axon. Spasticity is related to increased muscle reactivity to stretch. Muscle strength gains during the first 10 days of rehabilitation are due to improved neural firing patterns. Later strength gains are due to increases in ROM, muscle fiber size, muscle repair, and tendon repair. Trunk extensors are stronger than trunk flexors.

J. Immobilization—Changes the number of sarcomeres at the musculotendinous junction and accelerates granulation tissue response in the injured muscle. Immobilization in lengthened positions decreases contractures and maintains strength. Atrophy can result from disuse or altered nervous system recruitment. Electrical stimulation can help offset these effects.

II. Nervous System

A. Organization
   1. CNS—Patients may continue to improve up to 6 months after a **stroke** and up to 18 months after **traumatic brain injury.**
      a. Spinal cord injury—The most common mechanism of **spinal cord injury** in adults is motor vehicle accidents. **Spinal (neurogenic) shock** (a state of vasodilation presenting with paradoxical hypotension and bradycardia; the bulbocavernosus reflex is also absent) after cervical or upper thoracic spinal cord injury occurs because the descending sympathetic pathways are disrupted. Spinal shock is treated by positioning, pressor agents, and atropine. **Patients with spinal cord injury who present less than 8 hours after injury have the best chance to optimize their neurologic outcomes if given methylprednisolone: <3 hours from injury = an initial bolus of 30 mg/kg over 15 minutes followed by an infusion of 5.4 mg/kg per hour for 23 hours; between 3 and 8 hours from injury = an initial bolus of 30 mg/kg over 15 minutes followed by an infusion of 5.4 mg/kg per hour for 47 hours.** This regimen is associated with improved root function at the level of the injury, although improvement of spinal cord function may or may not occur. **The regimen is not indicated for nerve root deficits, brachial plexus deficits, or gunshot wounds.**
      b. Concussion—**Concussion** (Table 1–30) is a jarring injury to the brain that results in disturbance (to some degree) of cerebral function. Grade I injuries (mild): An athlete may return to play when asymptomatic. Grade II injuries (moderate): characterized by retrograde amnesia (persists for several minutes after injury) despite resolution of confusion and disorientation; a first-time grade II concussion allows return to play after a week without symptoms. Long periods without play (months) are required for a third-time grade I concussion, a second grade II concussion, or a first-time grade III (severe) concussion.
   2. Peripheral nervous system (PNS) (Fig. 1–67)
      a. Nerves—Bundles of axons enclosed in a connective tissue sheath
      b. Nerve fiber—Axon plus surrounding Schwann cell (myelin) sheath
         (1) Myelinated fibers—An axon 1-2 μm in diameter is considered myelinated. Each myelinated axon is associated with one Schwann cell. Conduction velocity is faster than that in unmyelinated fibers.
         (2) Unmyelinated fibers—One Schwann cell surrounds several axons. Conduction velocity is relatively slow.
         (3) Afferents—Transmit information from sensory receptors to the CNS. *Somatic afferents* originate in receptors in muscle, skin, and the sensory organs of the head

TABLE 1-30 CONCUSSION

Severity	Characteristics	Treatment
Grade I (mild)	No loss of consciousness No retrograde amnesia	Return to play as soon as asymptomatic Long-term suspension of play for a third-time grade I concussion
Grade II (moderate)	Loss of consciousness <5 min Retrograde amnesia (there is always some permanent loss of memory regarding the injury itself) Confusion and disorientation resolve rapidly.	*First episode*—Return to play after asymptomatic for 1 week *Repeat episode*—Long-term suspension of play
Grade III (severe)	Prolonged unconsciousness Permanent retrograde amnesia Confusion and disorientation persist	Long-term suspension of play

(vision, hearing, taste, smell). *Visceral afferents* originate in viscera.

(4) Efferents—Transmit information from the CNS to the periphery. Motor efferents innervate skeletal muscle fibers. *Somatic efferents* innervate skin, skeletal muscle, and joints. *Autonomic efferents* (splanchnics) innervate viscera.

B. Histology and signal generation
   1. Neuron (see Fig. 1–67)—Composed of four regions: cell body, axon, dendrites, and presynaptic terminal.
      a. Cell body—The metabolic center; accounts for <10% of neuron size; gives rise to a single axon.
      b. Axon—Primary conducting vehicle of the neuron; conveys electrical signals (over long distances) via action potentials.

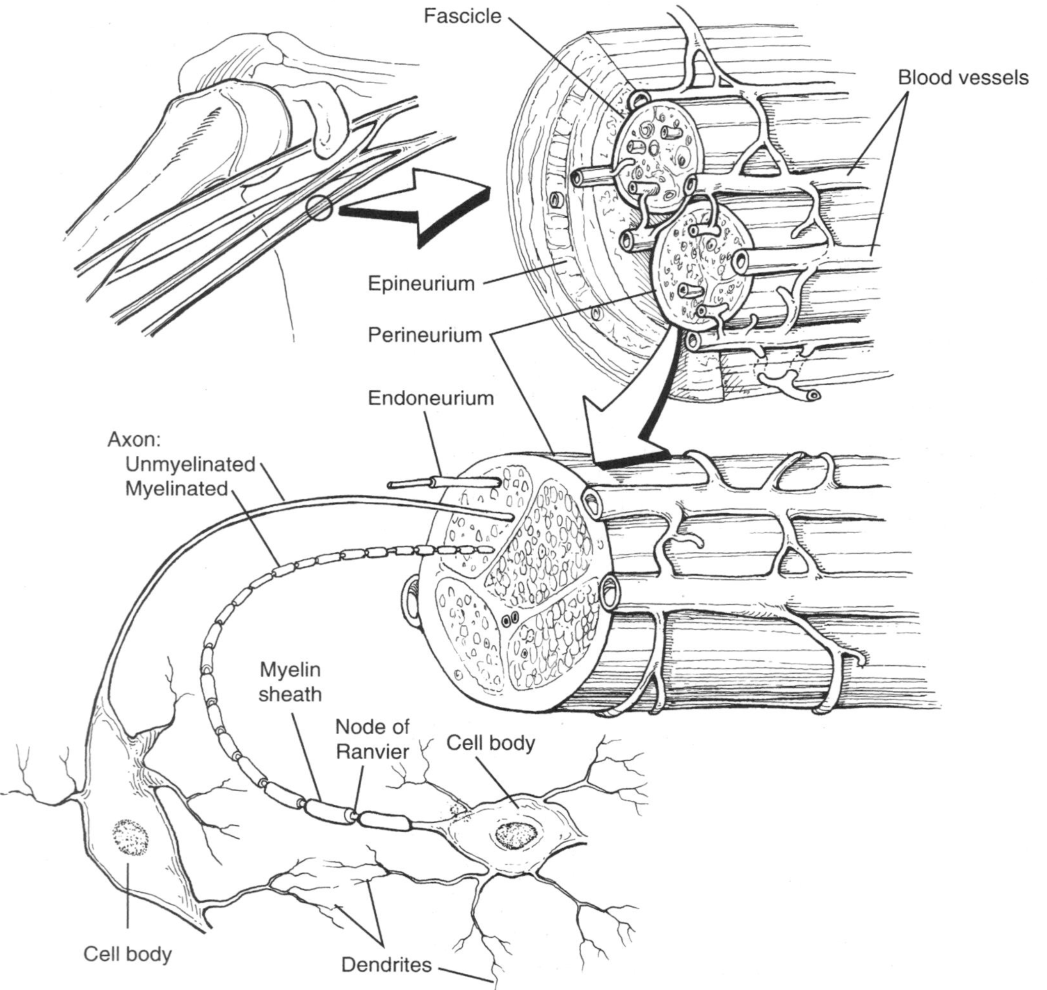

FIGURE 1–67 Nerve architecture. (From Brinker MR, Miller MD: Fundamentals of Orthopaedics, p 13. Philadelphia, WB Saunders, 1999.)

c. Dendrites—Thin processes branching from the cell body; receive input (synaptic) from surrounding nerve cells.
d. Presynaptic terminals—Transmit information from one neuron to another (i.e., to the cell body or dendrites of the "receiving" neuron).

2. Glial cells (Fig. 1–68)—Three basic types have been described: Schwann cells, oligodendrocytes, and astrocytes.
   a. Schwann cells—**Responsible for myelinating peripheral nerve axons** (forms an elongated double-membrane structure). Loss of the myelin sheath (demyelination) disrupts conduction of action potentials along the axon. Myelin is 70% lipid and 30% protein.
   b. Oligodendrocytes—Only in the CNS; form myelin.
   c. Astrocytes—Most common of the glial cells; only in the CNS. Astrocytes have many functions but serve primarily as a supporting structure of the brain.
3. Resting and action potentials
   a. Resting potential—Results from unequal distribution of ions on either side of the neuronal cell membrane (lipid bilayer). The four most plentiful ions around the cell membrane are Na^+, K^+, Cl^-, and a group of other organic ions (A^-). The resting potential of a neuron is −50 to −80 mV (cell inside is negative relative to outside) (Fig. 1–69).
   b. Action potential—Transmits signals rapidly via electrical impulses to other neurons or effector organs (e.g., muscle). Depolarization and the action potential result from an increase in cell membrane permeability to Na^+ in response to a stimulus. This process is related to the three types of gated ion channels (Fig. 1–70): voltage-gated channels, mechanically gated channels, and chemical transmitter–gated channels. Action potentials propagate via both passive current flow and active membrane changes (Fig. 1–71).

C. Sensory system—**Sensory receptors** (located peripherally) receive messages from the environment and other parts of the body and transmit them to the CNS. The four attributes of a stimulus are quality, intensity, duration, and location. Sensory receptor types include photoreceptors (vision), mechanoreceptors (hearing, balance, mechanical stimuli), thermoreceptors (temperature), chemoreceptors (taste, smell), and nociceptors (pain). Neurogenic pain (and inflammatory) mediators are identifiable within the dorsal root ganglion of the lumbar spine. The pain associated with an osteoid osteoma comes from prostaglandins secreted by the tumor itself.

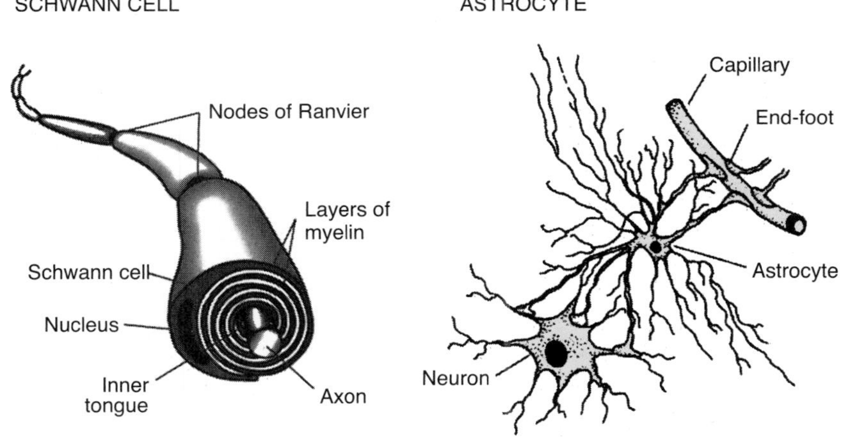

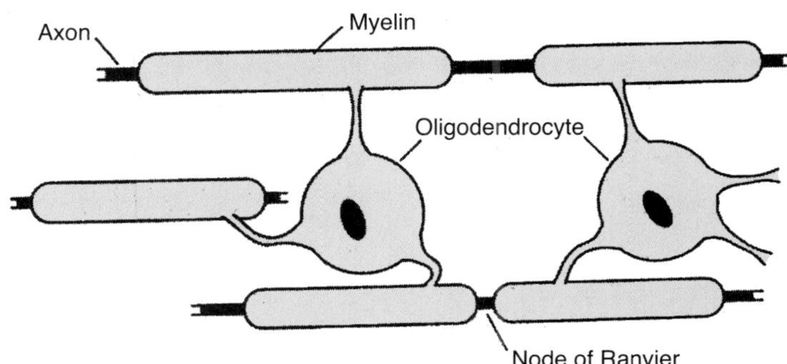

FIGURE 1–68 Glial cells include the Schwann cell, astrocytes, and oligodendrocytes. (From Simon SR, ed: Orthopaedic Basic Science, p 320. Rosemont, IL, American Academy of Orthopaedic Surgeons, 1994.)

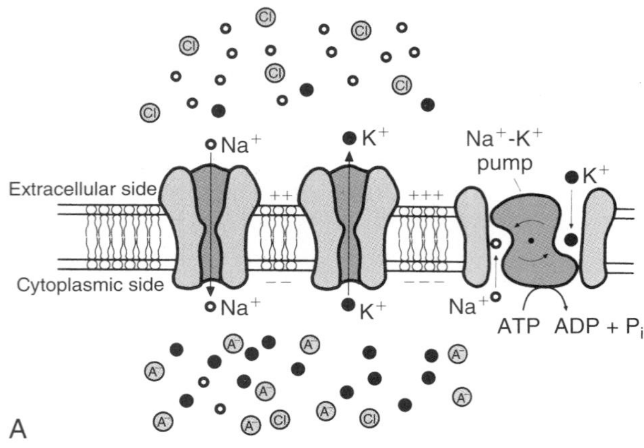

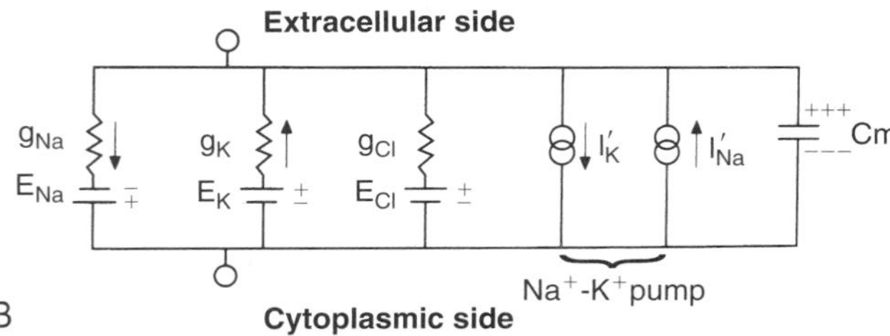

FIGURE 1–69 Electrolyte transport across cell walls. **A**, Passive fluxes of Na^+ and K^+ into and out of the cell are balanced by the energy-dependent sodium-potassium pump. **B**, Electrical circuit model of a neuron at rest. (From Simon SR, ed: Orthopaedic Basic Science, p 332. Rosemont, IL, American Academy of Orthopaedic Surgeons, 1994.)

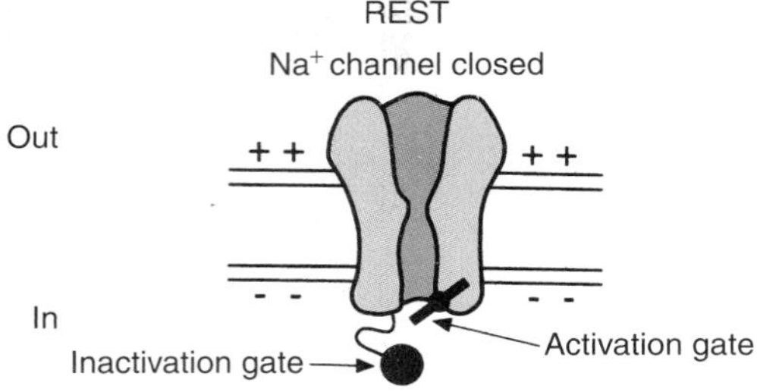

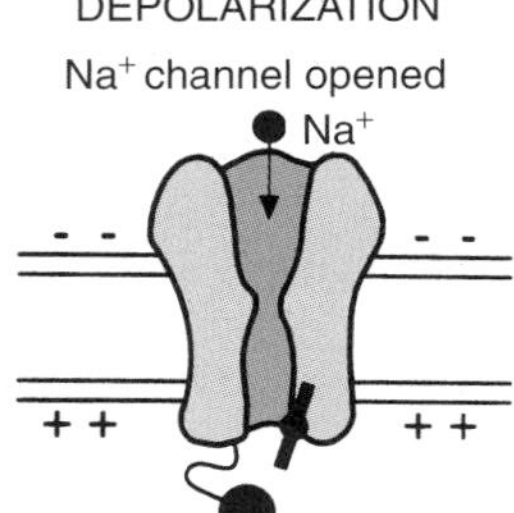

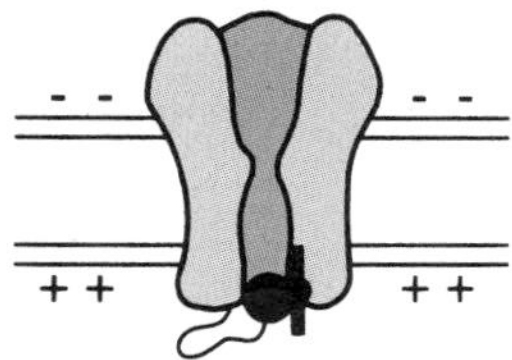

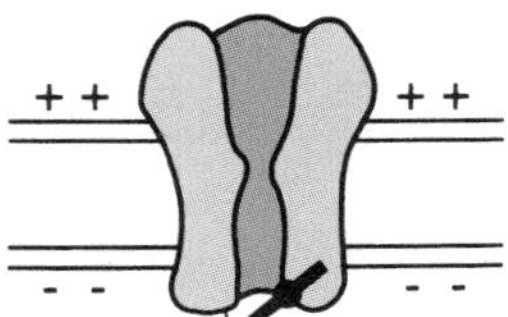

FIGURE 1–70 Gated sodium channel response during an action potential. (From Kandel ER, Schwartz JH, Jessell TM: Principles of Neural Science, 3rd ed, p 14. Norwalk CT, Appleton & Lange, 1991. Reproduced by permission of the McGraw-Hill Companies, Inc.)

1. Somatosensory system—Conveys three modalities: mechanical, pain, and thermal. Each of these is mediated by a specific type of sensory receptor (Table 1–31). Somatosensory input from each of these three modalities is transmitted to the spinal cord (or brainstem) via the **dorsal root ganglion** (Fig. 1–72).

D. Motor system—Organized into four areas: spinal cord, brainstem, motor cortex, and premotor cortical areas (basal ganglia and cerebellum).

1. Spinal cord (see Fig. 1–72)
   a. White matter (peripheral)—Ascending and descending fiber tracts; myelinated and unmyelinated axons.
   b. Gray matter (central)—Contains neuronal cell bodies, glial cells, dendrites, and axons (myelinated and unmyelinated); contains three types of neurons.
      (1) Motoneurons (α and γ)—Axons exit via ventral roots.
      (2) Interneurons—Axons remain in the spinal cord.
      (3) Tract cells—Axons ascend to supraspinal centers.
   c. Spinal cord reflexes (Table 1–32)—A reflex is a "stereotyped response" to a specific sensory stimulus. **A reflex pathway involves a sensory organ (receptor), an interneuron, and a motoneuron.**
      (1) Monosynaptic reflex—Only one synapse is involved between receptor and effector.
      (2) Polysynaptic reflex—Involves one or more interneurons. **Most human reflexes are polysynaptic.**
2. Motor unit—Composed of an α-motoneuron and the muscle fibers it innervates. Four types exist, based on physiologic demands (Table 1–33): type S (slow, fatigue resistant); type FR (fast, fatigue resistant); type FI (fast, fatigue intermediate); and type FF (fast fatigue).
3. Upper and lower motoneurons
   a. Upper motoneurons—Located in the descending pathways of the cortex, brainstem, and spinal cord.
   b. Lower motoneurons—Located in the ventral gray matter of the spinal cord.

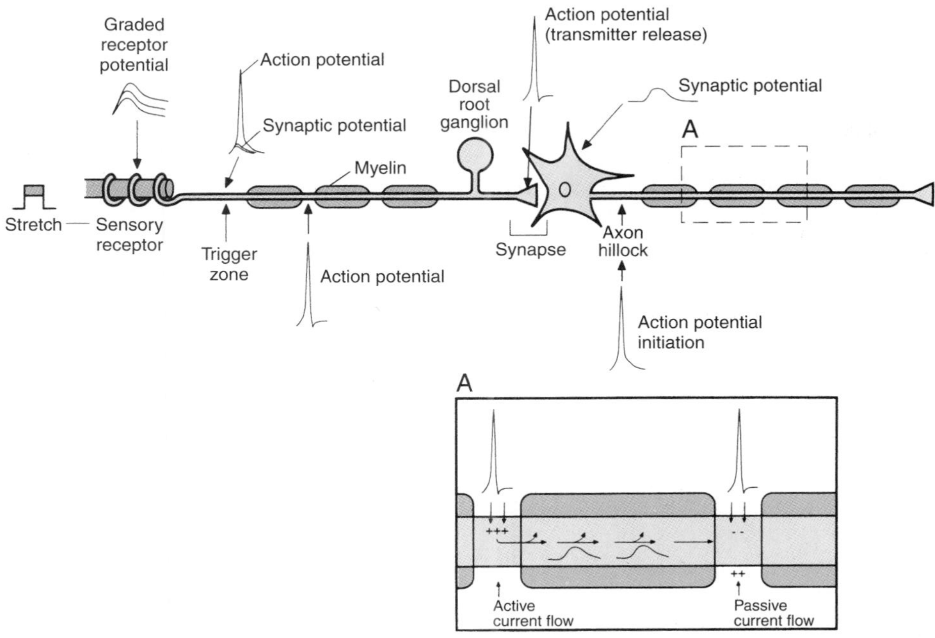

FIGURE 1–71 Action potential is propagated to the terminal region, where it triggers the release of a transmitter, which initiates a synaptic potential in the motoneuron. Action potential propagation results from the spread of local passive depolarizing currents between the nodes of Ranvier (**A**). At the nodes, voltage-gated channels open, producing an action potential. (From Simon SR, ed: Orthopaedic Basic Science, p 337. Rosemont, IL, American Academy of Orthopaedic Surgeons, 1994.)

c. Motoneuron lesions—**Table 1–34 shows findings associated with upper and lower motoneuron lesions. Spasticity** is common in patients with an **upper motoneuron lesion.**

E. Peripheral nerve
1. Morphology (see Fig. 1–67)—The peripheral nerve is a highly organized structure composed of nerve fibers, blood vessels, and connective tissues. Axons, coated with a fibrous tissue called **endoneurium,** group into nerve bundles called **fascicles,** which are covered with connective tissue called **perineurium.** Peripheral nerves are composed of one (mono-), a few (oligo-), or several (poly-) fascicles and surrounding areolar connective tissue **(epineurium)** enclosed within an epineural sheath.
2. Nerve fibers (axons) (2-25 μm in diameter)—Three types of nerve fiber are shown in Table 1–35.
3. Conduction—As has been previously discussed, myelinated axons conduct action potentials

TABLE 1-31 RECEPTOR TYPES

Receptor Type	Fiber Type	Quality
Nociceptors		
Mechanical	Aδ	Sharp, pricking pain
Thermal and mechanothermal	Aγ	Sharp, pricking pain
Thermal and mechanothermal	C	Slow, burning pain
Polymodal	C	Slow, burning pain
Cutaneous and Subcutaneous Mechanoreceptors		
Meissner's corpuscle	Aβ	Touch
Pacini's corpuscle	Aβ	Flutter
Ruffini's corpuscle	Aβ	Vibration
Merkel's receptor	Aβ	Steady skin indentation
Hair-guard, hair-tylotrich	Aβ	Steady skin indentation
Hair down	Aβ	Flutter
Muscle and Skeletal Mechanoreceptors		
Muscle spindle primary	Aα	Limb proprioception
Muscle spindle secondary	Aβ	Limb proprioception
Golgi tendon organ	Aα	Limb proprioception
Joint capsule mechanoreceptor	Aβ	Limb proprioception

From Kandel ER, Schwartz JH, Jessell TM, eds: Principles of Neural Science, 3rd ed, p 342. Norwalk, CT, Appleton & Lange, 1991.

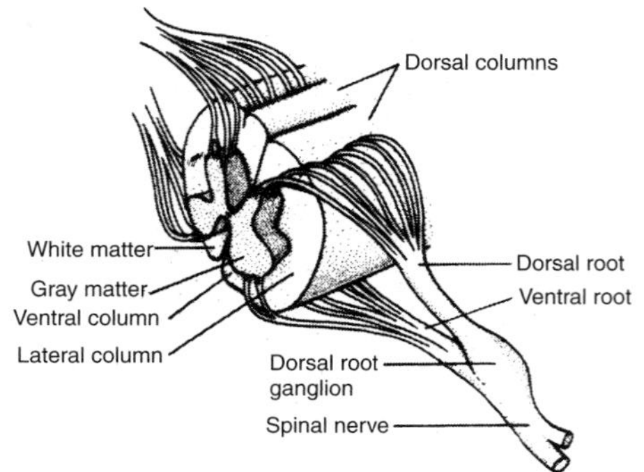

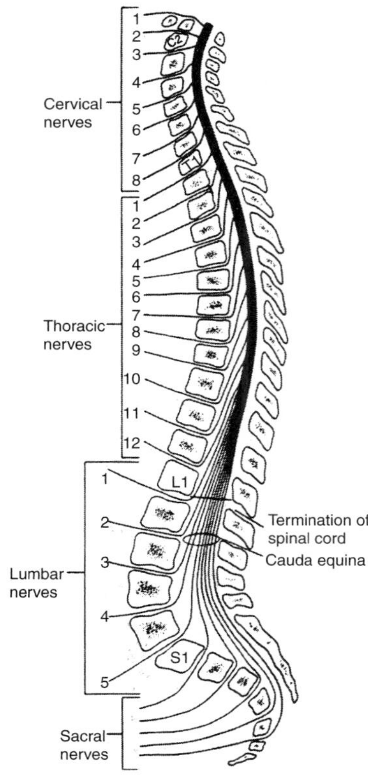

FIGURE 1–72 Spinal cord anatomy. *Left*, Each spinal nerve has a dorsal (sensory) and a ventral (motor) root. Dorsal roots are branches from dorsal root ganglia cells; ventral roots are motor axons from cells in the ventral horn. *Right*, Note that the spinal cord terminates at the L1 vertebra. The dorsal and ventral roots of the lumbar and sacral nerves are collectively called the cauda equina. (From Kandel ER, Schwartz JH, Jessell TM: Principles of Neural Science, 3rd ed, pp 285-286. Norwalk, CT, Appleton & Lange, 1991.)

rapidly, facilitated by **nodes of Ranvier** (gaps between Schwann cells).

4. Blood supply
   a. Extrinsic—Vessels run in loose connective tissue surrounding the nerve trunk.
   b. Intrinsic—Vascular plexuses in the epineurium, perineurium, and endoneurium (with interconnections between these three plexuses).

F. Injury to the nervous system

1. Types of injuries—**Peripheral nerve injury** leads to death of the distal axons and **wallerian degeneration** (of myelin), which extends distal to the somatosensory receptor. Nerve injury may be characterized as one of three types (Table 1–36). Mechanical deformation of a compressed peripheral nerve is greatest in superficial regions and in zones between compressed and uncompressed segments. **Nerve stretching** can also affect function: An 8% elongation diminishes a nerve's microcirculation; 15% elongation disrupts axons. **"Stingers"** (or "burners") refer to neurapraxia from a brachial plexus stretch injury, seen most commonly in football players; the time for recovery is variable, as are residual sequelae (e.g., permanent muscle atrophy). **Cauda equina syndrome** is discussed in Chapter 8, Spine. A double-level cauda equina nerve root compression (even at low pressures) results in a dramatic reduction in impulse conduction and blood flow compared with a single-level cauda equina compression. The nucleus pulposus induces an inflammatory response when in contact with the nerve roots; the response includes leukotaxis, increased vascular permeability, and decreased nerve conduction velocities.
2. Nerve regeneration—Proximal axonal budding occurs (after a 1-month delay) and leads to regeneration at the rate of about 1 mm/day (possibly 3-5 mm/day in children). Nerve regeneration is influenced by contact guidance (attraction to the basal lamina of the Schwann cell), neurotrophism (factors enhancing growth), and neurotropism

TABLE 1-32 SUMMARY OF SPINAL REFLEXES

Segmental Reflex	Receptor Organ	Afferent Fiber
Phasic stretch reflex	Muscle spindle (primary endings)	Type Ia (large myelinated)
Tonic stretch reflex	Muscle spindle (secondary endings)	Type II (intermediate myelinated)
Clasp-knife response	Muscle spindle (secondary endings)	Type II (intermediate myelinated)
Flexion withdrawal reflex	Nociceptors (free nerve endings), touch and pressure receptors	Flexor-reflex afferents: small unmyelinated cutaneous afferents (A-delta, C and muscle afferents, group III)
Autogenic inhibition	Golgi tendon organ	Type Ib (large myelinated)

From Simon SR: Orthopaedic Basic Science, p 350. Rosemont, IL, American Academy of Orthopaedic Surgeons, 1994.

TABLE 1-33 GENERAL CHARACTERISTICS OF MOTOR UNIT TYPES

Parameter	Motor Unit Types		
	FF	*FR*	*S*
Muscle unit physiology*			
Contraction time	Fastest	Slightly slower	Slowest
Sag	Present	Present	Absent
Maximum tension	Largest	Smaller	Smallest
Fatigue index	<0.25	<0.75-1.00	0.7-1.0
Muscle unit anatomy†			
Innervation ratio	2.9	2.1	1.0
Fiber cross-sectional area	1.3	0.98	1.0
Specific tension	1.4	1.2	1.0
Muscle unit metabolism			
Fiber type	FG	FOG	SO
Myosin heavy chain	IIB	IIA	I
Glycogen	High	High	Low
Hexokinase	Low	Intermediate	High
Glycolytic enzymes	High	High	Low
Oxidative enzymes	Low	High	High
Cytochrome c	Low	High	High
Capillary supply	Sparse	Rich	Very rich
Motoneuron			
Cell body size	Largest	Slightly smaller	Smallest
Conduction velocity	Fastest	Slightly slower	Slowest
After-hyperpolarization duration	Shortest	Slightly shorter	Longest
Input resistance	Lowest	Slightly higher	Highest

**Data relative to the FF unit.*
†Data relative to the slow unit.
FF, fast fatigable; FG, fast glycolytic; FOG, fast oxidative glycolytic; FR, fast fatigue-resistant; S, fatigue-resistant; SO, slow oxidative.
From Simon SR: Orthopaedic Basic Science, p 344. Rosemont, IL, American Academy of Orthopaedic Surgeons, 1994; reprinted by permission.

(preferential attraction toward nerves rather than other tissues). **Pain is the first modality to return.**

3. Testing—Neurologic studies (electromyography/nerve conduction study [EMG/NCS]) may be useful to document the extent of injury in patients with muscle atrophy or motor weakness. Cortical evoked potential testing is the most sensitive method of predicting neural compression. In a patient with an injury of the brachial plexus, a **positive histamine response** implies that there is an intact reflex arc (afferent nerve, efferent nerve, intervening cell body or ganglion), indicating that the lesion is proximal to the ganglion (preganglionic).

TABLE 1-34 FINDINGS IN UPPER AND LOWER MOTONEURON LESIONS

Findings	Upper Motoneuron Lesions	Lower Motoneuron Lesions
Strength	Decreased	Decreased
Tone	Increased	Decreased
Deep tendon reflexes	Increased	Decreased
Superficial tendon reflexes	Decreased	Decreased
Babinski's sign	Present	Absent
Clonus	Present	Absent
Fasciculations	Absent	Present
Atrophy	Absent	Present

From Simon SR: Orthopaedic Basic Science, p 354. Rosemont, IL, American Academy of Orthopaedic Surgeons, 1994.

TABLE 1-35 TYPES AND CHARACTERISTICS OF NERVE FIBERS

Type	Diameter (μm)	Myelination	Speed	Examples
A	10-20	Heavy	Fast	Touch
B	<3	Intermediate	Medium	ANS
C	<1.3	None	Slow	Pain

ANS, autonomic nervous system.

G. Nerve repair—Several methods are available. Younger patients have a better chance of recovery than older patients after an operative repair of a nerve transection. It is critical to properly align nerve ends during surgical repair in order to maximize the potential for functional recovery.
   1. Direct muscular neurotization—Insertion of the proximal nerve stump into the affected muscle belly; results in less than normal function but is indicated in selected cases.
   2. Epineural repair—Primary repair of the outer connective tissue layer of the nerve at the site of injury after resecting the proximal neuroma and distal glioma. Care is taken to ensure proper rotation and lack of tension on the repair.
   3. Grouped fascicular repair—Identical to epineural repair, but with reapproximation of individual fascicles under microscopic control. Used for large nerves, but no significant improvement in results over epineural repair has been demonstrated.

III. Connective Tissues

A. Tendons (Fig. 1–73)—Dense, regularly arranged tissues that attach muscle to bone.
   1. Composition—Tendons are composed of fascicles (groups of collagen bundles), separated by **endotenon** and surrounded by **epitenon.** Tendons consist of fibroblasts (predominant cell type) arranged in parallel rows (Fig. 1–74) in fascicles (composed of fibrils) with surrounding loose areolar tissue (peritenon). Fibroblasts produce mostly **type I collagen** (85% of the dry weight of tendon) and a small amount of type III collagen (5% of dry weight). **Tendon inserts**

TABLE 1-36 TYPES AND CHARACTERISTICS OF NERVE INJURIES

Injury	Pathophysiology	Prognosis
Neurapraxia	Reversible conduction block characterized by local ischemia and selective demyelination of the axon sheath	Good
Axonotmesis	More severe injury, with disruption of the axon and myelin sheath but leaving the epineurium intact	Fair
Neurotmesis	Complete nerve division, with disruption of the endoneurium	Poor

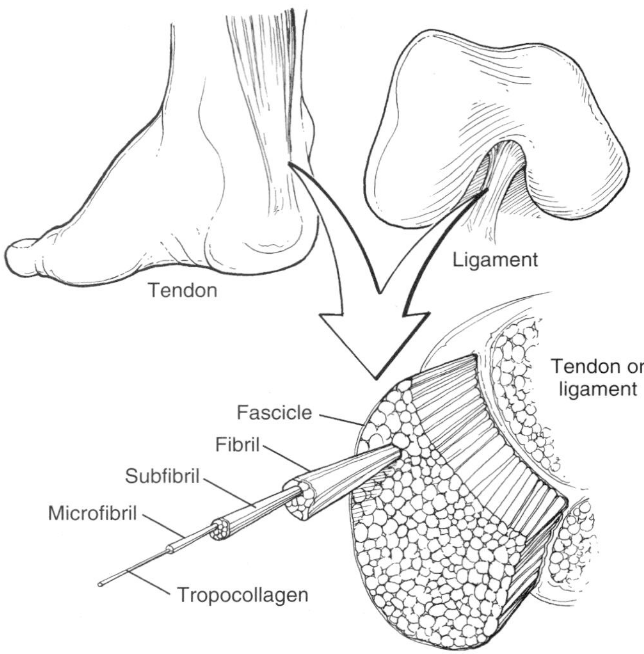

FIGURE 1–73 Tendon and ligament architecture. (From Brinker MR, Miller MD: Fundamentals of Orthopaedics, p 15. Philadelphia, WB Saunders, 1999.)

into bone via four transitional tissues (for force dissipation): tendon, fibrocartilage, mineralized fibrocartilage (Sharpey's fibers), and bone.

2. Types—Two types of tendons exist: (1) paratenon-covered tendons and (2) sheathed tendons. Paratenon-covered tendons (vascular tendons) have many vessels supplying a rich capillary system (Fig. 1–75). With a sheathed tendon, a mesotenon (vincula) carries a vessel that supplies only one tendon segment; avascular areas receive nutrition via diffusion from vascularized segments (Fig. 1–76). Because of these vascular differences, paratenon-covered tendons heal better. Tendinous structures tend to orient themselves along stress lines.
3. Treatment and healing—Tendinous healing after injury is initiated by fibroblasts from the epitenon and macrophages that initiate healing and remodeling. Treatment affects the repair process. Tendon healing occurs in large part through intrinsic capabilities. Tendon repairs are the **weakest at 7-10 days;** they regain most of their original strength at 21-28 days and achieve **maximum strength at 6 months.** Early mobilization allows increased ROM but results in decreased tendon repair strength. Immobilization leads to increased tendon substance strength at the expense of ROM but tends to decrease the strength at the tendon–bone interface. Bony avulsions of tendon insertions heal more rapidly than midsubstance tears. Animal experiments (goats) have demonstrated no significant benefit from the creation of a trough (exposing the tendon to cancellous bone) for a tendon repair compared with direct repair to cortical bone.

B. Ligaments (see Fig. 1–73)
1. Composition—Composed primarily of type I collagen (**90% of the dry weight of ligament**) with small amounts of type III collagen and elastin, these structures attach bone to bone to stabilize joints. Their ultrastructure is similar to that of tendons, but the fibers are more variable and have **higher elastin content. Unlike tendons, ligaments have a "uniform microvascularity" that receives its supply at the insertion site.** They also contain mechanoreceptors and free nerve endings that may play a role in stabilizing joints.
2. Insertion—Collagen sliding plays an important role in changes in ligament length (during growth and contracture). **Ligament insertion into bone** represents a transition from one material to another and can be classified into two types: **indirect insertion** (more common) and **direct insertion.**
   a. Indirect insertion—Superficial ligament fibers insert at acute angles into the periosteum.

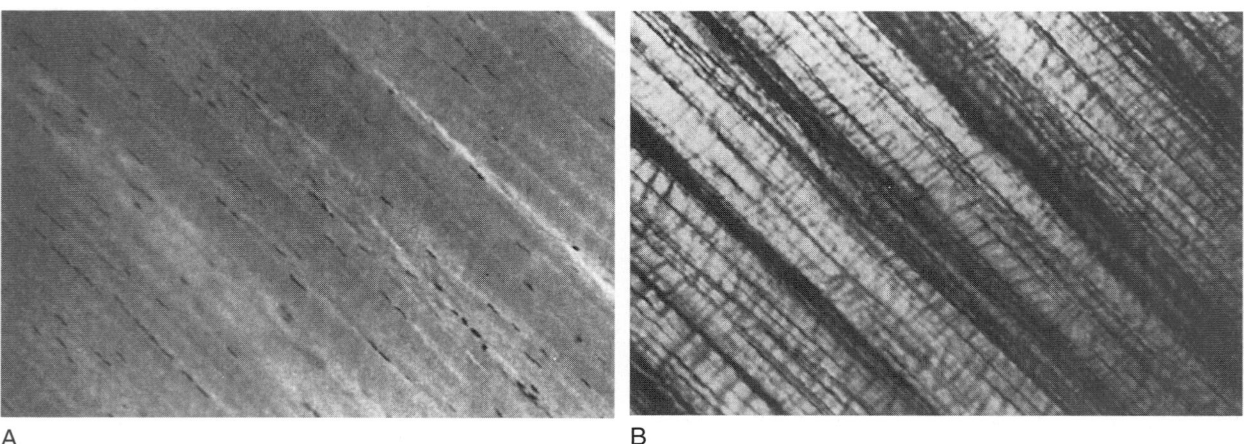

FIGURE 1–74 **A**, Photomicrograph of a flexor tendon with parallel rows of fibroblasts and collagen bundles. **B**, Polarized light photograph of the same section illustrating parallel, longitudinally arranged collagen bundles. (From Simon SR, ed: Orthopaedic Basic Science, p 49. Rosemont, IL, American Academy of Orthopaedic Surgeons, 1994.)

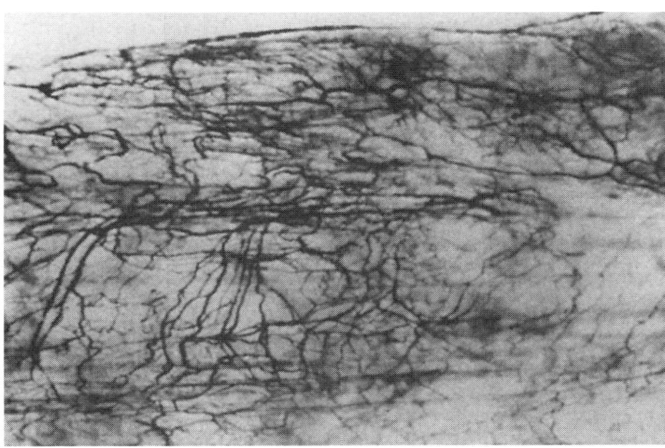

FIGURE 1–75 India ink injection of rabbit calcaneal tendon (Spalteholz technique) demonstrating the vasculature of the paratenon. (From Simon SR, ed: Orthopaedic Basic Science, p 50. Rosemont, IL, American Academy of Orthopaedic Surgeons, 1994.)

b. Direct insertion—Has both superficial and deep fibers; the deep fibers attach to bone at 90-degree angles, and the transition from ligament to bone occurs in four phases: ligament, fibrocartilage, mineralized fibrocartilage, and bone.

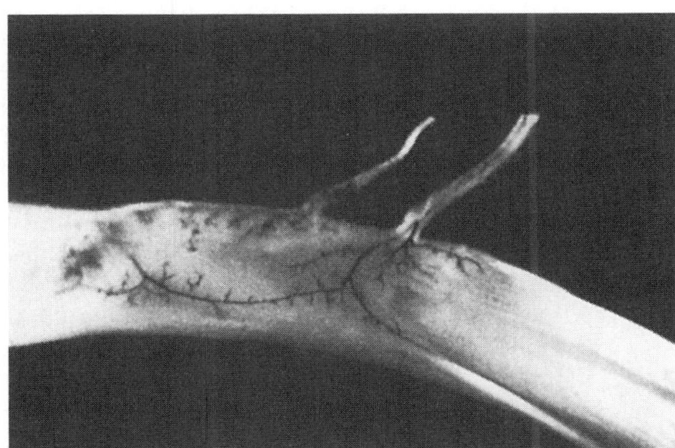

A

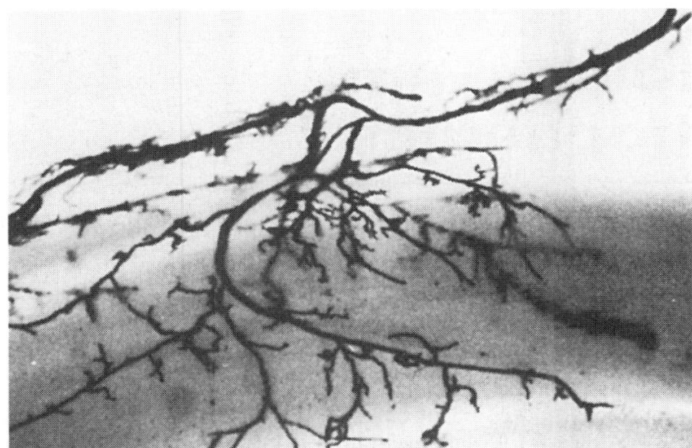

B

FIGURE 1–76 **A**, India ink specimens demonstrating the vascular supply of the flexor tendons via vincula. **B**, Close-up of the specimen. (From Simon SR, ed: Orthopaedic Basic Science, 2nd ed, p 51. Rosemont, IL, American Academy of Orthopaedic Surgeons, 1994.)

3. **Injury— The most common mechanism of ligament failure is rupture of sequential series of collagen fiber bundles** distributed throughout the body of the ligament and not localized to one specific area. **Ligaments do not plastically deform** ("they break, not bend"). **Midsubstance ligament tears are common in adults; avulsion injuries are more common in children. Ligamentous avulsion typically occurs between the unmineralized and mineralized fibrocartilage layers. The major blood supply for the cruciate ligaments is the middle genicular artery.**
4. Postinjury considerations—Healing (three phases, as in bone) benefits from normal stress and strain across the joint. Local injection of corticosteroids at the site of an injured ligament is detrimental to the healing process. **Early ligament healing occurs with type III collagen that is later converted to type I collagen.** Immobilization adversely affects the strength (elastic modulus decreases) of an intact ligament and ligament repair. In animal studies (rabbit), the breaking strength of the medial collateral ligament (MCL) was reduced dramatically (66%) after 9 weeks of cast immobilization. The negative effects of immobilization reverse slowly upon remobilization. The mechanical properties of a ligament return to normal much more rapidly than those of an insertion site. The fixation site is the most common location for an immediate postoperative failure of a bone–patellar tendon–bone ACL reconstruction. Exercise increases ligaments' mechanical and structural properties.

C. Intervertebral discs—Allow spinal motion and stability. Two components: central nucleus pulposus (a hydrated gel with compressibility; high GAG/low collagen) and a surrounding annulus fibrosis (extensibility and increased tensile strength; high collagen/low GAG). **Composed of water (85%), proteoglycans, and collagen type I in the annulus fibrosis and collagen type II in the nucleus pulposus.** The **disc is avascular** and receives nutrients and fluid via diffusion through pores in the hyaline cartilage end plates, which separate it from the vertebral body. The aging disc shows decreased water content (as a result of a lack of large proteoglycans and aggrecans and decreased proteoglycan concentration, but keratin sulfate concentration increases with age) and increased collagen. The superficial layer of the annulus contains nerve fibers. Various neuropeptides, believed to be involved in sensory transmission, nociceptive transmission, neurogenic inflammation, and skeletal metabolism, include substance P, calcitonin gene-related peptide (CGRP), vasoactive intestinal peptide (VIP), and the c-flanking peptide of neuropeptide Y (CPON). Cigarette smoking is a predisposing factor in degenerative disc disease.

D. Soft tissue healing
1. Four phases of soft tissue healing have been described.

a. Hemostasis—Primary platelet plug is formed within 5 minutes of injury. Secondary clotting via the coagulation cascade and fibrin occurs within 10-15 minutes. Fibronectin, a large glycoprotein, binds fibrin to cells and acts as a chemotactic factor. Platelets release factors that activate the next phase of healing.
b. Inflammation—Involves débridement of injured/necrotic tissue via macrophages and occurs within the first week. It has three stages: (1) activation (immediate), (2) amplification (48-72 hours), and (3) débridement (by means of bacteria, phagocytosis, and matrix [biochemical]). Prostaglandins help to mediate the inflammatory response.
c. Organogenesis—Occurs at 7-21 days and consists of tissue modeling. Mesenchymal precursors differentiate into myofibroblasts. Angiogenesis occurs. Further differentiation leads to the final stage of healing.
d. Remodeling (of individual tissue lines)—Continues for up to 18 months. Realignment and cross-linking of collagen fibers allow increased tensile strength.

2. Growth factors—Require activation, are redundant, and function through feedback loop mechanisms.
   a. Chemotactic factors—Attract cells. The factors include prostaglandins (PMNs), prostanoids (PMNs), complement (PMNs and macrophages), PDGF (macrophages and fibroblasts), and angiokines (endothelial cells).
   b. Competence factors—Activate dormant (G_0) cells. Include PDGF and prostaglandins.
   c. Progression factors—Allow cell growth. Induce epidermal growth factor, IL-1, and somatomedins.
   d. Inductive factors—Stimulate differentiation. Include angiokines, bone morphogenetic protein, and specific tissue growth factors.
   e. Transforming factors—Cause dedifferentiation and proliferation.
   f. Permissive factors—Enhancing factors; include fibronectin and osteonectin.

E. Soft tissue implants
   1. Introduction—Usually used around the knee (ACL, meniscus); implants can be allografts, autografts, and synthetics.
   2. Allografts—Have no donor-site morbidity but incite an immune response and may transmit infection **(risk of HIV exposure from a ligament allograft is 1:1,000,000).** Freeze-drying reduces the immunogenic response but also decreases strength (deep freezing without drying does not significantly affect strength). If not harvested under sterile conditions, treatment with cold ethylene oxide gas may have adverse affects **(graft failure),** particularly if >3 mega rad irradiation is used in conjunction (2 mega rad with ethylene oxide does not appear to significantly decrease the mechanical properties). Allograft ligaments exhibit slower, less predictable histologic recovery than autografts.
   3. Synthetic ligaments—Unlike autografts or allografts, these structures have no initial period of weakness. However, they suffer from wear (debris) and are associated with **sterile joint effusions,** with increased levels of neutral proteinases (**collagenase** and gelatinase) and chondrocyte activation factor (IL-1).

F. Miscellaneous—Fibroblastic proliferation in Dupuytren's contracture is associated with PDGF, TGF-β, and epidermal growth factor. A **fibrillin** (a component of the elastic fiber system) metabolism defect has been demonstrated in some patients with adolescent idiopathic scoliosis, and fibrillin abnormalities have been demonstrated in most patients with Marfan's syndrome.

SECTION 4 Cellular and Molecular Biology, Immunology, and Genetics of Orthopaedics

The fields of molecular biology, immunology, and genetics are rapidly expanding, including advances specific to the field of musculoskeletal science. This section introduces the basic concepts of these fields.

I. Cellular and Molecular Biology

A. Chromosomes—Human chromosomes are located in the nucleus of every cell (46 chromosomes; 23 pairs [22 pairs of autosomes and 1 pair of sex chromosomes]). Each chromosome contains more than 150,000 **genes.** The genes are regulated so that a relatively small number of genes can be expressed for any given cell. Regulation of **gene expression** determines the unique biologic qualities of each cell. Chromosomes contain both deoxyribonucleic acid (DNA) and ribonucleic acid (RNA).

B. DNA—All nuclear DNA resides in the 23 chromosome pairs. Located within the chromosome (in the cell nucleus), DNA is responsible for regulating cellular functions via **protein synthesis.** DNA has been classically described as a double helix (double-stranded) that contains **two sugar molecules** (each strand of DNA represents one sugar molecule), each of which has one of four nitrogenous bases (adenine, guanine, cytosine, thymine) (Fig. 1–77). The nitrogenous bases from one strand are linked to those of the other strand via hydrogen bonds. (In DNA, adenine is always linked to thymine, and

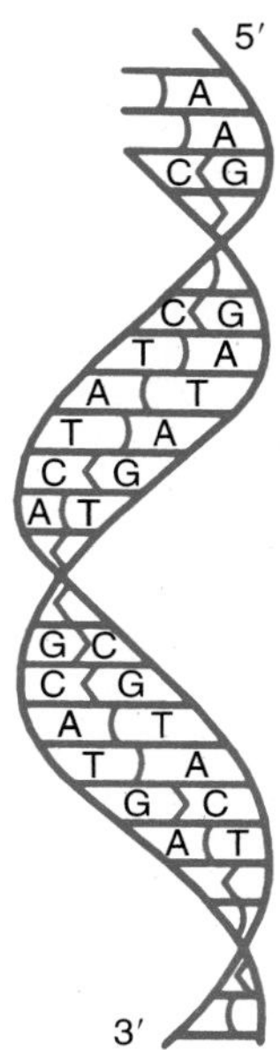

FIGURE 1–77 DNA structure. The two deoxyribose strands are connected by a pair of nucleotides (which form the rung of the ladder) that are in turn connected by hydrogen bonds. A, adenine; T, thymine; C, cytosine; G, guanine. (From Simon SR, ed: Orthopaedic Basic Science, p 221. Rosemont, IL, American Academy of Orthopaedic Surgeons, 1994.)

guanine is always linked to cytosine.) DNA is important for three cellular processes: (1) DNA replication, (2) transcription of messenger RNA (mRNA), and (3) regulation of cell division and the production of mRNA.

C. Nucleotide—The sugar molecule plus one nitrogenous base. The nucleotide sequence in one strand of DNA determines the complementary nucleotide sequence in the other strand. The genetic message is grouped into three-letter words known as **codons.** The codon specifies one of the 20 amino acids that are the building blocks of all proteins (Fig. 1–78).

D. Gene—Portion of DNA that codes for a specific enzyme ("one gene equals one enzyme").

E. Transcription (Fig. 1–79)—To produce a specific protein, the DNA of the gene for that specific protein must be transcribed to an mRNA molecule (via RNA polymerase).

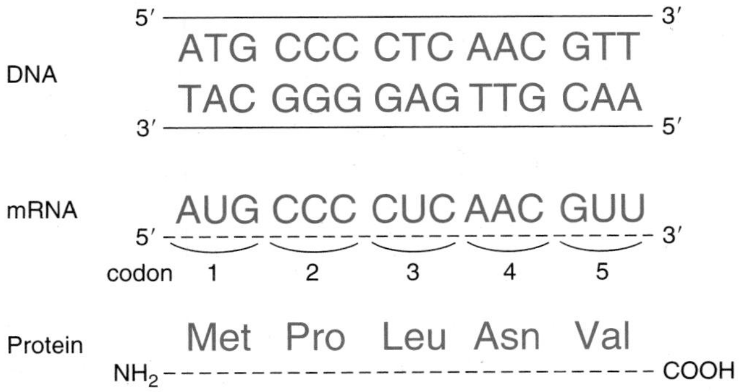

DNA
5′ ATG CCC CTC AAC GTT 3′
3′ TAC GGG GAG TTG CAA 5′

mRNA
5′ AUG CCC CUC AAC GUU 3′
codon 1 2 3 4 5

Protein
NH_2 Met Pro Leu Asn Val COOH

FIGURE 1–78 A genetic message begins as a double-stranded DNA molecule, which serves as the template for messenger RNA (mRNA). The mRNA, in groups of three nucleotides to a codon, directs the order of amino acids in protein. (From Ross DW, ed: Introduction to Molecular Medicine, 2nd ed, p 4. New York, Springer-Verlag, 1996.)

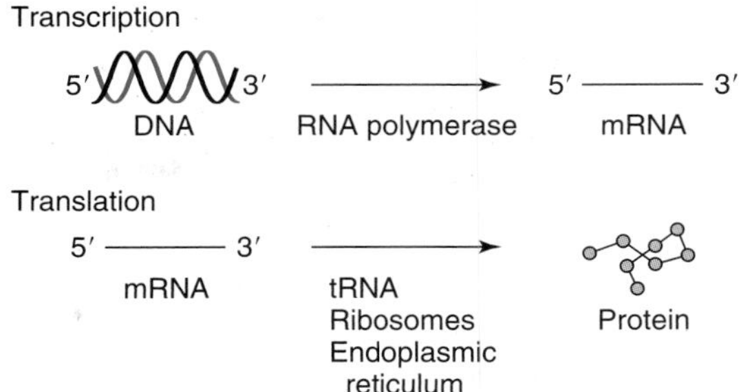

FIGURE 1–79 DNA information is transcribed into RNA in the nucleus. mRNA is then transported to the cytoplasm, where translation into proteins occurs in the endoplasmic reticulum. DNA, deoxyribonucleic acid; RNA, ribonucleic acid; mRNA, messenger RNA; tRNA, transfer RNA. (From Simon SR, ed: Orthopaedic Basic Science, p 222. Rosemont, IL, American Academy of Orthopaedic Surgeons, 1994.)

F. Translation (see Fig. 1–79)—Process by which mRNA builds proteins from amino acids.

G. Protein coding and regulation—Each **codon** is a sequence of three nucleotides in DNA or RNA that provide the genetic code information for one of the 20 amino acids that are the building blocks of all proteins (see Fig. 1–78; Fig. 1–80). Between functional coding sequences are large noncoding sequences known as **regulating DNA.** The **gene promoter** is part of the regulatory DNA and is required for transcription. **Consensus sequences** (named for a specific nucleotide sequence) serve as binding sites for specific proteins involved in gene regulation. **Gene enhancers** are binding sites for proteins (transcription factors) that are involved in the regulation of transcription. Protein coding and regulation are shown in Figure 1–81.

H. Techniques used to study genetic (inherited) disorders
   1. Restriction enzymes—Used to cut DNA at a precise, reproducible cleavage location. Fragments of DNA that have been cleaved this way are called **restriction fragments. Linkage analysis** uses statistical methods to estimate the probability that a

1st	2nd: U	2nd: C	2nd: A	2nd: G	3rd
U	Phe	Ser	Tyr	Cys	U
	Phe	Ser	Tyr	Cys	C
	Leu	Ser	STOP	STOP	A
	Leu	Ser	STOP	Trp	G
C	Leu	Pro	His	Arg	U
	Leu	Pro	His	Arg	C
	Leu	Pro	Gln	Arg	A
	Leu	Pro	Gln	Arg	G
A	Ile	Thr	Asn	Ser	U
	Ile	Thr	Asn	Ser	C
	Ile	Thr	Lys	Arg	A
	Met	Thr	Lys	Arg	G
G	Val	Ala	Asp	Gly	U
	Val	Ala	Asp	Gly	C
	Val	Ala	Glu	Gly	A
	Val	Ala	Glu	Gly	G

FIGURE 1–80 The genetic code for translation of the triplet nucleotide codons of mRNA into amino acids in proteins. (From Ross DW, ed: Introduction to Molecular Medicine, 2nd ed, p 7. New York, Springer-Verlag, 1996.)

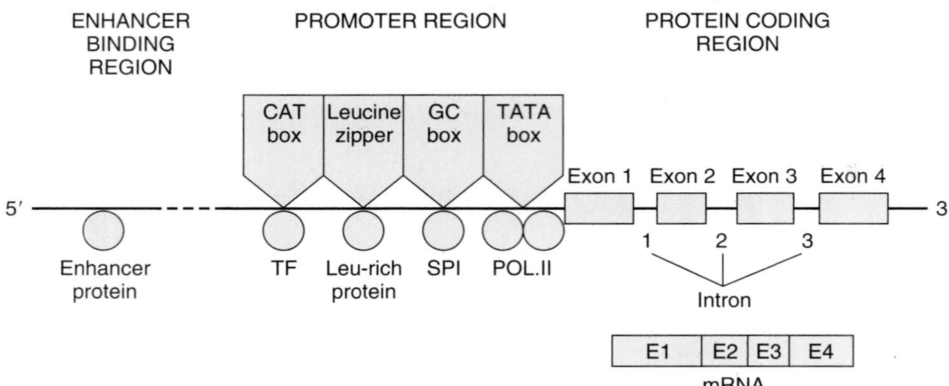

FIGURE 1–81 Protein coding and regulation. mRNA, messenger ribonucleic acid; TF, transcription factor; POL. II, RNA polymerase II; SPI, serum promoter. (From Simon SR, ed: Orthopaedic Basic Science, p 223. Rosemont, IL, American Academy of Orthopaedic Surgeons, 1994.)

genetic trait or disease is associated with various polymorphisms (alternative gene expressions) identified in the restriction fragments.

2. Agarose gel electrophoresis—When exposed to an electrical field, negatively charged DNA suspended in agarose gel moves through the gel toward the positive pole of the field. The gel acts as a "sieve:" Small DNA fragments move more easily (farther in a given time) than large fragments. Agarose gel electrophoresis is commonly used after (and in conjunction with) restriction enzymes.
3. DNA ligation—Process of attaching genes removed from human DNA to pieces of nonhuman DNA known as **plasmids** to facilitate the study of specific genes. Two DNA fragments linked via ligation form **recombinant DNA.**
4. Plasmid vectors—Used to produce large quantities of a gene to be studied. The gene is ligated to a plasmid (which is then known as a **recombinant plasmid**) and inserted into a bacterium (the vector) by a process called **transformation.** The recombinant plasmid replicates inside the bacterium and thus increases the recombinant DNA and the gene it carries.
5. Genomic screening (Fig. 1–82)
6. Transgenic animals (Fig. 1–83)—Used to investigate the function of cloned genes. A transgenic animal is produced by inserting a foreign gene **(transgene)** into a single-cell embryo, which then replicates and carries the transgene to every cell in the body.
7. Southern blotting (hybridization)—Technique that uses restriction enzymes and agarose gel electrophoresis to identify a particular **DNA sequence** in an extract of mixed DNA.
8. Northern blotting (hybridization)—Technique that uses restriction enzymes and agarose gel electrophoresis to identify a particular **RNA sequence** in an extract of mixed RNA.
9. Western blotting—Technique that uses sodium dodecyl sulfate–polyacrylamide gel electrophoresis (SDS-PAGE) to identify a particular **protein** in an extract of mixed proteins.
10. Polymerase chain reaction (PCR) amplification—**Method used to repetitively synthesize (amplify) a specific DNA sequence** in vitro such that the number of DNA copies doubles each cycle. PCR amplification has gained widespread use and has been employed for the prenatal diagnosis of sickle cell disease and as a means of screening DNA for gene mutations.

I. Cloning
1. Definition—Cloning is the making of identical biologic entities.
2. Types
   a. Therapeutic cloning—DNA is removed from a patient and inserted into an embryo. Stem cells are then removed from the growing embryo (which then dies) and stimulated so that they differentiate into a specific tissue. The goal of therapeutic cloning is to produce a specific type of tissue or an organ that will be transplanted back into the patient to avoid transplantation of an organ from another person, thus avoiding organ rejection and the associated complications of immunosuppressive agents.
   b. Reproductive cloning—DNA is removed from a host and inserted into an embryo. The embryo is then implanted into a healthy womb and allowed to develop. The goal of reproductive cloning is to produce an animal that is genetically identical to the host.
   c. Embryo cloning—One or more cells are removed from a fertilized embryo and stimulated to develop in utero. The goal of embryo cloning is to produce several genetically identical animals (such as twins or triplets).

II. Immunology

A. Overview—Immunology is the study of the body's defense mechanisms. Areas of particular relevance to the musculoskeletal system are infection, transplantation, tumors, autoimmune disorders (e.g., RA), and bone remodeling. Two types of immune responses have been described: nonspecific and specific.

B. Nonspecific immune response—**Inflammatory reaction** that begins when a foreign antigen is recognized. May arise as a result of a fracture, soft tissue injury, or foreign body. Histamine is released and results in local vasodilation (exudate), with phagocytic cells that enzymatically digest "offending material." The inflammatory response may be enhanced by

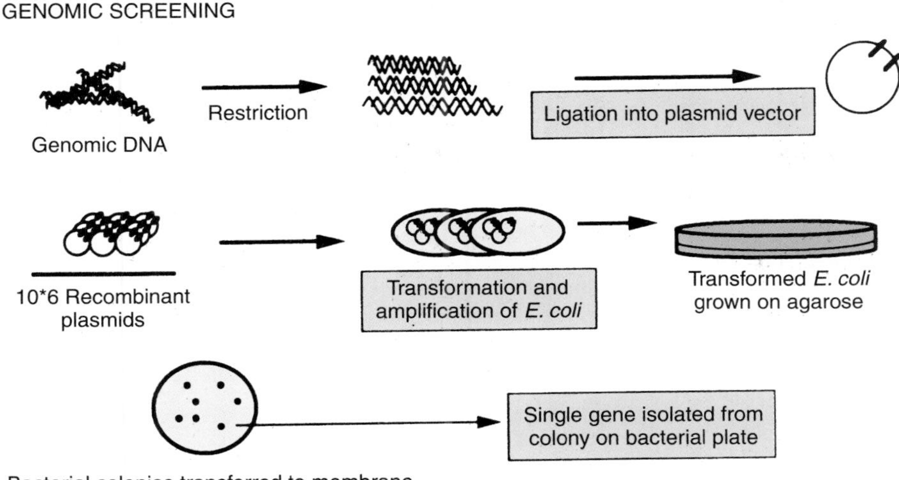

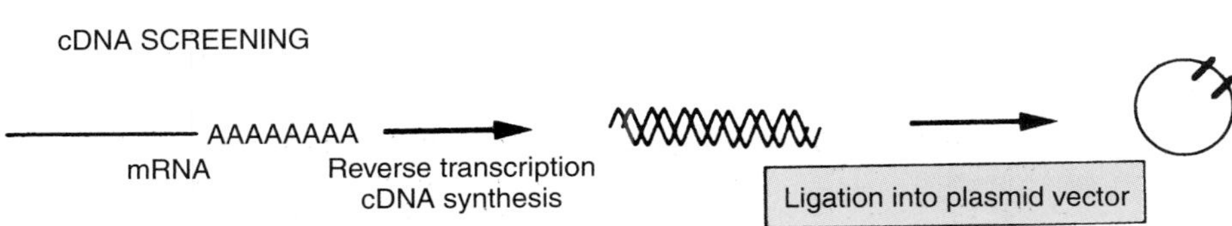

FIGURE 1–82 Genomic library of recombinant plasmids with fragments of all the DNA in the chromosome. The entire genome, restricted into small fragments, is ligated into plasmid vectors restricted by the same enzymes. These recombinant plasmids transform bacteria, which can be screened to isolate specific genes of interest. (From Simon SR, ed: Orthopaedic Basic Science, p 227. Rosemont, IL, American Academy of Orthopaedic Surgeons, 1994.)

activation of the complement system or suppressed by anti-inflammatory medication.

C. Specific immune response (Fig. 1–84)—Includes **cell-mediated** and **humoral antibody–mediated** immune responses. The cells involved in specific immune responses (B and T cells) arise from primitive mesenchymal cells from the bone marrow (Fig 1–85) B lymphocytes mature in the lymph nodes; T lymphocytes originate in the bone marrow and pass

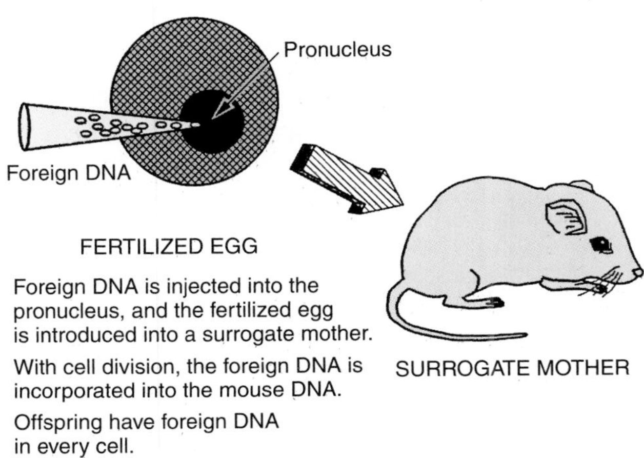

Pronucleus
Foreign DNA
FERTILIZED EGG
Foreign DNA is injected into the pronucleus, and the fertilized egg is introduced into a surrogate mother.
With cell division, the foreign DNA is incorporated into the mouse DNA.
Offspring have foreign DNA in every cell.
SURROGATE MOTHER

FIGURE 1–83 Transgenic mice. Recombinant DNA is injected into a fertilized mouse egg. The foreign DNA is incorporated into the chromosome, with cell division. As the egg develops into an embryo, every cell in the animal contains the foreign DNA. (From Simon SR, ed: Orthopaedic Basic Science, p 228. Rosemont, IL, American Academy of Orthopaedic Surgeons, 1994.)

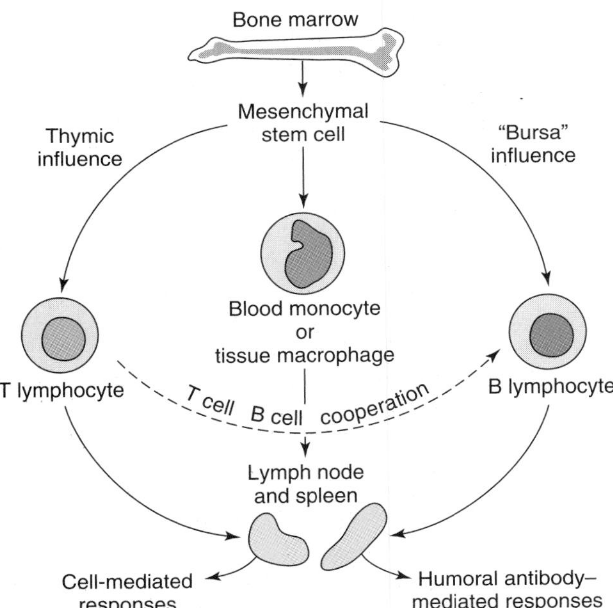

FIGURE 1–84 Bone marrow primitive mesenchymal cells differentiate into Band T lymphocytes and macrophages and cooperate in cell-mediated and humoral responses. (From Friedlaender GE: Immunology. In Albright, JA, and Brand, RA, eds: The Scientific Basis of Orthopaedics, 2nd ed, p 484. Norwalk, CT, Appleton & Lange, 1987. Reproduced with permission of the McGraw-Hill Companies, Inc.)

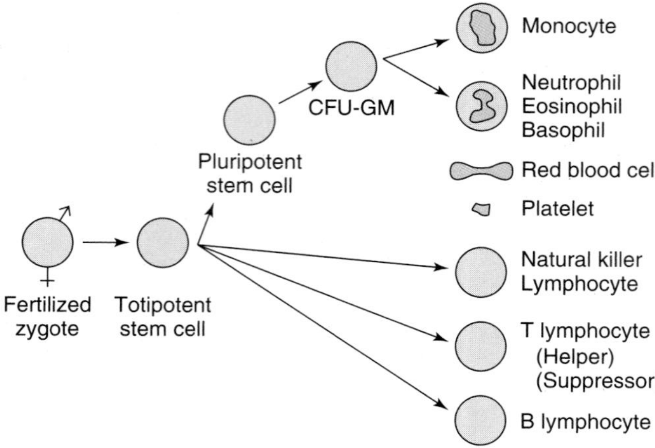

FIGURE 1–85 Stem cells generate all the cell types of the blood and immune systems by a process of proliferation and differentiation in response to growth signals. CFU-GM, colony-forming unit of the granulocyte/macrophage. (From Ross DW, ed: Introduction to Molecular Medicine, 2nd ed, p 112. New York, Springer-Verlag, 1996.)

through the thymus during fetal development before moving to the lymph nodes and blood. T cells include helper T cells, suppressor T cells, and killer T cells. **Antigens** evoke an immune response. **Macrophages and monocytes** are responsible for processing antigen so that it will be able to stimulate lymphocytes. Lymphocytes have the unique ability to mount specific reactions to millions of potential antigens. They do this by rearranging their genes (which no other cell can do) to achieve antigenic diversity and thus produce millions of antibodies.

1. **Cell-mediated immune response** (Fig. 1–86)—Involves T lymphocytes. The protein produced by the gene rearrangement of T cells stays fixed to the surface of the T cells and acts as a receptor molecule. The T-cell receptor acts indirectly on a foreign antigen (it does not bond directly, as seen with B lymphocytes).
2. **Humoral antibody–mediated immune response** (Fig. 1–87)—Involves B lymphocytes, which differentiate into **plasma cells** to produce immunoglobins against specific antigens. **B lymphocytes are associated with immunoglobulins and the HLA system,** whereas T lymphocytes are not. Immunoglobulins are produced by plasma cells in a "Y" configuration (Fig. 1–88). Five classes of immunoglobulins have been described.
   a. IgA—Mucosal surfaces
   b. IgM—Produced earliest by fetus; largest; RF is an IgM
   c. IgG—Most common; arises in response to infection
   d. IgD—Acts as a receptor
   e. IgE—Allergic responses

D. Cytokines—Proteins (or glycoproteins) that are cell products secreted in response to a foreign antigen. They are produced by T cells and regulate inflammatory and immune responses. Cytokines have been described in four broad categories.
   1. Interferons
   2. Growth factors
   3. Colony-stimulating factors
   4. Interleukins

E. Complement system (Fig. 1–89)—A group of 25 proteins that act in a "cascading sequence" to amplify an immune response.

F. Immunogenetics—HLAs contribute to the "specificity of immune recognition" and are associated

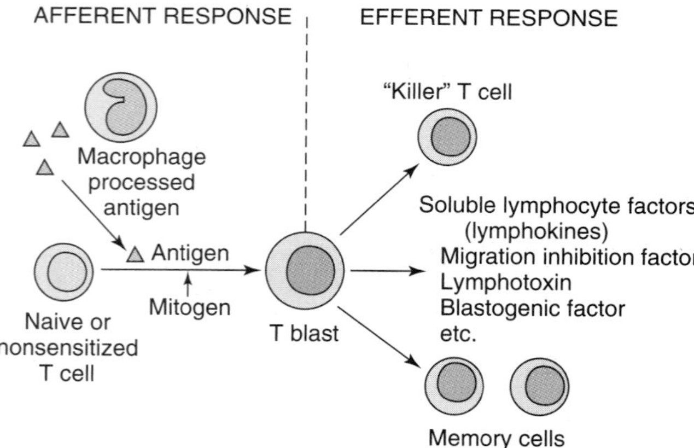

FIGURE 1–86 The cell-mediated immune response. (From Friedlaender GE: Immunology. In Albright JA, Brand RA, eds: The Scientific Basis of Orthopaedics, 2nd ed, p 493. Norwalk, CT, Appleton & Lange, 1987. Reproduced with permission of the McGraw-Hill Companies, Inc.)

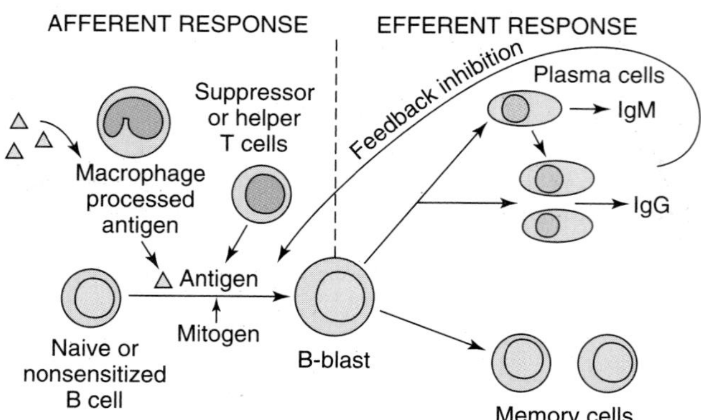

FIGURE 1–87 The humoral antibody response; activation of B cells and immunoglobulin production. (From Friedlaender GE: Immunology. In Albright JA, Brand RA, eds: The Scientific Basis of Orthopaedics, 2nd ed, p 492. Norwalk, CT, Appleton & Lange, 1987.)

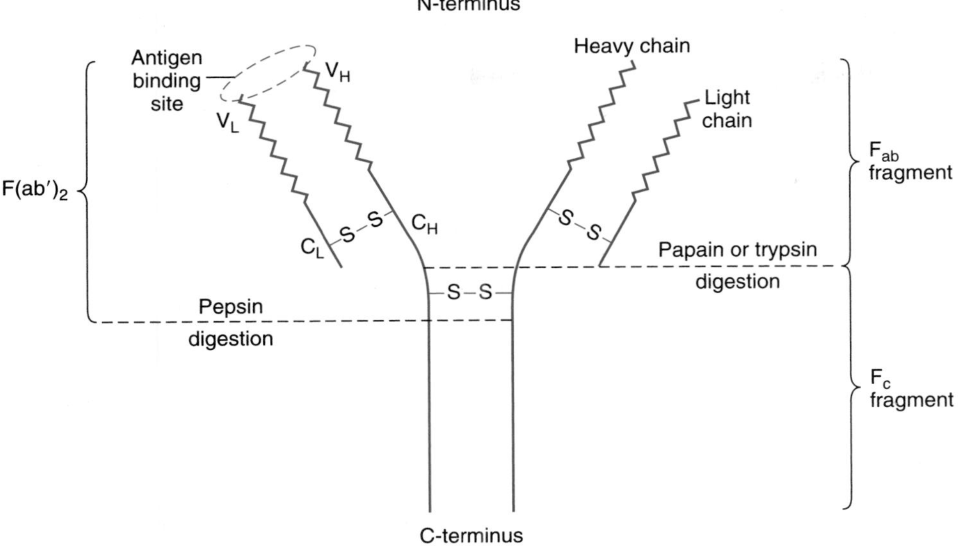

FIGURE 1–88 Basic subunit structure of the immunoglobulin molecule. (From Friedlaender GE: Immunology. In Albright JA, Brand RA, eds: The Scientific Basis of Orthopaedics, 2nd ed, p 486. Norwalk, CT, Appleton & Lange, 1987.)

with a variety of rheumatologic diseases. The HLA gene is located on chromosome 6 (short arm); there are 6 class I loci and 14 class II loci.

G. Transplantation
1. Allogenic grafting—Transplantation between non-identical members of the same species
2. Xenografting—Transplantation of tissues across species
3. Graft preparation
   a. Freezing—Cellular response diminished
   b. Freeze-drying (lyophilization)—Cellular response nearly undetectable

Immunoglobulin
Antigen
Cell membrane
C1
C1
Increased vascular permeability
Ca^{++}
C4
Mg^{++} C2
C receptor
C4,2
Enhanced phagocytosis
Immune adherence
Opsonization
Anaphylatoxin, histamine release
C3
C4,2,3
C5,6,7
C4,2,3,5,6,7
Chemotactic factor
C8
C9
Membranolysis
C4,2,3,5,6,7,8,9

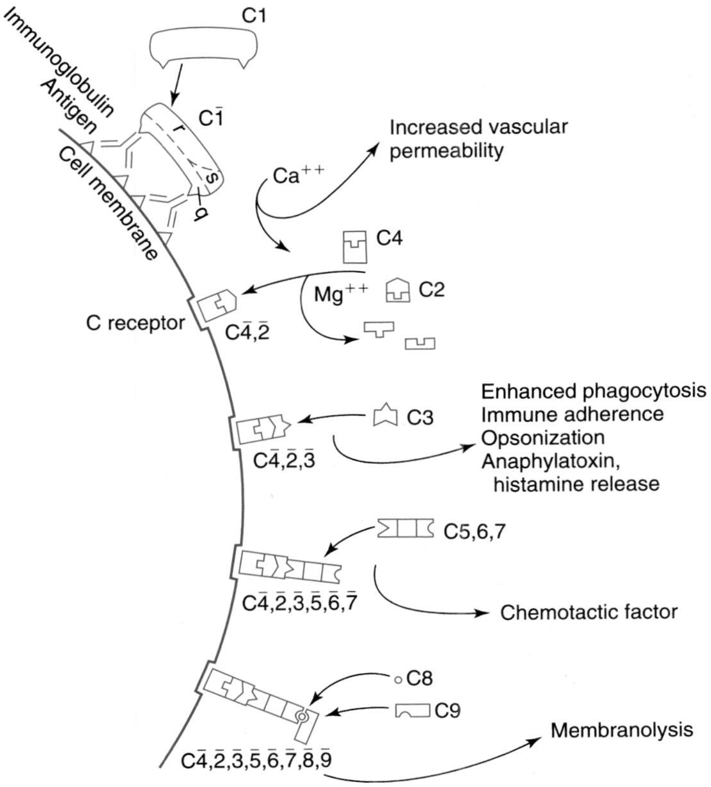

FIGURE 1–89 Complement cascade. (From Friedlaender GE: Immunology. In Albright JA, Brand RA, eds: The Scientific Basis of Orthopaedics, 2nd ed, p 491. Norwalk, CT, Appleton & Lange, 1987.)

H. Oncology (Fig. 1–90)—Cancer is a disease characterized by abnormal, uncontrolled cell growth due to damage to the cell's DNA. The molecular approach to cancer seeks to discover the mechanisms by which normal cells become cancer cells. Any of various mechanisms may damage normal cells and result in malignancy, such as a point mutation in DNA, a gene deletion, or a chromosomal translocation (which results in gene rearrangement).
1. **Oncogenes**—Growth control genes. Improper expression of an oncogene results in unregulated cell growth, as seen in cancer cells.

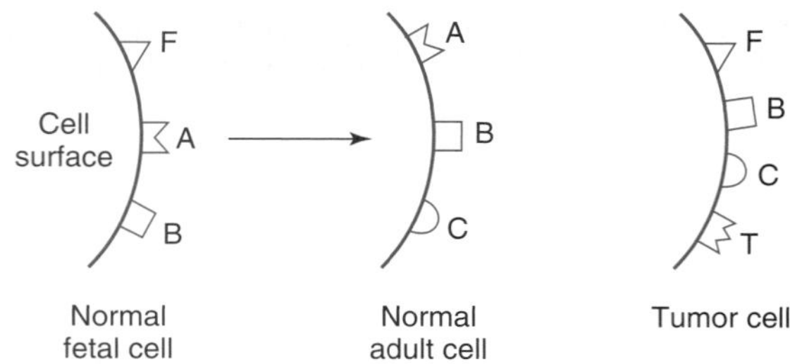

FIGURE 1–90 Tumor cells have cell-surface antigens common to other normal cells reflecting the tissue of origin (B and C). They may also demonstrate antigens normally present only on fetal cells (F) and loose antigens common to the cell type of origin (A). In addition, they acquire new tumor-associated antigens (T). (From Friedlander GE: Immunology. In Albright JA, Brand RA, eds: The Scientific Basis of Orthopaedics, 2nd ed, p 502. Norwalk, CT, Appleton & Lange, 1987. Reproduced with permission of the McGraw-Hill Companies, Inc.)

2. **Antioncogenes (tumor suppressor genes)**—Suppress growth in damaged cells to inhibit tumors.
3. Metastases—The sequence of events for primary tumor cells to metastasize to a distant organ.
   a. Sequence of events
      (1) Progressive growth of the primary tumor
      (2) Neovascularization of the tumor
      (3) Basement membrane erosion and invasion
         (a) **Matrix metalloproteinases have the capacity to degrade type IV collagen, which is present in the basement membrane** (see Table 1–20).
         (b) Matrix metalloproteinases are therefore believed to be important for tumor cell metastasis.
      (4) Entry of tumor cells into adjacent blood vessels
      (5) Detachment of cells from the primary tumor
      (6) Embolization of tumor cells into the general circulation
      (7) Attachment of tumor cells at a distant site
      (8) Invasion into vessel walls, with migration into surrounding parenchyma
      (9) Progressive tumor growth at the new site
   b. Types of tumors—**The most common tumors that metastasize to bone, in decreasing order of incidence, are those of the breast, prostate, lung, kidney, and thyroid.**
4. Miscellaneous—**Flow cytometry and cytofluorometry** are methods used to quantify the amount of DNA in cells. **These techniques are useful for determining the amount of abnormal (aneuploid) DNA in a malignant tumor. P-glycoprotein** is an energy-dependent cell-wall pump that functions to eliminate natural toxins (and some chemotherapeutic agents) from the cytoplasm. P-glycoprotein allows both cancer and normal cells to develop resistance to chemotherapeutic agents.

I. **Miscellaneous topics related to specific immune-related orthopaedic conditions—Latex allergy** has been reported as an intraoperative complication, particularly in patients with myelomeningocele. Latex allergy in these children is likely due to repetitive mucosal and parenteral latex exposure (e.g., operations, examinations). **Type I hypersensitivity to latex involves IgE antibodies** that are specific for proteins from the sap of the rubber tree (*Hevea brasiliensis*) used to make gloves. Preoperative prophylaxis (cimetidine and diphenhydramine) decreases the frequency of potentially catastrophic events (anaphylaxis). The development of RA is related to a reaction between T cells (helper/inducer) and antigen-presenting cell macrophage. The foreign-body response to particulate biomaterials appears to be initiated by macrophages. Lymphocytes do not appear to be essential for this response. Endosteal bone erosion (osteolysis; aggressive granulomatous lesions) surrounding an uninfected femoral stem after THA is associated with macrophage activity in response to particulate debris.

III. Genetics

A. Introduction—Although more than 3000 genetic disorders have been identified, very few genes responsible for musculoskeletal diseases and disorders have been identified.

B. Mendelian inheritance—Mendelian traits are those that follow specific patterns of inheritance controlled by a single gene pair ("monogenic"). A **genetic locus** is a gene's specific position on a chromosome. An **allele** is one of several possible alternative forms of a gene. Because the chromosomes are paired (46 chromosomes; 23 pairs [22 pairs of autosomes and 1 pair of sex chromosomes]), there are two copies (loci) for every gene. An individual is **homozygous** if the two alleles on each of the paired chromosomes are identical; the individual is **heterozygous** if the alleles differ. The term **phenotype** refers to the features exhibited by an individual due to genetic make-up; **genotype** refers to the presence or absence of particular genes, not the associated traits that are expressed. Mendelian traits may be inherited by one of four modes: autosomal dominant, autosomal recessive, X-linked dominant, and X-linked recessive. A detailed description of these four modes of mendelian inheritance is shown in Table 1–37. The overall incidence of mendelian disorders in humans is approximately 1%. Nonmendelian traits may be inherited via "polygenic" transmission (caused by the action of several genes).

C. Mutations—Genetic disorders arise from alterations (mutations) in the genetic material. Mutations may be passed from generation to generation, following mendelian inheritance, or they may represent new mutations **(sporadic mutations)** that occur in the sperm or egg of the parents or in the embryo.

D. Chromosomal abnormalities—Result from disruptions in the normal arrangement or number of chromosomes. These include
1. Aneuploidy—An abnormal number of chromosomes.
   a. Triploidy—Three copies of chromosomes (69 chromosomes)

TABLE 1–37 MENDELIAN INHERITANCE

Inheritance Pattern	Description	Punnett Square(s)
Autosomal dominant*	Typically represent **structural defects** Heterozygote state (Aa) manifests the condition 50% of offspring are affected (assuming that only one parent is affected) Normal offspring do not transmit the conditon There is no gender preference	| A | a a | Aa | aa a | Aa | aa
Autosomal recessive†	Typically represent **biochemical or enzymatic defects** Homozygote state (aa) manifests the condition Parents are unaffected (they are most commonly heterozygotes) 25% of offspring are affected (assuming that each parent is a heterozygote) There is no gender preference	| A | a A | AA | Aa a | Aa | aa
X-linked dominant‡	Heterozygotes (X'X or X'Y) manifest the condition Affected female (mating with unaffected male) transmits the X-linked gene to 50% of daughters and 50% of sons	| X | Y X' | X'X | X'Y X | XX | XY
	Affected male (mating with unaffected female) transmits the X-linked gene to all daughters and no sons	| X' | Y X | X'X | XY X | X'X | XY
X-linked recessive§	Heterozygote (X'Y) male manifests the condition Heterozygote (X'X) female is unaffected Affected male (mating with unaffected female) transmits the X-linked gene to all daughters (who are carriers) and no sons	| X' | Y X | X'X | XY X | X'X | XY
	Carrier female (mating with unaffected male) transmits the X-linked gene to 50% of daughters (who are carriers) and 50% of sons (who are affected)	| X | Y X' | X'X | X'Y X | XX | XY

*A is the mutant dominant allele.
†a is the mutant recessive allele.
‡X' is the mutant dominant X allele.
§X' is the mutant recessive X allele.

b. Tetraploidy—Four copies of chromosomes (92 chromosomes)
c. Monosomy—One chromosome of one pair is absent (45 chromosomes)
d. Trisomy—One chromosome pair has an extra chromosome (47 chromosomes)

2. Deletion—A section of one chromosome (in a chromosome pair) is absent.
3. Duplication—An extra section of one chromosome (in a chromosome pair) is present.
4. Translocation—A portion of one chromosome is exchanged with a portion of another chromosome.
5. Inversion—A broken portion of a chromosome reattaches to the same chromosome in the same location but in a reverse direction.

E. The genetics of musculoskeletal conditions and conditions associated with musculoskeletal abnormalities—Table 1–38 shows the inheritance pattern of the musculoskeletal (and related) disorders that appear most often on board examinations. Table 1–39 is a comprehensive compilation of the known genetic defects involved in disorders that display musculoskeletal manifestations.

TABLE 1-38 INHERITANCE PATTERNS OF SOME MUSCULOSKELETAL-RELATED DISORDERS

Autosomal Dominant	Autosomal Recessive	X-Linked Dominant	X-Linked Recessive
Achondroplasia Spondyloepiphyseal dysplasia (congenita form) Multiple epiphyseal dysplasia Metaphyseal chondrodysplasia (Schmid and Jansen types) Kniest's dysplasia Malignant hyperthermia Marfan's syndrome Ehlers-Danlos syndrome Osteogenesis imperfecta (types I and IV) Osteochondromatosis Polydactyly	Metaphyseal chondrodysplasia (McKusick type) Diastrophic dysplasia Laron's dysplasia Sickle cell anemia Hurler's syndrome Osteogenesis imperfecta (types II and III) Hypophosphatasia Hereditary vitamin D–dependent rickets Homocystinuria	Hypophosphatemic rickets	Spondyloepiphyseal dysplasia (tarda form) Hemophilia Hunter's syndrome Duchenne's muscular dystrophy

TABLE 1-39 COMPREHENSIVE COMPILATION OF INHERITANCE PATTERN, DEFECT, AND ASSOCIATED GENE OF MUSCULOSKELETAL-RELATED DISORDERS

Disorder	Inheritance Pattern	Defect	Associated Gene
Dysplasias			
Achondroplasia	Autosomal dominant	Defect in the fibroblast growth factor (FGF) receptor 3	FGF receptor 3 gene
Diastrophic dysplasia	Autosomal recessive	Mutation of a gene coding for a sulfate transport protein	Sulfate-transporter gene (chromosome 5)
Kniest's dysplasia	Autosomal dominant	Defect in type II collagen	COL 2A1
Laron's dysplasia (pituitary dwarfism)	Autosomal recessive	Defect in the growth hormone receptor	
McCune-Albright syndrome (polyostotic fibrous dysplasia, café-au-lait spots, precocious puberty)	Sporadic mutation	Germ line defect in the Gsα protein	Mutation of Gsα subunit of the receptor/adenylyl cyclase–coupling G proteins
Metaphyseal chondrodysplasia (Jansen form)	Autosomal dominant		
Metaphyseal chondrodysplasia (McKusick form)	Autosomal recessive		
Metaphyseal chondrodysplasia (Schmid-tarda form)	Autosomal dominant	Defect in type X collagen	COL 10A1
Multiple epiphyseal dysplasia	Autosomal dominant (most commonly)	Cartilage oligomeric matrix protein	
Spondyloepiphyseal dysplasia	Autosomal dominant (congenita form) X-linked recessive (tarda form)	Defect in type II collagen	Linked to X p22.12-p22.31 and COL 2A1
Achondrogenesis	Autosomal recessive	Fetal cartilage fails to mature	
Apert syndrome	Sporadic mutation/autosomal dominant		
Chondrodysplasia punctata (Conradi–Hünerman)	Autosomal dominant		
Chondrodysplasia punctata (rhizomelic form)	Autosomal recessive	Defect in subcellular organelles (peroxisomes)	
Cleidocranial dysplasia (dysostosis)	Autosomal dominant	Mutation of a gene coding for a protein related to osteoblast function	cbfal
Dysplasia epiphysealis hemimelica (Trevor's disease)	??		
Ellis-van Creveld syndrome (chondroectodermal dysplasia)	Autosomal recessive		

TABLE 1-39 COMPREHENSIVE COMPILATION OF INHERITANCE PATTERN, DEFECT, AND ASSOCIATED GENE OF MUSCULOSKELETAL-RELATED DISORDERS—cont'd

Disorder	Inheritance Pattern	Defect	Associated Gene
Fibrodysplasia ossifican progressiva	Sporadic mutation/autosomal dominant		
Geroderma osteodysplastica (Walt Disney dwarfism)	Autosomal recessive		
Grebe chondrodysplasia	Autosomal recessive		
Hypochondroplasia	Sporadic mutation/autosomal dominant		
Kabuki make-up syndrome	Sporadic mutation		
Mesomelic dysplasia (Langer type)	Autosomal recessive		
Mesomelic dysplasia (Nievergelt type)	Autosomal dominant		
Mesomelic dysplasia (Reinhardt-Pfeiffer type)	Autosomal dominant		
Mesomelic dysplasia (Werner type)	Autosomal dominant		
Metatrophic dysplasia	Autosomal recessive		
Progressive diaphyseal dysplasia (Camurati-Engelmann disease)	Autosomal dominant		
Pseudoachondroplastic dysplasia	Autosomal dominant		
Pyknodysostosis	Autosomal recessive		
Spondylometaphyseal chondrodysplasia	Autosomal dominant		
Spondylothoracic dysplasia (Jarcho-Levin syndrome)	Autosomal recessive		
Thanatophoric dwarfism	Autosomal dominant		
Tooth-and-nail syndrome	Autosomal dominant		
Treacher Collins syndrome (mandibulofacial dysostosis)	Autosomal dominant		
Metabolic Bone Diseases			
Hereditary vitamin D–dependent rickets	Autosomal recessive	See Table 1–15	
Hypophosphatasia	Autosomal recessive	See Table 1–15	
Hypophosphatemic rickets (vitamin D–resistant rickets)	X-linked dominant	See Table 1–15	
Osteogenesis imperfecta	Autosomal dominant (types I and IV) Autosomal recessive (types II and III)	Defect in type I collagen (abnormal cross-linking)	COL 1A1, COL 1A2
Albright hereditary osteodystrophy (pseudohypo-parathyroidism)	Uncertain	Parathyroid hormone has no effect at the target cells (in the kidney, bone, and intestine)	
Infantile cortical hyperostosis (Caffey's disease)	???		
Ochronosis (alkaptonuria)	Autosomal recessive	Defect in the homogentisic acid oxidase system	
Osteopetrosis	Autosomal dominant (mild, tarda form) Autosomal recessive (infantile, malignant form)		
Connective Tissue Disorders			
Marfan's syndrome	Autosomal dominant	Fibrillin abnormalities (some patients also have type I collagen abnormalities)	Fibrillin gene (chromosome 15)
Ehlers-Danlos syndrome (there are at least 13 varieties)	Autosomal dominant (most common)	Defects in types I and III collagen have been described for some varieties; lysyl oxidase abnormalities	COL 1A2 (for Ehlers-Danlos type VII)
Homocystinuria	Autosomal recessive	Deficiency of the enzyme cystathionine β-synthase	

Continued

TABLE 1-39 COMPREHENSIVE COMPILATION OF INHERITANCE PATTERN, DEFECT, AND ASSOCIATED GENE OF MUSCULOSKELETAL-RELATED DISORDERS—cont'd

Disorder	Inheritance Pattern	Defect	Associated Gene
Mucopolysaccharidosis			
Hunter's syndrome ("gargoylism")	X-linked recessive		
Hurler's syndrome	Autosomal recessive	Deficiency of the enzyme α-L-iduronidase	
Maroteaux-Lamy syndrome	Autosomal recessive		
Morquio's syndrome	Autosomal recessive		
Sanfilippo's syndrome	Autosomal recessive		
Scheie's syndrome	Autosomal recessive	Deficiency of the enzyme α-L-iduronidase	
Muscular Dystrophies			
Duchenne's muscular dystrophy	X-linked recessive	Defect on the short arm of the X chromosome	Dystrophin gene
Becker's dystrophy	X-linked recessive		
Fascioscapulohumeral dystrophy	Autosomal dominant		
Limb-girdle dystrophy	Autosomal recessive		
Steinert's disease (myotonic dystrophy)	Autosomal dominant		
Hematologic Disorders			
Hemophilia (A and B)	X-linked recessive	Hemophilia A–factor VIII deficiency Hemophilia B–factor IX deficiency	
Sickle cell anemia	Autosomal recessive	Hemoglobin abnormality (hemoglobin S)	
Gaucher's disease	Autosomal recessive	Deficient activity of the enzyme β-glucosidase (glucocerebrosidase)	
Hemochromatosis	Autosomal recessive		
Niemann-Pick disease	Autosomal recessive	Accumulation of sphingomyelin in cellular lysosomes	
Smith-Lemli-Opitz syndrome	Uncertain		
Thalassemia	Autosomal recessive	Abnormal production of hemoglobin A	
von Willebrand's disease	Autosomal dominant		
Chromosomal Disorders with Musculoskeletal Abnormalities			
Down syndrome		Trisomy of chromosome 21	
Angelman's syndrome		Chromosome 15 abnormality	
Clinodactyly		Associated with many genetic anomalies, including trisomy of chromosomes 8 and 21	
Edward's syndrome		Trisomy of chromosome 18	
Fragile X syndrome	X-linked trait (does not follow the typical pattern of an X-linked trait)		Xq27-Xq28
Klinefelter's syndrome (XXY)		Male has an extra X chromosome	
Langer-Giedion syndrome	Sporadic mutation	Chromosome 8 abnormality	
Nail-patella syndrome	Autosomal dominant	Chromosome 9 abnormality	
Patau's syndrome		Trisomy of chromosome 13	
Turner's syndrome (XO)		Female missing one of the two X chromosomes	
Neurologic Disorders			
Charcot-Marie-Tooth disease	Autosomal dominant (most common)		
Congenital insensitivity to pain	Autosomal recessive		
Dejerine-Sottas disease	Autosomal recessive		
Friedreich's ataxia	Autosomal recessive		
Huntington's disease	Autosomal dominant		
Menkes' syndrome	X-linked recessive	Inability to absorb and use copper	
Pelizaeus-Merzbacher disease	X-linked recessive	Defect in the gene for proteolipid (a component of myelin)	
Riley-Day syndrome	Autosomal recessive		

TABLE 1-39 COMPREHENSIVE COMPILATION OF INHERITANCE PATTERN, DEFECT, AND ASSOCIATED GENE OF MUSCULOSKELETAL-RELATED DISORDERS—cont'd

Disorder	Inheritance Pattern	Defect	Associated Gene
Spinal muscular atrophy (Werdnig-Hoffman disease and Kugelberg-Welander disease)	Autosomal recessive		
Sturge-Weber syndrome	Sporadic mutation		
Tay-Sachs disease	Autosomal recessive	Deficiency in the enzyme hexosaminidase A	
Diseases Associated with Neoplasias			
Ewing's sarcoma			11;22 chromosomal translocation (EWS/FL11 fusion gene)
Multiple endocrine neoplasia I (MEN I)	Autosomal dominant		RET
MEN II	Autosomal dominant		
MEN III	Autosomal dominant	Chromosome 10 abnormality	
Neurofibromatosis (von Recklinghausen's disease)	Autosomal dominant		NF1, NF2
Synovial sarcoma			X;18 chromosomal translocation (STT/SSX fusion gene)
Miscellaneous Disorders			
Malignant hyperthermia	Autosomal dominant		
Osteochondromatosis	Autosomal dominant		
Polydactyly	Autosomal dominant (a small number of cases of sporadic gene mutations have been reported)		
Captodactyly	Autosomal dominant		
Cerebro-oculofacioskeletal syndrome	Autosomal recessive		
Congenital contractural arachnodactyly			Fibrillin gene (chromosome 5)
Distal arthrogryposis syndrome	Autosomal dominant		
Dupuytren's contracture	Autosomal dominant (with partial sex limitation)		
Fabry's disease	X-linked recessive	Deficiency of α-galactosidase A	
Fanconi's pancytopenia	Autosomal recessive		
Freeman-Sheldon syndrome (craniocarpotarsal dysplasia; whistling face syndrome)	Autosomal dominant Autosomal recessive		
GM1 gangliosidosis	Autosomal recessive		
Hereditary anonychia	Autosomal dominant Autosomal recessive		
Holt-Oram syndrome	Autosomal dominant		
Humeroradial synostosis	Autosomal dominant Autosomal recessive		
Klippel-Feil syndrome		Faulty development of spinal segments along the embryonic neural tube	
Klippel-Trénaunay-Weber syndrome	Sporadic mutation		
Krabbe's disease	Autosomal recessive	Deficiency of galactocerebroside β-galactosidase	
Larsen's syndrome	Autosomal dominant Autosomal recessive		
Lesch-Nyhan disease	X-linked trait	Absence of the enzyme hypoxanthine guanine phosphoribosyl transferase	
Madelung's deformity	Autosomal dominant		
Mannosidosis	Autosomal recessive	Deficiency of the enzyme α-monosidase	
Maple syrup urine disease	Autosomal recessive	Defective metabolism of the amino acids leucine, isoleucine, and valine	
Meckel's syndrome (Gruber's syndrome)	Autosomal recessive		
Mobius' syndrome	Autosomal dominant		

Continued

TABLE 1-39 COMPREHENSIVE COMPILATION OF INHERITANCE PATTERN, DEFECT, AND ASSOCIATED GENE OF MUSCULOSKELETAL-RELATED DISORDERS—cont'd

Disorder	Inheritance Pattern	Defect	Associated Gene
Mucolipidosis (oligosaccharidosis)	Autosomal recessive	A family of enzyme deficiency diseases	
Multiple exostoses	Autosomal dominant		
Multiple pterygium syndrome	Autosomal recessive		
Noonan's syndrome	Sporadic mutation		
Oral-facial-digital (OFD) syndrome	OFD I—X-linked dominant OFD II (Mohr's syndrome)—autosomal recessive		
Osler-Weber-Rendu syndrome (hereditary hemorrhagic telangiectasia)	Autosomal dominant		
Pfeiffer's syndrome (acrocephalosyndactyly)	Sporadic mutation/autosomal dominant		
Phenylketonuria	Autosomal recessive	Enzyme deficiency characterized by the inability to convert phenylalanine to tyrosine due to a chromosome 12 abnormality	
Phytanic acid storage disease	Autosomal recessive		
Progeria (Hutchinson-Gilford progeria syndrome)	Autosomal dominant		
Proteus syndrome	Autosomal dominant		
Prune-belly syndrome	Uncertain	Localized mesodermal defect	
Radioulnar synostosis	Autosomal dominant		
Rett's syndrome	Sporadic mutation/X-linked dominant		
Roberts' syndrome (pseudothalidomide syndrome)	Sporadic mutation/autosomal recessive		
Russell-Silver syndrome	Sporadic mutation (possibly X-linked)		
Saethre-Chotzen syndrome	Autosomal dominant		
Sandhoff's disease	Autosomal recessive	Enzyme deficiency of hexosaminidase A and B	
Schwartz-Jampel syndrome	Autosomal recessive		
Seckel's syndrome (bird-headed dwarfism)	Autosomal recessive		
Stickler's syndrome (hereditary progressive arthro-ophthalmopathy)	Autosomal dominant	Collagen abnormality	
TAR syndrome (thrombocytopenia–aplasia of radius syndrome)	Autosomal recessive		
Tarsal coalition	Autosomal dominant		
Trichorhinophalangeal syndrome	Autosomal dominant		
Urea cycle defects	Argininemia—autosomal recessive Argininosuccinic aciduria—autosomal recessive Carbamyl phosphate synthetase deficiency—autosomal recessive Citrullinemia—autosomal recessive Ornathine transcarbamylase deficiency—X-linked	A group of enzyme disorders characterized by high levels of ammonia in the blood and tissues	
VATER association	Sporadic mutation		
Werner's syndrome	Autosomal recessive		
Zygodactyly	Autosomal dominant		

SECTION 5 Orthopaedic Infections and Microbiology

I. Musculoskeletal Infections

The following is an overview. Specific infections unique to particular orthopaedic areas are detailed in the chapters that follow. In general, the following initial treatment regimen recommendations are based on the presumed type of infection as determined by clinical findings and symptoms. Definitive treatment should be based on final culture results when available. **Glycocalyx** is an exopolysaccharide coating that envelops bacteria. Bacterial adherence to biologic implants is promoted by an inflammatory tissue interface and inhibited by a noninflammatory tissue interface.

A. Soft tissue infections (Table 1–40)

1. Bite injuries (Table 1–41)

B. Bone infections—Osteomyelitis is an infection of bone and bone marrow that may be caused by direct inoculation of an open traumatic wound or by blood-borne organisms (hematogenous). **It is not possible to determine the microscopic organism causing chronic osteomyelitis based on the clinical picture and patient age; thus, a specific microbiologic diagnosis via deep cultures is essential (organisms isolated from sinus tract drainage typically do not accurately reflect the organisms present deep within the wound and within bone).**

1. Acute hematogenous osteomyelitis
   a. Causes and clinical features—Bone and bone marrow infection caused by blood-borne organisms, commonly in children (boys more often than girls). In children, the infection is most common in the metaphysis or epiphysis of the long bones and more common in the lower extremity than the upper extremity. Radiographic changes of acute hematogenous osteomyelitis include soft tissue swelling (early), bone demineralization (10-14 days), and **sequestra** (dead bone with surrounding granulation tissue) and **involucrum** (periosteal new bone) later. Pain, loss of function of the involved extremity, and a soft tissue abscess may be present.
   b. Diagnosis—Patients commonly show an elevated WBC count and an elevated ESR; blood cultures may also be positive. **C-reactive protein is the most sensitive monitor of the course of infection in children with acute hematogenous osteomyelitis** because it has a short half-life and dissipates in about 1 week after effective treatment. Nuclear medicine studies may be helpful in equivocal cases. **MRI shows changes in bone and bone marrow before plain films: decreased T_1-weighted bone marrow signal intensity, increased postgadolinium fat-suppressed T_1-weighted signal intensity, and an increased T_2-weighted signal relative to normal fat.**
   c. Treatment—The treatment of acute osteomyelitis may be summarized as follows: (1) identify the organisms, (2) select appropriate antibiotics, (3) deliver antibiotics to the infected site, and (4) halt tissue destruction.
      (1) Empirical treatment—Before definitive cultures become available, empirical therapy is based on the patient's age and/or special circumstances.
         (a) **Newborn (up to 4 months of age)**—The most common organisms include *Staphylococcus aureus*, gram-negative bacilli, and group B streptococcus. Primary empirical therapy includes nafcillin or oxacillin plus a third-generation cephalosporin. Alternative antibiotic therapy includes vancomycin plus a third-generation cephalosporin. Newborns with hematogenous osteomyelitis may be afebrile, and the best predictors of the osteomyelitis are local signs in the extremity, including warmth. Almost 70% of newborn patients with hematogenous osteomyelitis have positive blood cultures.
         (b) **Children 4 years of age or older**—The most common organisms are *S. aureus*, group A streptococcus, and coliforms (uncommon). The empirical treatment of choice is nafcillin or oxacillin; alternative regimens include vancomycin or clindamycin. When the Gram stain shows gram-negative organisms, a third-generation cephalosporin should be added. **With recent immunization programs, *Haemophilus influenzae* bone infections causing hematogenous osteomyelitis have been almost completely eliminated.**
         (c) **Adults 21 years of age or older—The most common organism is *S. aureus*,** but a wide variety of other organisms have been isolated. Initial empirical therapy includes nafcillin, oxacillin, or cefazolin; vancomycin can be used as an alternative initial therapy.
         (d) Sickle cell anemia—*Salmonella* is a characteristic organism. The primary treatment is with one of the fluoroquinolones (only in adults); alternative treatment is with a third-generation cephalosporin.
         (e) Hemodialysis patients and intravenous drug abusers—*S. aureus, S. epidermidis*, and *Pseudomonas aeruginosa* are common organisms. The treatment of choice is one of the penicillinase-resistant

TABLE 1-40 SOFT TISSUE INFECTIONS

Type	Affected Tissues	Clinical Findings	Organisms	Treatment
Cellulitis	Subcutaneous; generally deeper and with less distinct margins than erysipelas	Erythema; tenderness; warmth; lymphangitis; lymphadenopathy	Group A strep (most common) *Staphylococcus aureus* (less common)	Initial antibiotic treatment is penicillinase-resistant synthetic penicillins (PRSPs [nafcillin or oxacillin]). Alternative therapies: erythromycin, first-generation cephalosporins, amoxicillin/ clavulanate (Augmentin), azithromycin, clarithromycin, dithromycin, and tigecycline
Erysipelas	Superficial; progressively enlarging, well demarcated, red, raised, painful plaque	Similar to cellulitis but more superficial and well demarcated	In diabetics: group A strep, *S. aureus*, Enterobacteriaceae, and clostridia	Same as cellulitis Second- or third-generation cephalosporin or amoxicillin for early and mild cases Severe cases may require imipenem (Primaxin), meropenem, or trovafloxacin Diabetics may require surgical débridement to rule out necrotizing fasciitis and obtain definitive cultures Septic patients should receive x-ray examinations to rule out gas in the soft tissues.
Necrotizing fasciitis	Muscle fascia	Aggressive, life-threatening; may be associated with an underlying vascular disease (particularly diabetes) Commonly occurs after surgery, trauma, or streptococcal skin infection	Many acute cases involve several organisms. Groups A, C, and G strep are the most common. Clostridia or polymicrobial infections (aerobic plus anaerobic) are also seen. Methicillin-resistant *S. aureus* (MRSA)	Requires emergent, extensive surgical débridement (involving the entire length of the overlying cellulitis) and IV antibiotics Initial antibiotic treatments: penicillin G for strep or clostridia; imipenem, cilastatin, or meropenem for polymicrobial infections Vancomycin if MRSA suspected
Gas gangrene	Muscle; commonly in grossly contaminated, traumatic wounds, particularly those that are closed primarily	Progressive, severe pain; edema (distant from the wound); foul-smelling, serosanguineous discharge; high fever; chills; tachycardia; confusion Clinical findings consistent with toxemia Radiographs typically show widespread gas in the soft tissues (facilitates rapid spread of the infection)	Classically caused by *Clostridium perfringens, Clostridium specticum*, or other histotoxic *Clostridium* species These gram-positive, anaerobic, spore-forming rods produce exotoxins that cause necrosis of fat and muscle and thrombosis of local vessels.	Surgical (radical) débridement with fasciotomies is the primary treatment. Hyperbaric oxygen may be a useful adjuvant therapy, although its effectiveness remains inconclusive. Initial antibiotic treatment is clindamycin plus penicillin G. Alternative therapies include ceftriaxone and erythromycin.
Toxic shock syndrome (TSS): staphylococcal	TSS is a form of toxemia, not a septicemia In orthopaedics, TSS is secondary to colonization of surgical or traumatic wounds (even after minor trauma). TSS can be associated with tampon use via colonization of the vagina with toxin-producing *S. aureus*	Fever, hypotension, an erythematous macular rash with a serous exudate (gram-positive cocci are present) The infected wound may look benign and may be misleading with regard to the seriousness of the underlying condition	Caused by toxins produced by *S. aureus*	Irrigation and débridement and IV antibiotics with IV immune globulin Initial antibiotic treatment is a PRSP (nafcillin or oxacillin), vancomycin if MRSA. Alternative therapies include first-generation cephalosporins. Patients may also require emergent fluid resuscitation.
Toxic shock syndrome (TSS): streptococcal	Toxemia is not septicemia Commonly associated with erysipelas or necrotizing fasciitis	Similar to *staph* TSS	Toxins from Group A, B, C, or G *Streptococcus pyogenes*	Initial antibiotic treatment is clindamycin plus penicillin G and IV immune globulin. Alternative therapies include erythromycin, or ceftriaxone and clindamycin.
Surgical wound infection	Varies		Most commonly, *S. aureus*, but Groups A, B, C, and G strep and Enterobacteriaceae are not uncommon. Methicillin-resistant *S. aureus*	MRSA species are best treated with vancomycin (alternatives to vancomycin for MRSA include teicoplanin, trimethoprim [Bactrim] plus sulfamethoxazole,

TABLE 1-40 SOFT TISSUE INFECTIONS—cont'd

Type	Affected Tissues	Clinical Findings	Organisms	Treatment
			(MRSA) species infections are also increasing. Vancomycin-methicillin–resistant *S. aureus* (VMRSA) has also been reported.	quinupristin/dalfopristin, linezolid, daptomycin, dalbavancin, fusidic acid, fosfomycin, rifampin, and novobiocin). VMRSA is currently treated with quinupristin/dalfopristin, linezolid, or daptomycin.
Marine injuries	Varies	History of fishing (or other marine activity) injury, with signs of infection Culture specimens at 30°C (6°F); cultures may take several weeks to grow on culture media	Marine injuries involve organisms that can cause indolent infections. *Vibrio vulnificus* is most likely the organism in infected wounds that were exposed to brackish water or shellfish; can cause a devastating infection. Consider atypical mycobacteria (e.g., *Mycobacterium marinum*) for injuries with indolent, low-grade infection.	*V. vulnificus* is best treated with ceftazidime (doxycycline for penicillin allergy or in addition to ceftazidime); cefotaxime and ciprofloxacin are alternatives. *M. marinum* is best treated with clarithromycin, minocycline, doxycycline, trimethoprim/sulfamethoxazole, or rifampin plus ethambutol.

synthetic penicillins (PRSPs) plus ciprofloxacin; an alternative treatment is vancomycin with ciprofloxacin.

(2) Operative treatment—Should be started after cultures have been obtained, either by aspiration or surgical drainage when indicated. The indications for operative intervention include (1) drainage of an abscess, (2) débridement of infected tissues to prevent further destruction, and (3) refractory cases that show no improvement after nonoperative treatment.

TABLE 1-41 BITE INJURIES

Source of Bite	Organism(s)	Primary Antimicrobial (or Drug) Regimen
Human	*Streptococcus viridans (100%)* *Bacteroides* *Staphylococcus epidermidis* *Corynebacterium* *S. aureus* *Peptostreptococcus* *Eikenella*	Early treatment (not yet infected): amoxicillin/clavulanate (Augmentin) With signs of infection: ampicillin/sulbactam (Unasyn), cefoxitin, ticarcillin/clavulanate (Timentin), or piperacillin-tazobactam Patients with penicillin allergy: clindamycin plus either ciprofloxacin or trimethoprim/sulfamethoxazole *Eikenella* is resistant to clindamycin, nafcillin/oxacillin, metronidazole, and possibly to first-generation cephalosporins and erythromycin; susceptible to fluoroquinolones and trimethoprim/sulfamethoxazole; treat with cefoxitin or ampicillin.
Dog	*S. aureus* *Pasteurella multocida* *Bacteroides* *Fusobacterium* *Capnocytophaga*	Amoxicillin/clavulanate (Augmentin), clindamycin (adults), or clindamycin plus trimethoprim/sulfamethoxazole (children) Consider antirabies treatment. Only 5% become infected.
Cat	*P. multocida* *S. aureus* Possibly tularemia	Amoxicillin/clavulanate, cefuroxime axetil, or doxycycline
Rat	*S. moniliformis* Spirillum minus	Amoxicillin/clavulanate or doxycycline Antirabies treatment not indicated
Pig	Polymicrobial (aerobes and anaerobes)	Amoxicillin/clavulanate, third-generation cephalosporin, ticarcillin/clavulanate (Timentin), ampicillin/sulbactam, or imipenem-cilastatin
Skunk, raccoon, bat	Varies	Amoxicillin/clavulanate or doxycycline Antirabies treatment is indicated.
Pit viper (snake)	*Pseudomonas* Enterobacteriaceae *S. epidermidis* *Clostridium*	Antivenom therapy Ceftriaxone Tetanus prophylaxis
Brown recluse spider	—	Dapsone
Catfish sting	Toxins (may become secondarily infected)	Amoxicillin/clavulanate

Adapted from Gilbert DN, Moellering RC, Eliopoulos GM, Sande MA: The Sanford Guide to Antimicrobial Therapy, p 38. Hyde Park, VT, Antimicrobial Therapy, Inc., 2006.

2. Acute osteomyelitis (after open fracture or open reduction with internal fixation)—Clinical findings may be similar to acute hematogenous osteomyelitis. Treatment includes radical irrigation and débridement with removal of orthopaedic hardware as necessary. Open wounds may require rotational or free flaps. The most common offending organisms are *S. aureus*, *P. aeruginosa*, and coliforms. Empirical therapy prior to definitive cultures is nafcillin with ciprofloxacin; alternative therapy is vancomycin with a third-generation cephalosporin. Patients with acute osteomyelitis and vascular insufficiency and those who are immunocompromised generally show a polymicrobial picture.
3. Chronic osteomyelitis—May arise as a result of an inappropriately treated acute osteomyelitis, trauma, or soft tissue spread, especially in the Cierny type C elderly host (Table 1–42), the immunosuppressed, diabetics, and intravenous drug abusers. Chronic osteomyelitis may be classified anatomically (Fig. 1–91). Skin and soft tissues are often involved, and the sinus tract may occasionally develop squamous cell carcinoma. Periods of quiescence (of the infection) are often followed by acute exacerbations.
   a. Diagnosis—Nuclear medicine studies are often helpful for determining the activity of the disease. **Operative sampling of deep specimens from multiple foci is the most accurate means of identifying the pathologic organisms.**
   b. Treatment— **Treatment is based on deep cultures and sensitivity testing; empirical therapy is not indicated for chronic osteomyelitis.** A combination of intravenous antibiotics (based on deep cultures), surgical débridement **(complete removal of compromised bone and soft tissue), and retained hardware is the most important factor in eliminating infection. It is almost impossible to eliminate implant-associated infection without removing the implant because organisms grow in a glycocalyx (biofilm) that shields them from antibodies and antibiotics.** After sterilization of the affected area, bone grafting and soft tissue coverage is often required. Unfortunately, amputations are still required in certain cases. *S. aureus*, Enterobacteriaceae, and *P. aeruginosa* are the most frequent offending organisms.
4. Subacute osteomyelitis
   a. Diagnosis—Usually discovered radiologically in a patient with a painful limp and no systemic (and often no local) signs or symptoms. Subacute osteomyelitis may arise secondary to a partially treated acute osteomyelitis or occasionally develops in a fracture hematoma. Unlike acute osteomyelitis, the WBC count and blood cultures are frequently normal. ESR, bone cultures, and radiographs are often useful. Subacute osteomyelitis most commonly affects the femur and tibia; and unlike acute osteomyelitis, it can cross the physis, even in older children. Radiographic changes include **Brodie's abscess** (localized radiolucency usually seen in the metaphyses of long bones). It is sometimes difficult to differentiate from Ewing's sarcoma.
   b. Treatment—Treatment of Brodie's abscess in the metaphysis includes surgical curettage. When localized to the epiphysis only, other lesions (e.g., chondroblastoma) must be ruled out. **Epiphyseal osteomyelitis is caused almost exclusively by *S. aureus*.** Epiphyseal osteomyelitis requires surgical drainage only if pus is present; otherwise, 48 hours of intravenous antibiotics followed by 6 weeks of oral antibiotics is curative.
5. Chronic sclerosing osteomyelitis—An unusual infection that primarily involves the diaphyseal bones of adolescents. Typified by intense proliferation of the periosteum leading to bony deposition, it may be caused by anaerobic organisms. An insidious onset; dense, progressive sclerosis on radiographs; and localized pain and tenderness are common. Malignancy must be ruled out.
6. Chronic multifocal osteomyelitis—Caused by an infectious agent, it appears in children without systemic symptoms. Except for an elevated ESR, normal laboratory values are common. Radiographs demonstrate multiple metaphyseal lytic lesions, especially in the medial clavicle, distal tibia, and distal femur. Usually resolves spontaneously, requiring only symptomatic treatment.
7. Osteomyelitis with unusual organisms—Several unusual organisms occur in certain clinical settings (Table 1–43). Radiographs show characteristic

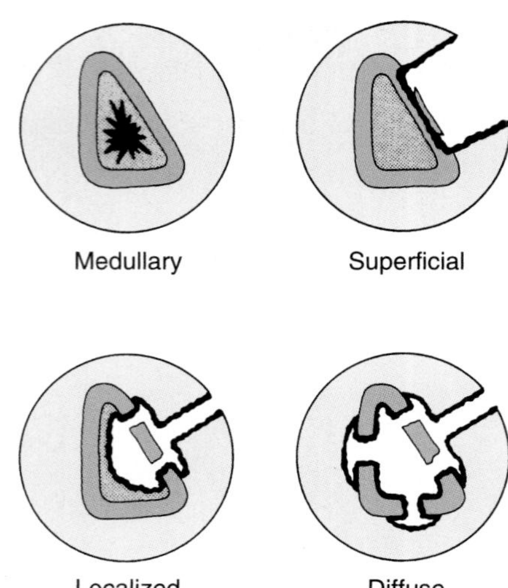

FIGURE 1–91 Cierny's anatomic classification of adult chronic osteomyelitis. (From Cierny G, III: Chronic osteomyelitis: Results of treatment. Instr Course Lect 39:495, 1990.)

TABLE 1-42 INFECTED HOST TYPES

Type	Description	Risk
A	Normal immune response; nonsmoker	Minimal
B	Local or mild systemic deficiency; smoker	Moderate
C	Major nutritional or systemic disorder	High

TABLE 1-43 UNUSUAL ORGANISMS THAT MAY BE FOUND IN OSTEOMYELITIS

Organism	Risk Factor(s)	Symptoms/Signs/Findings	Treatment
Serratia marcescens	IV drug abuse	Axial skeleton	Cotrimoxazole
Pseudomonas aeruginosa	IV drug abuse	Nonspecific	Aminoglycoside
Brucella (G−)	Meat handling	Flat bones	Tetracycline/Septra
Salmonella	Sickle cell disease	Asymptomatic	Ampicillin
Anaerobes	Skin contamination	Tissue culture	Clindamycin/cephalosporin
Fungi	Skin contamination	Special study	Amphotericin B
Treponema pallidum	Sexual contact	Nontender swelling	Penicillin
Mycobacteria	TB/leprosy/fishermen	PPD/granuloma/culture at 30°C	PAS, isoniazid

G−, gram negative; IV, intravenous; PPD, purified protein derivative; PAS, p-aminosalicylic acid; TB, tuberculosis.

features in syphilis (*Treponema pallidum*) (radiolucency in the metaphysis from granulation tissue) and tuberculosis (joint destruction on both sides of a joint). Histology can also be helpful (e.g., tuberculosis with granulomas).

C. Joint infections
  1. Septic arthritis
    a. Diagnosis—Commonly follows hematogenous spread or extension of metaphyseal osteomyelitis in children. Can also arise as a complication of a diagnostic or therapeutic procedure. Most cases involve infants (hip) and children. **The metaphyses of the proximal femur, proximal humerus, radial neck, and distal fibula are within their respective joint capsules; metaphyseal osteomyelitis can rupture into the joint in these areas. The most common site at which septic arthritis follows acute osteomyelitis is the proximal femur/hip.** RA (tuberculosis most characteristic, *S. aureus* most common) and intravenous drug abuse (*Pseudomonas* most characteristic) predispose adults to septic arthritis.
    b. Treatment
      (1) Empirical therapy prior to the availability of definitive cultures—Based on the patient's age and/or special circumstances.
        (a) **Newborn (up to 3 months of age)—The most common organisms include *S. aureus* and group B streptococcus; less common organisms include** Enterobacteriaceae and *Neisseria gonorrhoeae*. Adjacent bony involvement is seen in almost 70% of patients. Blood cultures are commonly positive. Initial treatment is with a PRSP plus a third-generation cephalosporin. Alternative treatment is with a PRSP plus an antipseudomonal aminoglycosidic antibiotic (APAG). If the organism is methicillin-resistant *Staphylococcus aureus* (MRSA), use vancomycin (instead of a PRSP) with an APAG.
        (b) **Children (3 months to 14 years of age)**—The most common organisms are as follows: *S. aureus, Streptococcus pyogenes, S. pneumoniae, H. influenzae* **(the incidence of *H. influenzae* septic arthritis has markedly decreased with vaccination programs),** and gram-negative bacilli. Initial treatment is with a PRSP plus a third-generation cephalosporin; alternative treatment is with vancomycin plus a third-generation cephalosporin.
        (c) **Acute monarticular septic arthritis in sexually active adults**—The most common organisms include *N. gonorrhoeae, S. aureus*, streptococci, and aerobic gram-negative bacilli (uncommon). Empirical drug therapy when the Gram stain is negative is ceftriaxone, cefotaxime, or ceftizoxime; when the Gram stain shows gram-positive cocci in clusters, the treatment is nafcillin or oxacillin.
        (d) **Acute monarticular septic arthritis in adults who are not sexually active**—The most common organisms are *S. aureus*, streptococci, and gram-negative bacilli. Antibiotic treatment is with a PRSP plus a third-generation cephalosporin or a PRSP plus ciprofloxacin.
        (e) **Chronic monarticular septic arthritis**—The most common organisms are *Brucella, Nocardia, Mycobacteria*, and fungi.
        (f) **Polyarticular septic arthritis**—The most common organisms are gonococci, *B. burgdorferi*, acute rheumatic fever, and viruses.
      (2) Surgical drainage or daily aspiration—The mainstay of treatment. Open (or arthroscopic) drainage is required for septic hip joints. SI joint sepsis is unusual and is best diagnosed by physical examination (flexion, abduction, and external rotation [FABER] most specific), ESR, a bone scan, a CT scan, and aspiration. A pannus (similar to that of inflammatory arthritis) can be seen in tuberculosis infections. Late sequelae of septic arthritis include soft tissue contractures that can sometimes be treated with soft tissue procedures (such as a quadricepsplasty).

2. Septic bursitis—Most commonly caused by an *S. aureus* infection. Treatment is with a PRSP.
3. Infected TJA—Covered in Chapter 5, Adult Reconstruction, but bears some mention here.
    a. Prevention—Perioperative intravenous antibiotics constitute the most effective method for decreasing its incidence, although a good operative technique, laminar flow (avoiding obstruction between the air source and the operative wound), and special "space suits" also have a role. Most patients who have undergone total joint replacement do not need prophylactic antibiotics when undergoing dental surgery. The most common organism infecting a TJA after a dental procedure is ***Peptostreptococcus*.** Preoperative aspiration of the knee joint prior to revision TKA appears to be useful to rule out infection.
    b. Diagnosis—***S. epidermidis* is the most common pathogen in infection associated with an implant or other foreign body (including allograft);** the next most frequent pathogens are *S. aureus* and group B streptococcus. The ESR is the most sensitive indicator of infection, but it is nonspecific. Culture of the hip aspirate is sensitive and specific C-reactive protein may also be helpful. Preoperative skin ulcerations are associated with an increased risk for infecting a TKA. The most accurate test for infection of a TJA is a tissue culture. Routine aspiration of all hip joints prior to revision THA results in a high incidence of false-positive cultures.
    c. Treatment—**Acute infections (within 2-3 weeks of arthroplasty) can usually be treated with prosthesis salvage, exchanging only polyethylene components (provided that the metallic components are stable).** Synovectomy for an acute TKA infection is also beneficial. **Delayed or chronic TJA infections require implant (and cement) removal.** A staged exchange arthroplasty may be performed later, depending on the virulence of the organism. Polymicrobial organisms may form an overlying glycocalyx, making infection control difficult without removing the prosthesis and vigorous débridement. However, according to Cierny, the host is more important than the organism in terms of risk (see Table 1–44). The use of antibiotic-impregnated cement in revision arthroplasties and antibiotic spacers/beads in infected total joints may be helpful. Reimplantation after thorough débridement and use of polymethylmethacrylate (PMMA) with antibiotics has been successful at variable intervals. Some advocate frozen sections at the time of reimplantation to ensure that local tissues have fewer than 5-10 PMNs per high-power field.
4. Lacerations resulting from a clenched fist to the mouth—Lacerations overlying the joints of the hand that has struck another person's mouth ("fight bite") should be considered a penetrating joint injury. These wounds should be operatively explored, and the patient should be treated with intravenous antibiotics.

D. Other infections

1. Tetanus—**A potentially lethal neuroparalytic disease caused by an exotoxin of *Clostridium tetani*.** Prophylaxis requires classifying the patient's wound (tetanus-prone or nontetanus-prone) and a complete history of the patient's immunizations. Tetanus-prone wounds are greater than 6 hours old; have an irregular configuration; have a depth greater than 1 cm or are the result of a projectile injury, crush injury, burn, or frostbite; have devitalized tissue; and are grossly contaminated. Patients with tetanus-prone wounds who have an unknown tetanus status or have received fewer than three immunizations require tetanus and diphtheria toxoids and tetanus immune globulin (human). Fully immunized patients with tetanus-prone wounds do not require immune globulin, but tetanus toxoid should be administered if the wound is severe or over 24 hours old or the patient has not received a booster within the past 5 years. The only type of patient with a nontetanus-prone wound who requires any treatment is one with an unknown immunization history or a history of fewer than three doses of tetanus immunization; these patients require tetanus toxoid. The treatment of established tetanus is primarily to control the patient's muscle spasms with diazepam. Initial antibiotic therapy includes penicillin G or doxycycline; alternative antibiotic therapy includes metronidazole.
2. Rabies—**An acute infection characterized by irritation of the CNS that may be followed by paralysis and death. The organism involved in rabies is a neurotropic virus that may be present in the saliva of rabid animals.** In dog or cat bites, healthy animals should be observed for 10 days; there is no need to start antirabies treatment. If the animal begins to experience symptoms, human rabies immune globulin with human diploid cell vaccine or rabies vaccine absorbed (inactivated) should be started. For bites from dogs and cats suspected or known to be rabid, vaccination of the patient should occur immediately. Bites from skunks, raccoons, bats, foxes, and most carnivores should be considered rabid, and the patient should be immunized immediately. Animals whose bites rarely require antirabies treatment include mice, rats, chipmunks, gerbils, guinea pigs, hamsters, squirrels, rabbits, and rodents.
3. Puncture wounds of the foot—**The most characteristic organism resulting from a puncture wound from a nail through the sole of an athletic shoe is *P. aeruginosa*** (unless the host is immunocompromised or diabetic). *Pseudomonas* infections (gram-negative rod) require aggressive débridement and appropriate antibiotics (often require a two-antibiotic regimen). The initial antibiotic regimen for an established infection should

include ceftazidime or cefepime; an alternative initial antibiotic regimen might include ciprofloxacin (except in children), imipenem, cilastatin, or a third-generation cephalosporin. The prophylactic antibiotic treatment for a recent (hours) puncture through the sole of an athletic shoe (without infection) remains controversial. **Osteomyelitis develops in 1-2% of children who sustain a puncture wound through the sole of an athletic shoe.**

4. Diabetic foot infections
   a. Limited in extent (no osteomyelitis, no previous history of foot infection)—The most common organism is aerobic gram-positive cocci. The antibiotic regimen of choice is clindamycin or a first-generation cephalosporin. Débridement of soft tissues is performed as clinically indicated.
   b. Chronic, recurrent, limb-threatening diabetic foot—These infections can be life threatening, **cultures** generally **show a polymicrobial picture** (including aerobic cocci, aerobic bacilli, and anaerobes). **In early cases or relatively milder cases** of a chronic, recurrent, limb-threatening diabetic foot, the initial antibiotic regimen can include ampicillin/sulbactam (Unasyn), piperacillin-tazobactam, ticarcillin/clavulanate (Timentin), or clindamycin plus one of the following: ceftriaxone/cefotaxime, ciprofloxacin, levofloxacin, or aztreonam. In cases of a **severe, chronic, recurrent, limb-threatening diabetic foot** or when the patient is septic, the antibiotic regimen of choice includes vancomycin plus one of the following: imipenem/cilastatin (Primaxin), meropenem, or trovafloxacin. Cultures from diabetic foot ulcers are unreliable. **Rapid surgical intervention with irrigation and débridement is essential.** Surgical débridement helps differentiate a diabetic foot from necrotizing fasciitis or gas gangrene.
5. Paronychia—Infection/inflammation of the paronychial fold on the side of the nail
   a. Nail biting and manicuring—The most common organism is *S. aureus;* anaerobes are also common. The initial antibiotic treatment includes clindamycin; erythromycin is an alternative initial antibiotic treatment.
   b. Dentists, anesthesiologists, wrestlers (those who are in contact with the oral mucosa of others)—The most common organism is herpes simplex (herpetic whitlow). Commonly presents with vesicles containing clear fluid. A Gram stain and routine cultures are negative. The treatment of choice is acyclovir; there is no need to débride the vesicles.
   c. Dishwashers or others who engage in activities that involve prolonged immersion in water—The most common organism is *Candida*, and the treatment is topical clotrimazole.
6. Fungal infections—Fungi are multicellular organisms with mycelia (branches) that induce a tissue hypersensitivity reaction, causing chronic granuloma, abscess, and necrosis. Surgical treatment and **amphotericin B** administration are often required. Oral ketoconazole is effective for some limited infections.
7. HIV infection
   a. Incidence—Incidence is high in the homosexual male population and is becoming increasingly common in heterosexual patients. Additionally, a large portion of the hemophiliac population is affected. HIV primarily affects the lymphocyte and macrophage cell lines and **decreases the number of T helper cells (formerly known as T4 lymphocytes but now known as CD4 cells).**
   b. Diagnosis—**The diagnosis of AIDS requires an HIV-positive test plus one of the following two scenarios: (1) one of the opportunistic infections (such as pneumocystis) or (2) a CD4 count of less than 200 (normal CD4 count = 700-1200).**
   c. Transmission—HIV has increased the importance of precautions for handling blood and body fluids during trauma management and surgery. The risk of seroconversion from a contaminated needle stick is 0.3% (increases if the exposure involves a larger amount of blood); the risk of seroconversion from mucous membrane exposure is 0.09%. The risk of HIV transmission via a large, frozen bone allograft is 1 in 1 million; **donor screening is the most important factor in preventing viral transmission. Blood donated for transfusion that tests negative for the HIV antibody may transmit HIV to the recipient because there is a delay (in the donor) between infection with HIV and development of a detectable antibody.** The risk of transmission of HIV via a blood transfusion is estimated to be 1 in 1,125,000 per unit transfused.
   d. Associated risks—HIV positivity is not a contraindication to performing required surgical procedures. Even if they are asymptomatic, HIV-positive patients with traumatic orthopaedic injuries (especially open fractures) or undergoing certain orthopaedic surgical procedures appear to be at increased risk for wound infections and non–wound-related complications (e.g., urinary tract infection, pneumonia). Patients with HIV can develop secondary rheumatologic conditions such as Reiter's syndrome. Fetal AIDS is transmitted across the placenta; affected children typically have a box-like forehead, wide eyes, a small head, and growth failure.
8. Hepatitis—Three types are commonly recognized.
   a. Hepatitis A—Common in areas with poor sanitation and public health concerns. Not a major problem regarding surgical transmission.
   b. Hepatitis B—Approximately 200,000 people are infected with the hepatitis B virus each year, and there are currently more than 12 million carriers in the United States and 350

million carriers worldwide. Screening and vaccination have reduced the risk of transmission for health care workers. Immune globulin is administered after exposure in nonvaccinated persons. Neither the vaccine nor immune globulin administration has been documented as causing HIV transmission.

c. Hepatitis C (non-A, non-B)—The offending virus has been identified (hepatitis C virus). Recent advances in screening methods have decreased the risk of hepatitis C as a cause of transfusion-associated hepatitis (1 in 1,935,000 transfusions). **Hepatitis C is also related to intravenous drug abuse. PCR is the most sensitive method for early detection of infection.**

9. Lyme disease—Discussed in the section on Arthroses. A Lyme disease vaccine, LYMErix (Recombinant OspA), is available for persons 15-70 years of age.
10. **Cat scratch fever (cat scratch disease)**—Infection of the lymphatic system by ***Bartonella henselae.*** The disease is transmitted via a wound inflicted by a cat. The patient presents with an erythematous, painful lymphadenitis. Treatment is with azithromycin; alternative treatment is supportive only (resolves in 2-6 months), with the use of needle aspiration of suppurative lymph nodes to relieve pain. **Do not perform incision and drainage on the lesions.**
11. Allograft infection—May involve up to 20% of allografts; requires aggressive measures to control.
12. Meningococcemia—Can develop in patients with multiple infarcts, such as those with **electrical burns.**
13. Marjolin's ulcer—Squamous cell carcinoma that develops in patients with chronic drainage from sinus tracts; seen in untreated chronic osteomyelitis.
14. Nutritional status and infection—Good nutrition decreases the incidence of postoperative infection. Malnutrition is common after multiple trauma.
15. Postsplenectomy patients—Susceptible to streptococcal infections and respond poorly to them.
16. Infections of the spine (discussed in Chapter 8, Spine)
    a. Diskitis—Children present with back pain and may have difficulty walking or sitting. Radiographs may appear normal; bone scans and MRI may show early changes. The initial treatment is immobilization and antibiotics. A biopsy is indicated if initial treatment fails.
    b. Vertebral osteomyelitis—Activity-related pain of insidious onset is the most common symptom. Neurologic signs are uncommon until late in the disease progression. Weight loss and chills are common. The lumbar spine is the most common site; diabetics are particularly prone. Both a bone scan and MRI are usually diagnostic. Recommended treatment is immobilization and antibiotics. Surgery (I&D and immediate spinal arthrodesis) is indicated if (1) nonoperative treatment fails or (2) vertebral collapse with a neurologic deficit occurs.
    c. Epidural abscess—The onset of symptoms may be rapid. There are often a history of recent trauma, generally markedly limited ROM to the lumbar spine, and a positive straight leg–raising test (indicating associated inflammation of the dura or nerve root sleeves). Bone scans are typically negative. MRI and contrast CT are excellent for imaging an epidural abscess. Antibiotics are generally ineffective, so surgical drainage is necessary.
    d. Postoperative spinal infections—Early diagnosis is difficult; clinical findings are often vague, and there are no excellent diagnostic tests. After spinal surgery, both the ESR and C-reactive protein peak at 2-3 days and may remain elevated for as long as 2 weeks. Fever spikes and a rising ESR indicate infection (blood cultures should be done). Treatment is with intravenous antibiotics, operative débridement, and retention of spinal implants.
    e. Other spinal infections—Pyogenic infections, tuberculous spondylitis, coccidioidomycosis spondylitis

II. Antibiotics

A. Introduction—Antibiotics in orthopaedics may be used in a variety of ways.

1. Prophylactic treatment—Used to prevent postoperative sepsis (for clean surgical cases, administer 1 hour preoperatively and continue for 24 hours postoperatively). Perioperative use of first-generation cephalosporins is efficacious in cases requiring hardware. **Using a shorter course of prophylactic antibiotics decreases the likelihood that bacteria will develop resistance.**
2. Initial care after an open traumatic wound—Types I and II open fractures require a first-generation cephalosporin (some authors have recently suggested the addition of an aminoglycoside or the use of a second-generation cephalosporin); type IIIA open fractures require a first-generation cephalosporin plus an aminoglycoside; penicillin is added for grossly contaminated (type IIIB) open fractures.
3. Treatment of established infections—Overall, *S. aureus* remains the leading cause of osteomyelitis and nongonococcal septic arthritis. In general, the virulence of *S. epidermidis* infections is closely related to orthopaedic hardware. **Clindamycin achieves the highest antibiotic concentrations in bone** (nearly equals serum concentrations after intravenous administration) **and is bacteriostatic.** To prevent the development of vancomycin-resistant strains, vancomycin should not be used in patients with a blood culture of coagulase-negative *S. aureus* that is not methicillin resistant.

B. Antibiotic-resistant bacteria—Two types of antibiotic resistance exist.

1. Intrinsic resistance—Inherent features of a cell that prevent antibiotics from acting on the cell (such as the absence of a metabolic pathway or enzyme). **MRSA has a gene (mecA) that produces penicillin-binding protein 2a (PBP2a), an enzyme that prevents the normal enzymatic acylation of antibiotics.**
2. Acquired resistance—A newly resistant strain emerges from a population that was previously sensitive (acquired resistance is mediated by plasmids [extrachromosomal genetic elements] and transposons).

C. Spectrum of antimicrobial agents (Box 1–3)
D. Antibiotic indications and side effects (Table 1–44)
E. Mechanism of action of antibiotics (Table 1–45)
F. Other forms of antibiotic delivery
1. Antibiotic beads or spacers—PMMA impregnated with antibiotics (usually an aminoglycoside); useful when treating infected TJA or osteomyelitis with bony defects. Antibiotic powder is mixed with cement powder; the antibiotic used is guided by the microorganism, and dosage depends on the selected antibiotic and type of PMMA. Antibiotics that have been used with

Box 1–3 Overview of Antimicrobial Agents

PENICILLINS

Natural

Penicillin G
Penicillin-VK

Penicillinase-Resistant (PRSP)

Methicillin (Staphcillin, Celbenin)
Nafcillin (Unipen, Nafcil)
Oxacillin (Prostaphlin, Bactocill)
Cloxacillin (Tegopen, Cloxapen)
Dicloxacillin (Dynapen, Pathocil)
Flucloxacillin (Floxapen, Ladropen, Staphcil)

Aminopenicillins

Ampicillin (Omnipen, Polycillin)
Amoxicillin (Amoxil)
Bacampicillin (Spectrobid)
Amoxicillin/clavulanate (Augmentin)
Ampicillin/sulbactam (Unasyn)
Antipseudomonal Agents
Indanyl carbenicillin (Geocillin)
Ticarcillin (Ticar)
Ticarcillin/clavulanate (Timentin)
Mezlocillin (Mezlin)
Piperacillin (Pipracil)
Piperacillin/tazobactam (Zosyn)

CEPHALOSPORINS

First Generation

Cephalothin (Keflin, Seffin)
Cefazolin (Ancef, Kefzol)
Cephapirin (Cefadyl)
Cephradine (Velosef)
Cephalexin (Keflex, Keftab)
Cefadroxil (Duricef, Ultracef)

Second Generation

Cefaclor (Ceclor)
Cefamandole (Mandol)
Cefoxitin (Mefoxin)
Cefuroxime (Zinacef, Kefurox)
Cefuroxime axetil (Ceftin)
Cefmetazole (Zefazone)
Cefotetan (Cefotan)
Cefprozil (Cefzil)
Cefonicid (Monocid)
Loracarbef (Lorabid)
Ceftibuten (Cedax)

Third Generation

Cefdinir (Omnicef)
Cefditoren pivoxil (Spectracef)
Cefetamet pivoxil (R. 15-8075)
Cefotaxime (Claforan)
Cefpodoxime proxetil (Vantin)
Cefoperazone (Cefobid, Claforan)
Ceftibuten (Cedax)
Ceftizoxime (Cefizox)
Ceftriaxone (Rocephin, Nitrocephin)
Ceftazidime (Fortaz, Tazicef, Tazidime)
Ceftriaxone (Rocephin)
Cefixime (Suprax)
Cefpodoxime proxetil (Vantin)

Fourth Generation

Cefpirome (HR 810)
Cefepime (Maxipime)

CARBAPENEMS

Ertapenem (Invanz)
Imipenem cilastatin (Primaxin)
Meropenem (Merrem)

MONOBACTAMS

Aztreonam (Azactam)

AMINOGLYCOSIDES

Amikacin (Amikin)
Gentamicin (Garamycin)
Kanamycin (Kantrex)
Neomycin
Netilmicin (Netromycin)
Tobramycin (Nebcin)

FLUOROQUINOLONES

Norfloxacin (Noroxin)
Ciprofloxacin (Cipro)
Ofloxacin (Floxin)
Enoxacin (Penetrex)
Gatifloxacin (Tequin)
Gemifloxacin (Factive)
Grepafloxacin (Raxar)
Lomefloxacin (Maxaquin)
Moxifloxacin (Avelox)
Pefloxacin
Levofloxacin (Levaquin)
Sparfloxacin (Zagam)
Trovafloxacin (Trovan)

Continued

Box 1–3 Overview of Antimicrobial Agents—cont'd

MACROLIDES, AZALIDES, LINCOSAMIDES, KETOLIDES

Azithromycin (Zithromax)
Clarithromycin (Biaxin)
Dirithromycin (Dynabac)
Erythromycin
Telithromycin (Ketek)
Clindamycin (Cleocin)

OTHER ANTIBACTERIAL AGENTS

Chloramphenicol (Chloromycetin)
Colistin
Dalbavancin
Daptomycin (Cubicin)
Linezolid (Zyvox)
Quinupristin/dalfopristin (Synercid)
Rifampin (Rifaclin, Rimactane)
Rifaximin (Xifaxan)
Tigecycline (Tygacil)
Vancomycin (Vancocin, Vancoled)
Teicoplanin (Targocid)
Doxycycline (Vibramycin)
Minocycline (Minocin)
Tetracycline (Terramycin)
Polymyxin B (Aerosporin)
Fusidic acid (Fucidin)
Fosfomycin (Monurol)
Sulfisoxazole (Gantrisin)
Trimethoprim/sulfamethoxazole (Bactrim, Septra)
Metronidazole (Flagyl)

ANTIFUNGAL AGENTS

Amphotericin B (Fungizone)
Fluconazole (Diflucan)
Flucytosine (Ancobon)
Ketoconazole (Nizoral)
Itraconazole (Sporanox)
Voriconazole
Capsofungin
Micafungin

ANTIMYCOBACTERIAL AGENTS

Amikacin (Amikin)
Capreomycin (Capastat)
Cycloserine (Seromycin)
Ethambutol (Myambutol)
Ethionamide
Isoniazid (INH [Nydrazid])
Pyrazinamide
Rifabutin (Mycobutin)
Rifampin (Rifadin)
Streptomycin
Thiacetazone

ANTIPARASITIC AGENTS

Albendazole (Zentel)
Atovaquone (Mepron)
Dapsone
Ivermectin (Stromectol)
Mefloquine (Lariam)
Nitrazoxanide (Alinia)
Proguanil (Paludrine)
Pentamidine (Pentam 300)
Pyrimethamine (Daraprim)
Praziquantel (Biltricide)
Quinine
Tinidazole

ANTIVIRAL AGENTS

Abacavir (Ziagen)
Acyclovir (Zovirax)
Adefovir (Hepsera)
Amantadine (Symmetrel)
Amprenvir (Agenerase)
Atazanavir (Reyataz)
Cidofovir (Vistide)
Delavirdine (Rescriptor)
Didanosine (Videx)
Efavirenz (Sustiva)
Emtricitabine (Emtriva)
Enfuvirtide (Fuzeon)
Entecavir (Baraclude)
Famciclovir (Famvir)
Fosamprenavir (Lexiva)
Foscarnet (Foscavir)
Ganciclovir (Cytovene)
Indinavir (Crixivan)
Lamivudine (Epivir, Epivir-HBV)
Lopinavir/ritonavir (Kaletra)
Nelfinavir (Viracept)
Nevirapine (Viramune)
Oseltamivir (Tamiflu)
Ribavirin (Virazole)
Rimantadine (Flumadine)
Ritonavir (Norvir)
Saquinavir (Invirase, Fortovase)
Stavudine (Zerit)
Tenofovir (Viread)
Tipranavir (Aptivus)
Valacyclovir (Valtrex)
Zalcitabine (Hivid)
Zidovudine [AZT (Retrovir)]

Adapted from Gilbert DN, Moellering RC, Eliopoulos GM, Sande MA: The Sanford Guide to Antimicrobial Therapy 2006, 36th ed, pp 59-81. Sperryville, VA, Antimicrobial Therapy, Inc., 2006.

PMMA for infection are tobramycin, gentamicin, cefazolin (Ancef) and other cephalosporins, oxacillin, cloxacillin, methicillin, lincomycin, clindamycin, colistin, fucidin, neomycin, kanamycin, and ampicillin. Chloramphenicol and tetracycline appear to be inactivated during polymerization. Antibiotics elute from PMMA beads, with an exponential decline over a 2-week period, and cease to be present locally in significant levels by 6-8 weeks. Much higher local tissue concentrations of antibiotic can be achieved than those obtained by systemic administration but do not seem to cause problems in the doses typically used. (Extremely high local concentrations of antibiotics can decrease cellular replication or even result in cell death.) Increased surface area of

TABLE 1-44 ANTIBIOTIC INDICATIONS AND SIDE EFFECTS

Antibiotics	Organisms	Complications/Other
Aminoglycosides	G–, PM	Auditory (most common) and vestibular toxicity is caused by destruction of the cochlear and vestibular sensory cells from drug accumulation in the perilymph and endolymph; renal toxicity; neuromuscular blockade
Amphotericin	Fung	Nephrotoxic
Aztreonam	G–, no anaerobes	
Carbenicillin/ticarcillin/piperacillin	Better against G–	Bleeding diathesis (carbenicillin)
Cephalosporins		
First generation	Prophylaxis (surgical)	Cephazolin is the drug of choice
Second generation	Some G+/G–	
Third generation	G–, fewer G+	Hemolytic anemia (bleeding diathesis [moxalactam])
Chloramphenicol	*Haemophilus influenzae*, anaerobes	Bone marrow aplasia
Ciprofloxacin	G–, methicillin-resistant *S. aureus*	Tendon ruptures; cartilage erosion in children; antacids reduce absorption of ciprofloxacin; theophylline increases serum concentrations of ciprofloxacin
Clindamycin	G+, anaerobes	Pseudomembranous enterocolitis
Erythromycin	G+ (PCN allergy)	Ototoxic
Imipenem	G+, some G–	Resistance, seizure
Methicillin/oxacillin/nafcillin	Penicillinase resistant	Same as penicillin; nephritis (methicillin); subcutaneous skin slough (nafcillin)
Penicillin	Strep, G+	Hypersensitivity/resistance; hemolytic
Polymyxin/nystatin	GU	Nephrotoxic
Sulfonamides	GU	Hemolytic anemia
Tetracycline	G+ (PCN allergy)	Stains teeth/bone (up to age 8)
Vancomycin	Methicillin-resistant *S. aureus, C. difficile*	Ototoxic; erythema with rapid IV delivery

G+, gram positive; G–, gram negative; GU, genitourinary; IV, intravenous; PM, polymicrobial; PCN, penicillin; Strep, streptococcus.

PMMA (e.g., with oval beads) enhances antibiotic elution. Beads are inserted only after thorough débridement.Because PMMA may cause a foreign body reaction, the beads should always be removed. Antibiotic powder in doses of 2 g/40 g of powdered PMMA (simplex P) does not appreciably affect the compressive strength of PMMA. Much higher concentrations (4-5 g antibiotic powder/40 g PMMA) significantly reduce the compressive strength (important in cemented joint arthroplasties). Antibiotic-impregnated cement spacers help prevent soft tissue contracture after removing an infected TKA.

2. Osmotic pump—Delivers high concentrations of antibiotics locally. Used mainly for osteomyelitis.
3. Home intravenous therapy—Cost-effective alternative for long-term intravenous antibiotics; facilitated by a Hickman or Broviac indwelling catheter.
4. Immersion solution—Contaminated bone from an open fracture may be sterilized (100% effective) by immersion in a chlorhexidine gluconate scrub and an antibiotic solution.

TABLE 1-45 MECHANISM OF ACTION OF ANTIBIOTICS

Class of Antibiotic	Examples	Mechanism of Action
β-lactam antibiotics	Penicillin Cephalosporins	Inhibits bacterial peptidoglycan synthesis (the mechanism is via binding to the penicillin-binding proteins on the surface of the bacterial cell membrane)
Aminoglycosides	Gentamicin Tobramycin	Inhibits protein synthesis (the mechanism is via binding to cytoplasmic ribosomal RNA)
Clindamycin and macrolides	Clindamycin Erythromycin Clarithromycin Azithromycin	Inhibit the dissociation of peptidyl-transfer RNA from ribosomes during translocation (the mechanism is via binding to 50S-ribosomal subunits)
Tetracyclines		Inhibit protein synthesis (on 70S and 80S ribosomes)
Glycopeptides	Vancomycin Teicoplanin	Interfere with the insertion of glycan subunits into the cell wall
Rifampin		Inhibits RNA synthesis in bacteria
Quinolones	Ciprofloxacin Levofloxacin Ofloxacin	Inhibit DNA gyrase
Oxazolidinones	Linezolid	Inhibits protein synthesis (blocks formation of the 70S ribosomal translation complex

SECTION 6 Perioperative Problems

I. Pulmonary Problems

A. General considerations—Pulmonary function tests and blood gas measurements are often helpful for evaluating baseline status. Thoracic and abdominal surgery can significantly affect these values.

B. Blood gas evaluation—The following simple working formula is useful for evaluating blood gases:

$$pO_2 = 7(FiO_2) - pCO_2$$

where pO_2 is the anticipated or normal pO_2 given FiO_2 in a normal person, FiO_2 is the percentage of inspired oxygen, and pCO_2 is the value obtained by the blood gas assay.

Example. A 63-year-old man has an acute onset of shortness of breath 12 hours after a THA. Assume that a blood gas assay obtained 15 minutes after placing the patient on 60% oxygen ($FiO_2 = 60$) reveals the following **observed values:**

$$pO_2 = 120$$

$$pCO_2 = 60$$

$$pO_2 = 7(60) - pCO_2 = 420 - pCO_2$$

With a pCO_2 of 60, the anticipated (normal) pO_2 would be

$$pO_2 = 420 - 60 = 360$$

Therefore, with 60% oxygen and a pCO_2 of 60, expected $pO_2 = 360$ if all were normal. The observed pO_2 (120) indicates an obvious problem with pulmonary status. To quantify the extent of the problem, calculate the **Aa gradient:**

$$\text{Aa gradient} = (\text{anticipated or normal } pO_2 \text{ [for a given } FiO_2\text{]}) - (\text{observed } pO_2)$$

Continuing with the example:

$$\text{Aa gradient} = (360) - (120) = 240$$

Finally, the **percent physiologic shunt** is calculated:

$$\text{Percent physiologic shunt} = \text{Aa gradient}/20$$

Continuing with the example:

$$\text{Percent physiologic shunt} = 240/20 = 12\%$$

C. Thromboembolism—Common in orthopaedic patients, especially those with procedures around the hip. Risk increases with a history of thromboembolism, obesity, malignancy, aging, congestive heart failure (CHF), use of a birth control pill, varicose veins, smoking, use of general anesthetics (in contrast with continuous epidural anesthesia), increased blood viscosity, immobilization, paralysis, and pregnancy.

1. Deep venous thrombosis (DVT)
   a. Diagnosis—Clinical suspicion is often more helpful than physical examination (pain, swelling, Homans sign) for DVT. Useful studies include **venography (the "gold standard"),** which is 97% accurate (70% for iliac veins); ^{125}I-labeled fibrinogen (operative-site artifact causes false positives); impedance plethysmography (poor sensitivity); duplex ultrasonography (B-mode)—90% accurate for DVT proximal to the trifurcation vessels; and Doppler imaging (immediate bedside tool, often best first study).
   b. Prophylaxis—Prophylaxis is the most important factor in decreasing morbidity and mortality; common methods are listed in Table 1–46. Because DVT is relatively uncommon after elective spinal surgery, only mechanical prophylaxis (such as compression stockings) is recommended; mechanical prophylaxis prevents venous stasis and increases the systemic release of endogenous fibrinolytic activity. **The anticoagulation effects of warfarin (Coumadin) result from the inhibition of hepatic enzymes, vitamin K epoxide, and perhaps vitamin K reductase. This inhibition results in decarboxylation of the vitamin K–dependent protein factors II (prothrombin), VII (the first to be affected), IX, and X. Warfarin does not directly bind vitamin K or the clotting factors but inhibits post-translational modification of vitamin K–dependent clotting factors. The anticoagulation effects of warfarin can be reversed with vitamin K or more rapidly with fresh-frozen plasma.** Rifampin **and phenobarbital** are antagonists to warfarin.
   c. Treatment—The diagnosis of DVT postoperatively requires initiation of heparin therapy (followed by later conversion to long-term [3 months] warfarin therapy). **Low-dose warfarin given to a patient with a DVT acts by interfering with the metabolism of factors II (prothrombin), VII, IX, and X.** Treatment is recommended for all thigh DVTs; however, treatment of DVTs occurring below the popliteal fossa is controversial. **Preoperative identification of a DVT in a patient with lower extremity or pelvic trauma is an indication for placement of a vena cava filter. Virchow's triad** of factors involved in venous thrombosis is venous stasis, hypercoagulability, and intimal injury. Thromboembolism formation is summarized in Figure 1–92.

TABLE 1-46 THROMBOEMBOLISM PROPHYLAXIS

Method	Effect	Advantages	Disadvantages
Heparin			
Intravenous	Coagulation cascade—antithrombin III inhibitor	Reversible, effective	Control, embolization
Subcutaneous	Antithrombin III inhibitor	Reversible	No effect in extremity surgery
Warfarin (Coumadin)*	Coagulation cascade—vitamin K–dependent clotting factors	Most effective, oral	3-5 days to full effect, control
Aspirin	Inhibits platelet aggregation; inhibits thromboxane A2 synthesis	Easy, no monitoring	Limited efficacy
Dextran	Dilutional	Effective	Fluid overload, bleeding
Pneumatic compression (and foot pumps)	Mechanical	Inexpensive, no bleeding	Bulky
Enoxaparin (Lovenox), a low-molecular-weight heparin	Inhibits clotting—forms complexes between antithrombin III and factors IIa and Xa	Fixed dose, no monitoring, improved bioavailability	Bleeding

See text for details.

2. Pulmonary embolism (PE)—PE should be suspected in postoperative patients with an acute onset of pleuritic pain, **tachypnea (90%),** and tachycardia (60%). Initial workup includes an ECG (right bundle branch block [RBBB], right axis deviation [RAD] in 25%; may also show ST depression or T wave inversion in lead III), a chest radiograph (hyperlucency rare), and arterial blood gases (ABGs) (normal pO_2 does not exclude PE). A nuclear medicine ventilation–perfusion scan may be helpful, but pulmonary angiography (the "gold standard") is required to make the diagnosis if there is any question. Once PE is diagnosed, heparin therapy (continuous intravenous infusion) is initiated and monitored by the partial thromboplastin time (PTT). More aggressive therapy (thrombolytic agents, vena cava filter, or other surgical measures) is required in select cases. Seven to 10 days of heparin therapy is followed by 3 months of oral warfarin (monitored by the prothrombin time [PT]). Approximately 700,000 people in the United States have an asymptomatic PE each year, of which 200,000 are fatal. The most important factor for survival is early diagnosis with prompt therapy initiation. The incidence of DVT and fatal PE in unprotected patients is summarized in Table 1–47.
3. Coagulation (Fig. 1–93)—A cascade of enzymatic reactions, beginning with prothrombin-converting activity and concluding with **fibrin** clot formation

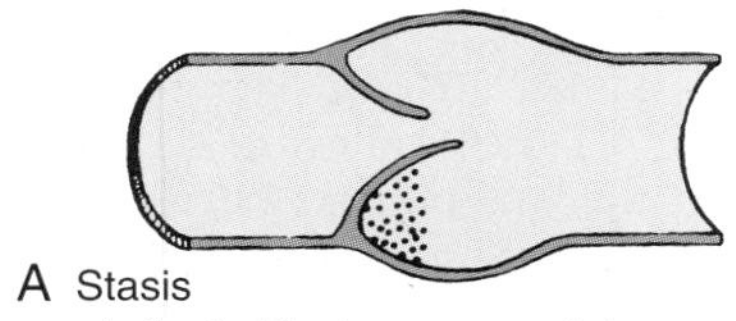

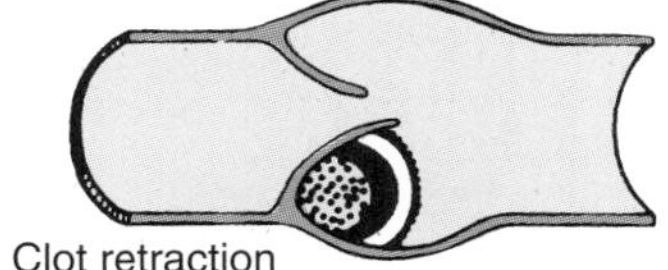

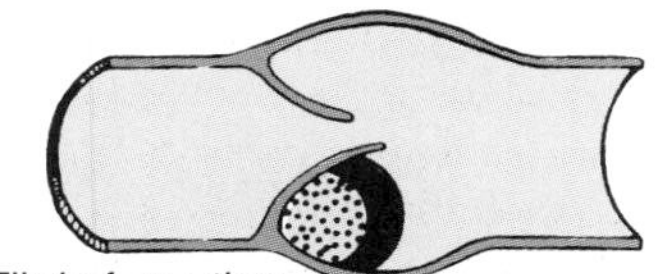

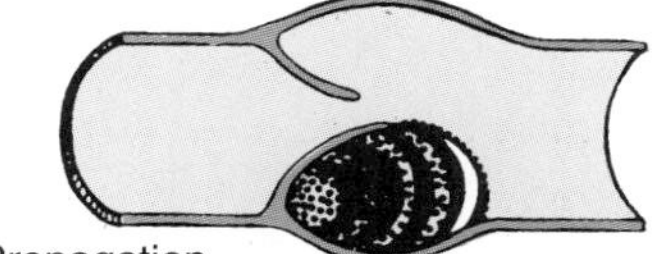

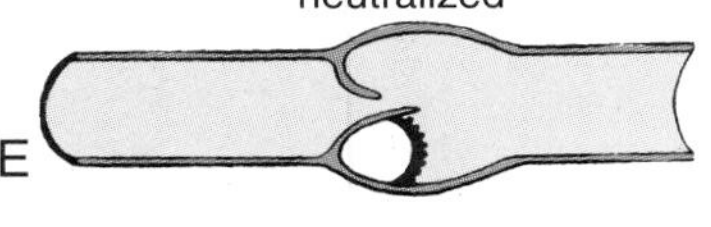

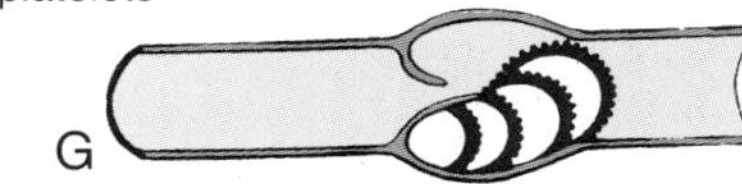

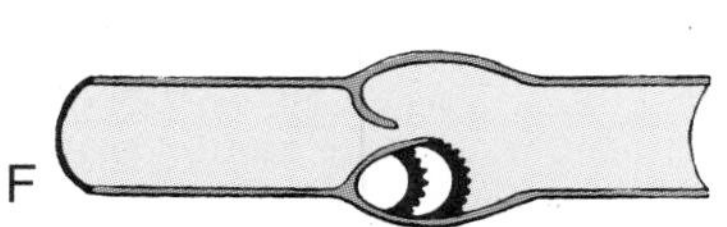

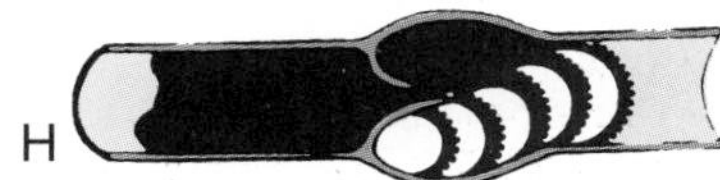

FIGURE 1–92 Venous thromboembolus formation. **A**, Stasis. **B**, Fibrin formation. **C**, Clot retraction. **D**, Propagation. **E** through **H**, This process continues until the vessel is effectively occluded. (From Simon SR, ed: Orthopaedic Basic Science, p 492. Rosemont, IL, American Academy of Orthopaedic Surgeons, 1994.)

TABLE 1-47 FREQUENCY OF DEEP VEIN THROMBOSIS AND FATAL PULMONARY EMBOLISM (DIAGNOSED BY VENOGRAPHY)

	Frequency (%)	
Unprotected Patients	*DVT*	*Fatal PE*
Elective hip arthroplasty	70	2
Elective knee arthroplasty	80	1
Open meniscectomy	20	?
Hip fracture	60	3.5
Spinal fracture with paralysis	100	~1
Polytrauma patients	35	?
Pelvic/acetabular fracture	20	?

From Simon SR: Orthopaedic Basic Science, p 489. Rosemont, IL, American Academy of Orthopaedic Surgeons, 1994.

(as fibrinogen is converted to fibrin). Two interconnecting pathways have been described.

a. Intrinsic pathway—Monitored by PTT. Activated when factor XII contacts the collagen of damaged vessels.
b. Extrinsic pathway—Monitored by PT. Activated by thromboplastin release into the circulation after cellular injury.
c. The **bleeding-time test measures platelet function**. The **fibrinolytic system** is responsible for dissolving clots. Plasminogen is converted to plasmin (with the help of tissue activators, factor XIIa, and thrombin); plasmin dissolves a fibrin clot.

D. Acute respiratory distress syndrome (ARDS)—Acute respiratory failure secondary to pulmonary edema after such events as trauma, shock, or infection. Causes of ARDS include pulmonary infection, sepsis, fat embolism, microembolism, aspiration, fluid overload, atelectasis, oxygen toxicity, pulmonary contusion, and head injury. Fluid overload, aspiration, and microscopic emboli may also contribute. Complement system activation leads to further progression. Signs include tachypnea, dyspnea, hypoxemia, and decreased lung compliance. **The clinical diagnosis of ARDS after a long-bone fracture is best made with the use of ABGs.** Normal supportive care is often unsuccessful; a 50% mortality rate is not uncommon. Ventilation with positive end-expiratory pressure (PEEP) is important; steroids have not been proven to be efficacious. Early stabilization of long-bone fractures (particularly the femur) decreases the risk of pulmonary complications.

E. Fat embolism (Fig. 1–94)—Usually seen 24-72 hours after trauma (3-4% of patients with long-bone fractures); fatal in 10-15% of cases. **Early skeletal stabilization decreases the incidence of clinically significant fat embolism** and is a key to prevention. **Onset may be heralded by hypoxemia ($PaO_2 < 60$ mm Hg), CNS depression, petechiae** (axillae, conjunctivae, palate), tachypnea, pulmonary edema, tachycardia, mental status changes, and confusion.

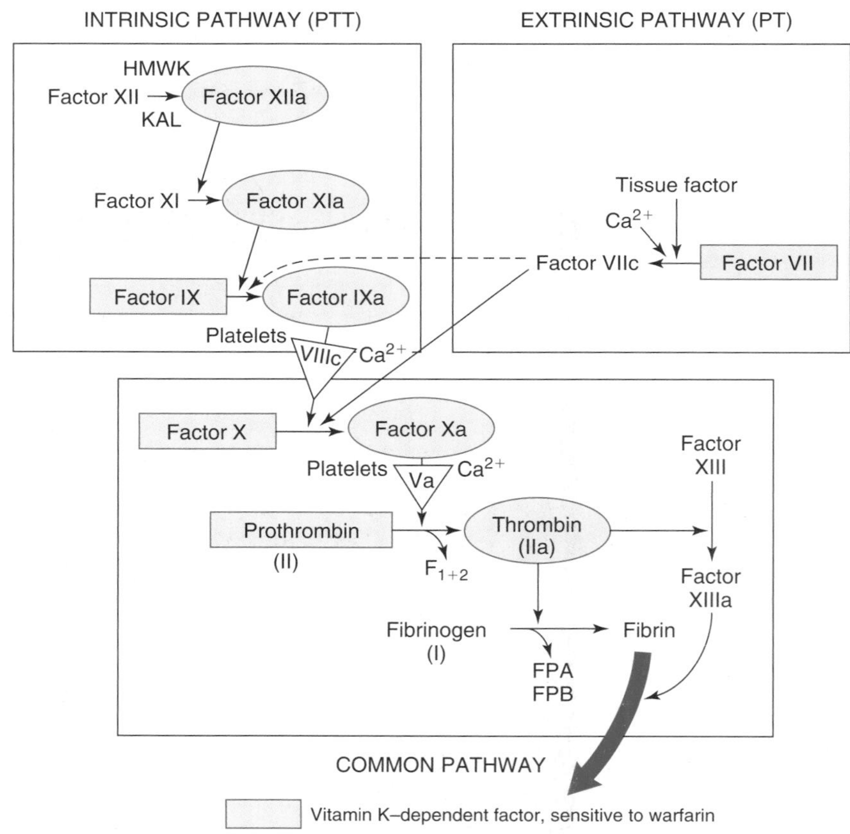

FIGURE 1–93 Coagulation cascade. (From Stead RB: Regulation of hemostasis. In Goldhaber SZ, ed: Pulmonary Embolism and Deep Venous Thromboembolism, p 32. Philadelphia, WB Saunders, 1985.)

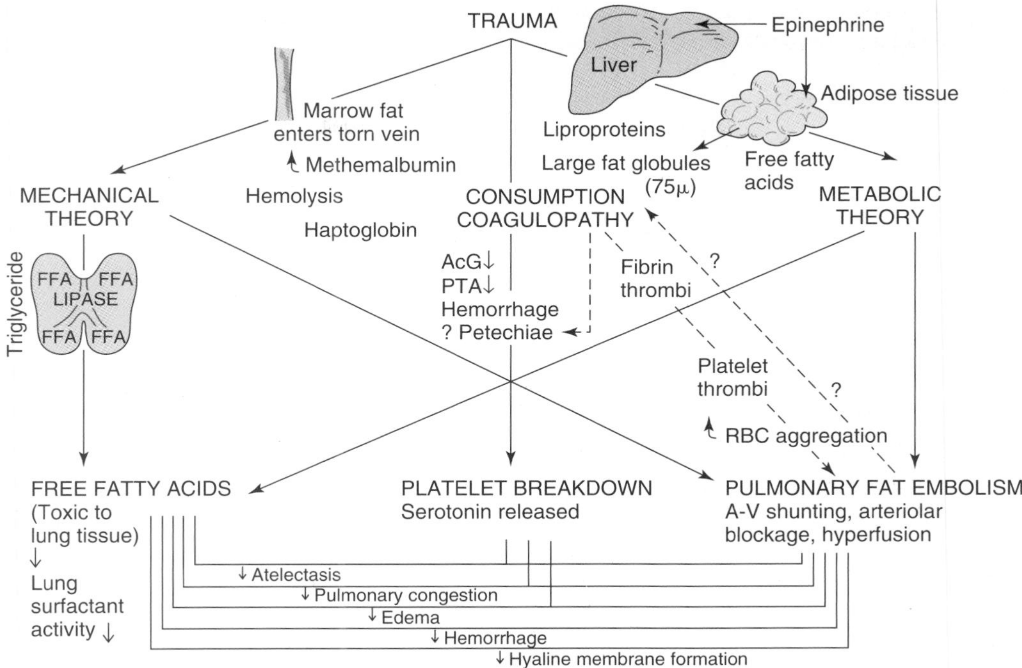

FIGURE 1–94 Pathologic events of fat embolism syndrome. (From Simon SR, ed: Orthopaedic Basic Science, p 502. Rosemont, IL, American Academy of Orthopaedic Surgeons, 1994.)

May be caused by bone marrow fat **(mechanical theory)**, chylomicron changes as a result of stress **(metabolic theory)**, or both. Metabolism to free fatty acids, initiation of the clotting cascade, pulmonary capillary leakage, bronchoconstriction, and alveolar collapse result in a **ventilation–perfusion deficit** (hypoxemia) consistent with ARDS. Treatment includes mechanical ventilation with **high levels of PEEP.** Steroids do not appear to have a prophylactic role. Over-reaming the femoral canal can decrease the incidence of fat embolism (embolization of marrow contents) during TKA. **Reamers that have a wider driver shaft increase the risk of fat emboli during femoral reaming.**

F. Pneumonia—Aspiration pneumonia can occur in patients with decreased mentation, supine positioning, and decreased GI motility. Simple measures (raising the head of the bed, using antacids and metoclopramide [Reglan]) can be preventive. Treated by appropriate intravenous antibiotics and pulmonary toilet.

G. Pulmonary complications of orthopaedic disorders—Scoliosis of significant magnitude can cause pulmonary dysfunction. Spontaneous pneumothorax is common in patients with Marfan's syndrome.

II. Other Medical Problems (Nonpulmonary)

A. Nutrition—Adequate nutrition should be ensured prior to elective surgery. Malnutrition may be present in 50% of patients on a surgical ward. Several indicators exist (e.g., anergy panels, albumin levels, transferrin level); the **measurement of arm muscle circumference is the best indicator of nutritional status.** Wound dehiscence and infection, pneumonia, and sepsis can result from poor nutrition. Lack of enteral feeding can lead to **atrophy of the intestinal mucosae, leading in turn to bacterial translocation.** Nutritional requirements are significantly elevated as a result of stress. Full enteral or parenteral nutrition (nitrogen 200 mg/kg per day) should be provided for patients who cannot tolerate normal intake. Early elemental feeding through a jejunostomy tube can decrease complications in the multiple-trauma patient. **Enteral protein supplements have proved effective in patients at risk of developing multiple organ system failure.** The metabolic changes of starvation and stress are compared in Table 1–48.

B. Myocardial infarction (MI)—Acute chest pain, radiation, and ECG changes are classic and warrant monitoring in an appropriate critical care environment, where cardiac enzymes and the ECG can be monitored on a continuing basis. Risk factors of MI include increased age, smoking, elevated cholesterol, hypertension, aortic stenosis, a history of coronary artery disease, and a variety of other factors.

C. GI complications—Can range from ileus (treated with nasogastric suction [NG tube] and antacids) to upper GI bleeding. Postoperative ileus is common in diabetics with neuropathy. Upper GI bleeding is more likely in patients with a history of ulcers, NSAID use, and smoking. Treatment includes lavage, antacids, and H_2-blockers. Vasopressin (left gastric artery) may be required for more serious cases. Ogilvie's syndrome, which includes cecal distention, can follow total joint replacement surgery. If the cecum is >10 cm on an abdominal flat plate radiograph, it must be decompressed (usually can be done colonoscopically).

D. Decubitus ulcers—Associated with advanced age, critical illness, and neurologic impairment. Common sites include the sacrum, heels, and

TABLE 1-48 METABOLIC CHANGES OF STARVATION AND STRESS

Metabolic Activity	Starvation		Stress	
	Early	*Late*	*Hypermetabolism*	*Multisystem*
Energy expenditure	↓	↓↓	↑↑	Organ failure
Mediator activation	None	None	++	++
Metabolic responsiveness	Intact	Intact	Abnormal	Abnormal
Primary fuel	CHO	KB	"Mixed" (no KB)	"Mixed" (no KB)
Hepatic gluconeogenesis	↓	↓	↑	↑ or ↓
Hepatic protein synthesis	↓	↓	↑	↑ or ↓
Whole-body protein catabolism	Slight ↑	Slight ↑	↑↑	↑↑↑
Urinary nitrogen excretion	Slight ↑	Slight ↑	↑↑	↑↑↑
Malnutrition	Slow	Slow	Rapid	Rapid

↓, decrease(d); ↑, increase(d); CHO, carbohydrate; KB, ketone bodies.
Adapted from Simon SR: Orthopaedic Basic Science, p 510. Rosemont, IL, American Academy of Orthopaedic Surgeons, 1994.

buttocks, which may be a source of infection and increased morbidity. Prevention with constant changing of position, special mattresses, and treatment of systemic illness and malnutrition is essential. Once established, débridement and sometimes soft tissue flaps are required for treatment.

E. Urinary tract infection (UTI)—Most common nosocomial infection (6-8%). Causes increased risk for joint sepsis after TJA (but may not be from direct seeding). Established UTIs should be adequately treated preoperatively. Perioperative catheterization (removed 24 hours postoperatively) may reduce the rate of postoperative UTI.

F. Prostatic hypertrophy—Causes postoperative urinary retention. If the history, physical examination (prostate), and urine flow studies (<17 mL/sec peak flow rate) are suggestive, urologic referral should be accomplished preoperatively.

G. Acute tubular necrosis—Can cause renal failure in trauma patients. Alkalization of urine is important during the early treatment of this disorder.

H. Genitourinary injury—NSAIDs can affect the kidney, and appropriate screening laboratories are required at regular intervals. A retrograde urethrogram best evaluates lower genitourinary injuries with displaced anterior pelvic fractures.

I. Shock—Capillary blood flow is insufficient for the perfusion of vital tissues and organs. There are four types of shock.
   1. Hypovolemic shock ("volume loss")—Decreased cardiac output (CO), increased peripheral vascular resistance (PVR), and venous constriction. The most reliable early clinical finding is tachycardia; a drop in systolic blood pressure is a late finding.
   2. Cardiogenic shock ("ineffective pumping")—Decreased CO, increased PVR, and venous dilation
   3. Vasogenic shock (PE or pericardial tamponade)—Arteriolar constriction and venous dilation
   4. Neurogenic shock/septic shock ("blood pooling")—Arteriolar, capillary, and venous dilation

J. Compartment syndrome—Covered in detail in Chapter 11, Trauma. (This subject matter is always tested heavily. Questions regarding the foot and thigh seem popular.)

K. Frostbite
   1. Superficial—Treat with general rewarming of the entire body plus immersion of the hands or feet in a warm-water bath (104°F, 40°C) for 15 to 30 minutes. Splinting, tetanus prophylaxis, analgesics, and antibiotics may also be indicated. Severe swelling may occur upon rewarming; monitor for compartment syndromes.
   2. Deep—Débridement is often necessary

L. **Wound healing—Adequate healing following surgery is promoted by**
   1. **Transcutaneous oxygen tension >30 mm Hg**
   2. **Ischemic index (such as the ankle-brachial systolic index) ≥0.45**
   3. Albumin >30 g/dL
   4. Total lymphocyte count of 1500/mm^3

M. **Anemia**—Physiologic effects include increased heart rate, increased cardiac output, increased coronary blood flow demand, decreased peripheral resistance, and decreased blood viscosity.

III. Intraoperative Considerations

A. Anesthesia
   1. Benefits—Regional anesthesia may (there is disagreement in the literature) allow quicker recovery, decreased blood loss, and fewer postoperative complications, including reduced blood loss and incidence of DVT/PE in THA patients. Controlled hypotension during surgery helps with blood loss and is a widely accepted technique, especially with THA and spinal arthrodesis (nitroprusside, nitroglycerine, and isoflurane are all effective). Patient positioning on a kneeling frame for spinal surgery decreases (1) intra-abdominal pressure, (2) pressure on the inferior vena cava, (3) pressure on the vertebral venous system, and (4) blood loss. Transient intraoperative decreases in blood pressure with PMMA insertion are well known. The use of the fiber-optic bronchoscope has benefited surgery on RA patients and others with cervical spine abnormalities. The use of local anesthetics for arthroscopy has also gained popularity.
   2. Drawbacks—**Malignant hyperthermia,** an autosomal dominant, hypermetabolic disorder of skeletal muscle, can be triggered by the use of

various anesthetics (especially halothane and succinylcholine) in susceptible patients (e.g., those with neuromuscular disorders). The disorder involves impaired function of the sarcoplasmic reticulum and calcium homeostasis. Patients with Duchenne's muscular dystrophy, arthrogryposis, and osteogenesis imperfecta are especially at risk. Cell membrane defects affect calcium transport, leading to muscle rigidity and hypermetabolism. Masseter muscle spasm, increased temperature, rigidity, and acidosis are the hallmarks of the disease. Early diagnosis and treatment with **dantrolene sodium (blocks calcium release by stabilizing the sarcoplasmic reticulum while permitting uptake of calcium and thus decreasing the intracellular concentration of calcium),** balancing of electrolytes, increasing urinary output, respiratory support, and cooling are essential. The **most accurate method for diagnosing malignant hyperthermia is muscle biopsy** (in vitro muscle fiber testing).

B. Spinal cord monitoring—Usually involves testing the posterior column, but monitoring of other areas is under investigation. Electrical monitoring includes the use of somatosensory cortical evoked potentials (SCEPs) to record summed input from stimulation of peripheral areas. Somatosensory spinal evoked potentials (SSEPs) are more invasive but can be more sensitive. Preoperative recordings are compared with readings (especially latency and amplitude) at critical times during the procedure. The (Stagnara) wake-up test is still the standard for monitoring and relies on the lightening of anesthesia and the patient moving selected extremities upon command.

C. Tourniquet—Can injure the nerves and muscles directly underneath the tourniquet; EMG abnormalities may occur in 70% of patients after routine surgery with the use of a tourniquet. Careful application, wide cuffs, lower pressures (200 mm Hg in the upper extremity and 250 mm Hg in the lower extremity [or 100-150 mm Hg above systolic blood pressure in the lower extremity]), and double cuffs help avoid these problems. Equilibrium can be re-established within 5 minutes after 90 minutes of tourniquet application but requires 15 minutes after the use of a tourniquet for 3 hours.

IV. Other Problems

A. Pain control—Acute pain implies the presence of potential tissue damage; chronic pain (3-6 months) does not. Nociceptors transduce stimuli through substances, allowing transmission along peripheral nerves (types A and C fibers) to the dorsal column, spinothalamic tract, and thalamus. Modulation occurs via brainstem centers and endogenous opiates. Postoperative pain control can be targeted at any step. Local prostaglandin inhibitors and long-acting local anesthetics target transduction of pain. Perispinal opiates affect modulation, and systemic opiates affect the perception and modulation of pain.

1. Local anesthetics—Result in a transient and reversible loss of sensation that is confined to a particular area. **Local anesthetics achieve their effects by interfering with nerve conduction.** Specifically, these agents interfere with the rate of rise of the depolarization phase of the action potential; cells fail to depolarize enough to fire after excitation, and the action potential is blocked. Examples of local anesthetics include
   a. Amides—Lidocaine (Xylocaine), bupivacaine (Marcaine), and others
   b. Esters of *p*-aminobenzoic acid—Procaine (Novocain), butethamine (Monocaine), and others
   c. Esters of meta-aminobenzoic acid—Cyclomethycaine (Surfacaine) and metabutoxycaine (Primacaine)
   d. Esters of benzoic acid—Cocaine, ethyl aminobenzoate (Benzocaine), and others
2. NSAIDs—Produce their anti-inflammatory, antipyretic, analgesic, and antiplatelet effects by inhibiting the synthesis and release of prostaglandins. **These drugs inhibit the enzyme cyclooxygenase (COX).** COX catalyzes the synthesis of cyclic endoperoxides, which are important in the formation of prostaglandins from arachidonic acid. Acetaminophen does not affect COX activity; it is an antipyretic analgesic drug that inhibits an IL-1β–dependent translocation, which in turn inhibits prostaglandin production.
   a. COX inhibitors—Two isoforms of COX have been identified (COX-1 and COX-2). In general, the acronym "NSAID" (and thus the entity it denotes) refers to an agent that inhibits both COX-1 and COX-2. Examples of NSAIDs include salicylates (such as aspirin), salicylate-like anti-inflammatory agents (such as ibuprofen), and analgesic combinations and mixtures (such as codeine plus aspirin). Several mechanisms exist by which NSAIDs inhibit COX, three of which are provided here: (1) Aspirin binds with a serine residue of COX, which results in irreversible steric hindrance of the active site; (2) ibuprofen is a reversible competitive inhibitor of COX; and (3) indomethacin acts at the lipoxygenase side of the arachidonic metabolism pathway, which results in inhibition of leukotriene inflammatory mediators.
   b. COX-2 specific inhibitors—One of the major benefits of COX-2 specific inhibitors is that they do not inhibit the beneficial functions of COX-1 (**maintaining gastric mucosa,** regulating renal blood flow, influencing platelet aggregation). COX-2 specific inhibitors can be used in the perioperative period because they do not affect platelet function. At the time of writing (2007), celecoxib (Celebrex) is the only COX-2 inhibitor available in the United States, and it carries a label warning

about increased risk of cardiovascular events. COX inhibitors may delay or inhibit fracture healing, although COX-2 specific inhibitors do so to a lesser extent.

3. Substance P—A sensory neurotransmitter that plays an important role in pain. Capsaicin (pepper cream, obtained from red pepper) is believed to produce analgesia via neuropeptide depletion in unmyelinated C fibers (and depletion of substance P from the spinal cord, which elevates the threshold to painful stimuli).

B. Transfusion—Because of the possibility of disease transmission, this has become an important issue.

1. Transfusion reactions—Include allergic, febrile, and hemolytic reactions
   a. Allergic reaction—Most common; occurs toward the end of transfusion and usually subsides spontaneously. Symptoms include chills, pruritus, erythema, and urticaria. Pretreatment with diphenhydramine (Benadryl) and hydrocortisone may be appropriate in patients with a history of allergic reactions.
   b. Febrile reaction—Also common; occurs after the initial 100-300 mL of packed RBCs have been transfused. Chills and fever are caused by antibodies to foreign WBCs. Treatment consists of stopping the transfusion and giving antipyretics, as for an allergic reaction.
   c. Hemolytic reaction—Less common but most serious. It occurs early in the transfusion, with symptoms that include chills, fever, tachycardia, chest tightness, and flank pain. Treatment comprises stopping the transfusion, administering intravenous fluids, performing appropriate laboratory studies, and monitoring the patient in an intensive care setting.
2. Transfusion risks—Include transmission of hepatitis (C [1 in 1,935,000 per unit transfused], B [1 in 205,000 per unit transfused]), cytomegalovirus (highest incidence, since over 70% of donors are positive, but not clinically important), human T-cell lymphotropic virus (HTLV-1) (1 in 2,993,000 per unit transfused), and HIV (1 in 1,125,000 per unit transfused). Donor deferral for high-risk persons and more effective screening methods are helping to manage these risks.
3. Alternatives to homologous (blood bank) blood transfusion (Table 1–49)

TABLE 1-49 ALTERNATIVES TO HOMOLOGOUS (BLOOD BANK) BLOOD TRANSFUSION

Type	Procedure	Notes
Autologous deposition	Requires a hemoglobin level of ~11 (and a hematocrit level of 33%) and some lead time Iron supplementation during donation is routine.	Allows storage of several units of blood prior to elective procedures, with significant blood loss anticipated Significant cardiac disease, such as unstable angina, is a contraindication. About 20% of THA patients who donate 2 units of autologous blood require a homologous (from another donor) blood transfusion. Significantly reduces hepatitis C risk Autologous blood that tests positive for hepatitis can be reinfused but requires warning labels and special handling and storage. **Autologous donation is not recommended unless the risk of transfusion is greater than 10%.**
"Cell saver"	Intraoperative autotransfusion	Usually requires 400 mL of blood loss to recover 1 unit (250 mL) Can be used for only 4 hours at one time
Autotransfusion	Allows postoperative drain recuperation and use	Reinfusion should begin within 6 hours of the beginning of collection to reduce febrile reaction risk.
Acute preoperative normovolemic hemodilution	Immediate preoperative storage of autologous blood for intra-/postoperative use	Replace withdrawn autologous blood with crystalloid.
Pharmacologic intervention	Desmopressin (antidiuretic hormone [ADH] analogue that increases levels of plasma factor VIII) Recombinant erythropoietin (stimulates erythrogenesis) Synthetic erythrocyte substitutes	
Judicious use of blood products	Platelet transfusion for massive bleeding or coagulopathies Fresh-frozen plasma is reserved for patients with massive bleeding and significantly abnormal coagulation tests Cryoprecipitate is used for hemophilia (less exposure than factor concentrates) and as a source of fibrinogen for consumptive coagulopathies	Platelet transfusion is based on clinical parameters rather than set platelet thresholds

C. Heterotopic ossification—See section above on Bone Injury and Repair and Chapter 5, Adult Reconstruction. Seen most commonly following THA, in head-injured patients, and in those with elbow injuries. **Indomethacin** is effective for prophylaxis in patients undergoing THA. Single-fraction, low-dose radiation therapy is recommended as prophylaxis for THA patients at high risk for HO. **Diphosphonates** do not prevent formation of an osteoid matrix; after discontinuation of medication, the matrix calcifies, and therefore diphosphonates are not good for prophylaxis. Etidronate sodium inhibits bone resorption at low doses and bone mineralization at high doses.

D. Corticosteroid injections—The most common complications of intra-articular or extra-articular injection of corticosteroids are subcutaneous fat atrophy and skin pigment changes.

SECTION 7 Imaging and Special Studies

I. Nuclear Medicine

A. Bone scan—Technetium-99m phosphate complexes reflect increased blood flow and metabolism and are absorbed onto the hydroxyapatite crystals of bone in areas of infection, trauma, and neoplasia, among others. Whole-body views and more detailed (pinhole) views can be obtained.

1. Uses—It is particularly useful for the diagnosis of subtle fractures, avascular necrosis (hypoperfused [diminished blood flow] early, increased uptake during the reparative phase), osteomyelitis (especially when a triple-phase study is performed or in conjunction with a gallium or indium scan), THA and TKA loosening (especially femoral components; a technetium scan can be used in conjunction with a gallium scan to rule out concurrent infection), and patellofemoral overload. A technetium scan is a useful means of evaluating a patient for osteochondritis dissecans of the talus.
2. Phase studies—Three-phase (or even four-phase) studies may be helpful for evaluating diseases such as reflex sympathetic dystrophy and osteomyelitis. A triple-phase bone scan is the most reliable test for assessing whether a nondisplaced scaphoid fracture exists.
   a. **First phase (blood flow, immediate)**—Displays blood flow through the arterial system.
   b. **Second phase (blood pool, 30 minutes)**—Displays equilibrium of tracer throughout the intravascular volume.
   c. **Third phase (delayed, 4 hours)**—Displays the sites at which the tracer accumulates. Delayed-phase scans may be negative in pediatric septic arthritis.

B. Gallium scan—**Gallium-67 citrate localizes in sites of inflammation and neoplasia, probably because of exudation of labeled serum proteins.** Requires delayed imaging (24-48 hours or more). Frequently used in conjunction with a bone scan—a "double-tracer" technique. Gallium is less dependent on vascular flow than technetium and may identify foci that would otherwise be missed. It is difficult to differentiate cellulitis from osteomyelitis on a gallium scan.

C. Indium scan—Indium-111–labeled WBCs (leukocytes) accumulate in areas of inflammation and do not collect in areas of neoplasia. Useful for evaluation of acute infections (such as osteomyelitis) and possibly TJA infections.

D. Technetium-labeled WBC scan—Similar to indium scan.

E. Radiolabeled monoclonal antibodies—May have a role in identifying primary malignancies and metastatic disease.

F. Other studies

1. Bone mineral analysis—Single-photon absorptiometry (usually of the distal radius and cortical bone; has limited utility) and dual-photon absorptiometry (vertebral bodies and femoral neck). (For further details see section on Measurement of Bone Density.)
2. DVT/PE scan—Radioactive iodine-labeled fibrinogen accumulates in clot and shows up on scanning; is inaccurate in areas of surgical wounds. Radioisotope lung scans may help in evaluating pulmonary blood flow but is also limited at present.
3. Single-photon emission computed tomography (SPECT)—Uses scintigraphy and CT to evaluate overlapping structures. Femoral head osteonecrosis, patellofemoral syndrome, and healing of spondylolytic defects have been evaluated with SPECT.

II. Arthrography (Table 1–50)

III. Magnetic Resonance Imaging

A. Introduction—Excellent study to evaluate soft tissues and bone marrow; MRI is not effective for the evaluation of trabecular bone and cortical bone (because these tissues have virtually no hydrogen nuclei and therefore generate no signal). MRI is frequently used to evaluate osteonecrosis, neoplasms, infection, and trauma. Allows both axial and sagittal representations. Contraindications: pacemakers, cerebral aneurysm clips, or shrapnel or hardware in certain locations.

B. Basic principles of MRI (Tables 1–51 through 1-53)—MRI uses radio frequency pulses on tissues in a magnetic field and displays images in any desired plane without the use of ionizing radiation. MRI aligns nuclei that have odd numbers of protons/

TABLE 1-50 ARTHROGRAPHY

Anatomic Location	Conditions	Description
Shoulder		Technique can be single or double contrast (better detail).
	Rotator cuff tear	Extravasation of contrast through the tear into the subacromial bursa
	Adhesive capsulitis	Demonstrates diminished joint capsule size and loss of the normal axillary fold May be therapeutic (distends the capsule)
	Recurrent dislocations	May demonstrate a distended capsule or disruption of the glenoid labrum Use with tomography or computed tomography (CT) to better demonstrate capsular or labral pathology.
	Other	Bicipital tendon abnormalities Articular pathology Impingement syndrome
Elbow	Articular cartilage defects/loose bodies Osteochondral fractures	Especially helpful when used with tomography
Wrist	Post-traumatic ligament disruption	Digital subtraction techniques are helpful in this area Communication between compartments is used to determine pathology, but remember that communication is common in asymptomatic patients >40 years Communication at the radiocarpal and midcarpal joints—suspect S-L or L-T ligament tear Communication at the radiocarpal and distal radioulnar joints—suspect a triangular fibrocartilage complex (TFCC) tear
Hip		
Infants and children	"Septic" hip	Obtain aspirate and assess joint damage
	Developmental dysplasia of the hip	Degree of joint incongruity—interposed limbus
	Legg-Calvé-Perthes disease	Severity of deformity
Adolescents and adults	Arthritis	Cartilage destruction and loose bodies
	Osteochondral fractures, chondrolysis, and THA loosening	Digital subtraction arthrography can be useful for suspected loose THAs
Knee	Meniscal tears (except posterior horn of the lateral meniscus) and discoid lateral menisci	Can be useful for screening patients with an equivocal history or findings Evaluation of cruciate ligaments is less accurate than evaluation of the menisci
	Articular cartilage evaluation	
	Loose bodies	Only air contrast is recommended for evaluation of loose bodies.
	Pathologic synovial tissue	PVNS, popliteal cysts, synovial chondromatosis, plicae
Ankle	Acutely torn ligaments Chronic osseous and osteocartilaginous abnormalities	
Spine	Facet joints	May be useful combined with therapeutic injections (anesthetics and steroids)

neutrons (with a normally random spin) parallel to a magnetic field. Most MRI magnets have a strength of 0.5-15 Tesla (1 Tesla = 10,000 Gauss). Radio frequency pulses deflect the nuclear magnetic moments of these particles, resulting in an image. The use of surface coils decreases the signal-to-noise ratio. Body coils are used for large joints; smaller coils are available for other studies. Sequences have been developed to demonstrate the differences in T_1 and T_2 relaxation between tissues. **T_1 images are weighted toward fat; T_2 images are weighted toward water.** Typically, T_1-weighted images have TR (time to repetition) values <1000, and T_2-weighted images have TR values >1000. Water, cerebrospinal fluid (CSF), acute hemorrhage, and soft tissue tumors appear dark on T_1 studies and bright

TABLE 1-51 MAGNETIC RESONANCE IMAGING (MRI) TERMINOLOGY

Term	Explanation
T1	Time constant of exponential growth of magnetism; T1 measures how rapidly a tissue gains magnetism (see Table 1–55)
T2	Time constant of exponential decay of signal after an excitation pulse; a tissue with a long T2 (such as that with a high water content) maintains its signal (is bright on T2-weighted image) (see Table 1–55)
T2*	Similar to T2 but includes the effects of magnetic field homogeneity
TR	Time to repetition; the time between successive excitation pulses; short TR is less than 80, long TR is greater than 80
TE	Time to echo; the time that an echo is formed by the refocusing pulse; short TE is less than 1000, long TE is greater than 1000
NEX	Number of excitations; higher NEX results in decreased noise with better images
FOV	Field of view
Spin-echo	A commonly used pulse sequence in MRI
FSE	Fast spin-echo; a type of pulse sequence
GRE	Gradient-recalled echo; a type of pulse sequence

TABLE 1-52 MAGNETIC RESONANCE IMAGING SIGNAL INTENSITIES

Tissue	Appearance on T1-Weighted Image	Appearance on T2-Weighted Image
Cortical bone	Dark	Dark
Osteomyelitis	Dark	Bright
Ligaments	Dark	Dark
Fibrocartilage	Dark	Dark
Hyaline cartilage	Gray	Gray
Meniscus	Dark	Dark
Meniscal tear	Bright	Gray
Yellow bone marrow (fatty-appendicular)	Bright	Gray
Red bone marrow (hematopoietic-axial)	Gray	Gray
Marrow edema	Dark	Bright
Fat	Bright	Gray
Normal fluid	Dark	Bright
Abnormal fluid (pus)	Gray	Bright
Acute blood collection	Gray	Dark
Chronic blood collection	Bright	Bright
Muscle	Gray	Gray
Tendon	Dark	Dark
Intervertebral disc (central)	Gray	Bright
Intervertebral disc (peripheral)	Dark	Gray

Modified from Brinker MR, Miller MD: Fundamentals of Orthopaedics, p 24. Philadelphia, WB Saunders, 1999.

on T_2 studies. Other tissues remain basically the same intensity on both images. Cortical bone, rapidly flowing blood, and fibrous tissue are all dark; muscle and hyaline cartilage are gray; and fatty tissue, nerves, slowly flowing (venous) blood, and bone marrow are bright. **T_1 images best demonstrate anatomic structure (high signal-to-noise ratio),** whereas T_2 images are best for contrasting normal and abnormal tissues. When tendon or ligament tissue is oriented near 55 degrees to the magnetic field, T1-weighted images may appear to have increased signal (brightness), thus creating a false appearance of pathology; this is called the "**magic angle phenomena**" and occurs most commonly in the shoulder, ankle, and knee. Contrast between fluid and nonfluid (bone, fat, etc.) is best demonstrated using STIR (spin tau inversion recovery) or fat-suppressed T_2-weighted images.

TABLE 1-53 IMAGING OF BONE MARROW DISORDERS

Disorder	Pathology	Examples	MRI Changes
Reconversion	Yellow→red	Anemia, metastasis	↓ T1 image
Marrow infiltration		Tumor, infection	↓ T1 image
Myeloid depletion		Anemia, chemotherapy	↓ T1 image
Marrow edema		Trauma, RSD	↓ T1, ↑ T2 images
Marrow ischemia		Osteonecrosis	↓ T1 image

↑, increased; ↓, decreased; MRI, magnetic resonance imaging; RSD, reflex sympathetic dystrophy.

C. Specific applications of MRI

1. Osteonecrosis—**MRI is the method with the highest sensitivity and specificity for early detection of ON** (detects early marrow necrosis and ingrowth of vascularized mesenchymal tissue). MRI is highly specific (98%) and reliable for estimating the age and extent of disease. T_1 images demonstrate diseased marrow as dark MRI allows direct assessment of overlying cartilage.
2. Infection and trauma—MRI has excellent sensitivity to increases in free water and demonstrates areas of infection and fresh hemorrhage (dark on T_1 and bright on T_2 studies). **MRI is an excellent (accurate and sensitive) method of evaluating patients for occult fractures (particularly in the elderly hip).**
3. Neoplasms—MRI has many applications in the study of primary and metastatic bone tumors. Primary tumors, particularly soft tissue components (extraosseous and marrow), are well demonstrated on MRI. Although nuclear medicine studies remain the procedure of choice for seeking metastatic foci in bone, MRI has a role in evaluating patients for skip lesions and spinal metastases. Benign, bony tumors are typically bright on T_1 images and dark on T_2 images. Malignant, bony lesions are often bright on T_2 images. Differential diagnosis, however, is best made based on plain films.
4. Spine—Disc disease is well demonstrated on T_2 images. Degenerated discs lose water content and become dark on T_2-weighted studies; the extent of herniated discs is also well shown. **Recurrent disc herniation is best diagnosed via an MRI scan with gadolinium** and can be differentiated from scar based on the following characteristics. On T_1 image: scar, decreased signal; free fragment, increased signal; extruded disc, decreased signal; on T_2 image: scar, increased signal; free fragment, increased signal; extruded disc, and decreased signal. Gadolinium–diethylenetriamine pentaacetic acid (DTPA) can also be used to differentiate a scar from a disc by enhancing edematous structures in T_1 images. MRI is the best (most sensitive) study for diagnosing early diskitis (decreased signal on T_1 and increased signal on T_2). **Recent studies have shown the following regarding MRI findings of the spine in asymptomatic persons:** (1) 28% of subjects over 40 years of age have an abnormality of the cervical spine on MRI, (2) 20-30% of subjects under 40 years of age show evidence of a lumbar disc herniation on MRI, and (3) 93% of subjects over 60 years of age show evidence of degeneration or bulging of one or more lumbar discs on MRI. Biochemical studies have shown that degenerative disc changes occur as early as the second decade of life.
5. Bone marrow changes—Best demonstrated by MRI (but nonspecific). Five groups of disorders have been described and are shown in Table 1–53.

6. Knee MRI—Arthrography with MRI can be accomplished with instillation of saline, creating an iatrogenic effusion. This technique can improve joint definition. Knee derangements are well demonstrated on MRI. ACL rupture is correctly diagnosed in 95% of cases.Meniscal pathology has been classified into four groups of myxoid changes (Lotysch) (Table 1–54). **MRI is the best radiologic test to demonstrate a posterior cruciate ligament (PCL) rupture** (physical examination is probably the best test overall).
7. Shoulder MRI
   a. Rotator cuff tears—Results are improving with use (sensitivity and specificity are about 90%). Grade 0 tears show a normal signal, and grades 1, 2, and 3 tears show an increased signal. The morphology of grades 0 and 1 tears is normal, grade 2 tears show abnormal morphology, and grade 3 tears show discontinuity.
   b. Capsular/labral tears—MRI is equal to CT arthrography in the presence of an effusion.
8. MRI spectroscopy—May help with the measurement of metabolic changes (especially ischemic changes).

IV. Other Imaging Studies

A. CT—Continues to be important for evaluating many orthopaedic areas. Hounsfield units are used to identify tissue types (−100 = air, −100 to 0 = fat, 0 = water, 100 = soft tissue, 1000 = bone). **Compared with the original CT technology, multiple-detector row arrays in the latest generation of CT have improved resolution in the longitudinal axis, decreased data acquisition times, improved spatial resolution and the quality of reconstructing algorithms, and reduced artifact due to hardware.** CT demonstrates details of bony anatomy better than any other study. It also shows herniated nucleus pulposus better than myelography alone and may be helpful in differentiating recurrent disc herniation from scar (like MRI). Intravenous contrast material is taken up in scar but not disc tissue. CT is frequently used in conjunction with contrast (e.g., arthrographic CT, myelographic CT). Sagittal and three-dimensional reconstruction techniques may expand its indications. Cine CT (and MRI) may be helpful for evaluating many joint disorders. CT digital radiography (CT scanogram) can be used for accurate demonstration of leg-length discrepancy with minimal radiation exposure. CT best demonstrates joint incongruity after closed reduction of a dislocated hip. **CT scanning is useful for measuring the cross-sectional dural area in the workup of cervical spinal stenosis; spinal stenosis is present if this area is less than 100 mm^2.** CT is also important for evaluating subtalar joint injuries and diagnosing tarsal coalitions; talocalcaneal tarsal coalitions are also well visualized via axial (Harris)-view plain radiographs. A dynamic CT scan is the test of choice for patients with atlantoaxial rotatory subluxation (Grisel's syndrome is spontaneous atlantoaxial subluxation occurring in conjunction with inflammation of the soft tissues of the neck [such as pharyngitis]). CT images can be distorted by metal implants.

TABLE 1-54 MAGNETIC RESONANCE IMAGING CHANGES OF MENISCAL PATHOLOGY

Group	Characteristics
I	Globular areas of hyperintense signal
II	Linear hyperintense signal
III	Linear hyperintense signal that communicates with the meniscal surface (tears)
IV	Vertical longitudinal tear/truncation

B. Ultrasonography—Has been used successfully in several areas of orthopaedics.
   1. Shoulder—May be useful for diagnosing rotator cuff tears.
   2. Hip—Effective in diagnosis and follow-up of developmental hip dysplasia and identifying iliopsoas bursitis in adults.
   3. Knee—Used to assess articular cartilage thickness and identify intra-articular fluid.
   4. Other areas—Helpful for evaluating soft-tissue masses, hematoma, tendon rupture, abscesses, foreign body location, intraspinal disorders in infants, and the aorta (in patients at increased risk for aortic dilation or rupture [such as Marfan's syndrome]).
   5. Fractures—May help evaluate progression of fracture healing.

C. Guided biopsies—Aspiration and core biopsy (using a trephine needle) is helpful in the workup of musculoskeletal lesions; commonly used in conjunction with CT.

D. Myelography—Still useful for evaluating cervical radiculopathy, subarachnoid cysts, and the failed back syndrome. **It is the procedure of choice for extramedullary intradural pathology.** It can be used in conjunction with other studies, such as CT.

E. Discography—Although its use is controversial, it is helpful for evaluating symptomatic disc degeneration. Reproduction of pain with injection and characteristic changes on discograms help identify pathologic discs. It is commonly used in conjunction with CT.

F. Measurement of bone density (noninvasive methods) —Several methods are available for measuring bone density and assessing the risk of fracture.
   1. Single-photon absorptiometry—The density of the cortical bone is inversely proportional to the quantity of photons passing through it. The radioisotope ^{125}I emits a single-energy beam of photons that passes through bone. A sodium iodide scintillation counter detects the transmitted photons. Where the bone is dense, the photon beam is attenuated and fewer photons pass through to the scintillation counter. Single-photon absorptiometry is best used in the

TABLE 1-55 NERVE CONDUCTION STUDY RESULTS

Condition	Latency	Conduction Velocity	Evoked Response
Normal study	Normal	Upper extremities: >45 m/sec; lower extremities: >40 m/sec	Biphasic
Axonal neuropathy	Increased	Normal or slightly decreased	Prolonged, decreased amplitude
Demyelinating neuropathy	Normal	Decreased (10-50%)	Normal or prolonged, with decreased amplitude
Anterior horn cell disease	Normal	Normal (rarely decreased)	Normal or polyphasic, with prolonged duration and decreased amplitude
Myopathy	Normal	Normal	Decreased amplitude; may be normal
Neurapraxia			
Proximal to lesion	Absent	Absent	Absent
Distal to lesion	Normal	Normal	Normal
Axonotmesis			
Proximal to lesion	Absent	Absent	Absent
Distal to lesion	Absent	Absent	Normal
Neurotmesis			
Proximal to lesion	Absent	Absent	Absent
Distal to lesion	Absent	Absent	Absent

Modified from Jahss MH: Disorders of the Foot. Philadelphia, WB Saunders, 1982.

appendicular skeleton (radius-diaphysis or distal metaphysis); it is unreliable in the axial skeleton (the depth of the soft tissues alters the beam).

2. Dual-photon absorptiometry—Like single-photon absorptiometry, dual-photon absorptiometry is an isotope-based means of measuring bone density. Dual-photon absorptiometry, however, allows for measurement of the axial skeleton and the femoral neck by accounting for the attenuation of the signal caused by the soft tissues overlying the spine and the hip.
3. Quantitative computed tomography—Allows preferential measurement of trabecular bone density (the bone that is at the greatest risk for early metabolic changes). Involves the simultaneous scanning of phantoms of known density, thus creating a standard calibration curve. Precision is excellent; accuracy is within 5-10%. The radiation dose with this technique is higher than that of dual-energy x-ray absorptiometry (DEXA).
4. DEXA—The most accurate and reliable method of predicting fracture risk, with a lower radiation dose than that with quantitative CT. DEXA measures bone mineral content and soft tissue composition.

G. Thermography—Maps body surface temperatures. Thermography has low specificity and is not recommended for clinical evaluation of disorders of the spine.

V. Electrodiagnostic Studies

A. Nerve conduction studies—Allow evaluation of peripheral nerves and their sensory and motor responses anywhere along their courses. Nerve impulses are stimulated and recorded by surface electrodes, allowing calculation of a conduction velocity. Latency (the time between the stimulus onset and response) and response amplitude are measured. Late responses (F and H) allow evaluation of proximal lesions (impulse travels to the spinal cord and returns). Somatosensory evoked potentials can be used to study brachial plexus injuries and for spinal cord monitoring.

B. Electromyography (EMG)—Uses intramuscular needle electrodes to evaluate muscle units. Most studies are done to evaluate patients for denervation, which demonstrates fibrillations (earliest sign usually at 4 weeks), sharp waves, and an abnormal recruitment pattern.

C. Interpretation—For peripheral nerve entrapment syndromes, distal motor and sensory latencies >35 m/sec, nerve conduction velocities of <50 m/sec, and changes over a distinct interval are considered abnormal (Tables 1–55 and 1–56).

TABLE 1-56 ELECTROMYOGRAPHIC FINDINGS

Condition	Insertional Activity	Activity at Rest	Minimal Contraction	Interference
Normal study	Normal	Silent	Biphasic and triphasic potentials	Complete
Axonal neuropathy	Increased	Fibrillations and positive sharp waves	Biphasic and triphasic potentials	Incomplete
Demyelinating neuropathy	Normal	Silent (occasional activity)	Biphasic and triphasic potentials	Incomplete
Anterior horn cell disease	Increased	Fibrillations, positive sharp waves, fasciculations	Large polyphasic potentials	Incomplete
Myopathy	Increased	Silent or increased spontaneous activity	Small polyphasic potentials	Early
Neurapraxia	Normal	Silent	None	None
Axonotmesis	Increased	Fibrillations and positive sharp waves	None	None
Neurotmesis	Increased	Fibrillations and positive sharp waves	None	None

Modified from Jahss MH: Disorders of the Foot. Philadelphia, WB Saunders, 1982.

SECTION 8 Biomaterials and Biomechanics

I. Basic Concepts

A. Definitions
1. Biomechanics—Science of the action of forces, internal or external, on the living body.
2. Statics—Study of the action of forces on rigid bodies that are in equilibrium (i.e., either rest or moving at a constant velocity).
3. Dynamics—Study of bodies that are accelerating and the related forces. There are two subtypes.
   a. Kinematics—Study of motion (displacement, velocity, and acceleration) without reference to the forces causing the motion.
   b. Kinetics—Relates the effects of forces to the motion of bodies.
4. Kinesiology—Study of human movements and motions, including kinematics, kinetics, anatomy, physiology, and motor control.

B. Principal quantities
1. Basic quantities—Described by the International System of Units (SI) or the metric system.
   a. Length—Meters (m)
   b. Mass—Amount of matter (kilograms [kg])
   c. Time—Seconds (sec)
2. Derived quantities—Derived from basic quantities
   a. Velocity—Time rate of change of displacement (m/sec). The rate of translation displacement is *linear velocity*; the rate of rotational displacement is *angular velocity*.
   b. Acceleration—Time rate of change of velocity (m/sec^2); can also be linear or angular.
   c. Force—Action causing acceleration of a mass (body) in a certain direction (kg·m/sec^2[N]).

C. Newton's laws
1. First law: Inertia—If the net external force acting on a body is zero, the body will remain at rest or move with a constant velocity. Allows static analysis via the equation $\Sigma F = 0$ (the sum of the external forces applied to a body equals zero).
2. Second law: Acceleration—The acceleration *(a)* of an object of mass *m* is directly proportional to the force (F) applied to the object: $F = ma$ Helps in dynamic analysis.
3. Third law: Reactions—For every action (force) there is an equal and opposite reaction (force). Leads to free-body analysis and assists in the study of interacting bodies.

D. Scalar and vector quantities
1. Scalar quantities—Have magnitude but no direction. Examples include volume, time, mass, and speed (not velocity).
2. Vector quantities—Have magnitude and direction. Examples include force and velocity. Vectors have four characteristics: (1) magnitude (length of the vector), (2) direction (head of the vector), (3) point of application (tail of the vector), and (4) line of action (orientation of the vector). Vectors can be added, subtracted, and split into components (resolved) for analysis. The result of two vectors follows the principle of "parallelogram of forces."
3. Tensors—Arrays of numbers or functions that represent the physical properties of a system. Scalar quantities (e.g., mass) are tensors of rank 0; vector quantities (e.g., force) are tensors of rank 1; stress is an example of a tensor of rank 2; stress has magnitude and direction and is also determined over a specific plane. Higher-order tensors are used to represent properties more complex than those that can be represented by vectors.

E. Free-body analysis—Uses forces, moments, and free-body diagrams to analyze the action of forces on bodies. **Know how to solve these problems!**
1. Force—A mechanical push or pull (load) causing external (acceleration) and internal (strain) effects. Force vectors can be split into independent components (usually in the *x* and *y* directions) for easier analysis. The unit of force is the Newton (N). Some elementary knowledge of trigonometry is helpful ($F_x = F \cos \theta$, $F_y = F \sin \theta$). Also remember the following simple approximations:

$$\sin 30^\circ = \cos 60^\circ \cong 05$$

$$\sin 45^\circ = \cos 45^\circ \cong 07$$

$$\sin 60^\circ = \cos 30^\circ \cong 09$$

   A normal force is perpendicular to the surface upon which it acts; a tangential force is parallel to the surface. A compressive force shrinks a body in the direction of the force; a tensile force elongates it.
2. Moment (*M*)—The rotational effect of a force acting at a distance from a specified point on a body. A moment is defined as the force (*F*) multiplied by the perpendicular distance from a specified point (the moment arm or lever arm = *d*): $M = F \times d$. *Torque* is a moment that occurs when a force acts perpendicular to the long axis of a body, causing rotation. A *bending moment* is one that occurs when a force acts parallel to the long axis, causing bending. ***Mass moment of inertia* is resistance of the body (or body segment) to rotation;** it is the product of the body's mass times the square of the distance from a specified point on the body (or body segment): $I = m \times d^2$. Mass moment of inertia affects angular acceleration.
3. Free-body diagram (FBD)—Sketch of a body (or portions thereof) isolated from all other bodies and showing all forces acting on it. The weights of objects act through the center of gravity (CG).

The CG for the human body is just anterior to S2.

4. Free body analysis—After all forces are represented on the FBD, apply the concept of equilibrium (sum of forces and moments both equal zero [$\Sigma F = 0$ and $\Sigma M = 0$]) and solve for unknowns. Assumes no change in motion, no deformation, and no friction. The following steps are used in the analysis:
   a. Identify the system (objective, knowns, assumptions)
   b. Select a coordinate system
   c. Isolate free bodies (FBD)
   d. Apply Newton's laws ($\Sigma F = 0$ and $\Sigma M = 0$)
   e. Solve for unknowns
5. Example—Calculate the biceps force necessary to hold the weight of the forearm (20 N), with the elbow flexed to 90 degrees; assume that the biceps insertion is 5 cm distal to the elbow and the CG of the forearm is 15 cm distal to the elbow (Fig. 1–95). (*Answer:* 60 N) Also solve for the joint force (*J*) (*Answer:* −40 N).

F. Finite element analysis—Used to model complex geometric forms and material properties. The structure is modeled as a finite number of simple geometric forms, typically triangular or trapezoidal elements, and a computer is used to match the forces and moments between neighboring elements. Finite element analysis is often used to estimate internal stresses and strains, such as those occurring at a bone–implant interface.

G. Other important basic concepts
1. Work—The product of a force and the displacement it causes. Work (*W*) = force (only the vector components parallel to the displacement) × distance (displacement produced by *F*). Units: N•m [joules]

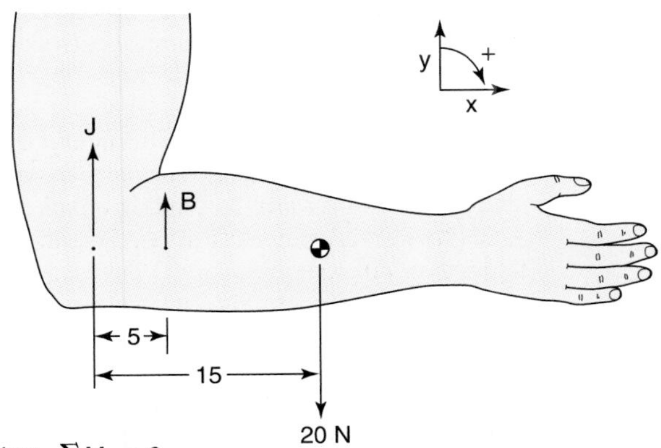

Solution: $\Sigma M_J = 0$

$- B(.05) \quad 20(.15) = 0$

$.05\,B = 3$

$B = 60N$

$\Sigma F_y = 0$

$+ J + B - 20 = 0$

$J = +20 - B$

$J = -40N$

FIGURE 1–95 Free-body diagram (see text for explanation).

2. Energy—Ability to perform work (unit is also joules). According to the law of conservation of energy, energy is neither created nor destroyed; it is transferred from one condition to another.
   a. Potential energy—Stored energy; the ability of a body to do work as a result of its position or configuration (strain energy)
   b. Kinetic energy—Energy of an object due to its motion ($KE = \frac{1}{2} mv^2$)
3. Friction (*f*)—Resistance to motion between two bodies when one slides over the other; produced at points of contact. Oriented opposite to the applied force. When the applied force exceeds *f*, motion begins. Frictional force is proportional to the coefficient of friction and the applied normal (perpendicular) load; *f* is independent of the area of contact and the shape of the surface.
4. Piezoelectricity—Electrical charge from deformation of crystalline structures when forces are applied. **Concave (compression) side is electronegative; convex (tension) side is electropositive.**

II. Biomaterials

A. Strength of materials
1. Definition—Branch of mechanics that deals with relations between externally applied loads and the resulting internal effects and deformations induced in the body subjected to these loads.
   a. Loads—Forces that act on a body (compression, tension, shear, torsion).
   b. Deformations—A temporary (elastic) or permanent (plastic) change in the shape of a body. Changes in load produce changes in deformation.
   c. Elasticity—Ability to return to resting length after undergoing lengthening or shortening.
   d. Extensibility—Ability to be lengthened.
2. Stress—Intensity of internal force: **Stress = force/area.** Used to analyze the *internal* resistance of a body to a load. Helps in selection of materials. Normal stresses (compressive or tensile) are perpendicular to the surfaces on which they act. Shear stresses are parallel to the surfaces on which they act, causing a part of a body to be displaced relative to another part. Stress has the units N/m^2 (pascals [Pa]). Stress is different than *pressure*, which is the distribution of an *external* force to a solid body, although the definition (= force/area) and unit (Pa) are the same.
3. Strain—Relative measure of the deformation (six components) of a body as a result of loading. **Strain = change in length/original length of an object.** It can also be normal or shear. Strain is a proportion and therefore has no units. *Strain rate* is the strain divided by the time that the load is applied (units = sec^{-1}).
4. Hooke's law—Basically, stress is proportional to strain up to a limit (the proportional limit).
5. Young's modulus (of elasticity [*E*])—Measure of the stiffness of material or its ability to resist

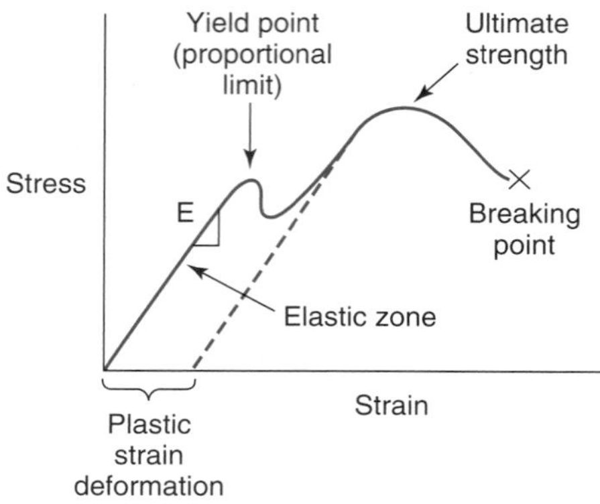

FIGURE 1–96 Stress-strain curve.

deformation in tension: E = stress/strain (in the elastic range of the stress–strain curve, E is the slope). **Modulus of elasticity is the critical factor in load-sharing capacity. Linearly perfect elastic material** has a straight stress–strain curve to the point of failure; the modulus is calculated by dividing the stress at failure (the ultimate stress) by the strain at failure (the ultimate strain). E is unique for every type of material. A material with a higher E can withstand greater forces than that with a smaller E.

6. Shear modulus—The ratio of shear stress to shear strain; a measure of stiffness. Unit: Pa.
7. Stress–strain curve—Derived by loading a body and plotting stress versus strain (Fig. 1–96); the shape of the curve varies by material.
   a. Proportional limit—Transition point at which stress and strain are no longer proportional, but the material will return to its original length if the stress is removed, which is still elastic behavior.
   b. Elastic limit (yield point)—Transition point from elastic to plastic behavior of the material. Beyond this point, the structure of the material is irreversibly changed. The elastic limit is usually 0.2% strain in most metals.
   c. **Plastic deformation—Irreversible change in length after removing the load in the plastic range** (after the elastic limit but before the breaking point).
   d. Ultimate strength—Maximum strength obtained by the material.
   e. Breaking point—Point at which the material fractures. If the deformation between the elastic limit and breaking point is large, the material is *ductile*; if this deformation is small, the material is *brittle*.
   f. **Strain energy—The capacity of material (such as bone) to absorb energy. On a stress–strain curve it is the area under the curve.** Total strain energy = recoverable strain energy (resilience) + dissipated strain energy. A measure of the toughness (ability to absorb energy before failure) of material.

B. Materials and structures
   1. Material—Related to a substance or element. Defined by mechanical properties (force, stress, strain) and rheologic properties (elasticity [ability to regain original shape], plasticity [permanent deformation], viscosity [resistance to flow or shear stress], and strength).
      a. **Brittle materials** (e.g., PMMA)—Exhibit a linear stress–strain curve up to the point of failure. Brittle materials undergo only **fully recoverable (elastic) deformation** prior to failure and have little or no capacity to undergo permanent (plastic) deformation prior to failure.
      b. **Ductile materials** (e.g., metal)—Undergo a large amount of plastic deformation prior to failure. Ductility is a measure of postyield deformation.
      c. **Viscoelastic materials** (e.g., bone and ligaments)—**Exhibit stress–strain behavior that is time-rate dependent (varies with the material); the material's deformation and properties depend on the load and the rate at which the load is applied.** Viscoelastic materials exhibit properties of both a fluid (viscosity; resistance to flow) and a solid (elasticity). **The modulus of viscoelastic material increases as the strain rate increases. Viscoelastic behavior is a function of the internal friction of the material.** Viscoelastic materials also exhibit **hysteresis: Loading and unloading curves differ because energy is dissipated during loading.** Most biologic tissues (bone, ligament, muscle, etc.) exhibit viscoelasticity.
      d. **Isotropic materials—Possess the same mechanical properties in all directions (e.g., a golf ball)**
      e. **Anisotropic materials—Have mechanical properties that vary with the direction of the applied load (e.g., bone is stronger axially than radially)**
      f. Homogeneous materials—Have a uniform structure or composition throughout.
   2. Structure—Related to both the material and the shape of an object and its loading characteristics. A load deformation curve can be constructed similarly to a stress–strain curve. The slope of the curve in the elastic range is referred to as the rigidity of the structure. **Bending rigidity of a rectangular structure** is proportional to the base multiplied by the height cubed ($bh^3/12$). **Bending rigidity of a cylinder** (e.g., intramedullary nails, half-pins) is related to the fourth power of the radius. Bending rigidity is **closely related to the area moment of inertia** (I [resistance to bending]), which is a function of the width and thickness of the structure, and the **polar moment of inertia** (J), which represents the resistance to torsion (twisting). ***I* and *J* are functions of the distribution of material in the cross section of the structure.** For more information, see section

on Intramedullary Nails. **Deflection associated with bending** is proportional to the applied force (*F*) divided by the elastic modulus (*E*) of the material being bent multiplied by the area moment of inertia (*I*).

$$\text{Deflection} \propto (F/E) \times (I)$$

3. Metals—Demonstrate stress–strain curves, as discussed earlier. Other important concepts follow.
   a. Fatigue failure—Occurs with repetitive loading cycles at stress below the ultimate tensile strength. Fatigue failure depends on the magnitude of the stress and number of cycles. If the stress is less than a predetermined amount, called the **endurance limit (the maximum stress under which the material will not fail regardless of how many loading cycles are applied),** the material may be loaded cyclically an infinite number of times ($>10^6$ cycles) without breaking. Above the endurance limit, the fatigue life of material is expressed by the stress (*S*) versus the number of loading cycles (*n*), or the *S-n* curve.
   b. **Creep (cold flow)—Progressive deformation of metals (or other materials [such as polyethylene]) in response to a constant force applied over an extended period of time.** If sudden stress followed by constant loading causes material to continue to deform over time, it demonstrates creep. Creep can produce a permanent deformity and may affect mechanical function (such as that occurring in a TJA).
   c. Corrosion—Chemical dissolving of metals as it may occur in the high-saline environment of the body. Several types of corrosion may occur (Table 1–57). **Stainless steel (316L) is the most susceptible metal to both crevice corrosion and galvanic corrosion. The risk of galvanic corrosion is the highest between 316L stainless steel and cobalt-chromium (Co-Cr) alloy.** Modular components of THA have direct contact between either similar or dissimilar metals (at the modular junctions) and thereby have corrosion products (metal oxides, metal chlorides, and others). Corrosion can be decreased by using similar metals (e.g., with plates and screws of similar metals), with proper design of implants, and with passivation by an adherent oxide layer (a thin layer that effectively separates the metal from the solution [e.g., stainless steel coated with chromium oxide]).
   d. Types of metals—Orthopaedic implants are typically made of 316L (L = low carbon) **stainless steel** (iron, chromium, and nickel), "supermetal" alloys (**e.g., Co-Cr-molybdenum (Mo)** [65% Co, 35% Cr, 5% Mo] made with a special forging process), and **titanium alloy** (Ti-6Al-4V). Each possesses a **different stiffness (*E*)** (Fig. 1–97). Problems associated with certain metals include wear, stress shielding (increased in metals with a higher *E*), and ion release (Co-Cr causes macrophage proliferation and synovial degeneration). **Titanium has poor resistance to wear (notch sensitivity),** particulates may incite a histiocytic response, and there is an uncertain association between titanium and neoplasms. Polishing, passivation, and ion implantation improve the fatigue properties of titanium alloy. **Titanium is extremely biocompatible material; it rapidly forms an adherent oxide coating (self-passivation) that covers its surface (a nonreactive ceramic coating). Another advantage of titanium is its relatively low *E* (most closely emulates the axial and torsional stiffness of bone) and high yield strength. Co-Cr alloy generates less metal debris (in THA) than titanium alloy does. Problems with orthosis fabrication: stainless steel is heavy and aluminum has a low endurance limit.**
4. Nonmetals—Include polyethylene, PMMA (bone cement), silicone, and ceramics.
   a. Polyethylene—Ultra–high-molecular-weight polyethylene (UHMWPE) polymer consists of long carbon chains; used in weight-bearing components of TJAs such as acetabular cups

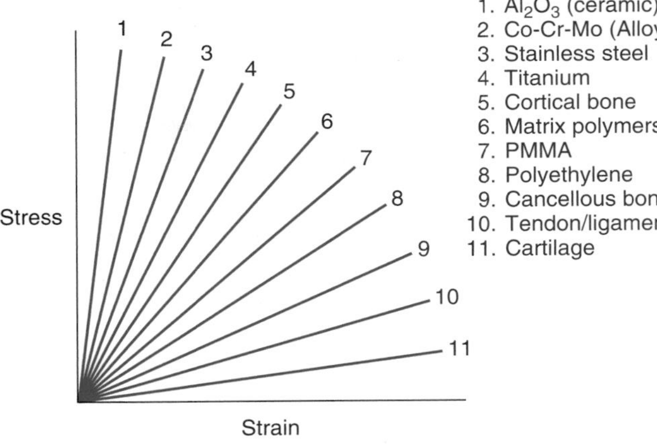

FIGURE 1–97 Comparison of Young's modulus (relative values, not to scale) for various orthopaedic materials.

TABLE 1–57 TYPES OF CORROSION

Corrosion	Description
Galvanic	Dissimilar metals*; electrochemical destruction
Crevice	Occurs in fatigue cracks with low O_2 tension
Stress	Occurs in areas with high stress gradients
Fretting	From small movements abrading outside layer
Other	Inclusion, intergranular, etc.

Metals such as 316L stainless steel and Co–Cr–Mo produce galvanic corrosion.

and tibial trays. These materials have wear characteristics superior to those of high-density polyethylene (HDP); they are tough, ductile, resilient, and resistant to wear, and they exhibit low friction. Polyethylenes are viscoelastic and highly susceptible to abrasion. **Wear damage to a UHMWPE articulating surface is most often caused by third-body inclusions. UHMWPE is also thermoplastic and may be altered by temperature or high-dose radiation.** The oxidative degradation of polyethylene after gamma irradiation in air is related to free radical formation (which increases susceptibility to oxidation); **gamma irradiation** increases polymer chain cross-links, which greatly **improves wear characteristics but reduces resistance to fatigue and fracture resistance** and decreases the elastic modulus, tensile strength, ductility, and yield stress. Polyethylenes are weaker than bone in tension and have a low *E*. Wear debris is associated with a histiocytic osteolytic response. Wear (and the associated osteolytic response) is increased with thinner (<6 mm), flatter, carbon fiber–reinforced polyethylene. Metal backing may help minimize plastic deformation of HDP (and loosening) but decreases its effective thickness (wear). Catastrophic wear of polyethylene tibial inserts is associated with varus knee alignment, thin inserts (<6 mm), flat, nonconforming inserts; and heat treatments of the insert. **Polyethylene wear debris is the main factor affecting the longevity of THAs.** Fatigue wear is more prevalent in TKA than in THA. **Volumetric wear is most affected by the relative motion between the two surfaces in contact**

b. PMMA (bone cement)—Used for fixation (as a grout, not an adhesive) and load distribution for implants. PMMA reaches its ultimate strength within 24 hours. PMMA can also be used as an internal splint for patients with poor bone stock; it should be thought of as a temporary internal splint until the bone heals (if the bone fails to heal, the PMMA will ultimately fail). **PMMA has poor tensile and shear strength. It is strongest in compression (however, it is not as strong as bone in compression) and has a low *E*.** Reduction in the number of voids (porosity) with insertion (vacuum mixing, centrifugation, good technique) increases cement strength and decreases cracking. **PMMA functions by mechanically interlocking with bone. Insertion can lead to a precipitous drop in blood pressure.** Wear particles can incite a macrophage response that leads to loosening of a prosthesis. **Cement failure is often caused by microfracture and fragmentation of cement.** PMMA may be used to minimize tumor contamination by filling defects in bone created by biopsy or curettage (this use has not been cleared by the Food and Drug Administration [FDA]).

c. Silicones—Polymers used for replacement in non–weight-bearing joints. Their poor strength and wear capabilities are responsible for frequent synovitis with extended use.

d. Ceramics—Broad class of materials that contain metallic and nonmetallic elements bonded ionically in a highly oxidized state; they are good insulators (poor conductors). Include biostable (inert) crystalline materials such as Al_2O_3 (alumina) and ZrO_2 (zirconium dioxide) and bioactive (degradable), noncrystalline substances such as bioglass. **Ceramics are typically brittle (no elastic deformation), have a high modulus (*E*), have high compressive strength, have low tensile strength, have a low yield strain, and exhibit poor crack resistance characteristics (low fracture toughness [low resistance to fracture]).** Ceramics have the best wear characteristics, with polyethylene and a low oxidation rate. **High surface wettability and high surface tension** make them highly conducive to tissue bonding and result in less friction and **diminished wear** ("smooth surface"). Small grain size also allows an ultrasmooth finish and less friction. Calcium phosphates (e.g., hydroxyapatite) may have application as a coating (plasma sprayed) to increase attachment strength and promote bone healing.

5. Other materials—Examples such as polylactic acid (PLA)–coated carbon, which serves as a biodegradable scaffolding, and new polymer composites, some with carbon fiber reinforcement, are still investigational. Fabrication of these newer devices involves assembling "piles" of carbon fibers impregnated with matrix polymer (polysulfone or polyetherketone). Difficulties with abrasion and impact resistance, radiolucency, and manufacturing are still present. Bioabsorbable polymer implants induce foreign body reactions in a large number of patients.
6. Biomaterials—Possess certain unique characteristics, including **viscoelasticity** (time-dependent stress–strain behavior), creep, and stress relaxation (internal stress decreases with time, although deformation remains constant). They are also capable of self-adaptation and repair; characteristics change with aging and sampling.
7. Comparison of common orthopaedic materials —Figure 1–97 compares Young's modulus of elasticity for various orthopaedic materials.

C. Orthopaedic structures
  1. Bone
     a. Mechanical properties—Bone is a composite of collagen and hydroxyapatite. Collagen has a low *E*, good tensile strength, and poor compressive strength. Calcium apatite is stiff, brittle material with good compressive strength.

The combination is **anisotropic** material that resists many forces; **bone is strongest in compression, weakest in shear, and intermediate in tension and resists rapidly applied loads better than slowly applied loads. The mineral content is the main determinant of the elastic modulus of cortical bone.** Cancellous bone is 25% as dense, 10% as stiff, and 500% as ductile as cortical bone. Cortical bone is excellent versus torque; cancellous bone is good versus compression and shear. Bone is dynamic material: able to self-repair, change with aging (becomes stiffer and less ductile), and change with prolonged immobilization (becomes weaker). **The material properties of bone decline with aging; to offset the loss in material properties, bone remodels its geometry to increase the inner and outer cortical diameters, which increases the area moment of inertia and thus decreases bone's bending stresses.** Stress concentration effects occur at defect points within bone or the implant-bone interface (stress risers) and reduce the overall loading strength of bone. Stress shielding by load-sharing implants induces osteoporosis in adjacent bone due to a decrease in normal physiologic stresses in the bone. This commonly occurs under plates and at the femoral calcar in high-riding THAs. A hole that is 20-30% of bone diameter reduces overall strength up to 50%, regardless of whether it is filled with a screw, and does not return to normal until 9-12 months after screw removal. Cortical defects can reduce strength 70% or more (oval defects less than rectangular defects due to a smaller stress riser).

b. Fracture—Type is based on mechanism of injury.
   (1) **Tension**—By muscle pull, typically transverse, perpendicular to the load and bone axis.
   (2) **Compression**—By axial loading of cancellous bone; results in a crush type of fracture.
   (3) **Shear**—Commonly around joints; the load is parallel to the bone surface, and the fracture is parallel to the load.
   (4) **Bending**—By eccentric loading or direct blows. **The fracture begins on the tension side of the bone and continues transversely/obliquely, eventually bifurcating to produce a butterfly fragment** (with high-velocity bending there will be a comminuted butterfly fracture).
   (5) **Torsion—Creates shear and tensile stresses around the longitudinal axis that are most likely to result in a spiral fracture.** Because torsional stresses are proportional to the distance from the neutral axis to the periphery of a cylinder, **a long bone under torsion experiences the greatest stresses on the outer (periosteal) surface.**

c. **Comminution**—A function of the amount of energy transmitted to bone

2. Ligaments and tendons—Can sustain 5-10% tensile strain before failure (versus 1-4% in bone), commonly from tension rupture of fibers and shear failure among fibers. Most ligaments can undergo plastic strain to the point that function is lost but structure remains in continuity. Soft tissue implants include stents, ligament augmentation devices, and scaffolding.
   a. **Tendons**—Strong in tension only; *E* is only 10% that of bone but increases with slower loading; parallel fiber orientation. Tendons demonstrate stress relaxation and creep.
   b. **Ligament fibers**—Oriented parallel if they resist major joint stress, more randomly if they resist forces from different directions. Stiffness = force/strain, as depicted on a force deformation graph (similar to *E* but does not consider cross-sectional area); the bone-ligament complex is softer (less stiff—decreased *E*). Prolonged immobilization lowers ligament yield point and tensile strength, and bone resorbs at the tendon insertion site.
   c. Stents—Internal splint devices: include Proplast Tendon Transfer Stabilizer with the use of synthetic polymers, Gore-Tex prosthetic ligaments, Xenotech (bovine tendon), and polyester implants. These do not allow adequate collagen ingrowth and therefore all eventually fail. Synthetic ligaments produce wear particles that increase the levels of proteinases, collagenase, gelatinase, and chondrocyte activation factor.
   d. Ligament augmentation devices (LADs)—Examples such as the Kennedy LAD (polypropylene yarn) and Dacron LADs do allow some fibrous ingrowth, but their use is limited.
   e. Biodegradable tissue scaffolding—Allows immediate stability and long-term replacement with host tissue. Carbon fiber and polylactic acid (PLA)-coated carbon fiber devices have been used, with limited success (slow ingrowth is improved with PLA coating).
3. Articular cartilage—The ultimate tensile strength of cartilage is only 5% that of bone, and *E* is 0.1% that of bone; nevertheless, because of its highly viscoelastic properties, it is well suited for compressive loading. Articular cartilage is said to be biphasic, with a solid phase that depends on the structural matrix and a fluid phase that depends on the deformation and shift of water within the solid matrix. The relatively soft and impermeable solid matrix requires high hydrodynamic pressure to maintain fluid flow; the significant support thus provided by the fluid component produces a stress-shielding effect on the matrix.
4. Metal implants
   a. **Screws**—Characterized by pitch (distance between threads), **lead** (distance advanced in

one revolution), **root diameter** (minimal/inner diameter ∝ tensile strength), and **outer diameter** (determines holding power [pullout strength]). **To maximize pullout strength, a screw should have a large outer diameter, a small root diameter, and a fine pitch.** Pullout strength of a pedicle screw is most affected by the degree of osteoporosis.

b. **Plates**—Strength varies with the material and moment of inertia. **The rigidity (bending stiffness) of a plate is proportional to the thickness (t) to the third power (t^3).** Thus, doubling plate thickness increases its bending stiffness eightfold. Plates are load-bearing devices and most effective when placed on a fracture's tension side. Types of plates include static compression (best in the upper extremity; can be stressed for compression), dynamic compression (e.g., tension band plate), neutralization (resists torsion), and buttress (protects bone graft). Stress concentration at open screw holes can lead to implant failure. **Screw holes that remain after removal of a plate and screws represent a stress riser and a site at risk for refracture.** Blade plates provide increased resistance to torsional deformation in subtrochanteric fractures. **Locking plates have been shown to have biomechanical advantages over standard plates for osteoporotic fractures without cortical contact.**

c. **Intramedullary (IM) nails**—Require a high polar moment of inertia to maximize torsional rigidity and strength. **In characterizing the mechanical characteristics of an intramedullary nail, we describe the torsional rigidity and the bending rigidity.**
   (1) **Torsional rigidity** is the amount of torque needed to produce torsional (rotational) deformation (a unit angle of torsional deformation). **Torsional rigidity of an intramedullary nail** (cylinder) depends on both material properties (shear modulus) and structural properties (polar moment of inertia).
   (2) **The bending rigidity of an intramedullary nail** is the amount of force required to produce a unit amount of deflection. This **bending rigidity** also depends on both material properties (elastic modulus) and structural properties (area moment of inertia, length). **The bending rigidity of an intramedullary nail is related to the fourth power of the nail's radius;** increasing nail diameter by 10% increases bending rigidity by 50%.
   (3) Reaming allows increased torsional resistance due to the increased contact area and allows use of a larger nail with increased rigidity and strength. Intramedullary nails are better at resisting bending than rotational forces. Unslotted nails allow stronger fixation and a smaller diameter (at the expense of flexibility). **The greatest mechanical advantage of closed-section intramedullary nails over slotted nails is increased torsional stiffness.** During IM nail insertion for a femoral shaft fracture, the hoop stresses are the lowest for a slotted nail with a thin wall made of titanium alloy. Posterior starting points for femoral nails decrease hoop stresses and iatrogenic comminution of fractures. Implant failure occurs more frequently with smaller-diameter, unreamed intramedullary nails. **Intramedullary nails are load-sharing devices.**

d. External fixators
   (1) **Conventional external fixators—The most important factor for stability of fixation of a fracture treated with external fixation is to allow the fracture ends to come into contact. Other factors of the external fixator that may be used to enhance stability (rigidity) are as follows:**
      (a) **Larger-diameter pins (the second most important factor)**—The bending rigidity of each pin is proportional to the fourth power of the pin diameter.
      (b) **Additional pins**
      (c) **Decreased bone-rod distance**—The bending stiffness of each pin is proportional to the third power of the bone-rod distance.
      (d) **Pins in different planes** (pins separated by more than 45 degrees)
      (e) **Increased mass of the rods or stacked rods** (a second rod in the same plane provides increased resistance to bending moments in the sagittal plane)
      (f) **Rods in different planes**
      (g) **Increased spacing between pins**—Place central pins closer to the fracture site and peripheral pins further from the fracture site (near-near, far-far). For tibial shaft fractures, the use of additional lag screws with external fixation is associated with a higher refracture rate than external fixation alone.
   (2) **Circular (Ilizarov) external fixators**—Thin wires (usually 18 mm in diameter) are fixed under tension (usually between 90 and 130 kg) to circular rings. Half-pins may also be used but offer better purchase in diaphyseal (not metaphyseal) bone. The optimum orientation of the implants on the ring is 90 degrees to each other to maximize stability (90 degrees is not always possible because of anatomic constraints [such as

neurovascular structures]). The bending stiffness of the frame is independent of the loading direction because the frame is circular. Each ring should have at least two implants (wires or half-pins); the most stable construct when two implants are used on a ring is an olive wire and a half-pin at 90 degrees to each other. When two wires are used on a ring, one wire should be positioned superior to the ring and one should be positioned inferior to the ring (two tensioned wires on the same side of a ring can cause the ring to deform). Factors that enhance stability of circular external fixators include (a) larger-diameter wires (and half-pins); (b) decreased ring diameter; (c) the use of olive wires; (d) additional wires and/or half-pins; (e) wires (and/or half-pins) crossing at 90 degrees; (f) increased wire tension (up to 130 kg); (g) placement of the two central rings close to the fracture site; (h) decreased spacing between adjacent rings; and (i) increased number of rings.

e. THA—Evolving design has reduced biomechanical constraints

(1) Cemented versus cementless—Femoral components are designed for use with or without cement. In cementless designs, the proximal porous coating should be circumferential to seal the diaphysis from wear debris. In cemented designs, a cement mantle less than 2 mm thick increases the incidence of crack formation.

(2) Stem length—Stem length is directly related to rigidity. Metal femoral heads have greater neck-length options than ceramics. A design with a broad medial surface, a broader lateral surface, and a large moment of inertia minimizes compressive and tensile stresses in adjacent structures.

(3) Moment arms—Femoral component design must account for rotational forces. Rotational torque in retroversion is the force most responsible for the initiation of loosening in cemented femoral stems; this rotational torque is increased in femoral stems with a higher offset. **The femoral component should be in neutral or slight valgus to decrease the moment arm, cement stress, and abductor length. Increasing femoral component offset moves the abductor attachment away from the joint center and increases the abductor moment arm; this reduces the abductor force required in normal gait and thus reduces the resulting hip joint reactive force. Unfortunately, increased offset also increases the bending moment on the implant (increased strain) and increases strain on the medial cement mantle.**

(4) **Femoral head size—Femoral head size should be a compromise between small (22-mm) components, which decrease friction and torque and polyethylene volumetric wear but also decrease ROM and stability, and large (36-mm) components, which increase friction and torque and polyethylene volumetric wear but also increase ROM and stability.** A 26- or 28-mm head seems to be the ideal size in most instances.

(5) Durability—The relatively poor survivorship of surface replacement hip arthroplasty is primarily due to volumetric wear of polyethylene, which is 4-10 times that of a THA when a 28-mm head is used. Metal backing of acetabular components decreases the stress in cement and cancellous bone. The use of different metal alloys and titanium (with *E* closer to cortical bone) is being investigated. **Polyethylene on titanium makes a poor bearing surface because of excessive volumetric wear. The use of titanium on weight-bearing surfaces (poor resistance to wear, notch sensitivity) may lead to fretting, wear debris, and blackening of the soft tissues.** Histiocyte injection of submicron polyethylene debris has been associated with wear synovitis in TJA. UHMWPE serves as a "shock absorber" and should be at least 6 mm thick to prevent creep. **The lowest coefficient of friction is for a ceramic femoral head on a ceramic acetabulum. The wear rate of UHMWPE in the acetabulum is about 0.1 mm (100 μm) per year. By comparison, the wear rate of metal-on-metal bearings for THA is approximately 0.002-0.005 mm (2-5 μm) per year. Ceramic bearing surfaces exhibit wear rates of only 0.0005-0.0025 mm (0.5-25 μm) per year**. Other new concepts include computer design of THA stems, modularity (increased corrosion at modular metallic junction sites [such as the junction of the head and stem]), custom designs, and more flexible stems. Forging of components appears to be superior to casting.

f. TKA—Design has evolved significantly after original design errors that did not take kinematics of the human knee into consideration (i.e., original hinge design). An appropriate compromise between total-contact designs (high conformity) with excess stability (and less motion) but less wear and a low-contact design with less stability and increased wear is being approached. Metal alloys are typically used. **Cemented, cruciate-substituting TKA designs are associated with low polyethylene wear rates and minimal osteolysis (due to the high degree of conformity of the tibiofemoral articulation).**

g. Compression hip screws—Demonstrate loading characteristics superior to blade plates. Higher-angled plates are subjected to lower bending loads but may be more difficult to insert. Sliding of the screw is proportional to the screw/side plate angle and the length of the screw in the barrel.

5. Implant fixation—Three basic forms exist: interference, interlocking, and biologic.
   a. Interference fit—Mechanical or press-fit components rely on the formation of a fibrous tissue interface. Loosening can occur if stability is not maintained and high-*E* substances (leading to increased bone resorption/remodeling) are used.
   b. Interlocking fit—PMMA (a grout with a low *E*) allows a gradual transfer of stress to bone (microinterlocking of cement within cancellous bone). Microinterlocking may not be achievable when a cemented revision of a previously cemented TKA is done. Aseptic loosening can occur over time. A careful technique with limiting of porosities and gaps and the use of a 3-5–mm cement thickness yields the best results. Other improvements include low-viscosity cement, better bone bed preparation, plugging and pressurization, and better (vacuum) cement mixing.
   c. Biologic fit—Tissue ingrowth makes use of fiber-metal composites, void metal composites, or microbeads to create **pore sizes of 100-400 μm (ideally 100-250 μm).** Mechanical stability is required for ingrowth, which is most typically limited to 10-30% of the surface area. Problems include fiber/bead loosening, increased cost, proximal bone resorption (monocyte/macrophage-mediated), corrosion, and decreased implant fatigue strength. Bone ingrowth in the tibial component of an uncemented TKA occurs adjacent to fixation pegs and screws. Bone ingrowth of uncemented TJA components depends on the avoidance of micromotion (may be seen on follow-up radiographs as radiodense reactive lines about the prosthesis) at the bone–implant interface. Canal filling (maximal endosteal contact) of more fully coated femoral stems is an important factor for bone ingrowth.

6. Bone-implant unit—The integrated unit is a composite structure that has shared properties. The more accurately the bone cross section is reconstructed with metallic support, the better the loading characteristics. Plates should act as tension bands. Materials with increased *E* may result in bone resorption, whereas materials with decreased *E* may result in implant failure. **Placement of the implant initiates a race between bone healing and implant failure.**

III. Biomechanics

A. Joint biomechanics—General

1. Degrees of freedom—Joint motion is described as rotations and translations occurring in the *x*, *y*, and *z* planes, thus requiring **six parameters, or degrees of freedom,** to describe motion. Fortunately, translations are usually relatively insignificant for most joints and can often be ignored in biomechanical analyses.
2. Joint reaction force (*R*)—Force generated within a joint in response to forces acting on the joint (both intrinsic and extrinsic). **Muscle contraction about a joint is the major factor contributing to the joint reaction force.** Values (of *R*) correlate with the predisposition to degenerative changes. Joint contact pressure (stress) can be minimized by decreasing *R* and increasing contact area.
3. Coupled forces—In certain joints, rotation about one axis is accompanied by an obligatory rotation about another axis; such movements (and associated forces) are said to be coupled. For example, lateral bending of the spine is accompanied by axial rotation, and these movements/forces are coupled.
4. Joint congruence—Relates to the fit of two articular surfaces and is a necessary condition for joint motion. It can be evaluated radiographically. High congruence increases joint contact area; low congruence decreases joint contact area. Movement out of a position of congruence causes increased stress in cartilage by allowing less contact area for distribution of the joint reaction force, predisposing the joint to degeneration.
5. **Instant center of rotation—Point about which a joint rotates. In joints such as the knee, the location of the instant center changes during the arc of motion (due to joint translation and morphology),** following a curved path. The instant center normally lies on a line perpendicular to the tangent of the joint surface at all points of contact.
6. Rolling and sliding (Fig. 1–98)—During range of motion, almost all joints undergo simultaneous rolling and sliding in order to remain in congruence. Pure rolling occurs when the instant center of rotation is at the rolling surfaces and the contacting points have zero relative velocity (no "slipping" of one surface on the other). Pure sliding occurs with pure translation or rotation about a stationary axis; there is no angular change in position and no instant center of rotation ("slipping" of one surface on the other).
7. Friction and lubrication—Friction is the resistance between two bodies as one slides over the other; it is not a function of the contact area. Lubrication decreases the coefficient of friction (0 = no friction) between surfaces. Articular

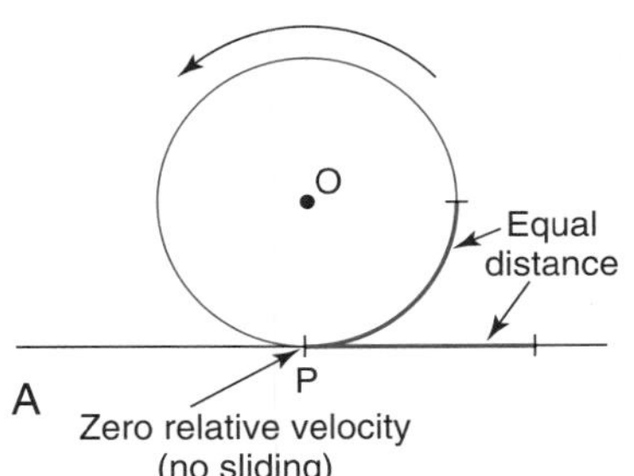

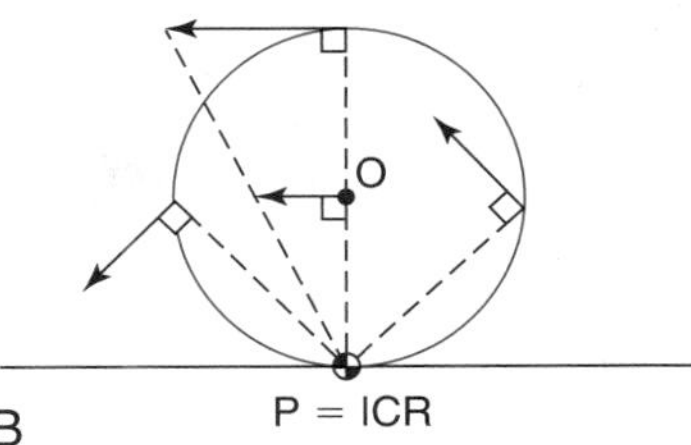

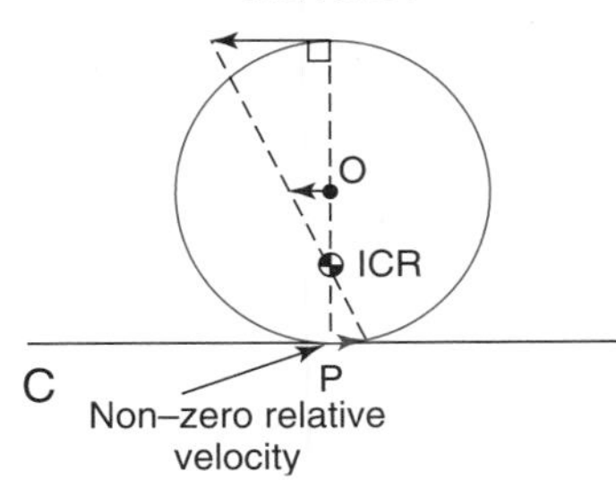

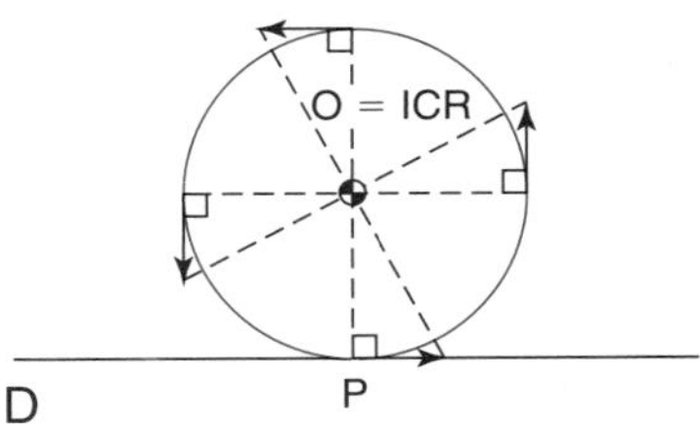

FIGURE 1–98 **A**, Rolling contact occurs when the circumferential distance of the rolling object equals the distance traced along the plane. This can only occur when there is no sliding, that is, the relative velocity at the point of contact (P) is zero. **B**, For rolling contact, the point P of the wheel has zero velocity because it is in contact with the ground. Therefore, P is the instant center of rotation (ICR) of the wheel. This diagram shows the actual velocity of points along the wheel as it rolls along the ground. **C**, Rolling and sliding contact occurs when the relative velocity at the contact point is not zero. **D**, Pure sliding occurs when the wheel rotates about a stationary axis (O). In this case, the wheel would have no forward motion. (From Buckwalter JA, Einhorn TA, Simon SR: Orthopaedic Basic Science: Biology and Biomechanics of the Musculoskeletal System, 2nd ed, p 145. Rosemont, IL, American Academy of Orthopaedic Surgeons, 2000.)

surfaces lubricated with synovial fluid have a coefficient of friction 10 times better than that of the best synthetic systems. **The coefficient of friction for human joints is 0.002–0.04 The coefficient of friction for joint arthroplasty (metal on UHMWP) is 0.05–0.15 (not as good as human joints). Elastohydrodynamic lubrication is the primary mechanism responsible for lubrication of articular cartilage during dynamic function.**

B. Hip biomechanics
1. Kinematics
   a. ROM (Table 1–58)
   b. Instant center—Simultaneous triplanar motion for this ball-and-socket joint makes analysis impossible.
2. Kinetics—**The joint reaction force (R) in the hip can reach three to six times body weight (W) and is primarily due to contraction of muscles crossing the hip**. This phenomenon can be demonstrated with the FBD in Figure 1–99. If $A = 5$ and $B = 125$, using standard FBD analysis:

$M = 0$ (the sum of the moments = 0)

$$-5\ M_y + 125\ W = 0$$

$$M_y = 25\ W$$

$F_y = 0$ (the sum of the forces = 0)

$$-M_y - W + R_y = 0$$

$$R_y = 35\ W$$

$$R = R_y/(\cos 30\ \text{degrees})$$

$$R = (\textit{approximately})\ 4\ W$$

An increase in the ratio of A/B (e.g., with medialization of the acetabulum, with a long-neck prosthesis, or with lateralization of the greater trochanter) decreases R. If $A = 75$ and $B = 10$, $R \approx 23\ W$. **Both joint reaction force (R) and abductor moment are reduced by shifting the body weight over the hip (Trendelenburg gait). A cane in the contralateral hand produces an additional moment and can reduce the joint reaction force up to 60% (carrying a load in the**

TABLE 1–58 HIP BIOMECHANICS: RANGE OF MOTION

Motion	Average Range (degrees)	Functional Range (degrees)
Flexion	115	90 (120 to squat)
Extension	30	
Abduction	50	20
Adduction	30	
Internal rotation	45	0
External rotation	45	20

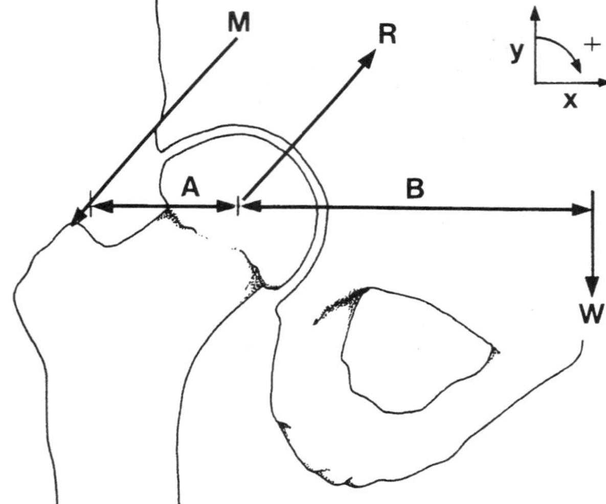

FIGURE 1–99 Free-body diagram of the hip (see text for explanation).

ipsilateral hand also decreases joint reaction force at the hip). Energy expenditure is 264% of normal with a resection arthroplasty of the hip (such as that occurring after a THA infection). The hip and trunk generate approximately 50% (the largest component) of the force generated during a tennis serve.

3. Other considerations
   a. Stability—Largely based on the intrinsic stability of the deep-seated "ball-and-socket" design.
   b. Sourcil—Condensation of subchondral bone under the superomedial acetabulum. At this point *R* is maximal (Pauwels).
   c. Gothic arch—Remodeled bone supporting the acetabular roof, with the sourcil at its base (Bombelli).
   d. Neck-shaft angle—Varus angulation decreases *R* and increases shear across the neck. **Varus also leads to shortening of the lower extremity and alters the muscle tension resting length of the hip abductors, which may cause a persistent limp.** Valgus angulation increases *R* and decreases shear. Neutral or valgus is better for a THA because PMMA resists shear poorly.
   e. Arthrodesis—**The position for hip arthrodesis should be 25-30 degrees of flexion and 0 degrees of abduction and rotation (external rotation is better than internal rotation). If the hip is fused in an abducted position, the patient will lurch over the affected lower extremity with an excessive trunk shift, which will later result in lower back pain.** Hip arthrodesis increases oxygen consumption, decreases gait efficiency (to approximately 50% of normal), and increases transpelvic rotation of the contralateral hip.

C. Knee biomechanics
   1. Kinematics
      a. ROM—ROM of the knee is from 10 degrees of extension (recurvatum) to about 130 degrees of flexion. Functional ROM is from nearly full extension to about 90 degrees of flexion (117 degrees is required for squatting and lifting). Approximately 110 degrees of flexion is required to rise from a chair after TKA. Rotation varies with flexion: At full extension there is minimal rotation; at 90 degrees of flexion, 45 degrees of external rotation and 30 degrees of internal rotation are possible. Abduction/adduction is essentially 0 degrees (a few degrees of passive motion is possible at 30 degrees of flexion). Motion about the knee is a complex series of movements about a changing instant center of rotation (i.e., polycentric rotation). There is 0.5 cm of excursion of the medial meniscus and 11 cm of excursion of the lateral meniscus during a 0- to 120-degree arc of knee motion.
      b. Joint motion—The instant center of rotation, when plotted, describes a J-shaped curve about the femoral condyle, moving posteriorly as the knee flexes. Flexion and extension of the knee involve both **rolling and sliding** motions. The femur internally rotates (external tibial rotation) during the last 15 degrees of extension (**"screw home" mechanism,** related to the size and convexity of the medial femoral condyle [MFC] and the musculature). **Posterior rollback of the femur on the tibia during knee flexion increases maximum knee flexion.** Normal femoral rollback is compromised when the PCL is sacrificed, as in some TKAs. The axis of rotation of the intact knee is in the MFC. The patellofemoral joint is a sliding articulation (patella slides 7 cm caudally with full flexion), with an instant center near the posterior cortex above the condyles.
   2. Kinetics—Extension via the quadriceps mechanism through the patellar apparatus; flexion via the hamstring muscles.
      a. Knee stabilizers—Although bony contours contribute to knee stability, it is the ligaments and muscles of the knee that play the major role (Table 1–59). The ACL is typically subjected to peak loads of 170 N during walking and up to 500 N with running. The ultimate

TABLE 1-59 KNEE STABILIZERS

Direction	Structures
Medial	Superficial MCL (1°), joint capsule, medial meniscus, ACL/PCL
Lateral	Joint capsule, IT band, LCL (mid), lateral meniscus, ACL/PCL (90°)
Anterior	ACL (1°), joint capsule
Posterior	PCL (1°), joint capsule; PCL tightens with IR
Rotatory	Combinations—MCL checks ER; ACL checks IR

ACL, anterior cruciate ligament; ER, external rotation; IR, internal rotation; IT, iliotibial; LCL, lateral collateral ligament complex; MCL, medial collateral ligament complex; PCL, posterior cruciate ligament.

strength of the ACL in young patients is about 1750 N. The ACL fails by serial tearing at 10-15% elongation. Cadaver studies have shown that sectioning the PCL increases contact pressures in the medial compartment and across the patellofemoral joint.

b. Joint forces
   (1) Tibiofemoral Joint—Knee joint surface loads are **three times body weight during level walking** and up to **four times body weight with stair walking.** Menisci help with load transmission (bear one third to one half body weight), and removal of these structures increases contact stresses (up to four times the load transfer to bone). The quadriceps muscle produces maximum anterior directed force on the tibia at knee flexion of 0-60 degrees.
   (2) Patellofemoral joint—The patella aids in knee extension by increasing the lever arm and in stress distribution. This joint has the thickest cartilage in the entire body because it must bear the greatest load—ranging from one half body weight with normal walking to seven times body weight with squatting and jogging. Loads are proportional to the quadriceps force/knee flexion ratio. **While descending stairs, the compressive force between the patella and the trochlea of the femur reaches two to three times body weight. After patellectomy, the length of the moment arm is decreased by the width of the patella (30% reduction), and the power of extension is decreased by 30%.** During TKA, the following enhance patella tracking: external rotation of the femoral component, lateral placement of the femoral and tibial components, medial placement of the patellar component, and avoidance of malrotation of the tibial component (avoid internal rotation).

c. Axes of the lower extremity (Fig. 1–100)
   (1) Mechanical axis of the lower extremity—From the center of the femoral head to the center of the ankle. The mechanical axis of a normal lower extremity passes just medial to the medial tibial spine.
   (2) Vertical axis—From the center of gravity to the ground.
   (3) Anatomic axes—Along the shafts of the femur and tibia. There is a normal valgus angle where these two axes intersect at the knee.
   (4) Mechanical axis of the femur—From the center of the femoral head to the center of the knee.
   (5) Mechanical axis of the tibia—From the center of the tibial plateau to the center of the ankle.

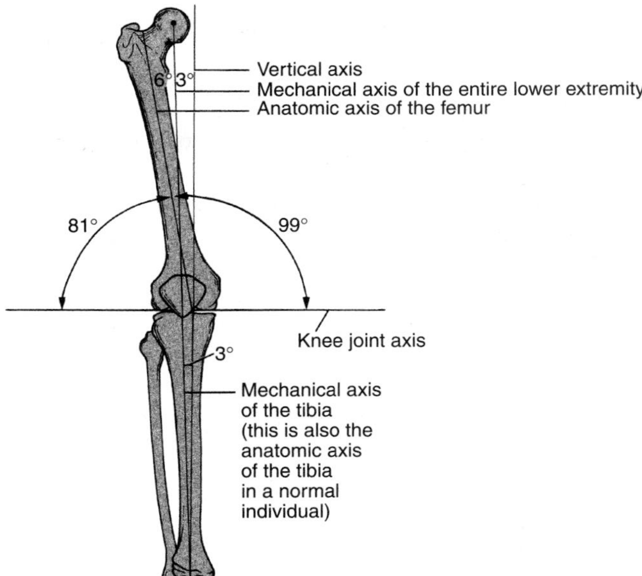

FIGURE 1–100 Axes of the lower extremity. (Modified from Helfet DL: Fractures of the distal femur. In Browner BD, Jupiter JB, Levine AM, et al, eds: Skeletal Trauma, p 1645. Philadelphia, WB Saunders, 1992.)

   (6) Relationships—The mechanical axis of the lower extremity is in 3 degrees of valgus from the vertical axis. The anatomic axis of the femur is in 6 degrees of valgus from the mechanical axis (9 degrees versus the vertical axis). The anatomic axis of the tibia is in 2-3 degrees of varus from the mechanical axis.

d. Arthrodesis—**The position for knee arthrodesis should be 0-7 degrees of valgus and 10-15 degrees of flexion.**

D. Ankle and foot biomechanics

1. Ankle
   a. Kinematics—Instant center of rotation is within the talus, and the lateral and posterior points are at the tips of the malleoli; they change slightly with movement. The talus is described as forming a cone, with the body and trochlea wider anteriorly and laterally. Therefore, the talus and fibula must externally rotate slightly with dorsiflexion. Ankle dorsiflexion and abduction are coupled movements in the ankle. Average ankle ROM is 25 degrees of dorsiflexion, 35 degrees of plantar flexion, and 5 degrees of rotation.
   b. Kinetics—The tibial/talar articulation is the major weight-bearing surface of the ankle, supporting compressive forces up to five times body weight (W) on level surfaces

TABLE 1-60 ARCHES OF THE FOOT

Arch	Components	Keystone	Ligament Support	Muscle Support
Medial longitudinal	Calcaneus, talus, navicular, three cuneiforms, first to third metatarsals	Talus head	Spring (calcaneonavicular)	Tibialis posterior, flexor digitorum longus, flexor hallucis longus, adductor hallucis
Lateral longitudinal	Calcaneus, cuboid, fourth and fifth metatarsals		Plantar aponeurosis	Abductor digiti minimi, flexor digitorum brevis
Transverse	Three cuneiforms, cuboid, metatarsal bases			Peroneus longus, tibialis posterior, adductor hallucis (oblique)

and shear (backward to forward) forces up to *W*. A large weight-bearing surface area allows for decreased stress (force/area) at this joint. The fibular/talar joint transmits about one sixth of the force. The highest net muscle moment at the ankle occurs during the terminal-stance phase of gait.

c. Other considerations—Stability is based on the shape of the articulation (a mortise that is maintained by the talar shape) and ligamentous support. The greatest stability is in dorsiflexion. During weight bearing (loaded), the tibial and talar articular surfaces contribute most to joint stability. A windlass action has been described in the ankle, where full dorsiflexion is limited by the plantar aponeurosis, and further tension on the aponeurosis (e.g., with toe dorsiflexion) causes the arch to rise. **A syndesmosis screw limits external rotation of the ankle. Arthrodesis of the ankle should be performed in neutral dorsiflexion, 5-10 degrees of external rotation, and 5 degrees of hindfoot valgus** (anticipate a loss of 70% of the sagittal plane motion of the foot).

2. Subtalar joint (talus-calcaneus-navicular)—The axis of rotation is 42 degrees in the sagittal plane and 16 degrees in the transverse plane. Described as functioning like an oblique hinge; its motions are also coupled with dorsiflexion, abduction, and eversion in one direction (pronation) and plantar flexion, adduction, and inversion (supination) in the other. Average ROM of pronation is 5 degrees; supination is 20 degrees Functional ROM is approximately 6 degrees.
3. Transverse tarsal joint (talus-navicular, calcaneal-cuboid)—Motion is based on foot position with two axes of rotation (talonavicular and calcaneocuboid). With eversion of the foot (such as that occurring during the early stance phase), the two joint axes are parallel and ROM is permitted. With foot inversion (late stance), external rotation of the lower extremity causes the joint axes to no longer be parallel, and motion is limited.
4. Foot—Transmits about 12 times body weight with walking and 3 times body weight with running. It is composed of three arches (Table 1–60). The second metatarsal (Lisfranc) joint is ''keylike'' and stabilizes the second metatarsal, allowing it to carry the most load with gait (the first metatarsal bears the most load while standing). The expected life span of a Plastazote shoe insert in an active adult is less than 1 month (fatigues rapidly in both compression and shear). Therefore, in a shoe insert, Plastazote should be replaced frequently and/or supported with other materials, such as Spenco or PPT.

E. Spine biomechanics

1. Kinematics—ROM varies with anatomic segment (Table 1–61). Analysis is based on the functional unit **(a motion segment consists of two vertebrae and their intervening soft tissues). Six degrees of freedom exist about all three axes. Coupled motion** (simultaneous rotation, lateral bending, and flexion or extension) is also demonstrated, especially axial rotation with lateral bending. The instant center of rotation lies within the disc. The normal sagittal alignment of the lumbar spine (55-60 degrees of lordosis) exists because of the disc spaces (not the vertebrae); most of the lordosis is between L4 and S1. Loss of disc space height can cause a significant loss of the normal lumbar lordosis. Iatrogenic flat

TABLE 1-61 RANGE OF MOTION OF SPINAL SEGMENTS

Level	Flexion/Extension (Degrees)	Lateral Bending (Degrees)	Rotation (Degrees)	Instant Center
Occiput-C1	13	8	0	Skull, 2-3 cm above dens
C1-C2	10	0	45	Waist of odontoid
C2-C7	10-15	8-10	10	Vertebral body below
T-spine	5	6	8	Vertebra below/disc centrum
L-spine	15-20	2-5	3-6	Disc annulus

C, cervical; L, lumbar; T, thoracic.

back syndrome of the lumbar spine is the result of a distraction force.

2. Supporting structures—Anterior supporting structures include the anterior longitudinal ligament, the posterior longitudinal ligament, and the vertebral disc. Posterior supporting structures include the intertransverse ligaments, capsular ligaments and facets, and ligamentum flavum (yellow ligament). The halo vest is the most effective device for controlling cervical motion (because of pin purchase in the skull).
   a. Apophyseal joints—Resist torsion during axial loading; the attached capsular ligaments resist flexion. They guide the motion of the motion segment. The direction of motion is determined by the orientation of the facets of the apophyseal joint, which varies with each level. **In the cervical spine the facets are oriented 45 degrees to the transverse plane and parallel to the frontal plane. In the thoracic spine the facets are oriented 60 degrees to the transverse plane and 20 degrees to the frontal plane. In the lumbar spine the facets are oriented 90 degrees to the transverse plane and 45 degrees to the frontal plane** (i.e., they progressively tilt up [transverse plane] and in [frontal plane]). **Cervical facetectomy of greater than 50% causes a significant loss of stability in flexion and torsion. Torsional load resistance in the lumbar spine has a 40% contribution by the facets and a 40% contribution by the disc; the ligamentous structures contribute the remaining 20% resistance to torsional load.**
3. Kinetics
   a. Disc—**Behaves viscoelastically and demonstrates creep (deforms with time) and hysteresis (absorbs energy with repeated axial loads and later decreases in function).** Compressive stresses are highest in the nucleus pulposus, and tensile stresses are highest in the annulus fibrosus. Stiffness of the disc increases with increasing compressive load. With higher loads, increased deformation and faster creep can be expected. Repeated torsional loading may separate the nucleus pulposus from the annulus and end plate, forcing nuclear material out through an annular tear (produced by shear forces). Loads increase with bending and torsional stresses. **After subtotal diskectomy, extension is the most stable loading mode. Disc pressures are lowest in the lying supine position on a flat surface, higher with standing, and highest with sitting. When loads are carried, disc pressures are lowest when the load** is carried close to the body.
   b. Vertebrae—Strength is related to the bone mineral content and vertebrae size (increased in the lumbar spine). Fatigue loading may lead to pars fractures. Compression fractures occur at the end plate. Decreased vertebral body stiffness in osteoporosis is caused by loss of horizontal trabeculae. Increasing implant stiffness for an implant-augmented spinal arthrodesis results in an increased probability of a successful fusion but an increased likelihood of decreased bone mineral content of the bridged vertebrae.

F. Shoulder biomechanics (Table 1–62)
   1. Kinematics—The scapular plane is 30 degrees anterior to the coronal plane and is the preferred reference for ROM. Abduction requires external rotation of the humerus to prevent greater tuberosity impingement. With internal rotation contractures, patients cannot abduct more than 120 degrees. Abduction is a result of glenohumeral motion (120 degrees) and scapulothoracic motion (60 degrees) in a 2:1 ratio (although this ratio varies over the first 30 degrees of motion). **Deceleration is the most violent phase of pitching; the rotator cuff is the principal decelerator and is susceptible to tensile failure from eccentric loading.** Movement at the acromioclavicular joint is responsible for the early part of scapulothoracic motion, and sternoclavicular movement is responsible for the later portion, with clavicular rotation along the long axis. Surface joint motion in the glenohumeral joint is a combination of rotation, rolling, and translation.

TABLE 1-62 SHOULDER BIOMECHANICS: MUSCLE FORCES

Motion	Muscle Forces	Comments
Glenohumeral		
Abduction	Deltoid, supraspinatus	Cuff depresses head
Adduction	Latissimus dorsi, pectoralis major, teres major	
Forward flexion	Pectoralis major, deltoid (anterior), biceps	
Extension	Latissimus dorsi	
Internal rotation	Subscapularis, teres major	
External rotation	Infraspinatus, teres minor, deltoid (posterior)	
Scapular		
Rotation	Upper trapezius, levator scapulae (anterior), serratus anterior, lower trapezius	Works through a force couple
Adduction	Trapezius, rhomboid, latissimus dorsi	
Abduction	Serratus anterior, pectoralis minor	

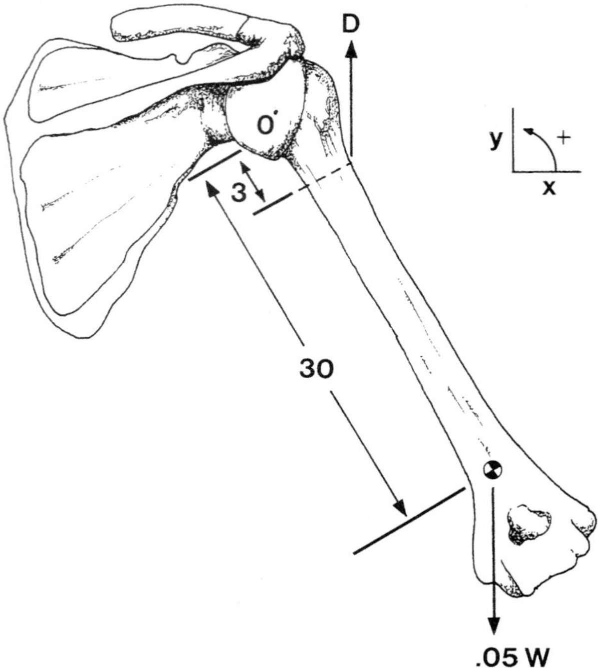

FIGURE 1–101 Free-body diagram of the deltoid force (see text for explanation).

2. Kinetics—The zero position (Saha), 165 degrees of abduction in the scapular plane, minimizes deforming forces about the shoulder. This position is ideal for reducing shoulder dislocations (or "fractures with traction"). Free-body analysis of the deltoid force (Fig 1–101) reveals the following:

$$M_0 = 0$$

$$3D - 005\ W(30) = 0$$

$$D = 05\ W$$

3. Stability—Limited about the glenohumeral joint. Humeral head surface area is larger than that for the glenoid (48 × 45 mm versus 35 × 25 mm). Bony stability is limited and relies only on inclination (125 degrees) and retroversion (25 degrees) of the humeral head and a slight retrotilt of the glenoid. **The inferior glenohumeral ligament (superior band) is the most important static stabilizer about the shoulder.** The superior and middle glenohumeral ligaments are stabilizers secondary to anterior humeral translation. **Inferior subluxation of the humeral head is prevented by the shoulder's negative intra-articular pressure. The rotator cuff muscles provide a dynamic contribution to shoulder stability.** Stress on the posterior shoulder capsule is greatest during follow-through of throwing. **The position for arthrodesis of the shoulder is 15-20 degrees of abduction, 20-25 degrees of forward flexion, and 40-50 degrees of internal rotation (avoid excessive external rotation).**
4. Other joints—The acromioclavicular joint allows scapular rotation (through the conoid and trapezoid ligaments) and scapular motion (through the acromioclavicular joint itself). The sternoclavicular joint allows clavicular protraction/retraction in a transverse plane (through the coracoclavicular ligament), clavicular elevation and depression in the frontal plane (also through the coracoclavicular ligament), and clavicular rotation around the longitudinal axis.

G. Elbow biomechanics

1. Introduction—The elbow serves three functions: (1) as a component joint of the lever arm when the hand is positioned, (2) as a fulcrum for the forearm lever, and (3) as a weight-bearing joint in patients using crutches. During throwing, the elbow functions primarily as a positioner and a means of transferring energy from the shoulder and trunk. Most activities of daily living can be performed with an elbow range of motion of 30-130 degrees of flexion, 50 degrees of supination, and 50 degrees of pronation.
2. Kinematics—Motion about the elbow includes flexion and extension (0-150 degrees, with a **functional ROM of 30-130 degrees;** the axis of rotation is the center of the trochlea) and pronation (P) and supination (S): P = 80 degrees and S = 85 degrees, with a **functional P and S of 50 degrees each;** the axis is a line from the capitellum through the radial head and to the distal ulna (defines a cone). The normal carrying angle (valgus angle at the elbow) is 7 degrees for males and 13 degrees for females. This angle decreases with flexion.
3. Kinetics—The forces that act about the elbow have short lever arms and are relatively inefficient, resulting in large joint reaction forces that subject the elbow to degenerative changes. Flexion is primarily by the brachialis and biceps, extension by the triceps, pronation by the pronators (teres and quadratus), and supination by the biceps and supinator. Static loads approach, and dynamic loads exceed, body weight (*W*). The FBD in Figure 1–102 demonstrates the inefficiency of elbow flexion.

$$M_0 = 0$$

$$-5B + 15W = 0$$

$$B = 3W$$

4. Stability—Provided partially by articular congruity. **The three necessary and sufficient constraints for elbow stability are the coronoid, lateral (ulnar) collateral ligament, and the anterior band of the MCL.** The **most important stabilizer is the MCL** (anterior oblique fibers). It stabilizes the elbow against both

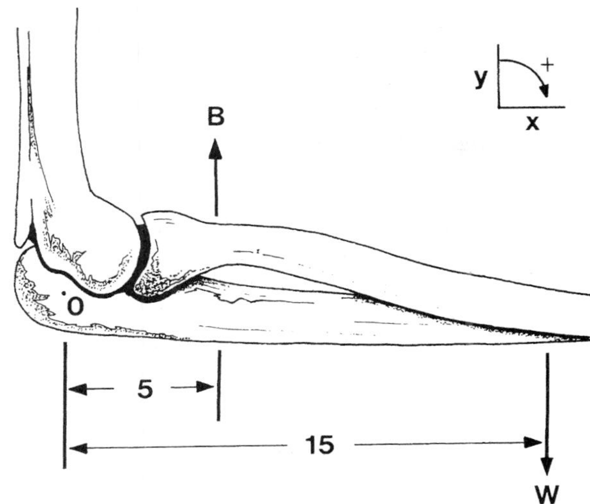

FIGURE 1–102 Free-body diagram of elbow flexion (see text for explanation).

valgus and distractional force with forearm flexion (90 degrees). **The most important secondary stabilizer against valgus stress at the elbow is the radial head,** which provides about 30% of valgus stability and is more important in 0-30 degrees of flexion and pronation. Valgus extension overload of the elbow occurs during the late cocking and early acceleration phases of throwing. In extension, the capsule is the primary restraint to distractional forces. Laterally, stability is provided by the lateral collateral ligament (LCL), anconeus, and joint capsule. The position for unilateral arthrodesis is about 90 degrees of flexion; for bilateral arthrodesis one elbow is placed at 110 degrees of flexion (to reach the mouth) and the other at 65 degrees of flexion (for perineal hygiene needs). Arthrodesis is difficult and (fortunately) rarely required.

5. Forearm—About 17% of the axial load is transmitted by the ulna. The line of the center of rotation runs from the radial head to the distal ulna.

H. Wrist and hand biomechanics

1. Wrist—Part of an intercalated link system
   a. Kinematics—Motion about the wrist includes flexion (65 degrees normal, 10 degrees functional), extension (55 degrees normal, 35 degrees functional), radial deviation (15 degrees normal, 10 degrees functional), and ulnar deviation (35 degrees normal, 15 degrees functional). Flexion and extension are primarily radiocarpal (two thirds), but intercarpal movement is also important (one third). Radial deviation is primarily due to intercarpal movement, whereas ulnar deviation relies on radiocarpal and intercarpal motion. The instant center for wrist motion is the head of the capitate but is variable.
   b. Columns—Three columns have been described for the wrist (Taleisnik) (Table 1–63).
   c. Link system—The carpus makes up a system of three links in a "chain" (Gilford): radius-lunate-capitate. This arrangement allows for less motion to be required at each link but adds to the instability of the chain. Stability, however, is enhanced by strong volar ligaments and the scaphoid, which bridges both carpal rows.

TABLE 1-63 COLUMNS OF THE WRIST

Column	Function	Comments
Central	Flexion-extension	Distal carpal row and lunate (link)
Medial	Rotation	Triquetrum
Lateral	Mobile	Scaphoid

   d. Relationships—Carpal collapse can be evaluated based on the ratio of carpal height/third metacarpal height (normally 0.54) Ulnar translation can be determined by using the ratio of ulna-to-capitate length to third metacarpal height (normal is 0.30) The distal radius normally bears about 80% of the distal radioulnar joint load and the distal ulna 20%. Ulnar load bearing can be increased with ulnar lengthening or decreased with ulnar shortening. Wrist arthrodesis is relatively common. A position of 10-20 degrees of dorsiflexion is good for unilateral fusion, and if bilateral fusion is necessary (avoid if possible), the other wrist should be fused in 0-10 degrees of palmar flexion.
2. Hand
   a. Kinematics—ROM at the MCP joint (universal joint, 2 degrees of freedom) includes 100 degrees of flexion and 60 degrees of abduction-adduction. PIP joints usually have about 110 degrees of flexion and DIP joints 80 degrees.
   b. Arches—The hand has two transverse arches (proximal through the carpus and distal through the metacarpal heads) and five longitudinal arches (through each of the rays).
   c. Stability—MCP joint stability is provided by the volar plate and the collateral ligaments. **The collateral ligaments of the MCP joints are taut in flexion and lax in extension.** The PIP joints and DIP joints rely more on joint congruity. There is also a large ligament/articular surface ratio in these joints.
   d. Other concepts—The pulleys in the hand prevent bowstringing and decrease tendon excursion. Bowstringing increases the moment arm to the joint instant center. The sagittal bands allow extension at the MCP joint. With hyperextension at the MCP joint, the intrinsics must function for PIP joint extension because the extensor tendon is lax. Normal grasp is 50 kg for males and 25 kg for females (only 4 kg is required for daily function). Normal pinch is 8 kg for males and 4 kg for females (1 kg is needed for daily activities).

e. Kinetics—Joint loading with pinch is mostly in the MCP joint, but because the MCP joints have a larger surface area, the contact pressures (joint load/contact area) at the MCP joints are less. The DIP joints have the most contact pressures and subsequently develop the most degenerative changes with time (Heberden's nodes). Grasping contact pressures are less but focus on the MCP joint; therefore, patients with MCP joint arthritis have frequently had occupations that required grasping activities. Compressive loads at the thumb with pinching include 3 kg at the interphalangeal joint, 5 kg at the MCP joint, and 12 kg at the thumb CMC joint (an unstable joint), which frequently leads to its degeneration.
f. Arthrodesis—Recommended positions of flexion for arthrodesis of joints in the hand are shown in Table 1–64.

TABLE 1-64 RECOMMENDED POSITIONS OF FLEXION FOR ARTHRODESIS OF THE JOINTS OF THE HAND

Joint	Degrees of Flexion	Other Factors
MCP	20-30	
PIP	40-50	Less radial than ulnar
DIP	15-20	
Thumb CMC		
Thumb MCP	25	MC in opposition
Thumb IP	20	

DIP, distal interphalangeal; IP, interphalangeal; CMC, carpometacarpal; MC, metacarpal; MCP, metacarpophalangeal.

Selected Bibliography

HISTOLOGY OF BONE

Recent Articles

Athanasou NA: Cellular biology of bone-resorbing cells. J Bone Joint Surg [Am] 78:1096–1112, 1996.

Brinker MR, Lippton HL, Cook SD, et al: Pharmacological regulation of the circulation of bone. J Bone Joint Surg [Am] 72:964–975, 1990.

Doherty W, DeRome ME, McCarthy E, et al: The effect of glucocorticoids on osteoblast function. J Bone Joint Surg [Am] 77:396, 1994.

Dunlap JN, Brinker MR, Cook SD: A new in vivo method for the direct measurement of nutrient artery blood flow. Orthopedics 20:613–619, 1997.

Eyre DR: Biochemical markers of bone turnover. In Primer on the Metabolic Bone Diseases and Disorders of Mineral Metabolism, 3rd ed, pp 114–118. Philadelphia, Lippincott-Raven, 1996.

Hosoda K, Kanzaki S, Eguchi H, et al: Secretion of osteocalcin and its propeptide from human osteoblastic cells: Dissociation of the secretory patterns of osteocalcin and its propeptide. J Bone Min Res 8:553–565, 1993.

Hupel TM, Aksenov SA, Schemitsch EH: Cortical bone blood flow in loose and tight fitting locked unreamed intramedullary nailing: A canine segmental tibia fracture model. J Orth Trauma 12:127–135, 1998.

Iannotti JP: Growth plate physiology and pathology. Orthop Clin North Am 21:1–17, 1990.

Iannotti JP, Brighton CP, Iannotti V, et al: Mechanism of action of parathyroid hormone–induced proteoglycan synthesis in the growth plate chondrocyte. J Orthop Res 8:136–145, 1990.

Jiranek WA, Machado M, et al: Production of cytokines around loosened cemented acetabular components: Analysis with immunohistochemical techniques and in situ hybridization. J Bone Joint Surg [Am] 75: 863–879, 1993.

Kaysinger KK, Nicholson NC, Ramp WK, et al: Toxic effects of wound irrigation solutions on cultured tibiae and osteoblasts. J Orthop Trauma 9:303–311, 1995.

Kitazawa S, Kitazawa R: RANK ligand is a prerequisite for cancer-associated osteolytic lesions. J Pathol 198:228–236, 2002.

Majeska R, Ryaby J, Einhorn T: Direct modulation of osteoblastic activity with estrogen. J Bone Joint Surg [Am] 76:713, 1994.

Mundy GR, Yoneda T: Facilitation and suppression of bone metastasis. Clin Orthop 312:34–44, 1995.

Schemitsch EH, Kowalski MJ, Swiontkowski MF, et al: Comparison of the effect of reamed and unreamed locked intramedullary nailing on blood flow in the callus and strength of union following fracture of the sheep tibia. J Orth Res 13:382–389, 1995.

Smith SR, Bronk JR, Kelly PJ: Effect of fracture fixation on cortical bone blood flow. J Orthop Res 8:471–478, 1990.

Stuecker R, Brinker MR, Bennett JT, et al: Blood flow to the immature hip—ultrasonic measurements in pigs. Acta Orthop Scand 68:25–33, 1997.

Yoo JU, Johnstone B: The role of osteochondral progenitor cells in fracture repair. Clin Orthop 355:S73–S81, 1998.

Classic Articles

Ash P, Loutit JF, Townsend KMS: Osteoclasts derived from haematopoietic stem cells. Nature 283:669–670, 1980.

Azuma H: Intraosseous pressure as a measure of hemodynamic changes in bone marrow. Angiology 15:396–406, 1964.

Branemark P: Experimental investigation of microcirculation in bone marrow. Angiology 12:293–306, 1961.

Bright RW, Burstein AH, Elmore SM: Epiphyseal-plate cartilage: A biomechanical and histological analysis of failure modes. J Bone Joint Surg [Am] 56:688–703, 1974.

Brighton CT: Clinical problems in epiphyseal plate growth and development. Instr Course Lect 23:105–122, 1974.

Brighton CT: Structure and function of the growth plate. Clin Orthop 136:22–32, 1978.

Brookes M: The blood supply of bone: An approach to bone biology. London, Butterworth and Company, 1971.

Buck BE, Malinin TI, Brown MD: Bone transplantation and human immunodeficiency virus: An estimate of risk of acquired immunodeficiency syndrome (AIDS). Clin Orthop 240:129–136, 1989.

Buckwalter JA: Proteoglycan structure in calcifying cartilage. Clin Orthop 172:207–232, 1983.

Houghton GR, Rooker GD: The role of the periosteum in the growth of long bones: An experimental study in the rabbit. J Bone Joint Surg [Br] 61:218–220, 1979.

McPherson A, Scales JT, Gordon LH: A method of estimating qualitative changes of blood-flow in bone. J Bone Joint Surg [Br] 43:791–799, 1961.

Ogden JA: Injury to the growth mechanisms of the immature skeleton. Skel Radiol 6:237–253, 1981.

Ponseti IV, McClintock R: Pathology of slipping of the upper femoral epiphysis. J Bone Joint Surg [Am] 38:71–83, 1956.

Rhinelander FW: Effects of medullary nailing on the normal blood supply of diaphyseal cortex. Instr Course Lect 22:161–187, 1973.

Rhinelander FW: Tibial blood supply in relation to fracture healing. Clin Orthop 105:34–81, 1974.

Rhinelander FW, Phillips RS, Steel WM, et al: Microangiography in bone healing. II: Displaced closed fractures. J Bone Joint Surg [Am] 50: 643–662, 1968.

Salter RB, Harris WR: Injuries involving the epiphyseal plate. J Bone Joint Surg [Am] 45:587–622, 1968.

Shim SS: Physiology of blood circulation. J Bone Joint Surg [Am] 50: 812–824, 1968.

Review Articles

Buckwalter JA, Glimcher MJ, Cooper RR, et al: Bone biology—Part II: Formation, form, modeling, remodeling, and regulation of cell function. J Bone Joint Surg [Am] 77:1276–1283, 1995.

Buckwalter JA, Glimcher MJ, Cooper RR, et al: Bone biology—Part I: Structure, blood supply, cells, matrix and mineralization. J Bone Joint Surg [Am] 77:1256–1272, 1995.

Frymoyer JW: Bone metabolism and metabolic bone disease. In Orthopaedic Knowledge Update 4: Home Study Syllabus, p 77. Rosemont, IL, American Academy of Orthopaedic Surgeons, 1993.

Book Chapters

Bostrum MPG, Boskey A, Kaufman JJ, Einhorn TA: Form and function of bone. In Buckwalter JA, Einhorn TA, Simon SR, eds: Orthopaedic Basic Science: Biology and Biomechanics of the Musculoskeletal System, 2nd ed, pp 319–370. Rosemont, IL, American Academy of Orthopaedic Surgeons, 2000.

Day SM, Ostrum RF, Chao EYS, et al: Bone injury, regeneration, and repair. In Buckwalter JA, Einhorn TA, Simon SR, eds: Orthopaedic Basic Science: Biology and Biomechanics of the Musculoskeletal System, 2nd ed, pp 371–400. Rosemont, IL, American Academy of Orthopaedic Surgeons, 2000.

Frassica FJ, Gitelis S, Sim FH: Metastatic bone disease: General principles, pathophyisology, evaluation, and biopsy. Instr Course Lect 41:293–300, 1992.

Guyton AC: Local control of blood flow by tissues, and nervous and humoral regulation. In Guyton AC, ed: Textbook of Medical Physiology, 7th ed, pp 230–243. Philadelphia, WB Saunders, 1986.

Iannotti JP, Goldstein S, Kuhn J, et al: The formation and growth of skeletal tissues. In Buckwalter JA, Einhorn TA, Simon SR, eds: Orthopaedic Basic Science: Biology and Biomechanics of the Musculoskeletal System, 2nd ed, pp 77–110. Rosemont, IL, American Academy of Orthopaedic Surgeons, 2000.

Simon MA, Springfield DS, eds: Surgery for Bone and Soft Tissue Tumors. Philadelphia, Lippincott-Raven, 1998.

Vaananen K: Osteoclast function: Biology and mechanisms. In Bilezikian JP, Raisz LG, Rodan GA, eds: Principles of Bone Biology, pp 103–113. San Diego, Academic Press, 1996.

BONE INJURY AND REPAIR

Recent Articles

Brinker MR, Cook SD, Dunlap JN, et al: Early changes in nutrient artery blood flow following tibial nailing with and without reaming: A preliminary study. J Orthop Trauma 13:129–133, 1999.

Bostrom MPG, Lane JM, Berberian WS, et al: Immunolocalization and expression of bone morphogenetic proteins 2 and 4 in fracture healing. J Orthop Res 13:357–367, 1995.

Cook SD, Salkeld SL, Brinker MR, et al: Use of an osteoinductive biomaterial (rhOP-1) in healing large segmental bone defects. J Orthop Trauma 12:407–417, 1998.

Cook SD, Wolfe MW, Salkeld SL: Effect of recombinant human osteogenic protein-1 on healing of segmental defects in non-human primates. J Bone Joint Surg [Am] 77:734–750, 1995.

Einhorn TA: Enhancement of fracture-healing. J Bone Joint Surg [Am] 77:940–956, 1995.

Heckman JD, Ryaby JP, McCabe J, et al: Acceleration of tibial fracture-healing by non-invasive, low-intensity pulsed ultrasound. J Bone Joint Surg [Am] 76:26–34, 1994.

Hietaniemi K, Paavolainen P, Penttinen R: Connective tissue parameters in experimental nonunion. J Orthop Trauma 10:114–118, 1996.

Holbein O, Neidlinger-Wilke C, Suger G, et al: Ilizarov callus distraction produces systemic bone cell mitogens. J Orthop Res 13:629–638, 1995.

Horowitz MC, Friedlaender GE: Induction of specific T-cell responsiveness to allogeneic bone. J Bone Joint Surg [Am] 73:1157–1168, 1991.

Iwasaki M, Nakahara H, Nakata K: Regulation of proliferation and osteochondrogenic differentiation of periosteum-derived cells by transforming growth factor-β and basic fibroblast growth factor. J Bone Joint Surg [Am] 77:543–554, 1995.

Jazrawi LM, Majeska RJ, Klein ML, et al: Bone and cartilage formation in an experimental model of distraction osteogenesis. J Orthop Trauma 12:111–116, 1998.

Kurdy NMG, Bowles S, Marsh DR, et al: Serology of collagen types I and III in normal healing of tibial shaft fractures. J Orthop Trauma 12:122–126, 1998.

Lieberman J, Daluiski A, Einhorn TA: The role of growth factors in the repair of bone: Biology and clinical applications. J Bone Joint Surg [Am] 84:1032–1044, 2002.

Murray JH, Fitch RD: Distraction histiogenesis: Principles and indications. J Am Acad Orthop Surg 4:317–327, 1996.

Porter SE, Hanley EN: The musculoskeletal effects of smoking. J Am Acad Orthop Surg 9:9–17, 2001.

Classic Articles

Friedlaender GE: Bone grafts: The basic science rationale for clinical applications. J Bone Joint Surg [Am] 69:786–790, 1987.

Lane JM, Suda M, von der Mark K, et al: Immunofluorescent localization of structural collagen types in endochondral fracture repair. J Orthop Res 4:318–329, 1986.

Mankin HJ, Doppelt SH, Tomford WW: Clinical experience with allograft implantation: The first ten years. Clin Orthop 174:69–86, 1983.

Mirels H: Metastatic disease in long bones: A proposed scoring system for diagnosing impending pathologic fractures. Clin Orthop 249:256–264, 1989.

McKibbin B: The biology of fracture healing in long bones. J Bone Joint Surg [Br] 60:150–162, 1978.

Rhinelander FW: Tibial blood supply in relation to fracture healing. Clin Orthop 105:34–81, 1974.

Springfield DS: Massive autogenous bone grafts. Orthop Clin North Am 18:249–256, 1987.

Stevenson S, Dannucci GA, Sharkey NA, et al: The fate of articular cartilage after transplantation of fresh and cryopreserved tissue-antigen–matched and mismatched osteochondral allografts in dogs. J Bone Joint Surg [Am] 71:1297–1307, 1989.

Stevenson S, Quing LX, Martin B: The fate of cancellous and cortical bone after transplantation of fresh and frozen tissue-antigen–matched and mismatched osteochondral allografts in dogs. J Bone Joint Surg [Am] 73:1143–1156, 1991.

Sumner DR, Turner TM, Purchio AF, et al: Enhancement of bone ingrowth by transforming growth factor-β. J Bone Joint Surg [Am] 77:1135–1147, 1995.

Review Articles

Brighton CT: Principles of fracture healing Part I: The biology of fracture repair. Instr Course Lect 33:60–87, 1984.

Burchardt H: The biology of bone graft repair. Clin Orthop 174:28–42, 1983.

Einhorn TA: Current concepts review enhancement of fracture-healing. J Bone Joint Surg [Am] 77:940–952, 1995.

Friedlaender GE: Immune responses to osteochondral allografts: Current knowledge and future directions. Clin Orthop 174:58–68, 1983.

O'Sullivan ME, Chao EYS, Kelly PJ: The effects of fixation on fracture-healing. J Bone Joint Surg [Am] 71:306–310, 1989.

Book Chapters

Bolander ME: Inducers of osteogenesis. In Friedlaender GE, Goldberg VM, eds: Bone and Cartilage Allografts, pp 75–83, Park Ridge, IL, American Academy of Orthopaedic Surgeons, 1991.

Buckwalter JA, Einhorn TA, Bolander ME: Healing of the musculoskeletal tissues. In Rockwood CA Jr, Green DP, Bucholz RW, et al, eds: Rockwood and Green's Fractures in Adults, 4th ed, pp 261–276. Philadelphia, Lippincott-Raven, 1996.

Day SM, Ostrum RF, Chao EYS, et al: Bone injury, regeneration, and repair. In Buckwalter JA, Einhorn TA, Simon SR, eds: Orthopaedic Basic Science: Biology and Biomechanics of the Musculoskeletal System, 2nd ed, pp 371–400. Rosemont, IL, American Academy of Orthopaedic Surgeons, 2000.

Friedlaender GE: Bone grafts. In Frymoyer JW, ed: Orthopaedic Knowledge Update 4: Home Study Syllabus, pp 233–243. Rosemont, IL, American Academy of Orthopaedic Surgeons, 1993.

Friedlaender GE, Mankin HJ, Sell KW, eds: Osteochondral Allografts: Biology, Banking, and Clinical Applications. Boston, Little, Brown, 1983.

CONDITIONS OF BONE MINERALIZATION, BONE MINERAL DENSITY, AND BONE VIABILITY

Recent Articles

Brinker MR, Rosenberg AG, Kull L, et al: Primary total hip arthroplasty using noncemented porous-coated femoral components in patients with osteonecrosis of the femoral head. J Arthroplasty 9:457–468, 1994.

Byers PH, Wallis GA, Willing MC: Osteogenesis imperfecta: Translation of mutation to phenotype. J Med Genet 28:433–442, 1991.

Delmas PD, Mennier PJ: The management of Paget's disease of bone. N Engl J Med 336:558–566, 1997.

Emery SE, Brazinski MS, Koka E, et al: The biological and biomechanical effects of irradiation on anterior spinal bone grafts in a canine model. J Bone Joint Surg [Am] 76:540–548, 1994.

Garland DE, Stewart CA, Adkins RH, et al: Osteoporosis after spinal cord injury. J Orthop Res 10:419–423, 1981.

Guerra JJ, Steinberg ME: Distinguishing transient osteoporosis from avascular necrosis of the hip. J Bone Joint Surg [Am] 77:616–624, 1995.

Healey JH: Corticosteroid osteoporosis. Curr Opin Orthop 8:1–7, 1997.

Heckman JD, Sassard R: Musculoskeletal considerations in pregnancy. J Bone Joint Surg [Am] 76:1720–1730, 1994.

Kaplan FS, Singer FR: Paget's disease of bone: Pathophysiology, diagnosis, and management. J Am Acad Orthop Surg 3:336–344, 1995.

Lane JM, Nydick M: Osteoporosis: Current modes of prevention and treatment. J Am Acad Orthop Surg 7:19–31, 1999.

Mankin HJ: Rickets, osteomalacia, and renal osteodystrophy: An update. Orthop Clin North Am 21:81–96, 1990.

Melton LJ: Epidemiology of spinal osteoporosis. Spine 22:2S–11S, 1997.

Mont MA, Hungerford DS: Non-traumatic avascular necrosis of the femoral head. J Bone Joint Surg [Am] 77:459–474, 1995.

Pellegrini VD, Gregoritch SJ: Preoperative irradiation for prevention of heterotopic ossification following total hip arthroplasty. J Bone Joint Surg [Am] 78:870–881, 1996.

Schipani E, Kruse K, Juppner H: A constitutively active mutant PTH-PTHrP receptor in Jansen-type metaphyseal chondrodysplasia. Science 268: 98–100, 1995.

World Health Organization: Assessment of fracture risk and its application to screening of postmenopausal osteoporosis: Report of a WHO study group. World Health Organ Tech Rep Ser 843:1–129, 1994.

Classic Articles

Evans GA, Arulanantham K, Gage JR: Primary hypophosphatemic rickets: Effect of oral phosphate and vitamin D on growth and surgical treatment. J Bone Joint Surg [Am] 62:1130–1138, 1980.

Glimcher MJ, Kenzora JE: The biology of osteonecrosis of the human femoral head and its clinical implications. I: Tissue biology. II: The pathological changes in the femoral head as an organ and in the hip joint. III: Discussion of the etiology and genesis of the pathological sequelae: Comments on treatment. Clin Orthop 138:284–309, 1979.

Kanis JA: Vitamin D metabolism and its clinical application. J Bone Joint Surg [Br] 64:542–560, 1982.

Kiel DP, Felson DT, Anderson JJ, et al: Hip fracture and the use of estrogens in postmenopausal women: The Framingham study. N Engl J Med 317:1169–1174, 1987.

Lane JM, Vigorita VJ: Osteoporosis. J Bone Joint Surg [Am] 65:274–278, 1983.

Mankin HJ: Rickets, osteomalacia, and renal osteodystrophy: Part II. J Bone Joint Surg [Am] 56:352–386, 1974.

Nordin BEC, Horsman A, Marshall DH, et al: Calcium requirement and calcium therapy. Clin Orthop 140:216–239, 1979.

Sillence D: Osteogenesis imperfecta: An expanding panorama of variants. Clin Orthop 159:11–25, 1981.

Wallach S: Hormonal factors in osteoporosis. Clin Orthop 144:284–292, 1979.

Review Articles

Barth RW, Lane JM: Osteoporosis. Orthop Clin North Am 19:845–858, 1988.

Boden SD, Kaplan FS: Calcium homeostasis. Orthop Clin North Am 21: 31–42, 1990.

Bullough PG, Bansal M, DiCarlo EF: The tissue diagnosis of metabolic bone disease: Role of histomorphometry. Orthop Clin North Am 21:65–79, 1990.

Kleerekoper MB, Tolia K, Parfitt AM: Nutritional endocrine and demographic aspects of osteoporosis. Orthop Clin North Am 12:547–558, 1981.

Lotke P, Ecker M: Current concepts review: Osteonecrosis of the knee. J Bone Joint Surg [Am] 70:470–473, 1988.

Mankin HJ: Rickets, osteomalacia, and renal osteodystrophy: An update. Orthop Clin North Am 21:81–96, 1990.

Mankin HJ: Metabolic bone disease. J Bone Joint Surg [Am] 76:760–788, 1994.

Mont MA, Hungerford DS: Current concepts review: Non-traumatic avascular necrosis of the femoral head. J Bone Joint Surg [Am] 77:459–469, 1995.

Book Chapters

Aglietti P, Bullough PG: Osteonecrosis. In Insall JN, ed: Surgery of the Knee, pp 527–549. New York, Churchill Livingstone, 1984.

Bilezikian JP: Primary hyperparathyroidism. In Favus MJ: Primer on the Metabolic Bone Diseases and Disorders of Mineral Metabolism, 3rd ed, p 181. Philadelphia, Lippincott-Raven, 1996.

Bostrum MPG, Boskey A, Kaufman JJ, Einhorn TA: Form and function of bone. In Buckwalter JA, Einhorn TA, Simon SR, eds: Orthopaedic Basic Science: Biology and Biomechanics of the Musculoskeletal System, 2nd ed, pp 319–370. Rosemont, IL, American Academy of Orthopaedic Surgeons, 2000.

Broadus AE: Mineral balance and homeostasis. In Favus MJ: Primer on the Metabolic Bone Diseases and Disorders of Mineral Metabolism, 3rd ed, p 57. Philadelphia, Lippincott-Raven, 1996.

Buckwalter JA, Cruess RL: Healing of the musculoskeletal tissues. In Rockwood CA Jr, Green DP, eds: Fractures in Adults, pp 181–264. Philadelphia, JB Lippincott, 1991.

Canale ST, King RE: Part II: Fractures of the hip. In Rockwood CA Jr, Wilkins KE, King RE, eds: Fractures in Children 3, pp 1046–1120. Philadelphia, JB Lippincott, 1991.

Day SM, Ostrum RF, Chao EYS, et al: Bone injury, regeneration, and repair. In Buckwalter JA, Einhorn TA, Simon SR, eds: Orthopaedic Basic Science: Biology and Biomechanics of the Musculoskeletal System, 2nd ed, pp 371–400. Rosemont, IL, American Academy of Orthopaedic Surgeons, 2000.

Frymoyer JW, ed: Bone metabolism and metabolic bone disease. In Orthopaedic Knowledge Update 4: Home Study Syllabus, p 77. Rosemont, IL, American Academy of Orthopaedic Surgeons, 1993.

Glorieux FH: Hypophosphatemic vitamin D–resistant rickets. In Favus MJ: Primer on the Metabolic Bone Diseases and Disorders of Mineral Metabolism, 3rd ed, p 316. Philadelphia, Lippincott-Raven, 1996.

Greech P, Martin TJ, Barrington NA, et al: Diagnosis of Metabolic Bone Disease. Philadelphia, WB Saunders, 1985.

Klein GL: Nutritional rickets and osteomalacia. In Favus MJ: Primer on the Metabolic Bone Diseases and Disorders of Mineral Metabolism, 3rd ed, p 301. Philadelphia, Lippincott-Raven, 1996.

Liberman UA, Marx SJ: Vitamin D–dependent rickets. In Favus MJ: Primer on the Metabolic Bone Diseases and Disorders of Mineral Metabolism, 3rd ed, p 311. Philadelphia, Lippincott-Raven, 1996.

Mankin HJ: Metabolic bone disease. Instr Course Lect 44:3–29, 1995.

Shane E: Hypercalcemia: Pathogenesis, clinical manifestations, differential diagnosis, and management. In Favus MJ: Primer on the Metabolic Bone Diseases and Disorders of Mineral Metabolism, 3rd ed, p 177. Philadelphia, Lippincott-Raven, 1996.

Whyte MP: Hypophosphatasia. In Favus MJ: Primer on the Metabolic Bone Diseases and Disorders of Mineral Metabolism, 3rd ed, p 326. Philadelphia, Lippincott-Raven, 1996.

ARTICULAR TISSUES

Recent Articles

Arnoczky SP, Warren RF, McDevitt CA: Meniscal replacement using a cryopreserved allograft: An experimental study in the dog. Clin Orthop 252:121–128, 1990.

Cannon WD, Morgan CD: Meniscal repair. Part II: Arthroscopic repair techniques. J Bone Joint Surg [Am] 76:294–311, 1994.

Chen FS, Frenkel SR, DiCesare PE: Repair of articular cartilage defects: Part I: Basic science of cartilage healing. Am J Orthop 28:31–33, 1999.

Chen FS, Frenkel SR, DiCesare PE: Repair of articular cartilage defects: Part II: Treatment options. Am J Orthop 28:88–96, 1999.

DeHaven KE, Arnoczky SP: Meniscal repair. Part I: Basic science, indications for repair and open repair. J Bone Joint Surg [Am] 76:140–152, 1995.

Hardingham TE, Fosang AJ: Proteoglycans: Many forms and many functions. FASEB J 6:861–870, 1992.

Jay GD, Tantravahi U, Britt DE, et al: Homology of lubricin and superficial zone protein (SZP): products of megakaryocyte stimulating factor (MSF) gene expression by human synovial fibroblasts and articular chondrocytes localized to chromosome 1q25. J Orthop Res 19:677–687, 2001.

Mente PL, Lewis JL: Elastic modulus of calcified cartilage is an order of magnitude less than that of subchondral bone. J Orthop Res 12: 637–647, 1994.

Müller FJ, Setton LA, Manicourt DH, et al: Centrifugal and biochemical comparison of proteoglycan aggregates from articular cartilage in experimental joint disuse and joint instability. J Orthop Res 12:498–508, 1994.

O'Driscoll SW, Recklies AD, Poole AR: Chondrogenesis in periosteal explants. J Bone Joint Surg [Am] 76:1042–1051, 1994.

Shapiro FR, Koide S, Glimcher MJ: Cell origin and differentiation in the repair of full-thickness defects of articular cartilage. J Bone Joint Surg [Am] 75:532–553, 1993.

Swoboda B, Pullig O, Kirsch T: Increased content of type VI collagen epitopes in human osteoarthritic cartilage: Quantitation by inhibition ELISA. J Orthop Res 16:96–99, 1998.

Verzijl N, DeGroot J, Thorpe SR, et al: Effect of collagen turnover on the accumulation of advanced glycation end products. J Biol Chem 275:39027–39031, 2000.

Wakitani S, Goto T, Pineda SJ, et al: Mesenchymal cell-based repair of large, full-thickness defects of articular cartilage. J Bone Joint Surg [Am] 76:579–592, 1994.

Walker GD, Fischer M, Gannon J, et al: Expression of type-X collagen in osteoarthritis. J Orthop Res 13:4–12, 1995.

Warman ML, Abbott M, Apte SS, et al: A type X collagen mutation causes Schmid metaphyseal chondrodysplasia. Nat Genet 5:79–82, 1993.

Classic Articles

Arnoczky SP, Warren RF: Miocrovasculature of the human meniscus. Am J Sports Med 10:90–95, 1982.

Buckwalter JA, Kuettner KE, Thonar EJ: Age-related changes in articular cartilage proteoglycans: Electron microscopic studies. J Orthop Res 3: 251–257, 1985.

Fairbank TJ: Knee joint changes after meniscectomy. J Bone Joint Surg [Br] 30:664–670, 1948.

Gannon JM, Walker G, Fischer M, et al: Localization of type X collagen in canine growth plate and adult canine articular cartilage. J Orthop Res 9:485–494, 1991.

Hardingham TE: The role of link-protein in the structure of cartilage proteoglycan aggregates. Biochem J 177:237–247, 1979.

Heinegard D, Oldberg A: Structure and biology of cartilage and bone matrix noncollagenous macromolecules. FASEB J 3:2042–2051, 1989.

Mankin HJ, Thrasher AZ: Water content and binding in normal and osteoarthritic human cartilage. J Bone Joint Surg [Am] 57:76–80, 1975.

Salter RB, Simmonds DF, Malcolm BW, et al: The biological effect of continuous passive motion on the healing of full-thickness defects in articular cartilage: An experimental investigation in the rabbit. J Bone Joint Surg [Am] 62:1232–1251, 1980.

Weiss C, Rosenberg L, Helfet AJ: An ultrastructural study of normal young adult human articular cartilage. J Bone Joint Surg [Am] 50:663–674, 1968.

Review Articles

Dehaven KE, Arnoczky SP: Meniscal repair. J Bone Joint Surg [Am] 76: 140–152, 1994.

Mankin HJ: Current concepts review: The response of articular cartilage to mechanical injury. J Bone Joint Surg [Am] 64:460–466, 1982.

Book Chapters

Arnoczky, S, Adams, M, DeHaven, K, et al: Meniscus. In Arnoczky, SP, and Warren, RF, eds: Miocrovasculature of the human meniscus. Am J Sports Med 10:90–95, 1982.

Arnoczky SP, McDevitt CA: The meniscus: Structure, function, repair, and replacement. In Buckwalter JA, Einhorn TA, Simon SR, eds: Orthopaedic Basic Science: Biology and Biomechanics of the Musculoskeletal System, 2nd ed, pp 531–546. Rosemont, IL, American Academy of Orthopaedic Surgeons, 2000.

Buckwalter JA, Hunziker EB: Articular cartilage biology and morphology. In Mow VC, Ratcliffe A, eds: Structure and Function of Articular Cartilage. Boca Raton, FL, CRC Press, 1993.

Buckwalter J, Rosenberg L, Coutts R, et al: Articular cartilage: Injury and repair. In Woo SL-Y, Buckwalter JA, eds: Injury and Repair of the Musculoskeletal Soft Tissues, pp 465–481. Park Ridge, IL, American Academy of Orthopaedic Surgeons, 1988.

Frymoyer JW, ed: Arthritis Orthopaedic Knowledge. Update 4: Home Study Syllabus, pp 89–106. Park Ridge, IL, American Academy of Orthopaedic Surgeons, 1993.

Iannotti JP, Goldstein S, Kuhn JL, et al: The formation and growth of skeletal tissues. In Buckwalter JA, Einhorn TA, Simon SR, eds: Orthopaedic Basic Science: Biology and Biomechanics of the Musculoskeletal System, 2nd ed, pp 77–110. Rosemont, IL, American Academy of Orthopaedic Surgeons, 2000.

Kasser JR, ed: Orthopaedic Knowledge Update 5, pp 163–175. Rosemont, IL, American Academy of Orthopaedic Surgeons, 1996.

Mankin HJ, Brandt KD: Biochemistry and metabolism of articular cartilage in osteoarthritis. In Moskowitz RW, Howell DS, Goldberg VM, et al, eds: Osteoarthritis: Diagnosis and Medical/Surgical Management, 2nd ed, pp 109–154. Philadelphia, WB Saunders, 1992.

Mankin HJ, Mow VC, Buckwalter JA, et al: Articular cartilage structure, composition, and function. In Buckwalter JA, Einhorn TA, Simon SR, eds: Orthopaedic Basic Science: Biology and Biomechanics of the Musculoskeletal System, 2nd ed, pp 443–470. Rosemont, IL, American Academy of Orthopaedic Surgeons, 2000.

Mayne R, Irwin MH: Collagen types in cartilage. In Kuettner KE, Schleyerbach R, Hascall VC, eds: Articular Cartilage Biochemistry, pp 23–38. New York, Raven Press, 1986.

Mow V, Rosenwasser M: Articular cartilage biomechanics. In Woo SL-Y, Buckwalter JA, eds: Injury and Repair of the Musculoskeletal Soft Tissues, pp 445–451. Park Ridge, IL, American Academy of Orthopaedic Surgeons, 1988.

Mow VC, Soslowsky LJ: Friction, lubrication, and wear of diarthrodial joints. In Mow VC, Hayes WC, eds: Basic Orthopaedic Biomechanics, p 263. New York, Churchill Livingstone, 1988.

Mow VC, Zhu W, Ratcliffe A: Structure and function of articular cartilage and meniscus. In Mow VC, Hayes WC, eds: Basic Orthopaedic Biomechanics, pp 143–198. New York, Raven Press, 1991.

Rosenberg LC, Buckwalter JA: Cartilage proteoglycans. In Kuettner KE, Schleyerbach R, Hascall VC, eds: Articular Cartilage Biochemistry, pp 39–58. New York, Raven Press, 1986.

Schenk RK, Eggli PS, Hunziker EB: Articular cartilage morphology. In Kuettner KE, Schleyerbach R, Hascall VC, eds: Articular Cartilage Biochemistry, pp 3–22. New York, Raven Press, 1986.

Woo SL-Y, An K, Frank CB, et al: Anatomy, biology, and biomechanics of tendon and ligament. In Buckwalter JA, Einhorn TA, Simon SR, eds: Orthopaedic Basic Science: Biology and Biomechanics of the Musculoskeletal System, 2nd ed, pp 581–616. Rosemont, IL, American Academy of Orthopaedic Surgeons, 2000.

Woo SL-Y, Buckwalter JA, eds: Injury and Repair of the Musculoskeletal Soft Tissues. Park Ridge, IL, American Academy of Orthopaedic Surgeons, pp 487–537, 1988.

ARTHROSES

Recent Articles

Brinker MR, Rosenberg AG, Kull L, et al: Primary noncemented total hip arthroplasty in patients with ankylosing spondylitis: Clinical and radiographic results at an average follow-up period of 6 years. J Arthroplasty 11:808–812, 1996.

Rivard GE, Girard M, Belanger R, et al: Synoviorthesis with colloidal 32P chromic phosphate for the treatment of hemophilic arthropathy. J Bone Joint Surg [Am] 76:482–488, 1994.

Schaller JG: Juvenile rheumatoid arthritis. Pediatr Rev 18:337–349, 1997.

Weinblatt ME, Kremer JM, Bankhurst AD, et al: A trial of etanercept, a recombinant tumor necrosis factor receptor: Fc fusion protein in patients with rheumatoid arthritis receiving methotrexate. N Engl J Med 340:253–259, 1999.

Classic Articles

Ahlberg AKM: On the natural history of hemophilic pseudotumor. J Bone Joint Surg [Am] 57:1133–1136, 1975.

Ansell BM, Swann M: The management of chronic arthritis of children. J Bone Joint Surg [Br] 65:536–543, 1983.

Byers PD, Cotton RE, Decon OW, et al: The diagnosis and treatment of pigmented villonodular synovitis. J Bone Joint Surg [Br] 50:290–305, 1968.

Chylack LT Jr: The ocular manifestations of juvenile rheumatoid arthritis. Arthritis Rheum 20:217–223, 1977.

Cofield RH, Morrison MJ, Beabout JW: Diabetic neuroarthropathy in the foot: Patient characteristics and patterns of radiographic change. Foot Ankle 4:15–22, 1983.

Culp RW, Eichenfield AH, Davidson RS, et al: Lyme arthritis in children: An orthopaedic perspective. J Bone Joint Surg [Am] 69:96–99, 1987.

Firooznia H, Seliger G, Genieser NB, et al: Hypertrophic pulmonary osteoarthropathy in pulmonary metastases. Radiology 115:269–274, 1975.

Ishikawa K, Masuda I, Ohira T, et al: A histological study of calcium pyrophosphate dihydrate crystal-deposition disease. J Bone Joint Surg [Am] 71:875–886, 1989.

Mankin HJ, Dorfman H, Lippiello L, et al: Biochemical and metabolic abnormalities in articular cartilage from osteo-arthritic human hips: II. Correlation of morphology with biochemical and metabolic data. J Bone Joint Surg [Am] 53:523–537, 1971.

Mankin HJ, Johnson ME, Lippiello L: Biochemical and metabolic abnormalities in articular cartilage from osteoarthritic human hips: III. Distribution and metabolism of amino sugar-containing macromolecules. J Bone Joint Surg [Am] 63:131–139, 1981.

Mankin HJ, Thrasher AZ: Water content and binding in normal and osteoarthritic human cartilage. J Bone Joint Surg [Am] 57:76–80, 1975.

McCarty DJ, Halverson PB, Carrera GR, et al: Milwaukee shoulder: Association of microspheroids containing hydroxyapatite, Active collagenase and neutral protease with rotator cuff defects: I. Clinical Aspects 24:464–473, 1981.

Neer CS, Craig EV, Fukuda H: Cuff-tear arthropathy. J Bone Joint Surg [Am] 65:1232–1244, 1983.

Resnick D: Radiology of seronegative spondyloarthropathies. Clin Orthop 143:38–45, 1979.

Simmon EH: The surgical correction of flexion deformity of the cervical spine in ankylosing spondylitis. Clin Orthop 86:132–143, 1972.

Williams B: Orthopaedic features in the presentation of syringomyelia. J Bone Joint Surg [Br] 61:314–323, 1979.

Review Articles

Alpert SW, Koval KJ, Zuckerman JD: Neuropathic arthropathy: Review of current knowledge. J Am Acad Orthop Surg 4:100–108, 1996.

Barry PE, Stillman JS: Characteristics of juvenile rheumatoid arthritis: Its medical and orthopaedic management. Orthop Clin North Am 6: 641–651, 1975.

Ford D: The clinical spectrum of Reiter's syndrome and similar postenteric arthropathies. Clin Orthop 143:59–65, 1979.

Book Chapters

Buchanan WW: Clinical features of rheumatoid arthritis. In Scott JT, ed: Copeman's Textbook of the Rheumatoid Diseases, 5th ed, pp 318–364. Edinburgh, Churchill Livingstone, 1978.

Calin A: Ankylosing spondylitis. In Kelley WN, Harris ED, Ruddy S, et al, eds: Textbook of Rheumatology, pp 1021–1037. Philadelphia, WB Saunders, 1989.

Currey HLF: Aetiology and pathogenesis of rheumatoid arthritis. In Scott JT, ed: Copeman's Textbook of the Rheumatoid Diseases, 5th ed, pp 261–272. Edinburgh, Churchill Livingstone, 1978.

Frymoyer JW, ed: Arthritis Orthopaedic Knowledge Update 4: Home Study Syllabus, pp 89–106. Rosemont, IL, American Academy of Orthopaedic Surgeons, 1993.

Gardner DL: Pathology of rheumatoid arthritis. In Scott JT, ed: Copeman's Textbook of the Rheumatoid Diseases, 5th ed, pp 273–317. Edinburgh, Churchill Livingstone, 1978.

Greene WB, McMillan CW: Nonsurgical management of hemophilic arthropathy. Instr Course Lect 38:367–381, 1989.

Guerra J, Resnick D: Radiographic and scintigraphic abnormalities in seronegative spondylarthropathies and juvenile chronic arthritis. In Calin A, ed: Spondylarthropathies, pp 339–382. New York, Grune & Stratton, 1984.

Hockberg MC: Epidemiology of rheumatoid disease. In Schumacher HR Jr, ed: Primer on the Rheumatic Diseases, 9th ed, pp 48–51. Atlanta, Arthritis Foundation, 1988.

Jacobs RL: Charcot foot. In Jahss MH, ed: Disorders of the Foot and Ankle, 2nd ed, vol 3, p 2164. Philadelphia, WB Saunders, 1991.

Kasser JR, ed: Orthopaedic Knowledge Update 5, pp 481–502. Rosemont, IL, American Academy of Orthopaedic Surgeons, 1996.

Kelley WN, Fox IH: Gout and related disorders of purine metabolism. In Kelley WN, Harris ED Jr, Ruddy S, et al, eds: Textbook of Rheumatology, 2nd ed, p 1382. Philadelphia, WB Saunders, 1985.

Mankin HJ, Brandt KD: Biochemistry and metabolism of articular cartilage in osteoarthritis. In Moskowitz RW, Howell VC, Goldberg VM, et al, eds: Osteoarthritis: Diagnosis and Medical/Surgical Management, 2nd ed, pp 109–154. Philadelphia, WB Saunders, 1992.

Mankin HJ, Mow VC, Buckwalter JA: Articular cartilage repair and osteoarthritis. In Buckwalter JA, Einhorn TA, Simon SR, eds: Orthopaedic Basic Science: Biology and Biomechanics of the Musculoskeletal System, 2nd ed, pp 471–488. Rosemont, IL, American Academy of Orthopaedic Surgeons, 2000.

Poss R, ed: Arthritis Orthopaedic Knowledge Update 3: Home Study Syllabus, p 63. Park Ridge, IL, American Academy of Orthopaedic Surgeons, 1990.

Rana NA: Rheumatoid arthritis, other collagen diseases, and psoriasis of the foot. In Jahss MH, ed: Disorders of the Foot, pp 1057–1058. Philadelphia, WB Saunders, 1982.

Rana NA: Rheumatoid arthritis, other collagen diseases, and psoriasis of the foot. In Jahss MH, ed: Disorders of the Foot and Ankle, 2nd ed, p 1745. Philadelphia, WB Saunders, 1991.

Rodnan GP, Schumacher HR, eds: Primer on the Rheumatic Diseases, 8th ed, pp 128–131. Atlanta, Arthritis Foundation, 1983.

Rogers LF: Diseases of the Joints, 6th ed, pp 125–127. Philadelphia, JB Lippincott, 1993.

Ryan LM, McCarty DJ: Calcium pyrophosphate crystal deposition disease; pseudogout; articular chondrocalcinosis. In McCarty DJ, Koopmen WJ, eds: Arthritis and Allied Conditions, 12th ed, vol 2, pp 1835–1855. Philadelphia, Lea & Febiger, 1993.

Sammarco GJ: Diabetic arthropathy. In Sammarco GJ, ed: The Foot in Diabetes, pp 153–172. Philadelphia, Lea & Febiger, 1991.

Schumacher RH, ed: Primer of Rheumatic Disease, 9th ed, p 149. Atlanta, Arthritis Foundation, 1988.

Smukler N: Arthritic disorders of the spine. In Rothman RH, Simeone FA, eds: The Spine, 2nd ed, pp 906–941. Philadelphia, WB Saunders, 1982.

Recklies AD, Poole AR, Banerjee S, et al: Pathophysiologic aspects of inflammation in diarthrodial joints. In Buckwalter JA, Einhorn TA, Simon SR, eds: Orthopaedic Basic Science: Biology and Biomechanics of the Musculoskeletal System, 2nd ed, p 489. Rosemont, IL, American Academy of Orthopaedic Surgeons, 2000.

Rosier RN, Reynolds PR, O'Keefe RJ: Molecular and cellular biology in orthopaedics. In Buckwalter JA, Einhorn TA, Simon SR, eds: Orthopaedic Basic Science: Biology and Biomechanics of the Musculoskeletal System, 2nd ed, pp 19–76. Rosemont, IL, American Academy of Orthopaedic Surgeons, 2000.

Westring D, Ries M, Dee R: Hematologic disorders. In Dee R, Mango E, Hurst LC, eds: Principles of Orthopaedic Practice, pp 290–294. New York, McGraw-Hill, 1998.

SKELETAL MUSCLE AND ATHLETICS

Recent Articles

American Academy of Orthopaedic Surgeons Position Statement: Anabolic Steroids to Enhance Athletic Performance. Park Ridge, IL, American Academy of Orthopaedic Surgeons, 1991.

Beiner JM, Jokl P, Cholewicki J, Panjabi MM: The effect of anabolic steroids and corticosteroids on healing of muscle contusion injury. Am J Sports Med 27:2, 1999.

Evans WJ: Effects of exercise on senescent muscle. Clin Orthop 403: S211–S220, 2002.

Hultman E, Soderlund K, Timmons JA, et al: Muscle creatine loading in men. J Appl Physiol 81:232–237, 1996.

Lutz GE, Palmitier RA, An KN, et al: Comparison of tibiofemoral joint forces during open-kinetic-chain and closed-kinetic-chain exercises. J Bone Joint Surg [Am] 75:732–739, 1993.

Nattiv A, Lynch L: Female athlete triad. Phys Sports Med 22:60–68, 1994.
Sapega AA: Muscle performance evaluation in orthopaedic practice. J Bone Joint Surg [Am] 72:1562–1574, 1990.
Sturmi JE, Diorio DJ: Anabolic agents. Clin Sports Med 17:261–282, 1998.
Thayer R, Collins J, Noble EG, et al: A decade of aerobic endurance training: Histological evidence for fibre type transformation. J Sports Med Phys Fitness 40:284–289, 2000.
Voss LA, Fadale PD, Hulstyn MJ: Exercise-induced loss of bone density in athletes. J Am Acad Orthop Surg 6:349–357, 1998.

Classic Articles

Baldwin KM, Winder WW, Holloszy JO: Adaptation of actomyosin ATPase in different types of muscle to endurance exercise. Am J Physiol 229: 422–426, 1975.
Booth FW: Physiologic and biochemical effects of immobilization on muscle. Clin Orthop 219:15–20, 1987.
Booth FW: Physiologic and biochemical effects in immobilization of muscle. Clin Orthop 219:25–27, 1987.
Faulkner JA: New perspectives in training for maximum performance. JAMA 205:741–746, 1968.
Gollnick PD, Armstrong RB, Saltin B, et al: Effect of training on enzyme activity and fiber composition of human skeletal muscle. J Appl Physiol 34:107–111, 1973.
Holloszy JO: Biochemical adaptations in muscle: Effects of exercise on mitochondrial oxygen uptake and respiratory enzyme activity in skeletal muscle. J Biol Chem 242:2278–2282, 1967.
Huxley HE: Electron microscope studies on the structure of natural and synthetic protein filaments from striated muscle. J Mol Biol 7:281–308, 1963.
Huxley HE: The mechanism of muscular contraction. Science 164: 1356–1365, 1969.
Lowey S, Risby D: Light chains from fast and slow muscle myosins. Nature 234:81–85, 1971.
MacDougall JD, Elder CG, Sale DG, et al: Effects of strength training and immobilization on human muscle fibres. Eur J Appl Physiol 43:25–34, 1980.

Review Articles

AMA Council on Scientific Affairs: Drug abuse in athletes: Anabolic steroids and human growth hormone. JAMA 259:1703–1705, 1988.
Haupt HA: Current concepts: Anabolic steroids and growth hormone. Am J Sports Med 21:468–474, 1993.
Kibler WB: Physiology of exercising muscle. AAOS Instr Course Lect 43:3–4, 1994.

Book Chapters

Asher MA, ed: Health maintenance of the musculoskeletal system, pp 1–8. Park Ridge, IL, American Academy of Orthopaedic Surgeons, 1984.
Best TM, Garret WE: Basic science of soft tissue: Muscle and tendon. In DeLee J, Drez D, eds: Orthopaedic Sports Medicine: Principles and Practice, vol 1, p 17. Philadelphia, WB Saunders, 1994.
Bodine SC, Lieber RL: Peripheral nerve physiology, anatomy, and pathology. In Buckwalter JA, Einhorn TA, Simon SR, eds: Orthopaedic Basic Science: Biology and Biomechanics of the Musculoskeletal System, 2nd ed, pp 617–682. Rosemont, IL, American Academy of Orthopaedic Surgeons, 2000.
Frymoyer JW, ed: Bone metabolism and bone metabolic disease. In Orthopaedic Knowledge Update 4, p 82. Rosemont, IL, American Academy of Orthopaedic Surgeons, 1993.
Garrett WE, Best TM: Anatomy, physiology, and mechanics of skeletal muscle. In Buckwalter JA, Einhorn TA, Simon SR, eds: Orthopaedic Basic Science: Biology and Biomechanics of the Musculoskeletal System, 2nd ed, pp 683–716. Rosemont, IL, American Academy of Orthopaedic Surgeons, 2000.
Kibler WB, Chandler TJ, Reuter BH: Advances in conditioning. In Griffin LY, ed: Orthopaedic Knowledge Update: Sports Medicine, pp 65–73. Rosemont, IL, American Academy of Orthopaedic Surgeons, 1994.
Poss R, ed: Exercise and athletic conditioning. In Orthopaedic Knowledge Update 3: Home Study Syllabus, pp 50–51. Park Ridge, IL, American Academy of Orthopaedic Surgeons, 1990.
Poss R, ed: Exercise and athletic conditioning: Drug use. In Orthopaedic Knowledge Update 3: Home Study Syllabus, p 50. Park Ridge, IL, American Academy of Orthopaedic Surgeons, 1990.
Poss R, ed: General knowledge: Exercise and athletic conditioning; effect of warm-up activities. In Orthopaedic Knowledge Update 3: Home Study Syllabus, p 47. Park Ridge, IL, American Academy of Orthopaedic Surgeons, 1990.
Simon SR: Anatomy: Muscle. In Orthopaedic Science: A Resource and Self-Study Guide for the Practitioner, p 28. Park Ridge, IL, American Academy of Orthopaedic Surgeons, 1986.
Simon RA, ed: Biomechanics: Biomechanics of materials; musculoskeletal tissues. In Orthopaedic Science: A Resource and Self-Study Guide for the Practitioner, p 163. Park Ridge, IL, American Academy of Orthopaedic Surgeons, 1986.
Waddler GI, Hainline B: Drugs in the Athlete, p 65. Philadelphia, FA Davis, 1989.

NERVOUS SYSTEM

Recent Articles

Bracken MB, Shepard MJ, Holford TR, et al: Administration of methylprednisolone for 24 or 48 hours or tirilazad mesylate for 48 hours in the treatment of acute spinal cord injury: Results of the Third National Acute Spinal Cord Injury Randomized Controlled Trial National Acute Spinal Cord Injury Study. JAMA 277:1597–1604, 1997.
Bracken MB, Shepard MJ, Collins WF, et al: A randomized controlled trial of methylprednisolone or naloxone in the treatment of spinal cord injury: Results of the Second National Acute Spinal Cord Injury Study. N Engl J Med 322:1405–1411, 1990.
Ditunno JF, Little JW, Tessler A, et al: Spinal shock revisited: A four-phase model. Spinal Cord 42:383–395, 2004.
Koman LA, Mooney JF, Smith B, et al: Management of cerebral palsy with botulinum-A toxin: Preliminary investigation. J Pediatr Orthop 13:489, 1993.
Olmarker K, Rydevik B: Single versus double-level nerve root compression. Clin Orthop 279:35–39, 1992.

Classic Articles

Seddon HJ: Three types of nerve injuries. Brain 66:238–283, 1943.

Review Articles

Battista A, Lusskin R: The anatomy and physiology of the peripheral nerve. Foot Ankle 7:65–70, 1986.
Bracken MB: Pharmacological treatment of acute spinal cord injury: Current status and future projects. J Emerg Med 11:43–48, 1993.
Bruno LA, Gennarelli TA, Torg JS: Management guidelines for head injuries in athletics. Clin Sports Med 6:17–29, 1987.

Book Chapters

Bodine SC, Lieber RL: Peripheral nerve physiology, anatomy, and pathology. In Buckwalter JA, Einhorn TA, Simon SR, eds: Orthopaedic Basic Science: Biology and Biomechanics of the Musculoskeletal System, 2nd ed, pp 617–682. Rosemont, IL, American Academy of Orthopaedic Surgeons, 2000.
Brown AG, ed: Organization in the Spinal Cord: The Anatomy and Physiology of Identified Neurones. Berlin, Springer-Verlag, 1981.
Lundborg G, ed: Nerve Injury and Repair, pp 149–195. New York, Churchill Livingstone, 1988.
Gelberman RH, Eaton RG, Urbaniak JR: Peripheral nerve compression. Instr Course Lect 33:31–53, 1994.
Gelberman RH, ed: Operative Nerve Repair and Reconstruction. Philadelphia, JB Lippincott, 1991.
Guskiewicz KM, Barth JT: Head injuries. In Schenk RC Jr, ed: Athletic Training and Sports Medicine, pp 143–167. Rosemont, IL, American Academy of Orthopaedic Surgeons, 1999.
Guyton AC: Basic Neuroscience: Anatomy and Physiology, 2nd ed. Philadelphia, WB Saunders, 1992.
McAfee PC: Cervical spine trauma. In Frymoyer JW, ed: The Adult Spine: Principles and Practice, vol 2, p 1079. New York, Raven Press, 1991.
Rall W: Core conductor theory and cable properties of neurons. In Kandel ER, ed: Handbook of Physiology, Section 1: The Nervous System, pp 39–97. Bethesda, MD, American Physiological Society, 1977.
Sutton DC, Siveri CP, Cotler JM: Initial evaluation and management of the spinal injured patient. In Cotler JM, Simpson JM, An HS, et al, eds: Surgery of Spinal Trauma, pp 113–126. Philadelphia, Lippincott, Williams & Wilkins, 2000.

CONNECTIVE TISSUES

Recent Articles

Terek RM, Jirnaek WA, Goldberg MJ, et al: The expression of platelet-derived growth factor gene in Dupuytren's contracture. J Bone Joint Surg [Am] 77:1–9, 1995.

Wiggins ME, Fadale PD, Ehrlich MG, et al: Effects of local injection of corticosteroids on the healing of ligaments. J Bone Joint Surg [Am] 77:1682–1691, 1995.

Classic Articles

Arnoczky SP: Anatomy of the anterior cruciate ligament. Clin Orthop 172:19–25, 1983.

Butler DL, Grood ES, Noyes FR, et al: Biomechanics of ligaments and tendons. Exerc Sports Sci Rev 6:125–181, 1976.

Kurosaka M, Yoshiya S, Andrish JT: A biomechanical comparison of different surgical techniques of graft fixation in anterior cruciate ligament reconstruction. Am J Sports Med 15:225–229, 1987.

Noyes FR, Butler DL, Grood ES, et al: Biomechanical analysis of human ligament grafts used in knee ligament repairs and reconstructions. J Bone Joint Surg [Am] 66:344–352, 1984.

Noyes FR, DeLucas JL, Torvik PJ: Biomechanics of anterior cruciate ligament failure: An analysis of strain-rate sensitivity and mechanisms of failure in primates. J Bone Joint Surg [Am] 56:236–253, 1974.

Book Chapters

Frymoyer JW, ed: Knee and leg: Soft-tissue trauma. In Orthopaedic Knowledge Update 4: Home Study Syllabus, pp 593–602. Rosemont, IL, American Academy of Orthopaedic Surgeons, 1993.

Poss R, ed: Soft tissue implants. In Orthopaedic Knowledge Update 3: Home Study Syllabus, pp 178–179. Park Ridge, IL, American Academy of Orthopaedic Surgeons, 1990.

Wood SL: Ligament, tendon, and joint capsule insertions to bone. In Woo SL-Y, Buckwalter JA, eds: Injury and Repair of the Musculoskeletal Soft Tissues. Park Ridge, IL, American Academy of Orthopaedic Surgeons, 1988.

Woo SL-Y, An K, Frank CB, et al: Anatomy, biology, and biomechanics of tendon and ligament. In Buckwalter JA, Einhorn TA, Simon SR, eds: Orthopaedic Basic Science: Biology and Biomechanics of the Musculoskeletal System, 2nd ed, pp 581–616. Rosemont, IL, American Academy of Orthopaedic Surgeons, 2000.

Woo SL-Y, Buckwalter JA, eds: Injury and Repair of the Musculoskeletal Soft Tissues. Park Ridge, IL, American Academy of Orthopaedic Surgeons, 1988.

CELLULAR AND MOLECULAR BIOLOGY, IMMUNOLOGY, AND GENETICS OF ORTHOPAEDICS

Recent Articles

D'Astous J, Drouin MA, Rhine E: Intraoperative anaphylaxis secondary to allergy to latex in children who have spina bifida: Report of two cases. J Bone Joint Surg [Am] 74:1084–1086, 1992.

Fuda C, Suvorov M, Vakulenko SB, et al: The basis for resistance to beta-lactam antibiotics by penicillin-binding protein 2a (PBP2a) of methicillin-resistant Staphyloccocus aureus. J Biol Chem 279:40802–40806, 2004.

Jiranek W, Jasty M, Wang JT: Tissue response to particulate polymethylmethacrylate in mice with various immune deficiencies. J Bone Joint Surg [Am] 77:1650–1661, 1995.

Giunta C, Superti-Furga A, Spranger S, et al: Ehlers-Danlos syndrome type VII: Clinical features and molecular defects. J Bone Joint Surg [Am] 81:225–238, 1999.

Lim D, Strynadka NC: Structural basis for the beta lactam resistance of PBP2a from methicillin-resistant Staphylococcus aureus. Nat Struct Biol 9: 870–876, 2002.

Meehan PL, Galina MP, Daftari T: Intraoperative anaphylaxis due to allergy to latex: Report of two cases. J Bone Joint Surg [Am] 74:1087–1089, 1992.

Miyasaka M: Cancer metastasis and adhesion molecules. Clin Orthop 312:10–18, 1995.

Rousseau F, Bonaventure J, Legeai-Mallet L, et al: Mutations in the gene encoding fibroblast growth factor receptor-3 in achondroplasia. Nature 371:252–254, 1994.

Shiang R, Thompson LM, Zhu YZ, et al: Mutations in the transmembrane domain of FGFR3 cause the most common genetic form of dwarfism, achondroplasia. Cell 78:335–342, 1994.

Tsipouras P, Del Mastro R, Sarfarazi M, et al: Genetic linkage of the Marfan syndrome, ectopia lentis, and congenital contractural arachnodactyly to the fibrillin genes on chromosomes 15 and 5: The International Marfan Syndrome Collaborative Study. N Engl J Med 326:905–909, 1992.

Classic Articles

Antonarakis SE: Diagnosis of genetic disorders at the DNA level. N Engl J Med 320:151–163, 1989.

Harrod MJ, Friedman JM, Currarino G, et al: Genetic heterogeneity in spondyloepiphyseal dysplasia congenita. Am J Med Genet 18:311–320, 1984.

McKusick VA: Mapping and sequencing the human genome. N Engl J Med 320:910–915, 1989.

Turc-Carel C, Aurias A, Mugneret F, et al: Chromosomes in Ewing's sarcoma: An evaluation of 85 cases of remarkable consistency of t(11;22)(q24;q12). Cancer Genet Cytogenet 32:229–238, 1988.

White R, Lalouel J-M: Chromosome mapping with DNA markers. Sci Am 258:40–48, 1988.

Veitch JM, Omer GE: Case report: Treatment of cat bite injuries of the hand. J Trauma 19:201–202, 1989.

Wahlig H, Dingeldein E, Bergmann R, et al: The release of gentamycin from polymethylmethacrylate beads: An experimental and pharmacokinetic study. J Bone Joint Surg [Br] 60:270–275, 1978.

Review Articles

Beals RK, Horton W: Skeletal dysplasias: An approach to diagnosis. J Am Acad Orthop Surg 3:174–181, 1995.

Evans CH, Robbins PD: Current concepts review—possible orthopaedic applications of gene therapy. J Bone Joint Surg [Am] 77:1103–1111, 1995.

Jaffurs BS, Evans C: The Human Genome Project: Implications for the treatment of musculoskeletal disease. Am Acad Orthop Surg 6:1–14, 1998.

Tolo VT: Spinal deformity in short stature syndromes. AAOS Instr Course Lect 39:399–405, 1990.

Book Chapters

Alberts B, Bray D, Lewis J, et al, eds: Molecular Biology of the Cell, 2nd ed. New York, Garland Publishing, 1989.

DiDonato S, DiMauro S, Mamoli A, et al: Molecular Genetics of Neurological and Neuromuscular Disease, vol 48. New York, Advances in Neurology, 1988.

Dietz FR, Murray JC: Update on the genetic basis of disorders with orthopaedic manifestations. In Buckwalter JA, Einhorn TA, Simon SR, eds: Orthopaedic Basic Science: Biology and Biomechanics of the Musculoskeletal System, 2nd ed, pp 111–132. Rosemont, IL, American Academy of Orthopaedic Surgeons, 2000.

Rosier RN, Reynolds PR, O'Keefe RJ: Molecular and cellular biology in orthopaedics. In Buckwalter JA, Einhorn TA, Simon SR, eds: Orthopaedic Basic Science: Biology and Biomechanics of the Musculoskeletal System, 2nd ed, pp 19–76. Rosemont, IL, American Academy of Orthopaedic Surgeons, 2000.

Ross DW: Introduction to Molecular Medicine, 2nd ed. New York, Springer-Verlag, 1996.

Watson JD, Tooze J, Kurtz DT: Recombinant DNA: A Short Course. New York, Scientific American Books, 1983.

Wynbrandt J, Ludman MD: The Encyclopedia of Genetic Disorders and Birth Defects. "Facts on File," New York, 1991.

MUSCULOSKELETAL INFECTIONS

Recent Articles

Barrack R, Harris W: The value of aspiration of the hip joint before revision total hip arthroplasty. J Bone Joint Surg [Am] 75:66–76, 1993.

Bass JW, Vincent JM, Person DA: The expanding spectrum of Bartonella infections: II Cat-scratch disease. Pediatr Infect Dis 16: 163–179, 1997.

Brodsky JW, Schneidler C: Diabetic foot infections. Orthop Clin North Am 22:473–489, 1991.

Chiang SR, Chuang YC: Vibrio vulnificus infection: Clinical manifestations, pathogenesis, and antimicrobial therapy. J Microbiol Immunol Infect 36:81–88, 2003.

Clarke HJ, Jinnah RH, Byank RP, et al: Clostridium difficile infection in orthopaedic patients. J Bone Joint Surg [Am] 72:1056–1059, 1990.

Feldman DS, Lonner JH, Desai P, et al: The role of intraoperative frozen sections in revision or total joint arthroplasty. J Bone Joint Surg [Am] 77:1807–1813, 1995.

Gristina AG: Implant failure and the immuno-incompetent fibro-inflammatory zone. Clin Orthop 298:106–118, 1994.

Hollmann MW, Horowitz M: Femoral fractures secondary to low velocity missiles: Treatment with delayed intramedullary fixation. J Orthop Trauma 4:64–69, 1990.

Holton PD, Mader J, Nelson CL, et al: Antibiotics for the practicing orthopaedic surgeon. Instr Course Lect 44:36–42, 2000.

Hospital Infection Control Practices Advisory Committee: Recommendations for preventing the spread of vancomycin resistance. Infect Control Hosp Epidemiol 16:105–113, 1995.

Miclau T, Edin ML, Lester GE, et al: Bone toxicity of locally applied aminoglycosides. J Orthop Trauma 9:401–406, 1995.

Mills WJ, Swiontkowski MF: Fatal group A streptococcal infection with toxic shock syndrome: Complicating minor orthopedic trauma. J Orthop Trauma 10:149–155, 1996.

Nelson JP, Fitzgerald RH Jr, Jaspers MT, et al: Prophylactic antimicrobial coverage in arthroplasty patients [editorial]. J Bone Joint Surg [Am] 72:1, 1990.

Paiement GD, Hymes RA, LaDouceur MS, et al: Postoperative infections in asymptomatic HIV seropositive orthopaedic trauma patients. J Trauma 37:545–551, 1994.

Patzakis MJ, Wilkins J, Kumar J, et al: Comparison of the results of bacterial cultures from multiple sites in chronic osteomyelitis of long bones. J Bone Joint Surg [Am] 76:664–666, 1994.

Sullivan PM, Johnston RC, Kelky SS: Late infection after total hip replacement, caused by an oral organism after dental manipulation. J Bone Joint Surg [Am] 72:121–123, 1990.

Thelander U, Larsson S: Quantitation of C-reactive protein levels and erythrocyte sedimentation rate after spinal surgery. Spine 17:400–404, 1992.

Tomford WW: Transmission of disease through transplantation of musculoskeletal allografts. J Bone Joint Surg [Am] 77:1742–1754, 1995.

Travis J: Reviving the antibiotic miracle. Science 264:360–362, 1994.

Unkila-Kallio L, Markku KJT, Peltola H: The usefulness of C-reactive protein levels in the identification of concurrent septic arthritis in children who have acute hematogenous osteomyelitis. J Bone Joint Surg [Am] 76: 848–853, 1994.

Wang KC, Shih CH: Necrotizing fasciitis of the extremities. J Trauma 32:179–182, 1992.

Wilson MG, Kelley K, Thornhill TS: Infection as a complication of total-knee replacement arthroplasty: Risk factors and treatment in sixty-seven cases. J Bone Joint Surg [Am] 72:878–883, 1990.

Windsor RE, Insall JN, Urs WK, et al: Two-stage reimplantation for the salvage of total knee arthroplasty complicated by infection: Further follow-up and refinement of indications. J Bone Joint Surg [Am] 72:272–278, 1990.

Classic Articles

Aalto K, Osterman K, Peltola H, et al: Changes in erythrocyte sedimentation rate and C-reactive protein after total hip arthroplasty. Clin Orthop 184:118–120, 1984.

Bailey JP Jr, Stevens SJ, Bell WM, et al: Mycobacterium marinum infection: A fishy story. JAMA 247:1314, 1982.

Bartlett P, Reingold AL, Graham DR, et al: Toxic shock syndrome associated with surgical wound infections. JAMA 247:1448–1451, 1982.

Brand RA, Black H: Pseudomonas osteomyelitis following puncture wounds in children. J Bone Joint Surg [Am] 56:1637–1642, 1974.

Buck BE, Malinin TI, Brown MD: Bone transplantation and human immunodeficiency virus: An estimate of risk of acquired immunodeficiency syndrome (AIDS). Clin Orthop 240:129–136, 1989.

Buchholz HW, Elson RA, Engelbrecht E, et al: Management of deep infection of total hip replacement. J Bone Joint Surg [Br] 63:342–353, 1981.

Committee on Trauma, American College of Surgeons: Prophylaxis against tetanus in wound management. Am Coll Surg Bull 69:22–23, 1984.

Dalinka MK, Dinnenberg S, Greendyk WH, et al: Roentgenographic features of osseous coccidioidomycosis and differential diagnosis. J Bone Joint Surg [Am] 53:1157–1164, 1971.

Digby JM, Kersley JB: Pyogenic non-tuberculous spinal infection: An analysis of thirty cases. J Bone Joint Surg [Br] 61:47–55, 1979.

Eismont FJ, Bohlman HH, Soni PL, et al: Pyogenic and fungal vertebral osteomyelitis with paralysis. J Bone Joint Surg [Am] 65:19–29, 1983.

Fee NF, Dobranski A, Bisla RS: Gas gangrene complicating open forearm fractures: Report of five cases. J Bone Joint Surg [Am] 59:135–138, 1977.

Fielding JW, Hawkins RJ: Atlanto-axial rotatory fixation. J Bone Joint Surg [Am] 59:37–44, 1977.

Fitzgerald RH, Cowan JDE: Puncture wounds of the foot. Orthop Clin North Am 6:965–972, 1975.

Fitzgerald RH Jr, Peterson LF, Washington JA II, et al: Bacterial colonization of wounds and sepsis in total hip arthroplasty. J Bone Joint Surg [Am] 55:1242–1250, 1973.

Garcia A, Grantham SA: Hematogenous pyogenic vertebral osteomyelitis. J Bone Joint Surg [Am] 42:429–436, 1960.

Garvin KL, Salvati EA, Brause BD: Role of gentamicin-impregnated cement in total joint arthroplasty. Orthop Clin North Am 19:605–610, 1988.

Goulet JA, Pellicci PM, Brause BD, et al: Prolonged suppression of infection in total hip arthroplasty. J Arthroplasty 3:109–116, 1988.

Grogan TJ, Dorey F, Rollins J, et al: Deep sepsis following total knee arthroplasty: Ten-year experience at the University of California at Los Angeles Medical Center. J Bone Joint Surg [Am] 68:226–234, 1986.

Gustilo RB, Gruninger RP, Davis T: Classification of type III (severe) open fractures relative to treatment and results. Orthopaedics 10:1781–1788, 1987.

Hawkins LG: Pasteurella multocida infections. J Bone Joint Surg [Am] 51:362–366, 1969.

Hill C, Flamont R, Mazas F, et al: Prophylactic cefazolin versus placebo in total hip replacement: Report of a multicentre double-blind randomized trial. Lancet 1:795–796, 1981.

Insall J, Thompson F, Brause B: Two-stage reimplantation for the salvage of infected total knee arthroplasty. J Bone Joint Surg [Am] 65:1087–1098, 1983.

Lange RH, Bach AW, Hansen ST Jr, et al: Open tibial fractures with associated vascular injuries: Prognosis for limb salvage. J Trauma 25:203–208, 1985.

MacAusland WR Jr: The management of sepsis following intramedullary fixation for fractures of the femur. J Bone Joint Surg [Am] 44:1643–1653, 1963.

McDonald DJ, Fitzgerald RH, Ilstrup DM: Two-stage reconstruction of a total hip arthroplasty. J Bone Joint Surg [Am] 71:828–834, 1989.

Mallouh A, Talab Y: Bone and joint infection in patients with sickle cell disease. J Pediatr Orthop 5:158–162, 1985.

Nelson JD: Antibiotic concentrations in septic joint effusions. N Engl J Med 284:349–353, 1971.

Nelson JD, Koontz WC: Septic arthritis in infants and children: A review of 117 cases. Pediatrics 38:966–971, 1966.

O'Connor BT, Steel WM, Sanders R: Disseminated bone tuberculosis. J Bone Joint Surg [Am] 52:537–542, 1970.

Pappas AM, Filler RM, Eraklis AJ, et al: Clostridial infections (gas gangrene): Diagnosis and early treatment. Clin Orthop 76:177–184, 1971.

Patzakis MJ, Harvey JP Jr, Ivler F: The role of antibiotics in the management of open fractures. J Bone Joint Surg [Am] 56:532–541, 1974.

Patzakis MJ, Wilkins J, Bassett RL: Surgical findings in clenched-fist injuries. Clin Orthop 220:237–240, 1987.

Patzakis MJ, Wilkins J, Moor TM: Considerations in reducing the infection rate in open tibial fractures. Clin Orthop 178:36–41, 1983.

Patzakis MJ, Wilkins J, Wiss DA: Infection following intramedullary nailing of long bones. Clin Orthop 212:182–191, 1986.

Riegler HF, Rouston GW: Complications of deep puncture wounds of the foot. J Trauma 19:18–22, 1979.

Roberts JM, Drummond DS, Breed AL, et al: Subacute hematogenous osteomyelitis in children: A retrospective study. J Pediatr Orthop 2:249–254, 1982.

Rovner RA, Baird RA, Malerick MM: Fatal toxic shock syndrome as a complication of orthopaedic surgery: A case report. J Bone Joint Surg [Am] 66:952–954, 1984.

Salvati EA, Callaghan JJ, Brause BD, et al: Reimplantation in infection: Elution of gentamicin from cement and beads. Clin Orthop 207:83–93, 1986.

Wahlig H, Dingeldein E, Bergmann R, et al: The release of gentamicin from polymethylmethacrylate beads: An experimental and pharmacokinetic study. J Bone Joint Surg [Br] 60:270–275, 1978.

Wopperer JM, White JJ, Gillespie R, et al: Long term follow-up of infantile hip sepsis. J Pediatr Orthop 8:322–325, 1988.

Review Articles

Chang HJ, Luck JV Jr, Bell DM, et al: Transmission of human immunodeficiency virus infection in the surgical setting. J Am Acad Orthop Surg 4:279–286, 1996.

Cierny G III: Chronic osteomyelitis: Results of treatment. Instr Course Lect 39:495–508, 1990.

Del Curling O Jr, Gower JD, McWhorter JM: Changing concepts in spinal epidural abscess: A report of 29 cases. Neurosurgery 27:185–192, 1990.

Fitzgerald RH Jr, ed: Infection, pp 71–82. Park Ridge, IL, American Academy of Orthopaedic Surgeons, 1987.

Fitzgerald RH Jr: Orthopaedic sepsis in osteomyelitis: Antimicrobial therapy for the musculoskeletal system. Instr Course Lect 31:1–9, 1982.

Frymoyer JW, ed: Orthopaedic Knowledge Update 4: Home Study Syllabus, p 157. Rosemont, IL, American Academy of Orthopaedic Surgeons, 1993.

Garvis KL, Hanssen AD: Current concepts review—infection after total hip arthroplasty. J Bone Joint Surg [Am] 77:1576–1584, 1995.

Gustilo RB, Merkow RL, Templeman D: The management of open fractures: Current concepts. J Bone Joint Surg [Am] 72:299–304, 1990.

McLaughlin TP, Zemel L, Fisher RL, et al: Chronic arthritis of the knee in Lyme disease: Review of the literature and report of two cases treated by synovectomy. J Bone Joint Surg [Am] 68:1057, 1986.

Tomford WW: Current concepts review: Transmission of disease through transplantation of musculoskeletal allografts. J Bone Joint Surg [Am] 77:1742–1750, 1995.

Waldvogel FA, Papageorgiou PS: Osteomyelitis: The past decade. N Engl J Med 303:360–370, 1980.

Book Chapters

AAOS Task Force on AIDS and Orthopaedic Surgery: Recommendations for the Prevention of Human Immunodeficiency Virus (HIV) Transmission in the Practice of Orthopaedic Surgery. Park Ridge, IL, American Academy of Orthopaedic Surgeons, 1989.

Frymoyer JW, ed: Infection, p 162. Rosemont, IL, American Academy of Orthopaedic Surgeons, 1993.

Gavin KL, Luck JV, Rupp ME, Fey PD: Infections in orthopaedics. In Buckwalter JA, Einhorn TA, Simon SR, eds: Orthopaedic Basic Science: Biology and Biomechanics of the Musculoskeletal System, 2nd ed, pp 239–260. Rosemont, IL, American Academy of Orthopaedic Surgeons, 2000.

Gilbert DN, Moellering RC, Sande MA: The Sanford Guide to Antimicrobial Therapy 32nd ed. Hyde Park, VT, Antimicrobial Therapy, Inc, 2002.

Gristina AJ, Naylor PT, Webb LX: Molecular mechanisms in musculoskeletal sepsis: A race for the surface. Instr Course Lect 34:471–482, 1990.

Kind AC, Williams DN: Antibiotics in open fractures. In Gustillo RB, ed: Management of Open Fractures and Their Complications, pp 55–59. Philadelphia, WB Saunders, 1982.

Mader JT, Calhoun JH: Antimicrobial treatment of musculoskeletal infections. In Evarts CM, ed: Surgery of the Musculoskeletal System, 2nd ed. New York, Churchill Livingstone, 1990.

Morris CD, Einhorn TA: Principles of orthopaedic pharmacology. In Buckwalter JA, Einhorn TA, Simon SR, eds: Orthopaedic Basic Science: Biology and Biomechanics of the Musculoskeletal System, 2nd ed, pp 217–238. Rosemont, IL, American Academy of Orthopaedic Surgeons, 2000.

Morrissy RT: Bone and joint infections. In Morrissy RT, ed: Lovell and Winter's Pediatric Orthopaedics, vol 1, 3rd ed, pp 539–561. Philadelphia, JB Lippincott, 1990.

Sande MA, Kapusnik-Ulner JE, Mandell GL: Antimicrobial agents. In Gilman AG, ed: Goodman and Gilman's The Pharmacological Basis of Therapeutics, 8th ed, pp 1103–1107. New York, McGraw-Hill, 1990.

Sande MA, Mandell GL: Antimicrobial agents: The aminoglycosides. In Gilman AG, Goodman LS, Gilman A, eds: The Pharmacological Basis of Therapeutics, 6th ed, pp 1162–1180. New York, MacMillan, 1980.

Gilbert DN, Moellering RC, Sande MA: The Sanford Guide to Antimicrobial Therapy, 32nd ed. Hyde Park, VT, Antimicrobial Therapy, Inc., 2002.

Tachdjian MO: Pediatric Orthopaedics, vol 2, 2nd ed, pp 1415–1441. Philadelphia, WB Saunders, 1990.

PERIOPERATIVE PROBLEMS

Recent Articles

Bierbaum BE, Callaghan JJ, Galante JO, et al: An analysis of blood management in patients having a total hip or knee arthroplasty. J Bone Joint Surg [Am] 81:2, 1999.

Brinker MR, Reuben JD, Mull JR, et al: Comparison of general and epidural anesthesia in patients undergoing primary unilateral total hip replacement. Orthopedics 20:109–115, 1997.

Colwell CW, Spiro TE, Trowbridge AA, et al: Use of enoxaparin, a low-molecular-weight heparin, and unfractionated heparin for the prevention of deep venous thrombosis after elective hip replacement: A clinical trial comparing efficacy and safety. J Bone Joint Surg [Am] 76:3–14, 1995.

Fahmy N, Chandler H, Danylchuk K: Blood gas and circulatory changes during total knee replacement: Role of the intramedullary alignment rod. J Bone Joint Surg [Am] 72:19–26, 1990.

Faris PM, Ritter MA, Keating EM, et al: Unwashed filtered shed blood collected after knee and hip arthroplasties: A source of autologous red blood cells. J Bone Joint Surg [Am] 73:1169–1178, 1991.

Gerstenfeld LC, Thiede M, Seibert K, et al: Differential inhibition of fracture healing by non-selective and cyclooxygenase-2 non-steroidal anti-inflammatory drugs. J Orthop Res 21:670–675, 2003.

Lieberman JR, Geerts WH: Prevention of venous thromboembolism after total hip and knee arthroplasty. J Bone Joint Surg [Am] 76:1239–1250, 1994.

MacLennan DH, Phillips MS: Malignant hyperthermia. Science 256: 789–794, 1992.

Mancini F, Landolfi C, Muzio M, et al: Acetaminophen down-regulates interleukin-1-beta–induced nuclear factor-kappa B nuclear translocation in a human astrocyte cell line. Neurosci Lett 353:79–82, 2003.

Pape HC, Regel G, Dwenger A, et al: Influences of different methods of intramedullary femoral nailing on lung function in patients with multiple trauma. J Trauma 35:709–716, 1993.

Webb LX, Rush PT, Fuller SB, et al: Greenfield filter prophylaxis of pulmonary embolism in undergoing surgery for acetabular fractures. J Orthop Trauma 6:139–145, 1992.

Classic Articles

Aiach M, Michaud A, Balian JL, et al: A new low molecular weight heparin derivative: In vitro and in vivo studies. Thromb Res 31:611–621, 1983.

Amato JJ, Rheinlander HF, Cleveland RJ: Post-traumatic adult respiratory distress syndrome. Orthop Clin North Am 9:693–713, 1978.

Baker J, Deitch E, Berg R, et al: Hemorrhagic shock induces bacterial translocation from the gut. J Trauma 28:896–905, 1988.

Barnes RW, Shanik GD, Slaymaker EE: An index of healing in below-knee amputation: Leg blood pressure by Doppler ultrasound. Surgery 79: 13–20, 1976.

Culver D, Crawford JS, Gardiner JH, et al: Venous thrombosis after fractures of the upper end of the femur: A study of incidence and site. J Bone Joint Surg [Br] 52:61–69, 1970.

DeLee JC, Rockwood CA Jr: Current concepts review: The use of aspirin in thromboembolic disease. J Bone Joint Surg [Am] 62:149–152, 1980.

Duis JH, Nijsten MWN, Kalausen HJ, et al: Fat embolism in patients with an isolated fracture of the femoral shaft. J Trauma 28:383–390, 1988.

Einhorn TA, Bonnarens F, Burstein AH: The contributions of dietary protein and mineral to the healing of experimental fractures: A biomechanical study. J Bone Joint Surg [Am] 68:1389–1395, 1986.

Jardon OM, Wingard DW, Barak AJ, et al: Malignant hyperthermia: A potentially fatal syndrome in orthopaedic patients. J Bone Joint Surg [Am] 61:1064–1070, 1979.

Johnson KD, Cadambi A, Seibert GB: Incidence of adult respiratory distress syndrome in patients with multiple musculoskeletal injuries: Effect of early operative stabilization of fractures. J Trauma 24:375–384, 1985.

Kakkar VV, Hose CT, Flanc C, et al: Natural history of postoperative deep vein thrombosis. Lancet 2:230–232, 1969.

Knize DM, Weatherly-White RCA, Paton BC, et al: Prognostic factors in the management of frostbite. J Trauma 9:749–759, 1969.

Matsen FA, Clawson DK: The deep posterior compartmental syndrome of the leg. J Bone Joint Surg [Am] 57:34–39, 1975.

Matsen FA III, Winquist A, Krugmire RB Jr: Diagnosis and management of compartment syndromes. J Bone Joint Surg [Am] 62:286–291, 1980.

Review Articles

Gellman H, Nichols D: Reflex sympathetic dystrophy in the upper extremity. J Am Acad Orthop Surg 5:313–322, 1997.

Levy D: The fat embolism syndrome: A review. Clin Orthop 261:281–286, 1990.

Whitesides T Jr, Heckman MM: Acute compartment syndrome: Update on diagnosis and treatment. J Am Acad Orthop Surg 4:209–218, 1996.

Zimlich RH, Fulbright BM, Friedman RJ: Current status of anticoagulation therapy after total hip and total knee arthroplasty. J Am Acad Orthop Surg 4:54–62, 1996.

Book Chapters

Bone LB: Emergency treatment of the injured patient. In Browner BD, Jupiter JB, Levine AM, et al, eds: Skeletal Trauma: Fractures, Dislocations and Ligamentous Injuries, p 138. Philadelphia, WB Saunders, 1992.

Frymoyer JW: Multiple trauma: Pathophysiology and management. In Orthopaedic Knowledge Update 4: Home Study Syllabus, pp 141–153. Rosemont, IL, American Academy of Orthopaedic Surgeons, 1993.

Lotke PA, Elia EA: Thromboembolic disease after total knee surgery: A critical review. Instr Course Lect 34:409–412, 1990.

MacLean LD: Shock: Causes and management of circulatory collapse. In Sabiston DC Jr, ed: Davis-Christopher Textbook of Surgery, 12th ed, pp 58–90. Philadelphia, WB Saunders, 1981.

Morris CD, Creevy WS, Einhorn TA: Pulmonary distress and thromboembolitic conditions affecting orthopaedic practice. In Buckwalter JA, Einhorn TA, Simon SR, eds: Orthopaedic Basic Science: Biology and Biomechanics of the Musculoskeletal System, 2nd ed, pp 307–318. Rosemont, IL, American Academy of Orthopaedic Surgeons, 2000.

Mubarak SJ: Compartment syndromes in operative technique. In Chapman MW, ed: Operative Orthopaedics, pp 1–202. Philadelphia, JB Lippincott, 1988.

Poss R, ed: Polytrauma, p 88. Park Ridge, IL, American Academy of Orthopaedic Surgeons, 1990.

IMAGING AND SPECIAL STUDIES

Recent Articles

Clarke HD, Kitaoka HB, Berquist TH: Imaging of tendon injuries about the ankle. Orthopedics 20:639–643, 1997.

Genant HK, Engelke K, Fuerst T, et al: Review: Noninvasive assessment of bone mineral density and stature: State of the art. J Bone Miner Res 11:707–730, 1996.

Moed BR, Kim EC, van Holsbeeck M: Ultrasound for the early diagnosis of tibial fracture healing after static interlocked nailing without reaming: Histologic correlation using a canine model. J Orthop Trauma 12: 200–205, 1998.

Moed BR, Subramanian S, van Holsbeeck M, et al: Ultrasound for the early diagnosis of tibial fracture healing after static interlocked nailing without reaming: Clinical results. J Orthop Trauma 12:206–213, 1998.

Nerlich AG, Schleicher ED, Boos N: Immunohistologic markers for age-related changes of human lumbar intervertebral discs. Spine 22:2781–2795, 1997.

Rizzo PF, Gould ES, Lyden JP, et al: Diagnosis of occult fractures about the hip: Magnetic resonance imaging compared with bone scanning. J Bone Joint Surg [Am] 75:395–401, 1993.

Classic Articles

Gilmer PW, Herzenberg J, Frank JL, et al: Computerized tomographic analysis of acute calcaneal fractures. Foot Ankle 6:184–193, 1986.

Guyer BH, Levinsohn EM, Fredericksohn BE, et al: Computed tomography of calcaneal fractures: Anatomy, pathology, and clinical relevance. Am J Radiol 145:911–919, 1985.

Hauzeur JP, Pasteels JL, Schoutens A, et al: The diagnostic value of magnetic resonance imaging in nontraumatic osteonecrosis of the femoral head. J Bone Joint Surg [Am] 71:641–649, 1989.

Herzenberg JE, Goldner JL, Martinez S, et al: Computerized tomography of talocalcaneal coalition: A clinical and anatomic study. Foot Ankle 6:273–288, 1986.

Kneeland JB, Middleton WD, Carrera GF, et al: MR imaging of the shoulder: Diagnosis of rotator cuff tears. AJR Am J Roentgenol 149:333–337, 1987.

Marchisello PJ: The use of computerized axial tomography for the evaluation of talocalcaneal coalition. J Bone Joint Surg [Am] 69:609–611, 1987.

Pykett IL, Newhouse JH, Buonanno FS, et al: Principles of nuclear magnetic resonance imaging. Radiology 143:157–168, 1982.

Robinson HJ Jr, Hartleben PD, Lund G, et al: Evaluation of magnetic resonance imaging in the diagnosis of osteonecrosis of the femoral head: Accuracy compared with radiographs, core biopsy, and intra-osseous pressure measurements. J Bone Joint Surg [Am] 71:650–653, 1989.

Watanabe AT, Carter BC, Tettelbaum GP, et al: Common pitfalls in magnetic resonance imaging of the knee. J Bone Joint Surg [Am] 71:857–862, 1989.

Book Chapters

Aminoff MJ, ed: Electrodiagnosis in Clinical Neurology, 3rd ed. New York, Churchill Livingstone, 1992.

Fitzgerald RH Jr, ed: Imaging of the musculoskeletal system: Orthopaedic Knowledge Update 2: Home Study Syllabus, p 159. Park Ridge, IL, American Academy of Orthopaedic Surgeons, 1987.

Herzog RJ: Magnetic resonance imaging of the spine. In Frymoyer JW, ed: The Adult Spine: Principles and Practice, pp 457–510. New York, Raven Press, 1991.

Peterfy CG, Roberts TPL, Genant HK: Magnetic resonance imaging of the musculoskeletal system: Advances in musculoskeletal imaging. In Buckwalter JA, Einhorn TA, Simon SR, eds: Orthopaedic Basic Science: Biology and Biomechanics of the Musculoskeletal System, 2nd ed, pp 261–278. Rosemont, IL, American Academy of Orthopaedic Surgeons, 2000.

Lane JM, Healey JH: Fractures of the hip. In Lane JM, ed: Diagnosis and Management of Pathologic Fractures, pp 122–127. New York, Raven Press, 1993.

Schneider R, Rapuano B: Radioisotopes in orthopaedics. In Buckwalter JA, Einhorn TA, Simon SR, eds: Orthopaedic Basic Science: Biology and Biomechanics of the Musculoskeletal System, 2nd ed, pp 289–306. Rosemont, IL, American Academy of Orthopaedic Surgeons, 2000.

BIOMATERIALS AND BIOMECHANICS

Recent Articles

Ambrose CG, Clanton TO: Bioabsorbable implants: Review of clinical experience in orthopedic surgery. Ann Biomed Eng 32:171–177, 2004.

Clarke IC, Manaka M, Green DD, et al: Current status of zirconia used in total hip implants. J Bone Joint Surg [Am] 85:73–84, 2003.

Collier JP, Currier BH, Kennedy FE, et al: Comparison of cross-linked polyethylene materials for orthopaedic applications. Clin Orthop 414: 289–304, 2003.

Collier JP, Sutula LC, Currier BH, et al: Overview of polyethylene as a bearing material: Comparison of sterilization methods. Clin Orthop 333:76–86, 1996.

Dye SF, Chew MH: The use of scintigraphy to detect increased osseous metabolic activity about the knee. Instr Course Lect 43:453–469, 1994.

Ebramzadeh E, Sarmiento A, McKellop HA, et al: The cement mantle in total hip arthroplasty: Analysis of long-term radiographic results. J Bone Joint Surg [Am] 76:77–87, 1994.

Jasty M, Goetz DD, Bragdon CR, et al: Wear of polyethylene acetabular components in total hip arthroplasty: An analysis of one hundred and twenty-eight components retrieved at autopsy or revision operations. J Bone Joint Surg [Am] 79:349–358, 1997.

King GJ, Morrey BF, An KN: Stabilizers of the elbow. J Shoulder Elbow Surg 2:165–174, 1993.

McKellop HA, Campbell P, Park SH, et al: The origin of submicron polyethylene wear debris in total hip arthroplasty. Clin Orthop 311:3–20, 1995.

McKellop H, Shen FW, Lu B, et al: Development of an extremely wear-resistant ultrahigh molecular weight polyethylene for total hip replacements. J Orthop Res 17:157–167, 1999.

O'Donnell RJ, Springfield DS, Motwani HK, et al: Recurrence of giant-cell tumors of the long bones after curettage and packing with cement. J Bone Joint Surg [Am] 76:1827–1833, 1994.

Schmalzried TP, Callaghan JJ: Wear in total hip and knee replacements. J Bone Joint Surg [Am] 81:115–136, 1999.

Skyhar MJ, Warren RF, Oriz GJ, et al: The effects of sectioning of the posterior cruciate ligament and the posterolateral complex on the articular contact pressures within the knee. J Bone Joint Surg [Am] 75:694–699, 1993.

Tan V, Klotz MJ, Greenwald AS, Steinberg ME: Carry it on the bad side. Am J Orthop 27:673–677, 1998.

Urban RM, Jacobs JJ, Sumner DR, et al: The bone-implant interface of femoral stems with non-circumferential porous coating. J Bone Joint Surg [Am] 78:1068–1081, 1996.

Classic Articles

Bobyn JD, Pilliar RM, Cameron HU, et al: The optimum pore size for the fixation of porous-surfaced metal implants by bone ingrowth. Clin Orthop 150:263–270, 1980.

Burstein AJ, Currey J, Frankel VH, et al: Bone strength: The effect of screw holes. J Bone Joint Surg [Am] 54:1143–1156, 1972.

Callaghan JJ, Brand RA, Pedersen DR: Hip arthrodesis: A long-term follow-up. J Bone Joint Surg [Am] 67:1328–1335, 1985.

Carter DR, Spengler DM: Mechanical properties and composition of cortical bone. Clin Orthop 135:192–217, 1978.

Freedman L, Munro RH: Abduction of the arm in the scapular plane: Scapular and glenohumeral movements. J Bone Joint Surg [Am] 18:1503–1510, 1966.

Hawkins RJ, Neer CS: A functional analysis of shoulder fusions. Clin Orthop 223:65–76, 1987.

Krettek C, Haas N, Tscherne H: The role of supplemental lag-screw fixation for open fractures of the tibial shaft treated with external fixation. J Bone Joint Surg [Am] 73:893–897, 1991.

McKellop HA, Sarmiento A, Schwinn CP, et al: In vivo wear of titanium-alloy hip prostheses. J Bone Joint Surg [Am] 72:512–517, 1990.

Morrey BF, Askew LJ, Chao EY: A biomechanical study of normal elbow motion. J Bone Joint Surg [Am] 63:872–877, 1981.

Morrey BF, Wiedeman GP: Complications and long-term results of ankle arthrodeses following trauma. J Bone Joint Surg [Am] 62:777–784, 1980.

Nachemson A. Lumbar intradiscal pressure. Acta Orthop Scand (Suppl) 43:1–104, 1960.

Perry J: Anatomy and biomechanics of the hindfoot. Clin Orthop 177:9–15, 1983.

Rowe CR: Re-evaluation of the position of the arm in arthrodesis of the shoulder in the adult. J Bone Joint Surg [Am] 56:913–922, 1974.

Review Articles

Friedman RJ, Black J, Galante JO, et al: Current concepts in orthopaedic biomaterials and implant fixation. J Bone Joint Surg [Am] 75:1086–1109, 1993.

Li S, Burstein AH: Current concepts review—ultra-high molecular weight polyethylene: The material and its use in total joint implants. J Bone Joint Surg [Am] 76:1080–1089, 1994.

Book Chapters

Black J: Orthopaedic Biomaterials in Research and Practice, pp 57–81. New York, Churchill Livingstone, 1988.

Burstein AH, Wright TM: Fundamentals of Orthopaedic Biomechanics, pp 171–187. Baltimore, Williams & Wilkins, 1994.

Chao EYS, Aro HT: Biomechanics of fracture fixation. In Mow VC, Hayes WC, eds: Basic Orthopaedic Biomechanics. New York, Raven Press, 1991.

Charnley J: Acrylic Cement in Orthopaedic Surgery. Baltimore, Williams & Wilkins, 1970.

Frankel VH, Burstein AH: Orthopaedic Biomechanics. Philadelphia, Lea & Febiger, 1970.

Frankel VH, Nordin M: Basic Biomechanics of the Skeletal System. Philadelphia, Lea & Febiger, 1980.

Fung YC: Biomechanics: Mechanical Properties of Living Tissues. New York, Springer-Verlag, 1981.

Fung YC: Biomechanics: Motion, Flow, Stress and Growth. New York, Springer-Verlag, 1990 pp. 95–125.

Hipp JA, Cheal EJ, Hayes WC: Biomechanics of fractures. In Browner BJ, Jupiter JB, Levine AM, et al, eds: Skeletal Trauma. Philadelphia, WB Saunders, pp 95–125, 1992.

Lemons JE: Metals and alloys. In Petty W, ed: Total Joint Replacement, pp 21–27. Philadelphia, WB Saunders, 1991.

Mow VC, Flatow EL, Ateshian GA: Biomechanics. In Buckwalter JA, Einhorn TA, Simon SR, eds: Orthopaedic Basic Science: Biology and Biomechanics of the Musculoskeletal System, 2nd ed, pp 133–180. Rosemont, IL, American Academy of Orthopaedic Surgeons, 2000.

Mow VC, Soslowsky LJ: Friction, lubrication and wear of diarthrodial joints. In Mow VC, Hayes WC, eds: Basic Orthopaedic Biomechanics, pp 256–257. New York, Raven Press, 1991.

Park JB: Biomaterials Science and Engineering. New York, Plenum Press, 1984.

Pauwels F. In Biomechanics in the Normal and Diseased Hip, p 26. Berlin, Springer-Verlag, 1976.

Simon SR, Alaranta H, An KN, et al: Kinesiology. In Buckwalter JA, Einhorn TA, Simon SR, eds: Orthopaedic Basic Science: Biology and Biomechanics of the Musculoskeletal System, 2nd ed, pp 730–827. Rosemont, IL, American Academy of Orthopaedic Surgeons, 2000.

Timoshenko S, Young DH. In Elements of Strength of Materials, 5th ed, pp 70–74. New York, Nostrand Reinhold, 1968.

White AA, Panjabi MM: Clinical Biomechanics of the Spine. Philadelphia, JB Lippincott, 1978.

Wright TM, Li SL: Biomaterials. In Buckwalter JA, Einhorn TA, Simon SR, eds: Orthopaedic Basic Science: Biology and Biomechanics of the Musculoskeletal System, 2nd ed, pp 181–216. Rosemont, IL, American Academy of Orthopaedic Surgeons, 2000.

CHAPTER 2

Anatomy

Franklin D. Shuler

CONTENTS

SECTION 1 Introduction

I. Introduction

A. Osteology—The human skeleton has 206 bones: 80 in the axial skeleton and 126 in the appendicular skeleton. **Ossification**, the formation of bone, can be intramembranous (without a cartilage model, as in the skull) or enchondral (with a cartilage model [most bones]). Enchondral growth begins in the diaphyses of long bones at primary ossification centers, most of which are present at birth (Table 2–1). Secondary ossification centers usually develop in the periphery of bones and are important for growth and the treatment of childhood fractures. Anatomic landmarks of the skeleton and their related structures are listed in Table 2–2.

B. Arthrology—Joints are commonly classified into three types based on their freedom of movement: (1) synarthroses, (2) amphiarthroses, and (3) diarthroses.
   1. Synarthroses—Although synarthroses, such as the sutures in the skull, may have motion during early childhood, they usually have no motion at maturity and simply serve to join two bony elements.
   2. Amphiarthroses—Amphiarthrodial joints, such as the symphysis pubis, have hyaline cartilage and intervening discs. Limited motion is possible.
   3. Diarthroses—In true diarthrodial joints, motion is enhanced and is characterized by hyaline cartilage, synovial membranes, capsules, and ligaments. Diarthrodial joints are further classified based on degrees of freedom of motion and their shape.
      a. Uniaxial joints (ginglymus [i.e., hinge] and trochoid [i.e., pivot])—Allow movement in one plane.
      b. Biaxial joints (e.g., condyloid, ellipsoid, saddle joints)—Allow movement in two planes.
      c. Polyaxial joints (spheroidal [ball and socket])—Allow movement in any direction.
      d. Plane (gliding) joints—Allow only slight sliding of one joint surface over another.

C. Myology—Several arrangements of fibers allow classification of muscles into the following categories.
   1. Parallel (e.g., rhomboids)
   2. Fusiform (e.g., biceps brachii)
   3. Oblique (with tendinous interdigitation)—Further classified as pennate, bipennate, multipennate
   4. Triangular (e.g., pectoralis minor)
   5. Spiral (e.g., latissimus dorsi)

TABLE 2-1 SUMMARY OF OSSIFICATION PATTERNS

Bone	Ossification Center	Age at Appearance	Age at Fusion
Scapula	Body (primary)	8 wk (fetal)	
	Coracoid (tip)	1 yr	
	Coracoid	15 yr	
	Acromion	15 yr	
	Acromion	16 yr	
	Inferior angle	16 yr	
	Medial border	16 yr	
Clavicle	Medial (primary)	5 wk (fetal)	
	Lateral (primary)	5 wk (fetal)	25 yr
	Sternal	19 yr	
Humerus	Body (primary)	8 wk (fetal)	Blends at 6 yr and unites at 20 yr
	Head	1 yr	
	Greater tuberosity	3 yr	
	Lesser tuberosity	5 yr	
	Capitulum	2 yr	Blends and unites with body at 16-18 yr
	Medial epicondyles	5 yr	
	Trochlea	9 yr	
	Lateral epicondyles	13 yr	
Ulna	Body (primary)	8 wk (fetal)	
	Distal ulna	5 yr	20 yr
	Olecranon	10 yr	16 yr
Radius	Body (primary)	8 wk (fetal)	
	Distal radius	2 yr	17-20 yr
	Proximal radius	5 yr	15-18 yr
Pelvis	Ilium (primary)	2 mo	15 yr
	Ischium (primary)	4 mo	15 yr
	Pubis (primary)	6 mo	15 yr
	Acetabulum	12 yr	15 yr
Tibia	Body (primary)	7 wk (fetal)	
	Proximal (secondary)	Birth	20 yr
	Distal (secondary)	2 yr	18 yr
Fibula	Body (primary)	8 wk (fetal)	
	Proximal (secondary)	3 yr	25 yr
	Distal (secondary)	2 yr	20 yr

TABLE 2-2 SKELETAL GROOVES, NOTCHES, AND POINTS

Region	Groove or Notch	Important Related Structures
Hand	Hook of hamate	Ulnar nerve
	Trapezial groove	FCR tendon
Wrist	Distal ulna	ECU
	Radial styloid	EPL
Elbow	Medial supracondylar process	Median nerve, brachial artery
Shoulder	Scapular notch	Suprascapular nerve
	Supraglenoid tubercle	Long head of biceps brachii
	Infraglenoid tubercle	Long head of triceps brachii
Hip	ASIS	Sartorius
	AIIS	Direct head of rectus femoris
	Ischial spine	Coccygeus, levator ani
	Lesser sciatic foramen	Pudendal nerve
	Piriformis fossa	Obturator externus
	Tip of greater trochanter	Piriformis
	Quadrate tubercle	Quadratus femoris
	Lesser trochanter	Psoas minor
Knee	Hunter's canal	Femoral artery becomes popliteal artery
	Adductor tubercle	Adductor magnus
	Gerdy tubercle	IT band
	Fibular neck	Common peroneal nerve
Foot	Henry knot	FDL–FHL intersection
	Sustentaculum tali	Spring ligament (FHL [inferior])
	Base of fifth metatarsal	Peroneus brevis/plantar aponeurosis
	Tuberosity of navicular	Tibialis posterior
	Cuboid groove	Peroneus longus
	Sinus tarsi	Ligamentum cervis tali and EDB

AIIS, anterior inferior iliac spine; ASIS, anterior superior iliac spine; ECU, extensor carpi ulnaris; EDB, extensor digitorum brevis; EPL, extensor pollicis longus; FCR, flexor carpi radialis; FDL, flexor digitorum longus; FHL, flexor hallucis longus; IT, iliotibial.

D. Nerves

1. Peripheral nerves—Most peripheral nerves originate from the ventral rami of spinal nerves and are distributed via several plexuses (cervical, brachial, lumbosacral). The mnemonic SAME can be used to help understand the function of nerves: **S**ensory = **A**fferent; **M**otor = **E**fferent. Efferent (motor) fibers carry impulses from the central nervous system to muscles; afferent (sensory) fibers carry information toward the central nervous system.
2. Autonomic nerves—The autonomic nervous system controls visceral structures and consists of the parasympathetic (craniosacral) and sympathetic (thoracolumbar) divisions.
   a. Preganglionic neurons of parasympathetic nerves—Arise in the nuclei of **cranial nerves** (CNs) III, VII, IX, and X and in the S2, S3, and S4 segments of the spinal cord; they synapse in peripheral ganglia.
   b. Preganglionic neurons in the sympathetic system—Are located in the spinal cord (T1-L3) and synapse in chain ganglia adjacent to the spine and collateral ganglia along major abdominal blood vessels.

E. Vessels—These structures consist of arteries, veins, and lymphatics. Of primary concern to the orthopaedist is avoiding major injury to these structures. Their courses and relationships are important and are highlighted in this chapter.

Table 2–3 summarizes upper extremity innervation. Table 2–4 summarizes standard surgical approaches to the upper extremity.

I. Shoulder

A. Osteology—The shoulder girdle is composed of the scapula and clavicle and attaches the upper limb to the trunk. The shoulder (glenohumeral) joint is the attachment of the upper humerus (see the following discussion on the arm) to the shoulder girdle.

1. Scapula—The scapula spans the second through seventh ribs and serves as an attachment for 17 muscles and four ligaments. The scapular glenoid is retroverted approximately 5 degrees. Key anatomic processes are the scapular spine, coracoid, and acromion. Attachments to the coracoid include the coracoacromial ligament, coracoclavicular ligaments (conoid and trapezoid [lateral]), conjoined tendon (coracobrachialis and short head of biceps), and pectoralis minor. The suprascapular notch is distinct from the spinoglenoid notch. The **suprascapular notch** has the superior transverse scapular ligament separating the suprascapular artery (superior) from the suprascapular nerve (inferior). The **spinoglenoid notch** has both the artery and nerve inferior to the inferior transverse scapular ligament. Long-term nerve compression at the spinoglenoid notch (i.e., ganglion [think labral pathology]) results in infraspinatus atrophy.
2. Clavicle—This structure acts as a fulcrum for lateral movement of the arm. It has a double curvature (sternal-ventral, acromial-dorsal) and serves as an attachment for the upper extremity. The clavicle is the first bone in the body to ossify (at 5 weeks of gestation) and the last to fuse (medial epiphysis at 25 years of age). Fracture of the clavicle is the most common musculoskeletal birth injury.

TABLE 2-3 SUMMARY OF UPPER EXTREMITY INNERVATION

Nerves	Muscles Innervated
Musculocutaneous (lateral cord)	Coracobrachialis, biceps, brachialis
Axillary (posterior cord)	Deltoid, teres minor
Radial (posterior cord)	Triceps, brachioradialis, extensor carpi radialis longus and brevis
Posterior interosseous	Supinator, extensor carpi ulnaris, extensor digitorum, extensor digiti minimi, abductor pollicis longus, extensor pollicis longus and brevis, EI
Median (medial and lateral cord)	PT, flexor carpi radialis, palmaris longus, flexor digitorum superficialis, abductor pollicis longus, supinator head of flexor pollicis brevis, OP, first and second lumbrical muscles
Anterior interosseous	Flexor digitorum profundus (first and second), flexor pollicis longus, pronator quadratus
Ulnar (medial cord)	Flexor carpi ulnaris, flexor digitorum profundus (third and fourth), PB, abductor digiti minimi, ODM, flexor digiti minimi, third and fourth lumbrical muscles, interossei, adductor pollicis, deep head of flexor pollicis brevis

EI, extensor indicis proprius; ODM, opponens digiti minimi; OP, opponens pollicis; PB, palmaris brevis; PT, pronator teres.

B. Arthrology—The shoulder area has one major articulation (glenohumeral joint) and several minor articulations (sternoclavicular, acromioclavicular, scapulothoracic joints). Additionally, numerous ligaments are associated with each articulation.

1. Glenohumeral joint (Fig. 2–1)—This joint is spheroidal (ball-and-socket). The articular surface of the glenoid is thickest at the periphery. This joint has the greatest range of motion of any joint, but motion is at the expense of stability. There are static and dynamic restraints of shoulder motion. Static restraints include the articular anatomy, glenoid labrum, negative pressure, capsule, and ligaments. Dynamic restraints include the rotator cuff, biceps tendon, and scapulothoracic motion. Important shoulder-stabilizing structures are summarized in Table 2–5.
2. Sternoclavicular joint—This joint is double-gliding, with an articular disc. Its ligaments include the capsule, anterior and posterior sternoclavicular ligaments, an interclavicular ligament, and a costoclavicular ligament. The sternoclavicular joint rotates 30 degrees with shoulder motion.
3. Acromioclavicular joint—This joint has plane/gliding characteristics and also possesses a fibrocartilaginous disc. Its ligaments (Fig. 2–2) include the capsule, acromioclavicular ligament, and coracoclavicular ligament (with trapezoid [anterolateral] and conoid [posteromedial and stronger] component ligaments). The acromioclavicular ligaments prevent anteroposterior displacement of the distal clavicle. The coracoclavicular ligaments prevent superior displacement of the distal clavicle. When the arm is maximally elevated, there is about 5-8 degrees of rotation at the acromioclavicular joint, although the clavicle rotates approximately 40-50 degrees.
4. Scapulothoracic joint—Though not a true joint, this attachment allows scapular movement against the posterior rib cage. It is fixed primarily by the scapular muscular attachments. Glenohumeral motion compared with scapulothoracic motion is a 2:1 ratio.
5. Intrinsic ligaments of the scapula—These ligaments include the superior transverse scapular ligament (which separates the suprascapular nerve [inferior] and vessels [superior] at the suprascapular notch—"water over the bridge"), the inferior transverse scapular ligament (spinoglenoid notch), and the coracoacromial ligament (which is a

TABLE 2-4 SUMMARY OF STANDARD UPPER EXTREMITY ORTHOPAEDIC SURGICAL APPROACHES

Region	Approach	Eponym	Muscular Interval 1 (Nerve)	Muscular Interval 2 (Nerve)	Structures at Risk
Shoulder	Anterior	Henry	Deltoid (axillary)	Pectoralis major (medial/lateral pectoral)	Musculocutaneous n./cephalic v.
	Lateral		Deltoid (splitting) (axillary)	Deltoid (splitting) (axillary)	Axillary n.
	Posterior		Infraspinatus (suprascapular)	Teres minor (axillary)	Axillary n./posterior circumflex humeral a.
Proximal humerus	Anterolateral		Deltoid/pectoralis major (axillary/ medial/lateral pectoral)	Radial and axillary n./anterior circumflex humeral a.	
Distal humerus	Anterolateral		Triceps/brachialis (radial/ musculocutaneous)	Brachioradialis (radial)	Radial n.
	Lateral		Lateral triceps/brachioradialis (radial)	Radial n.	
Humerus	Posterior		Long triceps (radial)	Radial n./brachial a.	
Elbow	Anterolateral	Henry	Brachialis/pronator teres (musculocutaneous/median)	Brachioradialis (radial)	Lateral ABC n./radial n.
	Posterolateral	Kocher	Anconeus (radial)	ECU (PIN)	PIN
	Medial		Brachialis (musculocutaneous)	Triceps/pronator teres (radial/ median)	Ulnar n.
Forearm	Anterior	Henry	Brachioradialis (radial)	Pronator teres/FCR (median)	PIN
	Dorsal	Thompson	ECRB (radial)	ED/EPL (PIN)	PIN
	Ulnar		ECU (PIN)	FCU (ulnar)	Ulnar n. and a.
Wrist	Dorsal		Third compartment (PIN)	Fourth compartment (PIN)	
Scaphoid	Volar	Russé	FCR or through sheath (median)	Radial a.	Radial a.
	Dorsolateral	Matti	First compartment (PIN)	Third compartment (PIN)	Superior radial n./radial a.

a, artery; ABC, antebrachial cutaneous; ECRB, extensor carpi radialis brevis; ECU, extensor carpi ulnaris; ED, extensor digitorum; n., nerve; EPL, extensor pollicis longus; FCR, flexor carpi radialis; FCU, flexor carpi ulnaris; PIN, posterior interosseous nerve; v., vein.

frequent cause of impingement). The coracoacromial ligament is important to superoanterior restraint in rotator cuff deficiencies and should be preserved when painful massive rotator cuff tears that cannot be surgically repaired are débrided. The acromial branch of the thoracoacromial artery runs on the medial aspect of the coracoacromial ligament.

C. Muscles (Fig. 2–3)
   1. Muscles connecting the upper limb to the vertebral column—Trapezius, latissimus, both rhomboids, and levator scapulae
   2. Muscles connecting the upper limb to the thoracic wall—Both pectoralis muscles, subclavius, and serratus anterior
   3. Muscles acting on the shoulder joint itself—Deltoid, teres major, and the four rotator cuff muscles [supraspinatus, infraspinatus, teres minor, subscapularis]). The rotator cuff muscles depress and stabilize the humeral head against the glenoid. The greater tuberosity of the humerus serves as an attachment for three rotator cuff muscles: the supraspinatus, infraspinatus, and teres minor. The lesser tuberosity of the humerus serves as the

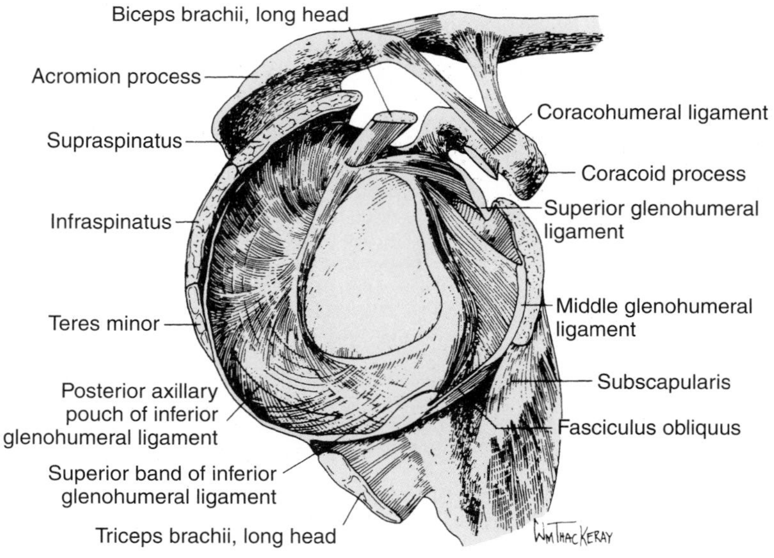

FIGURE 2–1 Glenohumeral ligaments and rotator cuff muscles. The rotator interval is between the anterior border of the supraspinatus and the superior border of the subscapularis. This interval helps limit flexion and external rotation of the shoulder. Within the rotator interval is the superior glenohumeral ligament, the primary restraint to inferior translation in the adducted shoulder and the primary restraint to external rotation in the adducted or slightly abducted arm. The middle glenohumeral ligament, absent in up to 30% of shoulders, is the primary stabilizer to anterior translation, with the arm slightly abducted (45 degrees). The inferior glenohumeral ligament complex is the primary stabilizer for anterior and inferior instability in abduction. The inferior coracohumeral ligament complex is composed of posterior-inferior and anterior-inferior glenohumeral ligaments. (From Turkel SJ, Panio MW, Marshall JL, et al: Stabilizing mechanisms preventing anterior dislocation of the glenohumeral joint. J Bone Joint Surg [Am] 63:1209, 1981.)

TABLE 2-5 GLENOHUMERAL STABILIZERS

Structure	Function
Coracohumeral ligament	Primary restraint to inferior translation of the adducted arm and to ER
Glenoid labrum	Increases surface area, static stabilizer
SGHL	Primary restraint to ER in adducted or slightly abducted arm Primary restraint to inferior translation in the adducted arm
MGHL (absent up to 30%)	Primary stabilizer to anterior translation, with the arm abducted to 45 degrees
IGHLC	Primary stabilizer for anterior and inferior instability in abduction

ER, external rotation; IGHLC, inferior glenohumeral ligament complex; MGHL, middle glenohumeral ligament; SGHL, superior glenohumeral ligament.

attachment site for the subscapularis muscle (shoulder internal rotator). The shoulder internal rotators (pectoralis major, latissimus dorsi, and subscapularis) are stronger than the external rotators (teres minor and infraspinatus), which is why posterior shoulder dislocations are more common than anterior dislocations after electrical shock and

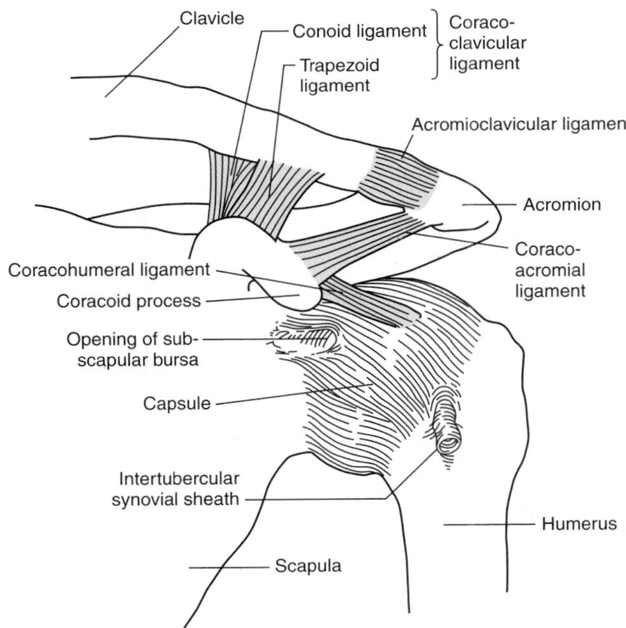

FIGURE 2–2 Ligaments about the shoulder. The acromioclavicular ligaments (superior, inferior, anterior, and posterior) prevent anteroposterior translation of the distal clavicle. The superior ligament is the most important and is reinforced by fibers from the trapezius and deltoid muscles. The coracoclavicular ligaments (conoid [posteromedial] and trapezoid [anterolateral]) prevent superior translation of the distal clavicle. The coracoacromial (CA) ligament should be preserved in massive rotator cuff defects because it provides superior restraint to the humeral head. Bleeding encountered during release of the CA ligament comes from the acromial branch of the thoracoacromial artery (second part of axillary artery [see Fig. 2-6]). (Adapted from Jenkins DB: Hollinshead's Functional Anatomy of the Limbs and Back, 6th ed, p 71. Philadelphia, WB Saunders, 1991.)

seizures. Table 2–6 presents the specifics on these muscles, and Figure 2–4 and Table 2–7 demonstrate the four layers of shoulder musculature.

D. Nerves
1. Anatomy of brachial plexus—The brachial plexus (Fig. 2–5) is formed from the ventral primary rami of C5-T1 and lies under the clavicle between the scalenus anterior and scalenus medius. The dorsal rami of C5-T1 innervate the dorsal neck musculature and skin. The brachial plexus consists of roots, trunks, divisions, cords, and branches (remember the mnemonic **R**on **T**aylor **d**rinks **c**old **b**eer).
   a. Five roots (C5-T1, although C4 and T2 can have small contributions)
   b. Three trunks (upper, middle, lower)
   c. Six divisions (two from each trunk)
   d. Three cords (named because of their anatomic relationship to the axillary artery [posterior, lateral, medial]). The termination of each cord is shown in Table 2–8.
   e. Multiple branches—Four preclavicular branches (from roots and upper trunk):
      Dorsal scapular nerve
      Long thoracic nerve
      Suprascapular nerve
      Nerve to the subclavius
2. Muscle innervation—Innervation of all rotator cuff muscles is derived from C5-C6 of the brachial plexus (Table 2–9). See also Table 2–3.
3. Brachial plexus injury
   a. Preganglionic (proximal to the dorsal root ganglion) brachial plexus lesions—Produce scapular winging (because of paralysis of the preclavicular long thoracic nerve) and Horner syndrome (injury to brachial plexus at C8-T1 involving the inferior/stellate ganglion)
   b. Postganglionic brachial plexus injuries—Do not produce Horner syndrome, a winged scapula, diaphragmatic paralysis, or rhomboid paralysis
   c. Summary of obstetric brachial plexus palsy—Table 2–10
   d. Injury to the spinal accessory nerve—Causes scapular-trapezius winging, resulting in shoulder depression with scapular translation laterally and the inferior angle rotated laterally because of the unopposed pull of the serratus anterior.
   e. Injury to the long thoracic nerve—Causes serratus anterior scapular winging, resulting in superior elevation with scapular translation medially and the inferior angle rotated medially.

E. Vessels
1. Subclavian artery—The subclavian artery arises either directly from the aorta (left subclavian) or from the brachiocephalic trunk (right subclavian). It then emerges between the scalenus anterior and medius muscles and becomes the axillary artery at the outer border of the first rib.
2. Axillary artery (Table 2–11 and Fig. 2–6)—The axillary artery is divided into three portions based on its physical relationship to the pectoralis minor (the first is medial to it, the second is under it, and

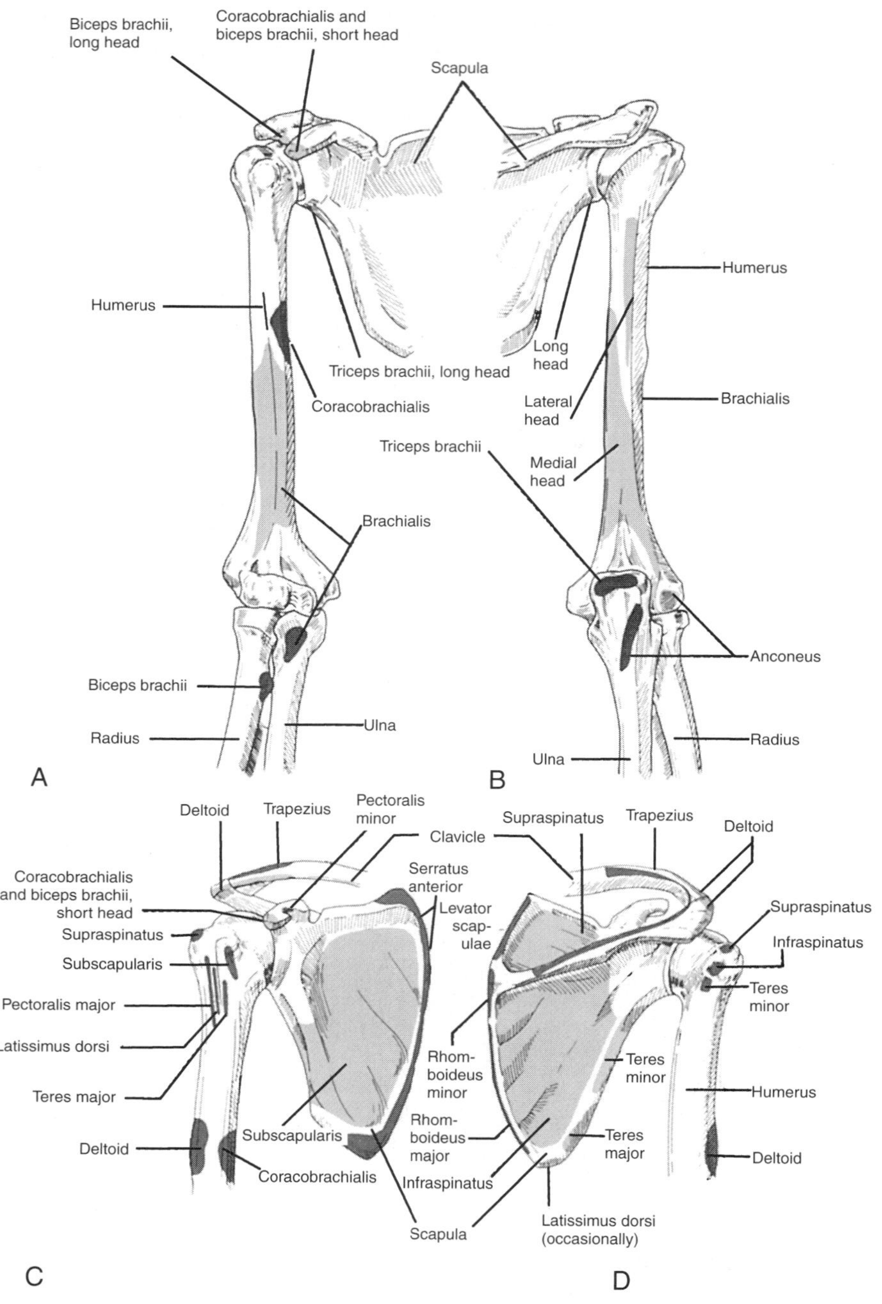

FIGURE 2–3 Origins and insertions of the muscles about the shoulder girdle. **A**, Anterior view. **B**, Posterior view. **C**, Anterior view. **D**, Posterior view. (From Jenkins DB: Hollinshead's Functional Anatomy of the Limbs and Back, 6th ed, Fig. 5-3. Philadelphia, WB Saunders, 1991.)

the third is lateral to it). Each part of the artery has as many branches as the number of that portion (e.g., the second part has two branches: thoracoacromial and lateral thoracic). The third part of the axillary artery, at the origin of the anterior and posterior humeral circumflex arteries, is the most vulnerable to traumatic vascular injury.

F. Surgical approaches to the shoulder (see Table 2–4)—Include the anterior approach (reconstructions and arthroplasties), lateral approach (acromioplasty and cuff repair), and posterior approach (posterior reconstruction). A summary is shown in Table 2–12.
   1. Anterior (Henry's) approach (Fig. 2–7)—This approach explores the interval between the deltoid (axillary nerve) and the pectoralis major (medial and lateral pectoral nerves). The cephalic vein is dissected and retracted laterally with the deltoid, and the underlying subscapularis is exposed. The subscapularis is then divided (preserving the most inferior fibers in order to protect the axillary nerve), and the shoulder capsule is visualized. Division of the subscapularis does not lead to denervation because innervation enters medially. A leash of three vessels (one artery and the superior and inferior venae comitantes) marks the lower border of the subscapularis. Protect the musculocutaneous nerve (lateral cord brachial plexus) by avoiding vigorous retraction of the conjoined tendon and avoiding dissection

TABLE 2-6 MUSCLES OF THE SHOULDER

Muscle	Origin	Insertion	Action	Innervation
Trapezius	SP C7-T12	Clavicle, scapula (AC, SP)	Rotate scapula	CN XI
Latissimus dorsi	SP T6-S5, ilium	Humerus (ITG)	Extend adduct, internally rotate humerus	Thoracodorsal
Rhomboid major	SP T2-T5	Scapula (medial border)	Adduct scapula	Dorsal scapular
Rhomboid minor	SP C7-T1	Scapula (medial spine)	Adduct scapula	Dorsal scapular
Levator scapulae	TP C1-C4	Scapula (superior medial)	Elevate, rotate scapula	C3,C4
Pectoralis major	Sternum, ribs, clavicle	Humerus (L-ITG)	Adduct, internally rotate arm	Medial and lateral pectoral nerves
Pectoralis minor	Ribs 3-5	Scapula (coracoid)	Protract scapula	Medial pectoral nerve
Subclavius	Rib 1	Inferior clavicle	Depress clavicle	Upper trunk
Serratus anterior	Ribs 1-9	Scapula (ventral medial)	Prevent winging	Long thoracic
Deltoid	Lateral clavicle, scapula	Humerus (deltoid tuberosity)	Abduct arm (2)	Axillary
Teres major	Inferior scapula	Humerus (M-ITG)	Adduct, internally rotate, extend	Lower subscapular
Subscapularis	Ventral scapula	Humerus (LT)	Internally rotate arm, anterior stability	Upper and lower subscapular
Supraspinatus	Superior scapula	Humerus (GT)	Abduct (1), externally rotate arm, stability	Suprascapular
Infraspinatus	Dorsal scapula	Humerus (GT)	Stability, externally rotate arm	Suprascapular
Teres minor	Scapula (dorsolateral)	Humerus (GT)	Stability, externally rotate arm	Axillary

AC, acromion; CN, cranial nerve; GT, greater tuberosity; ITG, intertubercular groove; L-ITG, lateral intertubercular groove; LT, lesser tuberosity; M-ITG, medial intertubercular groove; SP, spinous process; TP, transverse process.

medial to the coracobrachialis. This nerve usually penetrates the biceps/coracobrachialis 5-8 cm below the coracoid, but it enters these muscles proximal to this 5-cm "safe zone" almost 30% of the time. Palsy of the musculocutaneous nerve would affect the coracobrachialis, biceps brachii, and brachialis muscles and sensation in the lateral antebrachial cutaneous nerve (termination of the musculocutaneous nerve). The axillary nerve (posterior cord brachial plexus), which is just inferior to the shoulder capsule, must be protected during procedures in this area. Adduction and external rotation of the arm will help displace the axillary nerve from the surgical field.

2. Lateral approach—This approach involves splitting the deltoid muscle or subperiosteal dissection of the muscle from the acromion. The deltoid should not be split more than 5 cm below the acromion in order to avoid injury to the axillary nerve (posterior cord brachial plexus exiting from quadrangular space). If dissection extends more than 5 cm inferiorly, denervation of the deltoid can occur in a location anterior to the muscle split because of the posterior innervation of the muscle. The supraspinatus tendon is exposed and allows for repairs of the rotator cuff.
3. Posterior approach (Fig. 2–8)—In this approach, the interneural plane between the infraspinatus (suprascapular nerve) and teres minor (axillary nerve) is used. This plane can be approached by detaching the deltoid from the scapular spine or by splitting the deltoid (Rockwood). After this interval is found, the posterior capsule lies immediately

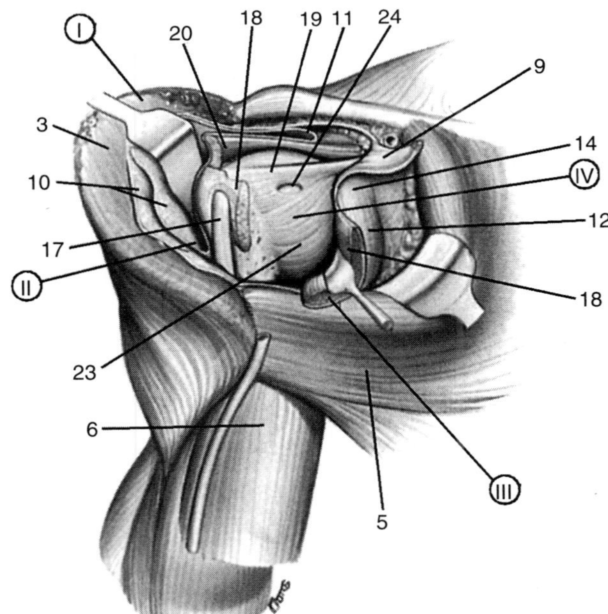

FIGURE 2–4 Anterior aspect of the right shoulder depicting the four layers (circled roman numerals). The lateral retractor is placed deep to layer II, demonstrating the ease of dissection in the plane of the bursa around the lateral aspect of the proximal humerus. The subscapularis and supraspinatus (layer III) have been reflected, disclosing layer IV (capsule and coracohumeral ligament). The usual shape and position of the defect in the rotator interval (if present) are depicted and show variability. 3, deltoid; 5, pectoralis major; 6, biceps; 9, coracoacromial ligament; 10, fasciae (II); 11, deep layer of subdeltoid bursa; 12, conjoined tendon; 14, tip of coracoid process; 17, biceps long head; 18, deep layer subdeltoid bursa and subscapularis; 19, coracohumeral ligament; 20, supraspinatus under deep bursa layer; 23, joint capsule; 24, hiatus in capsule. (From Cooper DE, O'Brien SJ, Warren RF: Supporting layers of glenohumeral joint. Clin Orthop 289:151, 1993.)

TABLE 2-7 SHOULDER-SUPPORTING LAYERS

Layer	Structures
I	Deltoid; pectoralis major
II	Clavipectoral fascia; conjoined tendon, short head of biceps, and coracobrachialis
III	Deep layer of subdeltoid bursa; rotator cuff muscles (supraspinatus, infraspinatus, teres minor, subscapularis [SITS])
IV	Glenohumeral joint capsule; coracohumeral ligament

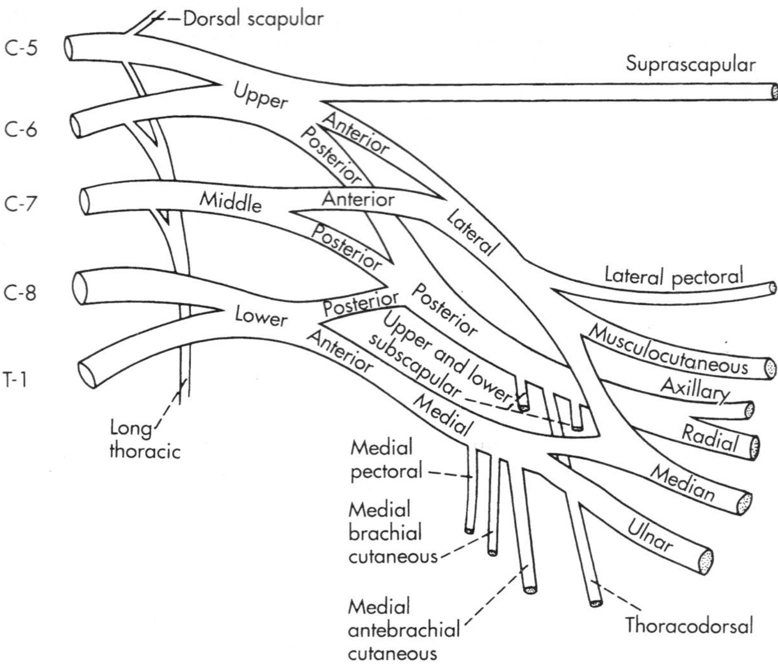

FIGURE 2–5 Brachial plexus. Remember the four preclavicular/supraclavicular branches: the long thoracic nerve (serratus anterior muscle), dorsal scapular nerve (rhomboid muscle), suprascapular nerve (supraspinatus and infraspinatus muscles), and nerve to the subclavius (not shown). (From Jenkins DB: Hollinshead's Functional Anatomy of the Limbs and Back, 6th ed, Fig. 5-7. Philadelphia, WB Saunders, 1991.)

below it. Both the axillary nerve and the posterior circumflex humeral artery run in the quadrangular space below the teres minor, so it is important to stay above this muscle. Excessive medial retraction of the infraspinatus can injure the suprascapular nerve.

G. Arthroscopy—The portals for arthroscopy (discussed in Chapter 4, Sports Medicine) include the anterior superior (musculocutaneous nerve at risk, with portals medial to it), the anterior inferior (must be above the subscapularis and lateral to the conjoined tendon), and the posterior (inferior portals may risk the axillary nerve).

II. Arm

A. Osteology—The humerus is the only bone of the arm and the largest and longest bone of the upper extremity. It is composed of a shaft and two articular extremities. The hemispheric head, directed superiorly, medially, and slightly dorsally, articulates with the much smaller scapular glenoid cavity. The anatomic neck, directly below the head, serves as an attachment for the shoulder capsule. The surgical neck is lower and is more often involved in fractures. The greater tuberosity, which is lateral to the head, serves as the attachment for the supraspinatus, infraspinatus, and teres minor muscles (anterior to posterior, respectively). The lesser tuberosity, located anteriorly, has only one muscular insertion: the last rotator cuff muscle, the subscapularis. The bicipital groove (for the tendon of the long head of the biceps) is situated between the two tuberosities. The shaft of the humerus has a posterior spiral groove adjacent to the deltoid tuberosity. This groove is approximately 13 cm above the articular surface of the trochlea. Distally, the humerus flares into medial and lateral epicondyles and forms half of the elbow joint with a medial spool-shaped trochlea (which articulates with the olecranon of the ulna) and a globular capitellum (which opposes the radial head). The normal articular alignment of the distal humerus has a 7-degree valgus tilt (carrying angle).

TABLE 2-8 BRACHIAL PLEXUS CORD TERMINATIONS

Cord	Termination
Lateral	**Musculocutaneous nerve**
	Lateral pectoral nerve
Posterior	**Radial and axillary nerve**
	Upper and lower subscapular nerve
	Thoracodorsal nerve
Medial	**Ulnar nerve**
	Medial pectoral nerve
	Medial brachial cutaneous nerve
	Medial antebrachial cutaneous nerve
Medial and lateral	**Median nerve**

Major branches are ***boldface****.*

TABLE 2-9 ROTATOR CUFF MUSCLE INNERVATION—ALL C5,C6 MUSCLE INNERVATION

Muscles Innervated	Nerves
External Rotators	
Supraspinatus	Suprascapular nerve (C5,C6)
Infraspinatus	Suprascapular nerve (C5,C6)
Teres minor	Axillary nerve (C5,C6)
Internal Rotator	
Subscapularis	Upper (C5) and lower (C5,C6) subscapular nerve

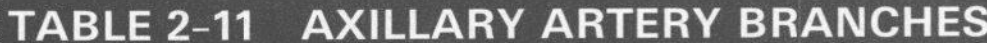

TABLE 2-10 SUMMARY OF OBSTETRIC BRACHIAL PLEXUS PALSY

Palsy	Roots	Deficit	Prognosis
Erb-Duchenne	C5,C6	Deltoid, rotator cuff, elbow flexors, wrist and hand extensors "Waiter's tip"	Best
Klumpke	C8,T1	Wrist flexors, intrinsics, Horner syndrome	Poor
Total plexus	C5-T1	Flaccid arm	Worst

TABLE 2-11 AXILLARY ARTERY BRANCHES

Part	Branch	Course
I	Supreme thoracic	Medial to serratus anterior and pectorals
II	Thoracoacromial	Four branches (deltoid, acromial, pectoralis, clavicular)
	Lateral thoracic	Descends to serratus anterior
III	Subscapular	Two branches (thoracodorsal and circumflex scapular [triangular space])
	Anterior humeral circumflex	Blood supply to humeral head—arcuate artery lateral to bicipital groove
	Posterior humeral circumflex	Branch in the quadrangular space accompanying the axillary nerve

Additionally, the humeral head is retroverted approximately 30 degrees relative to the transepicondylar axis of the humerus, with the scapular glenoid retroverted approximately 5 degrees.

B. Arthrology
1. Joints—The humerus articulates with the scapula on its upper end, forming the glenohumeral joint (discussed earlier), and with the radius and ulna on its lower end, forming the elbow joint. The elbow is composed of a compound ginglymus (hinge) joint (the humeroulnar articulation) and a trochoid (pivot) joint (the humeroradial articulation) (Table 2–13). The axis of rotation for the elbow is centered through the trochlea and capitellum and passes through a point anteroinferior on the medial epicondyle. The elbow joint has capsuloligamentous tissues (Fig. 2–9) that are a key source of testable material. The elbow capsule allows maximum distention at approximately 70-80 degrees of flexion, which is why patients with effusion hold their arms in this most comfortable position. Also, the anterior capsule attaches at a point approximately 6 mm distal to the tip of the coronoid. Because of this, the coronoid tip is an intra-articular structure that is visualized during elbow arthroscopy.
2. Ligaments (Table 2–14)—Other testable coronoid attachments include the anterior bundle of the **medial collateral ligament** (MCL) (18 mm distal to the coronoid tip) and brachialis (11 mm distal to the coronoid tip). The MCL (anterior, posterior, and transverse bundles) arises from the anteroinferior portion of the medial humeral epicondyle and provides stability to valgus stress. The anterior bundle is the most important in helping resist valgus forces. Valgus stability with the arm in pronation suggests an intact anterior bundle of the MCL. The lateral or radial collateral ligament

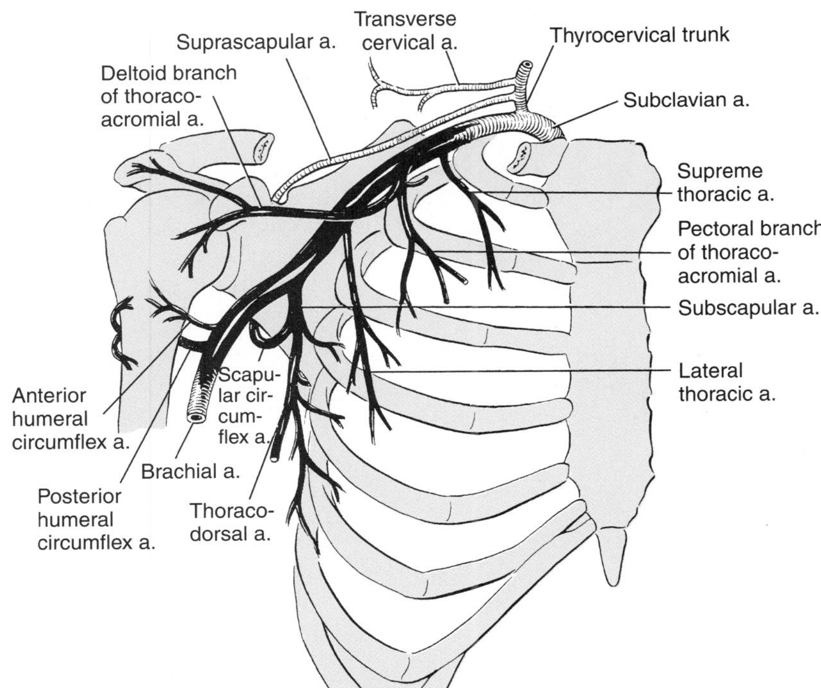

FIGURE 2–6 Branches of the axillary artery. When the subclavian artery passes beneath the clavicle, it becomes the axillary artery. The axillary artery is divided into three sections based on their relationship to the pectoralis minor muscle (not shown, but it attaches to coracoid). The first part of the axillary artery is medial to the pectoralis minor and supplies the supreme thoracic artery. The second part is beneath the muscle and supplies the thoracoacromial artery and the lateral thoracic artery. The third part is lateral to the pectoralis minor and supplies the subscapular artery and the posterior and anterior humeral circumflex arteries. The third part of the axillary artery at the origin of the anterior and posterior humeral circumflex arteries is the most vulnerable to traumatic vascular injury. (From Jenkins DB: Hollinshead's Functional Anatomy of the Limbs and Back, 6th ed, p. 77. Philadelphia, WB Saunders, 1991.)

TABLE 2-12 SHOULDER SURGICAL APPROACHES

Approach	Interval	Structures at Risk
Anterior (Henry)	Deltoid (axillary nerve) and pectoralis major (medial and lateral pectoral nerve)	Axillary nerve limits inferior exposure (place arm in adduction and external rotation). Musculocutaneous nerve—avoid vigorous retraction and medial dissection to the conjoined tendon/coracobrachialis.
Lateral	Deltoid splitting (axillary nerve)	Avoid deltoid split >5 cm below acromion to avoid damaging axillary nerve.
Posterior	Infraspinatus (suprascapular nerve) and teres minor (axillary nerve)	Dissection inferior to the teres minor risks quadrangular space structures: axillary nerve and posterior humeral circumflex artery. Avoid excessive medial retraction on infraspinatus, which can injure suprascapular nerve.

(annular, radial, and ulnar parts) originates on the lateral humeral epicondyle near the axis of elbow rotation. The **lateral ulnar collateral ligament** (LUCL) is an essential elbow stabilizer and runs from the lateral epicondyle to the ulna crista supinatoris (supinator crest). A deficiency of the LUCL is manifested as posterolateral rotatory instability of the elbow (see Table 2–14).

C. Muscles—There are four muscles of the arm (Table 2–15). The muscles controlling elbow motion include

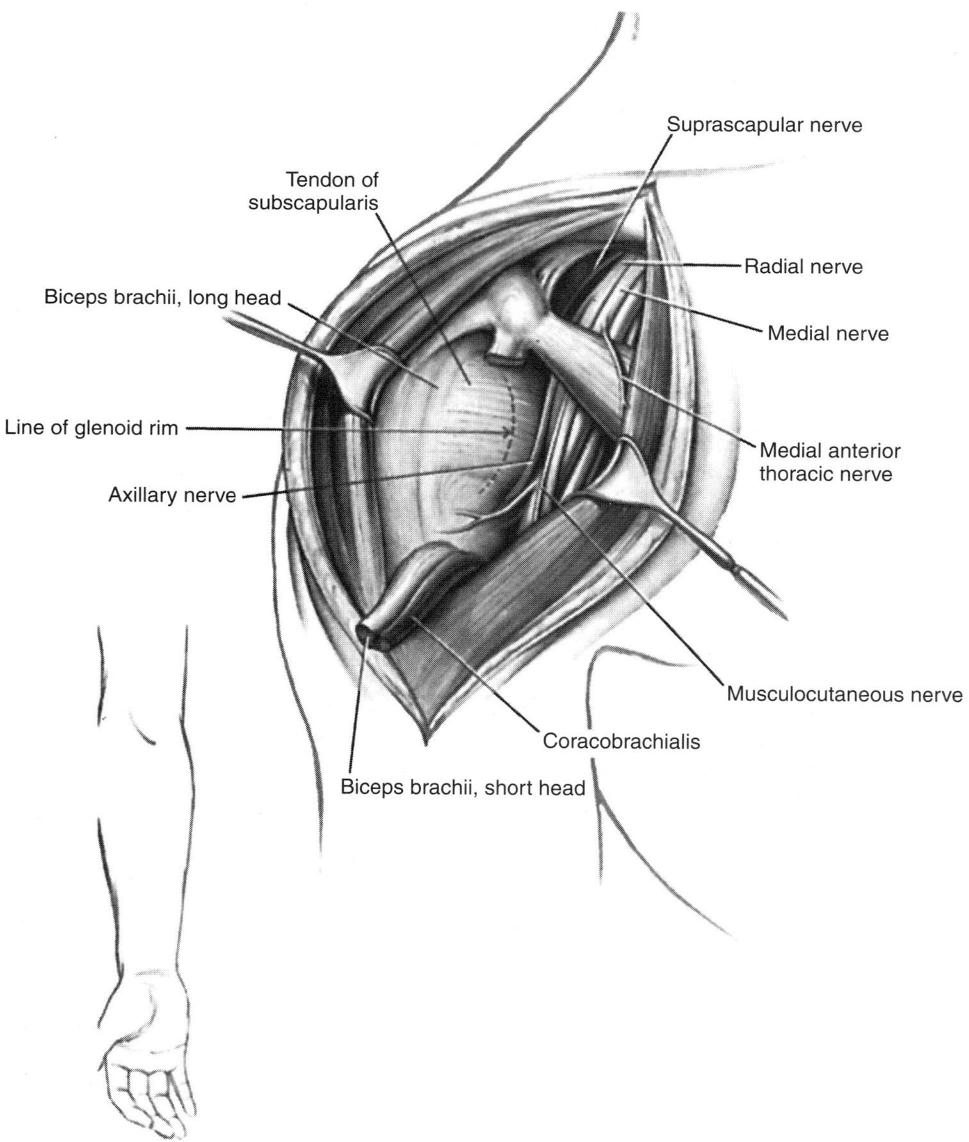

FIGURE 2–7 Anterior (Henry's) approach to the shoulder. The interval between the deltoid (axillary nerve) and the pectoralis major (medial and lateral pectoral nerves) is explored. Avoid excessive medial retraction (see medial retractor) on the coracobrachialis or dissection medial to this muscle to prevent injury to the musculocutaneous nerve. Avoid the axillary nerve, which is inferior to the shoulder capsule. Positioning the arm in adduction and external rotation helps displace the axillary nerve from the surgical field. (From Kaplan EB: Surgical Approaches to the Neck, Cervical Spine, and Upper Extremity, p 57. Philadelphia, WB Saunders, 1966.)

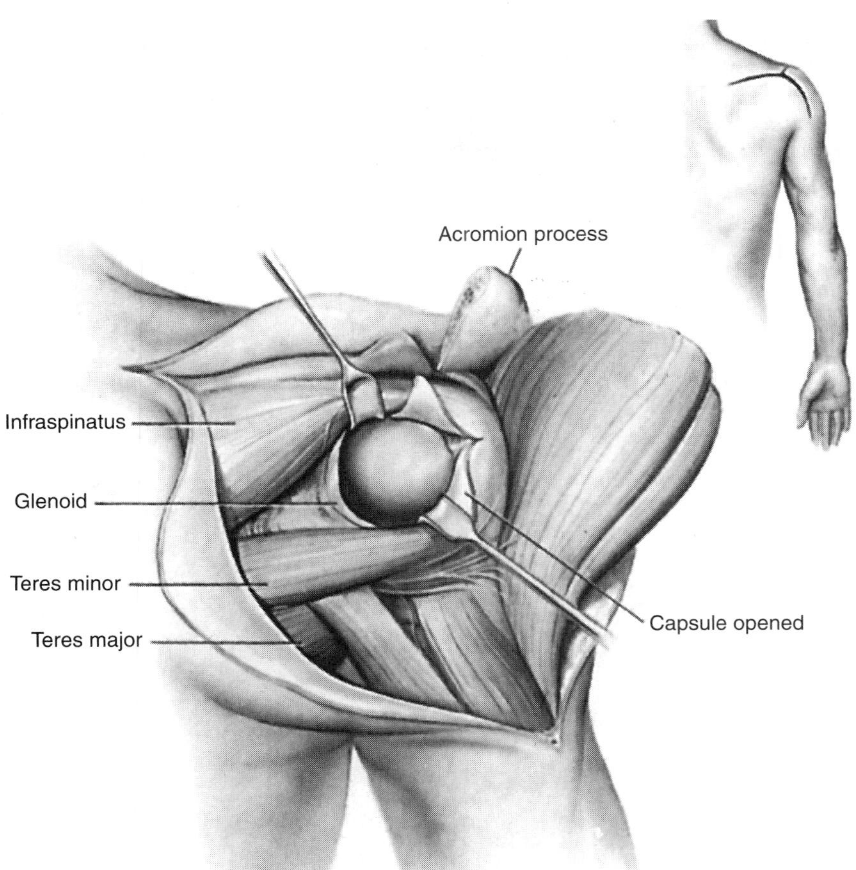

FIGURE 2–8 Posterior approach to the shoulder. The interval between the infraspinatus (suprascapular nerve) and the teres minor (axillary nerve) is explored. Do not dissect below the teres minor. Dissections below the teres minor risk injury to the structures in the quadrangular space: the posterior humeral circumflex artery and the axillary nerve. The axillary nerve divides into the deep (deltoid) and superficial (teres minor and cutaneous branch [Hilton's law]) branches within the quadrangular space. Also avoid excessive retraction of the infraspinatus to avoid suprascapular nerve palsy. (From Kaplan EB: Surgical Approaches to the Neck, Cervical Spine, and Upper Extremity, p 61. Philadelphia, WB Saunders, 1966.)

the flexors (biceps, brachialis, and brachioradialis) and extensors (triceps). Tennis elbow (lateral epicondylitis) primarily involves the **extensor carpi radialis brevis** (ECRB). The triceps muscle helps form borders for three important spaces—the triangular space, the quadrangular (quadrilateral) space, and the triangular interval (Fig. 2–10 and Table 2–16).

1. Triangular space—This space is bordered by the teres minor (superiorly), teres major (inferiorly), and long head of the triceps (laterally); it contains the circumflex scapular vessels.
2. Quadrangular space—This space is bordered by the teres minor (superiorly) and teres major (inferiorly), with the long head of the triceps forming the medial border and the humerus forming the lateral border. The quadrangular space transmits the posterior humeral circumflex vessels and the axillary nerve.
3. Triangular interval—This is immediately inferior to the quadrangular space and is bordered by the teres major (superiorly), long head of the triceps (medially), and lateral head of the triceps or the humerus (laterally). Through this interval, the profunda brachii artery and radial nerve can be seen.

TABLE 2-13 ELBOW JOINT ARTICULATIONS

Articulation	Components
Humeroulnar	Trochlea and trochlear notch
Humeroradial	Capitulum and radial head
Proximal radioulnar	Radial notch and radial head

D. Nerves
1. Anatomy—Four major nerves traverse the arm, two giving off branches to arm musculature and two innervating the distal musculature (Fig. 2–11). Most of the cutaneous innervation of the arm arises directly from the brachial plexus.
   a. Musculocutaneous nerve (lateral cord)—This nerve pierces the coracobrachialis 5-8 cm distal to the coracoid and then branches to supply this muscle, the biceps, and the brachialis. It also gives off a branch to the elbow joint before it becomes the lateral antebrachial cutaneous nerve of the forearm, which is located lateral to the cephalic vein.
   b. Radial nerve (posterior cord)—The radial nerve spirals around the humerus (medial to lateral) in the spiral groove at a distance of approximately 13 cm from the trochlea. It emerges on the lateral side of the arm after piercing the lateral intermuscular septum approximately 7.5 cm above the trochlea between the brachialis and brachioradialis anterior to the lateral epicondyle (where it supplies the anconeus muscle).

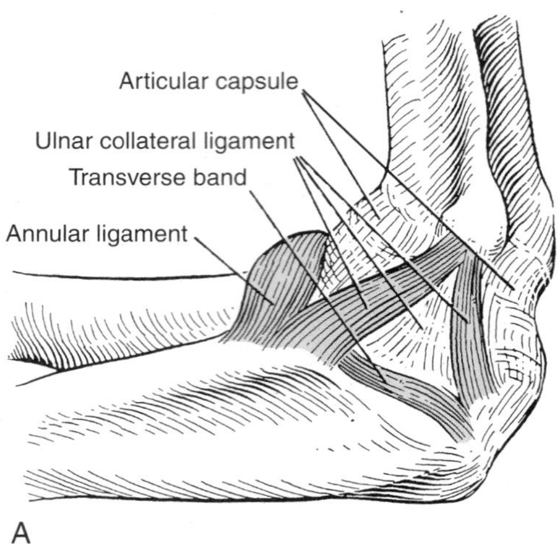

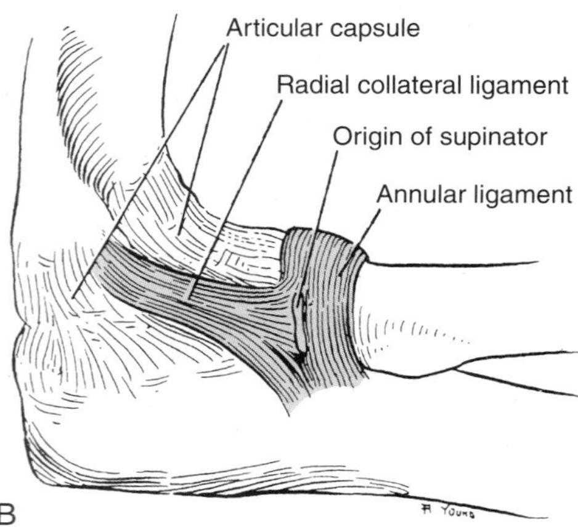

FIGURE 2–9 Elbow ligaments. **A**, Medial view. The most important portion of the medial collateral ligament is the anterior bundle or ulnar collateral ligament. **B**, Lateral view. The most important portion of the lateral collateral ligament complex is the lateral ulnar collateral ligament (LUCL) or radial collateral ligament. A deficiency of the LUCL results in posterolateral rotatory instability. (From Jenkins DB: Hollinshead's Functional Anatomy of the Limbs and Back, 6th ed, p 108. Philadelphia, WB Saunders, 1991.)

c. Median nerve (medial and lateral cords)—This nerve accompanies the brachial artery along the arm, crossing it during its course (lateral to medial). It supplies some branches to the elbow joint but has no branches in the arm itself.

TABLE 2-14 ELBOW LIGAMENTS

Ligament	Components	Comments
Medial collateral	Anterior bundle of MCL (ulnar collateral); posterior bundle; transverse bundle (Cooper ligament)	Anterior bundle (strongest of all elbow ligaments): anterior band taut from 60 degrees of flexion to full extension, posterior band taut from 60-120 degrees of flexion
Lateral collateral	LUCL; annular ligament; quadrate (annular ligament to radial neck) and oblique cord	Deficiency of LUCL results in posterolateral rotator instability

LUCL, lateral ulnar collateral ligament; MCL, medial collateral ligament.

d. Ulnar nerve (medial cord)—The ulnar nerve passes medial to the brachial artery in the arm and then runs behind the medial epicondyle of the humerus, where it is superficial. It also has branches to the elbow, but no arm branches.

e. Cutaneous nerves—The supraclavicular nerve (C3, C4) supplies the upper shoulder. The axillary nerve supplies the shoulder joint and the overlying skin (in accordance with the Hilton law). The medial, lateral, and dorsal brachial cutaneous nerves supply the balance of the cutaneous innervation of the arm. The lateral antebrachial cutaneous nerve is the termination of the musculocutaneous nerve (see Fig. 2–40 for a summary of dermatome patterns).

2. Compressive neuropathies (Table 2–17)
3. Muscle innervation (see Table 2–3)

E. Vessels—The brachial artery originates at the lower border of the tendon of the teres major and continues to the elbow, where it bifurcates into the radial and ulnar arteries (see Fig. 2–11). Lying medial in the arm, the brachial artery curves laterally to enter the cubital fossa (formed by the distal humerus proximally, the brachioradialis laterally, and the pronator teres medially). Its principal branches include the deep brachial (also known as the profunda, this artery accompanies the radial nerve posteriorly in the triangular interval), the superior and inferior ulnar collaterals, and the nutrient and muscular branches.

TABLE 2-15 MUSCLES OF THE ARM

Muscle	Origin	Insertion	Action	Innervation
Coracobrachialis	Coracoid	Mid-humerus (medial)	Flexion, adduction	Musculocutaneous
Biceps brachii	Coracoid (SH) Supraglenoid (LH)	Radial tuberosity	Supination, flexion	Musculocutaneous
Brachialis	Anterior humerus	Ulnar tuberosity (anterior)	Flexes forearm	Musculocutaneous, radial
Triceps brachii	Infraglenoid (LH) Posterior humerus (lat H) Posterior humerus (MH)	Olecranon	Extends forearm	Radial

lat H, lateral head; LH, long head; MH, medial head; SH, short head.

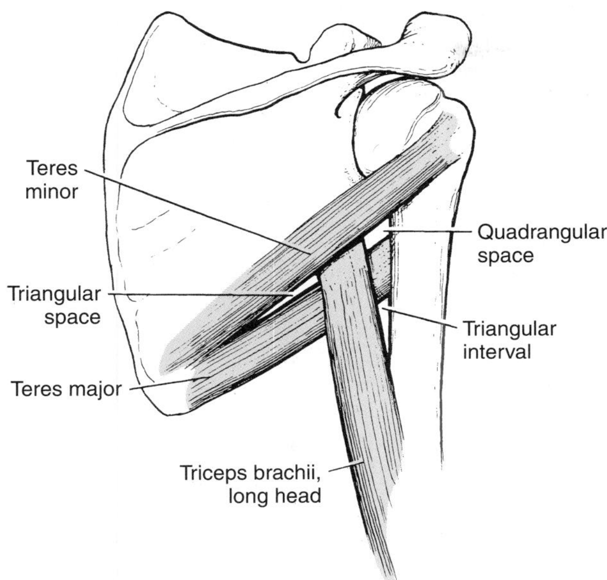

FIGURE 2–10 Borders of key spaces and intervals from posterior: quadrangular space (axillary nerve and posterior humeral circumflex artery), triangular space (circumflex scapular vessels), and triangular interval (radial nerve and profunda brachii artery). (From Kaplan EB: Surgical Approaches to the Neck, Cervical Spine, and Upper Extremity, p 53. Philadelphia, WB Saunders, 1966.)

The supratrochlear artery is the least flexible branch; these collateral vessels can bind up the brachial artery with distal humerus fractures.

F. Surgical approaches to the arm—A summary is provided in Table 2–18.
   1. Anterolateral approach to the proximal humerus (Fig. 2–12)—This approach depends on the internervous plane between the deltoid (axillary nerve) and pectoralis major (medial and lateral pectoral nerves) proximally and between the fibers of the brachialis (radial and musculocutaneous nerves) distally. The radial and axillary nerves are at risk mainly because of forceful retraction. The anterior circumflex humeral vessels may need to be ligated with a proximal approach.
   2. Posterior approach to the humerus (Fig. 2–13)—With the posterior approach, the interval between the lateral and long heads of the triceps superficially and a muscle-splitting approach for the medial (deep) head are used. The radial nerve (which limits proximal extension of this approach) and deep brachial artery must be identified and protected. The ulnar nerve is jeopardized unless subperiosteal dissection of the humerus is meticulous.
   3. Anterolateral approach to the distal humerus (Fig. 2–14)—In this approach, the interval between the brachialis (musculocutaneous and radial nerves) and brachioradialis (radial nerve) is used. The radial nerve must be identified and protected.
   4. Lateral approach to the distal humerus—By means of the lateral approach, the interval between the triceps and brachioradialis is exploited by elevating a portion of the common extensor origin from the lateral epicondyle. Proximal extension jeopardizes the radial nerve.

G. Surgical approaches to the elbow—Standard approaches are discussed below, and a summary table is provided (Table 2–19).
   1. Posterior approach to the elbow (Fig. 2–15)—Detachment of the extensor mechanism of the elbow gives excellent exposure for many elbow fractures. The olecranon osteotomy (best done with a chevron cut 2 cm distal to the tip) should be predrilled and the ulnar nerve protected. An alternative approach splits the triceps and leaves the olecranon intact.
   2. Medial approach to the elbow—With this approach, the interval between the brachialis (musculocutaneous nerve) and the triceps (radial nerve) proximally and the brachialis and pronator teres (median nerve) distally is exploited. The ulnar and medial antebrachial cutaneous nerves are in the field and must be protected.
   3. Anterolateral approach to the elbow (Henry)—An extension of the same approach to the distal humerus, it is a brachialis (musculocutaneous nerve) splitting approach proximally and is between the pronator teres (median nerve) and brachioradialis distally. The lateral antebrachial cutaneous nerve must be protected superficially and the radial nerve (and its branches) must be protected deep (supinate the forearm). Additionally, the brachial artery (which lies under the biceps aponeurosis) must be carefully protected. Branches of the recurrent radial artery must be ligated with this approach.

TABLE 2-16 SHOULDER SPACES AND INTERVALS

Space	Borders	Nerve	Vessel
Quadrangular (quadrilateral) space	Superior—lower border of teres minor Lateral—surgical neck of humerus Medial—long head of triceps Inferior—upper border of teres major	Axillary	Posterior humeral circumflex artery
Triangular space	Superior—lower border of teres minor Lateral—long head of triceps; medial—teres major		Circumflex scapular artery
Triangular interval	Superior—lower border of teres major Lateral—shaft of humerus; medial—long head of triceps	Radial	Profunda brachii artery

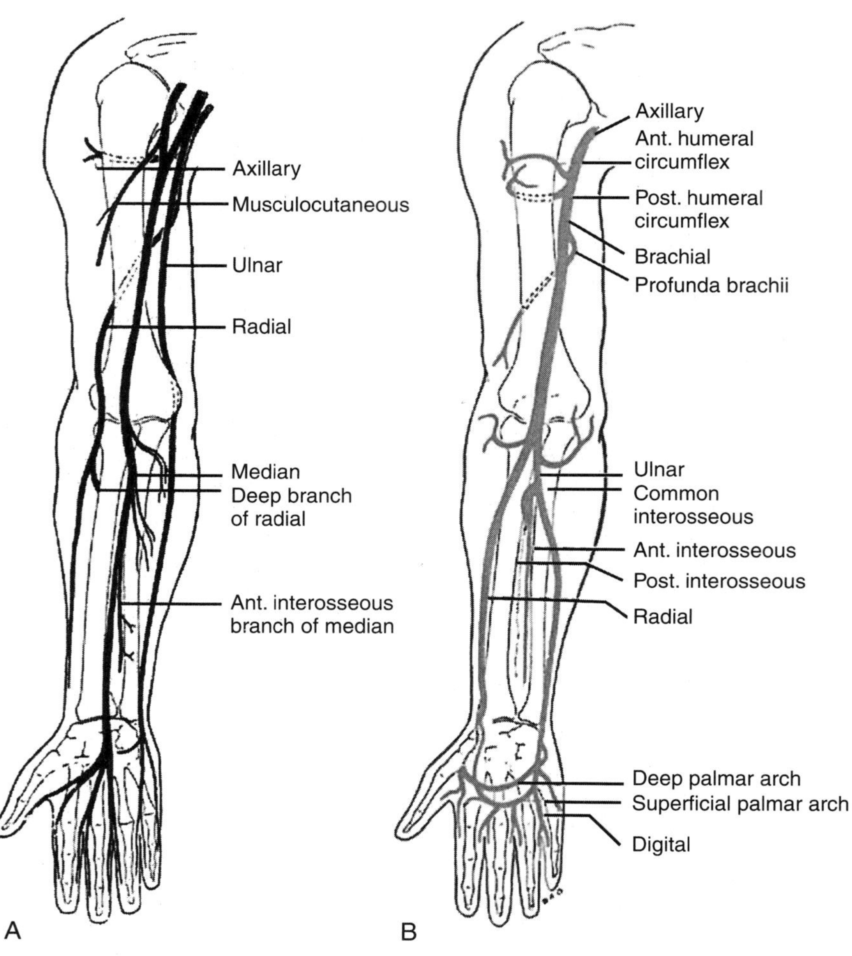

FIGURE 2–11 Principal nerves (**A**) and arteries (**B**) of the upper extremity. (From Jenkins DB: Hollinshead's Functional Anatomy of the Limbs and Back, 6th ed, p 62. Philadelphia, WB Saunders, 1991.)

TABLE 2–17 NERVE COMPRESSION SYNDROMES OF THE ARM AND FOREARM

Syndrome	Nerve Involved	Sites of Compression
Pronator	Median	Supracondylar process of humerus and ligament of Struthers Lacertus fibrosis (bicipital aponeurosis) Pronator teres Arch of flexor digitorum superficialis (FDS)
Anterior interosseous nerve (AIN)	AIN of median	Deep head of pronator teres (PT) FDS Aberrant vessels Accessory muscles (i.e., Gantzer)
Cubital tunnel	Ulnar	Arcade of Struthers Medial intermuscular septum Medial epicondyle Cubital tunnel Proximal edge of flexor carpi ulnaris (Osborne fascia) Deep flexor pronator aponeurosis
Posterior interosseous nerve (PIN) Radial tunnel	PIN of radial	Fibrous bands Recurrent leash of Henry Extensor carpi radialis brevis Arcade of Frohse (proximal edge of superficial head of supinator) Supinator distal margin
Superficial radial nerve	Superficial radial	Between the brachioradialis and extensor carpi radialis longus

4. (Postero)lateral (Kocher) approach to the elbow (Fig. 2–16)—This approach uses the interval between the anconeus (radial nerve) and origin of the main extensor (**extensor carpi ulnaris** [ECU], **posterior interosseous nerve** [PIN]). Pronation of the arm moves the PIN anteriorly

TABLE 2–18 HUMERAL SURGICAL APPROACHES

Approach	Interval	Structures at Risk
Anterolateral—proximal	Proximal—deltoid (axillary nerve) and pectoralis major (medial and lateral pectoral nerve) Distal—brachialis (radial and musculocutaneous nerve)	Radial nerve; axillary nerve; anterior humeral circumflex artery
Posterior	Triceps (radial nerve); lateral and long heads	Radial nerve; deep brachial artery
Anterolateral—distal	Brachialis (musculocutaneous and radial nerve) and brachioradialis (radial nerve)	Radial nerve
Lateral	Triceps (radial nerve) and brachioradialis (radial nerve)	Radial nerve with proximal extension

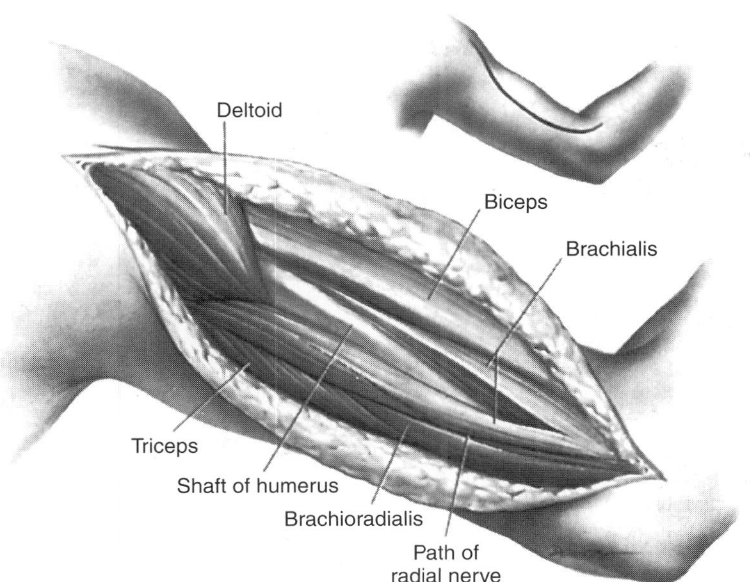

FIGURE 2–12 Lateral approach to the arm. (From Kaplan EB: Surgical Approaches to the Neck, Cervical Spine, and Upper Extremity, p 74. Philadelphia, WB Saunders, 1966.)

and radially, and the radial head is approached through the proximal supinator fibers. Extending this approach distal to the annular ligament increases the risk to the PIN.

H. Arthroscopy—Portals for elbow arthroscopy include the anterolateral portal (risk to the radial nerve), the anteromedial portal (risks to the medial antebrachial cutaneous and median nerves), and the posterolateral portals.

III. Forearm

A. Osteology—The forearm includes two long bones: the ulna and radius, which articulate with the humerus (principally the ulna) and carpi (principally the radius).

1. Ulna—Proximally, the ulna is composed of two curved processes, the olecranon and the coronoid processes, with an intervening trochlear notch. Distally, the ulna tapers and

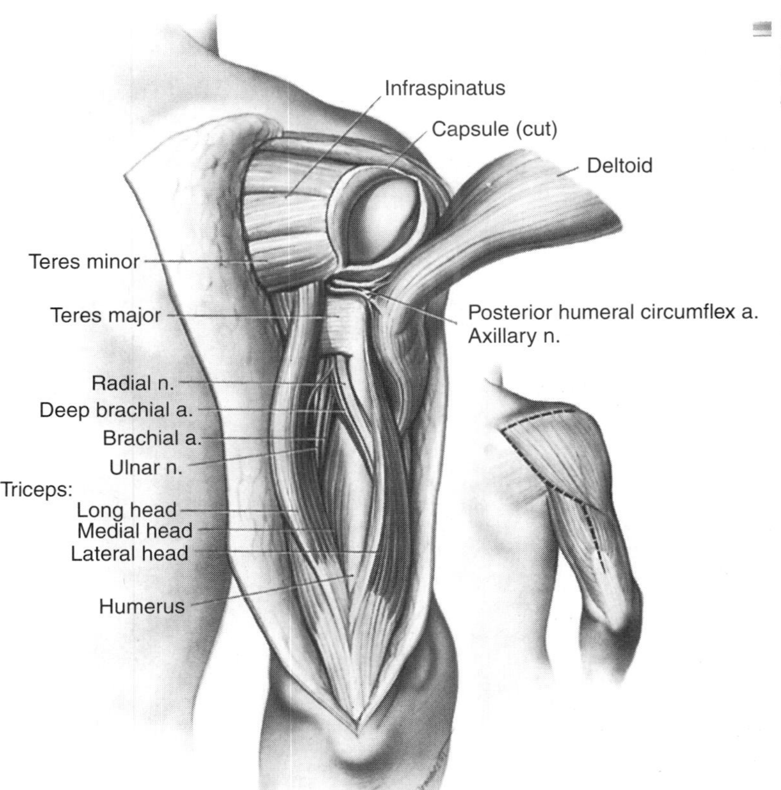

FIGURE 2–13 Posterior approach to the arm. The medial (deep) head of the triceps is split in this approach. (From Kaplan EB: Surgical Approaches to the Neck, Cervical Spine, and Upper Extremity, p 73. Philadelphia, WB Saunders, 1966.)

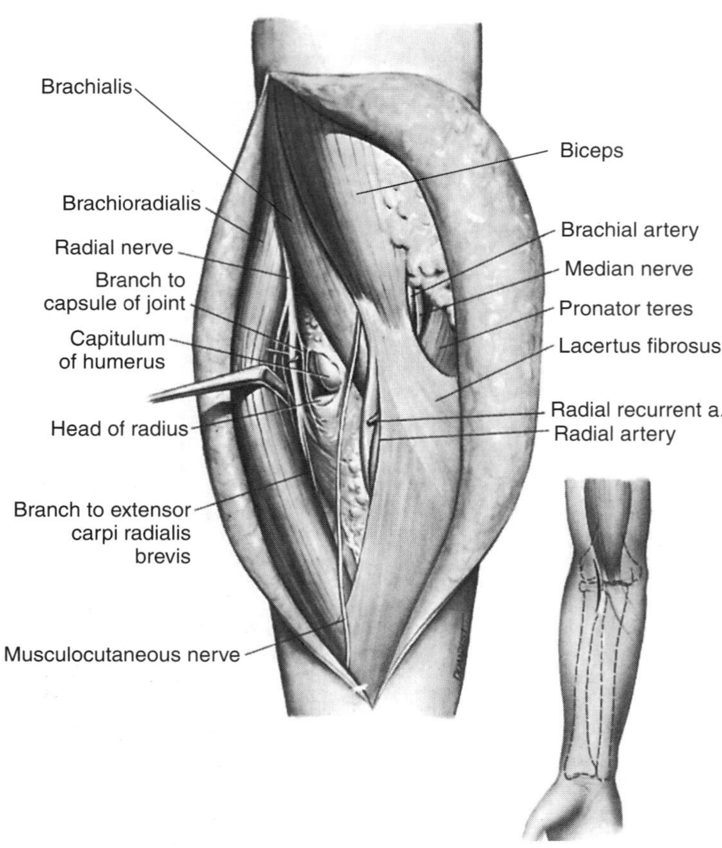

FIGURE 2–14 Anatomy of the anterior elbow. For exposure of the lateral distal humerus, the interval between the brachioradialis (radial nerve) and the brachialis (radial and musculocutaneous nerves) is explored while protecting the radial nerve. (From Kaplan EB: Surgical Approaches to the Neck, Cervical Spine, and Upper Extremity, p 77. Philadelphia, WB Saunders, 1966.)

TABLE 2–19 ELBOW SURGICAL APPROACHES

Approach	Interval	Structures at Risk
Posterior	Detach triceps or olecranon osteotomy	Ulnar nerve Olecranon nonunion
Medial	Proximally—brachialis (musculocutaneous nerve) and triceps (radial nerve) Distally—brachialis and pronator teres (median nerve)	Ulnar nerve; medial antebrachial cutaneous n.
Anterolateral (Henry)	Proximally—brachialis (musculocutaneous nerve) splitting Distally—pronator teres (median nerve) and brachioradialis (radial nerve)	Lateral antebrachial cutaneous nerve; radial nerve Ligation of radial recurrent artery; protect brachial artery To reduce risk: supinate forearm
Posterolateral (Kocher)	Anconeus (radial nerve) and extensor carpi ulnaris (PIN of radial nerve)	PIN (pronation moves PIN anteriorly and radially) To reduce risk: pronate forearm

PIN, posterior interosseous nerve.

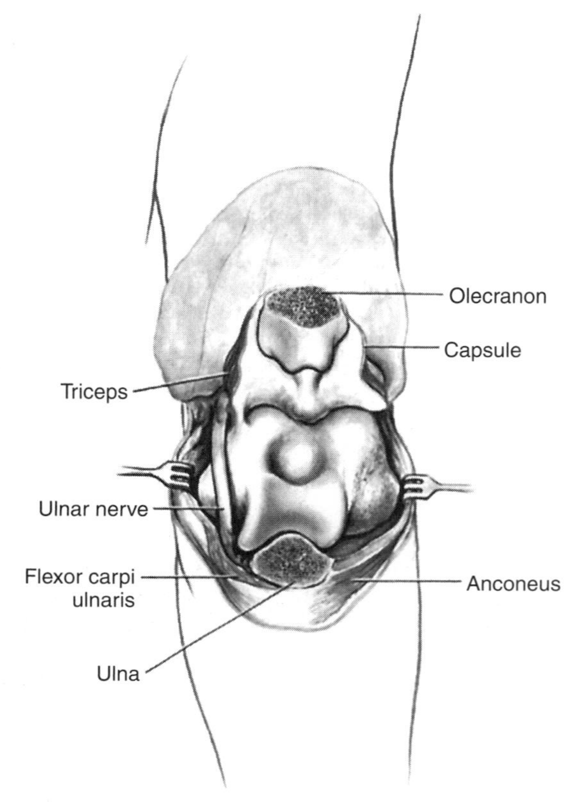

FIGURE 2–15 Posterior approach to the elbow. An olecranon osteotomy is shown. (From Kaplan EB: Surgical Approaches to the Neck, Cervical Spine, and Upper Extremity, p 82. Philadelphia, WB Saunders, 1966.)

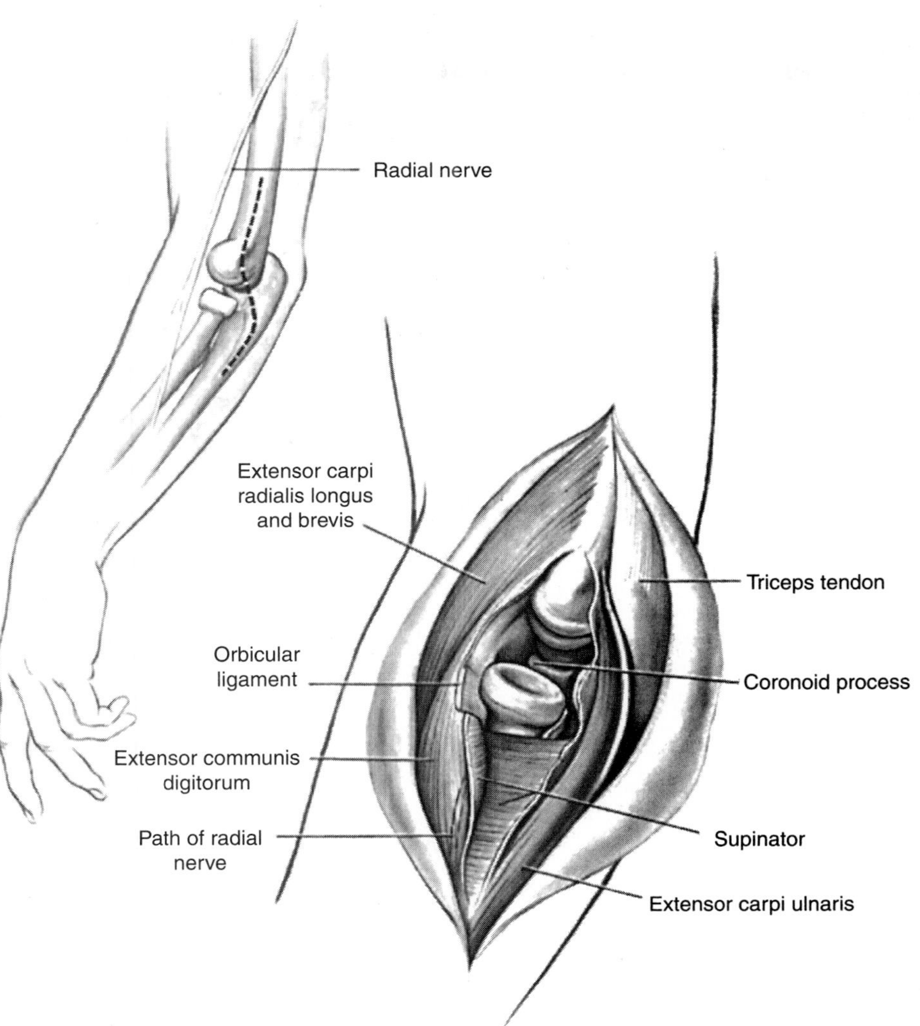

FIGURE 2–16 Lateral approach to the elbow. This approach explores the interval between the anconeus (radial nerve) and the extensor carpi ulnaris (posterior interosseous nerve [PIN]). Arm pronation helps move the PIN away from the surgical field. (From Kaplan EB: Surgical Approaches to the Neck, Cervical Spine, and Upper Extremity, p 83. Philadelphia, WB Saunders, 1966.)

ends in a lateral head and a medial styloid process.

2. Radius—The proximal radius is composed of a head with a central fovea, neck, and proximal medial radial tuberosity (for insertion of the biceps tendon). The radius has a gradual bend (convex laterally) and gradually increases in size distally. Restoration of the radial bow is important in the fixation of radial shaft fractures. The distal extremity of the radius is composed of the carpal articular surface, an ulnar notch, a dorsal tubercle (Lister tubercle, which is at the level of the scapholunate joint), and a lateral styloid process.

B. Arthrology—The radius and ulna articulate proximally at the elbow joint (discussed earlier) and distally at the wrist. The wrist consists primarily of the radiocarpal joint but also includes the distal radioulnar articulation (the most stable in supination), with its **triangular fibrocartilage complex** (TFCC).

1. Radiocarpal joint—This joint is ellipsoid and involves the distal radius and the scaphoid, lunate, and triquetrum. It is usually located at the level of the crease of the proximal wrist flexion. Covered by a loose capsule, the wrist relies heavily on ligaments, especially volar ligaments, for stability. They include the volar and dorsal radiocarpal ligaments and the ulnar and radial collateral ligaments.

2. TFCC (Fig. 2–17)—This structure originates from the most ulnar portion of the radius and extends into the caput ulnae and the ulnar wrist to the base of the fifth metacarpal. It includes the components listed in Table 2–20.

C. Muscles (Fig. 2–18)—The arrangement of these muscles is based on both location and function and is divided into volar flexors (superficial and deep) and dorsal extensors (superficial and deep) (Table 2–21).

D. Nerves

1. Anatomy—The nerves of the upper arm continue into the forearm (Fig. 2–19 and Table 2–22).

a. Radial nerve—Anterior to the lateral epicondyle, the radial nerve runs between the brachialis and brachioradialis and divides into the anterior and deep (PIN) branches. The PIN splits the supinator and supplies all of the extensor muscles, except the mobile wad (brachioradialis, **extensor carpi radialis brevis** [ECRB], **extensor carpi radialis**

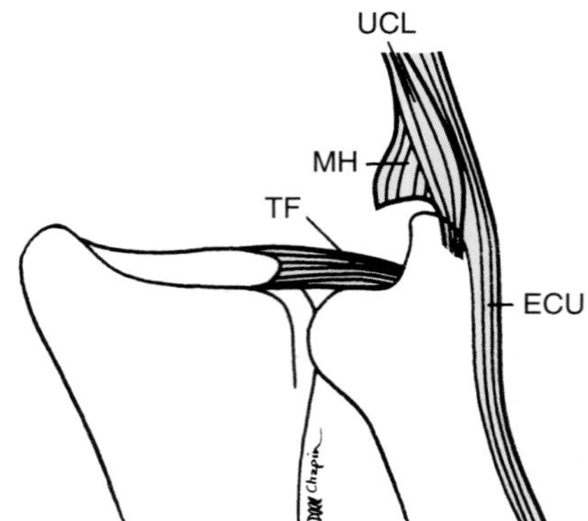

FIGURE 2–17 Triangular fibrocartilage complex. ECU, extensor carpi ulnaris; MH, meniscal homologue; TF, transverse fibers (radioulnar ligament); UCL, ulnar collateral ligament. (From Weissman BN, Sledge CB: Orthopedic Radiology, p 115. Philadelphia, WB Saunders, 1986.)

longus [ECRL]). Compression of the PIN can occur at six places (see under Summary of Compressive Neuropathies of the Forearm). The superficial branch of the radial nerve passes to the dorsal radial surface of the hand in the distal third of the forearm by passing between the brachioradialis and ECRL.

b. Median nerve—This nerve lies medial to the brachial artery at the elbow, superficial to the brachialis muscle. In the forearm the median nerve splits the two heads of the pronator teres and then runs between the **flexor digitorum superficialis** (FDS) and **flexor digitorum profundus** (FDP), becoming more superficial at the flexor retinaculum, where it continues into the hand. It has branches to all the superficial flexor muscles of the forearm except the **flexor carpi ulnaris** (FCU). Its anterior interosseous branch, which runs between the **flexor pollicis longus** (FPL) and FDP, supplies all the deep flexors except the ulnar half of the FDP.

c. Ulnar nerve—This nerve enters the forearm between the two heads of the FCU, which it supplies, and then runs between the FCU and FDP, innervating the ulnar half of this muscle. It lies more superficial at the wrist and enters the hand through the Guyon canal.

TABLE 2-20 COMPONENTS OF THE TRIANGULAR FIBROCARTILAGE COMPLEX

Component	Origin	Insertion
Dorsal and volar radioulnar ligament	Ulnar radius	Caput ulna
Articular disc	Radius/ulna	Triquetrum
Prestyloid recess	Disc	Meniscus homologue
Meniscus homologue	Ulna/disc	Triquetrum/UCL
Ulnar collateral ligament (UCL)	Ulna	Fifth metacarpal

d. Cutaneous nerves—The forearm has the lateral antebrachial cutaneous nerve (the continuation of the musculocutaneous nerve that passes lateral to the cephalic vein after emerging laterally from between the biceps and brachialis at the elbow), the medial antebrachial cutaneous nerve (a branch from the medial cord of the brachial plexus), and the posterior antebrachial cutaneous nerve (a branch of the radial nerve given off in the arm) (see Fig. 2–40).

2. Compressive neuropathies of the forearm (see Table 2–18)—An example of key testable material on compressive neuropathies would be to determine which muscle is last to return after the release of PIN palsy. Because the PIN innervates the supinator, ECU, **extensor digitorum** (ED), **extensor digiti minimi** (EDM), **abductor pollicis longus** (APL), **extensor pollicis longus** (EPL), **extensor pollicis brevis** (EPB), and **extensor indices proprius** (EIP), in that order, the last muscle to return to function (EIP) is the most distally innervated muscle.
3. Innervation of the forearm (Table 2–23)

E. Vessels (see Fig. 2–19)—At the elbow, the brachial artery enters the cubital fossa (bordered by the two epicondyles, the brachioradialis, and the pronator teres and overlying the brachialis and supinator). It then divides at the level of the radial neck into the radial and ulnar arteries (Table 2–24).

1. Radial artery—The radial artery initially runs on the pronator teres, deep to the brachioradialis, and continues to the wrist between this muscle and the **flexor carpi radialis** (FCR). Forearm branches include the recurrent radial (see earlier discussion) and muscular branches.
2. Ulnar artery—The larger of the two branches, the ulnar artery is covered by the superficial flexors proximally (between the FDS and FDP). Distally, the artery lies on the FDP, between the tendons of the FCU and FDS. Forearm branches include the anterior and posterior recurrent ulnar (discussed earlier), the common interosseous (with anterior and posterior branches), and several muscular and nutrient arteries.

F. Surgical approaches to the forearm (Table 2–25)

1. Anterior (Henry's) approach (Fig. 2–20)—The anterior approach uses the interval between the brachioradialis (radial nerve) and pronator teres (or FCR distally) (median nerve). It is necessary to isolate and ligate the leash of Henry (radial artery branches) proximally and to strip the supinator from its insertion subperiosteally. It is essential to protect the superficial branch of the radial nerve (retract laterally) and the brachioradialis. It is necessary to dissect off the FPL and pronator quadratus distally. Supination of the forearm displaces the PIN ulnarly.
2. Dorsal (posterior) (Thompson's) approach (Fig. 2–21)—In the posterior approach, the interval between the ECRL (radial nerve) and ED (or EPL distally) (PIN) is employed.

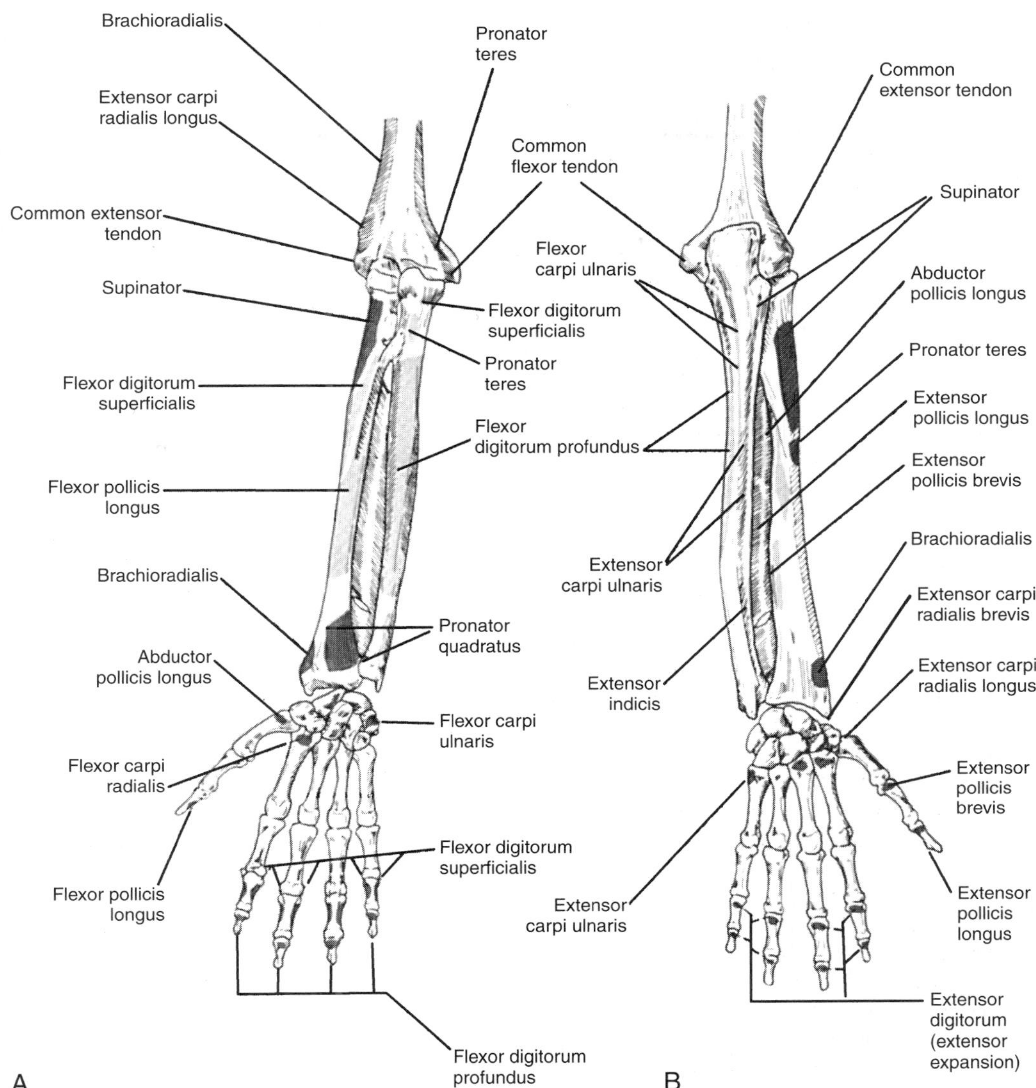

FIGURE 2–18 Origins and insertions of muscles of the forearm. **A**, Anterior. **B**, Posterior. (From Jenkins DB: Hollinshead's Functional Anatomy of the Limbs and Back, 6th ed, Fig. 8-4. Philadelphia, WB Saunders, 1991.)

The PIN must be identified and protected when this surgical approach is used. Excessive retraction of the supinator can injure the PIN.

3. Exposure of the ulna—The ulna is exposed via the interval between the ECU (PIN) and the FCU (ulnar nerve).
4. Cross-sectional diagrams of mid-forearm (Fig. 2–22) and distal forearm (Fig 2–23).

IV. Wrist and Hand*

A. Osteology

1. Carpal bones—Each carpal bone has six surfaces, with proximal, distal, medial, and lateral surfaces for articulation and palmar and dorsal surfaces for ligamentous insertion. Ossification begins at the capitate (usually present at 1 year of age) and proceeds in a counterclockwise direction. Therefore, the hamate is the second carpus to ossify (by 1-2 years), followed by the triquetrum (by 3 years), lunate (by 4-5 years), scaphoid (by 5 years), trapezium (by 6 years), and trapezoid (by 7 years). The pisiform, which is a large sesamoid bone, is the last to ossify (by 9 years). Several key features are important to recognize in the individual carpal bones (Table 2–26).
2. Metacarpals—The metacarpals have two ossification centers: one for the body (primary center of ossification), which ossifies at 8 weeks of fetal life (like most long bones), and one at the neck, which usually appears before 3 years of age. The first metacarpal is a primordial phalanx and has its secondary ossification center located at the base (like the phalanges). Several characteristics allow the identification of the individual metacarpals (Table 2–27).
3. Phalanges—The 14 phalanges (three for each finger and two for the thumb) are similar. They

*See Chapter 7, Hand, Upper Extremity, and Microvascular Surgery.

TABLE 2-21 MUSCLES OF THE FOREARM

Muscle	Origin	Insertion	Action	Innervation
Superficial Flexors				
Pronator teres	Medial epicondyle and coronoid	Mid-lateral radius	Pronate, flex forearm	Median
Flexor carpi radialis	Medial epicondyle	Second and third metacarpal bases	Flex wrist	Median
Palmaris longus	Medial epicondyle	Palmar aponeurosis	Flex wrist	Median
Flexor carpi ulnaris	Medial epicondyle and posterior ulna	Pisiform	Flex wrist	Ulnar
Flexor digitorum superficialis	Medial epicondyle and anterior radius	Base of middle phalanges	Flex PIP	Median
Deep Flexors				
Flexor digitorum profundus	Anterior and medial ulna	Base of distal phalanges	Flex DIP	Median-anterior interosseous/ulnar
Flexor pollicis longus	Anterior and lateral radius	Base of distal phalanges	Flex IP, thumb	Median-anterior interosseous
Pronator quadratus	Distal ulna	Volar radius	Pronate hand	Median-anterior interosseous
Superficial Extensors				
Brachioradialis	Lateral supracondylar humerus	Lateral distal radius	Flex forearm	Radial
Extensor carpi radialis longus	Lateral supracondylar humerus	Second metacarpal base	Extend wrist	Radial
Extensor carpi radialis brevis	Lateral epicondyle of humerus	Third metacarpal base	Extend wrist	Radial
Anconeus	Lateral epicondyle of humerus	Proximal dorsal ulna	Extend forearm	Radial
Extensor digitorum	Lateral epicondyle of humerus	Extensor aponeurosis	Extend digits	Radial-posterior interosseous
Extensor digiti minimi	Common extensor tendon	Small finger extensor carpi ulnaris	Extend small finger	Radial-posterior interosseous
Extensor carpi ulnaris	Lateral epicondyle of humerus	Fifth metacarpal base	Extent/adduct hand	Radial-posterior interosseous
Deep Extensors				
Supinator	Lateral epicondyle of humerus, ulna	Dorsolateral radius	Supinate forearm	Radial-posterior interosseous
Abductor pollicis longus	Dorsal ulna/radius	First metacarpal base	Abduct thumb, extend	Radial-posterior interosseous
Extensor pollicis brevis	Dorsal radius	Thumb proximal phalanx base	Extend thumb MCP	Radial-posterior interosseous
Extensor pollicis longus	Dorsolateral ulna	Thumb dorsal phalanx base	Extend thumb IP	Radial-posterior interosseous
Extensor indicis proprius	Dorsolateral ulna	Index finger extensor apparatus (ulnarly)	Extend index finger	Radial-posterior interosseous

DIP, distal interphalangeal joint; IP, interphalangeal joint; PIP, proximal interphalangeal joint; MCP, metacarpophalangeal joint.

all have secondary ossification centers at their bases that appear at ages 3 years (proximal), 4 years (middle), and 5 years (distal). The bases of the proximal phalanges are oval and concave, with the smaller heads ending in two condyles. The middle phalanges have two concave facets at their bases and pulley-shaped heads. The distal phalanges are smaller and have palmar ungual tuberosities distally.

B. Arthrology

1. Radiocarpal (wrist) joint—This joint is ellipsoid and is made up of the distal radius, scaphoid, lunate, triquetrum, and ligamentous structures (Table 2–28). The palmar/volar radiocarpal ligament is the strongest supporting structure, although it has a weak area on the radial side (the space of Poirier) that lends less support to the scaphoid, lunate, and trapezoid (Fig. 2–24).
2. Intercarpal joints
   a. Proximal row—The scaphoid, lunate, and triquetrum form gliding joints. Two dorsal intercarpal ligaments connect the scaphoid and lunate and the lunate and triquetral bones. Two palmar intercarpal ligaments connect the scaphoid and lunate and the lunate and triquetral bones. The dorsal intercarpal ligaments are stronger. The interosseous ligaments are narrow bundles connecting the scaphoid and lunate and the lunate and triquetral bones.
   b. Pisiform articulation—The pisotriquetral joint has a thin articular capsule. The

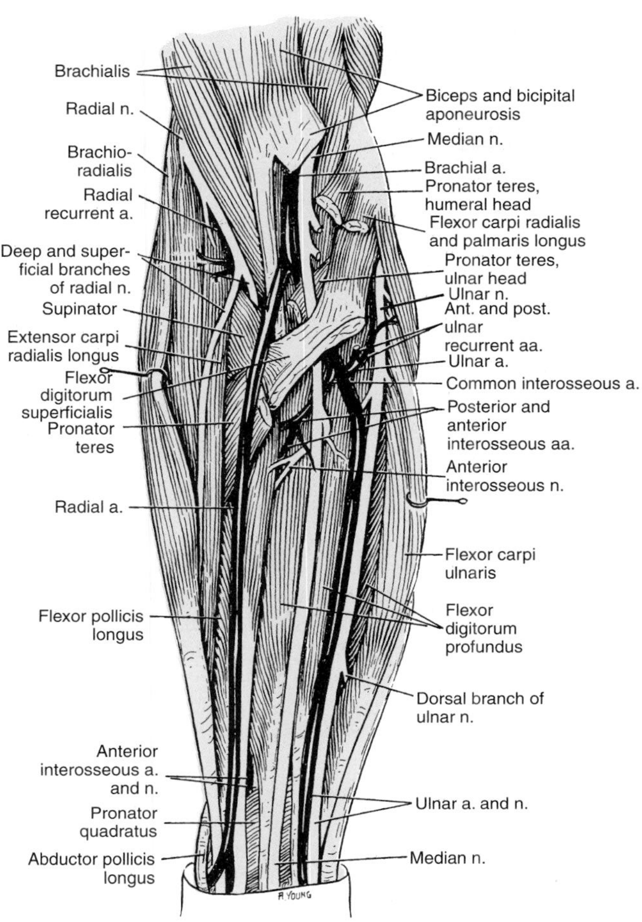

FIGURE 2–19 Arteries (black) and nerves of the forearm. (From Jenkins DB: Hollinshead's Functional Anatomy of the Limbs and Back, 6th ed, p. 131. Philadelphia, WB Saunders, 1991.)

TABLE 2-22 FOREARM NEUROANATOMIC RELATIONSHIPS

Nerve	Relationships
Radial	Between brachialis and brachioradialis
Posterior interosseous	Splits supinator
Superficial radial	Between brachioradialis and extensor carpi radialis longus
Median	Medial to brachial artery at elbow
Anterior interosseous	Splits pronator teres and runs between flexor digitorum superficialis and flexor digitorum profundus
	Between flexor pollicis longus and flexor digitorum profundus
Ulnar	Between flexor carpi ulnaris and flexor digitorum profundus

TABLE 2-23 INNERVATION OF THE FOREARM

Nerves	Muscles Innervated
Radial Nerve	
Radial (posterior cord)	Triceps, brachioradialis, extensor carpi radialis longus, extensor carpi radialis brevis
Posterior interosseous	Supinator, extensor carpi ulnaris, extensor digitorum, extensor digiti minimi, abductor pollicis longus, extensor pollicis longus, extensor pollicis brevis, extensor indicis proprius
Median Nerve	
Median (medial and lateral cord)	Tibialis posterior, flexor carpi radialis, palmaris longus, flexor digitorum superficialis, abductor pollicis brevis, supinator head of flexor pollicis brevis, opponens pollicis, first and second lumbricals
Anterior interosseous	Flexor digitorum profundus (first and second), flexor pollicis longus, pronator quadratus
Ulnar Nerve	
Ulnar (medial cord)	Flexor carpi ulnaris, flexor digitorum profundus (third and fourth), pollicis brevis, abductor digiti minimi, ODM, flexor digiti minimi, third and fourth lumbrical muscles, interossei, adductor pollicis, deep head of flexor pollicis brevis

TABLE 2-24 FOREARM VASCULAR ANATOMIC RELATIONSHIPS

Artery	Relationships
Radial	On pronator teres deep to brachioradialis
	Enters wrist between brachioradialis and flexor carpi radialis
Ulnar	Proximally between flexor digitorum superficialis (FDS) and flexor digitorum profundus (FDP)
	Distally on FDP between flexor carpi ulnaris and FDS

TABLE 2-25 FOREARM SURGICAL APPROACHES

Approach	Interval	Structures at Risk
Anterior (Henry)	Brachioradialis (radial nerve) and pronator teres (median nerve)	Ligate leash of Henry (radial artery branches)
	Distally—flexor carpi radialis (median nerve)	Superficial branch of radial nerve
Dorsal posterior (Thompson)	Extensor carpi radialis brevis (radial nerve) and extensor digitorum communis (PIN)	Posterior interosseous nerve (PIN)—avoid excessive retraction of supinator
	Distally—extensor pollicis longus	
Ulnar	Extensor carpi ulnaris (PIN) and flexor carpi ulnaris (ulnar nerve)	

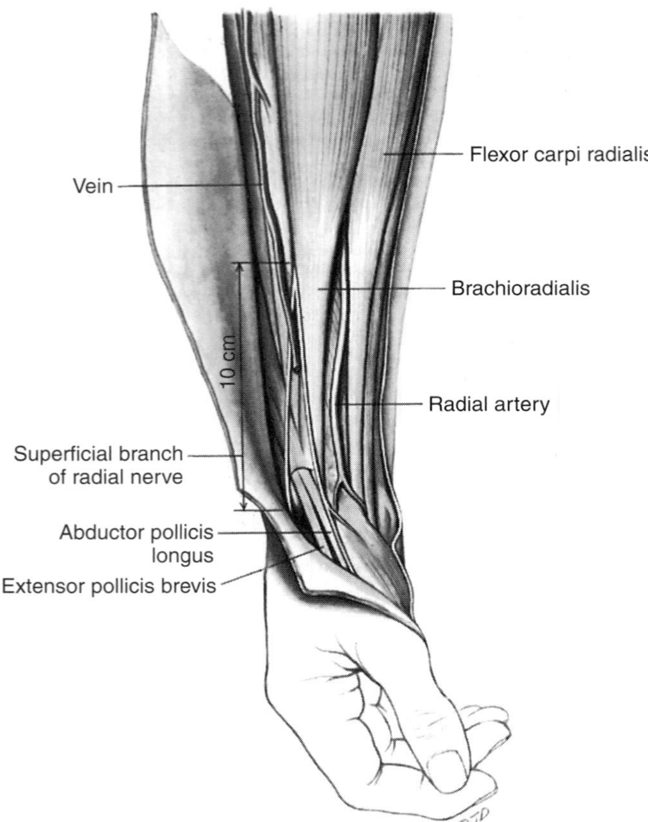

FIGURE 2–20 Anterior (Henry's) approach to the forearm. The interval between the brachioradialis (radial nerve) and the pronator teres or flexor carpi radialis (median nerve) is explored. Protect the superficial radial nerve, which lies underneath the brachioradialis. (From Kaplan EB: Surgical Approaches to the Neck, Cervical Spine, and Upper Extremity, p 92. Philadelphia, WB Saunders, 1966.)

ulnar collateral and palmar radiocarpal ligaments also connect the pisiform proximally. The pisohamate ligament and pisometacarpal ligaments help extend the pull of the FCU.

c. Distal row—The distal row comprises the trapezium, trapezoid, capitate, and hamate gliding joints. The dorsal intercarpal ligaments connect the trapezium with the trapezoid, the trapezoid with the capitate, and the capitate with the hamate. The palmar ligaments do the same. The interosseous ligaments are much thicker in the distal row, connecting the capitate and hamate (strongest), the capitate and trapezoid, and the trapezium and trapezoid (weakest).
d. Midcarpal joint—The transverse articulations between the proximal and distal rows are reinforced by palmar and dorsal intercarpal ligaments and carpal collateral ligaments (radial is stronger).

3. **Carpometacarpal** (CMC) joints
   a. Thumb CMC joint—This is a highly mobile saddle joint. It is supported by a capsule and radial, palmar, and dorsal CMC ligaments.
   b. Finger CMC joints—These are gliding joints with capsules, dorsal CMC ligaments (strongest), palmar CMC ligaments, and interosseous CMC ligaments.
4. Metacarpophalangeal joints—These joints are ellipsoid and covered by palmar (volar plate), collateral, and deep transverse metacarpal ligaments.
5. Interphalangeal joints—These are hinge joints, with capsules and obliquely oriented collateral ligaments.
6. Other important structures
   a. Extensor retinaculum—This structure covers the dorsum of the wrist and contains six synovial sheaths (Figs. 2–25 and 2–26). Orientation of the extensor tendons at the wrist is a key test (Table 2–29). The first dorsal compartment contains the APL and the **extensor pollicis brevis** (EPB). The EPB tendon is ulnar to the APL tendon (the APL frequently has multiple tendon slips, which should be addressed during release for de Quervain's tenosynovitis). In the second dorsal compartment, the ECRL tendon is radial to the ECRB tendon. Thus, the EPL tendon is ulnar to the ECRB tendon at the wrist level. The anatomic snuffbox is bordered by tendons of the first and third dorsal wrist compartments, with the EPB tendon serving as the radial snuffbox border and the EPL tendon as the ulnar border. The posterior interosseous nerve is contained within the floor of the fourth dorsal wrist compartment.
   b. **Transverse carpal ligament** ([TCL])—The TCL is actually one component of the flexor retinaculum, which serves as the roof of the carpal tunnel (see Fig. 2–25). The flexor retinaculum is attached medially to the pisiform and the hook of the hamate and laterally to the tuberosity of the scaphoid and the ridge of the trapezium. The carpal tunnel decreases in volume with wrist flexion. This tunnel contains the median nerve and nine tendons (1 FPL, 4 FDS, and 4 FDP). In the tunnel, the FDS tendons of the long and ring fingers are volar to the tendons of the index and small fingers. The flexor retinaculum also forms the floor of the Guyon canal, which is bordered as well by the hook of the hamate and the pisiform and is covered by the volar carpal ligament. Entrapment of the ulnar nerve in this canal is possible (Fig. 2–27).
   c. TFCC—This structure is formed by the triangular fibrocartilage, ulnocarpal ligaments (volar ulnolunate and ulnotriquetral ligaments), and a meniscal homologue. Injury to this structure is a common cause of ulnar wrist pain (see Fig. 2–17).
   d. Intrinsic apparatus (Table 2–30)—The intrinsic apparatus is a complex arrangement of structures that surround the digits (Fig. 2–28).

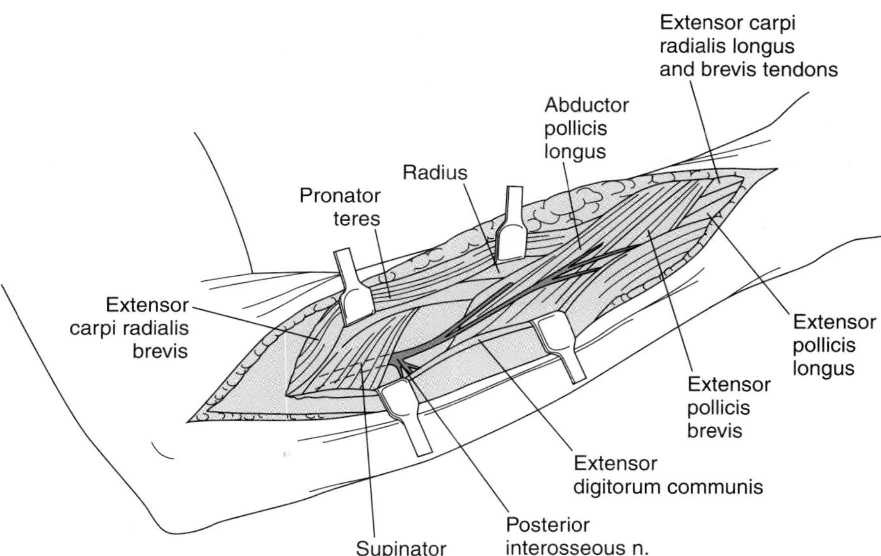

FIGURE 2–21 Dorsal (Thompson's) approach to the forearm. The interval between the extensor carpi radialis brevis (radial nerve) and the extensor digitorum communis (PIN) is explored.

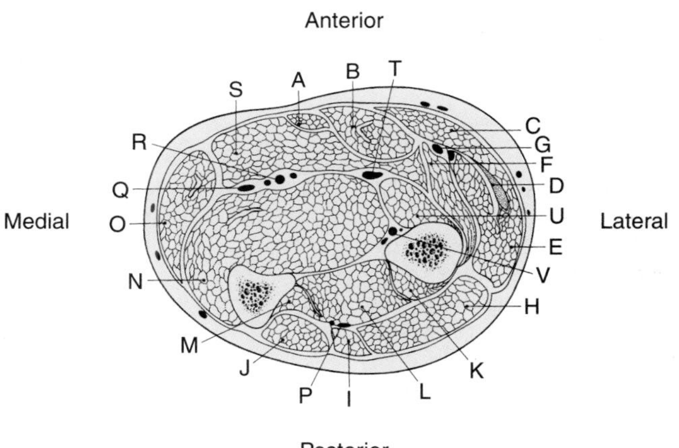

FIGURE 2–22 Cross section of the mid-forearm. (From Callaghan JJ, ed: Anatomy Self-Assessment Examination, Fig. 39. Park Ridge, IL, American Academy of Orthopaedic Surgeons, 1991.)

A—Palmaris longus m.
B—Flexor carpi radialis m.
C—Brachioradialis m.
D—Extensor carpi radialis longus m.
E—Extensor carpi radialis brevis m.
F—Pronator teres m.
G—Superficial branch of radial n.
H—Extensor digitorum m.
I—Extensor digiti minimi m.
J—Extensor carpi ulnaris m.
K—Abductor pollicis longus m.
L—Extensor pollicis brevis m.
M—Extensor pollicis longus m.
M—also Extensor indicis proprius m.
N—Flexor digitorum profundus m.
O—Flexor carpi ulnaris m.
P—Posterior interosseous n. and a.
Q—Ulnar n.
R—Ulnar a.
S—Flexor digitorum superficialis m.
T—Median n.
U—Flexor pollicis longus m.
V—Anterior interosseous a. and n.

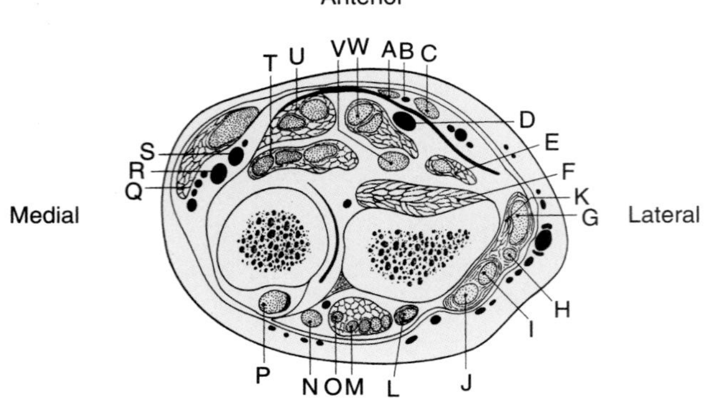

FIGURE 2–23 Cross-section of the distal forearm proximal to the distal radioulnar joint. (From Callaghan JJ, ed: Anatomy Self-Assessment Examination, Fig. 38. Park Ridge, IL, American Society of Orthopaedic Surgeons, 1991.)

A—Palmaris longus m.
B—Palmar branch of median n.
C—Flexor carpi radialis m.
D—Median n.
E—Flexor pollicis longus m.
F—Pronator quadratus m.
G—Abductor pollicis longus m.
H—Extensor pollicis brevis m.
I—Extensor carpi radialis longus m.
J—Extensor carpi radialis brevis m.
K—tendon of brachioradialis m.
L—Extensor pollicis longus m.
M—Extensor digitorum m.
N—Extensor digiti minimi m.
O—Extensor indicis proprius m.
P—Extensor carpi ulnaris m.
Q—Flexor carpi ulnaris m.
R—Ulnar n.
S—Ulnar a.
T—Flexor digitorum profundus m.
U—Flexor digitorum superficialis m.
V—Flexor digitorum profundus m.
W—Flexor digitorum superficialis m.

TABLE 2-26 CARPAL FEATURES

Carpal	Distinctive Features	Number of Articulations
Scaphoid	Tubercle (transverse carpal ligament [TCL], abductor pollicis brevis [APB]) distal vascular supply	5
Lunate	Lunar shape	5
Triquetrum	Pyramid shape	3
Pisiform	Spheroidal (TCL, flexor carpi radialis [FCR])	1
Trapezium	FCR groove, tubercle (opponens, APB, flexor pollicis brevis, TCL)	4
Trapezoid	Wedge shape	4
Capitate	Largest bone, central location	7
Hamate	Hook (TCL)	5

TABLE 2-27 METACARPAL FEATURES

Metacarpal	Distinctive Features
I (thumb)	Short, stout; base is saddle shaped
II (index)	Longest, largest base; medial at base
III (middle)	Styloid process
IV (ring)	Small quadrilateral base, narrow shaft
V (small)	Tubercle at base (extensor carpi ulnaris)

e. Flexor sheath (Fig. 2–29)—This structure covers the flexor tendons in the finger, protecting and nourishing the tendons (vincula). It also forms five pulleys (A1-A5) with three intervening cruciate attachments (C1-C3). The A2 pulley, overlying the proximal phalanx, is the most important one, followed by A4, which covers the middle phalanx. The A1 pulley is involved in trigger digits.

C. Muscles (Table 2–31); origins and insertions (Fig. 2–30)

D. Nerves (Fig. 2–31)

1. Anatomy
   a. Median nerve—The median nerve enters the wrist just under the TCL between the FDS and FCR. The palmar cutaneous branch, which arises proximal to the TCL between the palmaris longus and FCR, supplies the thenar skin. The deep (muscular) branch runs radially and supplies the thenar muscles. The digital nerves supply the lumbrical muscles and the volar aspect of the radial 3⅓ digits.
   b. Ulnar nerve—This nerve enters the wrist through the Guyon canal and divides into a superficial branch (palmaris brevis and skin) and a deep branch. The deep branch travels with the deep palmar arch and passes between the abductor digiti minimi and flexor digiti minimi brevis, giving off motor branches to the deep musculature (three

TABLE 2-28 RADIOCARPAL WRIST LIGAMENTS

Structure	Attachments	Distinctive Features
Articular capsule	Surrounds joint	Reinforced by volar and dorsal radiocarpal ligament (RCL)
Volar (RCL)	Radius, ulna, scaphoid, lunate, triquetrum, capitate	Oblique ulnar, strong
Dorsal radiocarpal ligament	Radius, scaphoid, lunate, triquetrum	Oblique radial, weak
Ulnar collateral ligament	Ulna, triquetrum, pisiform, transverse carpal ligament (TCL)	Fan-shaped, two fascicles
Radial collateral ligament	Radius, scaphoid, trapezium, TCL	Radial artery adjacent

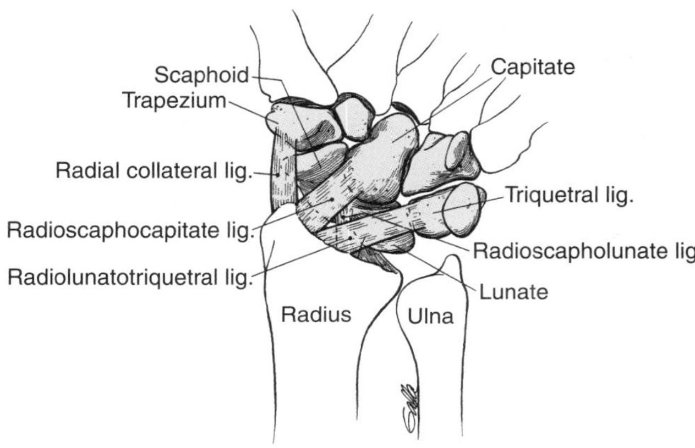

FIGURE 2–24 Extrinsic radiocarpal ligaments. (From Mooney JF, Siegel DB, Koman LA: Ligamentous injuries of the wrists in athletes. Clin Sports Med 11:129–139, 1992.)

hypothenar muscles, two ulnar lumbrical muscles, all interossei, and the adductor pollicis) and terminating in digital nerves for the ulnar 1½ digits. The dorsal cutaneous branch swings dorsally at the wrist and can be injured by either arthroscopic portal placement or surgical incision.

c. Sensation to the thumb—Thumb sensation is provided by five branches: the lateral antebrachial cutaneous nerve, superficial and dorsal digital branches of the radial nerve, and digital and palmar branches of the median nerve.

2. Innervation of the wrist and hand (Table 2–32)

E. Vessels (see Fig. 2–31)

1. Radial artery—At the wrist, the radial artery reaches the dorsum of the carpus by passing between the FCR and the APL and EPB tendons (snuffbox). Before that, it gives off a superficial palmar branch that communicates with the superficial arch (ulnar artery). In the hand, it forms the deep palmar arch. The dorsal carpal branch of the radial artery enters the scaphoid dorsally and distally.
2. Ulnar artery—At the wrist the ulnar artery lies on the TCL, gives off a deep palmar branch (which anastomoses with the deep arch), and then forms the superficial palmar arch (which is distal to the deep arch).
3. Digital arteries—These arteries arise from the superficial palmar arch and run dorsal to the nerves.

F. Surgical approaches (Table 2–33)

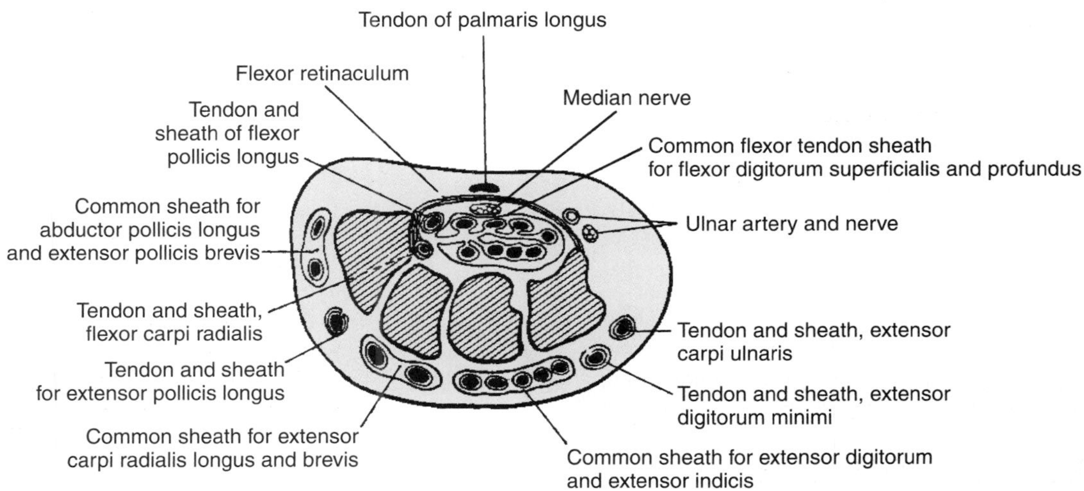

FIGURE 2–25 Components of the carpal tunnel. The roof of the carpal tunnel is the flexor retinaculum, which is composed of the deep forearm fascia, the transverse carpal ligament (TCL), and the distal aponeurosis between the thenar and hypothenar muscles. The carpal tunnel contains the median nerve and nine tendons (flexor pollicis longus [FPL] and four each of flexor digitorum superficialis and flexor digitorum profundus). The flexor carpi radialis (FCR) passes under the TCL and is not considered a tendon within the carpal tunnel. The FPL is located volar to the FCR, which is the most dorsal radial tendon passing under the flexor retinaculum. (From Jenkins DB: Hollinshead's Functional Anatomy of the Limbs and Back, 6th ed, p 162. Philadelphia, WB Saunders, 1991.)

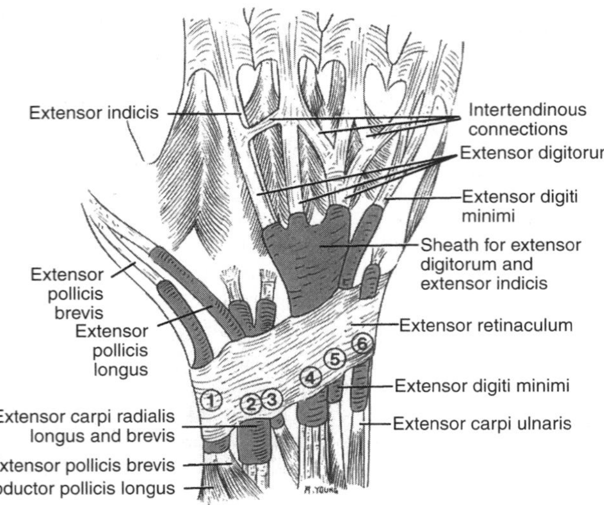

FIGURE 2–26 Extensor compartments of the wrist (1-6). See Table 2-29. (From Jenkins DB: Hollinshead's Functional Anatomy of the Limbs and Back, 6th ed, p 174. Philadelphia, WB Saunders, 1991.)

TABLE 2-29 DORSAL WRIST COMPARTMENTS

Compartment	Contents	Pathologic Condition
I	Abductor pollicis longus, extensor pollicis brevis	De Quervain's tenosynovitis
II	Extensor carpi radialis longus, brevis	Extensor tendinitis (intersection syndrome)
III	Extensor pollicis longus	Rupture at Lister tubercle (after wrist fractures) Drummer's wrist
IV	Extensor digitorum communis, extensor indicis proprius	Extensor tenosynovitis
V	Extensor digiti minimi	Rupture (RA—Vaughn-Jackson syndrome)
VI	Extensor carpi ulnaris	Snapping at ulnar styloid

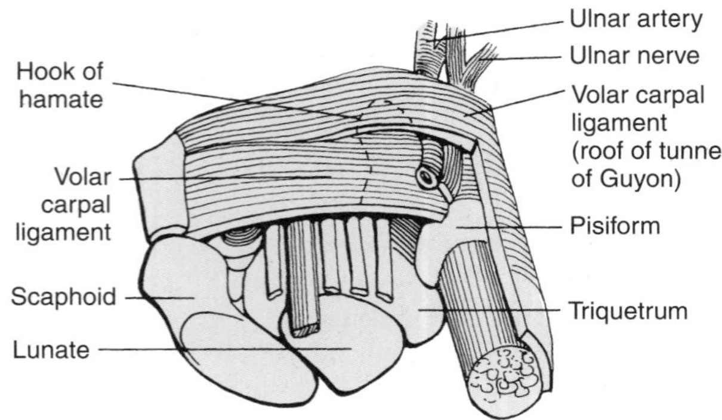

FIGURE 2–27 The carpal tunnel is formed by the transverse carpal ligament on the volar side and the carpal bones on the floor and sides. Guyon's canal is formed by the volar carpal ligament (roof), the hamate (lateral wall), and the pisiform (medial wall). (From DeLee JC, Drez D Jr.: Orthopaedic Sports Medicine: Principles and Practice, vol 1, p 932. Philadelphia, WB Saunders, 1994.)

TABLE 2-30 INTRINSIC APPARATUS

Structure	Attachments	Significance
Sagittal bands	Covers metacarpo-phalangeal (MCP)	Allows MCP extension
Transverse (sagittal)	Volar plate fibers	Allows MCP flexion (interossei)
Lateral bands	Covers proximal interphalangeal (PIP)	Allows PIP extension (lumbrical muscles)
Oblique retinacular ligament (Landsmeer)	A4 pulley, terminal tendon	Allows DIP extension (passive)

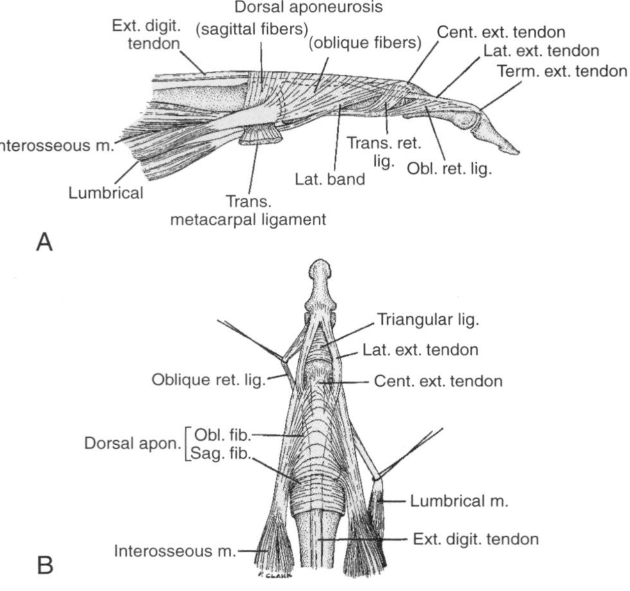

FIGURE 2–28 Dorsal extensor apparatus. **A**, Lateral view. **B**, Dorsal view. (Adapted from Bora FW: The Pediatric Upper Extremity, p 93. Philadelphia, WB Saunders, 1986.)

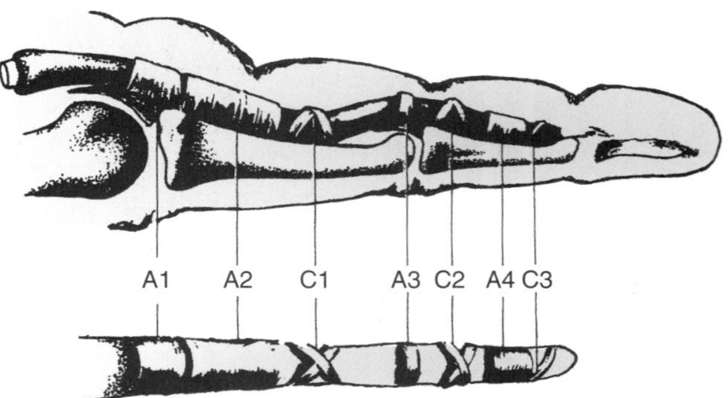

FIGURE 2–29 Flexor pulleys. The A1 pulley is the source of trigger digits. (From Tubiana R: The Hand, vol 3, p 173. Philadelphia, WB Saunders, 1985.)

TABLE 2-31 MUSCLES OF THE HAND AND WRIST

Muscle	Origin	Insertion	Action	Innervation
Thenar Muscles				
Abductor pollicis brevis	Scaphoid, trapezoid	Base of proximal phalanx, radial side	Abduct thumb	Median
Opponens pollicis	Trapezium	Thumb metacarpal	Abduct, flex, rotate (medially)	Median
Flexor pollicis brevis	Trapezium, capitate	Base of proximal phalanx, radial side	Flex metacarpophalangeal MCP)	Median, ulnar
Adductor pollicis	Capitate, second and third metacarpals	Base of proximal phalanx, ulnar side	Adduct thump	Ulnar
Hypothenar Muscles				
Palmaris brevis	Transverse carpal ligament (TCL), palmar aponeurosis	Ulnar palm	Retract skin	Ulnar
Abductor digiti minimi	Pisiform	Base of proximal phalanx, ulnar side	Abduct small finger	Ulnar
Flexor digiti minimi brevis	Hamate, TCL	Base of proximal phalanx, ulnar side	Flex MCP	Ulnar
Opponens digiti minimi	Hamate, TCL	Small-finger metacarpal	Abduct, flex, rotate (laterally)	Ulnar
Intrinsic Muscles				
Lumbricals	Flexor digitorum profundus	Lateral bands (radial)	Extend proximal interphalangeal	Median, ulnar
Dorsal interosseous	Adjacent metacarpals	Proximal phalanx base/extensor apparatus	Abduct, flex MCP	Ulnar
Volar interosseous	Adjacent metacarpals	Proximal phalanx base/extensor apparatus	Abduct, flex MCP	Ulnar

1. Dorsal approach to the wrist (Fig. 2–32)—The wrist is approached through the third and fourth extensor compartments (EPL and ED). Protecting and retracting these tendons allows access to the distal radius and the dorsal radiocarpal joint.
2. Volar approach to the wrist (Fig. 2–33)—Used most often for carpal tunnel release, the incision is usually made in line with the fourth ray to avoid the palmar cutaneous branch of the median nerve. Careful dissection through the TCL is necessary in order to avoid injury to the median nerve or its motor branch. The median nerve and flexor tendons can be retracted to allow access to the distal radius and carpus.
3. Volar (Russé's) approach to the scaphoid (Fig. 2–34)—With this approach, the interval between the FCR and radial artery is used. An approach

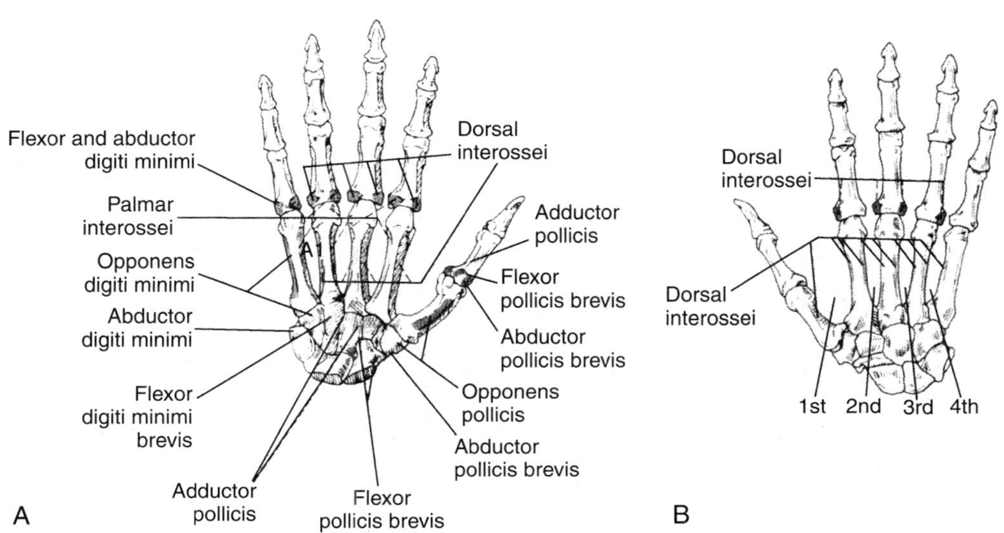

FIGURE 2–30 Origins and insertions of muscles of the wrist and hand. **A**, Dorsal view. **B**, Volar view. (From Jenkins DB: Hollinshead's Functional Anatomy of the Limbs and Back, 6th ed, Fig. 11-9. Philadelphia, WB Saunders, 1991.)

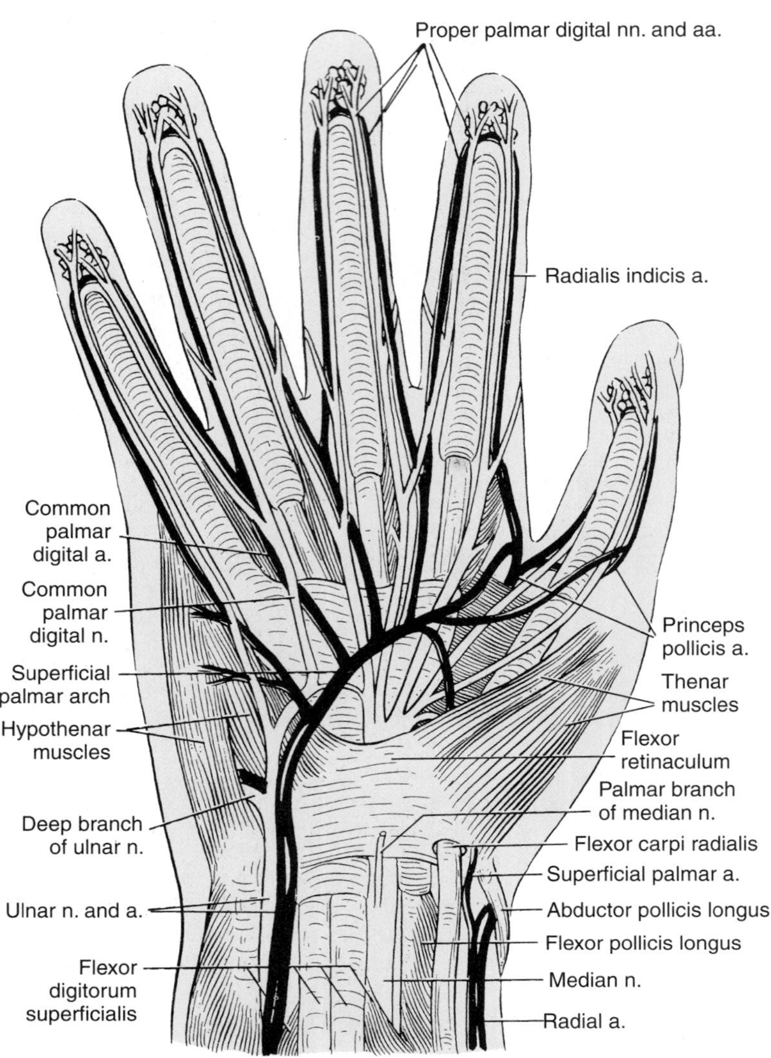

FIGURE 2–31 Nerves and vessels of the hand. (From Jenkins DB: Hollinshead's Functional Anatomy of the Limbs and Back, 6th ed, Fig. 11-11. Philadelphia, WB Saunders, 1991.)

TABLE 2-32 INNERVATION OF THE WRIST AND HAND

Nerve	Muscles Innervated
Median (medial and lateral cord)	Abductor pollicis brevis, supinator head of flexor pollicis brevis, opponens pollicis, first and second lumbricals
Ulnar (medial cord)	Abductor digiti minimi, opponens digiti minimi, flexor digiti minimi, third and fourth lumbricals, interossei, adductor pollicis, deep head of flexor pollicis brevis

TABLE 2-33 WRIST SURGICAL APPROACHES

Approach	Interval	Structures at Risk
Dorsal wrist	Third (extensor pollicis longus) and fourth (extensor digitorum communis) compartments	Transection of the innervation of the posterior interosseous nerve to the wrist capsule can be performed.
Volar wrist	Flexor carpi radialis (FCR)	Palmar cutaneous branch of median nerve
Volar scaphoid	FCR and radial artery	Radial artery
Dorsolateral scaphoid	First and third compartments	Superficial radial nerve and radial artery

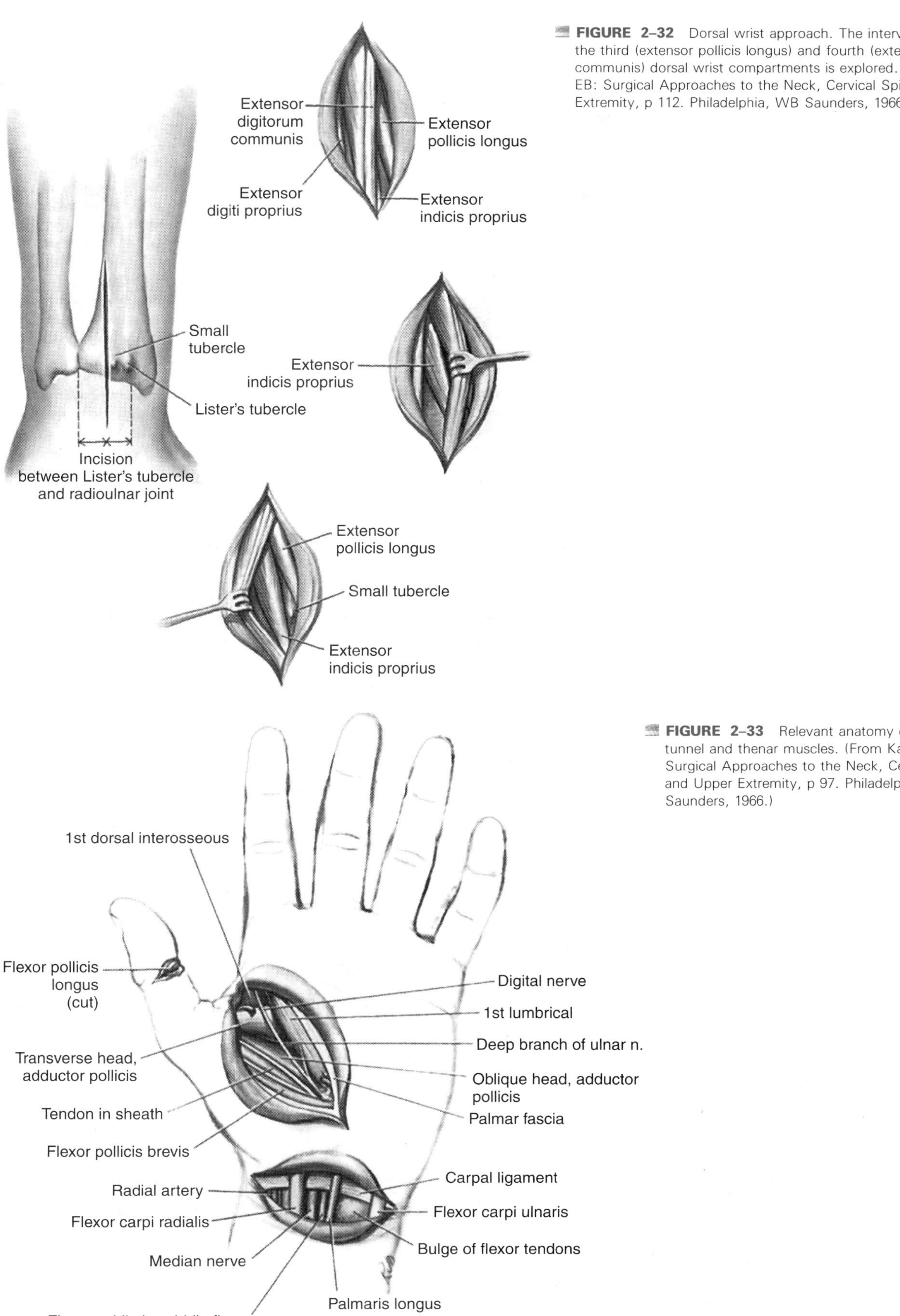

FIGURE 2–32 Dorsal wrist approach. The interval between the third (extensor pollicis longus) and fourth (extensor digitorum communis) dorsal wrist compartments is explored. (From Kaplan EB: Surgical Approaches to the Neck, Cervical Spine, and Upper Extremity, p 112. Philadelphia, WB Saunders, 1966.)

FIGURE 2–33 Relevant anatomy of the carpal tunnel and thenar muscles. (From Kaplan EB: Surgical Approaches to the Neck, Cervical Spine, and Upper Extremity, p 97. Philadelphia, WB Saunders, 1966.)

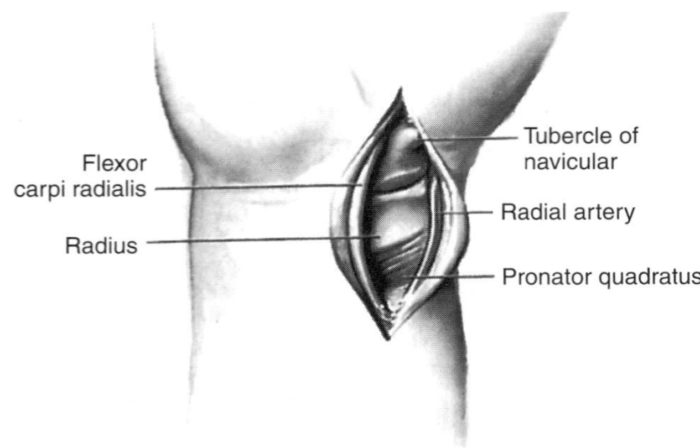

FIGURE 2–34 Russé's approach to the scaphoid. The interval between the flexor carpi radialis and radial artery is used. (From Kaplan, EB: Surgical Approaches to the Neck, Cervical Spine, and Upper Extremity, p 101. Philadelphia, WB Saunders, 1966.)

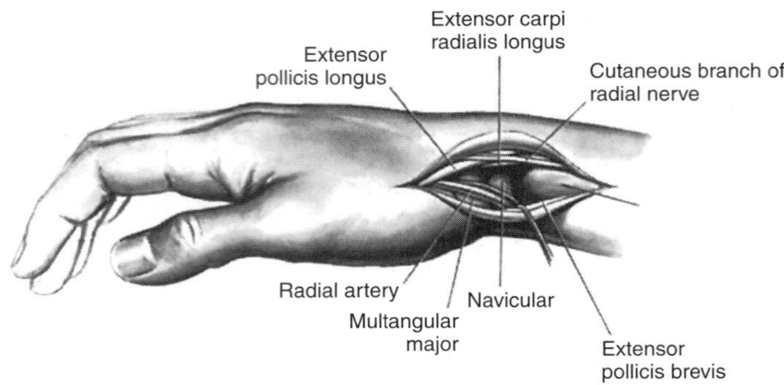

FIGURE 2–35 Dorsal approach to the scaphoid. The interval between the first and third dorsal wrist compartments is explored. (From Kaplan EB: Surgical Approaches to the Neck, Cervical Spine, and Upper Extremity, p 107. Philadelphia, WB Saunders, 1966.)

through the radial aspect of the FCR sheath is often easier and protects the radial artery.

4. Dorsolateral approach to the scaphoid (Fig. 2–35)—This approach uses an incision within the anatomic snuffbox (first and third dorsal wrist compartment), protecting the superficial radial nerve and radial artery (deep).
5. Volar approach to the flexor tendons (Bunnell)—Zigzag incisions across the flexor creases help to expose the flexor sheaths. The digital sheaths should be avoided.
6. Midlateral approach to the digits—Good for stabilization of fractures and neurovascular exposure, this approach requires a laterally placed incision at the dorsal extent of the interphalangeal creases. Exposure of the digital neurovascular bundle is carried out volar to the incision.

G. Arthroscopy—The portals used for wrist arthroscopy are based on the dorsal compartments. The 1-2 portal (risk to radial artery), 6-R, and 6-U portals (radial and ulnar to the sixth compartment; risks the ulnar nerve and artery) are the most dangerous. The commonly used 3-4 and 4-5 portals are safer.

SECTION 3 Spine

I. Spine

A. Osteology

1. Introduction—The spine contains 33 vertebrae: 7 cervical, 12 thoracic, 5 lumbar, 5 fused sacral, and 4 fused coccygeal. Normal curves include cervical lordosis, thoracic kyphosis, lumbar lordosis, and sacral kyphosis. The vertebral bodies generally increase in width craniocaudad, with the exception of T1-T3. The locations of important topographic landmarks are given in Table 2–34.
2. Cervical spine—The atlas (C1) has no vertebral body and no spinous process. C1 has two concave superior facets that articulate with the occipital condyles. The highest percentage of neck flexion and extension occurs at the occiput-C1 articulation (50% of the total). The axis (C2) develops from five ossification centers, with an initial cartilaginous junction between the dens and vertebral body (subdental synchondrosis) that fuses at 7 years of age. The base of the dens narrows because of the transverse ligament. The atlantoaxial articulation is responsible for the majority of neck rotation, with 50% of total rotation occurring at the C1-C2 articulation. The atlantoaxial joint is diarthrodial, which explains why pannus in rheumatoid arthritis can affect this articulation and result in instability (see Chapter 8, Spine). The C2-C7 vertebrae have foramina in each transverse process and bifid spinous processes (except for the C7 nonbifid posterior spinous process [vertebral prominens]). The vertebral artery travels in the transverse foramina of C1-C6. The carotid (Chassaignac) tubercle is found at C6. The diameter of the cervical spine canal is normally 17 mm, and the cervical cord may become compromised when the diameter is reduced to less than 13 mm.
3. Thoracic spine—Unique features include costal facets (present on all 12 vertebral bodies and the transverse processes of T1-T9) and a rounded vertebral foramen. The thoracic vertebrae articulation with the rib cage makes this the most rigid region of the axial skeleton.
4. Lumbar spine—These vertebrae are the largest and are higher anteriorly than posteriorly, significantly contributing to the lumbar lordosis. In most cases, lumbar lordosis ranges from 55-60 degrees with

TABLE 2-34 SPINE VERTEBRAL BODIES

Topographic Landmark	Spinal Level
Mandible	C2-C3
Hyoid cartilage	C3
Thyroid cartilage	C4-C5
Cricoid cartilage	C6
Vertebra prominens	C7
Scapular spine	T3
Distal tip of scapula	T7
Iliac crest	L4-L5

the apex at L3. The majority of cases of lumbar lordosis (66%) are situated in the region from L4 to the sacrum. Lumbar vertebrae contain short laminae and pedicles. They also have mammillary processes (separate ossification centers) that project posteriorly from the superior articular facet. Spondylolysis is a defect in the pars interarticularis and the most common cause of back pain in children and adolescents.

5. Sacrum—In the sacrum there is fusion of five spinal elements. The sacral promontory is the anterosuperior portion that projects into the pelvis. There are usually four pairs of pelvic sacral foramina located both anteriorly and posteriorly that transmit respective ventral and dorsal branches of the upper four sacral nerves. There is also a sacral canal, which opens caudally into the sacral hiatus.
6. Coccyx—In the coccyx there is fusion of the lowest four spinal elements. The coccyx attaches dorsally to the gluteus maximus, the external anal sphincter, and the coccygeal muscles.

B. Arthrology—Spinal ligaments include the anterior and posterior longitudinal ligaments; the ligamentum flavum; and the supraspinous, interspinous, and intertransverse ligaments.

1. General arrangement—The vertebral bodies are bound together by the strong **anterior longitudinal ligament** (ALL) and the weaker **posterior longitudinal ligament** (PLL). The ALL is usually the thickest at the center of the vertebral body and thins at the periphery. Separate fibers extend from one to five levels. The ALL resists hyperextension. The PLL extends from the occiput (tectorial membrane) to the posterior sacrum. It is separated from the center of the vertebral body by a space that allows passage of the dorsal branches of the spinal artery and veins. The PLL is hourglass shaped, with the wider (yet thinner) sections located over the discs. Ruptured discs tend to occur lateral to these expansions. Ligamentous capsules overlying the zygapophyseal joints and the intertransverse ligaments contribute little to interspinous stability. The ligamentum flavum is a strong, yellow, elastic ligament connecting the laminae. It runs from the anterior surface of the superior lamina to the posterior surface of the inferior lamina and is constantly in tension. Hypertrophy of the ligamentum flavum is said to contribute to nerve root compression. The supraspinous and interspinous ligaments lie dorsal to and between the spinous processes, respectively. The supraspinous ligament begins at C7 and is in continuity with the ligamentum nuchae (which runs from C7 to the occiput).
2. Spine stability (Denis)—The three-column system is summarized in Table 2–35.
3. Specialized ligaments
   a. Atlanto-occipital joint—This joint consists of two articular capsules (anterior and posterior) and the tectorial membrane (a cephalad extension of the PLL). It is further stabilized by the ligamentous attachments to the dens.
   b. Atlantoaxial joint—The transverse ligament is the major stabilizer of the median atlantoaxial joint. This articulation is further stabilized by the apical ligament (longitudinal), which together with the transverse axial ligament composes the cruciate ligament. Additionally, a pair of alar ("check") ligaments runs obliquely from the tip of the dens to the occiput (Fig. 2–36). An atlanto–dens interval of greater than 7-10 mm or a posterior space of less than 13 mm is a relative contraindication to elective orthopaedic surgery, and the spine should be stabilized first. Common measurements in C1-C2 disorders are covered in Fig. 8–2.
   c. Iliolumbar ligament—This stout ligament connects the transverse process of L5 with the ilium. Tension on this ligament in patients with unstable vertical shear pelvic fractures can lead to avulsion fractures of the transverse process.
4. Facet (apophyseal) joints—The orientation of the facets of the spine dictates the plane of motion at each relative level. The facet orientation varies with the spinal level and is summarized in Table 2–36. In the cervical spine the superior articular facet is anterior and inferior to the inferior articular process of the vertebra above. The nerve roots exit near the superior articulating process. In the lumbar spine, the superior articular facet is anterior and lateral to the inferior articular facet.

TABLE 2-35 DENIS SPINE COLUMNS

Column	Composition
Anterior	Anterior longitudinal ligament, anterior two thirds of annulus and vertebral body
Middle	Posterior third of body and annulus, posterior longitudinal ligament
Posterior	Pedicles, facets and facet capsules, spinous processes, posterior ligaments that include interspinous and supraspinous ligaments, ligamentum flavum

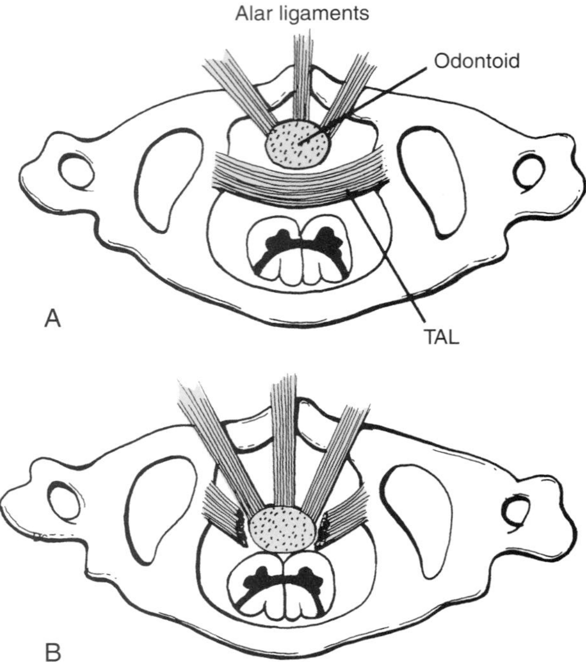

FIGURE 2–36 The atlantoaxial complex as seen from above (**A**). The disruption of the transverse axial ligament (TAL) with intact alar ligaments results in C1-C2 instability without cord compression (**B**). (From DeLee JC, Drez D Jr: Orthopaedic Sports Medicine: Principles and Practices, vol 1, p 432. Philadelphia, WB Saunders, 1994; **B** redrawn from Hensinger RN: Congenital anomalies of the atlantoaxial joint. The Cervical Spine Research Society Editorial Committee. The Cervical Spine, 2nd ed, p 242. Philadelphia, JB Lippincott, 1989.)

5. Intervertebral discs—The intervertebral discs are fibrocartilaginous, with an obliquely oriented annulus fibrosus composed of type I collagen and a softer central nucleus pulposus made of type II collagen. The nucleus pulposus has a high polysaccharide content and is approximately 88% water. Aging results in the loss of water and conversion to fibrocartilage. The discs account for 25% of the total height of the spinal column. They are attached to the vertebral bodies by hyaline cartilage, which is responsible for the vertical growth of the column. Intradisc pressure is position dependent: pressure is the lowest while lying supine and the highest while sitting and flexed forward with weights in the hands.

C. Muscles (Table 2–37)
   1. Neck
      a. Functional classification—For functional purposes, the neck is divided into the anterior and posterior regions.
         (1) Anterior—The anterior neck muscles include the superficial platysma muscle (CN VII innervated), stylohyoid and digastric muscles (CN XII innervated) above the hyoid, and "strap" muscles below the hyoid. Important strap muscles include the sternohyoid and omohyoid in the superficial layer and the thyrohyoid and sternohyoid in the deep layer; all are innervated by the ansa cervicalis (C1-C3). Laterally, the sternocleidomastoid (CN XI and ansa) runs obliquely across the neck, rotating the head to the contralateral side. The anterior triangle (borders: sternocleidomastoid, midline of the neck, and lower border of the mandible) is the largest area. Three smaller triangles include the submandibular; the carotid (bordered by the posterior aspect of the digastric and omohyoid and used for the anterior approach to C5); and the posterior (bordered by the trapezius, sternocleidomastoid, and clavicle).
         (2) Posterior—The posterior neck muscles form the borders of the suboccipital triangle. The superior and inferior heads of the obliquus capitis muscle and the rectus capitis posterior major muscle form this triangle. The vertebral artery and the first cervical nerve are within this triangle, and the greater occipital nerve (C2) is superficial.
      b. Frequently tested relationships—The contents of the carotid sheath include the internal carotid artery, common carotid artery, internal jugular vein, and CN X (vagus).
   2. Back—The back is blanketed by the trapezius (superiorly) and latissimus dorsi (inferiorly). The rhomboids and levator scapulae are deep to this layer. The deep muscles of the back are arranged into two groups: the erector spinae and transversospinalis. The erector spinae run from the

TABLE 2-36 ORIENTATION OF SPINE FACETS

Spinal Level	Orientation of Sagittal Facet	Orientation of Coronal Facet
Cervical	35 degrees at C2, increasing to 55 degrees at C7	Neutral, 0 degrees
Thoracic	60 degrees at T1, increasing to 70 degrees at T12	20 degrees posterior
Lumbar	137 degrees at L1, decreasing to 118 degrees at L5	45 degrees anterior

TABLE 2-37 SPINAL MUSCLE RELATIONSHIPS

Muscle	Relationships
Longus capitis	Anterior to longus colli Posterior to sympathetic chain
Longus colli	Anterior to vertebral artery Posterior to longus capitis

transverse and spinous processes of the inferior vertebrae to the spinous processes of the superior vertebrae. They stabilize and extend the back. All of the deep back musculature is innervated by dorsal primary rami of the spinal nerves.

D. Nerves

1. Spinal cord

a. General anatomy—The cord extends from the brainstem to the inferior border of L1, where it terminates as the conus medullaris. It is enclosed within the bony spinal canal with variable amounts of space (greatest in the upper cervical spine). The cord also varies in diameter (widest at the origin of the plexuses). In cross-section, the cord has both geographic and functional boundaries (Fig. 2–37). It is divided in the midline anteriorly by a fissure and posteriorly by the sulcus.

b. Functional anatomy—The functions of the ascending (sensory) and descending (motor) tracts are summarized in the Table 2–38. The posterior funiculi (dorsal columns) are located dorsally and receive ascending fibers, which deliver deep tactile, proprioceptive, and vibratory sensations. The lateral spinothalamic tract transmits pain and temperature. (It is the site for chordotomy to alleviate intractable pain.) Descending in the lateral corticospinal tract are fibers that transmit instructions for voluntary muscle contraction. Sacral structures are the most peripheral in the lateral corticospinal tracts, with cervical structures more medial. (This is why central cord syndrome affects the upper extremities more than the lower extremities.) The ventral (anterior) spinothalamic tract transmits light tactile sensation, and the ventral (anterior) corticospinal tract delivers cortical messages of voluntary contraction. Deficits associated with patterns of incomplete spinal cord injury are predicted by the anatomy of the ascending and descending tracts. The prognosis with incomplete spinal cord injury is unaffected by the bulbocavernosus reflex. A summary is provided in Table 2–39. The spinal cord tapers at L1 (conus medullaris), and a small filum terminale continues, with the surrounding nerve roots contained within a common dural sac (cauda equina) to its termination in the coccyx. Spinal cord injury at this level may permanently interrupt the bulbocavernosus reflex.

2. Nerve roots (Fig. 2–38)

a. Anatomy—There are 31 pairs of spinal nerves: 8 cervical, 12 thoracic, 5 lumbar, 5 sacral, and 1 coccygeal. Within the subarachnoid space, the dorsal root (and ganglia) and ventral roots converge to form the spinal nerve. The nerve becomes "extradural" as it approaches the intervertebral foramen (the dura becomes epineurium) at all levels above L1. Below this level, the nerves are contained within the cauda equina. After exiting the foramen the spinal nerve delivers dorsal primary rami, which

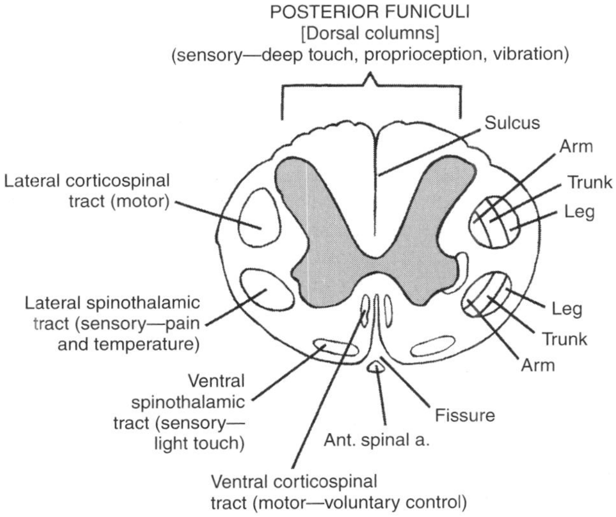

FIGURE 2–37 Cross section of the spinal cord illustrating functions of the ascending and descending tracts. Ascending tracts (sensory): dorsal columns, lateral spinothalamic, and ventral or anterior spinothalamic. Descending tracts (motor): lateral corticospinal and ventral or anterior corticospinal.

TABLE 2-38 SPINAL CORD TRACTS

	Tracts	Function
Ascending (sensory)	Dorsal columns	Deep touch, proprioception, vibratory
	Lateral spinothalamic	Pain and temperature
	Anterior spinothalamic	Light touch
Descending (motor)	Lateral corticospinal	Voluntary motor
	Anterior corticospinal	Voluntary motor

TABLE 2-39 PATTERNS OF INCOMPLETE SPINAL CORD INJURY

Pattern of Injury	Functional Deficit	Recovery
Central (most common)	UE affected more than LE, usually quadriparetic with sacral sparing. Flaccid paralysis of UE and spastic paralysis of LE	75%
Anterior	Complete motor deficit	10% (worst prognosis)
Brown-Séquard	Unilateral cord injury with ipsilateral motor deficit, contralateral pain, and temperature deficit (two levels below injury)	>90% recovery

UE, upper extremity; LE, lower extremity.

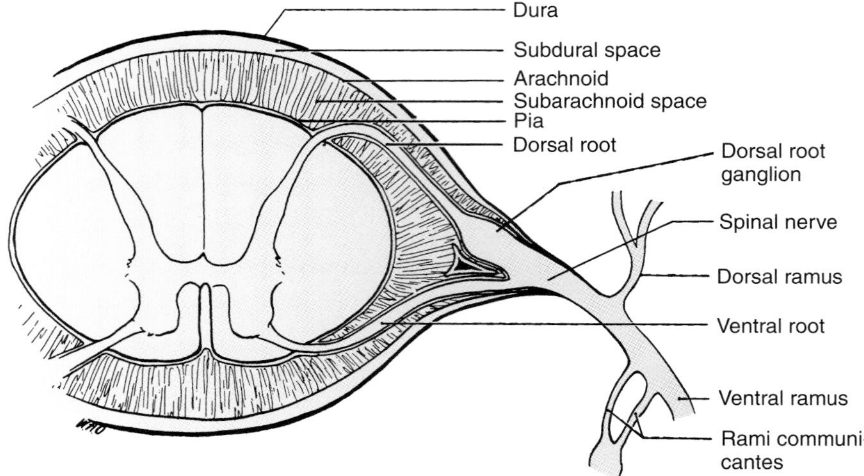

FIGURE 2–38 Spinal nerves. The facet joints are innervated by the medial branch of the dorsal primary ramus and sinovertebral nerve. (From Jenkins DB: Hollinshead's Functional Anatomy of the Limbs and Back, 6th ed, p 205. Philadelphia, WB Saunders, 1991.)

supply the muscles and skin of the neck and back regions. The innervation of structures within the spinal canal, including the periosteum, meninges, vascular structures, and articular connective tissue, is from the sinuvertebral nerve. The ventral rami supply the anteromedial trunk and limbs. With the exception of the thoracic nerves, the ventral rami are grouped in plexuses before delivering sensorimotor functions to a general region. In the cervical spine, the numbered nerve exits at a level above the pedicle of the corresponding vertebral level (e.g., C2 exits at C1-C2). In the lumbar spine, the nerve root traverses the respective disc space above the named vertebral body and exits the respective foramen under the pedicle (Fig. 2–39). Herniated discs usually impinge on the traversing nerve root and facet joint. For example, a disc herniation at L4-L5 would cause compression of the traversing L5 nerve root, resulting in a positive tension sign (straight-leg raise) and diminished strength in the hip abductors and **extensor hallucis longus** (EHL) and pain and numbness in the lateral leg to the dorsum of the foot (Fig. 2–40). A far lateral L4-L5 disc herniation would compress the exiting L4 nerve root, resulting in a positive tension sign (femoral nerve stretch test) and L4 compromise. The L5 nerve root is relatively fixed to the anterior sacral ala and can be damaged by sacral fractures and errant, anteriorly placed iliosacral screws.

b. Key testable neurologic levels (Table 2–40)
c. Nerve root compression—A summary of the findings of nerve root compression is highlighted in Chapter 8, Spine (Tables 8–2 [cervical] and 8–7 [lumbar]). Dermatomes are key testable items (see Fig. 2–40).

3. Sympathetic chain—The cervical sympathetic chain lies posterior and medial to the carotid sheath. It is anterior to the longus capitis muscle. The cervical sympathetic chain has three ganglia: the superior, middle, and inferior (Table 2–41). Disruption of the inferior ganglia can lead to Horner syndrome. There are 11 sympathetic ganglia in the thoracic region, four in the lumbar region, and four in the sacral region.

E. Vessels—Spinal blood supply is usually derived from the segmental arteries located at vertebral midbodies via the aorta (which lies on the left side of the vertebral

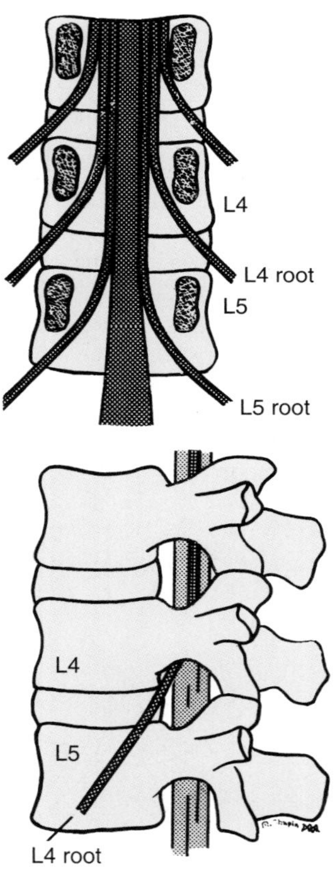

FIGURE 2–39 Locations of the lumbar spine nerve root in relation to vertebral landmarks. Central disc herniation between L4-L5 would compress the traversing root and therefore affect L5. A far lateral disc herniation between L4-L5 would affect the L4 exiting root. In the cervical spine the numbered nerve exists at a level above the pedicle of the corresponding vertebral level. (From Weissman BN, Sledge CB: Orthopedic Radiology, p 283. Philadelphia, WB Saunders, 1986.)

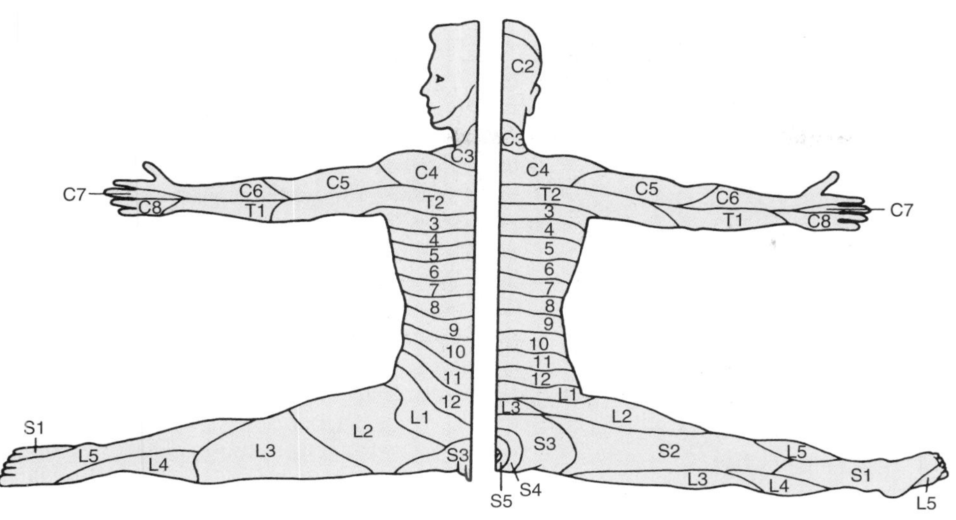

FIGURE 2–40 Dermatomal patterns.

column; the inferior vena cava and azygos vein are on the right). The primary supply to the dura and posterior elements is from the dorsal branches. The ventral branches supply the vertebral bodies via the ascending and descending branches, which are delivered underneath the PLL in four separate ostia. The vertebral artery (a branch of the subclavian) ascends through the transverse foramina of C1-C6 (anterior to and not through C7) posterior to the longus colli muscle and then posterior to the lateral masses, courses along the cephalic surface of the posterior arch of C1 (atlas), and passes ventromedially around the spinal cord and through the foramen magnum before uniting at the midline basilar artery. The distance from the spinous process of C1 laterally to the vertebral artery is 2 cm (a safe distance for dissections would therefore be less than 2 cm). The artery of Adamkiewicz (great anterior medullary artery) enters through the left intervertebral foramen in the lower thoracic spine from T8 to T12. It supplies the interior two thirds of the anterior cord. The arterial supply to the spinal cord is from the anterior and posterior spinal arteries and segmental branches of the vertebral artery and dorsal arteries, which travel via the dorsal and ventral rootlets to the respective dorsal and anterolateral portions of the cord. The venous drainage of the vertebral bodies is primarily through the central sinusoid located on the dorsum of each vertebral body.

F. Surgical approaches to the spine (Table 2–42)
   1. Anterior approach to the cervical spine—A transverse incision is based on the desired level (e.g., for C5, the carotid triangle should be entered). The platysma is retracted with the skin. The pretracheal fascia is exposed to explore the interval between the carotid sheath (which contains the internal and common carotid arteries, the internal jugular vein, and the vagus nerve [CN X]) and the trachea. The prevertebral fascia is sharply incised and the longus colli muscle gently retracted (protecting the recurrent laryngeal nerve [a branch of the vagus nerve that lies outside the sheath]) to expose the vertebral body. There is an increased risk of injury to the recurrent laryngeal nerve with right-sided approaches (paralysis is identified by a hoarse, scratchy voice from unilateral vocal cord paralysis visualized with direct laryngoscopy). The recurrent laryngeal nerve arises from the vagus at the level of the subclavian artery on the right, with the left arising at the level of the aortic arch. Lower-left–sided anterior cervical approaches risk injury to the thoracic duct that is posterior to the carotid sheath. By dissecting the longus muscles subperiosteally, the stellate ganglion is also protected (avoiding Horner syndrome). The anterior surface of the vertebral body is exposed (Fig. 2–41).
   2. Posterior approach to the cervical spine—After a midline approach through the ligamentum

TABLE 2-40 KEY TESTABLE NEUROLOGIC LEVELS

Neurologic Level	Representative Motor	Reflex
C5	Deltoid	Biceps
C6	Wrist extension	Brachioradialis
C7	Wrist flexion	Triceps
C8	Finger flexion	
T1	Interossei	
L4	Tibialis anterior	Patellar
L5	Toe extensors	
S1	Peroneal	Achilles

TABLE 2-41 CERVICAL SYMPATHETIC GANGLIA

Ganglion	Location	Comments
Superior	C2-C3	Largest
Middle	C6	Variable
Inferior	C7-T1	Stellate

TABLE 2-42 SURGICAL APPROACHES TO THE SPINE

Approach	Interval	Structures at Risk
Anterior cervical	Carotid sheath and the trachea	Recurrent laryngeal nerve Sympathetic ganglion
Posterior cervical	Midline approach between paracervical muscle	Vertebral artery
Anterior thoracic	Transverse between ribs two levels above surgical site	Dissect over top of rib to avoid intercostal neurovascular bundle
Posterior thoracolumbar	Midline approach over spinous processes	Posterior primary rami and segmental vessels. Protect nerve root
Anterior lumbar (transperitoneal)	Between segmentally innervated rectus abdominis	Presacral plexus of parasympathetic nerve

nuchae, the superficial (trapezius) and intermediate (splenius, semispinalis, longissimus capitis) layers are reflected laterally and the vertebrae exposed. The vertebral artery is especially vulnerable as it leaves the foramen transversarium and travels superiorly and medially to pierce the atlanto-occipital membrane at its lateral angle. The greater occipital nerve (C2) and the third occipital nerve (C3) should also be protected in the suboccipital region. Access to the spinal canal is via laminectomy or facetectomy.

3. Anterior (transthoracic) approach to the thoracic spine—A transverse incision is made approximately two ribs above the level of interest. Dissection over the top of the rib is carried out to avoid injuring the intercostal neurovascular bundle (which lies on the inferior internal surface of the rib). The rib is further dissected and removed from the field. The right-sided approach is favored in order to avoid the aorta, segmental arteries, artery of Adamkiewicz, and thoracic duct (in the upper thoracic spine on the left side of the esophagus and behind the carotid sheath). The esophagus, aorta, vena cava, and pleura of the lungs should be identified and protected.
4. Posterior approach to the thoracolumbar spine—A straight midline incision is made over the spinous processes and carried down through the thoracolumbar fascia. The plane between the two segmentally innervated erector spinae muscles is used. The paraspinal musculature is subperiosteally dissected from the attached spinous processes, exposing the posterior elements. The structures at risk include the posterior primary rami (near the facet joints) and segmental vessels (anterior to the plane connecting the transverse processes). Partial laminectomy allows greater exposure of the cord and discs. Pedicle screws are placed at the junction of the lateral border of the superior facet and the middle of the transverse process. These screws should be angled 15 degrees medially and in line with the slope of the vertebra, as seen on lateral radiographs.
5. Anterior approach to the lumbar spine (transperitoneal)—In this approach, a longitudinal incision is made from below the umbilicus to just above the pubic symphysis. The rectus abdominis muscles are split and the peritoneum is incised. Protect and retract the bladder distally and bowel cephalad and incise the posterior peritoneum longitudinally over the sacral promontory. The aortic bifurcation is revealed and the middle sacral artery ligated. Expose the L5-S1 disc space. Injury to the lumbar plexus, particularly the superior hypogastric plexus of the sympathetic plexus that lies over the L5 vertebral body, can cause sexual dysfunction and retrograde ejaculation. (Ejaculation is predominantly a sympathetic nervous system function and erection predominantly a parasympathetic nervous system function.)
6. Anterolateral approach to the lumbar spine (retroperitoneal)—This approach provides access from L1 to the sacrum. An oblique incision is centered over the 12th rib to the lateral border of the rectus abdominis muscle. The external oblique, internal oblique, and transversus abdominis

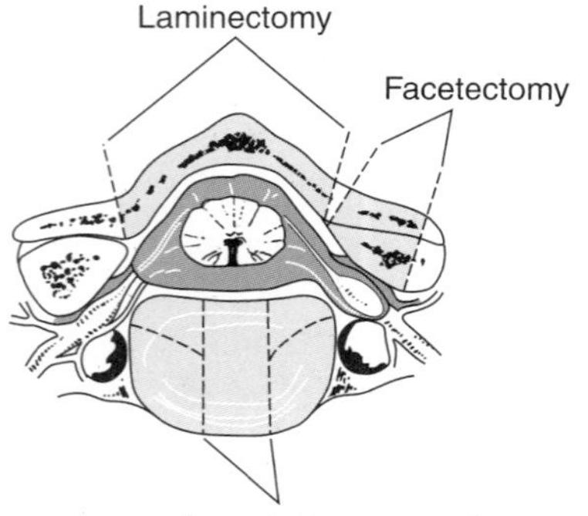

FIGURE 2–41 Surgical procedures on the cervical spine. (From Rothman RH, Simeon FA: The Spine, 2nd ed, p 484. Philadelphia, WB Saunders, 1982.)

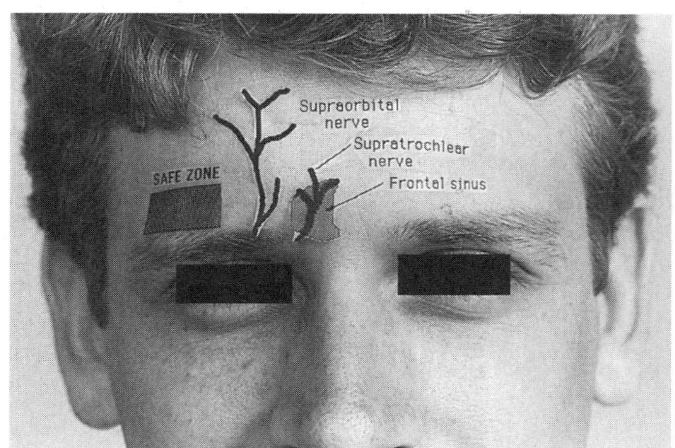

FIGURE 2–42 Safe placement of halo pins. The safe zone for halo pin placement is highlighted. From lateral to medial are the supraorbital nerve and the supratrochlear nerve, which overlies the frontal sinus.

muscles are incised in line with the skin incision. The retroperitoneal fat is elevated, revealing the psoas major muscle and genitofemoral nerve. The segmental lumbar vessels are ligated, and the aorta and vena cava are mobilized to expose the desired vertebral level. Protect the sympathetic chain (medial to the psoas and lateral to the vertebral body) and ureters (between the peritoneum and psoas fascia).

7. Anatomy important to placement of halo pins—The optimum position for the placement of anterolateral halo pins is approximately 1 cm superior to the orbital rim in the outer two thirds of the orbit below the equator of the skull (Fig. 2–42). With this pin position, the temporal fossa and temporalis muscle will be situated laterally and the supraorbital nerve, supratrochlear nerve, and frontal sinus medially. The supraorbital nerve is lateral to the supratrochlear nerve, which lies anterior to the frontal sinus. The most commonly injured cranial nerve with halo traction is the abdu-cens (CN VI), which is identified by the loss of lateral gaze.

SECTION 4 Lower Extremity and Pelvis

Table 2–43 summarizes lower extremity neurology. Table 2–44 summarizes lower extremity innervation. Table 2–45 summarizes standard surgical approaches to the lower extremity.

I. Pelvis and Hip

A. Osteology—The pelvic girdle is composed of two innominate (coxal) bones that articulate with the sacrum. Each innominate bone is composed of three united bones: the ilium, ischium, and pubis. The ilium has two important anterior prominences: the **anterior superior iliac spine** (ASIS) and **anterior inferior iliac spine** (AIIS). The ASIS is palpable at the lateral edge of the inguinal ligament. It is the origin of the sartorius muscle and the transverse and internal abdominal muscles. The AIIS is less prominent and provides the origin of the direct head of the rectus femoris and the iliofemoral ligament (Y ligament of Bigelow). The ilium also has a **posterior superior iliac spine** (PSIS), which is usually located 4-5 cm lateral to the S2 spinous process. The greater sciatic notch is located posterior and superior to the acetabulum. The iliopectineal eminence is an anteriorly raised region that represents the union of the ilium and pubis. The iliopsoas muscle traverses a groove between this eminence and the AIIS. The acetabulum is anteverted (15 degrees) and obliquely oriented (45 degrees caudally). The posterosuperior articular surface is thickened to accommodate weight bearing. The inferior surface is deficient and contains the acetabular, or cotyloid, notch bound by the transverse acetabular ligament. The proximal femur is composed of the femoral head, neck, and greater and lesser trochanters. The femoral neck is anteverted approximately 14 degrees in relation to the femoral condyles. The angle of the femoral neck shaft averages 127 degrees. The hip trabecular architecture is illustrated in Figure 2–43.

B. Arthrology

1. Hip—The hip joint is a spheroidal, ball-and-socket type of diarthrodial joint. Its stability is based primarily on the bony architecture. The acetabulum is deepened by the fibrocartilaginous labrum. The joint capsule extends anteriorly across the femoral neck to the trochanteric crest; however, it extends posteriorly only partially across the femoral neck, leaving the basocervical and intertrochanteric crest regions extracapsular (Fig. 2–44). Three ligaments compose the capsule anteriorly. The iliofemoral ligament (Y ligament of Bigelow) is the strongest ligament in the body and attaches the AIIS to the

TABLE 2-43 SUMMARY OF IMPORTANT LOWER EXTREMITY NEUROLOGY

Joint	Function	Neurologic Level
Hip	Flexion	T12-L3
	Extension	S1
	Adduction	L2-L4
	Abduction	L5
Knee	Flexion	L5,S1
	Extension	L2-L4
Ankle	Dorsiflexion	L4,L5
	Plantar flexion	S1,S2
	Inversion	L4
	Eversion	S1

TABLE 2-44 SUMMARY OF LOWER EXTREMITY INNERVATION

Nerves	Muscles Innervated
Femoral	Iliacus, psoas, quadriceps femoris (rectus femoris and the vastus lateralis, intermedius, and medialis)
Obturator	Adductor brevis, longus, and magnus (along with tibial nerve), gracilis
Superior gluteal	Gluteus medius and minimus, tensor fascia lata
Inferior gluteal	Gluteus maximus
Sciatic	Semitendinosus, semimembranosus, biceps femoris (long head [tibial division] and short head [peroneal division]), adductor magnus (with obturator nerve)
Tibial	Gastrocnemius, soleus, tibialis posterior, flexor digitorum longus, flexor hallucis longus, medial and lateral plantar nerve
Deep peroneal	Tibialis anterior, extensor digitorum longus, extensor hallucis longus, tibialis posterior, extensor digitorum brevis
Superficial peroneal	Peroneus longus and brevis

TABLE 2-45 SUMMARY OF STANDARD LOWER EXTREMITY ORTHOPAEDIC SURGICAL APPROACHES

Region	Approach	Eponym	Muscular Interval 1 (Nerve)	Muscular Interval 2 (Nerve)	Structures at Risk
Iliac crest	Posterior		Gluteus maximus (inferior gluteal)	Latissimus dorsi (thoracodorsal)	Clunial n, SGA, sciatic n
	Anterior		TFL/gluteus medius and minimus (superior gluteal)	External abdominal oblique (segmental)	ASIS/LFCN
Hip	Anterior	Smith-Peterson	Sartorius/rectus femoris (femoral)	TFL/gluteus medius (superior gluteal)	LFCN, femoral n, ascending. Branch of LFCA
	Anterolateral	Watson-Jones	Tensor fasciae latae (superior gluteal)	Gluteus medius (superior gluteal)	Femoral NAV/profunda a
	Lateral	Hardinge	Splits gluteus medius (superior gluteal)	Splits vastus lateralis (femoral)	Femoral NVA/LFCA (transverse branch)
	Posterior	Moore-Southern	Splits gluteus maximus (inferior gluteal)	N/A	Sciatic, inferior gluteal a
	Medial	Ludloff	Adductor longus/adductor brevis (anterior division of obturator)	Gracilis/adductor magnus (obturator/tibial)	Anterior division of obturator n/MFCA
Thigh	Lateral		Vastus lateralis (femoral)	Vastus lateralis (femoral)	Perforating branch of profundus a
	Posterolateral		Vastus lateralis (femoral)	Hamstrings (sciatic)	Perforating branch of profundus a
	Anteromedial		Rectus femoris (femoral)	Vastus medialis (femoral)	Medial superior geniculate a
Distal femur	Posterior		Biceps femoris (sciatic)	Vastus lateralis (femoral)	Sciatic n/PFCN
Knee	Medial parapatellar		Vastus medialis (femoral)	Rectus femoris (femoral)	Infrapatellar branch of saphenous n
	Medial		Vastus medialis (femoral)	Sartorius (femoral)	Infrapatellar branch of saphenous n
	Lateral		Iliotibial band (superior gluteal)	Biceps femoris (sciatic)	Peroneal n/popliteus ten.
	Posterior		Semimembranosus/lateral gastrocnemius (tibial)	Biceps/lateral gastrocnemius (tibia)/(tibia)	Medial sural cutaneous n/ tibial n/peroneal n
	Lateral		Vastus lateralis (femoral)	Biceps femoris (sciatic)	Peroneal n/lateral superior geniculate a
Tibia	Posterolateral		GS, soleus, FHL (tibial)	Peroneus brevis/longus (superior peroneal)	Lesser saphenous v/posterior tibial a
	Anterior		Tibialis anterior (peroneal)	Periosteum	Long saphenous v
Ankle	Anterior		EHL (deep peroneal)	EDL (deep peroneal)	S and D peroneal n/anterior tibial a
Medial malleolus	Posterior		Tibialis posterior	FDL	Saphenous n and v
Ankle	Posterolateral		Peroneus brevis (superior peroneal)	FHL (tibial)	Sural n/small saphenous v
Distal fibula	Lateral		Peroneus tertius (deep peroneal)	Peroneus brevis (superior peroneal)	Sural n
Foot	Anterolateral		Peroneal muscles (superior peroneal)	ED and peroneus tertius (deep peroneal)	Deep peroneal n/anterior tibial a
	Posteromedial		TP or FDL	FDL or FHL	Posterior tibial a/tibial n

a, artery; ASIS, anterior superior iliac spine; D, decreased; ED, extensor digitorum; EDL, extensor digitorum longus; EHL, extensor hallucis longus; FDL, flexor digitorum longus; FHL, flexor hallucis longus; GS, gastrocnemius soleus; LFCA, lateral femoral circumflex artery; LFCN, lateral femoral cutaneous nerve; MFCA, medial femoral circumflex artery; n, nerve; N/A, not applicable; PFCN, posterior femoral cutaneous nerve; S, superficial; SGA, superior gluteal artery; TFL, tensor fascia lata; TP, tibialis posterior; V, vein.

intertrochanteric line in an inverted Y fashion. The remaining anterior ligaments, the ischiofemoral and pubofemoral ligaments, are weaker but lend additional stability. Inside the joint, the ligamentum teres arises from the apex of the cotyloid notch and attaches to the fovea of the femoral head. It transmits an arterial branch of the posterior division of the obturator artery to the femoral head (less significant in adults). The blood supply to the femoral head changes with age; the key points are highlighted in Table 2–46, which helps explain why the standard starting point for antegrade femoral nailing is undesirable for pediatric femur fractures. Using the piriformis starting point would damage the posterosuperior retinacular vessels, causing avascular necrosis of the femoral head. Moreover, in adults, completely transecting the quadratus femoris muscle in the posterior acetabular approach should be avoided in order to avert damage to the main blood supply to the femoral head–medial femoral circumflex artery.

2. Sacroiliac joint—This structure is a true diarthrodial, gliding joint supported by three groups of ligaments: posterior and anterior sacroiliac ligaments and interosseous ligaments.
3. Symphysis pubis—The symphysis pubis connects the two hemipelvises anteriorly and is united with a fibrocartilaginous disc and supported by the superior and arcuate pubic ligaments.

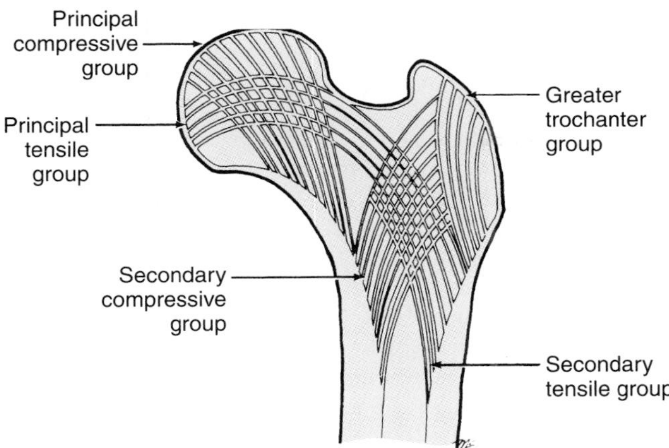

FIGURE 2–43 Hip trabeculae. Trabecular patterns help determine the presence of osteopenia (Singh index). If all trabecular groups are visualized, a Singh grade VI is established (normal). In addition, the difference between Garden types III and IV displaced femoral neck fractures is determined by the alignment of trabecular patterns of the femoral head and acetabulum. Alignment occurs in type IV because the femoral head assumes a normal position in the acetabulum. (From DeLee JC: Fractures and dislocations of the hip. In Rockwood CA Jr, Green DP, Buchholz RW, eds: Fractures in Adults, 3rd ed, p 1488. Philadelphia, JB Lippincott, 1991.)

4. Other ligaments—These include the sacrospinous and sacrotuberous ligaments, which outline the boundaries for the greater and lesser sciatic foramina. The sacrospinous ligament (anterior sacrum of the ischial spine) constitutes the inferior border of the greater sciatic foramen and the superior border of the lesser sciatic foramen. The lesser sciatic foramen is bordered inferiorly by the sacrotuberous ligament (anterior sacrum of the ischial tuberosity). The piriformis, sciatic nerve, and other important structures exit the greater sciatic foramen. The short external rotators of the hip exit the lesser sciatic foramen.

C. Muscles (Table 2–47; Fig. 2–45)—The principal hip flexor muscles are the iliopsoas, rectus femoris, and sartorius. The hip extensor muscles are the gluteus maximus and hamstrings (semitendinosus, semimembranosus, and long head of biceps femoris). Hip abduction results primarily from the actions of the gluteus medius and minimus. The tensor fasciae latae also helps with abduction in a flexed hip. Hip adduction results primarily from the actions of the adductor brevis, longus, and magnus, the pectineus, and the gracilis. Hip external rotation results from the action of the obturator internus, obturator externus, superior and inferior gemellus, quadratus femoris, and piriformis. Hip internal rotation is provided by secondary actions of the anterior fibers of the gluteus medius and minimus and by the tensor fasciae latae, semimembranosus, semitendinosus, pectineus, and posterior part of the adductor magnus.

D. Nerves (see Table 2–44)
   1. Lumbosacral plexus (Fig. 2–46; Table 2–48)—The lumbosacral plexus is composed of ventral rami from T12-S3 and lies posterior to the psoas muscle. The sciatic nerve (L4-S3) has an anterior preaxial tibial nerve division and a postaxial peroneal nerve division. The spatial orientation of the sciatic nerve also places the peroneal division more lateral than the tibial division. This orientation makes it more vulnerable to injury at the time of surgery. For example, the most common neural injury at the time of primary total hip arthroplasty is the peroneal division of the sciatic nerve. The only muscle innervated by the peroneal division of the sciatic nerve above the level of the fibular neck is the short head of the biceps femoris. The peroneal division of the sciatic nerve runs on the deep surface of the long head of the biceps femoris.
   2. Anatomic spatial relationships
      a. The lumbar plexus is found on the anterior surface of the quadratus lumborum under (and within) the substance of the psoas major muscle.
      b. The genitofemoral nerve pierces the psoas and then lies on the anteromedial surface of the psoas.
      c. The femoral nerve lies between the iliacus and psoas muscles.
      d. The lateral femoral cutaneous nerve lies on the surface of the iliacus muscle and exits the pelvis under the lateral attachment of the inguinal ligament.

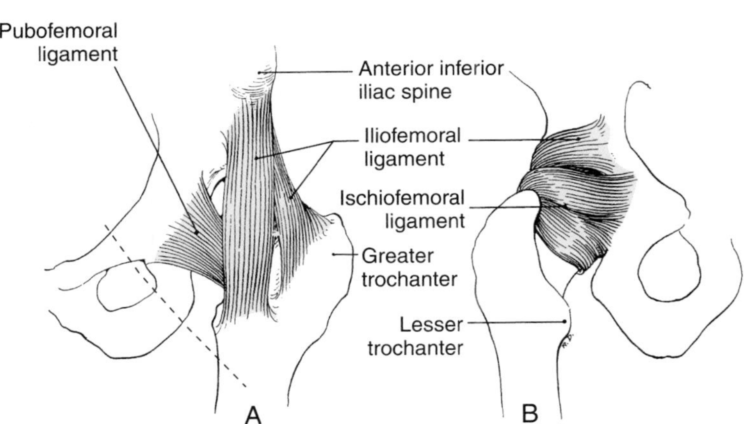

FIGURE 2–44 Hip capsuloligamentous structures. **A**, Anterior view. The anterior femoral neck is intracapsular. **B**, Posterior view. Because the posterior capsule extends only partially across the femoral neck, the posterior basicervical and intertrochanteric crest regions are extracapsular. (From Jenkins DB: Hollinshead's Functional Anatomy of the Limbs and Back, 6th ed, p 230. Philadelphia, WB Saunders, 1991.)

TABLE 2-46 AGE-DEPENDENT CHANGES TO FEMORAL HEAD BLOOD SUPPLY

Age	Blood Supply
Birth to 4 yr	Primary medial and lateral circumflex arteries (from deep femoral artery)
	Ligamentum teres with posterior division of obturator artery
4 yr to adult	Negligible lateral circumflex artery
	Minimum ligamentum teres
	Posterosuperior and posteroinferior retinacular from medial femoral circumflex artery
Adult	Medial femoral circumflex to lateral epiphyseal artery

e. Virtually all the important nerves about the hip leave the pelvis by way of the sciatic foramen.

f. The major reference point for the greater sciatic nerve and related structures in the hip is the piriformis muscle (the "key" to the sciatic foramen). The superior gluteal nerve and artery lie above the piriformis, and virtually everything else leaves below the muscle (remember POP'S IQ [lateral to the medial nerves]: **p**udendal, **o**bturator internus, **p**ostfemoral cutaneous, **s**ciatic, **i**nferior gluteal, **q**uadratus femoris).

g. Two nerves leave the greater sciatic foramen and re-enter the pelvis via the lesser foramen: the pudendal nerve and the nerve to the obturator internus.

h. Anteriorly, the great nerves and vessels enter the thigh (and into the femoral triangle) under the inguinal ligament (Fig. 2–47). The borders of this triangle include the sartorius laterally, the pectineus medially, and the inguinal ligament superiorly. Within the triangle, from a lateral to medial direction, are the femoral **n**erve, **a**rtery, and **v**ein and the **l**ymphatic vessels (remember NAVAL). The floor of the femoral triangle (again from a lateral to medial direction) is made up of the iliacus, psoas, pectineus, and adductor longus.

i. The femoral nerve descends between the iliacus and psoas and delivers numerous branches to muscle, overlying skin, and the hip joint (in accordance with the Hilton law). A spontaneous iliacus hematoma may irritate the femoral nerve due to its proximity. In addition, hip pain can also present as a result of Pott's

TABLE 2-47 MUSCLES OF THE PELVIS AND HIP

Muscle	Origin	Insertion	Nerve	Segment
Flexors				
Iliacus	Iliac fossa	Lesser trochanter	Femoral	L2-L4 (P)
Psoas	Transverse processes of L1-L5	Lesser trochanter	Femoral	L2-L4 (P)
Pectineus	Pectineal line of pubis	Pectineal line of femur	Femoral	L2-L4 (P)
Rectus femoris	Anterior inferior iliac spine, acetabular rim	Patella and tibial tubercle	Femoral	L2-L4 (P)
Sartorius	Anterior superior iliac spine	Proximal medial tibia	Femoral	L2-L4 (P)
Adductors				
Posterior adductor magnus	Inferior pubic ramus/ischial tuberosity	Linea aspera/adductor tubercle	Obturator (P) and sciatic (tibial)	L2-L4 (A)
Adductor brevis	Inferior pubic ramus	Linea aspera/pectineal line	Obturator (P)	L2-L4 (A)
Adductor longus	Anterior pubic ramus	Linea aspera	Obturator (A)	L2-L4 (A)
Gracilis	Inferior symphysis/pubic arch	Proximal medial tibia	Obturator (A)	L2-L4 (A)
External Rotators				
Gluteus maximus	Ilium, posterior gluteal line	Iliotibial band/gluteal sling (femur)	Inferior gluteal	L5-S2 (P)
Piriformis	Anterior sacrum/sciatic notch	Proximal greater trochanter	Piriformis	S12 (P)
Obturator externus	Ischiopubic rami/obturator	Trochlear fossa	Obturator	L2-L4 (A)
Obturator internus	Ischiopubic rami/obturator membrane	Medial greater trochanter (MGT)	Obturator internus	L5-S2 (A)
Superior gemellus	Outer ischial spine	MGT	Obturator internus	L5-S2 (A)
Inferior gemellus	Ischial tuberosity	MGT	Obturator femoris	L4-S1 (A)
Quadratus femoris	Ischial tuberosity	Quadrate line of femur	Obturator femoris	L4-S1 (A)
Abductors				
Gluteus medius	Ilium between posterior and anterior gluteal lines	Greater trochanter	Superior gluteal	L4-S1 (P)
Gluteus minimus	Ilium between anterior and inferior gluteal lines	Anterior border of greater trochanter	Superior gluteal	L4-S1 (P)
Tensor fasciae latae (tensor fasciae femoris)	Anterior iliac crest	Iliotibial band	Superior gluteal	L4-S1 (P)

A, anterior; P, posterior.

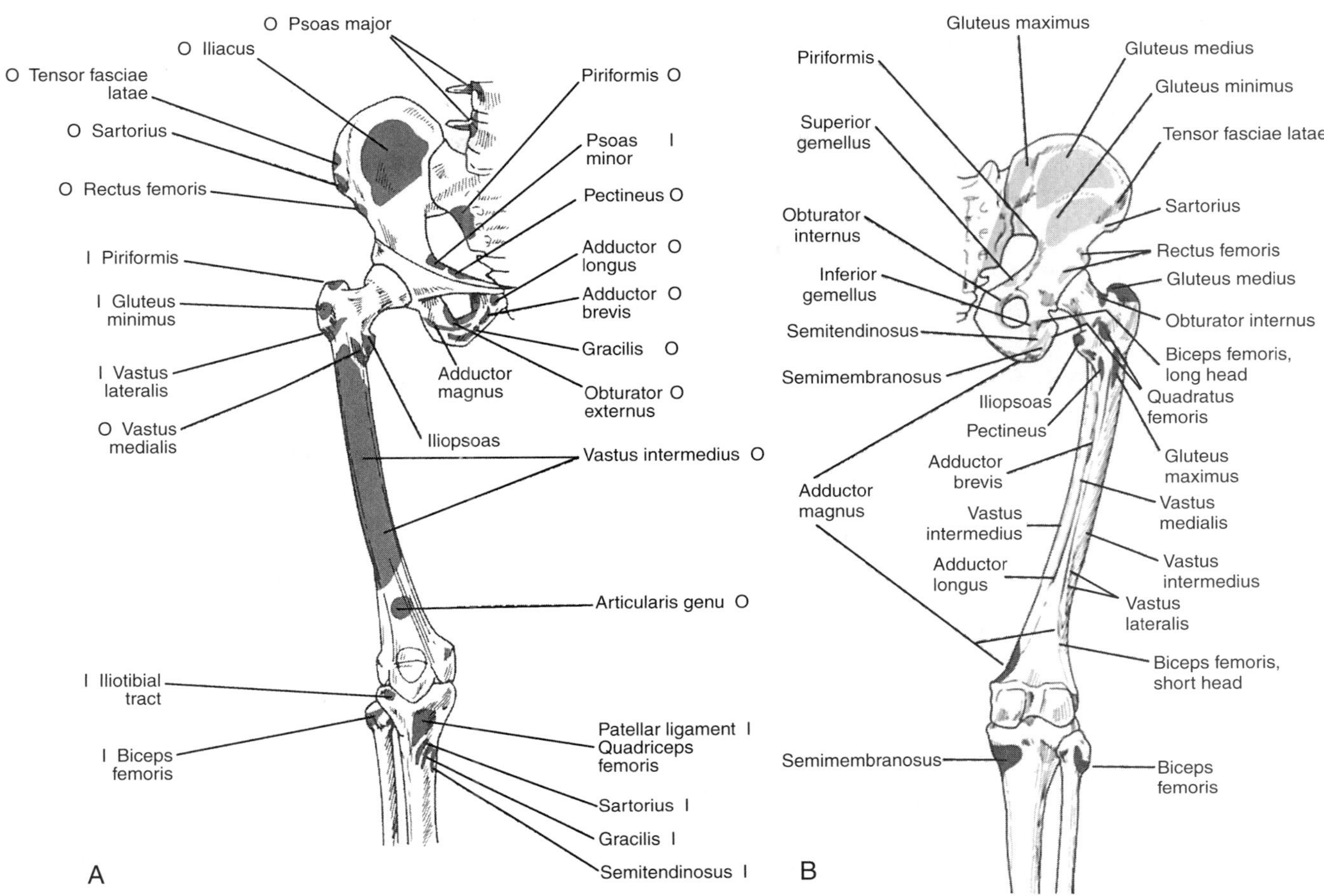

FIGURE 2–45 Origins and insertions of muscles of the hip and leg. **A**, Anterior view. **B**, Posterior view. O, origin (light areas). I, insertion (dark areas). (Adapted from Jenkins DB: Hollinshead's Functional Anatomy of the Limbs and Back, 6th ed, Figs. 16-7 and 17-3. Philadelphia, WB Saunders, 1991.)

disease (tuberculous spondylitis) of the spine because of the attachment of the iliopsoas to the lumbar spine.

j. At the apex of the femoral triangle, the saphenous nerve branches off and travels under the sartorius muscle.

k. The obturator nerve exits the pelvis via the obturator canal. It splits into anterior and posterior divisions within the canal. The anterior division proceeds anteriorly to the obturator externus and posteriorly to the pectineus, supplying the adductor longus and brevis and the gracilis; it then delivers cutaneous branches to the medial thigh. The posterior division supplies the obturator externus, adductor brevis, and upper part of the adductor magnus, and it delivers other branches to the knee joint. Referred pain from the hip to the knee can result from the continuation of the obturator nerve anteriorly, which can provide sensation to the medial side of the knee. Retractors placed behind the transverse acetabular ligament can injure the obturator nerve and artery.

E. Vessels (Fig. 2–48)

1. The aorta branches into the common iliac arteries anterior to the L4 vertebral body.
2. The common iliac vessels in turn divide into the internal (or hypogastric [medial]) and external (lateral) iliac vessels at the S1 level.
3. Important internal iliac artery branches include the obturator (the posterior branch supplies the transverse acetabular ligament), superior gluteal (can be injured in the sciatic notch), inferior gluteal (supplies the gluteus maximus and the short external rotators), and internal pudendal (re-enters the pelvis through the lesser sciatic notch) (Fig. 2–49). Anteroinferior screws and acetabular retractors jeopardize the obturator artery and vein.
4. The external iliac artery continues under the inguinal ligament to become the femoral artery. It can be injured by the placement of acetabular screws in the anterosuperior quadrant during total hip arthroplasty. A summary of the key issues for acetabular screw placement is shown in Table 2–49 (see Fig. 5–13).
5. The femoral artery enters the femoral triangle and delivers the profunda femoris, which supplies the anteromedial portion of the thigh and the perforators; these perforators pierce the lateral intermuscular septum to supply the vastus lateralis muscle. The profunda has two other important branches: the lateral and medial femoral circumflex arteries.

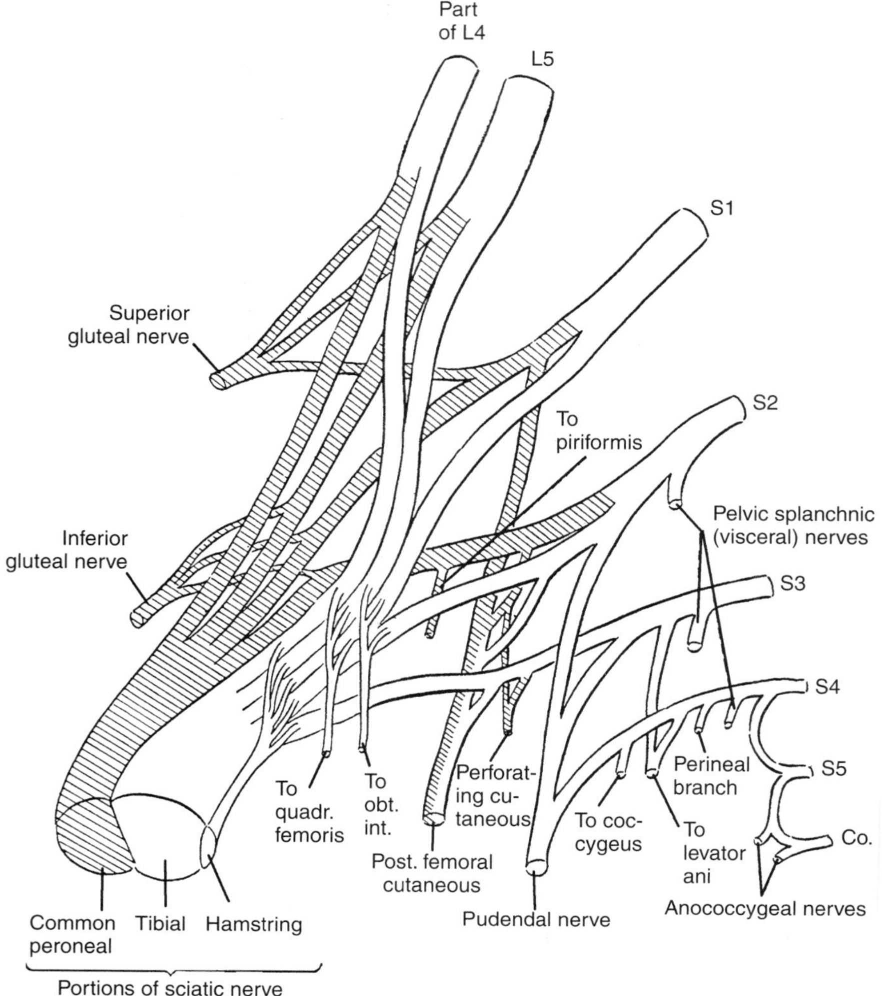

FIGURE 2–46 Sacral plexus. The anterior division is unshaded and the posterior division shaded. (From Jenkins DB: Hollinshead's Functional Anatomy of the Limbs and Back, 6th ed, p 256. Philadelphia, WB Saunders, 1991.)

TABLE 2–48 LUMBOSACRAL PLEXUS DIVISIONS AND INNERVATIONS

Nerve	Level	Muscles Innervated
Anterior Division		
Tibia	L4-S3	Semimembranosus/semitendinosus/biceps (long head)/adductor magnus/superior gemellus/soleus/ plantaris/popliteus/tibialis posterior/flexor digitorum longus/flexor hallucis longus
Quadratus femoris	L4-S1	Quadratus femoris/inferior gemellus
Obturator internus	L5-S2	Obturatorius internus/superior gemellus
Pudendal	S2-S4	Sensory: perineal Motor: bulbocavernosus/urethra/urogenital diaphragm
Coccygeus	S4	Coccygeus
Levator ani	S3-S4	Levator ani
Posterior Division		
Peroneal	L4-S2	Biceps (short head)/tibialis anterior/extensor digitorum longus/peroneus tertius/extensor hallucis longus Peroneus longus and brevis/extensor hallucis brevis/extensor digitorum brevis
Superior gluteal	L4-S1	Gluteus medius and minimus/tensor fascia lata
Inferior gluteal	L5-S2	Gluteus maximus
Piriformis	S2	Piriformis
Posterior femoral cutaneous	S1-S3	Sensory: posterior thigh

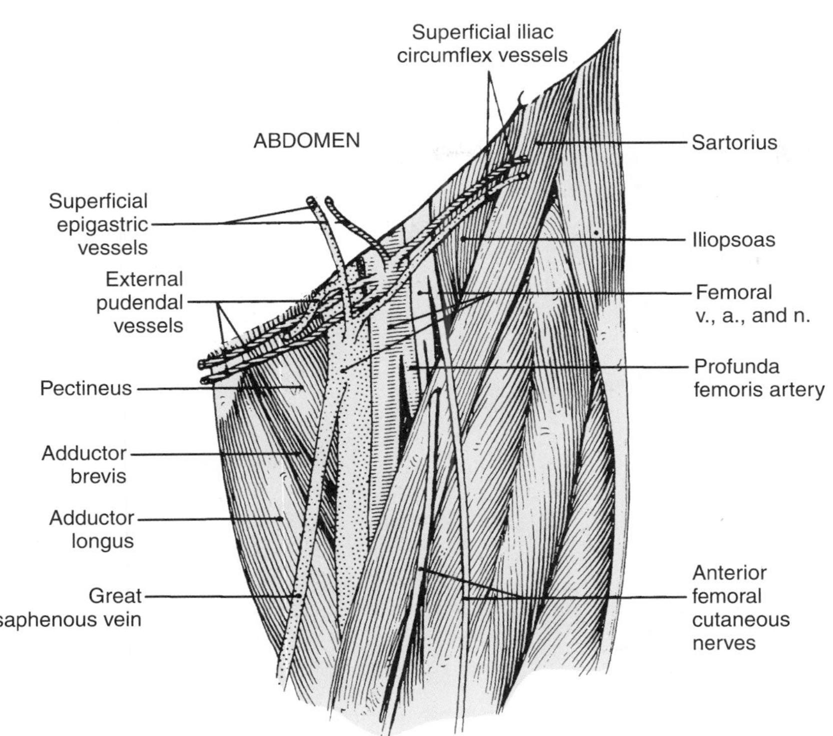

FIGURE 2–47 Femoral triangle. The order of structures of the femoral canal from lateral to medial: iliopsoas/iliacus, femoral nerve, femoral artery, femoral vein, and pectineus. (From Jenkins DB: Hollinshead's Functional Anatomy of the Limbs and Back, 6th ed, p 243. Philadelphia, WB Saunders, 1991.)

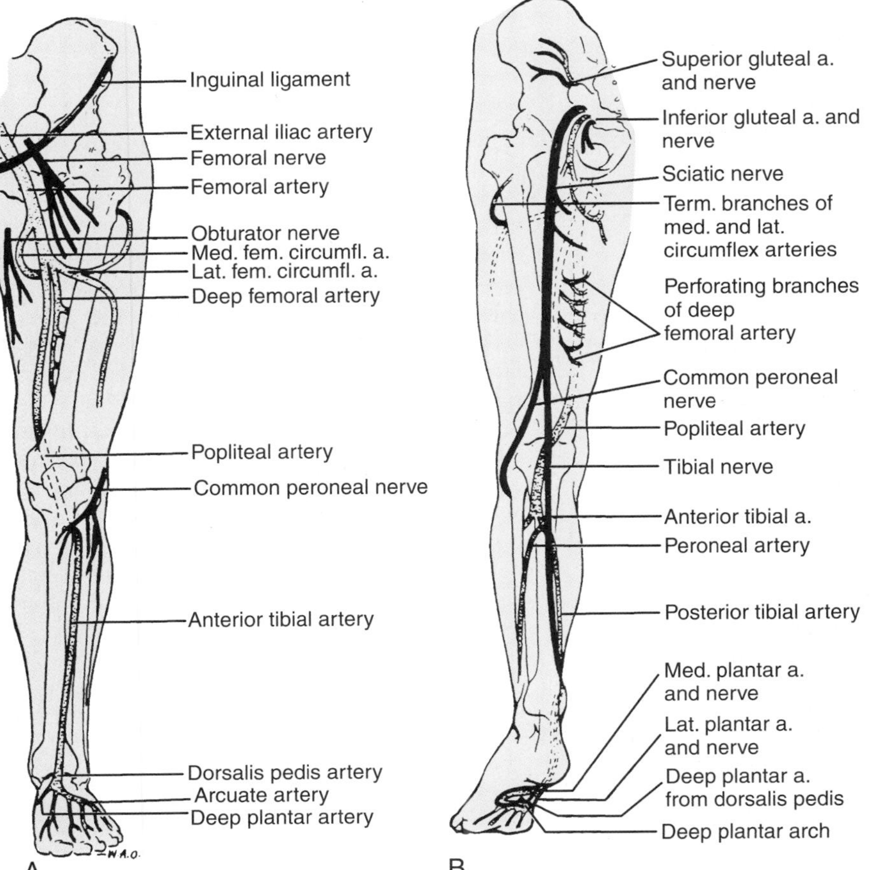

FIGURE 2–48 Nerves and vessels of the lower extremity. **A**, Anterior view. **B**, Posterior view. (From Jenkins DB: Hollinshead's Functional Anatomy of the Limbs and Back, 6th ed, p 221. Philadelphia, WB Saunders, 1991.)

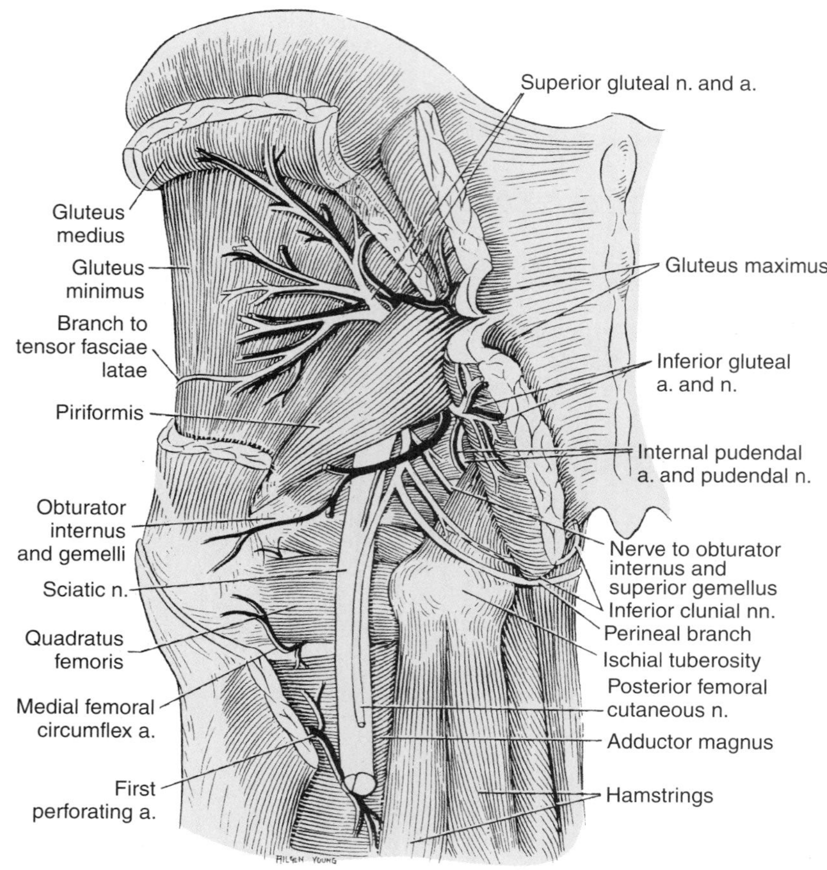

FIGURE 2–49 Posterior hip anatomy. Note relationship of structures to the piriformis muscle. (From Jenkins DB: Hollinshead's Functional Anatomy of the Limbs and Back, 6th ed, p 260. Philadelphia, WB Saunders, 1991.)

a. The lateral femoral circumflex travels obliquely and deep to the sartorius and rectus femoris. It delivers an ascending branch (at risk during anterolateral approaches) that proceeds to the greater trochanteric region and a descending branch that travels laterally under the rectus femoris.
b. The medial femoral circumflex, which supplies most of the blood to the femoral head, runs between the pectineus and iliopsoas, then in the interval between the obturator externus and adductor brevis muscles, and finally in the interval between the adductor magnus and brevis. It proceeds distally anterior to the quadratus femoris on its cranial edge just distal to the obturator externus.

TABLE 2-49 ACETABULAR SCREW PLACEMENT ZONES

Acetabular Zone	Structures at Risk
Posterior superior	None (safe zone)
Posterior inferior	None (safe zone)
Anterior superior	External iliac artery and vein
Anterior inferior	Anterior inferior obturator nerve, obturator artery and vein

6. The cruciate anastomosis is the confluence of the ascending branch of the first perforating artery, the descending branch of the inferior gluteal artery, and the transverse branches of the medial and lateral femoral circumflex arteries. It lies at the inferior margin of the quadratus femoris muscle.
7. The superficial femoral artery continues on the medial side of the thigh (between the vastus medialis and adductor longus) toward the adductor (Hunter) canal. It becomes the popliteal artery in the popliteal fossa in the posteromedial thigh.

F. Surgical approaches to the pelvis and hip (Table 2–50)
1. Posterior approach to the iliac crest—A curvilinear incision is made just inferior to the crest, beginning at the PSIS. After the iliac crest is identified, the gluteus maximus fibers are subperiosteally dissected from the outer table. The risks of this approach include injury to the greater sciatic notch (superior gluteal artery and sciatic nerve) and the cluneal nerves (8 cm anterolateral to the PSIS).
2. Anterior approach to the iliac crest—An oblique incision is made lateral to the ASIS, and the crest is exposed through the interval between the external oblique and the gluteus medius. There are risks to the greater sciatic notch, the inguinal ligament, and the lateral femoral cutaneous nerve.
3. Anterior (Smith-Peterson) approach to the hip (Fig. 2–50)—This approach takes advantage of the interneural plane between the sartorius (femoral nerve)

TABLE 2-50 HIP SURGICAL APPROACHES

Approach	Interval	Structures at Risk
Anterior (Smith-Peterson)	Sartorius/rectus femoris (femoral nerve) and tensor fasciae latae/ gluteus medius (superior gluteal nerve)	Lateral femoral cutaneous nerve (6-8 cm below anterior inferior iliac spine anterior or medial to sartorius) Ligation of ascending branch of lateral femoral circumflex artery (lies superficial to rectus femoris muscle)
Anterolateral (Watson-Jones)	Between tensor fasciae latae (supinator gluteal nerve) and gluteal branch of medius (supinator gluteal nerve)	Femoral nerve because of excessive medial retraction Injury to descending lateral femoral circumflex artery
Lateral (Hardinge)	Gluteus medius (supinator gluteal nerve) and vastus lateralis (femoral nerve)	Femoral nerve, artery, vein Lateral femoral circumflex artery
Posterior (Moore-Southern)	Gluteus maximus (inferior gluteal nerve) and gluteus medius/tensor fasciae latae (supinator gluteal nerve)	Sciatic nerve and inferior gluteal artery during the gluteus maximus muscle split If quadratus femoris transected, ligation of medial femoral circumflex artery
Medial (Ludloff)	Adductor longus and adductor brevis (obturator nerve) and gracilis/adductor magnus (obturator/tibial nerve)	Anterior division of obturator nerve Medial femoral circumflex artery Deep external pudendal artery

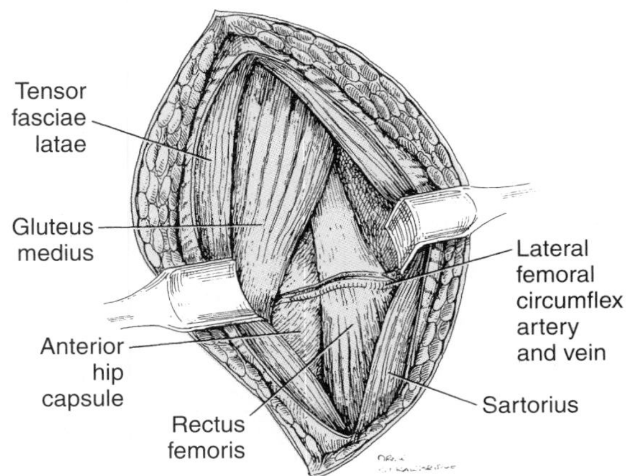

FIGURE 2–50 Anterior (Smith-Peterson) approach to the hip. The interval between the sartorius/rectus femoris (femoral nerve) and the tensor fasciae latae/gluteus medius (superior gluteal nerve) is explored. The ascending branch of the lateral femoral circumflex artery is ligated. (From Steinberg ME: The Hip and Its Disorders, p 92. Philadelphia, WB Saunders, 1991.)

and tensor fasciae latae (superior gluteal nerve). It is useful for operative procedures such as hemiarthroplasty and open reduction of the congenitally dislocated hip. The lateral femoral cutaneous nerve is retracted anteriorly, and the ascending branch of the lateral femoral circumflex artery (which lies superficial to the rectus) is ligated. For deeper dissection, approach the interval between the gluteus medius and rectus femoris. Detach the origin of both heads of the rectus femoris. Reflection of the conjoined rectus tendon too distally can risk injury to the descending branch of the lateral femoral circumflex artery. Retract the rectus medially and the gluteus medius laterally. Dissect any attachments of the iliopsoas to the inferior capsule and perform a capsulotomy. There is a risk to the lateral femoral cutaneous nerve, which is located anterior or medial to the sartorius about 6-8 cm below the ASIS. The superficial circumflex artery penetrates the tensor fasciae latae just anterior to the lateral femoral cutaneous nerve. The femoral nerve and vessels can sometimes be injured by aggressive medial retraction of the sartorius.

4. Anterolateral (Watson-Jones) approach to the hip (Fig. 2–51)—This approach can be used for total hip arthroplasty, as popularized by Watson-Jones. There is no true interneural plane, but the intermuscular plane between the tensor fasciae femoris and gluteus medius is used. After the incision and superficial dissection, the fasciae latae is split to expose the vastus lateralis. Detach the anterior third of the gluteus medius from the greater trochanter and the entire gluteus minimus. Dissect the reflected head of the rectus femoris (and capsular attachment of the iliopsoas if necessary) and retract medially. Perform a capsulotomy. The risks of this approach include damage to the femoral nerve by excessive medial retraction, denervation of the tensor fascia femoris if the intermuscular interval is exploited too superiorly (the superior gluteal nerve lies about 5 cm above the acetabular rim), and injury to the descending branch of the lateral femoral circumflex artery with anterior and inferior dissection.

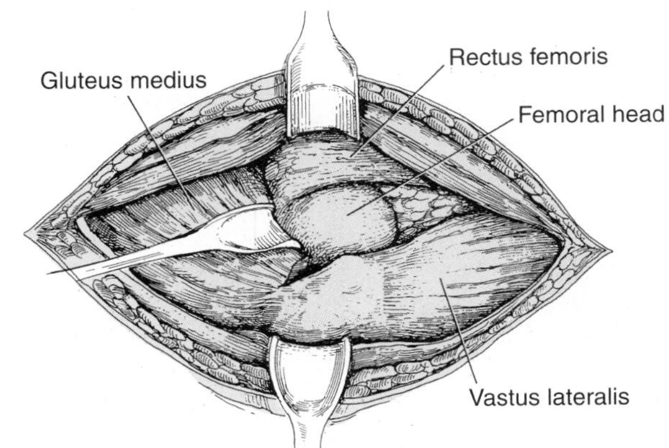

FIGURE 2–51 Anterolateral (Watson-Jones) approach to the hip. The interval between the tensor fasciae latae (superior gluteal nerve) and the gluteus medius (superior gluteal nerve) is explored. (From Steinberg ME: The Hip and Its Disorders, p 93. Philadelphia, WB Saunders, 1991.)

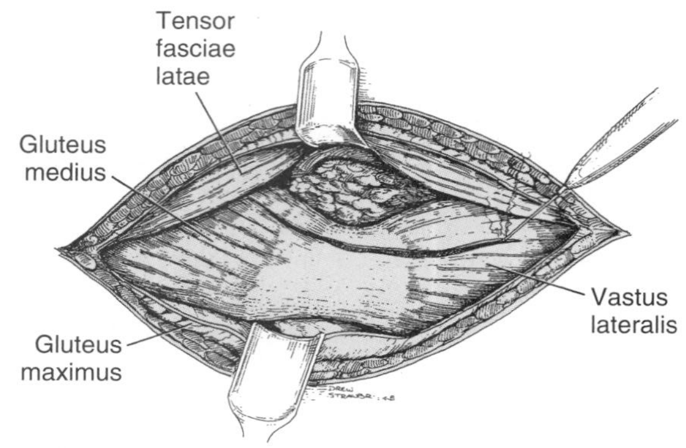

FIGURE 2–52 Lateral (Hardinge's) approach to the hip. The interval between the gluteus medius (superior gluteal nerve) and the vastus lateralis (femoral nerve) is explored. (From Steinberg ME: The Hip and Its Disorders, p 95. Philadelphia, WB Saunders, 1991.)

5. Lateral (Hardinge's) approach to the hip (Fig. 2–52)—This approach is useful for total hip arthroplasty, bipolar hemiarthroplasty, and revision work. It uses an incision that splits the gluteus medius and vastus lateralis in tandem. Incise the skin and the fascia lata to expose the gluteus medius and the vastus lateralis. Incise the gluteus medius from the greater trochanter, leaving a cuff of tissue and the posterior one half to two thirds attached. Extend this incision to split the gluteus medius proximally. Split the vastus lateralis distally along its anterior one fourth down to the femoral shaft. Detach the gluteus minimus from its insertion. The hip capsule is now exposed for further dissection. The risks include injury to the femoral nerve and possible denervation of the gluteus medius (superior gluteal nerve) if the split is too proximal (more than 5 cm proximal to the greater trochanter).
6. Posterior (Moore's or Southern's) approach to the hip (Fig. 2–53)—In one version, the interneural plane is between the gluteus maximus (inferior gluteal nerve) and the gluteus medius and tensor fasciae latae (superior gluteal nerve). However, most surgeons approach the hip by splitting the fibers of the gluteus maximus. Incise the skin and the fascia lata along the posterior border of the femur and then split the fibers of the gluteus maximus bluntly. Next, expose the short external rotators close to their insertions into the greater trochanter. Reflect them laterally to protect the sciatic nerve and expose the posterior hip capsule. A portion of the quadratus femoris may be taken down with the short external rotators, but one must be aware of the significant bleeding that can come from the inferior portion of this muscle (ascending branches of the medial femoral circumflex artery). The risk includes sciatic neurapraxia if the sciatic nerve is not properly protected by the short external rotators. Additional trouble may be encountered if the inferior gluteal artery is damaged during the splitting of the gluteus maximus.
7. Medial (Ludloff's) approach to the hip (Fig. 2–54)—Used occasionally for pediatric adductor release and open reduction, this approach explores the interval between the adductor longus and gracilis. The interval is deep between the adductor brevis and magnus. Structures at risk include the anterior division of the obturator nerve and medial femoral circumflex artery (between the adductor brevis and the adductor magnus/pectineus). The deep external pudendal artery (anterior to the pectineus near the adductor longus origin) is also at risk proximally.
8. Acetabular approaches—Used primarily for open reduction with internal fixation (ORIF) of pelvic fractures, these approaches are basically extensions of incisions for exposure of the hip (discussed earlier).
   a. The Kocher-Langenbeck incision—This is a posterolateral approach that provides access to the posterior column/acetabulum (Fig. 2–55).
   b. The ilioinguinal incision—This incision relies on mobilization of the rectus abdominis

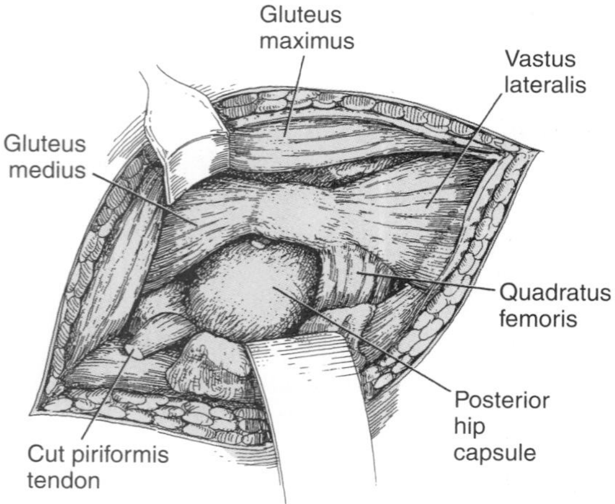

FIGURE 2–53 Posterior (Moore's or Southern's) approach to the hip. The interval between the gluteus maximus (inferior gluteal nerve) and the gluteus medius/tensor fascia lata (superior gluteal nerve) is explored. (From Steinberg ME: The Hip and Its Disorders, p 95. Philadelphia, WB Saunders, 1991.)

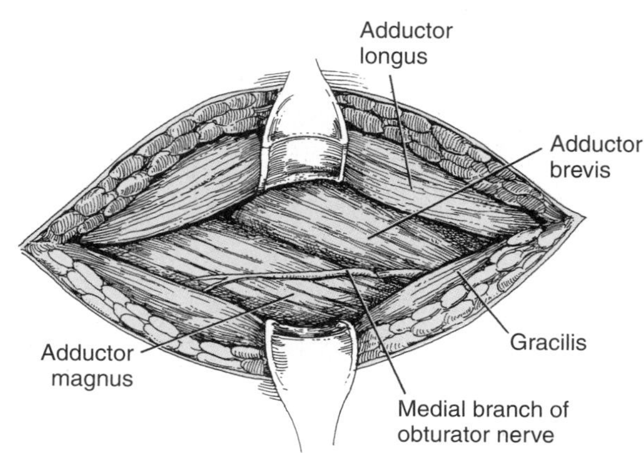

FIGURE 2–54 Medial (Ludloff's) approach to the hip. The interval between the adductor longus (obturator nerve) and the gracilis (obturator nerve) is explored. (From Steinberg ME: The Hip and Its Disorders. Philadelphia, WB Saunders, 1991, p 99.)

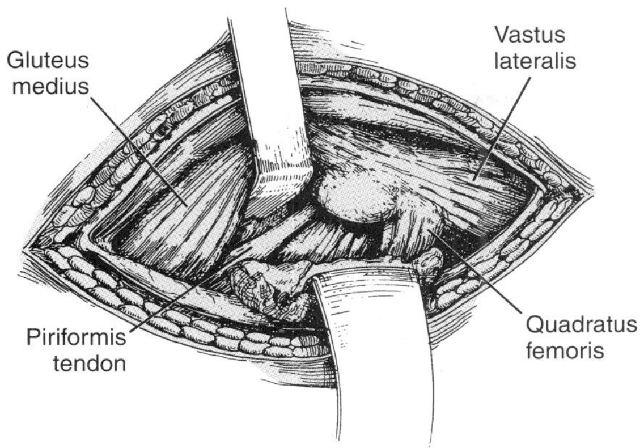

FIGURE 2–55 Posterolateral approach to the hip. (From Steinberg ME: The Hip and Its Disorders, p 96. Philadelphia, WB Saunders, 1991.)

and iliacus, exposing the anterior column (Fig. 2–56). Three windows are available with this approach. The first gives access to the internal iliac fossa and the anterior sacroiliac joint. The second (between the iliopectineal fascia and the external iliac vessels) gives access to the pelvic brim and part of the superior pubic ramus. The third (below the vessels and the spermatic cord) provides access to the quadrilateral plate and retropubic space.

c. The extended iliofemoral incision—This incision allows access to both columns by reflecting the gluteal muscles and tensor posteriorly and dividing the obturator internus and piriformis.

G. Arthroscopy—The portals for hip arthroscopy include the anterolateral and posterolateral portals (adjacent to the superior border of the greater trochanter) and the anterior portal (risk to the femoral and lateral femoral cutaneous nerves).

II. Thigh

A. Osteology of the femur

1. Introduction—The femur is the largest bone of the body. The neck–shaft angle averages approximately 127 degrees, although it begins at 141 degrees in the fetus. The anteversion varies from 1 to 40 degrees but averages 14 degrees. The femur has an anterior bow. There are two femoral condyles; the medial condyle is larger. The more prominent medial epicondyle supports the adductor tubercle.
2. Ossification—The important areas of femoral ossification include the head and the distal femur. The femoral head is usually not present at birth but appears as one large physis that includes both

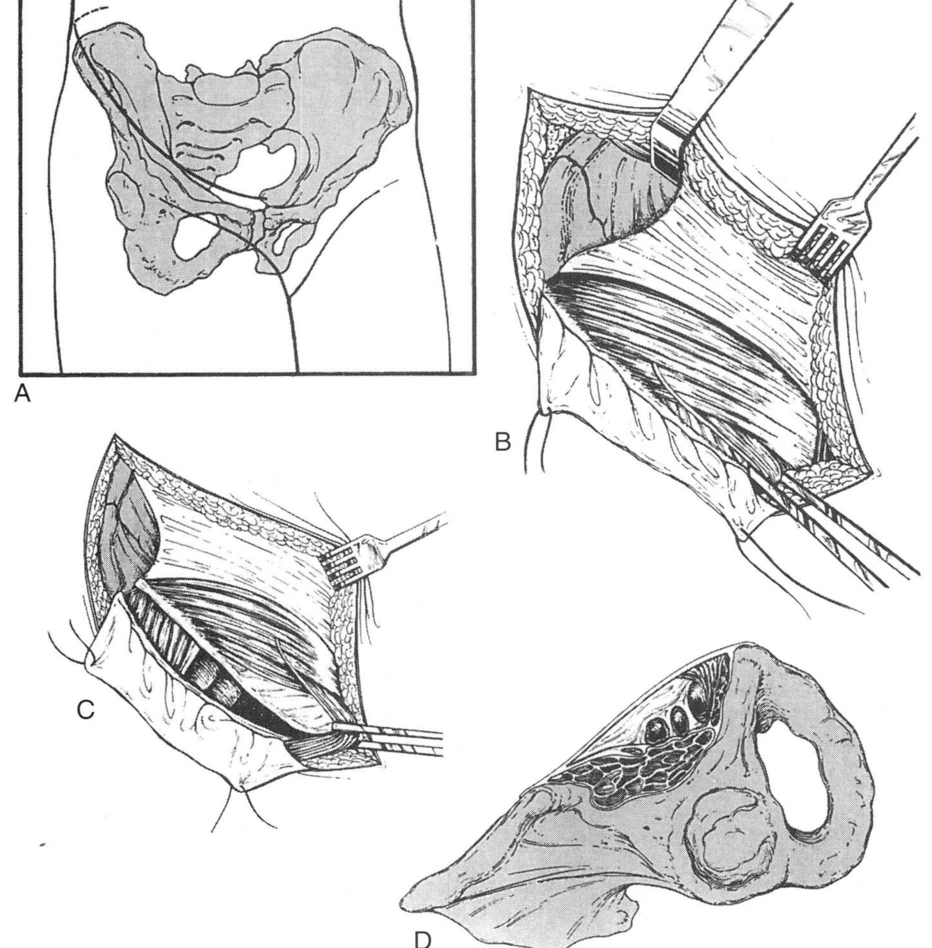

FIGURE 2–56 The ilioinguinal approach. **A**, The skin incision. **B**, The internal iliac fossa has been exposed, and the inguinal canal has been unroofed by distal reflection of the external oblique aponeurosis. **C**, An incision along the inguinal ligament detaches the abdominal muscles and transversalis fascia, giving access to the psoas sheath, the iliopectineal fascia, the external aspect of the femoral vessels, and the retropubic space of Retzius. **D**, An oblique section through the muscular and vascular lacunae at the level of the inguinal ligament.

Continued

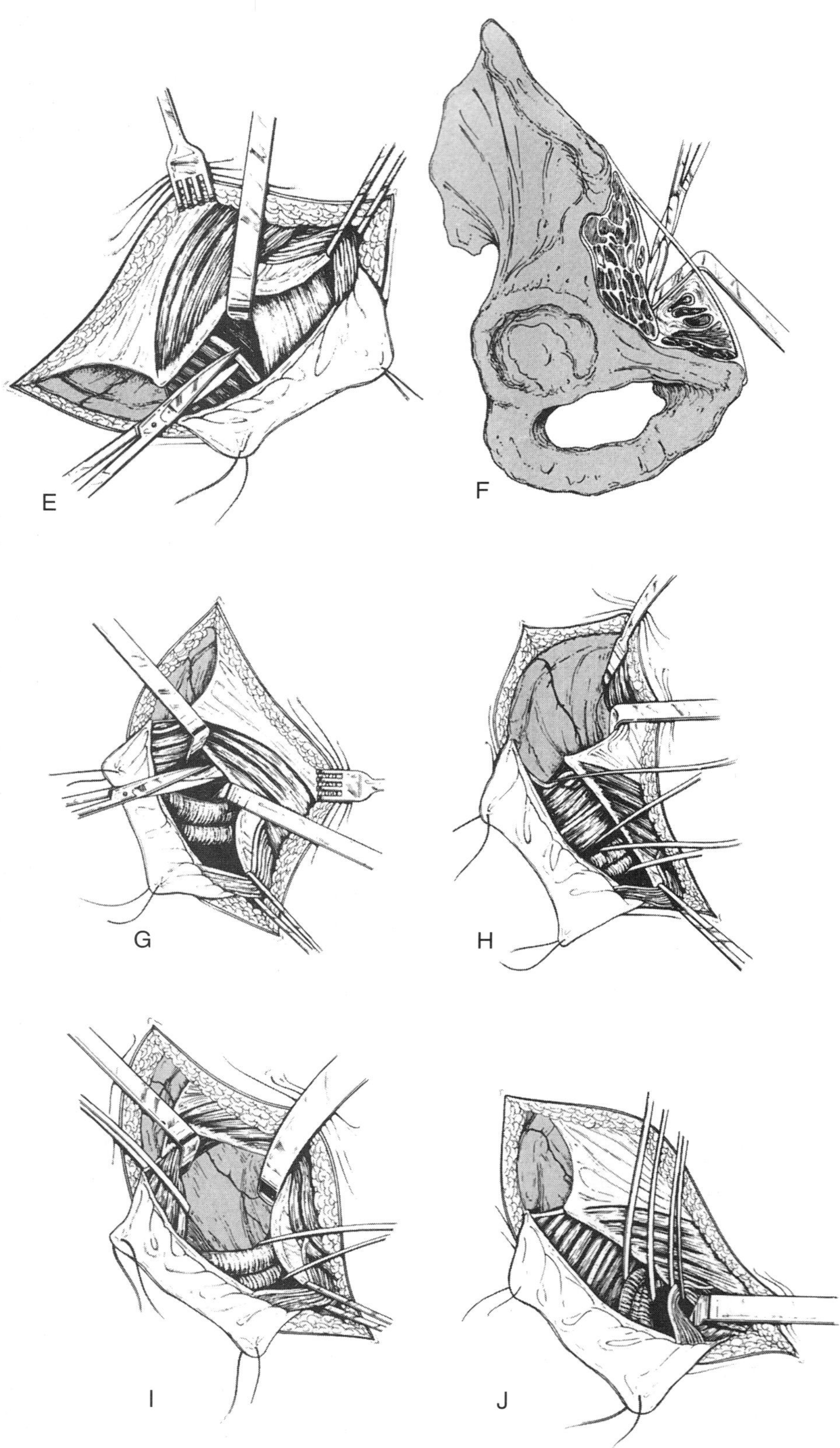

FIGURE 2-56, cont'd E, Division of the iliopectineal fascia to the pectineal eminence. **F**, An oblique section that demonstrates division of the iliopectineal fascia. **G**, Proximal division of the iliopectineal fascia from the pelvic brim to allow access to the true pelvis. **H**, The first window of the ilioinguinal approach, which gives access to the internal iliac fossa, the anterior sacroiliac joint, and the upper portion of the anterior column. **I**, The second window of the ilioinguinal approach, giving access to the pelvic brim from the anterior sacroiliac joint to the lateral extremity of the superior pubic ramus. The quadrilateral surface and posterior column are accessible beyond the pelvic brim. **J**, Access to the symphysis pubis and retropubic space of Retzius, medial to the spermatic cord and femoral vessels. (From Browner BD, Jupiter JB, Levine AM, Trafton PG: Skeletal Trauma: Fractures, Dislocations, Ligamentous Injuries, Fig. 32-5A-J, pp 907-909. Philadelphia, WB Saunders, 1992.)

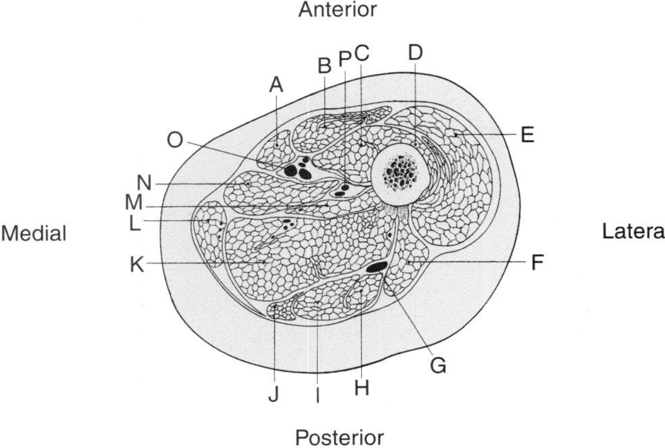

FIGURE 2–57 Cross section of the proximal thigh. (From Callaghan JJ, ed: Anatomy Self-Assessment Examination, Fig. 53. Park Ridge, IL, American Academy of Orthopaedic Surgeons, 1991.)

A—Sartorius m.
B—Rectus femoris m.
C—Vastus medialis m.
D—Vastus intermedius m.
E—Vastus lateralis m.
F—Short head of biceps femoris m.
G—Sciatic n.
H—Long head of biceps femoris m.
I—Semitendinosus m.
J—Semimembranosus m.
K—Adductor magnus m.
L—Gracilis m.
M—Adductor brevis m.
N—Adductor longus m.
O—Femoral a. and v.
P—Deep femoral a. and v.

trochanters at about 11 months and fuses at 18 years. Slipped capital femoral epiphysis occurs through the femoral head epiphysis (zone of hypertrophy). The distal femoral physis appears at birth and fuses at 19 years. Knee stress examinations should be included for the evaluation of distal femoral physeal fractures in pediatric patients.

B. Muscles (Fig. 2–57 and Table 2–51)
   Anterior thigh
   Medial thigh (see Table 2–47 for adductors)
   Posterior thigh

C. Nerves (also see the preceding discussion on the pelvis and hip and the following discussion on the knee and leg)
   1. Anatomy
      a. The sciatic nerve (L4-S3) emerges from its foramen anterior to the piriformis muscle (through the piriformis in 2% of people) and lies posterior to the other short external rotators. It descends below the gluteus maximus and proceeds posteriorly to the adductor magnus and between the long head of the biceps and semimembranosus. Before it emerges from the popliteal fossa, it divides into the common peroneal nerve and the tibial nerve. The peroneal division has one innervation in the thigh—the short head of the biceps femoris. The common peroneal nerve diverges laterally and traverses the lateral knee region under cover of the biceps femoris. The tibial nerve emerges into the popliteal fossa laterally, proceeds posteriorly to the vessel, and then descends between the heads of the gastrocnemius.
      b. The femoral nerve (L2-L4) is the largest branch of the lumbar plexus and supplies the thigh muscles. The largest branch of the femoral nerve is the saphenous nerve. The infrapatellar branch of the saphenous nerve supplies the skin of the medial side of the front of the knee and patellar ligament and can be damaged during total knee replacement surgery.
      c. The lateral femoral cutaneous nerve (L2-L3) supplies the skin and fascia on the surface of the anterolateral thigh from the greater trochanter to the knee. It can be damaged by acetabular approaches that dissect around its course underneath the lateral end of the inguinal ligament.

TABLE 2-51 MUSCLES OF THE THIGH

Muscle	Origin	Insertion	Innervation
Anterior Thigh			
Vastus lateralis	Iliotibial line/greater trochanter/lateral linea aspera	Lateral patella	Femoral
Vastus medialis	Iliotibial line/medial linea aspera/supracondylar line	Medial patella	Femoral
Vastus intermedius	Proximal anterior femoral shaft	Patella	Femoral
Posterior Thigh			
Biceps (long head)	Medial ischial tuberosity	Fibular head/lateral tibia	Tibial
Biceps (short head)	Lateral linea aspera/lateral intermuscular septum	Lateral tibial condyle	Peroneal
Semitendinosus	Distal medial ischial tuberosity	Anterior tibial crest	Tibial
Semimembranosus	Proximal lateral ischial tuberosity	Oblique popliteal ligament Posterior capsule Posterior/medial tibia Popliteus Medial meniscus	Tibial

TABLE 2-52 INNERVATION OF THE THIGH

Nerve	Components	Muscles Innervated
Femoral	L2-L4	Iliacus, psoas major (lower part), sartorius, pectineus, quadriceps, articularis genus muscles
Obturator	L2-L4	Obturator externus, hip adductors (brevis, longus, magnus), gracilis
Sciatic	L4-S3	Peroneal division—short head of biceps femoris Tibial division—hamstrings (semitendinosus, semimembranosus), part of adductor magnus, long head of biceps femoris

TABLE 2-53 THIGH VESSELS AT RISK DURING SURGICAL PROCEDURES

Approach	Vascular Structures at Risk
Anterior hip (Smith-Peterson)	Ascending branch of lateral femoral circumflex artery (superficial to rectus femoris muscle)
Anterolateral hip (Watson-Jones)	Descending branch of lateral femoral circumflex artery
Medial hip (Ludloff)	Medial femoral circumflex artery and deep external pudendal artery (at risk during percutaneous tenotomy of adductor longus)
Lateral and posterolateral thigh	Perforators from profunda femoris artery
Anteromedial distal femur	Medial superior geniculate artery

d. The obturator nerve (L2-L4) can be damaged during various hip and acetabular approaches (screw placement in the anteroinferior quadrant), resulting in a decrease in sensation in the medial thigh and loss of hip adductor function. The obturator nerve has two branches after it passes through the obturator foramen: the anterior branch (adductor longus, adductor brevis, gracilis) and the posterior branch (obturator externus, adductor magnus, adductor brevis [variable]). The anterior branch of the obturator nerve can provide sensation to the medial side of the knee and can be a source of referred pain from hip pathology. Always clinically and radiographically evaluate a joint above and below a patient's complaint.

2. Innervation (Table 2–52) (see also Table 2–44)

D. Vessels (also see the preceding discussion on the pelvis and hip and the following discussion on the knee and leg)

1. Anatomy
   a. The external iliac artery becomes the femoral artery after it traverses the inguinal ligament, arriving at the femoral triangle.
   b. The femoral artery branches to become the deep femoral artery and the superficial femoral artery. The deep femoral artery gives rise to the medial and lateral femoral circumflex arteries.
   c. The medial femoral circumflex artery is the major blood supply to the femoral head in the adult and lies anterior to the quadratus femoris muscle. After supplying the profundus (described earlier), the superficial femoral artery descends under cover of the sartorius muscle and proceeds between the adductor group and the vastus medialis into the adductor canal. At the level above the medial femoral condyle, the artery supplies a descending geniculate branch, then passes through a defect in the adductor magnus (adductor hiatus), and finally emerges in the popliteal fossa. The vein is usually posterior to the artery.
   d. The obturator artery is a branch of the internal iliac artery, and its posterior branch supplies the ligamentum teres acetabular artery. This artery is an important source of blood to the femoral head from birth to 4 years old. The internal iliac artery also supplies the superior and inferior gluteal arteries.
2. Vessels at risk (Table 2–53)

E. Surgical approaches to the thigh (Table 2–54)

1. Lateral approach to the thigh—The lateral approach is used for ORIF of intertrochanteric and femoral neck fractures. This approach can be extended for access to shaft and supracondylar fractures. There is no true interneural plane. Split the fascia lata in line with the femoral shaft. If necessary, include part of the tensor fasciae femoris. Then bluntly dissect the vastus lateralis in line with its fibers or dissect the fibers of the intermuscular septum. Identify and coagulate the various perforators from the profunda femoris.
2. Posterolateral approach to the thigh—This approach may be used for exposure of the entire length of the femur through an interneural plane. It exploits the interval between the vastus lateralis (femoral nerve) and the hamstrings (sciatic nerve). Incise the fascia under the iliotibial band and retract the vastus superiorly. Continue anteriorly to the lateral intermuscular septum with blunt dissection until the periosteum over the linea aspera is reached. The risk of this dissection lies in the series of perforating vessels from the profundus that pierce the lateral

TABLE 2-54 THIGH SURGICAL APPROACHES

Approach	Interval	Structures at Risk
Lateral	Vastus lateralis (femoral nerve)	Perforators from the profunda femoris artery
Posterolateral	Vastus lateralis (femoral nerve) and hamstrings (sciatic nerve)	Perforators from the profunda femoris artery
Anteromedial (distal)	Rectus femoris (femoral nerve) and vastus medialis (femoral nerve)	Medial superior geniculate artery, infrapatellar branch of saphenous nerve
Posterior	Biceps femoris (sciatic nerve) and vastus lateralis (femoral nerve)	Posterior femoral cutaneous nerve (between biceps and semitendinosus) and sciatic nerve

intermuscular septum to reach the vastus. If they are approached without care, these vessels can retract and bleed underneath the septum.

3. Anteromedial approach to the distal femur—This approach may be used for ORIF of distal femoral and femoral shaft fractures. Explore the interval between the rectus femoris and vastus medialis (femoral nerve) and extend to a point medial to the patella. Retract the rectus laterally. Explore the interval to reveal the vastus intermedius. It may be necessary to open the knee joint. If so, incise the medial patellar retinaculum and split a portion of the quadriceps tendon just lateral to the medial border. After identifying the vastus intermedius, split it along its fibers to expose the femur. The risk includes injury to the medial superior geniculate artery and the infrapatellar branch of the saphenous nerve because both cross the site of exposure. Additionally, one must leave an adequate cuff of tissue for a strong patellar retinacular repair or risk lateral subluxation of the patella.
4. Posterior approach to the thigh—This rare approach may be used for exploration of the sciatic nerve. It makes use of the interneural interval between the biceps femoris (sciatic nerve) and vastus lateralis (femoral nerve). Identify and protect the posterior femoral cutaneous nerve (between the biceps and semitendinosus). Next, explore the interval between the biceps and the lateral intermuscular septum. Detach the origin of the short head of the biceps from the linea aspera. This maneuver allows exposure of the femur at the midshaft level. In the lower thigh, retract the long head of the biceps laterally to expose the sciatic nerve. It lies on the surface of the adductor magnus and may be retracted laterally to expose this portion of the femur.

III. Knee and Leg

A. Osteology

1. Patella—The patella is the largest sesamoid bone. It serves three functions: It is a fulcrum for the quadriceps; it protects the knee joint; and it enhances lubrication and nutrition of the knee. An accessory or "bipartite" patella may represent failure of fusion of the superolateral corner of the patella and is commonly confused with patellar fractures.
2. Tibia—The tibia articulates with the distal femur by means of proximal medial facet (oval and concave) and lateral facet (circular and convex). The Gerdy tubercle lies on the lateral side of the proximal tibia and is the insertion of the iliotibial tract. The tibial shaft is triangular in cross-section and tapers to its thinnest point at the junction of the middle and distal thirds before widening again to form the tibial plafond. Distally, the tibia forms an inferior quadrilateral surface for articulation with the talus and the pyramid-shaped medial malleolus. Laterally, the fibular notch forms an articulation with the fibula.
3. Fibula—The styloid process of the head serves as the attachment for the fibular collateral ligament and the biceps tendon. Lying just below the head, the neck of the fibula is grooved by the common peroneal nerve. The expanded distal fibula is known as the lateral malleolus and extends beyond the distal margin of the medial malleolus. Together with the inferior distal surface of the tibia, these structures make up the ankle mortise.

B. Arthrology

1. Knee—The knee is a compound joint consisting of two condyloid joints and one sellar joint (patellofemoral articulation). The knee is enclosed in a capsule that has posteromedial and posterolateral recesses extending 15 mm distal to the subchondral surface of the tibial plateau (be careful to avoid intra-articular pin placement). The medial and lateral femoral condyles articulate with the corresponding tibial facets.
   a. Menisci—Intervening menisci serve to deepen the concavity of the facets, help protect the articular surface, and assist in rotation of the knee (Fig. 2–58). The peripheral third of the menisci are vascular and can be repaired; the inner two thirds are nourished by synovial fluid. The medial meniscus tears three times more often than the more mobile lateral meniscus. Protect the saphenous nerve during repairs to the medial meniscus. The lateral meniscus is associated with meniscal cysts and discoid menisci and is the most common site of tears in acute injuries to the **anterior cruciate ligament** (ACL). Protect the peroneal nerve during repairs to the lateral meniscus.
   b. Ligaments—The stability of the knee is enhanced by a complex arrangement of ligaments (Table 2–55; Fig. 2–59). The cruciate ligaments are crucial to anteroposterior stability, and the collateral ligaments provide varus/valgus stability. Each cruciate ligament is made up of two portions, or bundles. The anterior bundles of the ACL and **posterior cruciate ligament** (PCL) are tight in flexion. The PCL has an anterolateral bundle and the ACL an anteromedial bundle. Remember PAL: **P**CL has **a**ntero**l**ateral. Thus, the ACL is composed of an anteromedial portion that is tight in flexion and a posterolateral portion that is tight in extension. The PCL has an anterolateral portion that is tight in flexion and a posteromedial portion that is tight in extension. The PCL lies between the ligament of Humphrey (anterior) and the Wrisberg ligament (posterior). The **posterolateral corner** (PLC) comprises the arcuate ligament, popliteus, posterolateral capsule, **lateral collateral ligament** (LCL), popliteofibular ligament, and lateral head of the gastrocnemius. Injuries to the PCL and PLC

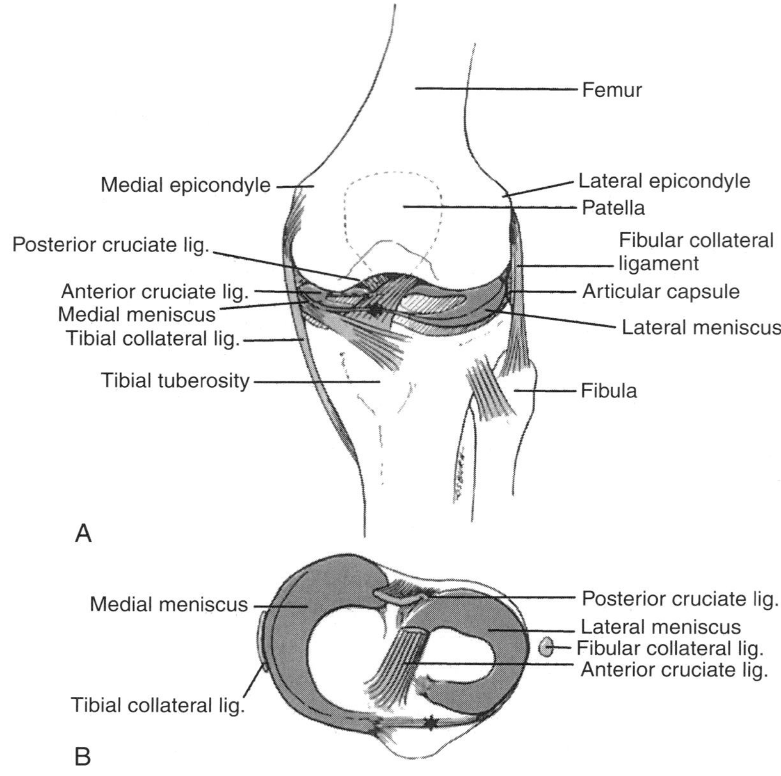

FIGURE 2–58 Menisci and ligaments of the knee. **A**, Anterior view. **B**, Superior view. (From Jenkins DB: Hollinshead's Functional Anatomy of the Limbs and Back, 6th ed, Fig 16-1. Philadelphia, WB Saunders, 1991.)

provide key testable material. Isolated injuries to the PCL cause the greatest instability at 90 degrees of knee flexion. Combined PCL and PLC injuries result in increasing instability as the knee is flexed from 30-90 degrees. Isolated PLC injuries result in increasing instability that is most notable at 30 degrees, with instability decreasing as the knee is flexed to 90 degrees.

c. Muscles and tendons—Several muscles and tendons traverse the knee, giving it dynamic stability. The hamstring tendons used for autograft ACL reconstruction are the gracilis and semitendinosus.

2. Superior tibiofibular joint—This is a plane or gliding joint that is strengthened by the anterior and posterior ligaments of the head of the fibula.

C. Muscles of the leg—These muscles are commonly divided into groups based on compartments (anterior, lateral, superficial posterior, and deep posterior) (Table 2–56). The posterior compartments are supplied by the tibial nerve and contain preaxial muscles. The anterior and lateral compartments are supplied by the common peroneal nerve (anterior supplied by the deep peroneal nerve, and lateral supplied by the superficial peroneal nerve) and contain postaxial muscles. The origins and insertions are noted in Figure 2–60. The popliteal fossa is bordered

TABLE 2-55 LIGAMENTS OF THE KNEE

Ligament	Origin	Insertion	Function
Retinacular	Vastus medialis and lateralis	Tibial condyles	Forms anterior capsule
Posterior fibers	Femoral condyles	Tibial condyles	Forms posterior capsule
Oblique popliteal	Semimembranosus tendon	Lateral femoral condyle/posterior capsule	Strengthens capsule
Deep medial collateral (MCL)	Medial epicondyle	Medial meniscus	Holds medial meniscus to femur
Superficial MCL	Medial epicondyle	Medial condyle of tibia	Resists valgus force
Arcuate	Lateral femoral condyle, over popliteus	Posterior tibia/fibular head	Posterior support
Lateral collateral	Lateral epicondyle	Lateral fibular head	Resists varus force
Anterior cruciate	Anterior intercondylar tibia	Posteromedial lateral femoral condyle	Limits hyperextension/sliding
Posterior cruciate (PCL)	Posterior sulcus of tibia	Anteromedial femoral condyle	Prevents hyperflexion/sliding
Coronary	Meniscus	Tibial periphery	Meniscal attachment
Wrisberg	Posterolateral meniscus	Medial femoral condyle (behind PCL)	Stabilizes lateral meniscus
Humphrey	Posterolateral meniscus	Medial femoral condyle (in front)	Stabilizes lateral meniscus
Transverse meniscal	Anterolateral meniscus	Anteromedial meniscus	Stabilizes menisci

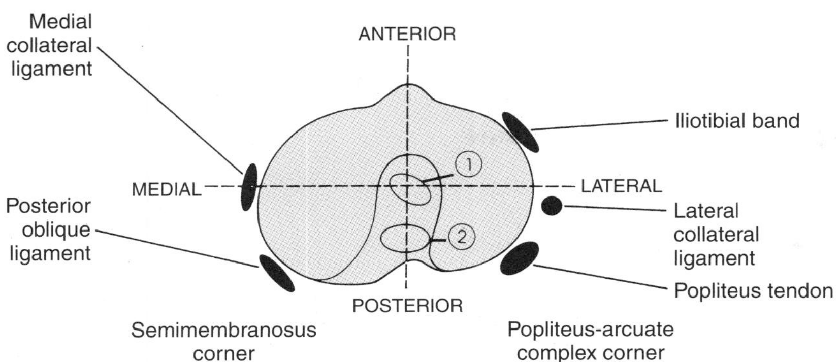

FIGURE 2–59 Ligaments of the knee. 1, Anterior cruciate ligament; 2, posterior cruciate ligament. (From Magee DJ: Orthopedic Physical Assessment, p 285. Philadelphia, WB Saunders, 1987.)

by the gastrocnemius muscles, semimembranosus, and biceps. The plantaris muscle makes up the floor of the fossa. Four compartment releases of the leg are key testable material and are summarized in Table 2–57. The saphenous nerve (termination of the femoral nerve) is subcutaneous.

D. Nerves (Fig. 2–61)
   1. Anatomy
      a. Tibial nerve (L4-S3) (see Table 2–45)—This nerve continues in the thigh deep to the long head of the biceps and enters the popliteal fossa. It then crosses over the popliteus muscle and splits the two heads of the gastrocnemius, passing deep to the soleus on its course to the posterior aspect of the medial malleolus. It terminates as the medial and lateral plantar nerves. Muscular branches supply the posterior leg along its course (superficial and deep posterior compartments).
      b. Common peroneal nerve (L4-S2)—The smaller terminal division of the sciatic nerve, this nerve runs laterally along the popliteal fossa in the interval between the medial border of the biceps and the lateral head of the gastrocnemius. Then it winds around the neck of the fibula and runs deep to the peroneus longus, where it divides into the superficial and deep branches. This nerve can be injured with traction and by lateral meniscal repair.
         (1) Superficial peroneal nerve—This nerve runs along the border between the lateral

TABLE 2-56 MUSCLES OF THE LEG

Muscle	Origin	Insertion	Action	Innervation
Anterior Compartment				
Tibialis anterior	Lateral tibia	Medial cuneiform, first metatarsal	Dorsiflex, invert foot	Deep peroneal (L4)
Extensor hallucis longus	Mid-fibula	Great toe, distal phalanx	Dorsiflex, extend toe	Deep peroneal (L5)
Extensor digitorum longus (EDL)	Tibial condyle/fibula	Toe, middle and distal phalanges	Dorsiflex, extend toe	Deep peroneal (L5)
Peroneus tertius	Fibula and EDL tendon	Fifth metatarsal	Evert, plantar flex, abduct foot	Deep peroneal (S1)
Lateral Compartment				
Peroneus longus	Proximal fibula	Medial cuneiform, first metatarsal	Evert, plantar flex, abduct foot	Superficial peroneal (S1)
Peroneus brevis	Distal fibula	Tuberosity of fifth metatarsal	Evert foot	Superficial peroneal (S1)
Superficial Posterior Compartment				
Gastrocnemius	Posterior medial and lateral femoral condyles	Calcaneus	Plantar flex foot	Tibial (S1)
Soleus	Fibula/tibia	Calcaneus	Plantar flex foot	Tibial (S1)
Plantaris	Lateral femoral condyle	Calcaneus	Plantar flex foot	Tibial (S1)
Deep Posterior Compartment				
Popliteus	Lateral femoral condyle, fibular head	Proximal tibia	Flex, internally rotate knee	Tibial (L5,S1)
Flexor hallucis longus	Fibula	Great toe, distal phalanx	Plantar flex great toe	Tibial (S1)
Flexor digitorum longus	Tibia	Second to fifth toes, distal phalanges	Plantar flex toes, foot	Tibial (S1,S2)
Tibialis posterior	Tibia, fibula, interosseous membrane	Navicular, medial cuneiform	Invert/plantar flex foot	Tibial (L4,L5)

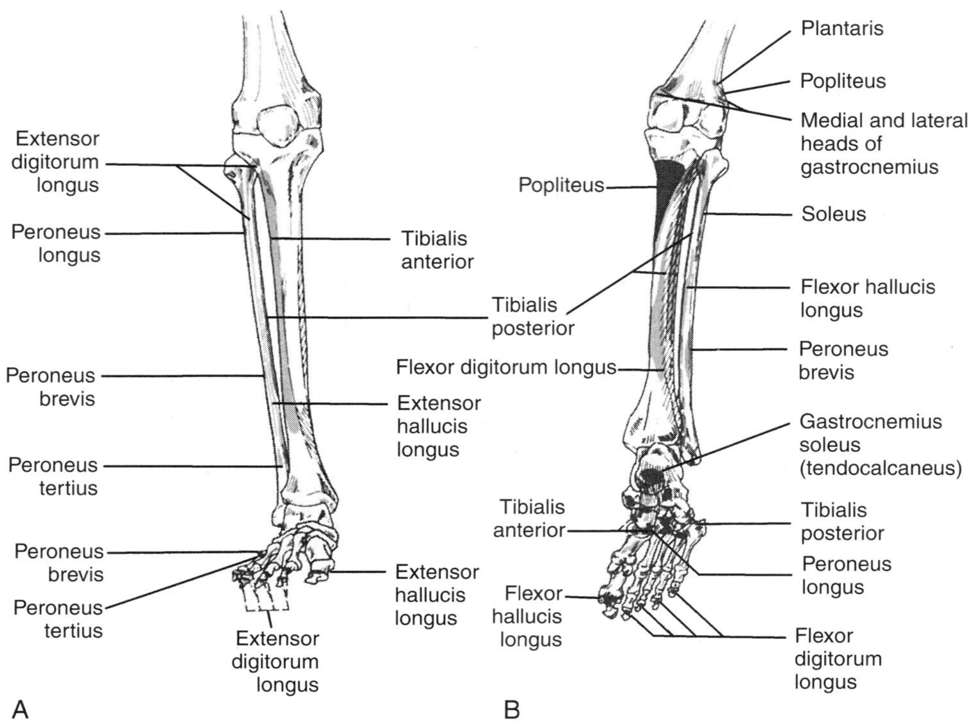

FIGURE 2–60 Origins and insertions of leg and foot muscles. **A**, Anterior view. **B**, Posterior view. (From Jenkins DB: Hollinshead's Functional Anatomy of the Limbs and Back, 6th ed, Fig. 19-3. Philadelphia, WB Saunders, 1991.)

and anterior compartments in the leg, supplying muscular branches to the peroneus longus and brevis (lateral compartment) (see Table 2–45). It terminates in two cutaneous branches (medial dorsal and intermediate dorsal cutaneous nerves) supplying the dorsal foot. The superficial peroneal nerve supplies dorsal medial sensation to the great toe.

(2) Deep peroneal nerve—Sometimes known as the anterior tibial nerve, this nerve runs along the anterior surface of the interosseous membrane, supplying the musculature of the anterior compartment (tibialis anterior [TA], EHL, extensor digitorum longus [EDL], tibialis posterior [TP]) (see Table 2–45). Sensation to the first web space is provided by the deep peroneal nerve.

c. Cutaneous nerves (see Fig. 2–40)—Important cutaneous nerves include the saphenous nerve (L3-L4) and the sural nerve (S1-S2). The saphenous nerve is the continuation of the femoral nerve of the thigh, and it becomes subcutaneous on the medial aspect of the knee between the sartorius and gracilis, where it is sometimes injured during procedures about the knee, for instance, meniscal repair. The saphenous nerve supplies sensation to the medial aspect of the leg and foot. The sural nerve, which is often used for nerve grafting and can cause painful neuroma when it is inadvertently cut, is formed by cutaneous branches of both the tibial (medial sural cutaneous) and common peroneal (lateral sural cutaneous) nerves. It lies on the lateral aspect of the leg and foot.

2. Innervation (see Table 2–45)

E. Vessels (see Fig. 2–61)—The branches of the popliteal artery (the continuation of the femoral artery) supply the leg. The artery enters the popliteal fossa between the biceps and semimembranosus and descends underneath the tibial nerve, terminating between the medial and lateral heads of the gastrocnemius and dividing into the anterior and posterior tibial arteries. Several genicular branches are given off in the popliteal fossa, including the medial and lateral geniculate arteries (which supply the menisci) and the middle geniculate artery (which supplies the cruciate ligaments). The superior lateral geniculate artery

TABLE 2-57 COMPARTMENT RELEASES OF LEG

Compartment	Muscles	Neurovascular Structures Released
Anterior	Tibialis anterior, extensor hallucis longus, extensor digitorum longus, tibialis posterior	Deep peroneal nerve and anterior tibial artery
Lateral	Peroneus longus and brevis	Superficial peroneal nerve
Superficial posterior	Gastrocsoleus complex, plantaris	Sural nerve
Deep posterior	Popliteus, flexor hallucis longus, flexor digitorum longus, tibialis posterior	Posterior tibial artery and vein, tibial nerve, peroneal artery and vein

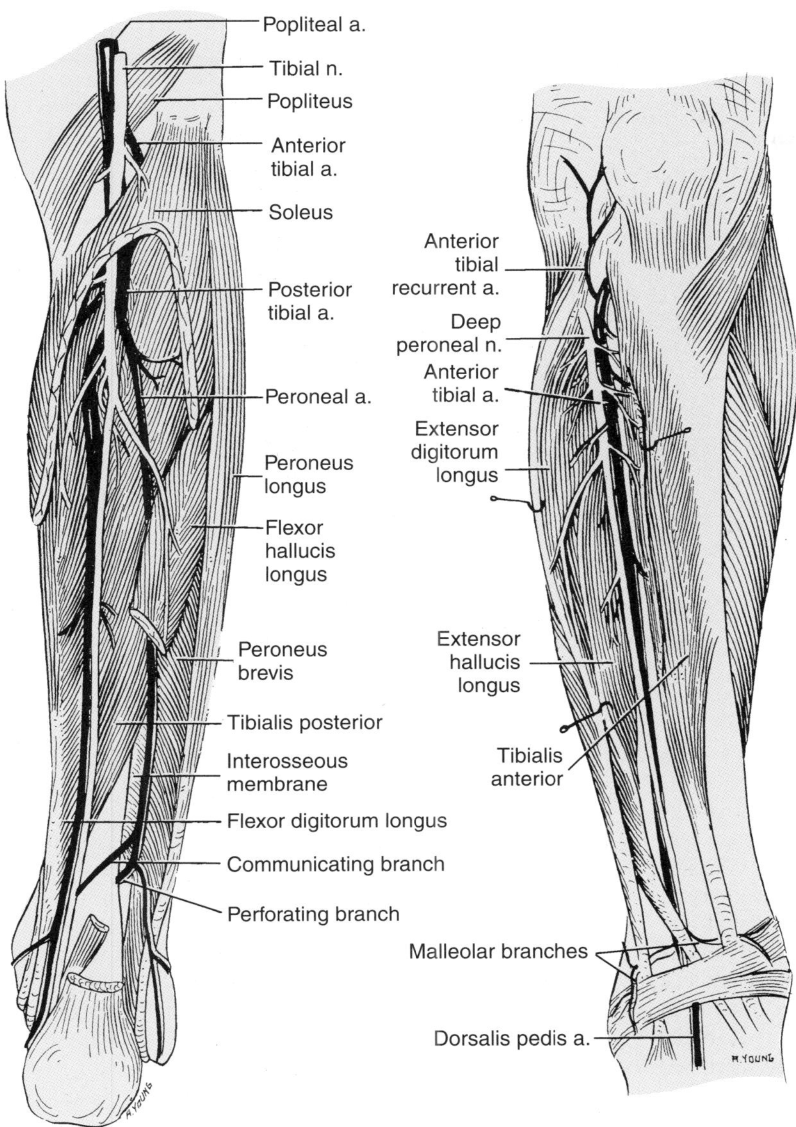

FIGURE 2–61 Nerves and vessels of the leg. **A**, Posterior. **B**, Anterior. (From Jenkins DB: Hollinshead's Functional Anatomy of the Limbs and Back, 6th ed, pp 292, 296. Philadelphia, WB Saunders, 1991.)

can be injured during lateral-release procedures. The descending geniculate artery (a branch of the femoral artery proximal to the Hunter canal) supplies the vastus medialis at the anterior border of the intermuscular septum. The inferior geniculate artery passes between the popliteal tendon and fibular collateral ligament in the posterolateral corner of the knee.

1. Anterior tibial artery—The first branch of the popliteal artery, this vessel passes between the two heads of the tibialis posterior (TP) and the interosseous membrane to lie on the anterior surface of that membrane between the TA and EHL until it terminates as the dorsalis pedis artery.
2. Posterior tibial artery—This artery continues in the deep posterior compartment of the leg, coursing obliquely to pass behind the medial malleolus, where it terminates by dividing into the medial and lateral plantar arteries. Its main branch, the peroneal artery, is given off 2.5 cm distal to the popliteal fossa and continues in the deep posterior compartment lateral to its parent artery between the TP and flexor hallucis longus (FHL), eventually terminating in the calcaneal branches.

F. Surgical approaches to the knee and leg (Table 2–58)

1. Medial parapatellar approach to the knee—Frequently used in operative procedures for total knee arthroplasty, this approach uses a midline incision and a medial parapatellar capsular incision. The infrapatellar branch of the saphenous nerve is sometimes cut with incisions that stray too far medially, leading to painful neuroma.
2. Medial approach to the knee (Fig. 2–62)—Used for repair of the MCL and capsule, this approach is in the interval between the sartorius and medial patellar retinaculum. The saphenous

TABLE 2-58 KNEE AND LEG SURGICAL APPROACHES

Approach	Interval	Structures at Risk
Medial parapatellar knee	Through quadriceps tendon	Infrapatellar branch of saphenous nerve
Medial knee	Sartorius and medial patellar retinaculum	Saphenous nerve and vein
Lateral knee	Iliotibial band (supinator gluteal nerve) and biceps femoris (sciatic nerve)	Common peroneal nerve Popliteus tendon Lateral inferior geniculate artery
Anterior tibia	Elevation of tibialis anterior	
Posterolateral tibia	Soleus and FHL (tibial nerve) and peroneal muscles (peroneal nerve)	Peroneal artery

nerve and vein must be identified and protected. Three layers are commonly recognized (from superficial to deep): (1) the pes anserinus tendons, (2) the superficial MCL, and (3) the deep MCL and capsule.

3. Lateral approach to the knee (Fig. 2–63)—Primarily used for exploring and repairing damaged ligaments, this approach uses the plane between the iliotibial band (superior gluteal nerve) and the biceps (sciatic nerve). The common peroneal nerve, located near the posterior border of the biceps, must be isolated and retracted. The popliteus tendon is also at risk and should be identified. The lateral inferior geniculate artery is posterior to the LCL between the lateral head of the gastrocnemius and the posterolateral capsule; it must also be identified and coagulated. The superior lateral geniculate artery is located between the femur and vastus lateralis.
4. Posterior approach to the knee—Occasionally required to address posterior capsular pathology, with this approach an S-shaped incision is used, beginning laterally and ending medially (distally). The popliteal fossa is exposed by using the small saphenous vein and medial sural cutaneous nerves as landmarks. The two heads of the gastrocnemius can be detached if greater exposure is necessary. An alternative approach is to mobilize the medial head of the gastrocnemius (lateral to the semimembranosus) and retract it laterally, with its muscle belly being used to protect the neurovascular structures.
5. Anterior approach to the tibia—This approach may be used for ORIF of fractures and bone grafting; it relies on subperiosteal elevation of the TA.
6. Posterolateral approach to the tibia—Typically used for bone grafting of tibial nonunions, this approach uses the interneural plane between the soleus and the FHL (tibial nerve) and the peroneal muscles (superficial peroneal nerve). The FHL is detached from its origin on the fibula, and the TP is detached from its origin along the interosseous membrane to reach the tibia. The neurovascular structures in the posterior compartment (including the peroneal artery) are protected by the muscle bellies of the FHL and TP.
7. Approach to the fibula—This approach is through the same interval as the posterolateral approach to the tibia, but it stays more anterior and relies on isolation and protection of the common peroneal nerve in the proximal dissection.

G. Arthroscopy—The arthroscopic portals for knee arthroscopy commonly include the inferomedial and inferolateral portals and a proximal (medial or lateral) portal. Posterior portals can place certain neurovascular structures at risk (lateral, common peroneal nerve; medial, saphenous nerve and vein).

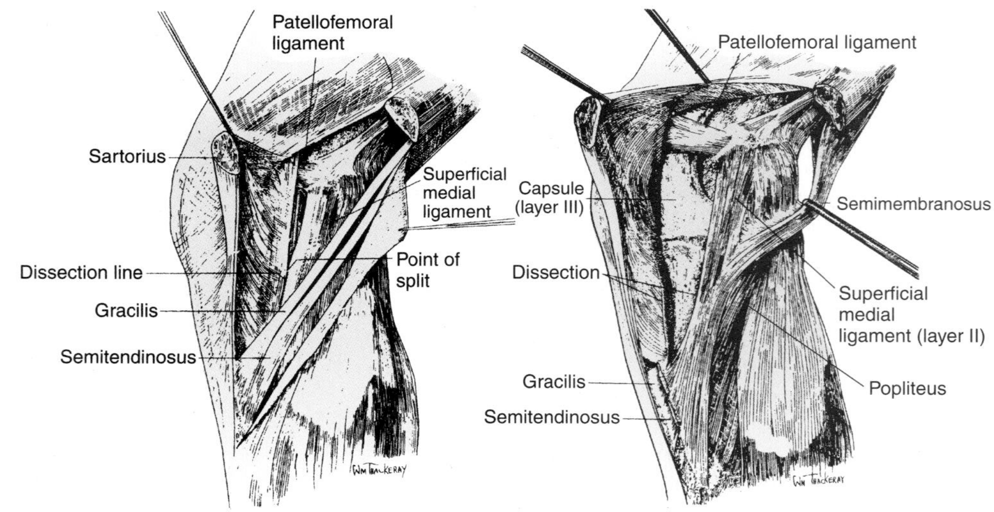

FIGURE 2–62 Medial structures of the knee. **A**, Superficial exposure. **B**, Deep exposure. (From Warren LF, Marshall JL: The supporting structures and layers of the medial side of the knee. J Bone Joint Surg [Am] 61:58, 1979.)

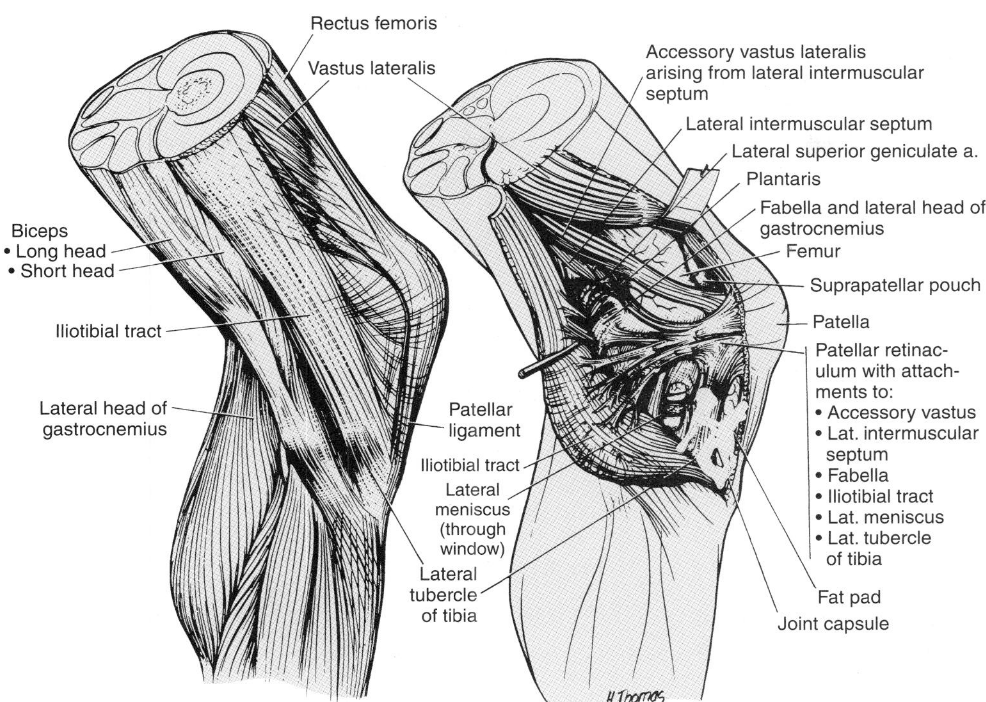

FIGURE 2–63 Lateral structures of the knee. **A**, Superficial exposure. **B**, Deep exposure. (From Seebacher JR, Inglis AE, Marshall JL, Warren RF: The structure of the posterolateral aspect of the knee. J Bone Joint Surg [Am] 64:533, 1982.)

IV. Ankle and Foot

A. Osteology

1. Anatomy—The 26 bones of the foot include 7 tarsal bones, 5 metatarsals, and 14 phalanges. The foot is divided into the hindfoot (talus and calcaneus), midfoot (navicular, cuboid, and three cuneiforms), and forefoot (metatarsals and phalanges).
   a. Tarsals—This network of bones includes the talus, calcaneus, cuboid, navicular, and three cuneiforms.
      (1) Talus—The talus articulates with the tibia and fibula in the ankle mortise and with the calcaneus and navicular distally. It is made up of a body that is wider anteriorly, with three articular surfaces (the trochlea [including surfaces for the malleoli articulations], and the posterior and middle calcaneal facets) and a posterior process (for the posterior talofibular ligament). The neck of the talus connects with the head, which in turn articulates with the navicular distally and the calcaneus inferiorly. The talus has no muscular attachments but has a groove posteriorly for the tendon of the FHL. Additionally, two thirds of the talus is covered with cartilage. The primary blood supply to the talar body is from the artery of the tarsal canal (posterior tibial artery). The other blood supplies include the superior neck vessels (anterior tibial artery) and the artery of the tarsal sinus (dorsalis pedis).
      (2) Calcaneus—The calcaneus is the largest and strongest bone in the foot. It has three surfaces that articulate with the talus: a large posterior facet, an anterior facet, and a middle facet. Distally, there is an articular surface that receives the cuboid bone. The sustentaculum tali is an overhanging horizontal eminence on the anteromedial surface of the calcaneus. The sustentaculum tali supports the middle articular surface above it and has an inferior groove for the FHL tendon.
      (3) Cuboid—Lying on the lateral aspect of the foot, the cuboid is grooved on the plantar surface by the peroneus longus and has four facets for articulation with the calcaneus, the lateral cuneiform, and the fourth and fifth metatarsals.
      (4) Navicular—The most medial tarsal bone, the navicular lies between the talus and the cuneiforms. Proximally, the surface is oval and concave for its articulation with the head of the talus. Distally, the navicular has three articular surfaces, one for each of the cuneiforms. The medial plantar projection serves as the insertion for the posterior tibial tendon.
      (5) Cuneiforms—These three bones (medial, intermediate, and lateral) articulate with the navicular and posterior cuboid (lateral cuneiform) and the first three metatarsals. The intermediate cuneiform does not extend as far distally as the medial

cuneiform, allowing the second metatarsal to "key" into place.

b. Metatarsals—Five bones, numbered from a medial to lateral direction, span the distance between the tarsal bones and phalanges. In general, their shape and function are similar to those of the metacarpals of the hand. The first metatarsal has a plantar cristae that articulates with the fibular and tibial sesamoids contained within the **flexor hallucis brevis** (FHB) tendon.

c. Phalanges—The phalanges of the foot are similar to those of the hand. The great toe has two phalanges, and the remaining digits have three.

2. Ossification—Each tarsal has a single ossification center except for the calcaneus, which has a second center posteriorly. The calcaneus, talus, and usually the cuboid are present at birth. The lateral cuneiform appears during the first year, the medial cuneiform during the second year, and the intermediate cuneiform and navicular during the third year. The posterior center for the calcaneus usually appears during the eighth year. The second through fifth metatarsals have two ossification centers: a primary center in the shaft and a secondary center for the head, which appears at age 5-8 years. The phalanges and first metatarsal have secondary centers at their bases that appear during the third or fourth year proximally and the sixth or seventh year distally.

B. Arthrology

1. Inferior tibiofibular joint—Formed by the medial distal fibula and the notched lateral distal tibia, this joint is supported by four ligaments: the anterior and posterior inferior tibiofibular ligaments, a transverse tibiofibular ligament, and an interosseous ligament. The anteroinferior tibiofibular ligament is an oblique band that connects the bones anteriorly. Avulsion of this ligament may result in a **Tillaux fracture**.

2. Ankle joint (Fig. 2–64; Table 2–59)—A ginglymus joint is formed by the malleoli and talus. The MCL (deltoid) comprises two layers: (1) the superficial-tibionavicular and tibiocalcaneal and (2) the deep anterior and posterior tibiotalar. The lateral fibular ligaments are the **anterior talofibular ligament** (ATFL), **calcaneofibular ligament** (CFL), and **posterior talofibular ligament** (PTFL). The ATFL is the weakest and is intracapsular (intracapsular thickening). The position of the ankle is critical when the lateral ligament complex is tested: plantar flexion tightens the ATFL and inversion with neutral flexion tightens the CFL.

3. Subtalar joint—Talar plantar facets articulate with the calcaneus. Stability is derived from four ligaments: the medial ligament, the lateral ligament, the interosseous talocalcaneal ligament, and the cervical ligament.

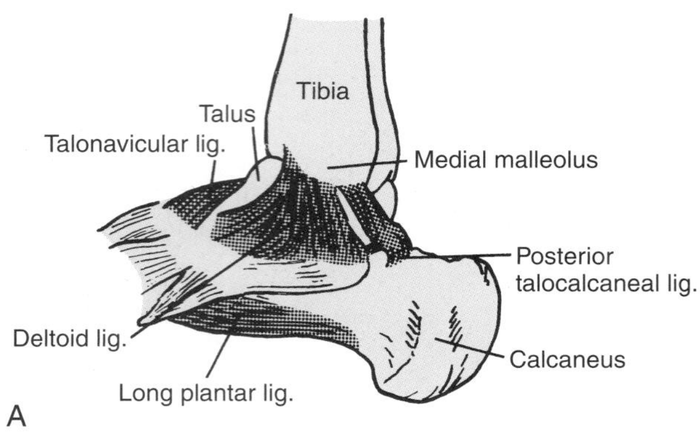

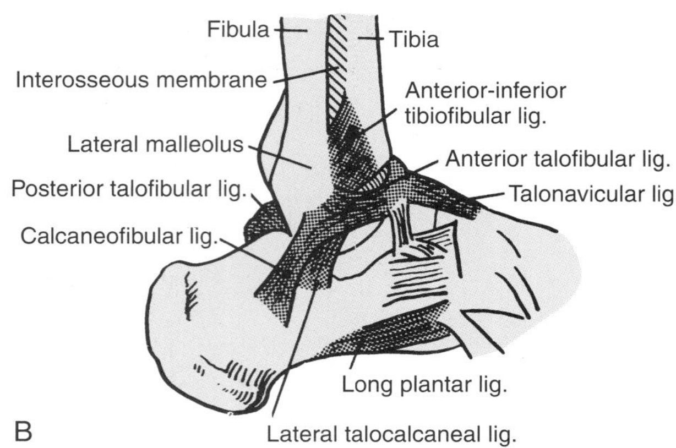

FIGURE 2–64 Ankle ligaments. **A**, Medial view. **B**, Lateral view. (From Weissman BN, Sledge CB: Orthopedic Radiology, pp 593-594. Philadelphia, WB Saunders, 1986.)

4. Intertarsal joints (Fig. 2–65)—There are several ligamentous structures that deserve notice (Table 2–60).

5. Other joints—Tarsometatarsal joints are gliding joints supported by dorsal, plantar, and interosseous ligaments. The base of the first metatarsal is not ligamentously connected to the second metatarsal. The Lisfranc ligament connects the medial (shortest) cuneiform to the second (longest) metatarsal; in about 20% of patients, it exists as

TABLE 2-59 ANKLE JOINT LIGAMENTS

Ligament	Origin	Insertion
Capsule	Tibia	Talus
Deltoid		
Tibionavicular	Medial malleolus	Navicular tuberosity
Tibiocalcaneal	Medial malleolus	Sustentaculum tali
Posterior tibiotalar	Medial malleolus	Inner side of talus
Anterior tibiotalar	Medial malleolus	Medial surface of talus
Anterior tibiofibular	Lateral malleolus	Transversely to talus anteriorly
Posterior tibiofibular	Lateral malleolus	Transversely to talus posteriorly
Calcaneofibular	Lateral malleolus	Obliquely to calcaneus posteriorly

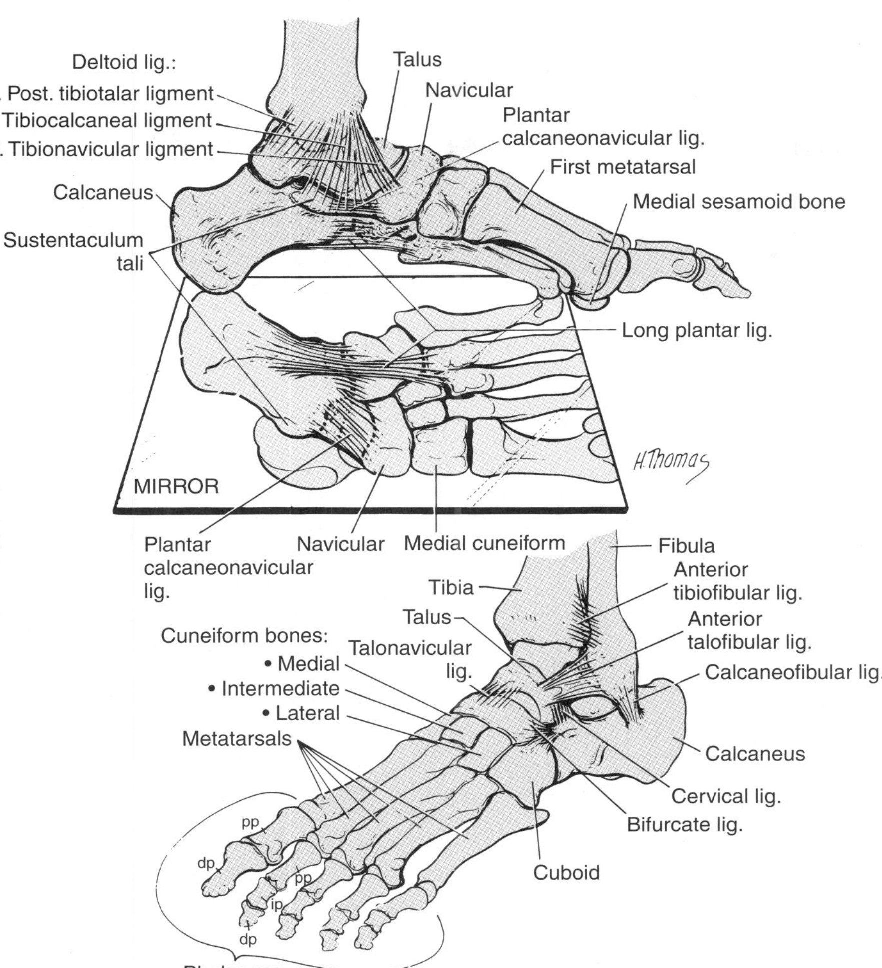

FIGURE 2–65 Ligaments of the foot. **A**, Medial view with inferior view highlighted with mirror. **B**, Lateral oblique view. (From Jahss MH: Disorders of the Foot, p 14. Philadelphia, WB Saunders, 1982.)

a plantar and dorsal structure. The deep transverse metatarsal ligaments interconnect the metatarsal heads. The digital nerve courses in a plantar direction under the transverse metatarsal ligament and is the spot where interdigital neuritis (Morton neuroma, usually the second or third interdigital space) occurs. Additionally, the transverse metatarsal ligament attaches the second metatarsal head to the fibular sesamoid. This ligament holds the hallucal sesamoids in place and gives the appearance of sesamoid subluxation when the first metatarsal moves medially in hallux valgus. The plantar and collateral ligaments support the metatarsophalangeal joints. The primary stabilizing structure of the metatarsophalangeal joint is the plantar plate. Interphalangeal joints are supported mainly by their capsules.

C. Muscles

1. Anatomy—The origins and insertions of muscles are shown in Figure 2–66, and the muscles and tendons about the foot and ankle are shown in Figure 2–67. The tendons are arranged about the toe as shown in Figure 2–68. The major tendons crossing the ankle joint include the following:

Posterior: Achilles

Lateral: peroneals with longus (superficial) and brevis (deep)

Anterior (from a lateral to medial direction): peroneus tertius, EDL, EHL, TA

Medial (**T**om, **D**ick, and **H**arry): **T**P, FD**L**, and F**H**L

TABLE 2-60 LIGAMENTS OF THE INTERTARSAL JOINTS

Ligament	Common Name	Origin	Insertion
Interosseous talocalcaneal	Cervical	Talus	Calcaneus
Calcaneocuboid/ calcaneonavicular	Bifurcate	Calcaneus	Cuboid and navicular
Calcaneocuboid-metatarsal	Long plantar	Calcaneus	Cuboid and first to fifth metatarsals
Plantar calcaneocuboid	Short plantar	Calcaneus	Cuboid
Plantar calcaneonavicular	Spring	Sustentaculum tali	Navicular
Tarsometatarsal	Lisfranc	Medial cuneiform	Second metatarsal base

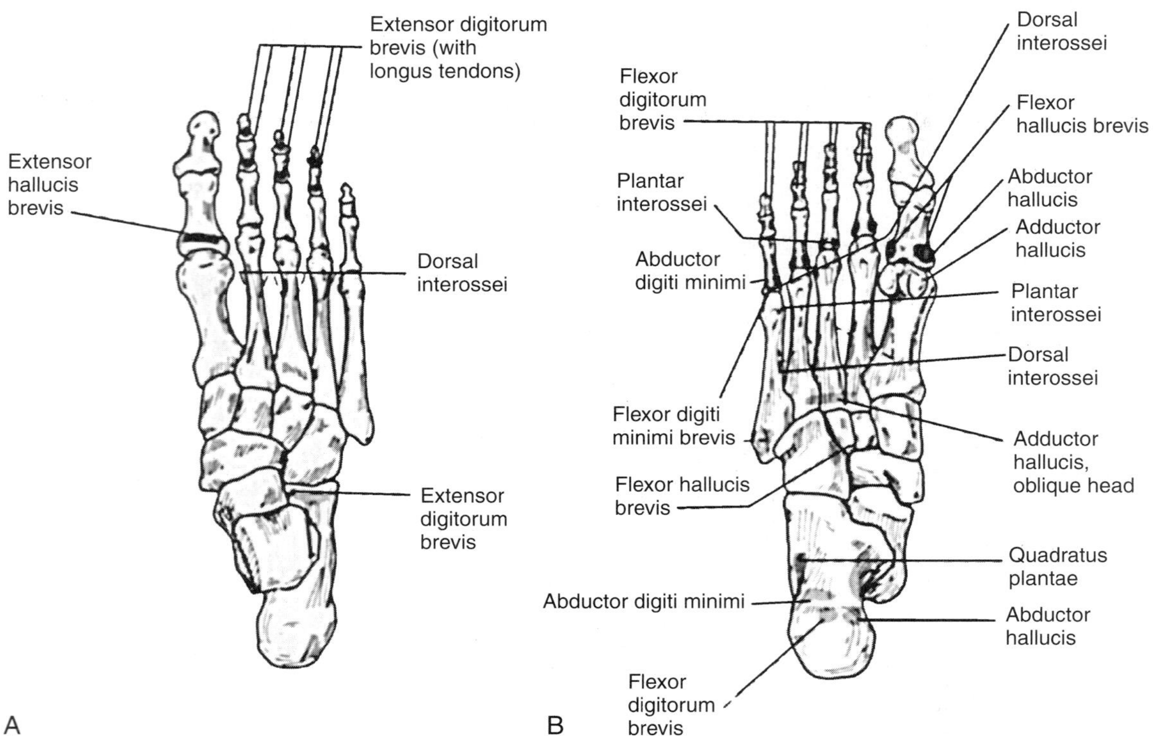

FIGURE 2–66 Origins and insertions of the muscles of the foot. **A**, Dorsal view. **B**, Plantar view. (From Jenkins DB: Hollinshead's Functional Anatomy of the Limbs and Back, 6th ed, Fig. 20-7. Philadelphia, WB Saunders, 1991.)

The Achilles tendon's maximum anteroposterior dimension on magnetic resonance imaging is 8 mm. The arrangement of muscles and tendons in the foot is best considered in layers (Table 2–61). On the plantar surface the intrinsic muscles dominate the first and third layers, and extrinsic tendons are more important in the second and fourth layers. There is one dorsal intrinsic muscle of the foot, which is the **extensor digitorum brevis** (EDB) (the lateral terminal branch of the deep peroneal nerve). Plantar heel spurs originate in the **flexor digitorum brevis** (FDB) (medial plantar nerve innervation). The lumbrical muscles are located plantar to the transverse metatarsal ligament, and interosseous tendons are dorsal. Key testable material comes from understanding which muscles are active during the different periods of the gait cycle (see Chapter 10, Rehabilitation: Gait, Amputations, Prostheses, Orthoses, and Neurologic lnjury). The posterior tibial tendon is the initiator of hindfoot inversion during gait (Chapter 10). This explains why a person cannot perform a single-stance toe rise with posterior tibial tendon deficiency and a normal Achilles tendon.

2. Neuromuscular interactions (Table 2–62)

D. Nerves (see Fig. 2–47)

1. Anatomy—The nerves of the ankle and foot are branches of the proximal nerves, discussed earlier.

a. Tibial nerve—The tibial nerve supplies all intrinsic foot muscles except the EDB (deep peroneal nerve). The tibial nerve splits into two branches (the medial and lateral plantar nerves) under the flexor retinaculum. Both of these nerves run in the second layer of the foot. The medial plantar nerve runs deep to the abductor hallucis, and the lateral plantar nerve runs obliquely under the cover of the quadratus plantae. The most proximal branch of the lateral plantar nerve is the nerve to the abductor digit quinti (Baxter nerve). The distribution of the sensory and motor branches of the plantar nerves is similar to that in the hand. The medial plantar nerve (like the median nerve of the hand) supplies plantar sensation to the medial 3½ digits and motor sensation to only a few plantar muscles (FHB, abductor hallucis, FDB, and the first lumbrical muscle). The lateral plantar nerve (like the ulnar nerve in the hand) supplies plantar sensation to the lateral 1½ digits and the remaining intrinsic muscles of the foot (Table 2–63). The digital nerve of the third web space consists of branches from both the medial and lateral plantar nerves.

b. Common peroneal nerve—This nerve splits into the superficial and deep branches in the leg and has terminal branches in the foot as well. The lateral terminal branch of the deep peroneal nerve ends in the proximal dorsal foot by supplying the EDB muscle. The medial terminal branch of the deep peroneal nerve supplies sensation to the first web space. The medial and intermediate dorsal cutaneous nerves of the superficial peroneal

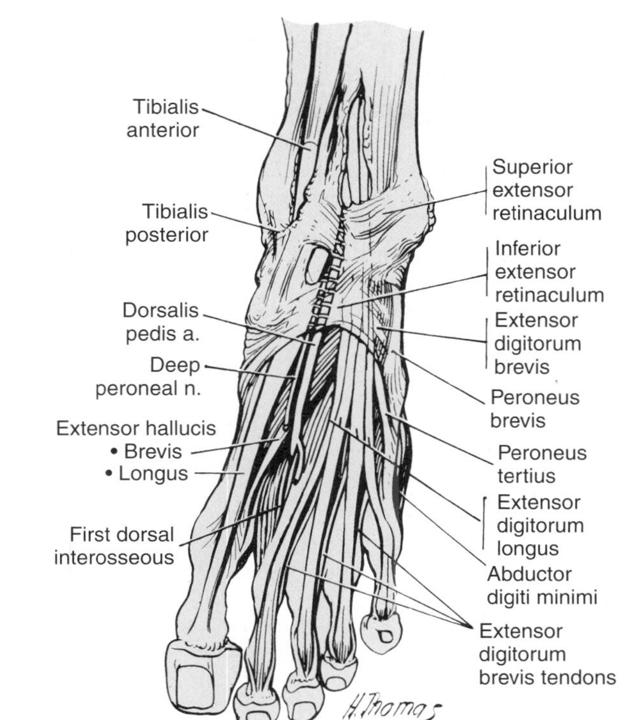

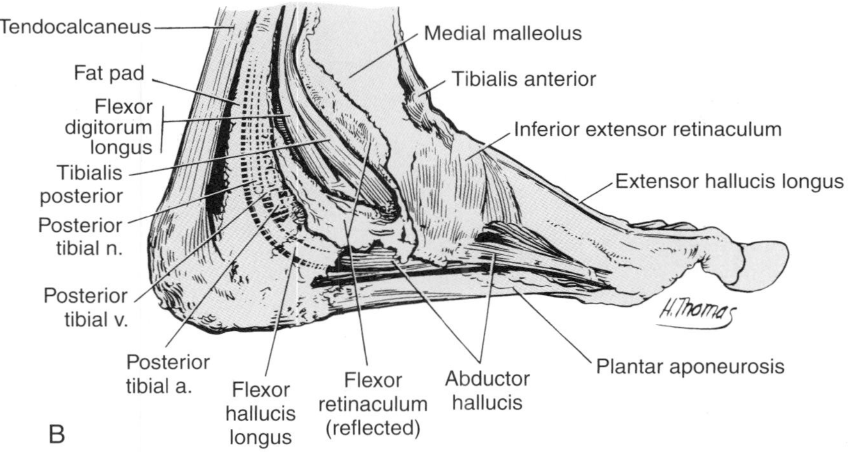

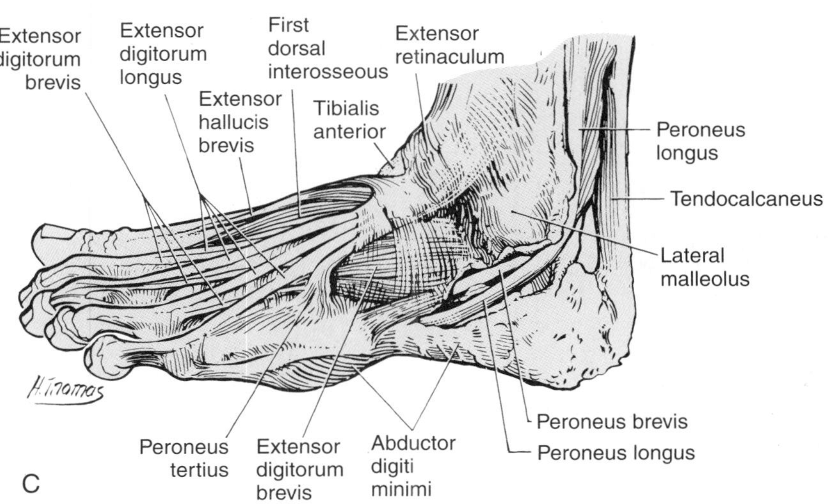

FIGURE 2–67 Muscles and tendons of the foot and ankle. **A**, Dorsal view. **B**, Medial view. **C**, Lateral view. (From Jahss MH: Disorders of the Foot, pp 18-20. Philadelphia, WB Saunders, 1982.)

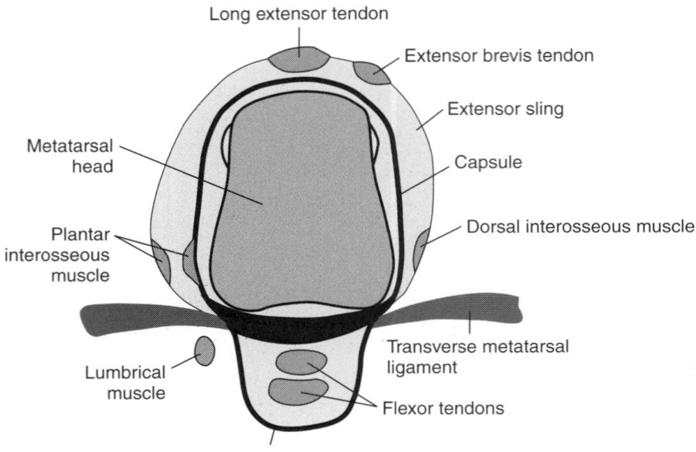

FIGURE 2–68 Cross section of the toe at the metatarsal base. The lumbricals are plantar to the transverse metatarsal ligament, and the interossei are dorsal to this ligament. The interossei and lumbricals (except the first lumbrical [medial plantar nerve]) are innervated by the lateral plantar nerve. (From Jahss MH: Disorders of the Foot, p 623. Philadelphia, WB Saunders, 1982.)

nerve supply the bulk of the remaining sensation to the dorsal foot. The dorsal intermediate branch is at risk during placement of the arthroscopic portal of the anterolateral ankle (discussed below). All sensation in the foot (except in the medial ankle and foot) is supplied by the sciatic nerve (saphenous nerve [termination of femoral nerve]). The dorsal medial cutaneous nerve (a branch of the superficial peroneal nerve) crosses the EHL from a lateral to medial direction and supplies sensation to the dorsomedial aspect of the great toe.

2. Neuromuscular interactions are summarized in Table 2–62.
3. Innervation—See Tables 2–44 and 2–63.

E. Vessels—Like the nerves that run with them, there are two main arteries that supply the ankle and foot.
   1. Dorsalis pedis artery—A continuation of the anterior tibial artery of the leg, this artery provides the blood supply to the dorsum of the foot via its lateral tarsal, medial tarsal, arcuate, and first dorsal metatarsal branches. Its largest branch, the deep plantar artery, runs between the first and second metatarsals and contributes to the plantar arch (see Fig. 2–67A).
   2. Posterior tibial artery—This artery divides into the medial and lateral plantar branches under the abductor hallucis muscle. The larger lateral branch receives the deep plantar artery and forms the plantar arch in the fourth layer of the plantar foot.

TABLE 2-61 MUSCLES OF THE ANKLE AND FOOT

Muscle	Origin	Insertion	Action	Innervation
Dorsal Layer				
Extensor digitorum brevis	Superolateral calcaneus	Base of proximal phalanges	Extend	Deep peroneal
First Plantar Layer				
Abductor hallucis	Calcaneal tuberosity	Base of great toe, proximal phalanx	Abduct great toe	Medial plantar
Flexor digitorum brevis (FDB)	Calcaneal tuberosity	Distal phalanges of second to fifth toes	Flex toes	Medial plantar
Abductor digiti minimi	Calcaneal tuberosity	Base of fifth toe	Abduct small toe	Lateral plantar
Second Plantar Layer				
Quadratus plantae	Medial and lateral calcaneus	FDL tendon	Helps flex distal phalanges	Lateral plantar
Lumbrical muscles	FDL tendon	Extensor digitorum longus tendon	Flex metatarsophalangeal, extend interphalangeal	Medial and lateral plantar
Flexor digitorum longus (FDL) and flexor hallucis longus	Tibia/fibula	Distal phalanges of digits	Flex toes/invert foot	Tibial
Third Plantar Layer				
Flexor hallucis brevis	Cuboid/lateral cuneiform	Proximal phalanx of great toe	Flex great toe	Medial plantar
Adductor hallucis	Oblique: second to fourth metatarsals	Proximal phalanx of great toe (lateral)	Adduct great toe	Lateral plantar
Flexor digiti minimi brevis	Base of fifth metatarsal head	Proximal phalanx of small toe	Flex small toe	Lateral plantar
Fourth Plantar Layer				
Dorsal interosseous	Metatarsal	Dorsal extensors	Abduct	Lateral plantar
Plantar interosseous (peroneus	Third to fifth metatarsals	Proximal phalanges medially	Adduct toes	Lateral plantar
longus and tibialis posterior)	Fibula/tibia	Medial cuneiform/navicular	Evert/invert foot	Superficial peroneal/tibial

Note: For abduction and adduction in the foot, the second toe serves as the reference.

TABLE 2-62 FOOT NEUROMUSCULAR INTERACTIONS

Foot Function	Muscle	Innervation
Inversion	Tibialis anterior	Deep peroneal nerve (L4)
	Tibialis posterior	Tibial nerve (S1)
Dorsiflexion	Tibialis anterior, extensor digitorum longus (EDL), extensor hallucis longus (EHL)	Deep peroneal nerve: TA (L4), EDL, and EHL (L5)
Eversion	Peroneus longus and brevis	Superficial peroneal nerve (S1)
Plantar flexion	Gastrocsoleus complex, flexor digitorum longus, flexor hallucis longus, tibialis posterior (also hindfoot inverter)	Tibial nerve (S1)

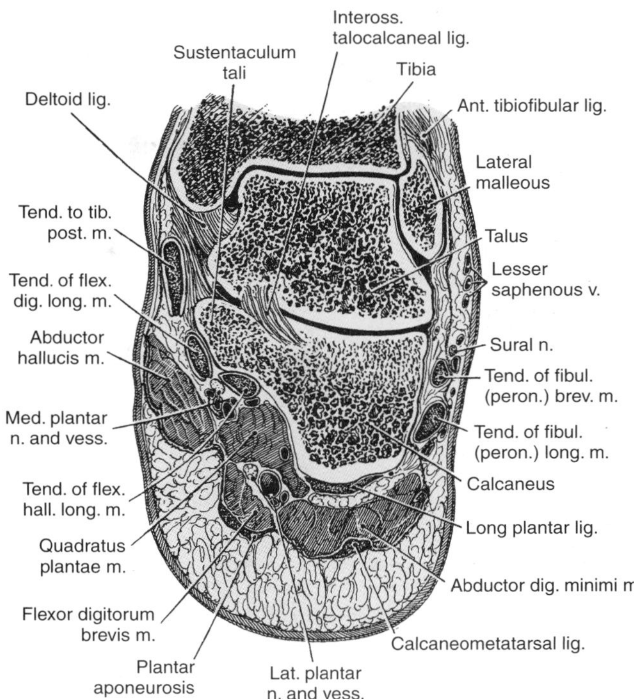

FIGURE 2–69 Vertical (coronal) section of the ankle. Note the groove of the flexor hallucis longus under the sustentaculum tali of the calcaneus. (From Woodburne RT, Burkel WE: Essentials of Human Anatomy, 9th ed. 1957, 1994 by Oxford University Press, Inc. Used by permission of Oxford University Press, Inc.)

F. Important neurovascular relationships—These may be seen in a coronal section (Fig. 2–69).

G. Surgical approaches (Table 2–64)

1. Anterior approach to the ankle—Primarily used for ankle fusion, this approach explores the interval between the EHL and EDL (both deep peroneal nerve). Before incising the extensor retinaculum, care must be taken to protect the superficial peroneal nerve. The deep peroneal nerve and anterior tibial artery, which lie directly in this interval, must be retracted medially along with the EHL.
2. Approach to the medial malleolus—This approach is commonly used for ORIF of ankle fractures. It is superficial and can be approached anteriorly or posteriorly. The anterior approach jeopardizes the saphenous nerve and the long saphenous vein; the posterior approach places at risk the structures running behind the medial malleolus in the following order: posterior **t**ibial tendon, F**D**L, posterior tibial **v**ein, posterior tibial **a**rtery, posterior tibial **n**erve, and FHL. (Use the **T**om, **D**ick and **v**ery **a**ngry **n**ervous **H**arry.) A posteromedial approach behind the medial malleolus can be made through the tendon sheath of the posterior tibialis.
3. Posteromedial approach to the ankle and foot—Used for clubfoot release in children, this approach begins medial to the Achilles tendon and curves distally along the medial border of the foot. Care must be taken to protect the posterior tibial nerve and artery and their branches. The posterior tibialis tendon is a landmark for the location of the subluxated navicular in the clubfoot.
4. Lateral approach to the ankle—Used for ORIF of distal fibula fractures, this approach is

TABLE 2-63 INNERVATION OF THE ANKLE AND FOOT

Nerves	Muscles Innervated
Medial plantar	Flexor hallucis brevis, abductor hallucis, flexor digitorum brevis, first lumbrical muscle
Lateral plantar	Pronator quadratus, abductor digiti minimi, flexor digiti minimi, adductor hallucis, interossei, second to fourth lumbrical muscles

TABLE 2-64 FOOT AND ANKLE SURGICAL APPROACHES

Approach	Interval	Structures at Risk
Anterior ankle	Extensor hallucis longus (deep peroneal nerve)	Superficial and deep peroneal nerve
	Extensor digitorum longus (deep peroneal nerve)	Anterior tibial artery
Anterior medial ankle		Saphenous nerve and vein
Distal fibula		Sural nerve (posterolateral) and superficial peroneal nerve (anterior with variable position)
Lateral hindfoot	Peroneus tertius (deep peroneal nerve) and peroneal tendons (supinator peroneal nerve)	Lateral branch of deep peroneal nerve
Anterolateral midfoot	Release of extensor digitorum brevis	Calcaneal navicular ligament

subcutaneous. The sural nerve (posterolateral) and the superficial peroneal nerve (anterior) must be avoided.

5. Lateral approach to the hindfoot—Used for triple arthrodesis, this approach explores the interneural plane between the peroneus tertius (deep peroneal nerve) and peroneal tendons (superficial peroneal nerve). The fat pad covering the sinus tarsi is removed, and the EDB is reflected from its origin to expose the joints. The lateral branch of the deep peroneal nerve (which supplies the EDB) must be protected in this approach. Deep penetration with an instrument used in this approach can injure the FHL.
6. Anterolateral approach to the midfoot—This approach requires release of the EDB. The risk of this approach, which is commonly used for excision of a calcaneonavicular bar, is to the calcaneal navicular (spring) ligament.
7. Approach to the midfoot and digits—This approach is direct and is consequently not discussed in detail. In general, care must be taken to protect the digital nerves and arteries.

H. Arthroscopy (Table 2–65)—The portals used in ankle arthroscopy can put important structures at risk. The anterolateral portal can jeopardize the dorsal intermediate cutaneous branch of the superficial peroneal nerve. The anteromedial portal can damage the greater saphenous vein. Anterior central portals are no longer recommended because of the risk to the dorsalis pedis artery. Posterior medial portals can injure the posterior tibial artery and are consequently not recommended, and posterior lateral portals can injure the sural nerve.

TABLE 2-65 PORTALS FOR ANKLE ARTHROSCOPY

Portal	Location	Structures at Risk
Anterolateral	Medial to lateral malleolus, lateral to peroneus tertius	Dorsal intermediate cutaneous branch of superficial peroneal nerve
Anteromedial	Medial to tibialis anterior tendon, lateral to medial malleolus	Saphenous nerve and vein
Posterolateral	Medial to peroneal tendons, lateral to Achilles tendon	Sural nerve and small saphenous vein
Anterocentral	Medial to extensor digitorum communis, lateral to extensor hallucis longus	Deep peroneal nerve and anterior tibial artery

Selected Bibliography

Arnoczky SP, Warren RF: Microvasculature of the human. Am J Sports Med 10:90–95, 1982.

Bohlman HH: The Neck. In D'Ambrosia R, ed: Musculoskeletal Disorders. Philadelphia, JB Lippincott, 1977.

Bora FW: The Pediatric Upper Extremity. Philadelphia, WB Saunders, 1986.

Browner BD, Jupiter JB, Levine AM, et al: Skeletal Trauma. Philadelphia, WB Saunders, 1992.

Callaghan JJ, ed: Anatomy Self-Assessment Examination. Park Ridge, IL, American Academy of Orthopaedic Surgeons, 1991.

Callaghan JJ, ed: Anatomy Self-Assessment Examination. Park Ridge, IL, American Academy of Orthopaedic Surgeons, 1996.

Cervical Spine Research Education Committee: The Cervical Spine, 2nd ed. Philadelphia, JB Lippincott, 1989.

Chapman MW, ed: Operative Orthopaedics. Philadelphia, JB Lippincott, 1988.

Chapman MW, ed: Gray's Anatomy, 30th Am ed. Philadelphia, Lea & Febiger, 1985.

Cohen MS, Bruno RJ: The collateral ligaments of the elbow. Clin Orthop 383:123–130, 2001.

Cooper DE, O'Brien SJ, Warren RF: Supporting layers of the glenohumeral joint. Clin Orthop 289:1441–1455, 1993.

Corley FG, ed: Shoulder and Elbow Self-Assessment Examination. Park Ridge, IL, American Academy of Orthopaedic Surgeons, 1996.

Corley FG, ed: Shoulder and Elbow Self-Assessment Examination. Park Ridge, IL, American Academy of Orthopaedic Surgeons, 1999.

Crock HV: An atlas of the arterial supply of the head and neck of the femur in man. Clin Orthop Relat Res 152:17–27, 1980.

DeCoster TA, ed: Anatomy Self-Assessment Examination. Park Ridge, IL, American Academy of Orthopaedic Surgeons, 1999.

DeCoster TA, ed: Anatomy Self-Assessment Examination. Park Ridge, IL, American Academy of Orthopaedic Surgeons, 2002.

DeLee JC, Drez D Jr.: Orthopaedic Sports Medicine: Principles and Practice. Philadelphia, WB Saunders, 1994.

Doyle JR: Anatomy of the finger flexor tendon sheath and pulley system. J Hand Surg [Am] 13:4734–4784, 1988.

Girgis FG, Marshall JL, Monajem ARS: The cruciate ligaments of the knee joint: Anatomical, functional, and experimental analysis. Clin Orthop 106:216–231, 1975.

Green DP, Hotchkiss RN, Pederson WC: Green's Operative Hand Surgery, 4th ed. New York, Churchill Livingstone, 1999.

Harding K: The direct lateral approach to the hip. J Bone Joint Surg [Br] 64:171–179, 1982.

Henry AK: Extensive Exposure, 2nd ed. New York, Churchill Livingstone, 1973.

Hollinshead, WH: Anatomy for Surgeons, vol 3, 2nd ed. New York, Harper & Row, 1969.

Hoppenfeld S: Orthopaedic Neurology: A Diagnostic Guide to Neurological Levels. Philadelphia, Lippincott-Raven, 1997.

Hoppenfeld S, DeBoer P: Orthopaedics: The Anatomic Approach. Philadelphia, J.B Lippincott, 1984.

Jahss MH: Disorders of the Foot. Philadelphia, WB Saunders, 1987.

Jenkins DB: Hollinshead's Functional Anatomy of the Limbs and Back, 6th ed. Philadelphia, WB Saunders, 1991.

Kaplan EB: Surgical Approaches to the Neck, Cervical Spine, and Upper Extremity. Philadelphia, WB Saunders, 1966.

Ludloff K: The open reduction of the congenital hip dislocation by an anterior incision. Am J Orthop Surg 10:438, 1913.

Magee DJ: Orthopaedic Physical Assessment. Philadelphia, WB Saunders, 1987.

Mooney JF, Siegel DB, Koman LA: Ligamentous injuries of the wrist in athletes. Clin Sports Med 11:129–139, 1992.

Morrey BF, An KN: Articular and ligamentous contributions to the stability of the elbow joint. J Sports Med 11:315–319, 1983.

Morrey BF, An KN: Functional anatomy of the ligaments of the elbow. Clin Orthop 210:84–90, 1985.

Myerson MS, ed: Foot and Ankle Self-Assessment Examination. Park Ridge, IL, American Academy of Orthopaedic Surgeons, 1997.

Myerson MS, ed: Foot and Ankle Self-Assessment Examination. Park Ridge, IL, American Academy of Orthopaedic Surgeons, 2000.

Netter, FH: The CIBA Collection of Medical Illustrations, vol 8: Musculoskeletal System, Part I Summit, NJ, Ciba-Geigy, 1987.

Orthopaedic Knowledge Update Home Study Syllabus I, II, and III. Chicago, American Academy of Orthopaedic Surgeons, 1984, 1987, 1990.
Place HM, ed: Adult Spine Self-Assessment Examination. Park Ridge, IL, American Academy of Orthopaedic Surgeons, 1997.
Place HM, ed: Adult Spine Self-Assessment Examination. Park Ridge, IL, American Academy of Orthopaedic Surgeons, 2000.
Rockwood CA Jr, Green DP, eds: Fractures in Adults, 3rd ed. Philadelphia, JB Lippincott, 1991.
Rothman RH, Simeon FA: The Spine, 2nd ed. Philadelphia, WB Saunders, 1982.
Ruge D, Wiltse LL, eds: Spinal Disorders: Diagnosis and Treatment. Philadelphia, Lea & Febiger, 1977.
Sarrafian SK: Anatomy of the Foot and Ankle. Philadelphia, JB Lippincott, 1983.
Seebacher JR, Inglis AE, Marshall JL, et al: The structure of the posterolateral aspect of the knee. J Bone Joint Surg [Am] 64:536–541, 1982.
Steinberg ME: The Hip and Its Disorders. Philadelphia, WB Saunders, 1991.
Tubiana R: The Hand. Philadelphia, WB Saunders, 1985.
Turkel SJ, Panio MW, Marshall JL, Girgis FG: Stabilizing mechanisms preventing anterior dislocation of the gleno-humeral joint. J Bone Joint Surg [Am] 63:1208–1217, 1981.
Verbiest HA: Lateral approach to the cervical spine: Technique and indications. J Neurosurg 28:191–203, 1968.
Warren IF, Marshall JL: The supporting structures and layers on the medial side of the knee. J Bone Joint Surg [Am] 61:56–62, 1979.
Watkins RG: Surgical Approaches to the Spine. New York, Springer-Verlag, 1983.
Weissman BN, Sledge CB: Orthopedic Radiology. Philadelphia, WB Saunders, 1986.
Wilson FC, Dirschl DR: Orthopaedics: Pre-Test and Self-Assessment and Review. New York, McGraw-Hill, 1996.
Woodburne RT, Burkel WE: Essentials of Human Anatomy, 9th ed. New York, Oxford University Press, 1994.

CHAPTER 3

Pediatric Orthopaedics

Todd A. Milbrandt AND Daniel J. Sucato

CONTENTS

I. Bone Dysplasias (Dwarfism)

A. Introduction—By definition, dysplasia means abnormal development. Bone dysplasias typically cause shortening of the involved bones, affecting specific portions of the growing bone (Fig. 3–1), thereby leading to the term *dwarfism*. *Proportionate dwarfism* implies a symmetrical decrease in both trunk and limb length (e.g., mucopolysaccharidoses). *Disproportionate dwarfing* conditions are subdivided into the short-trunk variety (e.g., Kniest's syndrome–spondyloepiphyseal dysplasia) or the short-limb variety (e.g., achondroplasia, diastrophic dysplasia). Short-limb dwarfism can be subdivided by the region of the limb that is short (e.g., rhizomelic-proximal, mesomelic-middle, acromelic-distal). The summation of all the dwarfisms is found in Table 3–1.

B. Achondroplasia

1. Introduction and etiology—Achondroplasia is the most common form of disproportionate dwarfism. It is an autosomal dominant (AD) condition, with an 80% prevalence of a spontaneous mutation in the **fibroblast growth factor receptor 3** (FGFR3). This disproportionate, short-limbed form of dwarfism is caused by abnormal endochondral bone formation that is more affected than appositional growth. Anatomically, achondroplasia is categorized as a physeal dysplasia. The defect involves a failure in the cartilaginous proliferative zone of the physis. Achondroplasia is a quantitative, not a qualitative, cartilage defect. It may be associated with advanced paternal age.

2. Signs and symptoms—Clinical features include a normal trunk and short limbs (rhizomelic). Typically, these patients have frontal bossing, button noses, small nasal bridges, trident hands (inability to approximate extended middle and ring fingers) (Fig. 3–2), thoracolumbar kyphosis (which usually resolves around the age of ambulation), lumbar stenosis (most likely to cause disability) and excessive lordosis (short pedicles with decreased interpedicular distances), radial head subluxation, and hypotonia during the first year of life. Involved children have normal intelligence but delayed motor milestones. Although sitting height may be normal, standing height is below the third percentile. Radiographs show increasingly narrowed interpedicular distance in the distal spine (L1-S1), with pedicular shortening, T12/L1 wedging, generalized posterior vertebral scalloping, delayed appearance of growth plates, and a pelvis that is wider than it is deep (''champagne glass'' pelvic outlet). Achondroplasia may also be associated with radial or tibial bowing, coxa valga, genu varum (with a disproportionately long fibula), and metaphyseal flaring, with an inverted V-shaped distal femoral physis. Neurologic symptoms are usually related to nerve root or spinal cord compression, which can occur at any level, including the foramen magnum (which may cause periods of apnea).

3. Treatment—Surgical options for symptomatic lumbar stenosis include decompression and

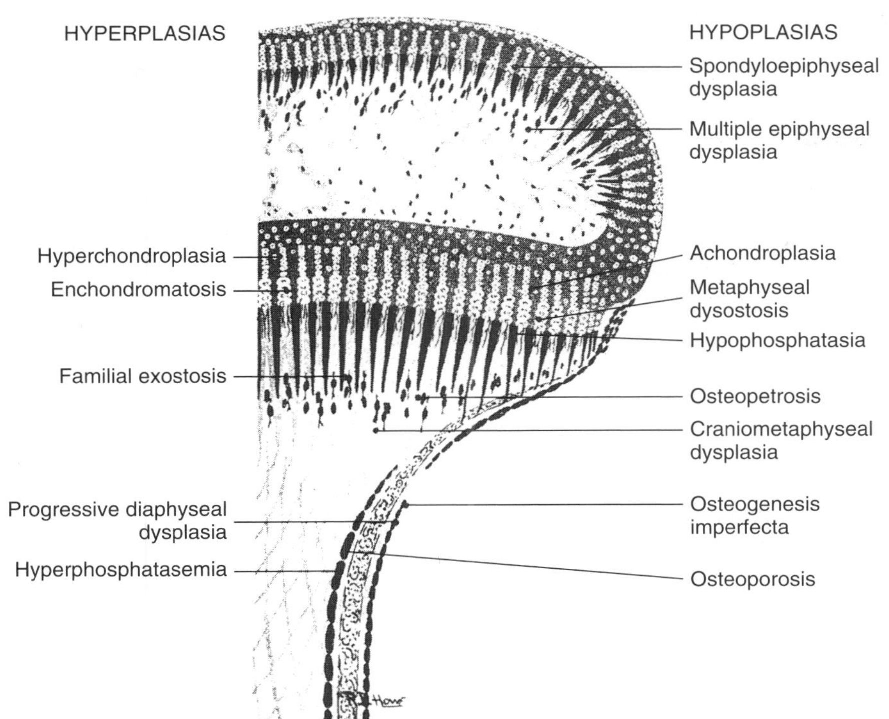

FIGURE 3–1 Location of abnormalities leading to dysplasias. (Adapted from Rubin P: Dynamic Classification of Bone Dysplasias. Chicago, Year Book Medical Publishers, 1964.)

fusion of the spine for a developing neurologic deficit (usually in children older than age 10). Symptomatic stenosis at the foramen magnum may require decompression. In rare cases, young children have progressive kyphosis without neurologic problems that fail bracing. In such cases, anterior fusion with strut grafting and posterior fusion are indicated for residual kyphosis greater than 60 degrees by age 5 years. Tibial osteotomies or hemiepiphyseodesis are indicated for genu varum. Limb-lengthening procedures via callodiastasis (lengthening through a metaphyseal corticotomy) have been well described, with a high rate of complications. The patients still have the other underlying problems, however, and limb-lengthening procedures remain controversial in achondroplastic patients.

4. Pseudoachondroplasia—This disorder is clinically similar to achondroplasia. The inheritance pattern is AD with a defect on chromosome 19 within the **cartilage oligometric matrix protein** (COMP). In contrast to achondroplasia, the affected children have normal facies. Radiographs demonstrate metaphyseal flaring and delayed epiphyseal ossification. Orthopaedic manifestations include cervical instability; scoliosis with increased lumbar

TABLE 3-1 SUMMATION OF MAJOR DWARFISMS

Dwarfism	Genetic Defect	Inheritance	Pathopneumonic Feature
Achondroplasia	FGFR3	AD	Trident hands and lumbar kyphosis
Pseudoachondroplasia	COMP	AD	Normal facies and cervical instability
Spondyloepiphyseal dysplasia	Type II collagen	Congenita—AD; tarda—X-linked recessive	Epiphyseal fragmentation with spine involvement
Kniest's syndrome	Type II collagen	AD	Retinal detachment and dumbbell-shaped bone
Jansen's metaphyseal chondroplasia	PTHRP	AD	Hypercalcemia with metaphyseal expansion
Schmid's metaphyseal chondroplasia	Type X collagen	AD	Coxa vara with proximal femur involvement
McKusick's metaphyseal chondroplasia	Unknown COMP	AR	Odontoid hypoplasia
Multiple epiphyseal dysplasia	Type II collagen	AD	Bilateral hip involvement
Mucopolysaccharidosis (see Table 3–2)			
Diastrophic dysplasia	Sulfate transport protein	AR	Cauliflower ears and kyphoscoliosis
Cleidocranial dysplasia	CBFA1	AD	Aplasia of clavicles and coxa vara

AD, autosomal dominant; AR, autosomal recessive; CBFA1, transcription factor for osteocalcin; COMP, cartilage oligomeric matrix protein; FGFR3, fibroblast growth factor receptor 3; PTHRP, parathyroid hormone–related peptide.

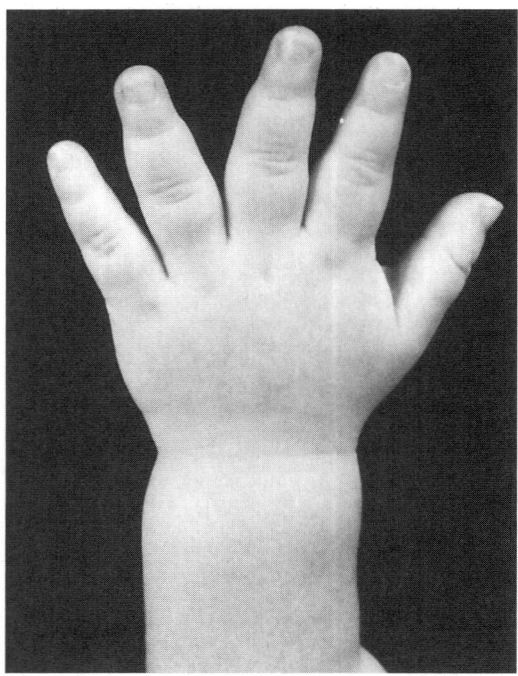

FIGURE 3–2 Trident hand characteristic of achondroplasia. Note the space between the middle and ring fingers. (From Herring JA: Tachdjian's Pediatric Orthopaedics, 4th ed, p 1685. Philadelphia, WB Saunders, 2008.)

lordosis; significant lower extremity bowing; and hip, knee, and elbow flexion contractures with precocious osteoarthritis.

C. Spondyloepiphyseal dysplasia—Two forms are generally recognized and must be differentiated from **multiple epiphyseal dysplasia** (MED). MED and spondyloepiphyseal dysplasia involve abnormal epiphyseal development in the upper and lower extremities. The distinguishing feature of spondyloepiphyseal dysplasia is the added typical spine involvement, and the genetic defect is within the gene encoding **type II collagen**.
   1. Congenita form—Short-trunked dwarfism associated with primary involvement of the vertebra (beaking) and epiphyseal centers (affects the proliferative zone), clinical heterogenicity, and AD inheritance. Clinically more severe than the tarda form. Delayed appearance of the epiphysis, flattened facies, platyspondyly (delayed ossification), kyphoscoliosis, odontoid hypoplasia, coxa vara, and genu valgum are common. Patients should also be screened for associated retinal detachment and myopia.
   2. Tarda form—These patients have an X-linked recessive inheritance and late (ages 8-10) manifestations of the disorder, which affects primarily the spine and large joints. Clinically less severe than the congenita form. Hips may be dislocated, and affected children are often susceptible to premature osteoarthritis (osteotomies may be helpful) and scoliosis (treated like idiopathic scoliosis). No lower extremity angular deformities.

D. Chondrodysplasia punctata—Characterized by multiple punctate calcifications seen on radiographs during infancy. The AD form (Conradi-Hünermann) has a wide variation of clinical expression. The severe, autosomal recessive (AR), rhizomelic form is usually fatal during the first year of life. Cataracts, asymmetrical limb shortening that may require surgical correction, and spinal deformities are common.

E. Kniest's syndrome—AD; short-trunked, disproportionate dwarfism with joint stiffness/contractures, scoliosis, kyphosis, dumbbell-shaped femora, and hypoplastic pelvis and spine. The genetic abnormality is within the gene for type II collagen. Radiographs show osteopenia and dumbbell-shaped bones. Respiratory problems and cleft palate are common. Associated retinal detachment and myopia require an ophthalmology consultation. Early therapy for joint contractures is required. Reconstructive procedures may be required for early hip degenerative arthritis. Otitis media and hearing loss are frequent.

F. Metaphyseal chondrodysplasia—Heterogeneous group of disorders characterized by metaphyseal changes of tubular bones with normal epiphyses. The defect appears to be in the proliferative and hypertrophic zones of the physis. Several types are recognized, including the following.
   1. Jansen's (rare)—Most severe form. The genetic defect is in **parathyroid hormone–related peptide** (PTHRP). AD, retarded, markedly short-limbed dwarf with wide eyes, monkey-like stance, and hypercalcemia. Striking bulbous metaphyseal expansion of long bones is a distinctive radiographic finding.
   2. Schmid's—More common, less severe form. The genetic defect is in **type X collagen**. AD, short-limbed dwarf not diagnosed until patient is older, due to coxa vara and genu varum. Predominantly involves the proximal femur. Gait is often Trendelenburg, and patients have increased lumbar lordosis. Often confused with rickets, but laboratory test results are normal.
   3. McKusick's—AR, cartilage-hair dysplasia (hypoplasia of cartilage and small diameter of hair) is seen most commonly among the Amish population and in Finland. Atlantoaxial instability is common (odontoid hypoplasia). Ankle deformity develops due to fibular overgrowth distally. These patients may have abnormal immunologic competence and have an increased risk for malignancies. In addition, they may have intestinal malabsorption and megacolon.

G. MED—Short-limbed, disproportionate dwarfism that often is not manifested until between the ages of 5 and 14. Must be differentiated from spondyloepiphyseal dysplasia. A mild form (Ribbing's) and a more severe form (Fairbanks') exist. MED is characterized by irregular, delayed ossification at multiple epiphyses (Fig. 3–3). Short, stunted metacarpals/metatarsals, irregular proximal femora, abnormal ossification (tibial "slant sign" and flattened femoral condyles, patella with double layer), valgus knees (consider early osteotomy), waddling gait, and early hip arthritis are common. The proximal femoral involvement can be confused with Perthes' disease; MED is bilateral

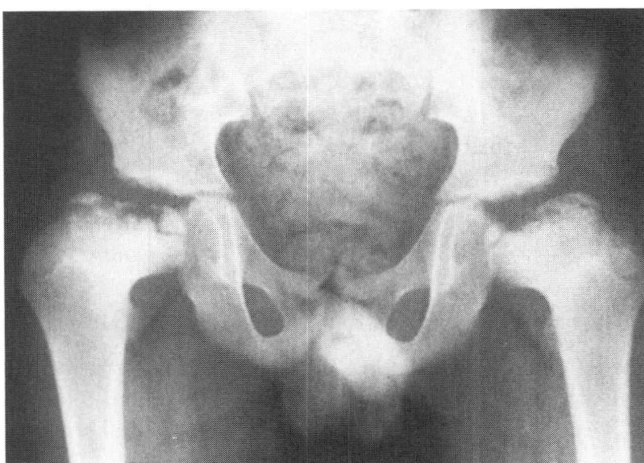

FIGURE 3–3 Multiple epiphyseal dysplasia. Radiographs of the pelvis at 6 years old show abnormal bilateral femoral heads. (From Benson M, Fixen J, Macnicol M: Children's Orthopaedics and Fractures, p 52. New York, Churchill Livingstone, 1994.)

and symmetrical, has early acetabular changes, and does not have metaphyseal cysts.

H. Dysplasia epiphysealis hemimelica (Trevor's disease)—Essentially an epiphyseal osteochondroma. Calcifications are seen within the joint. Most commonly seen at the knee. Usually affects only one joint. Partial excision of the prominent overgrowth (if symptomatic) and later osteotomies may be required. Recurrence is a common complication.

I. Progressive diaphyseal dysplasia (Camurati-Engelmann disease)—AD; affected children are often "late walkers" (because of associated muscle weakness), with symmetrical cortical thickening of long bones. Radiographs demonstrate widened, fusiform diaphyses with increased bone formation and sclerosis. The tibia, femur, and humerus are most often involved (in that order), affecting only the diaphyseal portion of bone. Symptomatic treatment includes salicylates, nonsteroidal anti-inflammatory drugs (NSAIDs), and steroids for refractory cases. Watch for leg-length inequality.

J. Mucopolysaccharidosis—In contrast to the aforementioned conditions, these forms of dwarfism are easily differentiated based on the presence of complex sugars found in the urine. They produce a proportionate dwarfism caused by accumulation of mucopolysaccharides due to a hydrolase enzyme deficiency. The four main types are **Morquio's, Hurler's, Hunter's,** and **Sanfilippo's** syndromes (Table 3–2).

1. Morquio's syndrome (AR) is the most common form and presents by age 18 months to 2 years with waddling gait, knock-knees, thoracic kyphosis, cloudy corneas, and normal intelligence. Morquio's syndrome is associated with urinary excretion of keratan sulfate. Bony changes include a thickening skull; wide ribs; anterior beaking of vertebrae; a wide, flat pelvis; coxa vara with unossified femoral heads; and bullet-shaped metacarpals. C1-C2 instability (due to odontoid hypoplasia) can be seen with Morquio's syndrome presenting with myelopathy and requiring decompression and cervical fusion.
2. Hurler's syndrome (AR) is the most severe form and is associated with urinary excretion of dermatan/heparan sulfate. Associated with mental retardation. Bone marrow transplantation has increased the life span for patients with this disorder.
3. Hunter's syndrome (sex-linked recessive) is associated with urinary excretion of dermatan/heparan sulfate. Associated with mental retardation. Bone marrow transplantation has increased the life span for patients with this disorder.
4. Sanfilippo's syndrome (AR) is associated with urinary excretion of heparan sulfate. Associated with mental retardation. Bone marrow transplantation has increased the life span for the patients with this disorder.

K. Diastrophic dysplasia—AR; severe, short-limbed dwarfism associated with a deficiency in sulfate transport protein. This "twisted" dwarf classically has a cleft palate (59%), severe joint contractures (especially hip and knee), cauliflower ears (80%), hitchhiker thumb, rigid clubfeet, **cervical kyphosis** (often severe, requiring immediate treatment), thoracolumbar kyphoscoliosis (83%), spina bifida occulta, and atlantoaxial instability. Risk of quadriplegia is a major concern. Surgical release of clubfoot deformities, osteotomies for contractures, and spinal fusion are often required.

L. Cleidocranial dysplasia (dysostosis)—AD; proportionate dwarfism that affects bones formed by intramembranous ossification. Defect in CBFA1 (transcription factor for osteocalcin). Patients present with dwarfism and aplasia of a portion of or the entire clavicle (Fig. 3–4). Usually the unilateral but often the lateral part of the clavicle is missing (no intervention necessary), and there are delayed skull suture closure, frontal bossing, coxa vara (consider intertrochanteric valgus osteotomy if neck–shaft angle is less than

TABLE 3-2 MUCOPOLYSACCHARIDOSES

Syndrome	Inheritance	Intelligence	Cornea	Urinary Excretion	Other
Hurler's	AR	MR	Cloudy	Dermatan/heparan sulfate	Worst prognosis
Hunter's	XR	MR	Clear	Dermatan/heparan sulfate	
Sanfilippo's	AR	MR	Clear	Heparin sulfate	Normal until 2 yr old
Morquio's	AR	Normal	Cloudy	Keratan sulfate	Most common

AR, autosomal recessive; MR, mentally retarded; XR, x-linked recessive.

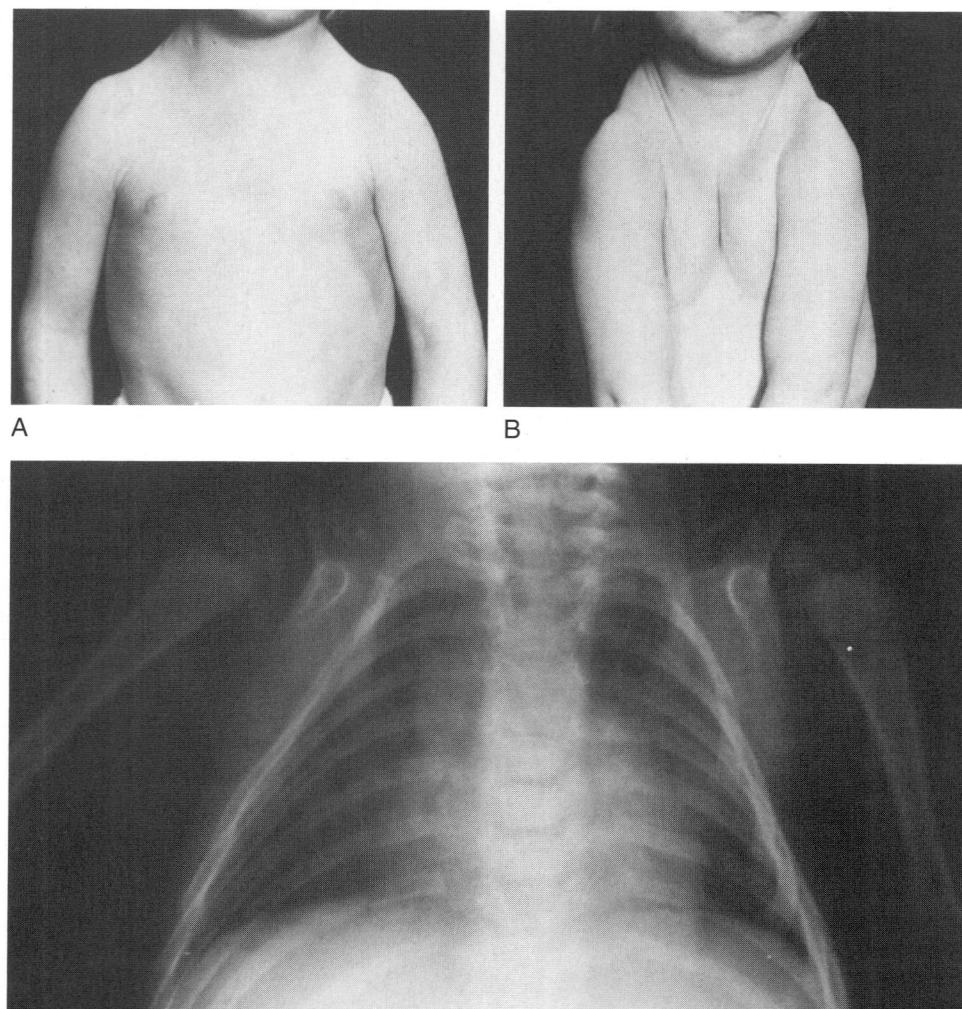

FIGURE 3–4 **A**, Clinical photograph of cleidocranial dysostosis, with the shoulders in normal position. **B**, Clinical photograph with the shoulders approximated. **C**, Radiograph of the chest and shoulders showing aplasia of the clavicles bilaterally. (From Benson M, Fixen J, Macnicol M: Children's Orthopaedics and Fractures, p 364. New York, Churchill Livingstone, 1994.)

100 degrees), delayed ossification of the pubis, and wormian-type bone.

M. Dysplasias associated with benign bone growth—Include multiple hereditary exostosis (osteochondromatosis), fibrous dysplasia, Ollier's disease (enchondromatosis), and Maffucci's syndrome (enchondromatosis and hemangiomas). These entities are discussed in Chapter 9, Orthopaedic Pathology.

II. Chromosomal and Teratologic Disorders

A. Down syndrome (trisomy 21)—Most common chromosomal abnormality; its incidence increases with maternal age. Usually associated with ligamentous laxity, hypotonia, mental retardation, heart disease (50%), endocrine disorders (hypothyroidism and diabetes), and premature aging. Orthopaedic problems include metatarsus primus varus, pes planus, spinal abnormalities (**atlantoaxial instability** [Fig. 3–5], scoliosis [50%], spondylolisthesis [6%]), hip instability (open reduction with or without osteotomy usually required), slipped capital femoral epiphysis (look for hypothyroidism), patellar dislocation, and symptomatic planovalgus feet. Atlantoaxial instability may be subtle in its presentation but commonly presents as a loss or change in motor milestones. Atlantoaxial instability is evaluated with flexion-extension radiographs of the cervical spine. Asymptomatic children with instability should avoid contact sports, diving, and gymnastics.

B. Turner's syndrome—45,XO females with short stature, sexual infantilism, webbed neck, and cubitus valgus. Idiopathic scoliosis is common. Growth hormone therapy can exacerbate scoliosis. Watch for osteoporosis. Genu valgum and shortening of the fourth and fifth metacarpals usually require no treatment. Malignant hyperthermia is common with anesthetic use. Must be differentiated from Noonan's syndrome (shared appearance except for normal gonadal development, mental retardation, and more severe scoliosis).

C. Prader-Willi syndrome—Partial chromosome 15 deletion (missing portion from father) causing a floppy, hypotonic infant who becomes an intellectually impaired, obese adult with an insatiable appetite.

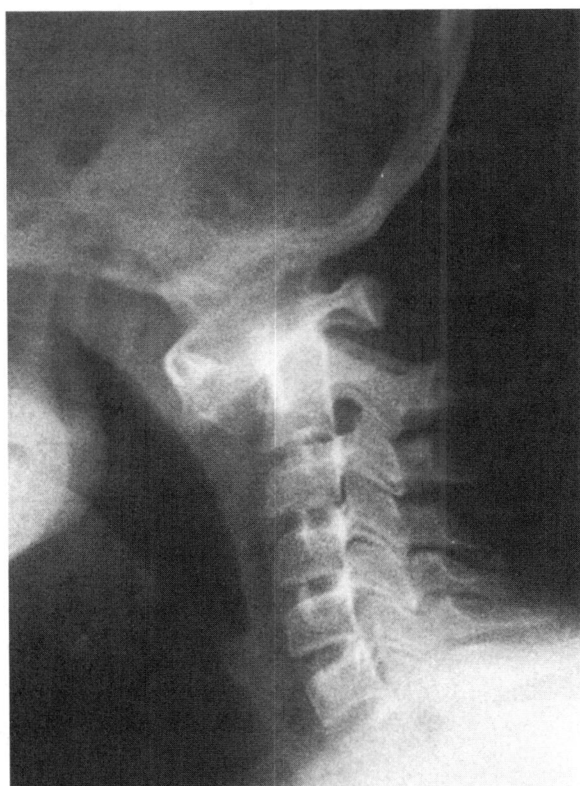

FIGURE 3–5 Eleven-year-old with Down syndrome showing gross atlantoaxial instability. His gait was clumsy, and he had poor coordination of his extremities. Therefore, he underwent posterior stabilization. (From Benson M, Fixen J, Macnicol M: Children's Orthopaedics and Fractures, p 590. New York, Churchill Livingstone, 1994.)

Growth retardation, hip dysplasia, hypoplastic genitalia, and juvenile-onset scoliosis are common.

D. Menkes' syndrome—Sex-linked recessive disorder of copper transport that affects bone growth and causes characteristic "kinky" hair. May be differentiated from occipital horn syndrome (which also affects copper transport) by the characteristic bony projections from the occiput of the skull in that disorder.

E. Rett's syndrome—Progressive impairment and stereotaxic, abnormal hand movements (like autism) characterize this disorder. It is seen in girls at 6-18 months of age, who present with rapid developmental delay that stabilizes. This is different from cerebral palsy (CP) because the infants have normal development for the first months of life and then decline. Affected children typically have scoliosis with a C-shaped curve unresponsive to bracing. Instrumentation must include all of the kyphosis and the scoliosis. Spasticity results in joint contractures, which are treated as they are in cerebral palsy patients.

F. Beckwith-Wiedemann syndrome—The triad of organomegaly, omphalocele, and a large tongue defines this disorder. Orthopaedic manifestations include hemihypertrophy with spastic cerebral palsy. The spasticity is thought to be the result of infantile hypoglycemic episodes secondary to pancreatic islet cell hypertrophy. There is a predisposition to Wilms' tumor (must be screened regularly by kidney ultrasound).

G. Teratogens
   1. Fetal alcohol syndrome—Maternal alcoholism can cause growth disturbances, central nervous system dysfunction, dysmorphic facies, hip dislocation, cervical spine vertebral and upper extremity congenital fusions, congenital scoliosis, and myelodysplasia. Contractures respond to physical therapy.
   2. Maternal diabetes—May lead to heart defects, sacral agenesis, and anencephaly. Careful management of pregnant diabetics is essential.
   3. Other teratogens—Include drugs (e.g., aminopterin, phenytoin, thalidomide), trace metals, maternal conditions, infections, and intrauterine factors; may also lead to orthopaedic manifestations in affected children.

III. Hematopoietic Disorders

A. Gaucher's disease—Aberrant AR lysosomal storage disease characterized by accumulation of cerebroside in cells of the reticuloendothelial system. The cause is a deficiency of the enzyme **β-glucocerebrosidase**. There are three different types: type I, most common; type II, infantile; and type III, chronic neuropathic. Type I is commonly seen in children of Ashkenazi Jewish descent; it is associated with osteopenia, metaphyseal enlargement (failure of remodeling), femoral head necrosis (may be confused with Perthes' disease or MED), "moth-eaten" trabeculae, patchy sclerosis, and "Erlenmeyer's flask" distal femora (70%). Affected patients may complain of bone pain (Gaucher crisis), and bleeding abnormalities are common. **Hepatosplenomegaly** is a characteristic finding. Histologic examination demonstrates characteristic lipid-laden histiocytes (Gaucher's cells). Treatment is supportive; new enzyme therapy is available but is extremely expensive.

B. Niemann-Pick disease—AR disorder. It is caused by an accumulation of sphingomyelin in reticuloendothelial system cells. Seen commonly in eastern European Jews. Marrow expansion and cortical thinning are common in long bones; coxa valga is also seen.

C. Sickle cell anemia—Sickle cell disease (affects 1% of African Americans) is more severe but less common than sickle cell trait (8% prevalence). Crises usually begin at age 2-3, are caused by substance P, and may lead to characteristic bone infarctions. Growth retardation/skeletal immaturity, osteonecrosis of femoral and humeral heads, osteomyelitis (often in diaphysis), biconcave "fish" vertebrae, and septic arthritis are commonly seen in this disorder. *Salmonella* is more commonly seen in children with sickle cell disease. Despite this tendency, *Staphylococcus aureus* is still the most common cause of osteomyelitis in sickle cell patients. Dactylitis (acute hand/foot swelling) is also common. Aspiration and culture may be necessary to differentiate infarction from osteomyelitis. Preoperative oxygenation and exchange transfusion are helpful for affected patients requiring surgery. Hydroxyurea has produced dramatic relief of pain when used for bone crises.

D. Thalassemia—It is similar to sickle cell anemia in presentation. Most commonly seen in people of Mediterranean descent. Common symptoms include bone pain and leg ulceration. Radiographs show long-bone thinning, metaphyseal expansion, osteopenia, and premature physeal closure.

E. Hemophilia—X-linked recessive disorder with decreased factor VIII (hemophilia A), abnormal factor VIII with platelet dysfunction (von Willebrand's disease), or factor IX (hemophilia B-Christmas disease); associated with bleeding episodes and skeletal/joint sequelae. Can be mild (5-25% of factor present), moderate (1-5% available), or severe (< 1% of factor present).

1. Presentation and diagnosis—Hemarthrosis presents with painful swelling and decreased range of motion (ROM) of affected joints. The knee is the most commonly affected joint. Deep intramuscular bleeding is also common and can lead to the formation of a pseudotumor (blood cyst), which can occur in soft tissue or bone. Intramuscular hematomas can lead to compression of adjacent nerves (e.g., an iliacus hematoma may cause femoral nerve paralysis and may mimic bleeding into the hip joint). Radiographic findings in hemophilia include squaring of the patellas and condyles, epiphyseal overgrowth with leg-length discrepancy, and generalized osteopenia with resulting fractures. Fractures heal in normal time with proper clotting. Cartilage atrophy due to enzymatic matrix degeneration and chondrocyte death is frequent.

2. Treatment—Home transfusion therapy has reduced the severity of the arthropathy with the advantage of treatment when bleeding occurs. Treatment of the sequelae includes contracture release, osteotomies, open synovectomy, arthroscopic synovectomy (better motion, shorter hospitalization), radiation synovectomy (useful in patients with antibody inhibitors and poor medical management), and total joint arthroplasty. Mild to moderate hemophilia A can be treated with desmopressin. Factor VIII levels should be increased for prophylaxis in the following situations: vigorous physical therapy (20%), treatment of hematoma (30%), acute hemarthrosis or soft tissue surgery (> 50%), and skeletal surgery (approach 100% preoperatively and maintain over 50% for 10 days postoperatively). Tourniquets, ligated vessels rather than cauterized vessels, and rigid fixation of fractures decrease postoperative bleeding. **Immunoglobulin G** (IgG) antibody inhibitors are present in 4-20% of hemophiliacs and are a relative contraindication to surgery. Because of the amount of blood component therapy required to treat this disorder, a large percentage of older hemophiliacs are positive for human immunodeficiency virus (HIV).

F. Leukemia—The most common malignancy of childhood. Acute lymphocytic leukemia (ALL) represents 80% of cases of leukemia. Peak incidence is at 4 years. Bony changes include demineralization of bones, periostitis, and occasionally lytic lesions. One fourth to one third of children have musculoskeletal complaints (back, pelvic, leg pains). Radiolucent "leukemia" lines may be seen in the metaphyses of affected bones in older children. Management of leukemia includes chemotherapy, which may predispose the patient to pathologic fractures.

IV. Metabolic Disease/Arthritides*

A. Rickets—Decrease in calcium (and sometimes phosphorus), affecting mineralization at the epiphyses of long bones. Classically, brittle bones with physeal cupping/widening, bowing of long bones, transverse radiolucent Looser's lines, ligamentous laxity, flattening of the skull, enlargement of costal cartilages (rachitic rosary), and dorsal kyphosis (cat back) characterize this disorder (Fig. 3–6). There are several varieties of rickets based on the underlying abnormality (e.g., gastrointestinal, kidney, diet, and organ); they are discussed in detail in Chapter 1, Basic Sciences. Histologically, widened osteoid seams and "Swiss cheese" trabeculae are characteristic in bone; at the growth plate there is gross distortion of the maturation zone (enlarged and distorted) and a poorly defined zone of provisional calcification.

B. Osteogenesis imperfecta—Defect in **type I collagen** (*COL 1A2* gene) that causes abnormal cross-linking and leads to decreased collagen secretion, bone fragility (brittle "wormian" bone), short stature, scoliosis, tooth defects (dentinogenesis imperfecta), hearing defects, and ligamentous laxity. Four types have been identified (Sillence), although the disorder is probably best considered as a continuum with different inheritance patterns and severity (Table 3–3).

1. Diagnosis—Radiographs demonstrate thin cortices and generalized osteopenia. Histologically, increased diameters of haversian canals and osteocyte lacunae, increased numbers of cells, and replicated cement lines are noted and result in the thin cortices seen on radiographs. Fractures are common; the initial healing is normal, but bone typically does not remodel. Fractures occur less frequently with advancing age (usually cease at puberty). Compression fractures (codfish vertebrae) are also common.

2. Treatment—The goal of treatment is fracture management and long-term rehabilitation. Bracing of extremities is indicated early to prevent deformity and minimize fractures. Sofield's osteotomies ("shish kebab" multiple long-bone osteotomies with either fixed-length Rush's rods or telescoping [Bailey-Dubow] intramedullary rods) are sometimes required for progressive bowing of long bones. Fractures in children

*See Chapter 1, Basic Sciences.

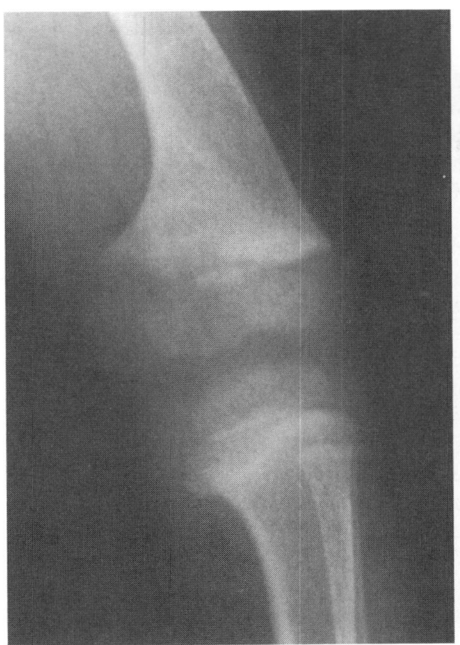
A

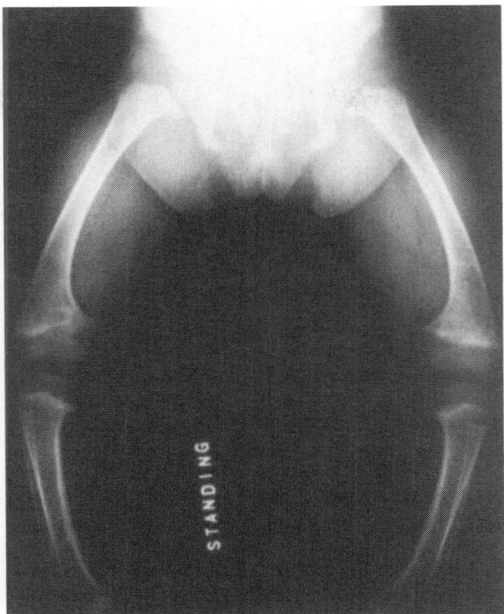

B

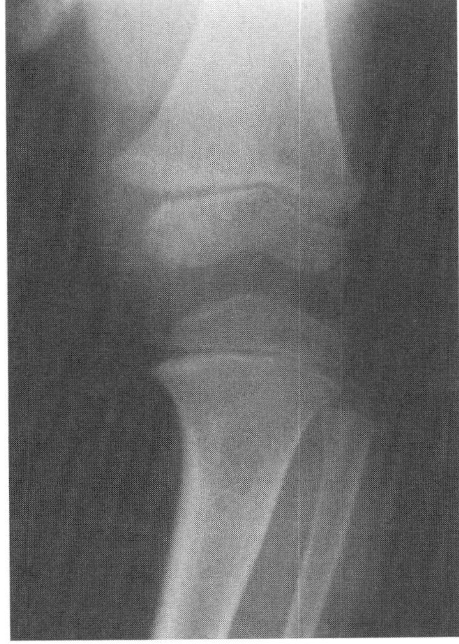
C

FIGURE 3–6 **A**, Hazy metaphysis with cupping in a young boy with rickets. **B**, Accentuated genu varum is present. **C**, With vitamin D replacement therapy, the bony lesions healed in 6 months. (From Herring JA: Tachdjian's Pediatric Orthopaedics, 4th ed, p 1921. Philadelphia, WB Saunders, 2008.)

TABLE 3-3 OSTEOGENESIS IMPERFECTA

Type	Inheritance	Sclerae	Features
IA, IB	AD	Blue	Preschool age (tarda), hearing loss (IA = teeth involved; IB = teeth not affected)
II	AR	Blue	Lethal, concertina femur beaded ribs
III	AR	Normal	Fractures at birth, progressively short stature
IVA, IVB	AD	Normal	Milder form, normal hearing (IVA = teeth involved; IVB = teeth not affected)

AD, autosomal dominant; AR, autosomal recessive.

younger than age 2 are treated similar to those in children without osteogenesis imperfecta. After age 2, telescoping intramedullary rods can be considered. Bisphosphonates have been shown to decrease the number of fractures in these patients. Scoliosis is common, and bracing is ineffective treatment. Surgery is necessary for scoliosis deformities exceeding 50 degrees, with a large blood loss to be expected.

C. Idiopathic juvenile osteoporosis—Rare, self-limiting disorder that appears between the ages of 8 and 14 with osteopenia, growth arrest, and bone and joint pain. Other manifestations can include multiple vertebral body microfractures that can be treated with bracing. Serum calcium and phosphorus levels are normal. Typically, there is spontaneous resolution 2-4 years after the onset of puberty. This disorder must be differentiated from other causes of osteopenia (e.g., osteogenesis imperfecta, malignancy, Cushing's disease).

D. Osteopetrosis—Failure of osteoclastic resorption, probably secondary to a defect in the thymus, leading to dense bone (marble bone), a "rugger jersey" spine (Fig. 3–7), marble bone, and an Erlenmeyer flask proximal humerus/distal femur. Loss of the medullary canal can cause anemias and encroachment on the optic and oculomotor nerves, causing blindness. Healing is normal, but time to healing may be prolonged. The mild form is AD; the "malignant" form is AR. **Bone marrow transplant** may be helpful for treating the malignant form (see Chapter 1, Basic Sciences).

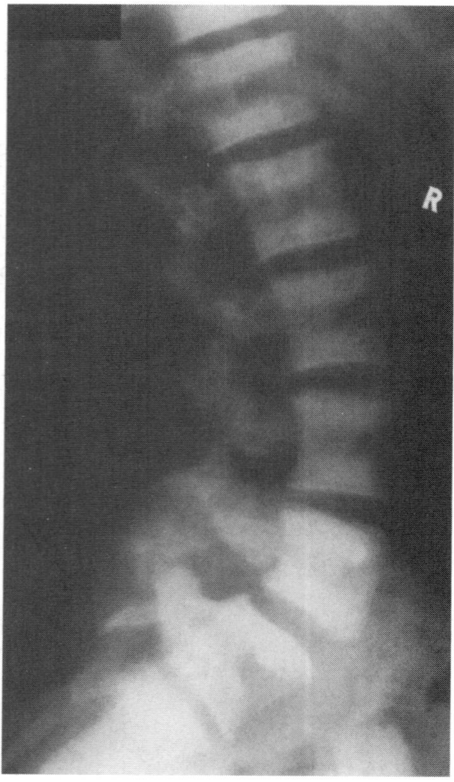

FIGURE 3–7 Spine radiographs in osteopetrosis showing the "rugger jersey" pattern of ossification. (From Benson M, Fixen J, Macnicol M: Children's Orthopaedics and Fractures, p 86. New York, Churchill Livingstone, 1994.)

E. Infantile cortical hyperostosis (Caffey's disease)—Soft tissue swelling and bony cortical thickening (especially the jaw and ulna) that follow a febrile illness in infants 0-9 months old. Radiographs show a characteristic periosteal reaction. This disorder may be differentiated from trauma (and child abuse) based on single-bone involvement. Infection, scurvy, and progressive diaphyseal dysplasia may also be in the differential diagnosis for children of all ages. The condition is benign and self-limiting.

F. Connective tissue syndrome—A heterogeneous group of disorders with a broad spectrum of features.
   1. Marfan's syndrome—AD disorder of fibrillin associated with arachnodactyly (long, slender fingers), pectus deformities, scoliosis (50%), acetabular protrusio, cardiac (aortic dilation) abnormalities, and ocular findings (superior lens dislocation in 60%). Other abnormalities may include dural ectasia and meningocele. Joint laxity is treated conservatively. Scoliosis and spondylolisthesis are common. Bracing is ineffective. The presence of kyphosis with scoliosis requires anterior diskectomy and fusion with posterior fusion and instrumentation.
   2. Ehlers-Danlos syndrome—AD disorder with hyperextensibility of "cigarette paper" skin, joint hypermobility and dislocation, soft tissue/bone fragility, and soft tissue calcification. Types II and III (of XI) are the most common and least disabling. Treatment consists of physical therapy, orthoses, and arthrodesis; soft tissue procedures fail.
   3. Homocystinuria—AR inborn error of methionine metabolism (decreased enzyme cystathionine β-synthase). Accumulation of the intermediate metabolite homocysteine in the production of the amino acid cysteine can lead to osteoporosis, a marfanoid-like habitus (but with stiffening joints), and inferior lens dislocation. The diagnosis is made by demonstrating increased homocysteine in urine (cyanide-nitroprusside test). This disorder is differentiated from Marfan's syndrome based on the direction of lens dislocation and the presence of osteoporosis in homocystinuria. Central nervous system effects, including mental retardation, are common in this disorder. Early treatment with vitamin B_6 and a decreased methionine diet is often successful.

G. Juvenile idiopathic arthritis (JIA)—Includes both juvenile rheumatoid arthritis (JRA) and juvenile chronic arthritis. Persistent noninfectious arthritis lasting 6 weeks to 3 months and diagnosed after other possible causes have been ruled out. To confirm the diagnosis, one of the following is required: rash, presence of rheumatoid factor, **iridocyclitis**, cervical spine involvement, pericarditis, tenosynovitis, intermittent fever, or morning stiffness. JIA affects girls more than boys and commonly involves the wrist (flexed and ulnar deviated) and hand (fingers extended, swollen, radially deviated). Cervical spine involvement can lead to kyphosis, facet ankylosis, and atlantoaxial subluxation. Lower extremity problems include flexion contractures (hip and knee flexed, ankle dorsiflexed), subluxation, and other deformities (hip protrusio, valgus knees, equinovarus feet). In 50% of patients, symptoms resolve without sequelae; 25% of patients are slightly disabled, and 20-25% have crippling arthritis/blindness. Medical therapy has moved away from high-dose steroids and salicylates and more toward more specific immunomodulating drugs (infliximab). Surgical interventions include joint injections and (rarely) synovectomy (for chronic swelling refractory to medical management). Arthrodesis and arthroplasty may be required for severe JIA. Slit-lamp examination is required twice yearly, as progressive iridocyclitis can lead to rapid loss of vision if left untreated.

H. Ankylosing spondylitis (AS)—Typically affects adolescent boys with asymmetrical, lower extremity, large-joint arthritis; heel pain; and sometimes eye symptoms. Hip and back pain (cardinal symptoms) may develop later. The HLA-B27 test is positive in 90-95% of patients with AS or Reiter's syndrome but is also positive in 4-8% of all white Americans and thus is limited as a screening tool. Limitation of chest wall expansion is more specific than HLA-B27. Radiographs show bilateral, symmetrical sacroiliac erosion, followed by joint space narrowing, subsequent ankylosis, and late vertebral scalloping (bamboo spine). NSAIDs and physical therapy are the mainstays of treatment.

V. Birth Injuries

A. Brachial plexus palsy—Decreasing in severity as a result of better obstetric management, yet 2 per 1000 births still have an injury associated with stretching or contusion of the brachial plexus. Occurs most often with large babies, shoulder dystocia, forceps delivery, breech position, and prolonged labor. Three types are commonly recognized (Table 3–4).

1. Treatment—The key to therapy is maintaining passive ROM and awaiting return of motor function (up to 18 months). Ninety percent or more of cases eventually resolve without intervention. However, lack of biceps function 6 months after injury and Horner's syndrome carry a poor prognosis. Late musculoskeletal surgery can improve functional motion. Options include releasing contractures (Fairbanks'), latissimus and teres major transfer to the shoulder external rotators (L'Episcopo's), tendon transfers for elbow flexion (Clarke's pectoral transfer and Steindler's flexorplasty), proximal humerus rotational osteotomy (Wickstrom's), and microsurgical nerve grafting. Reports have shown that release of the subscapularis tendon for internal rotation contracture, if performed by age 2 years, may result in improved active external rotation of the shoulder, with muscle transfer to assist in active external rotation. Watch for fixed posterior shoulder dislocation as a result of muscle imbalance.

B. Congenital muscular torticollis—A congenital deformity resulting from contracture of the sternocleidomastoid muscle. It is associated with other "molding disorders," such as hip dysplasia and metatarsus adductus (up to 20% association with hip dysplasia). The cause of congenital muscular torticollis remains uncertain, although most cases follow a difficult labor and delivery. Studies suggest that the muscle abnormality may be the result of an intrauterine compartment syndrome involving the sternocleidomastoid muscle. Fibrosis of the muscle and a palpable mass are noted within the first 4 weeks of life. Most patients (90%) respond to passive stretching within the first year. Surgery (Z-plasty of the sternocleidomastoid) may be required if torticollis persists beyond the first year. Torticollis may also be associated with congenital atlanto-occipital abnormalities.

C. Congenital pseudarthrosis of the clavicle—Failure of union of the medial and lateral ossification centers of the right clavicle (Fig. 3–8). The cause may be related to pulsations of the underlying subclavian artery. Presents as an enlarging, painless, nontender mass. Radiographs show rounded sclerotic bone at the pseudarthrosis site. Surgery (open reduction/internal fixation with bone grafting) is indicated for

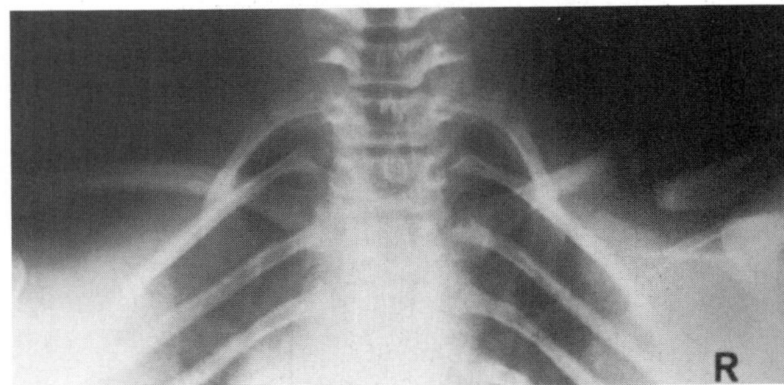

FIGURE 3–8 Radiograph of bilateral clavicles in a case of congenital pseudarthrosis of the clavicles. Note that the pseudarthrosis is on the right side. (From Benson M, Fixen J, Macnicol M: Children's Orthopaedics and Fractures, p 362. New York, Churchill Livingstone, 1994.)

TABLE 3-4 BRACHIAL PLEXUS PALSY

Type	Roots	Deficit	Prognosis
Erb-Duchenne palsy	C5, 6	Deltoid, cuff, elbow flexors, wrist and hand dorsiflexors; "waiter's tip" deformity	Best
Total plexus	C5, T1	Sensory and motor; flaccid arm	Worst
Klumpke	C8, T1	Wrist flexors, intrinsics; Horner's	Poor

unacceptable cosmetic deformities or with significant functional symptoms (mobility of the fragments and winging of the scapula) at ages 3-6. Successful union is predictable (in contrast to congenital pseudarthrosis of the tibia).

VI. Cerebral Palsy

A. Introduction—Nonprogressive neuromuscular disorder with onset before age 2 years, resulting from injury to the immature brain. The cause is usually not identifiable but can include prenatal intrauterine factors, perinatal infections (toxoplasmosis, other infections, rubella, cytomegalovirus infection, and herpes simplex), prematurity (most common), anoxic injuries, and meningitis. This upper motor neuron disease results in a mixture of muscle weakness and spasticity. Initially, the abnormal muscle forces cause dynamic deformity at joints. Persistent spasticity can lead to contractures, bony deformity, and ultimately joint subluxation/dislocation. MRI reveals periventricular leukomalacia.

B. Classification—CP can be classified based on physiology (according to the movement disorder) or anatomy (according to geographic distribution).

1. Physiologic classification
   a. Spastic—Characterized by increased muscle tone and hyperreflexia with slow, restricted movements because of simultaneous contraction of agonist and antagonist. This form of CP is the most common and is most amenable to improvement of musculoskeletal function by operative intervention.
   b. Athetosis—Characterized by a constant succession of slow, writhing, involuntary movements, this form of CP is less common and more difficult to treat.
   c. Ataxia—Characterized by an inability to coordinate muscles for voluntary movement, resulting in an unbalanced, wide-based gait. Also less amenable to orthopaedic treatment.
   d. Mixed—Typically involves a combination of spasticity and athetosis with total body involvement.
2. Anatomic classification
   a. Hemiplegia—Involves the upper and lower extremities on the same side, usually with spasticity. These children often develop early "handedness." All children with hemiplegia are eventually able to walk, regardless of treatment.
   b. Diplegia—Patients have more extensive involvement of the lower extremity than the upper extremity. Most diplegic patients eventually walk. IQ may be normal; strabismus is common.
   c. Total involvement—These children have extensive involvement, low IQ, and a high mortality rate; they are usually unable to walk.

C. Orthopaedic assessment—Based on examination and thorough birth and developmental history. A patient's locomotor profile is based on the persistence of primitive reflexes; the presence of two or more usually means the child will be a nonambulator. Commonly tested reflexes include the Moro startle reflex (normally disappears by age 6 months) and the parachute reflex (normally disappears by age 12 months). Surgery to improve function should be considered for a child more than 3 years old with spastic CP and voluntary motor control. Muscle imbalance yields later bony changes; therefore, the general surgical plan is to perform soft tissue procedures early and, if necessary, bony procedures later. Intramuscular botulinum A toxin can temporarily decrease dynamic spasticity. The mechanism of action of botulinum toxin is a postsynaptic blockade at the neuromuscular junction. The effectiveness of botulinum toxin is limited to 6 months; therefore, it is not a permanent cure for spasticity. Instead, it is used to maintain joint motion during rapid growth when a child is too young for surgery. Selective dorsal root rhizotomy is a neurosurgical procedure designed to decrease lower extremity spasticity. This treatment, indicated only for spastic CP, includes resection of dorsal rootlets not exhibiting a myographic or clinical response to stimulation. It may help reduce spasticity and complement orthopaedic management in spastic diplegic patients. It requires multilevel laminoplasty, which may lead to late instability and deformity. A discussion of hand disorders is included in Chapter 7, Hand, Upper Extremity, and Microvascular Surgery.

D. Gait disorders—Usually the cause of the orthopaedic consultation. Hemiplegics frequently present with toe walking only. The use of three-dimensional computerized gait analysis with dynamic electromyography and force-plate studies have allowed a more scientific approach to preoperative decision making and postoperative analysis of the results of CP surgery. Specific abnormal gait patterns have been identified, and surgical procedures have been devised to treat these patterns. The use of gait analysis has allowed a more individualized treatment plan for patients with CP. Lengthening of continuously active muscles and transfer of muscles out of phase are often helpful. Surgeries should usually be done at multiple levels to best correct the problem. In general, surgery is performed at 4-5 years old. A few generalized guidelines are given in Table 3–5.

E. Spinal disorders—Most commonly involve scoliosis, which can be severe, making proper wheelchair sitting difficult. The risk for scoliosis is highest in children with total body involvement (spastic quadriplegic). Surgical indications include curves greater than 45-50 degrees or worsening pelvic obliquity. Two groups of curves occur. Group I curves are double curves with thoracic and lumbar components and little pelvic obliquity. Group II curves are larger lumbar or thoracolumbar curves with marked pelvic obliquity (Fig. 3–9). Treatment is tailored to the needs of the patient. Custom-molded seat inserts allow better positioning but do not prevent curve progression. Small curves with no loss of function or large curves in severely involved patients may require

TABLE 3-5 SURGICAL OPTIONS FOR GAIT DISORDERS

Problem	Diagnosis	Surgical Option
Hip flexion	Positive Thomas test	Psoas tenotomy or recession
Spastic hip	Decreased abduction/uncovered head	Adductor release, osteotomy (late)
Hip adduction	Scissoring gait	Adductor release
Femoral anteversion	Prone internal rotation increased	Osteotomy, VDRO, hamstring lengthening
Knee flexion	Increased popliteal angle	Hamstring lengthening
Knee hypertension	Recurvatum	Rectus femoris lengthening
Stiff-leg gait	Electromyography—hamstring quadriceps continuous passive knee flexion decreased with hip extension	Distal rectus transfer to hamstrings
Talipes equinus	Toe walking	Achilles lengthening
Talipes varus	Standing position	Split anterior or posterior tibialis transfer (based on EMG findings)
Talipes valgus	Standing position	Peroneal lengthening, Grice's subtalar fusion, calcaneal lengthening osteotomy
Hallux valgus	Examination/radiographs	Osteotomy, metatarsophalangeal fusion

EMG, electromyographic; VDRO, varus derotation osteotomy.

observation alone. Group I curves in ambulators are treated as idiopathic scoliosis with posterior fusion and instrumentation. Group I curves in sitters and group II curves require anterior and posterior fusion with segmental posterior instrumentation from the upper thoracic spine to the pelvis (Luque-Galveston technique). The decision for one-stage or two-stage anterior and posterior fusion is based on the surgeon's skill and speed, blood loss, and the facility capabilities. Kyphosis is also common and may require fusion and instrumentation. It is important to assess nutritional status (albumin < 3.5 g/dL and white blood cell [WBC] count < 1500/uL) preoperatively and consider gastrostomy tube placement before spinal surgery if indicated.

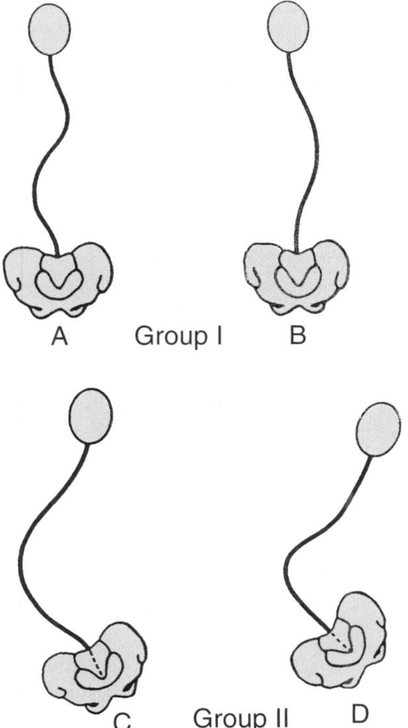

FIGURE 3–9 Curve patterns of cerebral palsy scoliosis. Group I curves are double curves with thoracic and lumbar components. **A**, There is little pelvic obliquity; the curve may be well balanced. **B**, If the thoracic curve is more significant, there may be some imbalance. Group II curves are large lumbar or thoracolumbar curves with marked pelvic obliquity. **C**, There may be a short fractional curve between the end of the curve and the sacrum. **D**, The curve may continue into the sacrum, with the sacral vertebrae forming part of the curve. (Adapted from Weinstein SL: The Pediatric Spine: Principles and Practice. New York, Raven Press, 1994.)

F. Hip subluxation/dislocation—Treated initially with a soft tissue release (adductor/psoas) plus abduction bracing. Later, hip subluxation/dislocation may require femoral and/or acetabular osteotomies (Dega's) to maintain hip stability. The goal is to keep the hip reduced. Spastic dislocation may lead to painful arthritis, which is difficult to treat. This entity is characterized by four stages.

1. Hip at risk—This situation is the only exception to the general rule of avoiding surgery in CP patients during the first 3 years of life. Characterized by abduction of < 45 degrees, with partial uncovering of the femoral head on radiographs. May benefit from adductor and psoas release. Neurectomy of the anterior branch of the obturator nerve is now rarely performed because, by converting an upper motor neuron lesion to a lower motor neuron lesion, the muscle is made stiff and fibrotic.
2. Hip subluxation—Best treated with adductor tenotomy in children with abduction of less than 20 degrees, sometimes with psoas release/recession. Femoral or pelvic osteotomies may be considered in femoral coxa valga and acetabular dysplasia, which is usually lateral and posterior.
3. Spastic dislocation—May benefit from open reduction, femoral shortening, varus derotation osteotomy, Dega's (Fig. 3–10), triple, or Chiari's osteotomy. The type of pelvic osteotomy indicated is best determined by obtaining a three-dimensional CT scan, which will demonstrate the area of acetabular deficiency (anterior, lateral, or posterior) and the congruency of the joint surfaces. Late dislocations may best be left out or treated with a Schanz abduction osteotomy

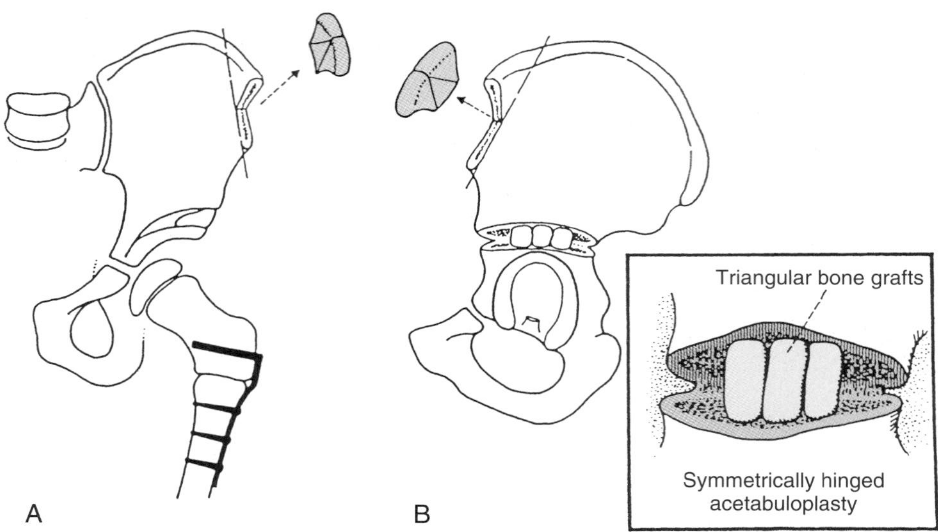

FIGURE 3–10 Placement of graft for Dega's acetabuloplasty. **A**, Bone graft is obtained from the anterosuperior iliac crest and converted to three small triangles, with the base measuring 1 cm. **B**, The grafts are placed in the osteotomy site, with the largest in the area where maximum improvement of coverage is desired. The triangular wedges are packed close to each other to prevent collapse, turning, or dislodgment; the result is a symmetrical hinging on the **triradiate cartilage** *(inset)*. With the medial wall of the pelvis maintained, the elasticity of the osteotomy keeps the wedges in place. No pins are necessary to maintain the osteotomy. (Adapted from Mubarak SJ, Valencia FG, Wenger DR: One-stage reconstruction of the spastic hip. J Bone Joint Surg [Am] 74:1352, 1992.)

or a modified Girdlestone resection arthroplasty (resection below the lesser trochanter).

4. Windswept hips—Characterized by abduction of one hip and adduction of the contralateral hip. Treatment is best directed at attempting to abduct the adducted hip with bracing or tenotomies and releasing the abduction contracture of the contralateral hip.

G. Knee abnormalities—Usually includes hamstring contractures and decreased ROM. Hamstring lengthening is often helpful (sometimes increases lumbar lordosis). Distal transfer of an out-of-phase rectus femoris muscle to semitendinosus or gracilis is indicated when there is loss of knee flexion during the swing phase of gait.

H. Foot and ankle abnormalities

1. Equinovalgus foot—More commonly seen in spastic diplegia. Caused by spastic peroneals, contracted heel cords, and ligamentous laxity. Peroneus brevis lengthening is often helpful in correcting moderate valgus. Lateral column-lengthening calcaneal osteotomy is used to correct hindfoot valgus.

2. Equinovarus foot—More common in spastic hemiplegia, caused by an overpulling of the posterior or anterior tibialis tendons (or both). Lengthening of the posterior tibialis is rarely sufficient. Likewise, transfer of an entire muscle (posterior or anterior tibialis) is rarely recommended. Split muscle transfers are helpful when the affected muscle is spastic during both the stance and swing phases of gait. The split posterior tibialis transfer (rerouting half of the tendon dorsally to the peroneus brevis) is used in cases with spasticity of the muscle, flexible varus foot, and weak peroneals. Complications include decreased foot dorsiflexion. Split anterior tibialis transfer (rerouting half of its tendon laterally to the cuboid) is used in patients with spasticity of the muscle and a flexible varus deformity. Most often it is coupled with Achilles tendon lengthening and posterior tibial tendon intramuscular lengthening (the Rancho procedure) to treat the fixed equinus contracture.

VII. Neuromuscular Disorders

A. Arthrogrypotic syndromes

1. Arthrogryposis multiplex congenita (amyoplasia) —Nonprogressive disorder with multiple congenitally rigid joints (Fig. 3–11). This disorder can be myopathic, neuropathic, or mixed and is associated with a decrease in anterior horn cells and other neural elements of the spinal cord. Intelligence is normal.

a. Evaluation—Evaluation should include neurologic studies, enzyme tests, and muscle biopsy (at 3-4 months). Affected patients typically have normal facies, normal intelligence, multiple joint contractures, and no visceral abnormalities. Upper extremity involvement usually includes adduction and internal rotation of the shoulder, extension of the elbow, and flexion and ulnar deviation of the wrist. The elbow has no creases.

b. Treatment—Treatment for the elbow deformities consists of passive manipulation and serial casting. Osteotomies are considered after 4 years of age to allow independent eating. One upper extremity should be left in extension at the elbow for positioning and perineal care and the other elbow in flexion for feeding. The lower extremity deformities

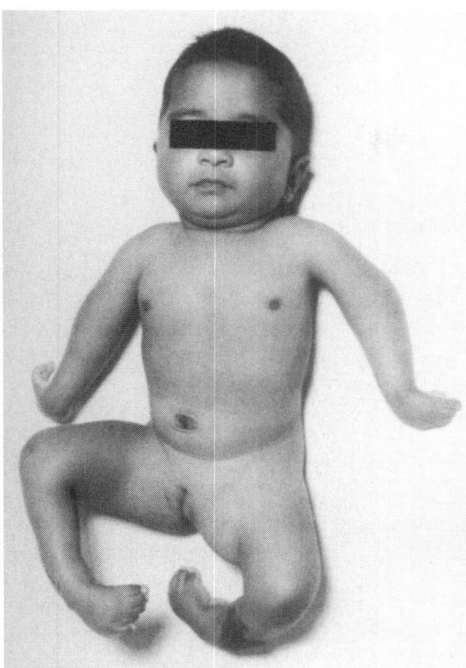

FIGURE 3–11 Typical appearance of a child with arthrogryposis in all four limbs. Note the lack of creases at the elbows, the flexion contractures at the knees, and the severe clubfoot deformities. (From Benson M, Fixen J, Macnicol M: Children's Orthopaedics and Fractures, p 321. New York, Churchill Livingstone, 1994.)

seen in arthrogryposis include teratologic hip dislocations, knee contractures, resistant clubfeet, and vertical talus. Treatment includes early (6-9 months) soft tissue releases (especially hamstrings) for knee contractures and medial open reduction with possible femoral shortening for hip dislocation. The foot deformities (clubfoot and vertical talus) are initially treated with a soft tissue release, but later recurrences may need bone procedures (talectomy). The goal is a stiff, plantigrade foot that enables shoe wear and possibly ambulation. Knee contractures should be corrected before hip reduction in order to maintain the reduction. The spine may be involved, with characteristic "C-shaped" (neuromuscular) scoliosis (33%). Fractures are also common (25%). These patients have an ability to adapt by using the feet as functional appendages.

2. Distal arthrogryposis syndrome—AD disorder that affects predominantly the hands and feet. Ulnarly deviated fingers (at metacarpal joints), metacarpal and proximal interphalangeal flexion contractures, and adducted thumbs with web space thickening are common. Clubfoot and vertical talus deformities are common in the feet.
3. Larsen's syndrome—Similar to arthrogryposis in clinical appearance, but joints are less rigid. The disorder is primarily associated with multiple joint dislocations (including bilateral congenital knee dislocations), flattened facies, scoliosis, clubfeet, and cervical kyphosis (watch for late myelopathy). These patients have normal intelligence.
4. Multiple pterygium syndrome—AR disorder that means "little wing" in Greek. It is characterized by cutaneous flexor surface webs (knee and elbow), congenital vertical talus, and scoliosis. Care must be taken when the webs are elongated because of the superficial nature of the neurovascular bundle.

B. Myelodysplasia (spina bifida)
   1. Introduction—Disorder of incomplete spinal cord closure or rupture of the developing cord secondary to hydrocephalus. Includes spina bifida occulta (defect in the vertebral arch, with confined cord and meninges), meningocele (sac without neural elements protruding through the defect), myelomeningocele (spina bifida; protrusion of the sac with neural elements), and rachischisis (neural elements exposed, with no covering). Can be diagnosed in utero (increased **α-fetoprotein**). Related to a folate deficiency in utero. Function is primarily related to the level of the defect and the associated congenital abnormalities. A type II Arnold-Chiari malformation is the most common comorbidity. Sudden changes in function (rapid increase of scoliotic curvature, spasticity, new neurologic deficit, or increase in urinary tract infections) can be associated with tethered cord, hydrocephalus (most common), or syringomyelia. Head CT scans (70% of myelodysplastic patients have hydrocephalus) and myelography or spinal MRI are required. Fractures are also common in myelodysplasia, most often about the knee and hip in children 3-7 years old, and can frequently be diagnosed only by noting redness, warmth, and swelling. Fractures are commonly misdiagnosed as infection in these patients. Fractures are treated conservatively, with a well-padded splint. Fractures usually heal, with abundant callus. The myelodysplasia level is based on the lowest functional level (Table 3–6). L4 is a key level because quadriceps can function and allow independent community ambulation (Fig. 3–12).
   2. Treatment principles—Careful observation of patients with myelodysplasia is important. Several myelodysplasia "milestones" have been developed to assess progress (Table 3–7). Treatment utilizes a team approach (urology, orthopaedics, neurosurgery, and developmental pediatrician) to allow maximum function consistent with the patient's level and other abnormalities. Proper use of orthoses is essential in myelodysplasia. The determination of ambulation potential is based on the level of the deficit and motivation of the child. Surgery for myelodysplasia focuses on balancing of muscles and correction of deformities. Increased attention has been focused on **latex sensitivity** in myelodysplastic patients. A latex-free environment is required to prevent life-threatening allergic reactions.

TABLE 3-6 MYELODYSPLASIA LEVELS

Level	Characteristics				
	Hip	*Knee*	*Feet*	*Orthosis*	*Ambulation*
L1	External rotation/flexed		Equinovarus	HKAFO	Nonfunctional
L2	Adduction/flexed	Flexed	Equinovarus	HKAFO	Nonfunctional
L3	Adduction/flexed	Recurvatum	Equinovarus	KAFO	Household
L4	Adduction/flexed	Extended	Cavovarus	AFO	Household plus
L5	Flexed	Limited flexion	Calcaneal valgus	AFO	Community
S1			Foot deformities	Shoes	Near normal

AFO, ankle-foot orthosis; HKAFO, hip-knee-ankle-foot orthosis; KAFO, knee-ankle-foot orthosis.

3. Hip problems—Flexion contractures commonly occur in patients with thoracic/high lumbar myelomeningocele resulting from unopposed hip flexors or in patients who sit most of the time. Treatment for these patients consists of anterior hip release with tenotomy of the iliopsoas, sartorius, rectus femoris, and tensor fasciae latae. For low-lumbar-level patients, the psoas should be preserved for independent ambulation. Hip abduction contracture can cause pelvic obliquity and scoliosis; it is treated with proximal division of the tensor fasciae latae and distal iliotibial band release (Ober-Yount procedure). Adduction contractures are treated with adductor myotomy. Hip dislocation frequently occurs in myelodysplastic patients because of paralysis of the hip abductors and extensors with unopposed hip flexors and adductors. Hip dislocation is most common at the L3-L4 level. Treatment of hip dislocation is controversial, but in general containment is considered essential only in patients with a functioning quadriceps. Redislocation may occur no matter what treatment is used to maintain the reduction. Late dislocation at the low lumbar level may be due to a tethered cord, which must be released before reducing the hip.
4. Knee problems—Usually include quadriceps weakness (usually treated with knee-ankle-foot orthoses). Flexion deformities are not important in wheelchair-bound patients but can be treated with hamstring release and posterior capsular release. Recurvatum is rarely a problem and can be treated early with serial casting and knee-ankle-foot orthoses. Tenotomies (quadriceps lengthening) are sometimes required. Valgus deformities are usually not a problem. Sometimes iliotibial band release or late osteotomies are needed.
5. Ankle and foot deformities—Objectives are to obtain braceable, plantigrade feet and muscle balance. Affected patients may present with a valgus foot. Ankle-foot orthoses are often helpful, but clubfoot release, tendon release (anterior tibialis, Achilles), posterior tibialis lengthening, and other procedures may be required. Triple arthrodesis should be avoided in most myelodysplastic patients and is used only for severe deformities with sensate feet. Rigid clubfoot secondary to retained activity or contracture of the tibialis posterior and tibialis anterior is common in L4-level patients. Treatment consists of complete subtalar release via a transverse (Cincinnati) incision, lengthening of the tibialis posterior and Achilles tendons, and transfer of the tibialis anterior tendon to the dorsal midfoot. Talectomy may be appropriate for recalcitrant clubfoot.

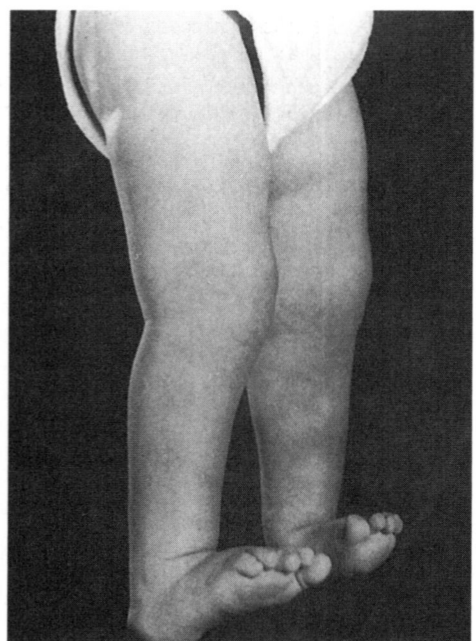

FIGURE 3–12 Typical posture of the legs and feet in a child with myelodysplasia below L5. The feet assume a progressive calcaneus posture that demands surgical correction. (From Benson M, Fixen J, Macnicol M: Children's Orthopaedics and Fractures, p 281. New York, Churchill Livingstone, 1994.)

TABLE 3-7 MILESTONES IN MYELODYSPLASIA

Age (mo)	Function	Treatment
4-6	Head control	Positioning
6-10	Sitting	Supports/orthoses
10-12	Prone mobility	Prone board
12-15	Upright stance	Standing orthosis
15-18	Upright mobility	Trunk/extremity orthosis

6. Spine problems—Deformity can be caused by the spine disorder itself, resulting in an upper lumbar kyphosis or other congenital malformation of the spine due to a lack of segmentation or formation (i.e., hemivertebrae, diastematomyelia, unsegmented bars). Scoliosis can also occur with severe lordosis as a result of muscular imbalance due to thoracic-level paraplegia. Spinal deformities are often severe and progressive. Nearly all patients with thoracic-level paraplegia develop scoliosis. Bracing is generally unsuccessful in treating these spinal deformities. Rapid curve progression can be associated with hydrocephalus or a **tethered cord**, which may be manifested as lower extremity spasticity or an increase in urinary tract infections. Severe, progressive curves require surgical treatment. Segmental Luque's sublaminar wiring with fixation to the pelvis (Galveston's technique) or fixation to the front of the sacrum (Dunn's technique) may be used. Kyphosis in myelodysplasia is a difficult problem. Resection of the kyphosis (kyphectomy) with local fusion (Figure 3–13 shows Lindseth's procedure) or fusion to the pelvis with instrumentation is required in severe cases. Infection rates are high because of frequent septicemia and poor skin quality over the lumbar spine.
7. Pelvic obliquity—Can occur in myelodysplasia as a result of prolonged unilateral hip contractures or scoliosis. Custom seat cushions, thoracolumbosacral orthosis, spinal fusion, and ultimately pelvic osteotomies may be required for treatment.

C. Myopathies (muscular dystrophies)—Noninflammatory, inherited disorders with progressive muscle weakness. Treatment focuses on physical therapy, orthoses, genetic counseling, and surgery. Several types of muscular dystrophy are classified based on their inheritance patterns.

1. Duchenne's—Sex-linked recessive abnormality of young boys manifested as clumsy walking, decreased motor skills, lumbar lordosis, calf pseudohypertrophy, a positive Gowers' sign

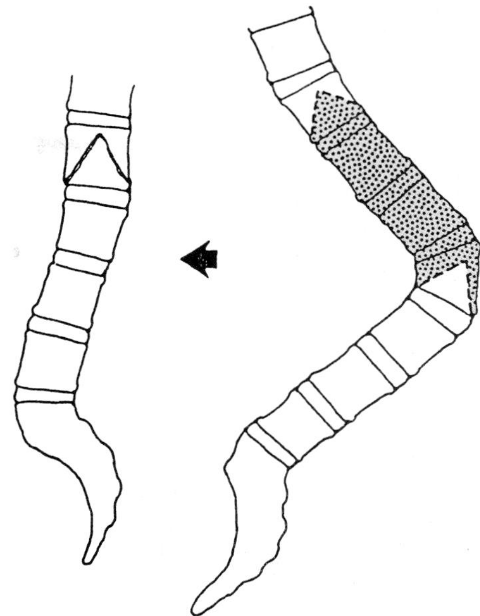

FIGURE 3–13 Rigid S-shaped kyphosis is corrected by excising the vertebrae between the apex of the kyphosis and the lordosis and fusing the apical vertebrae. (Adapted from Lindseth RE: Myelomeningocele. In Morrisey RT, ed: Lovell and Winters' Pediatric Orthopaedics, 3rd ed, p 522. Philadelphia, JB Lippincott, 1990.)

(rises by walking the hands up the legs to compensate for gluteus maximus and quadriceps weakness) (Fig. 3–14), markedly elevated **creatine phosphokinase** (CPK), and absent **dystrophin protein** on muscle biopsy and DNA testing. Hip extensors are typically the first muscle group affected. A muscle biopsy sample shows foci of necrosis and connective tissue infiltration. Treatment is based on keeping patients ambulatory as long as possible. Patients lose independent ambulation by age 10; although it is controversial, the use of knee-ankle-foot orthoses and release of contractures can extend walking ability for 2-3 years. Patients are usually wheelchair bound by age 15 years. With no muscle support, scoliosis progresses rapidly by age 14 years. Patients can become bedridden

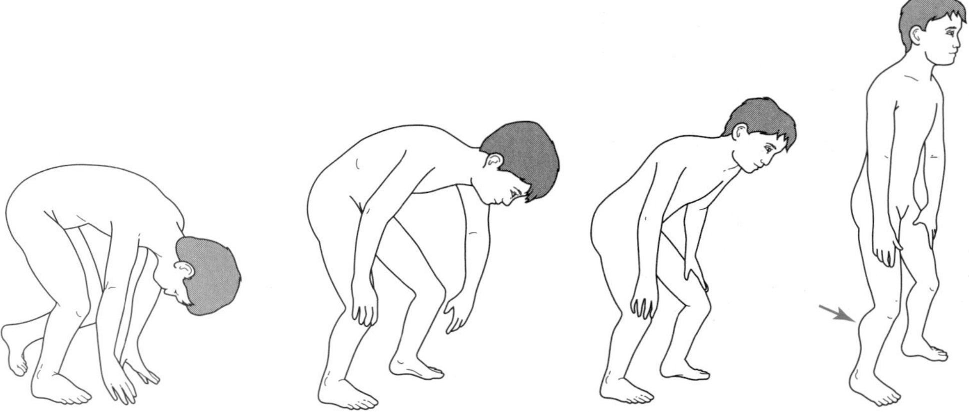

FIGURE 3–14 Gowers' sign. The child rises from the floor by "walking up the thighs with his hands—a functional test for quadriceps muscle weakness." Note the bulky calf *(arrow)*. (Redrawn from Herring JA: Tachdjian's Pediatric Orthopaedics, 3rd ed, p 85. Philadelphia, WB Saunders, 2002.)

by age 16 due to spinal deformity and are unable to sit for more than 8 hours. Scoliosis should be treated early (25-30 degrees of curvature) before pulmonary and cardiac function deteriorates. The surgical approach includes posterior spinal fusion with segmental instrumentation. These children usually die of cardiorespiratory complications before age 20. Newer medical treatment includes high-dose steroids, which have been shown to prevent scoliosis formation and prolong walking ability. Differential diagnosis includes **Becker's dystrophy** (also sex-linked recessive with a decrease in dystrophin), which is often seen in red/green color-blind boys with a similar but less severe picture. The diagnosis of Becker's dystrophy applies to those patients with the same examination findings but who live beyond 22 years without respiratory support. Newer medical therapies employing steroids have been shown to keep the patients ambulating longer and delaying the onset of scoliosis.

2. Fascioscapulohumeral—AD disorder typically seen in patients 6-20 years old with facial muscle abnormalities, normal CPK, and winging of the scapula (stabilized with scapulothoracic fusion).
3. Limb-girdle—AR disorder seen in patients 10-30 years old with pelvic or shoulder girdle involvement and increased CPK values.
4. Others—Gowers' (distal involvement; high incidence in Sweden); ocular, oculopharyngeal (high incidence in French Canadians).

D. Polymyositis, dermatomyositis—Characterized by a febrile illness that may be acute or insidious. Females predominate and typically exhibit photosensitivity and increased CPK and erythrocyte sedimentation rate (ESR) values. Muscles are tender, brawny, and indurated. Biopsy demonstrates the pathognomonic inflammatory response.

E. Hereditary neuropathies—Disorders associated with multiple central nervous system lesions, including the following:

1. Friedreich's ataxia—AR disorder with problems with the frataxin gene; spinocerebellar degenerative disease with mean onset between 7 and 15 years of age. Presents with staggering, wide-based gait; nystagmus; cardiomyopathy; a cavus foot (treated with plantar release with or without metatarsal and calcaneal osteotomies early, and triple arthrodesis later), and scoliosis. Involves motor and sensory defects, with an increase in polyphasic potentials by EMG. Ataxia forces use of a wheelchair by age 15, and death occurs between ages 40 and 50, usually from cardiomyopathy.
2. Hereditary sensory motor neuropathies (HSMNs)—A group of inherited neuropathic disorders with similar characteristics (Table 3–8).
3. Charcot-Marie-Tooth disease (peroneal muscular atrophy)—AD sensory motor demyelinating neuropathy. Two forms are described: a hypertrophic form with onset during the second decade of life, and a neuronal form with onset during the third or fourth decade but with more extensive foot involvement. Orthopaedic manifestations include pes cavus, hammer toes with frequent corns/calluses, peroneal weakness, and "stork legs." Low nerve conduction velocities with prolonged distal latencies are noted in peroneal, ulnar, and median nerves. Diagnosis is made most reliably by **DNA testing** for a duplication of a portion of chromosome 17. Intrinsic wasting is noted in hands. The most severely affected muscles are the tibialis anterior, peroneus longus, and peroneus brevis. Treatment includes plantar release, posterior tibial tendon transfer (if hindfoot varus is flexible), triple arthrodesis (poor long-term results) versus calcaneal and metatarsal osteotomies (if heel varus is fixed and the foot not too short), Jones' procedure for hammer toes, and intrinsic procedures for hand deformity. The Colman block test helps decide if calcaneal osteotomy is needed. Involves motor defects much more than sensory defects.

TABLE 3-8 MAJOR HEREDITARY MOTOR SENSORY NEUROPATHIES

Type	Terminology	Inheritance	Description
I	Charcot-Marie-Tooth syndrome (hypertrophic form)	AD	Peroneal weakness, slow nerve conduction, absent reflexes
II	Charcot-Marie-Tooth syndrome (neuronal form)	Variable	Peroneal weakness, normal nerve conduction, and normal reflexes
III	Dejerine-Sottas disease	AR	Begins in infancy and more severe

AD, autosomal dominant; AR, autosomal recessive.

4. Dejerine-Sottas disease—AR hypertrophic neuropathy of infancy. Delayed ambulation, pes cavus foot, footdrop, stocking-glove dysesthesia, and spinal deformities are common. The patient is confined to a wheelchair by the third or fourth decade.
5. Riley-Day syndrome (dysautonomia)—One of five inherited (AR) sensory and autonomic neuropathies. This disease is found only in patients of Ashkenazi Jewish ancestry. Clinical presentation includes dysphagia, alacrima, pneumonia, excessive sweating, postural hypotension, and sensory loss.

F. Myasthenia gravis—Chronic disease with insidious development of easy muscle fatigability after exercise. Caused by competitive inhibition of acetylcholine receptors at the motor end plate by antibodies produced in the thymus gland. Treatment consists of cyclosporin, anti-acetylcholinesterase agents, or thymectomy.

G. Anterior horn cell disorders

1. Poliomyelitis—Viral destruction of anterior horn cells in the spinal cord and brainstem motor

TABLE 3-9 SPINAL MUSCULAR ATROPHY

Type	Description	Age at Presentation	Prognosis
I	Acute Werdnig-Hoffman disease	< 6 mo	Poor
II	Chronic Werdnig-Hoffman disease	6-24 mo	May live into 5th decade
III	Kugelberg-Welander disease	2-10 yr	Good—may need respiratory support

nuclei; all but disappeared in the United States after vaccine was developed. Many surgical procedures still used were developed for the treatment of polio. The hallmark of polio is muscle weakness with normal sensation.

2. Spinal muscular atrophy—AR; loss of horn cells from the spinal cord. There are three types (Table 3–9). Often associated with progressive scoliosis that is best treated surgically like Duchenne's muscular dystrophy curves, except that fusion may be required while patient is still ambulatory (may result in loss of ambulatory ability). Patients have symmetrical paresis with more involvement of the lower extremity and proximal muscles.

H. Acute idiopathic postinfectious polyneuropathy (**Guillain-Barré syndrome**)—Symmetrical ascending motor paresis caused by demyelination after viral infection. Cerebrospinal fluid protein is typically elevated. Usually self-limiting; better prognosis with the acute form.

I. Overgrowth syndromes

1. Proteus syndrome—An overgrowth of the hands and feet, with bizarre facial disfigurement, scoliosis, genu valgum, hemangiomas, lipomas, and nevi. Must be differentiated from neurofibromatosis and McCune-Albright syndrome.
2. Klippel-Trénaunay syndrome—Overgrowth caused by underlying arteriovenous malformations. Associated with cutaneous hemangiomas and varicosities. Severely hypertrophied extremities often require amputation. Embolization is a treatment option in selected patients.
3. Hemihypertrophy—Can be caused by various syndromes, but most are idiopathic. The most commonly known cause is neurofibromatosis. This disorder is often associated with renal abnormalities (especially Wilms' tumor); best evaluated with serial ultrasound until age 5 years. Management of associated leg-length discrepancy is discussed below.

VIII. Congenital Disorders (Table 3–10)

TABLE 3-10 PEDIATRIC CONGENITAL DISORDERS AND ASSOCIATED GENETIC DEFECTS

Disorder	Genetic Defect
Achondroplasia	FGFR3
Hypochondroplasia	FGFR3
Thanatophoric dysplasia	FGFR3
Pseudoachondroplasia	COMP
Multiple epiphyseal dysplasia type I	COMP
Multiple epiphyseal dysplasia type II	Collagen type IX
Spondyloepiphyseal dysplasia congenita	Collagen type II
Kniest's syndrome	Collagen type II
Stickler syndrome (hereditary arthro-ophthalmopathy)	Collagen type II
Diastrophic dysplasia	Sulfate transporter gene
Schmid's metaphyseal chondrodysplasia	Collagen type X
Jansen's metaphyseal chondrodysplasia	PTHRP
Craniosynostosis	FGFR2
Cleidocranial dysplasia	CBFA1
Hypophosphatemic rickets	PEX
Marfan's syndrome	Fibrillin
Osteogenesis imperfecta	Collagen type I
Ehlers-Danlos syndrome	Types I and II: Collagen type V Type IV: Collagen type IV Types VI and VII: Collagen type I
Duchenne's/Becker's muscular dystrophies	Dystrophin
Limb-girdle dystrophies	Sarcoglycan and dystroglycan complex
Charcot-Marie-Tooth disease	PMP22
Spinal muscular atrophy	Survival motor neuron protein
Myotonic dystrophy	Myotonin
Friedreich's ataxia	Frataxin
Neurofibromatosis	Neurofibromin
McCune-Albright syndrome	cAMP

FGFR3/2, fibroblast growth factor receptor 3/2; COMP, cartilage oligomeric matrix protein; PTHRP, parathyroid hormone-related peptide; CBFA1, transcription factor for osteocalcin; PEX, period-extender gene; PMP22, peripheral myelin protein 22; cAMP, cyclic adenosine monophosphate.

Courtesy of Luke S. Choi, MD, Resident, Department of Orthopaedic Surgery, University of Virginia.

IX. Pediatric Spine

A. Idiopathic scoliosis

1. Introduction—A lateral deviation and rotational deformity of the spine without an identifiable cause. It may be related to a hormonal, brainstem, or proprioception disorder. Recent studies have suggested that hormonal factors (melatonin) may play a significant role in the cause. Most patients have a positive family history, but there is variable expression. The deformity is described as right or left based on the direction of the apical convexity. Right thoracic curves are the most common, followed by double major (right thoracic and left lumbar), left lumbar, and right lumbar curves. In adolescents left thoracic curves are rare, and evaluation of the spinal cord by MRI is suggested to rule out cord abnormalities. Idiopathic scoliosis is divided into three categories based on age: infantile (0-3 years), juvenile (4-10 years), and adolescent (> 10 years). The adolescent form is the most common. Risk factors for curve progression include **curve magnitudes** (> 20 degrees), **younger age** (< 12 years), and **skeletal immaturity** (**Risser** stage [0-1]) at presentation (Table 3–11). About 75% of immature

TABLE 3-11 INCIDENCE OF CURVE PROGRESSION AS RELATED TO THE MAGNITUDE OF THE CURVE AND RISSER'S STAGE

	Percent of Curves That Progressed	
Risser's Stage	*5-19 Degrees (Curves)*	*20-29 Degrees (Curves)*
0, 1	22%	68%
2, 3, 4	1.6%	23%

From Lonstein JE, Carlson JM: The prediction of curve progression in untreated idiopathic scoliosis during growth. J Bone Joint Surg [Am] 66:1067, 1984.

patients with curves of 20-30 degrees will progress at least 5 degrees. Peak growth velocity is the best predictor of progression occurring before the onset of menarche and the presence of Risser 1. Severe curves (> 90 degrees) may be associated with cardiopulmonary dysfunction, early death, pain, and a decreased self-image.

2. Diagnosis—Patients are often referred from school screening, in which rotational deformities may be noted on the Adams forward bend test with a scoliometer. A threshold level of **7 degrees** is thought to be an acceptable compromise between overreferral and a high false-negative rate and correlates best with a 20-degree coronal curve. Physical findings include shoulder elevation, waistline asymmetry, a trunk shift, limb-length inequality, spinal deformity, and rib rotational deformity (rib hump). Careful neurologic examination for potential spinal cord disorder is important (especially with left thoracic curves). An abnormal neurologic examination (especially asymmetrical abdominal reflexes from syringomyelia) warrant further workup (MRI). The lower extremities should be evaluated to ensure that cavus or cavovarus feet are not seen; these would warrant MRI evaluation. Standing posteroanterior and lateral radiographs are obtained and curves are measured based on the Cobb method (Fig. 3–15). Hypokyphosis of the apical vertebrae in the sagittal plane is seen with idiopathic scoliosis. If apical kyphosis is seen, an MRI should be obtained. The potential coexistence of spondylolisthesis can also be noted on the lateral x-ray film. Inclusion of the iliac crest on radiographs allows determination of skeletal maturity based on the Risser sign (ossification of the iliac crest apophysis and graded 0-5). An MRI scan is obtained for cases with noted structural abnormalities on plain films, excessive kyphosis, juvenile-onset scoliosis (age under 11 years), rapid curve progression, neurologic signs/symptoms, associated syndromes, and left thoracic/thoracolumbar curves or painful scoliosis.
3. Treatment—Based on the maturity of the patient (Risser stage and presence of menarche), magnitude of the deformity, and curve progression. Treatment options include observation, bracing, and surgery. Exercise and electrical stimulation have not been shown to affect the natural history of curve progression.
   a. Bracing—Bracing may help to halt or slow curve progression but does not reverse the magnitude of the deformity. Indications for bracing are curves > 30 degrees (or progression > 25 degrees while under direct observation) in skeletally immature patients (Risser 0-2). The Milwaukee brace (cervicothoracolumbosacral orthosis) or Boston underarm brace with Milwaukee superstructure is used for curves with the apex at or above T7 (poor tolerance). The Boston-type underarm thoracolumbosacral orthosis (TLSO) brace is used for curves with the apex at T8 or below. Patients with thoracic lordosis or hypokyphosis are poor candidates for bracing. The effectiveness of bracing patients with idiopathic scoliosis is dose related (the more the brace is worn each day, the more effective it is). Although the efficacy of full-time wear has been well demonstrated, long-term prospective studies on part-time brace wear have not been done.
   b. Surgical options—The basic options for the surgical treatment of idiopathic scoliosis are anterior spinal fusion (ASF) with instrumentation, posterior spinal fusion (PSF) with instrumentation, or combined ASF and PSF. ASF is most frequently used for thoracolumbar and lumbar curves

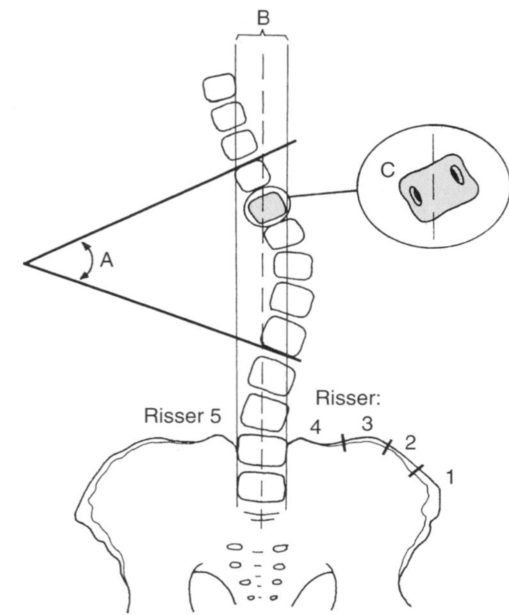

FIGURE 3–15 Measurements for idiopathic scoliosis. A, Cobb's angle; B, Harrington's stable zone; C, Moe's neutral vertebra; 1-5, Risser's staging.

because motion segments can be saved (end vertebra to end vertebra is fused), and outstanding three-dimensional correction is seen. The ASF may also be used for single thoracic curves, especially when hypokyphosis is seen and motion segments can be saved compared with PSF. PSF can be used in all curve patterns in adolescent idiopathic scoliosis (AIS) and is the most common approach used in AIS surgery. The indications for a combined ASF/PSF in idiopathic scoliosis are severe deformities (> 75 degrees) and crankshaft prevention (Risser stage 0; girls < 10 and boys < 13 years old, before or during peak growth velocity).

(1) Fusion levels—Successful surgery is based on choosing appropriate fusion levels, among other considerations. Several methods have been developed to select the correct levels. The goal is to fuse the spinal levels necessary to establish a well-balanced spine in the coronal and sagittal planes. Cochran identified a markedly increased incidence of late low-back pain, with fusion to L5 and some increase with fusion to L4. Therefore, efforts are made to avoid fusing below L3 and certainly L4. The **stable vertebra** is defined as the most proximal vertebra that is the most closely bisected by the center sacral line. It is almost never necessary to fuse to the pelvis in adolescent idiopathic scoliosis. King and colleagues identified five patterns and treatment options. These treatment options were developed in the Harrington instrumentation era (Fig. 3–16). The newer segmental spinal instrumentation systems allow more powerful correction of these three-dimensional deformities. A new classification by Lenke and associates define six curve types, three lumbar modifiers, and thoracic sagittal plane analysis. This classification provides a framework to define those curves which may require surgical arthrodesis and is always combined with the clinical appearance of the patient.

(2) Considerations for surgical fusion—In general, fusion levels for ASF surgery are to include the proximal and distal end vertebrae. For PSF, the proximal instrumented vertebra is typically the proximal end vertebra of the proximal or main thoracic curve. Selecting the lowest instrumented vertebra (LIV) is more challenging. In general, for single thoracic curves, the LIV is usually one or two levels proximal to the stable vertebra, and for double or triple major curves, the LIV is the distal end vertebra.

(3) Complications—The most disastrous complication of spinal surgery is a neurologic deficit, which is very rare. Successful surgical intervention is based on careful technique (intraoperative monitoring [somatosensory-evoked potentials and motor-evoked potentials] is helpful with or without Stagnara's wake-up test and clonus tests). It is especially useful in patients with congenital kyphoscoliosis. Attempting excessive correction or placement of sublaminar wires is associated with an increased risk of neurologic damage. Minimizing blood loss and maximizing the use of autologous blood are important in order to avoid transfusion-associated problems. Surgical complications include pseudarthrosis (1-2%), early wound infection (1-2%), and implant failure (early hook cutout, late rod breakage, and pain from prominent hardware). Late rod breakage frequently signifies failure of fusion. Only an asymptomatic pseudarthrosis (no pain or loss of curve correction) should be observed, because the results of the late repair do not differ from those performed earlier. Use of a compression implant facilitates pseudarthrosis repair.

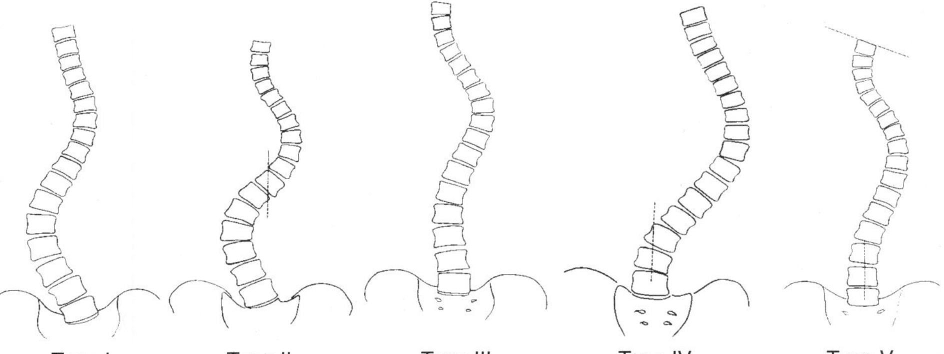

FIGURE 3–16 Five types of scoliotic curves (types I-V). See text for description. (Adapted from King HA, Moe JH, Bradford DS, et al: The selection of fusion levels in thoracic idiopathic scoliosis. J Bone Joint Surg [Am] 65:1302–1313, 1983.)

Creation of a "flat back syndrome," or early fatigability and pain due to loss of lumbar lordosis, can be minimized with rod contouring in the sagittal plane and effective use of compression and distraction devices. Treatment of this condition requires revision surgery with posterior closing wedge osteotomies. The results appear to be improved, with maintenance of correction, if anterior release and fusion precede the posterior osteotomies. The **crankshaft phenomenon** occurs in the setting of continued anterior spinal growth after posterior fusion in skeletally immature patients. It results in increased rotation and deformity of the spine because continued anterior growth causes a spin around the posterior tether (fusion mass). This situation is best avoided by anterior diskectomy and fusion coupled with PSF, as described previously.

4. Infantile idiopathic scoliosis—Presents at less than 3 years old with (more commonly) left-sided thoracic scoliosis, male predominance, plagiocephaly (skull flattening), and other congenital defects. The two factors most affecting progression are curve magnitude and the apical rib–vertebral angle difference (RVAD) of Mehta. Most curves less than 25 degrees with an RVAD less than 20 degrees tend to resolve spontaneously, and observation is appropriate in these patients. Surgical options for severe curves include instrumentation ("growing rods") without fusion or an ASF/PSF combination. Any child with infantile idiopathic scoliosis should have MRI preoperatively to rule out any possible spinal cord disease (20% incidence).
5. Juvenile idiopathic scoliosis (JIS)—Scoliosis in 3 to 10 year olds is similar to adolescent scoliosis in terms of presentation and treatment. A high risk of curve progression is seen; 70% require treatment, with 50% needing bracing and 50% requiring surgery. Fusion should be delayed until the onset of the adolescent growth spurt if possible (unless curve magnitude is > 50 degrees). The use of spinal instrumentation without fusion (as for infantile scoliosis) may facilitate this delay. In patients with severe deformities that require surgery, a careful assessment of their skeletal maturity should be done. In patients with multiple risk factors for skeletal immaturity, ASF and PSF with instrumentation should be performed to prevent the crankshaft phenomenon.

B. Neuromuscular scoliosis—Many children with neuromuscular disorders develop scoliosis or other spinal deformities.

1. Diagnosis—In contrast to idiopathic curves, neuromuscular curves are longer; involve more vertebrae; are less likely to have compensatory curves; progress more rapidly and may progress after maturity; and are often associated with **pelvic obliquity,** bony deformities, and cervical involvement. Pulmonary complications are also more frequent, including decreased pulmonary function, pneumonia, and atelectasis. For patients who are already wheelchair bound, curve progression may make them bedridden.
2. Treatment—Orthotic use is controversial for neuromuscular patients but can be used to improve sitting balance and delay surgical treatment. The surgical treatment of neuromuscular scoliosis often involves the fusion of more levels than those for idiopathic curves. Fusion to the pelvis is required for fixed pelvic obliquity in the nonambulatory patient. The **Galveston technique** of pelvic fixation has traditionally been used (bending the caudal end of the rods from the lamina of S1 to pass into the posterosuperior iliac spine and between the tables of the ilium just anterior to the sciatic notch). Other techniques include Dunn-McCarthy S rods (placed over the sacral ala) and sacral and iliac screws. The goal of treatment is stability and truncal balance with a level pelvis. Patients with upper motor neuron disease (cerebral palsy) are initially treated with wheelchair modifications or seat orthoses but require fusion for curve progression to greater than 50 degrees. Children with severe involvement require fusion from T2 to the sacrum, usually through a posterior approach only. Preoperative nutritional assessment is important and requires more than 1500 leukocytes and an albumin level greater than 3.5. Both anterior and posterior procedures for severe curve magnitude may be necessary for young patients to avoid the crankshaft phenomenon (delayed bone age is common in neuromuscular patients) and for those with large curves. Surgery is indicated in patients with Duchenne's muscular dystrophy for curves greater than 30 degrees and usually involves fusion from T2 to the pelvis. Preoperative assessment of pulmonary function (should be over 40% predicted) and cardiac function is necessary.

C. Congenital spinal disorders—Due to a developmental defect in the formation of the mesenchymal anlage during the fourth to sixth week of development. Three basic types of defects are noted: **failure of segmentation** (typically results in a vertebral bar), **failure of formation** (due to lack of material and may result in hemivertebrae), and **mixed.** Three-dimensional CT is helpful for defining the type of vertebral anomaly (Fig. 3–17). Spinal MRI scans should be obtained before any surgery to assess the patient for intraspinal anomalies. Associated anomalies include genitourinary (25%), cardiac (10%), and dysraphic (25%, usually diastematomyelia). Renal ultrasonography is used to rule out associated kidney abnormalities.

1. Congenital scoliosis—Most common congenital spinal disorder. The risk of progression is dependent on the morphology of the vertebrae. A fully segmented hemivertebra is free, with normal disc spaces on both sides (higher risk of progression), whereas an unsegmented hemivertebra is fused above and below (lower risk) (see Fig. 3–17).
   a. Prognosis—An incarcerated hemivertebra (within the lateral margins of the vertebrae above and below) has a better prognosis than an unincarcerated (laterally positioned) hemivertebra. A unilateral, unsegmented bar is a common disorder and is likely to progress. The best prognosis is with a block vertebra (bilateral failure of segmentation). The worst prognosis (most likely to progress) is seen with a unilateral, unsegmented bar with a contralateral, fully segmented hemivertebra and is an indication for surgery at presentation.
   b. Treatment—The treatment options include ASF and PSF in situ, convex anterior and posterior hemiepiphysiodesis, or resection of the hemivertebra. Other deformities should demonstrate progression before surgical options are considered. Bracing may be effective for compensatory curves or for smaller, supple curves above a vertebral anomaly, but it is ineffective for controlling congenital curves. Anterior and posterior hemivertebral excision may be indicated for lumbosacral hemivertebrae associated with progressive curves and an oblique takeoff (severe truncal imbalance). Isolated hemivertebral excision should be accompanied by anterior/posterior arthrodesis with instrumentation to stabilize the adjacent vertebrae. Anterior and posterior convex hemiepiphysiodesis/arthrodesis is safer, but correction of imbalance is less predictable. Posterior fusion in situ is the gold standard of treatment for most progressive curves. In young patients (girls < 10 and boys < 13 years old), the crankshaft phenomenon may occur because of continued anterior spinal growth; in these cases anterior/posterior fusion may be required. A summary of treatment recommendations for congenital scoliosis is found in Table 3–12.

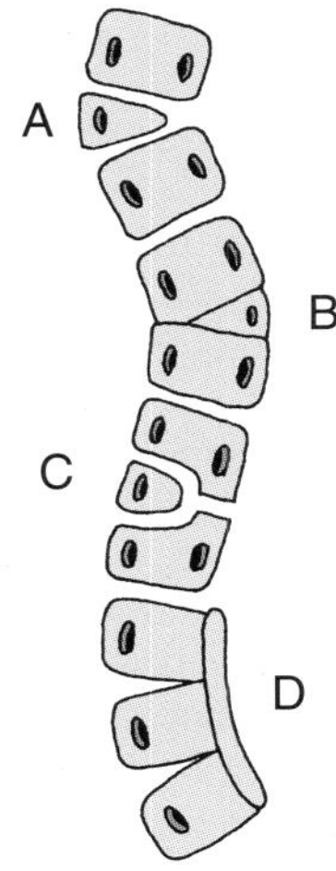

FIGURE 3–17 Vertebral anomalies leading to congenital scoliosis. A, Fully segmented hemivertebra; B, unsegmented hemivertebra; C, incarcerated hemivertebra; D, unilateral unsegmented bar.

2. Congenital kyphosis—May be secondary to failure of formation (**type I**), failure of segmentation (**type II**), or mixed abnormalities (**type III**). Failure of formation (type I, the most common) has the worst prognosis for progression (95%) and neurologic involvement of all spinal deformities. Type I congenital kyphosis is also the most likely to result in paraplegia (neurofibromatosis is second). The presence of significant congenital kyphosis secondary to failure of formation (type I) is an indication for surgery. Posterior fusion is favored in young children (< 5 years old) with curves less than 50 degrees. This is essentially a posterior (convex) hemiepiphysiodesis. Combined anterior/posterior fusion is reserved for older children or more severe curves. Anterior vertebrectomy, spinal cord decompression, and anterior fusion followed by posterior fusion are indicated for curves associated with neurologic deficits. A type II congenital kyphosis can be observed to document progression, but progressive curves should be fused posteriorly.

TABLE 3-12 PROGRESSION OF CONGENITAL SCOLIOSIS PATTERNS AND TREATMENT OPTIONS

Risk of Progression (Highest to Lowest)	Character of Curve Progression	Treatment Options
Unilateral unsegmented bar with contralateral hemivertebra	Rapid and relentless	Posterior spinal fusion (add anterior fusion for girls age < 10 yr, boys < 12 yr)
Unilateral unsegmented bar	Rapid	Same
Fully segmented hemivertebra	Steady	Anterior spinal fusion Hemivertebra excision
Partially segmented hemivertebra	Less rapid; curve usually < 40 degrees at maturity	Observation, hemivertebra excision
Incarcerated hemivertebra	May slowly progress	Observation
Nonsegmented hemivertebra	Little progression	Observation

D. Neurofibromatosis—AD disorder of neural crest origin, often associated with neoplasia and skeletal abnormalities.

1. Diagnosis—It is characterized by neurofibromas and café au lait spots. The spine is the most common site of skeletal involvement. Curves should be classified as nondystrophic (similar to idiopathic scoliosis) or dystrophic. Dystrophic curves are characterized by radiographic abnormalities such as vertebral scalloping; enlarged foramina; penciling of transverse processes or ribs; severe apical rotation; and short, tight curves. Spinal deformity secondary to neurofibromatosis is characteristically kyphoscoliosis in the thoracic region with dystrophic changes, but nondystrophic scoliosis or cervical involvement may also be noted.
2. Treatment—Nondystrophic scoliosis is treated similar to idiopathic scoliosis. However, dystrophic deformities should be treated more aggressively, especially when kyphosis is present, with surgical treatment indicated for any progression and when curves reach 40 degrees. For young patients and for those with associated kyphosis, a combined anterior/posterior surgery is necessary to prevent the crankshaft phenomenon and to ensure fusion because the incidence of pseudarthrosis is high. Isolated kyphosis of the thoracic spine is treated with anterior decompression of the kyphotic angular cord compression, followed by anterior and posterior fusion. Cervical spine involvement includes kyphosis or atlantoaxial instability. Posterior fusion with autologous grafting and halo immobilization is recommended for severe cervical spine deformity with instability. Neurologic involvement is common in neurofibromatosis and may be caused by the deformity itself, an intraspinal tumor, a soft tissue mass, or dural ectasia. Therefore, any patient with neurofibromatosis undergoing spinal surgery should have an MRI preoperatively. Because of a high pseudarthrosis rate, some authors recommend routine augmentation of the posterior fusion mass at 6 months postoperatively with a repeat iliac crest bone graft.

E. Other spinal abnormalities

1. Diastematomyelia—Fibrous, cartilaginous, or osseous bar creating a longitudinal cleft in the spinal cord (Fig. 3–18). More commonly occurs in the lumbar spine and can lead to tethering of the cord, with associated neurologic deficits. Intrapedicular widening on plain radiographs is suggestive, and myelographic CT or MRI is necessary to fully define the disorder. A diastematomyelia must be resected before correction of a spinal deformity, but if it is otherwise asymptomatic and without neurologic sequelae, it may be treated by observation.
2. Sacral agenesis—Partial or complete absence of the sacrum and lower lumbar spine. Highly associated with maternal diabetes, it is often accompanied by gastrointestinal, genitourinary, and cardiovascular abnormalities. Clinically, children have a prominent lower lumbar spine and atrophic lower extremities; they may sit in a "Buddha" position. Motor impairment is at the level of the agenesis, but sensory innervation is largely spared. Management may include amputation or spinal-pelvic fusion.

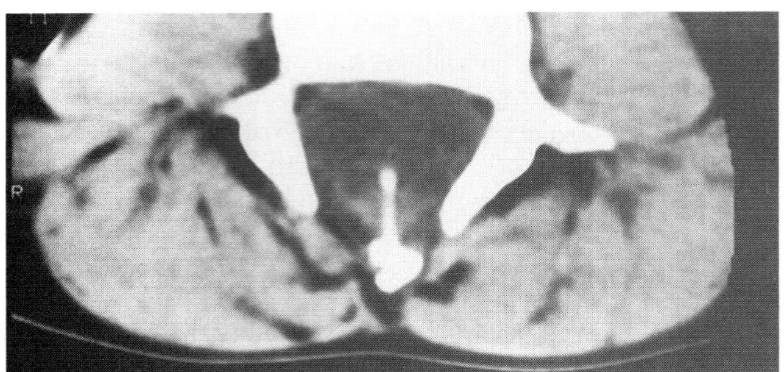

FIGURE 3–18 Ten-year-old girl with diastematomyelia. Note the incomplete bony spur between the hemicords. (From Benson M, Fixen J, Macnicol M: Children's Orthopaedics and Fractures, p 299. New York, Churchill Livingstone, 1994.)

F. Low-back pain (Table 3–13)—In children, complaints of low-back pain and especially painful scoliosis should be taken seriously.

1. Diskitis and osteomyelitis—Acute back pain can be associated with diskitis (presents as refusal to sit or walk; increased ESR; and subsequent disc space narrowing with preservation of the end plates, taking 3 weeks to appear on plain films) or osteomyelitis (systemic illness, leukocytosis). Rang and Wenger discussed the difficulty of differentiating between diskitis and osteomyelitis, and they recommended using the term **infectious spondylitis** to describe disc space infections in children.
2. Herniated nucleus pulposus—Occasionally, herniated nucleus pulposus, presenting as sciatica and back pain in older children, occurs and may require operative intervention, but most resolve with time.

TABLE 3–13 DIFFERENTIAL DIAGNOSIS FOR LOW-BACK PAIN IN CHILDREN

Category	Disease
Mechanical	Muscle strain Herniated nucleus pulposis
Infection and tumor	Diskitis osteomyelitis Eosinophilic granuloma Osteoid osteoma Osteoblastoma Ewing's spinal cord tumor Metastatic disease
Developmental	Spondylosis Spondylolisthesis Syringomyelia Tethered cord

3. Spondylolysis—Spondylolysis (stress fracture at the pars interarticularis) is common after athletic injuries, especially when engaging in activities involving repetitive hyperextension of the lumbosacral spine (gymnastics, football lineman), and is best visualized with a CT scan or single-photon emission computed tomography. Spondylolysis (pars defect) without slipping should be treated initially with nonoperative measures. If conservative measures fail, fusion (if at L5) or repair of the pars defect (if at L4 or higher) is appropriate.
4. Spondylolisthesis—Spondylolisthesis (forward slippage of the proximal vertebra on the distal vertebra) is most commonly seen at L5-S1. Can be lytic (from spondylolysis) or dysplastic (congenital absence or dysplasia of the facets) and is defined by the degree of forward translation (**Meyerding classification:** grade 1, 0-25%; grade 2, 25-50%; grade 3, 50-75%; and grade 4, 75-100%). Low-grade slips are Meyerding 1 and 2 while high-grade is defined as Myerding 3 and 4. Dysplastic spondylolisthesis is more at risk to progress, especially in the skeletally immature patient. The larger the slip, the greater the chance of progression. Asymptomatic, low-grade slips should be observed. Conservative treatment, including modification of exercise activity and occasionally bracing, is usually successful. Continued pain despite nonoperative methods and high-grade slips should have operative stabilization and fusion. In general, high-grade slips require L4-S1 fusion, while low-grade slips are often fused from L5 to S1. Decompression (**Gill procedure**) must also be considered for neurologic compromise. The use of instrumentation and reduction continues to be controversial and can be associated with neurologic injury.
5. Osteoma or spinal cord anomaly—Should be investigated aggressively. A bone scan is an excellent screening method for a child or adolescent with back pain.

G. Kyphosis
1. Congenital kyphosis—See the previous discussion of congenital spinal disorders.
2. Scheuermann's disease—Classic definition is increased thoracic kyphosis (> 45 degrees) with 5 degrees or more anterior wedging at three sequential vertebrae. Other radiographic findings include disc space narrowing, end plate irregularities, spondylolysis (30-50%), scoliosis (33%), and Schmorl's nodes (Sorenson) (Figs. 3–19 and 3–20).
   a. Diagnosis—Scheuermann's disease is more common in males and typically presents in adolescents with poor posture, often with pain over the kyphos or in the lumbar spine. Physical examination characteristically shows tight hamstrings and hyperkyphosis that does not reverse on attempts at hyperextension. Neurologic sequelae secondary to disc herniation or extradural spinal cysts are rare but have been reported.
   b. Treatment—Treatment consists of bracing (a modified Milwaukee brace) for a progressive curve in a patient with 1 year or more of skeletal growth remaining (Risser stage 2 or below), although it is not well tolerated

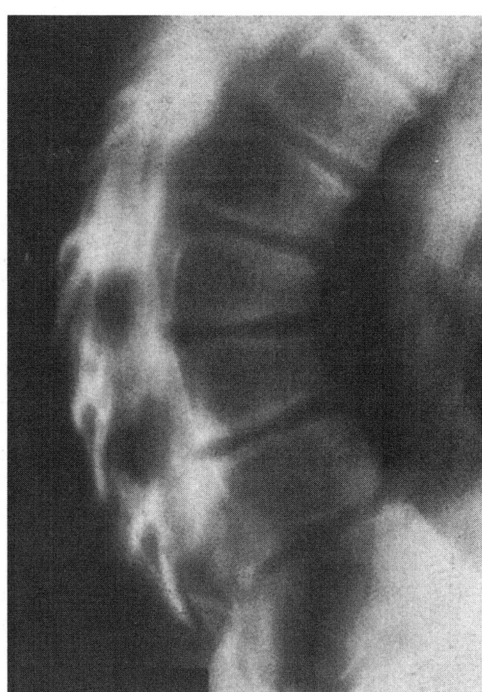

FIGURE 3–19 Lateral radiograph of a patient with Scheuermann's thoracic hyperkyphosis. Note the anterior wedging at three sequential vertebrae. (From Benson M, Fixen J, Macnicol M: Children's Orthopaedics and Fractures, p 19. New York, Churchill Livingstone, 1994.)

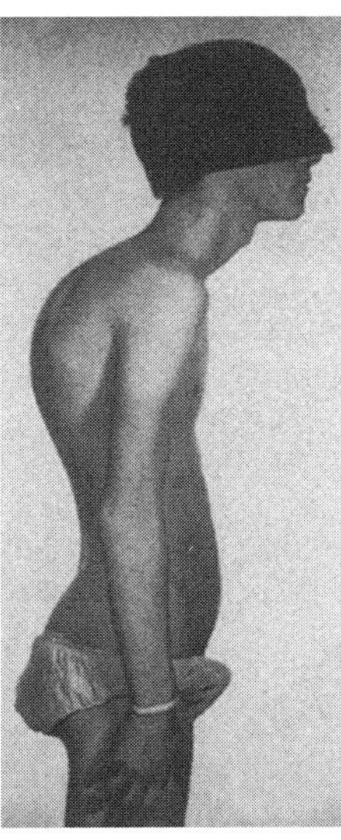

FIGURE 3–20 Clinical photograph of Scheuermann's thoracic kyphosis. (From Benson M, Fixen J, Macnicol M: Children's Orthopaedics and Fractures, p 610. New York, Churchill Livingstone, 1994.)

in these patients. For the skeletally mature patient with severe kyphosis (> 75 degrees), surgical correction is indicated for persistent pain despite physical therapy or curve progression. A relative indication for surgical treatment concerns cosmetics. Posterior fusion with segmental dual rod constructs is the treatment of choice for most patients. In general, fusion levels are from T2 proximally (more distal for lumbar Scheuermann's) and should include the first lordotic disc space distally. Multiple apical Smith-Peterson or chevron-type osteotomies provide room for compression of the posterior elements and correction of the deformity. Anterior release and interbody fusion are used less often, and only for very severe (> 90-degree) stiffness (fails to correct to < 60 degrees). Thoracoscopic anterior diskectomy and interbody fusion have decreased the morbidity associated with thoracotomy for anterior release and fusion.

c. Lumbar Scheuermann's disease—Less common than the thoracic variety but more often causes back pain on a mechanical basis (more common in athletes and manual laborers). The pain is often self-limiting. Lumbar Scheuermann's disease also demonstrates irregular vertebral end plates with Schmorl's nodes and decreased disc height, but it is not associated with vertebral wedging.

3. Postural round back—Also associated with kyphosis but does not demonstrate vertebral body changes. Forward bending demonstrates kyphosis, but there is no sharp angulation as in Scheuermann's disease. Correction with backward bending and prone hyperextension is typical. Treatment includes a hyperextension exercise program.

4. Other causes of kyphosis—Trauma, infections, spondylitis, bone dysplasias (mucopolysaccharidoses, Kniest's syndrome, diastrophic dysplasia), and neoplasms. Additionally, postlaminectomy kyphosis (most often for spinal cord abnormalities) can be severe and requires anterior and posterior fusion early. The performance of total laminectomy in immature patients without stabilization is contraindicated.

H. Cervical spine disorders

1. Klippel-Feil syndrome—Multiple abnormal cervical segments due to failure of normal segmentation or formation of cervical somites at 3-8 weeks of gestation. Often associated with congenital scoliosis, renal disease (aplasia, 33%), synkinesis (mirror motions), Sprengel's deformity (30%), congenital heart disease, brainstem abnormalities, and congenital cervical stenosis. The classic triad of **low posterior hairline, short "webbed" neck, and limited cervical ROM** is seen in fewer than 50% of cases. Most therapy is conservative, but chronic pain with myelopathy associated with instability may require surgery. Disc degeneration occurs in almost 100% of cases. Affected children should avoid collision sports.

2. Atlantoaxial instability

a. Anteroposterior instability—Associated with Down syndrome (trisomy 21), JRA, various osteochondrodystrophies, os odontoideum, and other abnormalities. In patients with Down syndrome and a normal neurologic examination, simple avoidance of contact sports is appropriate, but with any acute or progressive neurologic symptoms, posterior spinal fusion is indicated (high complication rate).

b. Rotatory atlantoaxial subluxation—May present with torticollis; can be caused by retropharyngeal inflammation (Grisel's disease). It is probably caused by secondary ligamentous laxity and is best treated with early traction and bracing. Current diagnosis is by CT scans at the C1-C2 level with the head straight forward, in maximum rotation to the right, and then in maximum rotation to the left (Fig. 3–21). Late diagnosis may require C1-C2 fusion. Traumatic atlantoaxial subluxation may present as torticollis, which can be treated initially with a soft collar for up to 1 week. If symptoms persist past this point, cervical traction

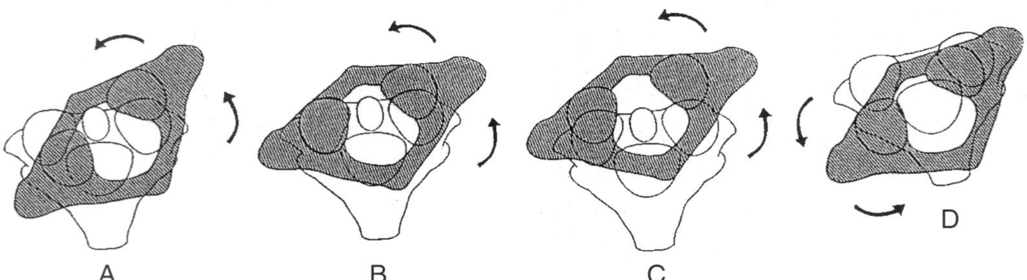

FIGURE 3–21 Four types of rotatory fixation. **A**, Type I: rotatory fixation with no anterior displacement and the odontoid acting as the pivot. **B**, Type II: rotatory fixation with anterior displacement of 3-5 mm, with one lateral process acting as the pivot. **C**, Type III: rotatory fixation with anterior displacement > 5 mm. **D**, Type IV: rotatory fixation with posterior displacement. (Adapted from Fielding JW, Hawkins RJ: Atlantoaxial rotatory fixation. J Bone Joint Surg [Am] 59:42, 1977.)

should be initiated. If it is discovered late (> 1 month), fusion may be required for fixed rotatory subluxation. Rotatory subluxation can also be seen in rheumatoid arthritis, Down syndrome, congenital anomalies, and cervical tumors.

3. Os odontoideum—Previously thought to be due to the failure of fusion of the base of the odontoid, it presents like a type II odontoid fracture. Evidence suggests that it may represent the residue of an old traumatic process. It is usually seen in place of the normal odontoid process (orthotopic type), but it may fuse to the clivus (dystopic type more often seen with neurologic compromise). Treatment is conservative unless there is instability (> 10 mm of the atlanto-dens interval [ADI] or < 13 mm space available for the cord [SAC]) or neurologic symptoms are present, which require a posterior C1-C2 fusion.
4. Pseudosubluxation of the cervical spine—Subluxation of C2 on C3 (and occasionally of C3 on C4) of up to 40%, or 4 mm, can be normal in children less than 8 years old because of the orientation of the facets. Rapid resolution of pain, relatively minor trauma, lack of anterior swelling, continued alignment of the posterior interspinous distances and the posterior spinolaminar line (**Schwischuk's line**) on radiographs (Fig. 3–22), and reduction of the subluxation with neck extension help differentiate this entity from more serious disorders.

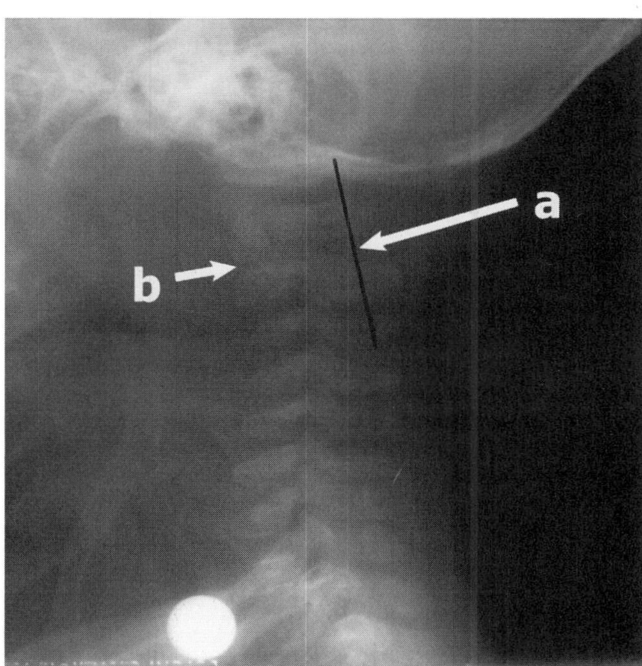

FIGURE 3–22 Physiologic subluxation of C2 and C3 confirmed by using the posterior cervical line (a). Synchondrosis between the odontoid and body of C2 is well demonstrated (b). (From Herring JA: Tachdjian's Pediatric Orthopaedics, 3rd ed, p 132. Philadelphia, WB Saunders, 2002.)

5. Intervertebral disc calcification syndrome—Pain, decreased ROM, low-grade fevers, increased ESR, and radiographic disc calcification (within the annulus) without erosion characterize this disorder, which usually involves the cervical spine. Conservative treatment is indicated for this self-limiting condition.
6. Basilar impression/invagination—Bony deformity at the base of the skull causes cephalad migration of the odontoid into the foramen magnum. A sagittal MRI scan best demonstrates impingement of the dens on the brainstem. Weakness, paresthesias, and hydrocephalus may result. Treatment is often operative and may include transoral resection of the dens, occipital laminectomy, and occipitocervical fusion and wiring.

X. Upper Extremity Problems*

A. Sprengel's deformity—Undescended scapula often associated with winging, hypoplasia, and omovertebral connections (30%) (Fig. 3–23). It is the most common congenital anomaly of the shoulder in children. Affected scapulae are usually small, relatively wide, and medially rotated. Increased association with Klippel-Feil syndrome, kidney disease, scoliosis, and diastematomyelia. Surgery for cosmetic or functional deformities (decreased abduction) includes distal advancement of the associated muscles and scapula (Woodward) or detachment and movement of the scapula (Schrock, Green). Clavicular osteotomy is often needed to avoid brachial plexus injury due to stretch. Surgery is best done on 3- to 8-year-olds.

B. Fibrotic deltoid problems—Short, fibrous bands replace the deltoid muscle and cause abduction contractures at the shoulder, with elevation and winging of the scapula when the arms are adducted. Surgical resection of these bands is often required.

XI. Lower Extremity Problems: General

A. Introduction—Lower extremity problems that are best considered as a whole are presented in this section to provide a basis for understanding and comparison.

B. Rotational problems of the lower extremities—Include femoral anteversion, tibial torsion, and metatarsus adductus. All of these problems may be a result of intrauterine positioning and commonly present with a pigeon-toed gait. These deformities are usually bilateral, and the clinician should be wary of asymmetrical findings. Evaluation should include the measurements noted in Table 3–14 and illustrated in Figure 3–24.

1. Metatarsus adductus—The forefoot is adducted at the tarsal-metatarsal joint. Usually seen during the first year of life. May be associated with hip

*See Chapter 7, Hand, Upper Extremity, and Microvascular Surgery.

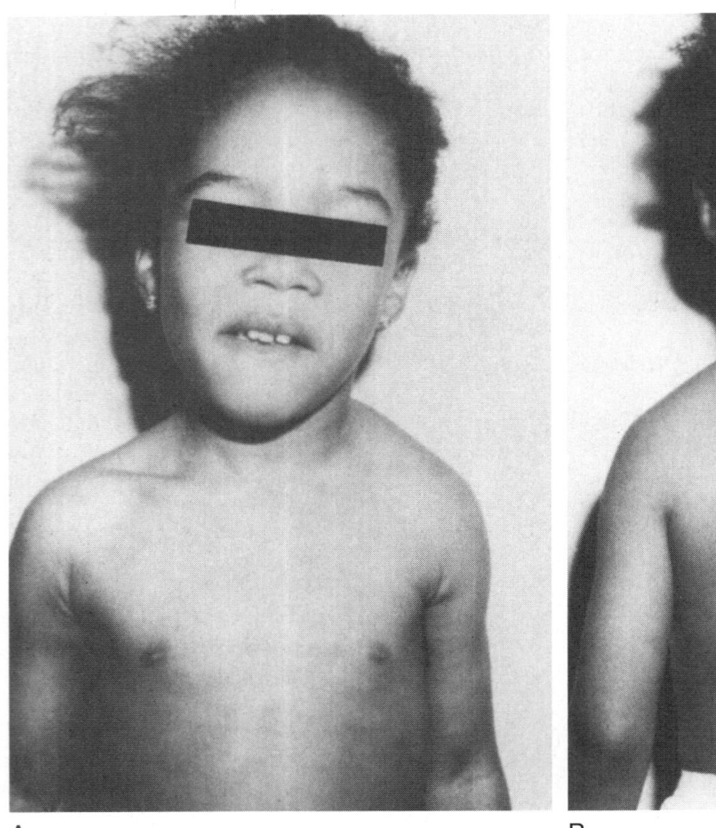

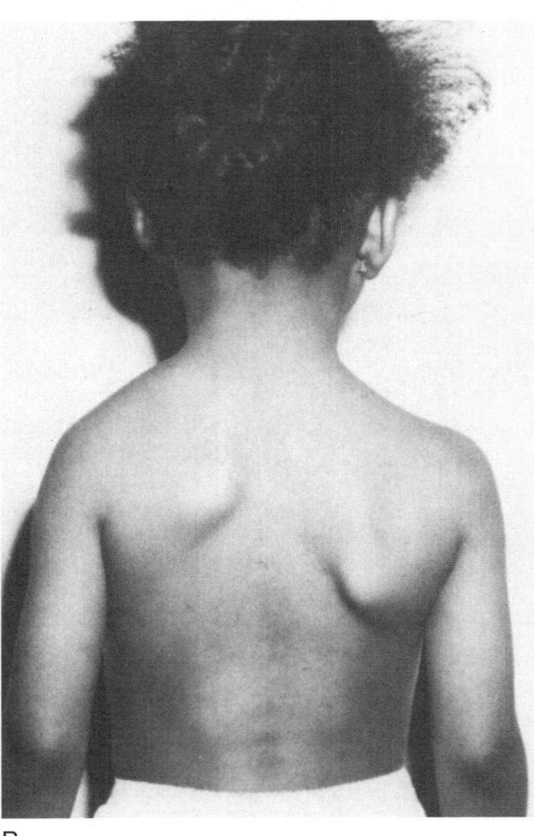

A B

FIGURE 3–23 Clinical photograph of a child with left Sprengel's shoulder. **A**, Anterior view. **B**, Posterior view. Note the elevation and rotation of the scapula. (From Benson M, Fixen J, Macnicol M: Children's Orthopaedics and Fractures, p 365. New York, Churchill Livingstone, 1994.)

dysplasia (10-15%). Approximately 85% of cases resolve spontaneously; feet that can be actively corrected to neutral require no treatment. Stretching exercises are used for feet that can be passively corrected to neutral (heel bisector line aligns with the second metatarsal). Though rare, feet that cannot be passively corrected usually respond to serial casting. Cuneiform osteotomies and limited medial release are indicated in resistant cases. The best results with osteotomies are seen when the surgery is performed after 5 years of age. Rigidity and heel valgus should be identified and treated with early casting.

2. Tibial torsion—The most common cause of the toes turned inward. Usually seen during the second year of life and can be associated with metatarsus adductus. It is often bilateral and may be secondary to excessive medial ligamentous tightness. Internal rotation of the tibia causes the pigeon-toed gait. This intrauterine "molding" deformity typically resolves spontaneously with growth. Operative correction is rarely necessary except in severe cases, which are addressed with a supramalleolar osteotomy.
3. Femoral anteversion—Internal rotation of the femur, seen in 3- to 6-year-olds. Increased internal rotation and decreased external rotation are noted on examination of a child with a pigeon-toed gait whose patellas are internally rotated. Children with this problem classically sit in a W position. If associated with tibial torsion, femoral anteversion may lead to patellofemoral problems. This disorder usually corrects spontaneously by age 10, but in the older child with less than 10 degrees of external rotation, femoral derotational osteotomy (intertrochanteric is best) may be

TABLE 3-14 EVALUATION OF ROTATIONAL PROBLEMS OF THE LOWER EXTREMITIES

Measurement	Technique	Normal Values (degrees)	Significance
Foot-progression angle	Foot vs. straight line	−5 to +20	Nonspecific rotation
Medial rotation	Prone hip ROM	20-60	> 70 degrees; femoral anteversion
Lateral rotation	Prone hip ROM	30-60	< 20 degrees; femoral anteversion
Thigh–foot angle	Knee bent; foot up	0-20	< −10 degrees; tibial torsion
Foot lateral border	Convex; medial crease	Straight; flexible	Metatarsus adductus

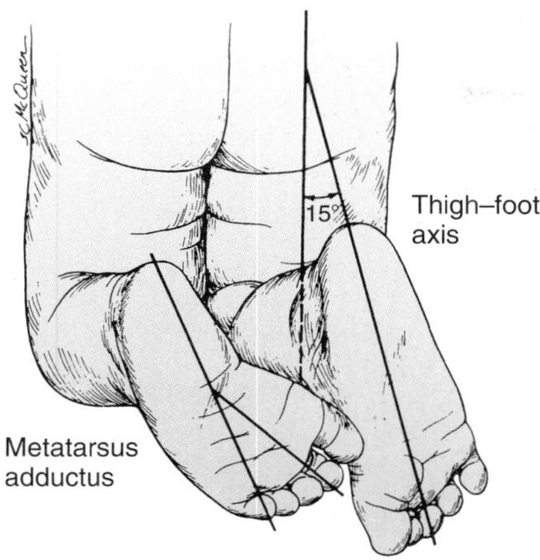

FIGURE 3–24 Deviation of the forefoot in metatarsus adductus. Note also the normal thigh-foot angle (15 degrees); negative thigh-foot angles (< 10 degrees) are seen in tibial torsion. (Adapted from Fitch RD: Introduction to pediatric orthopedics. In Sabiston DC Jr, ed: Sabiston's Essentials of Surgery. Philadelphia, WB Saunders, 1987.)

considered for cosmesis, although this is not a functional problem.

XII. Hip and Femur

A. Developmental dysplasia of the hip (DDH)

1. Introduction—Previously called congenital dysplasia of the hip, this disorder represents abnormal development or dislocation of the hip secondary to capsular laxity and mechanical factors (e.g., intrauterine positioning).
   a. Risk factors—Breech positioning, positive family history, female sex, and being a first-born child are risk factors (in that order). Less intrauterine space explains the increased incidence of DDH in the first-born child. DDH is seen most often in the left hip (67%) in females (85%) with a positive family history (20% or over), increased maternal estrogens, and breech births (30-50%).
   b. Related problems—Commonly associated with other "packaging problems," such as torticollis (20%) and metatarsus adductus (10%), it is partially characterized by increased amounts of type III collagen. This disorder includes the spectrum of complete dislocation, subluxation, instability, and acetabular dysplasia. If left untreated, muscles about the hip become contracted, and the acetabulum becomes more dysplastic and filled with fibrofatty tissue (**pulvinar**). Potential obstructions to obtaining a concentric reduction in DDH are an iliopsoas tendon, pulvinar, a contracted inferomedial hip capsule, the transverse acetabular ligament, and an inverted labrum. The teratologic form is most severe and usually requires early surgery. This form of DDH is defined as those hips that present with a pseudoacetabulum at or near birth. Teratologic hip dislocations commonly present in association with syndromes such as arthrogryposis and Larsen's syndrome.
2. Diagnosis
   a. Clinical findings and tests—Early diagnosis is possible with Ortolani's test (elevation and abduction of femur relocates a dislocated hip) and Barlow's test (adduction and depression of femur dislocates a dislocatable hip). Three phases are commonly recognized: (1) **dislocated** (Ortolani-positive, early; Ortolani-negative, late, when femoral head cannot be reduced), (2) **dislocatable** (Barlow-positive), and (3) **subluxatable** (Barlow-suggestive). Subsequent diagnosis is made with limitation of hip abduction in the affected hip as the laxity resolves and stiffness becomes more clinically evident. (Caution: Abduction may be decreased symmetrically with bilateral dislocations.) Another sign of dislocation includes a positive Galeazzi sign, demonstrated by the clinical appearance of foreshortening of the femur on the affected side. This clinical test is performed with the feet held together and knees flexed (a congenitally short femur can also cause a positive Galeazzi sign). Other clinical findings associated with DDH include asymmetrical gluteal folds (less reliable) and a positive Trendelenburg stance (older child). Repeat examination, especially in an infant, is important because a child's irritability can prevent proper evaluation.
   b. Other tests—Dynamic ultrasonography is useful for making the diagnosis in young children before ossification of the femoral head (which occurs at age 4-6 months) (Fig. 3–25). It is also useful for assessing reduction in a Pavlik harness and diagnosing acetabular dysplasia or capsular laxity; however, it is operator dependent. On the coronal view, the normal alpha angle is greater than 60 degrees and the femoral head is bisected by the line drawn down the ilium. Radiographs may be helpful in the older child (> 3 months), and measurement of the acetabular index (normal, < 25 degrees), measurement of Perkins' line (normally the ossific nucleus of the femoral head is medial to this line), and evaluation of Shenton's line are useful (Fig. 3–26). Later, delayed ossification of the femoral head on the affected side may be seen. Arthrography is helpful after closed reduction to determine concentric reduction.
3. Treatment (Fig. 3–27)—Based on achieving and maintaining early "concentric reduction" in order to prevent future degenerative joint disease.
   a. Pavlik harness—Specific therapy is based on the child's age and includes the Pavlik harness, which is designed to maintain infants (< 6 months) reduced in about 100 degrees

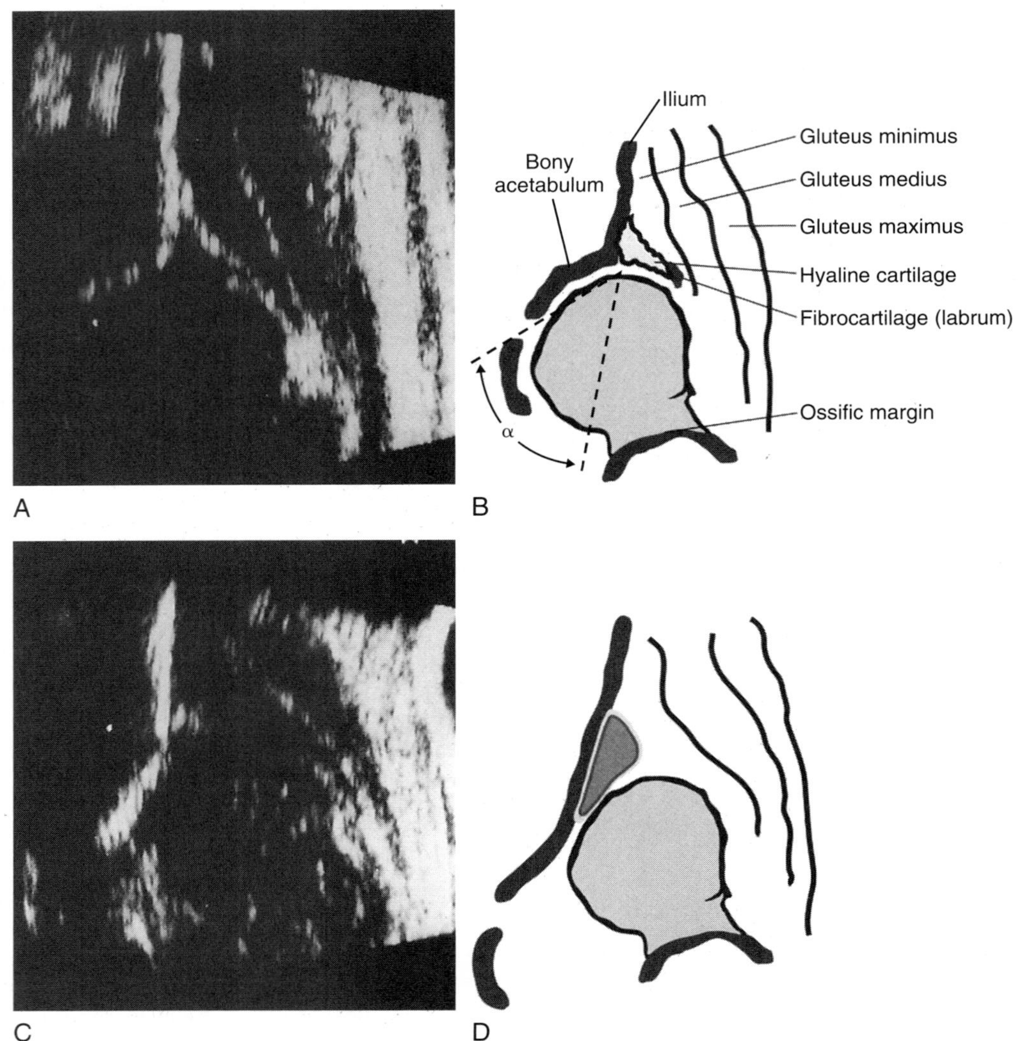

FIGURE 3–25 Ultrasound evaluation of the neonate's hip. **A**, Ultrasound of normal hip. **B**, Graphic representation of the ultrasound. **C**, Ultrasound of a dislocated hip with poor bony roof. **D**, Graphic illustration of the dislocated hip. (Modified from Benson M, Fixen J, Macnicol M: Children's Orthopaedics and Fractures, 2nd ed, p 364. Philadelphia, WB Saunders, 2002.)

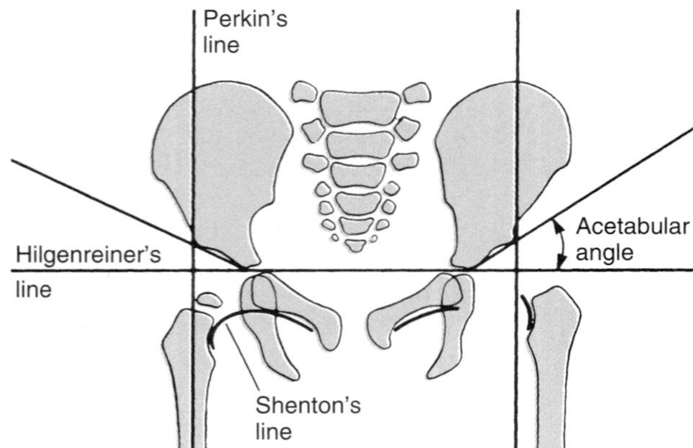

FIGURE 3–26 Common measurements used to evaluate developmental dysplasia of the hip. Note the delayed ossification, disruption of Shenton's line, and increased acetabular index on the left dislocated hip. (Adapted from Fitch RD: Introduction to pediatric orthopaedics. In Sabiston DC Jr, ed: Sabiston's Essentials of Surgery. Philadelphia, WB Saunders, 1987.)

of flexion and mild abduction (the "human position" [Salter]). The reduction should be confirmed by radiographs or ultrasound scans after placement in the harness and brace adjustment. The position of the hip should be within the "safe zone" of Ramsey (between maximum adduction before redislocation and excessive abduction, causing a high risk of avascular necrosis). Impingement of the posterosuperior retinacular branch of the medial femoral circumflex artery has been implicated in osteonecrosis associated with DDH treated in an abduction orthosis. Pavlik harness treatment is contraindicated in teratologic hip dislocations. A patient with a narrow safe zone (less than 40 degrees) should be considered for an adductor tenotomy. Excessive flexion may result in transient femoral nerve palsy. Failure to reduce a hip in 4 weeks should result in discontinuation of the Pavlik

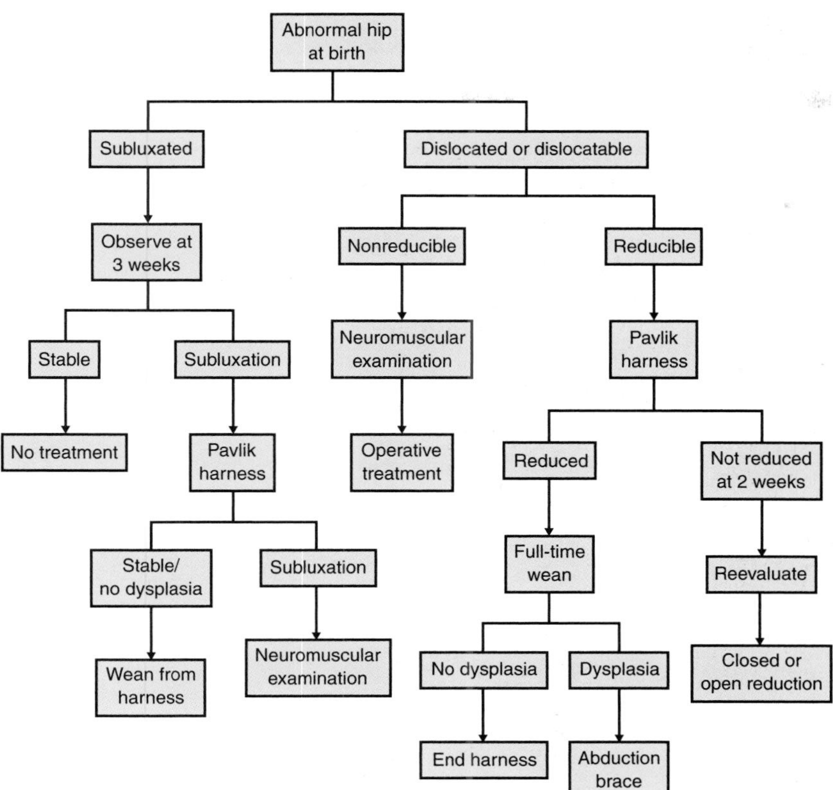

FIGURE 3–27 Algorithm for the treatment of developmental dysplasia of the hip. (Redrawn from Guille JT, Pizzutillo MD, MacEwen GD: Developmental dysplasia of the hip from birth to 6 months. JAAOS 8:232–242, 2000.)

harness to prevent "Pavlik disease"—erosion of the pelvis superior to the acetabulum. The Pavlik harness is usually worn 23 hours a day for at least 6 weeks after a reduction has been achieved and then an additional 6-8 weeks part-time (nights and naps).

b. Closed and open reduction
   (1) Closed reduction—Generally performed for patients who fail Pavlik treatment and for patients between 6 and 18 months. This is performed under general anesthesia with a physical examination, an arthrogram to assess reduction, and hip spica casting with the legs flexed to at least 90 degrees and in the stable zone of abduction. Confirmation by CT scan of a well-reduced hip is often performed, especially in questionable cases.
   (2) Open reduction—Reserved for children 6 to 18 months old who fail closed reduction, have an obstructive limbus, or have an unstable safe zone. Open reduction is also the initial treatment for children 18 months and older. It is usually done through an anterior approach, especially for patients older than 12 months (less risk to the **medial femoral circumflex artery**) and includes capsulorrhaphy, adductor tenotomy, femoral shortening to take tension off the reduction, and an acetabular procedure if severe dysplasia is present. The medial open reduction can be performed up to 12 months of age, results in less blood loss, directly addresses the obstacles to reduction but does not provide access for a capsulorrhaphy, and is more often associated with osteonecrosis.
   (3) Surgical risks—The major risk associated with both open and closed reductions is osteonecrosis (due to direct vascular injury or impingement versus disruption of the circulation from osteotomies). Failure of open reduction is difficult to treat surgically because of the high complication rate of revision surgery (50% osteonecrosis and 33% pain and stiffness in a recent study). Diagnosis after age 8 years (younger in patients with bilateral DDH) may contraindicate reduction because the acetabulum has little chance to remodel, although reduction may be indicated in conjunction with salvage procedures.

c. Osteotomy
   (1) Indications—May be required in toddlers and school-age children, usually for residual and persistent acetabular dysplasia. Osteotomies should be done only after a congruent reduction is confirmed on an abduction internal rotation

(AIR) view, with satisfactory ROM, and after reasonable femoral sphericity is achieved by closed or open methods. The choice of femoral versus pelvic osteotomy (Fig. 3–28) is sometimes a matter of the surgeon's choice. Some surgeons prefer to perform pelvic osteotomies after age 4 and femoral osteotomies before this age. In general, pelvic osteotomies should be done when severe dysplasia is accompanied by significant radiographic changes on the acetabular side (i.e., increased acetabular index, failure of lateral acetabular ossification), whereas changes on the femoral side (e.g., marked anteversion, coxa valga) are best treated by femoral osteotomies. These osteotomies rarely correct hip dysplasia successfully after age 5 years. Table 3–15 lists common reconstructive osteotomies.

(2) Procedures
   (a) The Salter osteotomy—May lengthen the affected leg up to 1 cm.
   (b) The Pemberton acetabuloplasty—A good choice for residual dysplasia because it reduces acetabular volume (bends on triradiate cartilage).
   (c) Acetabular reorientation procedures in older patients—Include the triple innominate osteotomy (Steel or Tönnis).
   (d) Dega-type osteotomies—Often favored for paralytic dislocations and in patients with posterior acetabular deficiency.
   (e) The Ganz periacetabular osteotomy—Provides improved three-dimensional correction because the cuts are close to the acetabulum, allow immediate weight bearing, spare stripping of the abductor muscles, allow for a capsulotomy to inspect the joint, and are performed through a single incision. However, the triradiate cartilage must be closed.
   (f) The Chiari osteotomy—A salvage procedure when a concentric reduction of the femoral head within the acetabulum cannot be achieved. This osteotomy shortens the affected leg and requires periarticular soft tissue metaplasia for success. It depends on metaplastic tissue (fibrocartilage) for a successful result.
   (g) The lateral shelf acetabular augmentation procedure—Done in patients over 8 years old with inadequate lateral coverage or trochanteric advancement and increased trochanteric overgrowth (improves hip abductor biomechanics). It depends on metaplastic tissue (fibrocartilage) for a successful result.

TABLE 3-15 COMMON PELVIC OSTEOTOMIES

Osteotomy	Procedure	Requirement
Femoral	Intertrochanteric osteotomy (VDRO)	Concentric reduction < 8 years of age
Salter's	Open wedge osteotomy through ileum	Concentric reduction < 8 years of age
Pemberton's	Through acetabular roof to triradiate cartilage	Concentric reduction < 8 years of age
Sutherland's (double)	Salter's + pubic osteotomy	Concentric reduction Open triradiate cartilage
Steel's (triple)	Salter's + osteotomy of both rami	Concentric reduction Open triradiate cartilage
Ganz	Periacetabular osteotomy	Surgeon's experience Closed triradiate cartilage
Chiari's	Through ilium above acetabulum (makes new roof)	Salvage procedure for asymmetrical incongruity
Shelf's	Slotted lateral acetabular augmentation	Salvage procedure for asymmetrical incongruity

VDRO, varus derotation osteotomy.

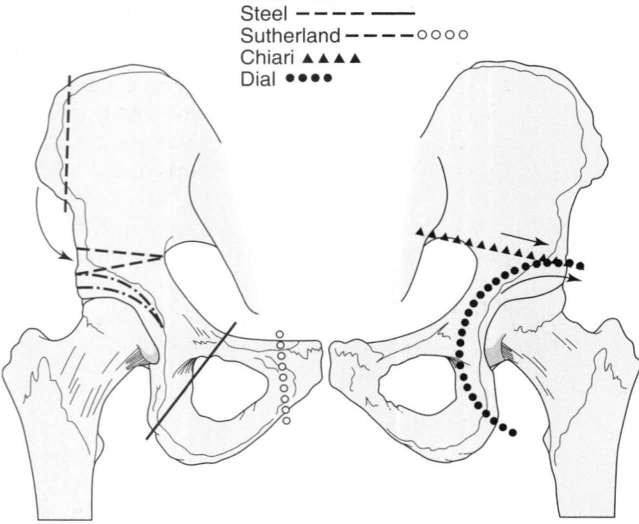

FIGURE 3–28 Common pelvic osteotomies for the treatment of developmental dysplasia of the hip.

B. Congenital coxa vara—Decreased neck–shaft angle due to a defect in ossification of the femoral neck.

1. Presentation—It is bilateral in one third to one half of cases. Coxa vara can be congenital (noted at birth and differentiated from DDH by MRI), developmental (AD, progressive), or acquired (e.g., trauma, Legg-Calvé-Perthes, slipped capital femoral epiphysis). May present with a waddling gait (bilateral) or a painless limp (unilateral). Radiographs classically demonstrate a triangular

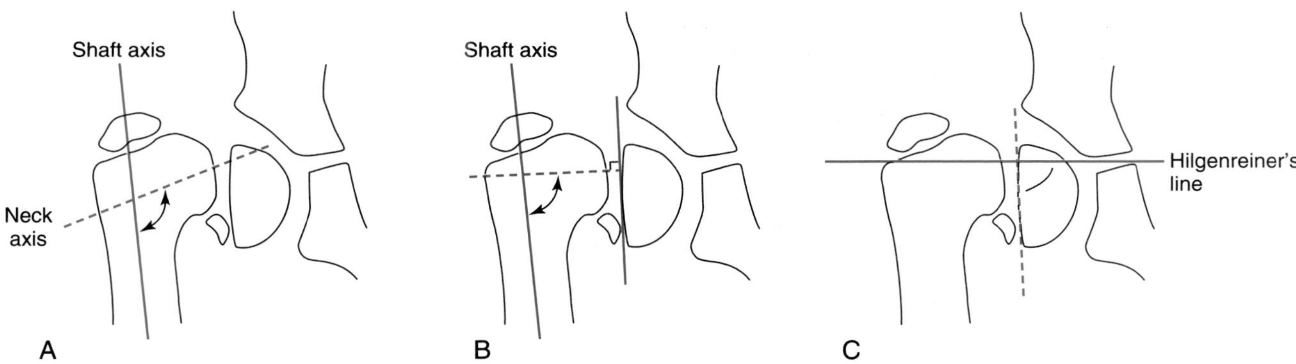

FIGURE 3–29 Quantification of the extent of radiographic deformity of the proximal femur in developmental coxa vara. **A**, The neck–shaft angle is the angle between the axis of the femoral shaft and the axis of the femoral neck. **B**, The head–shaft angle is the angle between the axis of the femoral shaft and a perpendicular line drawn to the base of the capital femoral epiphysis. **C**, The Hilgenreiner–epiphyseal angle is the angle between Hilgenreiner's line and a line drawn parallel to the capital femoral physis. (From Herring JA: Tachdjian's Pediatric Orthopaedics, 3rd ed, p 767. Philadelphia, WB Saunders, 2002.)

ossification defect in the inferomedial femoral neck in developmental coxa vara.

2. Treatment—The evaluation of **Hilgenreiner's epiphyseal angle** (the angle between Hilgenreiner's line and a line through the proximal femoral physis) is the key to treatment (Fig. 3–29). An angle of less than 45 degrees spontaneously corrects, whereas an angle of 45-60 degrees requires close observation, and over 60 degrees (with a neck–shaft angle of less than 110 degrees) usually requires surgery. The surgical treatment is a corrective valgus osteotomy of the proximal femur. Proximal femoral (valgus) with or without derotation osteotomy (Pauwels) is indicated for a neck–shaft angle of less than 90 degrees, a vertically oriented physeal plate, progressive deformities, or significant gait abnormalities. Concomitant distal/lateral transfer of the greater trochanter may also be indicated to restore more normal hip abductor mechanics.

C. Legg-Calvé-Perthes disease (coxa plana)—Noninflammatory deformity of the proximal femur secondary to a vascular insult of unknown etiology, leading to osteonecrosis of the proximal femoral epiphysis. Pathologically, the osteonecrosis is followed by revascularization and resorption via creeping substitution that eventually allows remodeling and fragmentation.

1. Presentation—Most common in boys 4-8 years old with delayed skeletal maturation, usually by 2 years of age, who are very active. There is an increased incidence with a positive family history, low birth weight, and abnormal birth presentation. Symptoms include pain (often knee pain), effusion (from synovitis), and a limp. Decreased hip ROM (especially abduction and internal rotation) and a Trendelenburg gait are also common. Prognosis is dependent on bone age and radiographic appearance during the fragmentation phase (**lateral pillar classification**). Patients who have a bone age over 6 years and a B or C lateral pillar have significantly poorer prognoses. Bilateral involvement may be seen in 12-15% of cases. However, in bilateral cases the involvement is asymmetrical and virtually never simultaneous. Bilateral involvement may mimic multiple epiphyseal dysplasia and warrants a skeletal survey. Radiographic findings vary with the stage of disease but include cessation of growth of the ossific nucleus, medial joint space widening, and development of a "crescent sign" representing subchondral fracture.

2. Classification
   a. Waldenstrom's classification determines the four stages that all cases follow: initial, fragmentation, reossification, and healed or reossified.
   b. The classification that is most prognostic is the Herring classification, or lateral pillar classification, which is based on the involvement of the lateral pillar of the capital femoral epiphysis (CFE) during the fragmentation stage (Table 3–16 and Fig. 3–30).

3. Differential diagnosis—Differential diagnosis includes septic arthritis, blood dyscrasias, hypothyroidism, and epiphyseal dysplasia.

4. Prognosis—Maintaining the sphericity of the femoral head is the most important factor in achieving a good result. The use of circular templates (Mose) is helpful for evaluating this parameter. Early degenerative hip joint disease results from aspherical femoral heads. Poor

TABLE 3-16 LATERAL PILLAR CLASSIFICATION

Group	Pillar Involvement	Prognosis
A	Little or no involvement of the lateral pillar	Uniformly good outcome
B	> 50% of lateral pillar height maintained	Good outcome in younger patients (bone age < 6 yr) but poorer outcome in older patients
C	< 50% of lateral pillar height maintained	Poor prognosis in all age groups

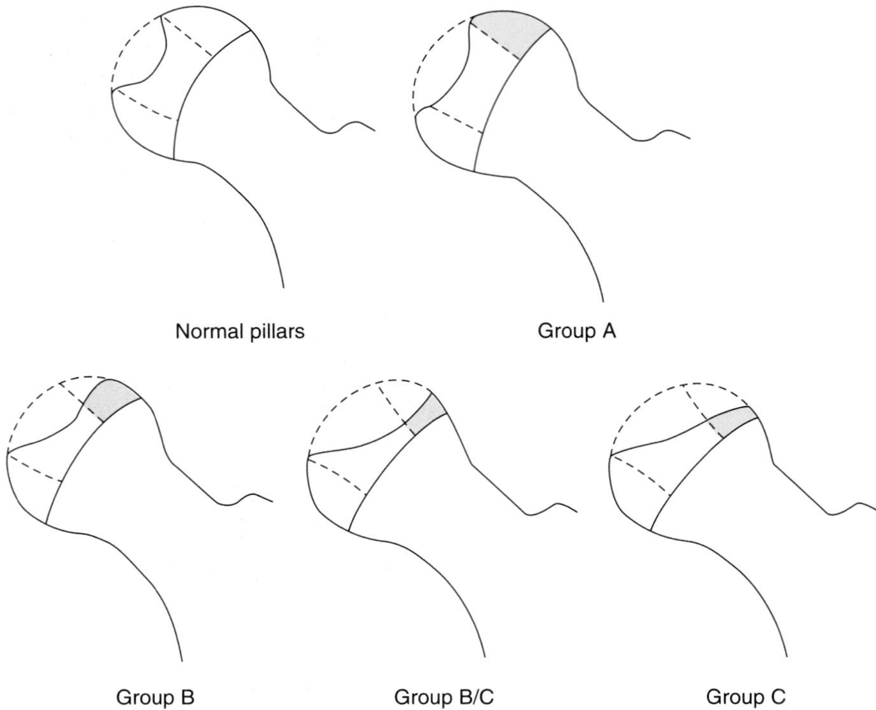

FIGURE 3–30 Lateral pillar classification of Legg-Calvé-Perthes disease. Normal pillars were derived by noting the lines of demarcation between the central sequestrum and the remainder of the epiphysis on the anteroposterior radiograph. In group A, the normal height of lateral pillar is maintained. In group B, more than 50% of height of lateral pillar is maintained. In the group B/C border, lateral pillar is less than or equal to 50% in height, but it (1) is very narrow (2 to 3 mm wide), (2) has very little ossification, or (3) has depressions relative to the central pillar. In group C, less than 50% of height of lateral pillar is maintained. (Adapted from Herring JA, Neustadt JB, Williams JJ, et al: The lateral pillar classification of Legg-Calvé-Perthes disease. J Pediatr Orthop 12:143–150, 1992.)

prognosis is associated with older children (bone age > 6 years), female sex, and decreased hip ROM (decreased abduction). Radiographic findings associated with poor prognosis (Catterall's "head at risk" signs) include (1) lateral calcification, (2) Gage's sign (V-shaped defect at lateral physis), (3) lateral subluxation, (4) metaphyseal cyst formation, and (5) a horizontal growth plate.

5. Treatment—In general, the goals of treatment are relief of symptoms, restoration of ROM, and containment of the hip. The use of outpatient or inpatient traction, anti-inflammatory medications, and partial weight bearing with crutches for periods of 1-2 days to several weeks is helpful for relieving symptoms. ROM is maintained with traction, muscle release, exercise, and/or the use of a Petrie cast. Containment of the hip by use of traction, muscle release, abduction bracing, and/or varus femoral versus pelvic osteotomy is helpful for maintaining hip sphericity. Herring has described a treatment plan based on age and the lateral pillar classification of disease involvement. Surgical treatment improves radiographic outcome at skeletal maturity for older patients (chronologic age > 8 years or bone age > 6 years) with lateral pillar B and B/C hips.

D. Slipped capital femoral epiphysis (SCFE)—Disorder of the proximal femoral epiphysis caused by weakness of the perichondrial ring and slippage through the hypertrophic zone of the growth plate. The femoral head remains in the acetabulum, and the neck is displaced anteriorly and externally rotates. SCFE is seen most often in African American, obese, adolescent boys (10-16 years old) occasionally with a positive family history. Up to 25% of cases are bilateral. It is related to puberty. May be associated with hormonal disorders in young children, such as hypothyroidism or renal osteodystrophy. Patients present with a coxalgic, externally rotated gait; decreased internal rotation; thigh atrophy; and **hip, thigh, or knee pain.** Symptoms vary with the acuteness of the slip. On physical examination, all patients have obligate external rotation with flexion of the hip.

1. Classification—Loder's classification of SCFE based on the patient's ability to bear weight at the time of presentation is prognostic for the severe complication of osteonecrosis of the femoral head. **Stable slips** are those in which weight bearing with or without crutches is possible. **Unstable slips** are those in which weight bearing is not possible because of severe pain. No patients with stable slips developed osteonecrosis, whereas 47% of the patients with unstable slips developed it. Radiographs show the slip, which is classified based on the percentage of slip: grade I, 0-33%; grade II, 34-50%; and grade III, > 50%. In mild cases, loss of the lateral overhang of the femoral ossific nucleus (Klein's line) and blurring of the proximal femoral metaphysis may be all that is seen on the anteroposterior film. A frog-leg pelvis should always be obtained and clearly defines the SCFE.
2. Treatment—Recommended treatment for stable and unstable slips is **pinning in situ.** Positioning on the table may partially reduce the acute component of an unstable slip. Forceful reduction before pinning is not indicated. Pin placement can be done percutaneously with one pin (Fig. 3–31). The pin should be started anteriorly on the femoral neck, ending in the central

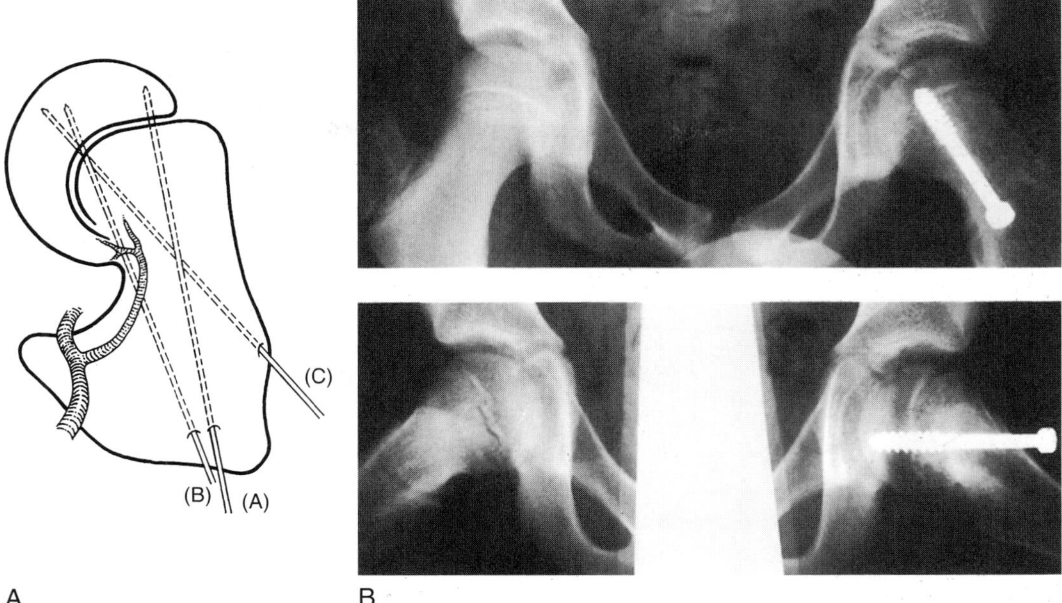

FIGURE 3–31 **A**, Percutaneous pinning or screw fixation for slipped capital femoral epiphysis. Note that the epiphysis slips posteriorly and inferiorly. The implant must be inserted into the anterior femoral neck and directed toward the center of the epiphysis. Pin C is optimally placed. **B**, Radiographs show satisfactory screw placement, with the screw entering the anterior femoral neck. (From Benson M, Fixen J, Macnicol M: Children's Orthopaedics and Fractures, p 464. New York, Churchill Livingstone, 1994.)

portion of the femoral head. The goal of treatment is to stabilize the epiphysis and promote closure of the proximal femoral physis. Patients presenting at less than 10 years of age should have an endocrine workup. Prophylactic pinning of the opposite hip is controversial but is generally recommended in patients diagnosed with an endocrinopathy and in young children (< 10 years old) or those with an open triradiate cartilage.

3. Prognosis and complications—In severe SCFE, the residual proximal femoral deformity may partially remodel with the patient's remaining growth. Intertrochanteric (Kramer's) or subtrochanteric (Southwick's) osteotomies may be useful in treating the deformities caused by SCFE that fail to remodel. Cuneiform osteotomy at the femoral neck has the potential to correct severe deformity but remains controversial due to the high reported rates of osteonecrosis (37%) and future osteoarthritis (37%). Complications associated with SCFE include chondrolysis (narrowed joint space, pain, and decreased motion), osteonecrosis (higher incidence in unstable slips), and degenerative joint disease (pistol-grip deformity of the proximal femur).

E. Proximal femoral focal deficiency (PFFD)—Developmental defect of the proximal femur recognizable at birth. Clinically, patients with PFFD have a short, bulky thigh that is flexed, abducted, and externally rotated. PFFD is often associated with coxa vara or fibular hemimelia (50%). Congenital knee ligamentous deficiency and contracture are also common. Treatment must be individualized based on leg-length discrepancy, adequacy of musculature, proximal joint stability, and the presence or absence of foot deformities. In general, prosthetic management is used when the femoral length is less than 50% of the opposite side, while lengthening with or without contralateral epiphysiodesis is used when it is greater than 50%. The percentage of shortening remains constant during growth. The Aiken classification divides PFFD into four groups (Fig. 3–32). Classes A and B have a femoral head, which potentially allows for reconstructive procedures that include limb lengthening. Classes C and D do not have a femoral head and present a more difficult treatment dilemma. Treatment options include amputation, femoral-pelvic fusion (Brown's procedure), Van Ness rotationplasty, and limb lengthening.

F. Leg-length discrepancy (LLD)

a. Causes and associated problems—There are many causes of LLD, such as congenital disorders (e.g., hemihypertrophy, dysplasias, PFFD, DDH), paralytic disorders (e.g., spasticity, polio), infection (pyogenic disruption of the physis), tumors, and trauma. Long-term problems associated with LLD include an inefficient gait, equinus contractures of the ankle, postural scoliosis, and low-back pain.

b. Measurement—The discrepancy must be measured accurately (e.g., with blocks of set height under the affected side, scanogram) and can be tracked with the Green-Anderson or Moseley graph (with serial leg-length films or CT scanograms and bone age determinations).

c. Treatment—In general, projected discrepancies at maturity of less than 2 cm are observed or treated with shoe lifts. Discrepancies of 2-5 cm

TYPE		FEMORAL HEAD	ACETABULUM	FEMORAL SEGMENT	RELATIONSHIP AMONG COMPONENTS OF FEMUR AND ACETABULUM AT SKELETAL MATURITY
A	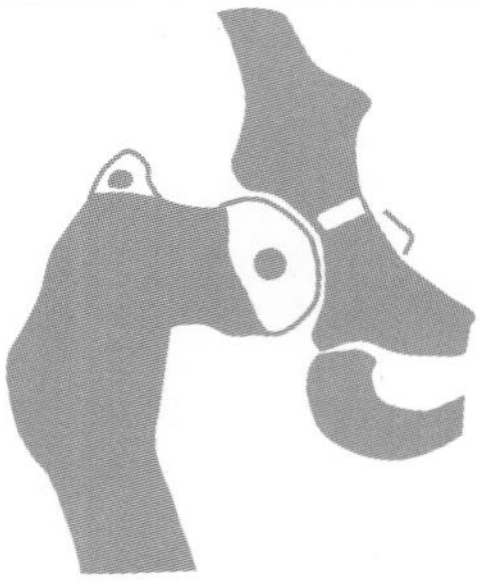	Present	Normal	Short	Bony connection between components of femur Femoral head in acetabulum Subtrochanteric varus angulation, often with pseudarthrosis
B	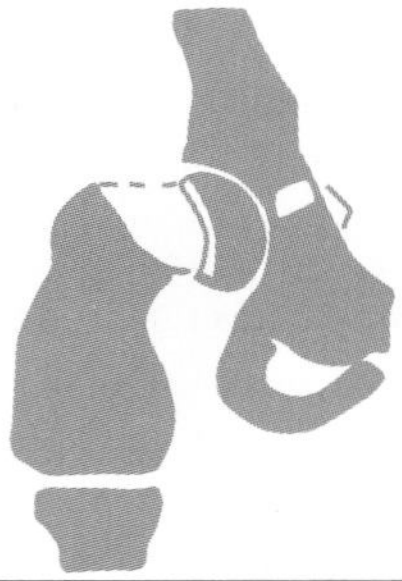	Present	Adequate or moderately dysplastic	Short, usually proximal bony tuft	No osseous connection between head and shaft Femoral head in acetabulum
C	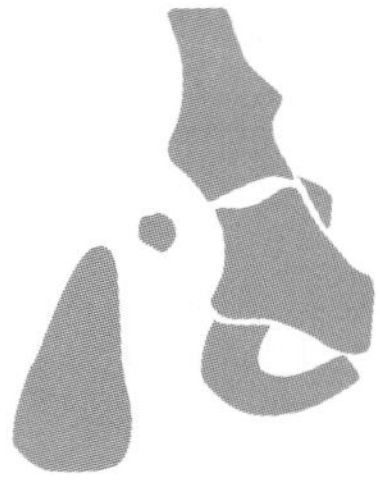	Absent or represented by ossicle	Severely dysplastic	Short, usually proximally tapered	May be osseous connection between shaft and proximal ossicle No articular relation between femur and acetabulum
D	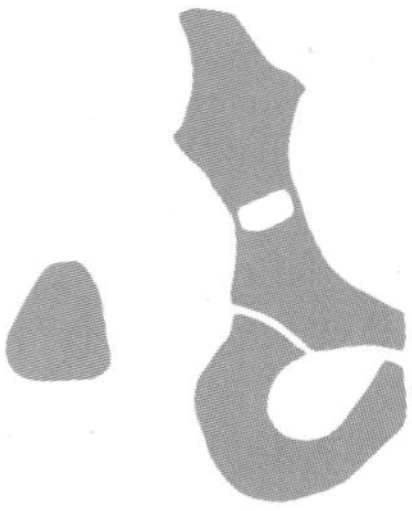	Absent	Absent Obturator foramen enlarged Pelvis squared in bilateral cases	Short, deformed	None

FIGURE 3–32 Aiken's classification of proximal femoral focal deficiency. Note lack of femoral head in types C and D. (From Herring JA: Tachdjian's Pediatric Orthopaedics, 4th ed, p 1998. Philadelphia, WB Saunders, 2008.)

can be treated with epiphysiodesis of the long side, shortening of the long side (ostectomy), or lengthening. Discrepancies of more than 5 cm are generally treated with lengthening. With the use of standard techniques, lengthening of 1 mm a day is typical. The Ilizarov principles are followed, including metaphyseal corticotomy (preserving the medullary canal and blood supply) followed by gradual distraction. On rare occasions, one can consider physeal distraction (chondrodiastasis). This procedure must be done near skeletal maturity because the physis almost always closes after this type of limb lengthening. A gross estimation of LLD can be made by using the following assumption of growth per year up to age 16 in boys and age 14 in girls: distal femur, ⅜ inch/year (9 mm); proximal tibia, ¼ inch/year (6 mm); and proximal femur, ⅛ inch/year (3 mm). Using the Moseley data gives more accurate results.

G. Lower extremity inflammation and infection (see Chapter 1, Basic Sciences)

1. Transient synovitis—Most common cause of painful hips during childhood, but it is a diagnosis of exclusion. Can be related to viral infection, allergic reaction, or trauma; however, the cause is unknown. The onset can be acute or insidious. The symptoms, which are self-limiting, include

voluntary limitation of motion and muscle spasm. With transient synovitis, the ESR is usually less than 20 mm/hour. Rule out septic hip with aspiration (especially in children with fever, leukocytosis, or elevated ESR); then observe the patient in Buck's traction for 24-48 hours.

2. Osteomyelitis—Occurs more often in children because of their rich metaphyseal blood supply and thick periosteum.
   a. Pathology—Most common organism is *Staphylococcus aureus* (except in neonates, in whom group B streptococcus is more common). With the advent of the *Haemophilus influenzae* vaccination, *H. influenzae* is now a much less common organism in musculoskeletal sepsis. A history of trauma is common in children with osteomyelitis. Osteomyelitis in children usually begins through hematogenous seeding of a bony metaphysis in the small arterioles that bend just beyond the physis, where blood flow is sluggish and phagocytosis is poor, creating a bone abscess (Fig. 3–33). Pus lifts the thick periosteum and puts pressure on the cortex, causing coagulation. Chronic bone abscesses may become surrounded by thick, fibrous tissue and sclerotic bone (Brodie's abscess).
   b. Diagnosis—Clinically, the child presents with a tender, warm, sometimes swollen area over a long-bone metaphysis. Fever may or may not be present. Laboratory tests may be helpful (blood cultures, white blood cell [WBC] count, ESR, C-reactive protein), and radiologic studies are also useful (radiographs with only soft tissue edema early, metaphyseal rarefaction late, and bone scans). Definitive diagnosis is made with aspiration (50% positive cultures).
   c. Treatment—Intravenous antibiotics are the best initial treatment if osteomyelitis is diagnosed early, before radiographic changes or the development of a subperiosteal abscess. Broad-spectrum antibiotics are initially chosen, followed by antibiotics specific for the organism cultured. Failure to respond to antibiotics, frank pus on aspiration, or the presence of a sequestered abscess (not accessible to antibiotics) requires operative drainage and débridement. Specimens should be sent for histology and culture. Antibiotics should be continued until the ESR (or C-reactive protein) returns to normal, usually at 4-6 weeks.

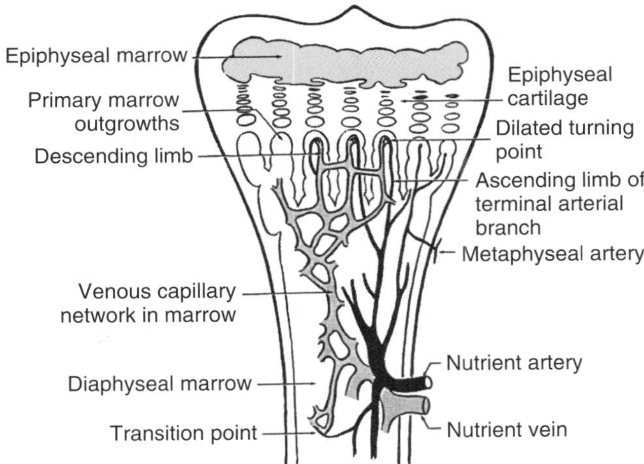

FIGURE 3–33 Metaphyseal sinusoids, where sluggish blood flow increases susceptibility to osteomyelitis. (From Tachdjian MO: Pediatric Orthopaedics, 2nd ed. Philadelphia, WB Saunders, 1990.)

3. Septic arthritis—Can develop from osteomyelitis (especially in neonates, in whom transphyseal vessels allow proximal spread into the joint) in joints with an intra-articular metaphysis (hip, elbow, shoulder, and ankle). Septic arthritis can also occur as a result of hematogenous spread of infection. Because pus is chondrolytic, septic arthritis in children is an acute surgical emergency. Organisms vary with age (Table 3–17).
   a. Diagnosis—Septic arthritis presents as a much more acute process than osteomyelitis. Decreased ROM and severe pain with passive motion may be accompanied by systemic symptoms of infection. Radiographs may show a widened joint space or even dislocation. Joint fluid aspirate shows a high WBC count (> 50,000/mm^3); a glucose level of 50 mg/dL less than serum levels; and in patients with gram-positive cocci or gram-negative rods, a high lactic acid level. Distinguishing septic arthritis of the hip from transient synovitis is a common problem; however, when three of four of the following criteria are present, the diagnosis of septic arthritis is over 90%: WBC > 12,000 cells/mL, ESR > 40, inability to bear weight, and fever higher than 101.5°F. Ultrasonography can be helpful in identifying the presence of an effusion. Lumbar puncture should be considered in a septic joint caused by *H. influenzae* because of the increased incidence of meningitis. The prognosis is usually good except in patients with a delayed diagnosis. Patients with *Neisseria gonorrhoeae* septic arthritis usually have a preceding migratory polyarthralgia; small, red

TABLE 3-17 COMMON ORGANISMS IN SEPTIC ARTHRITIS BY AGE

Age	Common Organisms	Empirical Antibiotics
< 12 mo	Staphylococcus, group B streptococcus	First-generation cephalosporin
6 mo-5 yr	Staphylococcus, *Haemophilus influenzae*	Second- or third-generation cephalosporin
5-12 yrs	*Staphylococcus aureus*	First-generation cephalosporin
12-18 yr	*S. aureus, Neisseria gonorrhoeae*	Oxacillin/cephalosporin

papules; and multiple joint involvement. This organism typically elicits less WBC response (< 50,000 cells/mL) and usually does not require surgical drainage. Large doses of penicillin are required to eliminate this organism.

b. Treatment—Aspiration should be followed by irrigation and débridement in major joints (especially in the hip; a culture of synovium is also recommended).

XIII. Knee and Leg

A. Leg—Genu varum (bowed legs) normally evolves naturally to genu valgum (knock-knees) by age 2.5 years, with a gradual transition to physiologic valgus by age 4 years.

1. Genu varum (bowed legs)—Normal in children less than 2 years old. Radiographs in physiologic bowing typically show flaring of the tibia and femur in a symmetrical fashion. Pathologic conditions that can cause genu varum include osteogenesis imperfecta, osteochondromas, trauma, various dysplasias, and (most commonly) **Blount's disease**. Blount's disease (tibia varum) is best divided into two distinct entities: infantile (0-4 years of age) and adolescent (over 10 years of age).

   a. Infantile Blount's disease—More common and usually affects both extremities. It occurs more often in the overweight child who begins walking at less than 1 year of age and is associated with internal tibial torsion. Radiographs may show a metaphyseal-diaphyseal angle abnormality and metaphyseal beaking. Drennan's angle of greater than 16 degrees is considered abnormal and is formed between the metaphyseal beaks (demonstrated in Fig. 3–34). The epiphyseal-metaphyseal angle is also useful (Fig. 3–35). Treatment is based on age and correlates with the stage of disease (Langinskiold's stages I-VI, with V and VI characterized by a metaphyseal-epiphyseal bony bridge). Bracing may be effective early in the disease, especially in unilateral cases. Proximal osteotomy for tibia/fibula valgus to overcorrect the deformity (because medial physeal growth abnormalities persist) is required for patients who do not respond to bracing or for a child older than age 4. Multiple procedures are often necessary to realign the lower extremities. Epiphysiolysis is also needed for stages V and VI disease.

   b. Adolescent Blount's disease—Less severe and more often unilateral. The initial treatment is lateral proximal tibial and fibular epiphysiodesis when growth remains. If residual deformity exists or the physes are closed proximally, tibial and fibular osteotomy is performed. When significant leg-length discrepancy is present, the Ilizarov technique allows for deformity correction and lengthening.

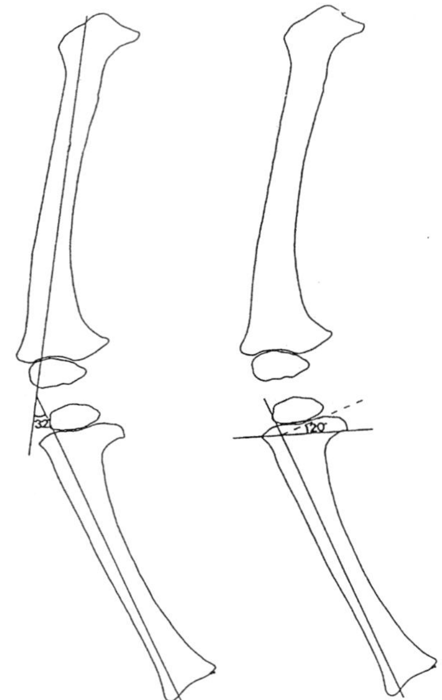

FIGURE 3–34 Comparison of tibiofemoral angle with Levine and Drennan's metaphyseal–diaphyseal angle in tibia vara. A line is drawn along the longitudinal axis of the tibia and the femur; the angle between the lines is the tibiofemoral angle (32 degrees). The metaphyseal–diaphyseal angle method is used to determine the metaphyseal–diaphyseal angle in the same extremity. A line is drawn perpendicular to the longitudinal axis of the tibia, and another is drawn through the two beaks of the metaphysis to determine the transverse axis of the tibial metaphysis. The metaphyseal–diaphyseal angle (12 degrees) is the angle bisected by the two lines. (Adapted from Levine AM, Drennan JC: Physiological bowing and tibia vara. J Bone Joint Surg [Am] 64:1159, 1982.)

2. Genu valgum (knock-knees)—Up to 15 degrees at the knee is common in 2- to 6-year-old children. Patients within this physiologic range

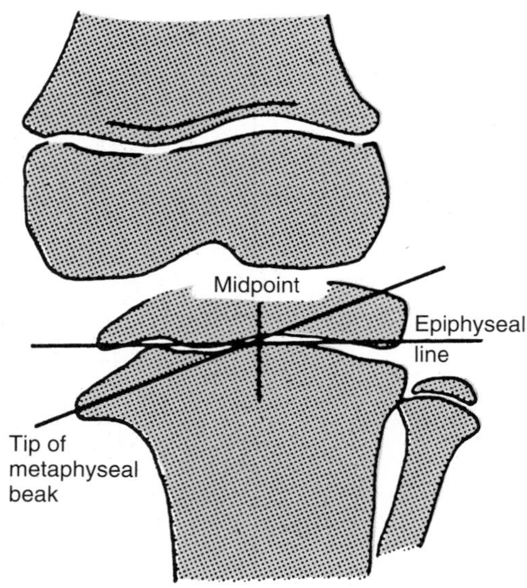

FIGURE 3–35 Blount's disease and measurement of the epiphyseal–metaphyseal angle. (Redrawn from Tachdjian MO: Pediatric Orthopaedics, 2nd ed. Philadelphia, WB Saunders, 1990.)

TABLE 3-18 TIBIAL BOWING

Type	Cause	Treatment
Posteromedial	Physiologic	Observation
Anteromedial	Fibular hemimelia	Bracing vs. amputation for severe deformities
Anterolateral	Congenital pseudarthrosis	Total-contact brace, intramedullary fixation, vascularized bone graft, or amputation

do not require treatment. For example, pathologic genu valgum may be associated with renal osteodystrophy (the most common cause if bilateral), tumors (e.g., osteochondromas), infections (may stimulate proximal asymmetrical tibial growth), or trauma. Conservative treatment is ineffective in pathologic genu valgum. Consider surgery at the site of the deformity in children over 10 years old with more than 10 cm between the medial malleoli or greater than 15 degrees of valgus. Hemiepiphysiodesis or physeal stapling of the medial side is effective before the end of growth for severe deformities.

B. Tibial bowing—Three types (Table 3–18) based on the apex of the curve.

1. Posteromedial-physiologic bowing—Usually of the middle and distal thirds of the tibia and may be the result of abnormal intrauterine positioning (Fig. 3–36). It is commonly associated with calcaneovalgus feet and tight anterior structures. Spontaneous correction is the rule, but follow the patient to evaluate LLD. The most common sequela of posteromedial bowing is an average LLD of 3-4 cm, which may require an age-appropriate epiphysiodesis of the long limb. Tibial osteotomies are not indicated.
2. Anteromedial tibial bowing—Typically caused by fibular hemimelia; a congenital longitudinal deficiency of the fibula is the most common long-bone deficiency. It is usually associated with anteromedial bowing, ankle instability, equinovarus foot (with or without lateral rays), tarsal coalition, and femoral shortening. Classically, skin dimpling is seen over the tibia. Significant LLD often results from this disorder. The fibular deficiency can be intercalary, which involves the whole bone (absent fibula) or terminal. Fibular hemimelia is frequently associated with femoral abnormalities such as coxa vara and PFFD. Radiographic findings include complete or partial absence of the fibula, a ball-and-socket ankle (secondary to tarsal coalitions), and deficient lateral rays in the foot. Treatment varies from a simple shoe lift or bracing to Syme's amputation. Treatment decisions are based on the degree of foot deformity, the number of rays, and the degree of shortening of the limb. Amputation is usually done to treat limbs with severe shortening and/or a stiff, nonfunctional foot at about 10 months of age. For less severe cases, reconstructive procedures, including lengthening, may be an alternative. This procedure should include resection of the fibular anlage to avoid future foot problems.
3. Anterolateral tibial bowing—**Congenital pseudarthrosis of the tibia** is the most common cause of anterolateral bowing. It is often accompanied by neurofibromatosis (50%, but only 10% of patients with neurofibromatosis have this disorder). Classification (Boyd's) is based on bowing and the presence of cystic changes, sclerosis, or dysplasia;

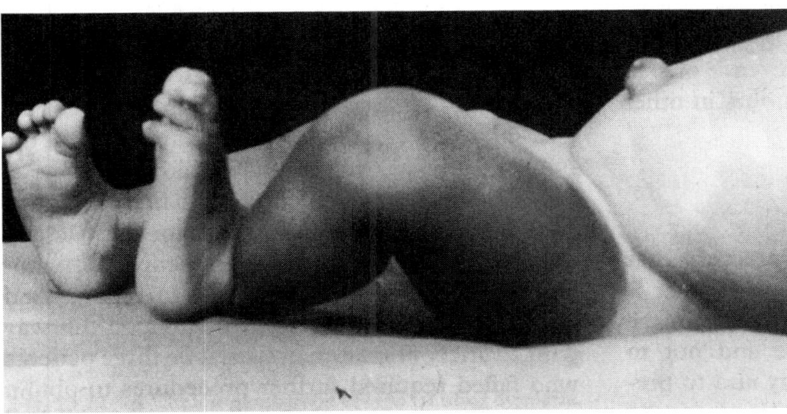

A

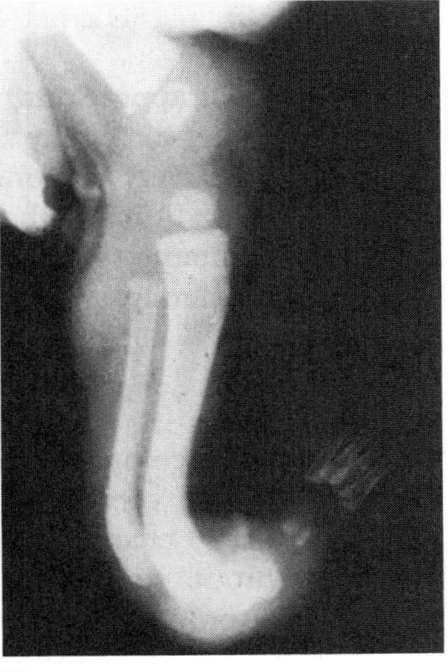

B

FIGURE 3–36 **A**, Clinical radiograph of a child age 5 months with posterior medial angulation of the tibia. **B**, Lateral radiograph of the same patient. The appearance is dramatic, but these deformities are best treated with stretching and splinting into equinus. (From Benson M, Fixen J, Macnicol M: Children's Orthopaedics and Fractures, p 408. New York, Churchill Livingstone, 1994.)

dysplasia and cystic changes are the most common. Initial treatment includes a total-contact brace to protect the patient from fractures. Intramedullary fixation with excision of hamartomatous tissue and autogenous bone grafting are options for nonhealing fractures. A vascularized fibular graft or Ilizarov's method should also be considered if bracing fails. Osteotomies to correct the anterolateral bowing are contraindicated. Amputation (Syme's) and prosthetic fitting are indicated after two or three failed surgical attempts. Syme's amputation is preferred to below-knee amputation in these patients because the soft tissue available at the heel pad is superior to that in the calf as a weight-bearing stump. The soft tissue in the calf in these patients is often scarred and atrophic.

4. Other lower limb deficiencies—Include tibial hemimelia, an AD disorder that is a congenital longitudinal deficiency of the tibia. Tibial hemimelia is the only long-bone deficiency with a known inheritance pattern (AD). It is much less common than fibular hemimelia and is often associated with other bony abnormalities (especially a lobster-claw hand). Clinically, the extremity is shortened and bowed anterolaterally with a prominent fibular head and an equinovarus foot, with the sole of the foot facing the perineum. The treatment for severe deformities with an entirely absent tibia is a knee disarticulation. Fibular transposition (Brown's) has been unsuccessful, especially with absent quadriceps function and an absent proximal tibia. When the proximal tibia and quadriceps functions are present, the fibula can be transposed to the residual tibia and create a functional below-knee amputation.

C. Osteochondritis dissecans—An intra-articular condition common in 10- to 15-year-olds that can affect many joints, especially the knee and elbow (capitellum). The lesion is thought to be secondary to trauma, ischemia, or abnormal epiphyseal ossification. The lateral portion of the medial femoral condyle is most frequently involved. Classified into three categories based on age at appearance (Pappas).

1. Diagnosis—Symptoms include activity-related pain, localized tenderness, stiffness, and swelling with or without mechanical symptoms. Radiographs should include the tunnel (notch) view to evaluate the condyles. MRI can determine if there is synovial fluid behind the lesion (the worst prognosis for nonoperative healing). Differential diagnosis includes anomalous ossification centers.
2. Treatment—Treatment consists of bracing and restricted weight bearing if the patient has significant growth remaining. Surgical therapy is reserved for the adolescent with minimal growth left or a loose lesion. Operative treatment includes drilling with multiple holes, fixation of large fragments, and bone grafting of large lesions. Osteochondritis dissecans is commonly treated arthroscopically. Poor prognosis is associated with lesions in the lateral femoral condyle and patella.

D. Osgood-Schlatter disease—An osteochondrosis, or fatigue failure, of the tibial tubercle apophysis due to stress from the extensor mechanism in a growing child (tibial tubercle apophysitis). Radiographs may show irregularity and fragmentation of the tibial tubercle. It is usually self-limiting and may require activity modification. Late excision of separate ossicles is occasionally required.

E. Discoid meniscus—Abnormal development of the lateral meniscus leads to the formation of a disk-shaped (or hypertrophic) rather than the normal crescent-shaped meniscus. Radiographs typically demonstrate widening of the cartilage space on the affected side (up to 11 mm). If symptomatic and torn, discoid meniscus can be arthroscopically débrided. If not torn, they should only be observed.

XIV. Foot (Fig. 3–37)

A. Clubfoot (congenital talipes equinovarus)—Forefoot adductus and supination; hindfoot equinus and varus. Talar neck deformity (medial and plantar deviation) with medial rotation of the calcaneus and medial displacement of the navicular and cuboid occurs. Clubfoot is more common in males, and half the cases are bilateral. It is associated with shortened/contracted muscles (intrinsics, Achilles tendon, tibialis posterior, flexor hallucis longus,

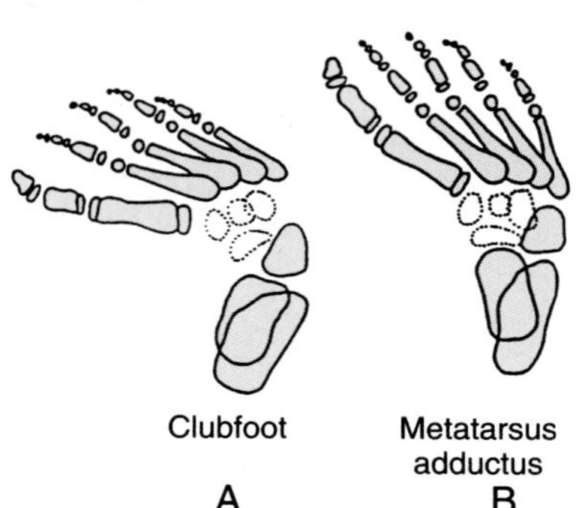

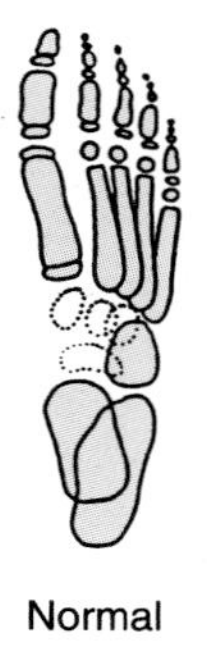

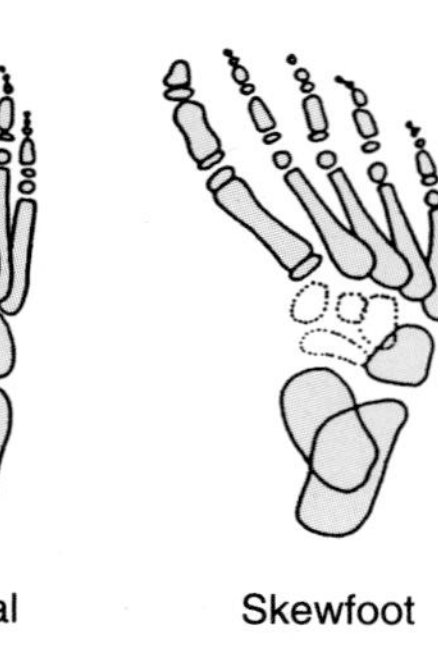

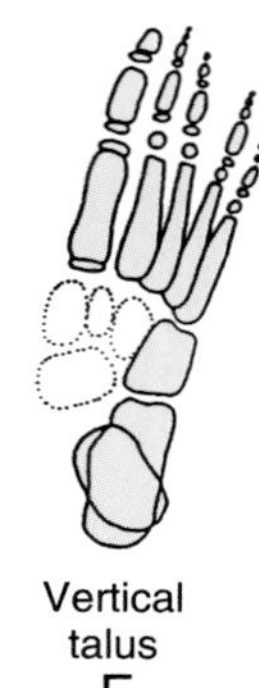

FIGURE 3–37 Anteroposterior view of common childhood foot disorders. **A**, Varus position of hindfoot and adducted forefoot in clubfoot. **B**, Normal hindfoot and adducted forefoot in metatarsus adductus. **C**, Normal foot. **D**, Valgus hindfoot (with increased talocalcaneal angle) and adducted forefoot in skewfoot. **E**, Increased talocalcaneal angle and lateral deviation of the calcaneus in congenital vertical talus.

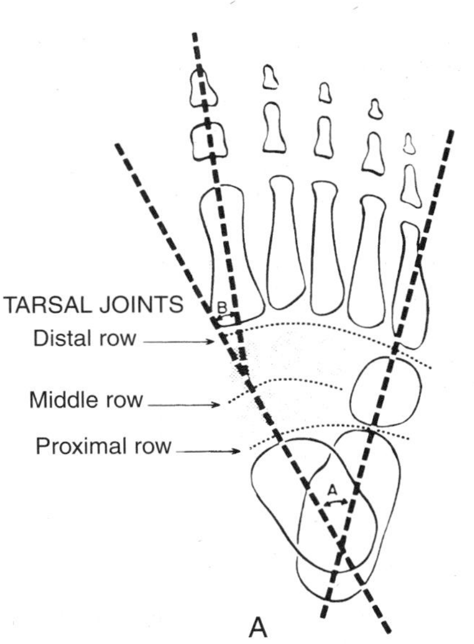

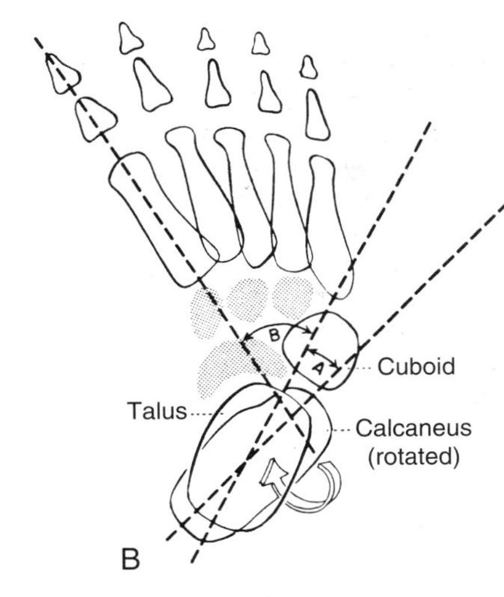

FIGURE 3–38 Radiographic evaluation of clubfoot. **A**, Normal foot. **B**, Note the "parallelism" of the talus and calcaneus, with a talocalcaneal angle (A) of < 20 degrees and a negative talus–first metatarsal angle (B) on the clubfoot side. (From Simons GW: Analytical radiology of club feet. J Bone Joint Surg [Br] 59:485–489, 1977.)

flexor digitorum longus), joint capsules, ligaments, and fascia, which lead to the associated deformities. Can be associated with hand anomalies (Streeter's dysplasia), diastrophic dwarfism, arthrogryposis, prune belly, tibial hemimelia, and myelomeningocele.

1. Radiography—Radiographs should include the dorsiflexion lateral view (Turco's), in which a talocalcaneal angle of greater than 35 degrees is normal; a smaller angle with a flat talar head is seen with clubfoot. On the anteroposterior view a talocalcaneal (Kite) angle of 20-40 degrees is normal (< 20 degrees is seen with clubfoot). The talus–first metatarsal angle is normally 0-20 degrees; a negative talus–first metatarsal angle is seen with clubfoot (Fig. 3–38). "Parallelism" of the calcaneus and talus is seen on both views.
2. Treatment
   a. The Ponseti method of serial weekly casting—Has recently become more popular because of the more favorable long-term results. This method requires a series of long-leg plaster casts and most often an Achilles release, and it is followed by external rotation of the feet in boots and bars for 2-3 years. Casting begins with correction of the cavus by aligning the first ray with the remaining metatarsals. Subsequent manipulation and casting uses lateral pressure on the distal talar head as a fulcrum to correct the forefoot adduction and heel varus. All deformities are corrected gradually. Residual equinus requires Achilles tendon release in over 90% of patients. Overcorrection of the foot in all planes is necessary at the completion of casting, and compliance in wearing the brace is essential for a successful outcome. Subsequent dynamic forefoot adduction/supination requires transfer of the anterior tibialis laterally in 15-20%.
   b. Resistant or refractory clubfeet—Surgical soft tissue release with tendon lengthening is favored in resistant feet, usually at age 6-9 months (Table 3–19). The posterior tibial artery must be carefully protected. The dorsalis pedis artery is often insufficient. Casting for several months is usually required postoperatively. In older patients (3-10 years old), a medial opening or lateral column–shortening osteotomy or cuboidal decancellization is recommended. For children who present with refractory clubfoot late (8-10 years old), triple arthrodesis is the only procedure possible for eliminating associated pain and deformity. Triple arthrodesis is contraindicated in patients with insensate feet because it causes a rigid foot that may lead to ulceration. Talectomy may be a better procedure in these patients.

B. Forefoot adduction (Fig. 3–39)
   1. Metatarsus adductus—See the discussion on rotational problems of lower extremities earlier under Lower Extremity Problems: General.

TABLE 3-19 STRUCTURES TO BE ADDRESSED IN THE SURGICAL CORRECTION OF CLUBFOOT

Structure	Procedure
Achilles tendon	Z-lengthening
Calcaneal-fibular ligament	Release
Posterior talofibular ligament	Release
Posterior tibialis tendon	Z-lengthening
Flexor digitorum longus tendon	Z-lengthening
Superficial deltoid	Release
Flexor hallucis longus tendon	Z-lengthening
Tibiotalar, subtalar capsule	Complete release
Talonavicular capsule	Release

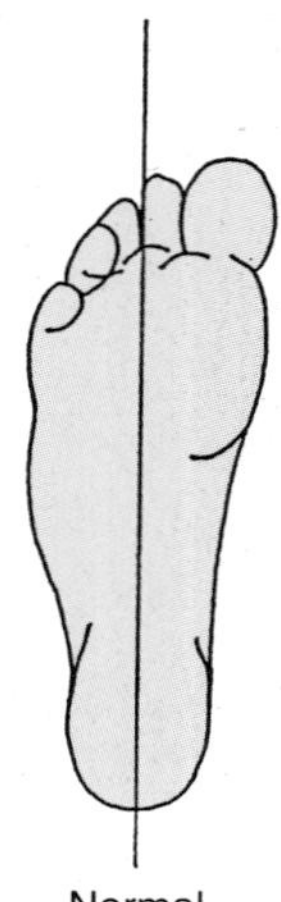

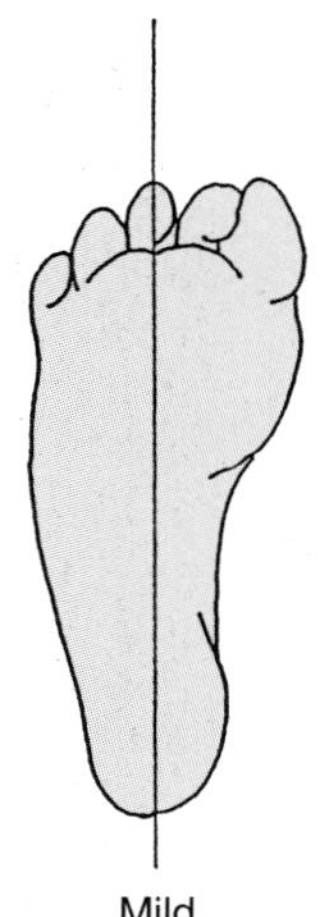

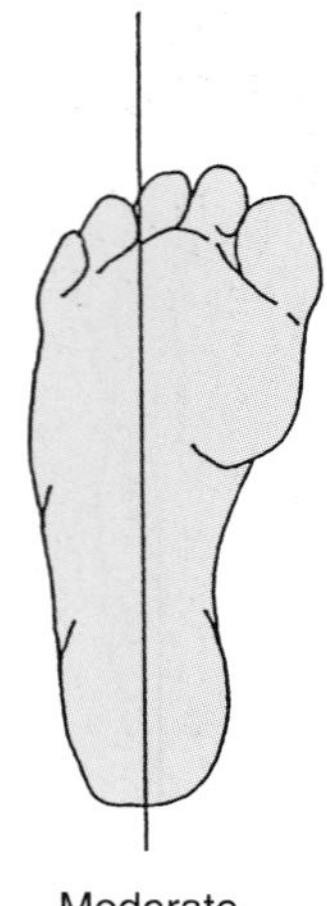

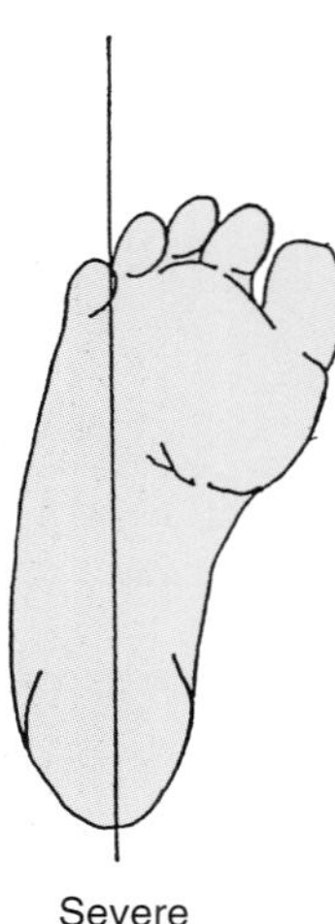

FIGURE 3–39 Classification of metatarsus adductus. (Adapted from Bleck EE: Metatarsus adductus: Classification and relationship to all kinds of treatment. J Pediatr Orthop 3:2–9, 1983.)

Adduction of the forefoot is commonly associated with DDH.

a. Grading—A simple clinical grading system has been described by Bleck, which is based on the heel bisector line (see Fig. 3–20). Normally, the heel bisector should align with the second/third toe web space. Four subtypes have been identified (Berg) (Table 3–20).
b. Treatment—If peroneal muscle stimulation corrects metatarsus adductus, it usually responds to stretching. Otherwise, manipulation and off-the-shelf orthoses or serial casting may be required. Surgical options in refractory cases (usually those with a medial skin crease) include abductor hallucis longus recession (for an atavistic first toe), medial capsular release with Evans' calcaneal osteotomy (lateral-column shortening), and medial-opening cuneiform and lateral-closing cuboid osteotomies with or without metatarsal osteotomies based on the severity of deformity.

2. Medial deviation of the talar neck—Benign disorder of the foot that generally corrects spontaneously.
3. Serpentine (Z) foot (complex skew foot)—Associated with residual tarsometatarsal adductus, talonavicular lateral subluxation, and hindfoot valgus. Nonoperative treatment is ineffective in correcting the deformity. Surgical treatment of this difficult problem is demanding and may include medial calcaneal sliding osteotomy (for hindfoot valgus), opening wedge cuboid osteotomy, and closing wedge cuneiform osteotomy (to correct midfoot lateral subluxation), and metatarsal osteotomy (to correct forefoot adductus). Most cases can be treated with observation.

TABLE 3-20 METATARSUS ADDUCTUS

Type	Features
Simple MTA	MTA
Complex MTA	MTA + lateral shift of midfoot
Skewfoot	MTA + valgus hindfoot
Complex skewfoot	MTA, lateral shift, valgus hindfoot

MTA, metatarsus adductus.

C. Pes cavus—Cavus deformity of the foot (elevated longitudinal arch) due to fixed plantar flexion of the forefoot. Pes cavus is commonly associated with neurologic disorders that include polio, CP, Friedreich's ataxia, and Charcot-Marie-Tooth disease (an imbalance between the tibialis anterior and peroneus longus muscles). Full neurologic workup is mandatory. The lateral block test (Coleman's) assesses hindfoot flexibility of the cavovarus foot (a flexible hindfoot corrects to neutral, with a lift placed under the lateral aspect of the foot) (Fig. 3–40). Nonoperative management is rarely successful. Surgical options in supple deformities include plantar release, metatarsal osteotomies, and tendon transfers. If the lateral block test is abnormal (rigid deformity), a calcaneal osteotomy is also done. In the past, triple arthrodesis has been used for rigid deformity in mature patients; the use of calcaneal sliding osteotomy, with multiple metatarsal extension osteotomies, may offer an alternative to subtalar fusion procedures.

D. Pes calcaneovalgus

1. Congenital vertical talus (convex pes valgus)—Irreducible dorsal dislocation of the navicular bone on the talus, with a fixed equinus hindfoot deformity.
   a. Diagnosis—Clinically, the talar head is prominent medially, the sole is convex, the forefoot is abducted and in dorsiflexion, and the hindfoot is in equinovalgus (Persian slipper foot) (Fig. 3–41). Patients may demonstrate a "peg-leg" gait (awkward gait with limited forefoot push-off). It is caused by a rigid flatfoot, which can be isolated or occur with chromosomal abnormalities, myeloarthropathies, or neurologic disorders. **Plantar-flexion lateral radiographs** show that a line along

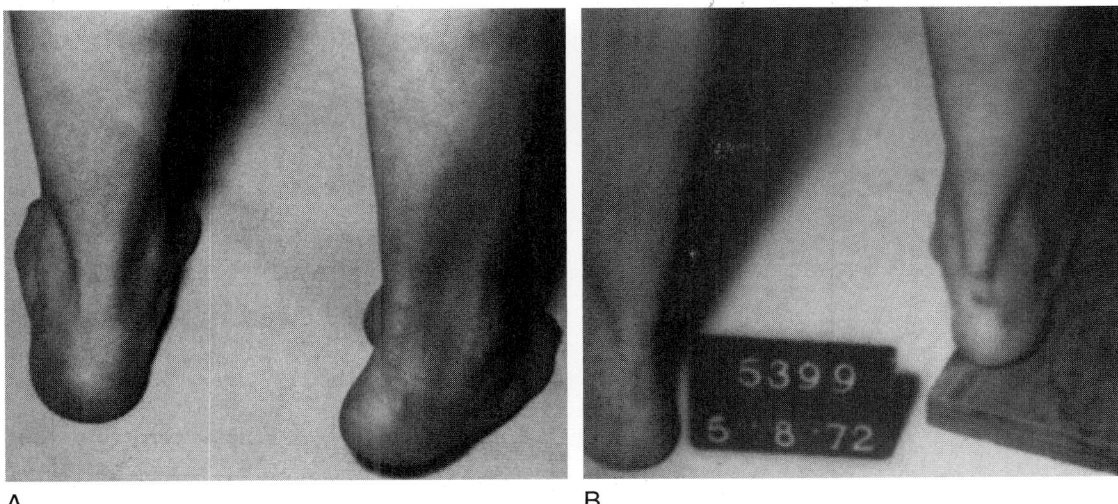

A B

FIGURE 3–40 Illustration of the Coleman block test to document hindfoot flexibility in a cavovarus foot. Posterior view of the foot of a 9-year-old boy with Charcot-Marie-Tooth disease. **A**, Note the heel varus. **B**, Placed on a 3-cm block, the heel assumes a normal position, thus sparing the calcaneus from an osteotomy during surgical correction. (From Benson M, Fixen J, Macnicol M: Children's Orthopaedics and Fractures, p 563. New York, Churchill Livingstone, 1994.)

the long axis of the talus passes below the first metatarsal–cuneiform axis (Meary's; tarsal–first metatarsal angle greater than 20 degrees [normal, 0-20 degrees dorsal tilt]). Anteroposterior radiographs show a talocalcaneal angle of greater than 40 degrees (normal, 20-40 degrees). Differential diagnosis includes an oblique talus (corrects with plantar flexion), tarsal coalition, and paralytic pes valgus.

b. Treatment—Three months of corrective casting (foot plantar flexed/inverted) or manipulative stretching is tried initially. Surgery when the patient is 6-12 months old includes soft tissue release/lengthening of the extensor tendons, peroneals, and Achilles tendon and reduction of the talonavicular joint with reconstruction of the spring ligament.

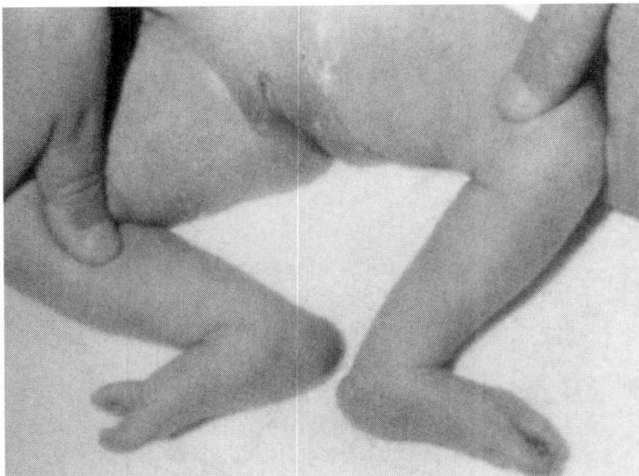

FIGURE 3–41 Clinical photograph of typical calcaneovalgus feet in a newborn infant. (From Benson M, Fixen J, Macnicol M: Children's Orthopaedics and Fractures, p 519. New York, Churchill Livingstone, 1994.)

2. Oblique talus—Talonavicular subluxation that reduces with plantar flexion of foot. Treatment consists of observation and sometimes a shoe insert (University of California, Berkeley, Laboratory [UCBL]). Some patients require pinning of the talonavicular joint in the reduced position and Achilles tendon lengthening.

E. Tarsal coalitions—A disorder of mesenchymal segmentation that leads to fusion of tarsal bones and rigid flatfoot. Occurs primarily as a talocalcaneal or calcaneonavicular coalition and is the leading cause of peroneal spastic flatfoot.

1. Diagnosis—The symptoms, which appear by age 10-12 years, include calf pain due to peroneal spasticity, flatfoot, and limited subtalar motion. Coalitions may be fibrous, cartilaginous, or osseous. **Calcaneonavicular coalition** is the most common in children ages 10-12, and **subtalar coalition** is more common in 12- to 14-year-olds. Lateral radiographs may demonstrate an elongated anterior process of the calcaneus ("anteater" sign). Talocalcaneal coalitions may demonstrate talar beaking on the lateral view (does not denote degenerative joint disease) or an irregular middle facet on Harris's axial view. The best study for identifying and measuring the cross-sectional area of a talocalcaneal coalition is a CT scan, which can also assess the patient for multiple coalitions (seen in 20% of cases).
2. Treatment—Initial treatment for either type involves immobilization (casting) or orthoses. Surgery is recommended in resistant cases. In calcaneonavicular coalitions, resection is commonly successful. For subtalar coalition, a symptomatic bar involving less than 50% of the middle facet should be resected; if over 50% of the middle facet is involved, then subtalar arthrodesis is preferred. Observation is

reasonable for asymptomatic bars in young children. Advanced cases and cases that fail attempts at resection often require triple arthrodesis.

F. Calcaneovalgus foot—Newborn condition associated with intrauterine positioning. It is common in first-born children. Presents with a dorsiflexed hindfoot, with eversion and abduction of the hindfoot that is passively correctable to neutral. Treatment consists of passive stretching and observation. Also seen with myelomeningocele at the L5 level due to muscular imbalance between foot dorsiflexors/everters (L4 and L5 roots) and plantar flexors/inverters (S1 and S2 roots).

G. Juvenile bunions—Are often bilateral and familial. This disorder is less common and usually less severe than the adult form. May be associated with ligamentous laxity and a hypermobile first ray. Usually found in adolescent girls. Optimal treatment is modification of shoe wear, with a wide toe box and arch supports. In general, surgery should be avoided because recurrence is frequent in the growing patient. If surgery is performed, symptomatic patients with an intermetatarsal angle of greater than 10 degrees (metatarsus primus varus) and a hallux valgus angle of greater than 20 degrees may require proximal metatarsal osteotomy, distal capsular reefing, and adductor tenotomy with a bunionectomy (modified McBride procedure). Complications include overcorrection and hallux varus.

H. Kohler's disease—Osteonecrosis of the tarsal navicular bone; usually presents at about 5 years old. Pain is the typical presenting complaint. Radiographs show sclerosis of the navicular bone. Symptoms usually resolve spontaneously with decreased activity with or without immobilization.

I. Flexible pes planus—Foot is flat only when standing and not with toe walking or foot hanging. This is frequently familial and almost always bilateral. Commonly associated with minor lower extremity rotational problems and ligamentous laxity.

1. Diagnosis—Symptoms can include an aching midfoot or pretibial pain. Lateral radiographic findings mimic those of vertical talus, but a plantar-flexed lateral view demonstrates that a line along the long axis of the talus passes above the metatarsal-cuneiform axis (Table 3–21).
2. Treatment—When the patient is symptomatic, arch supports and shoes with stiffer soles may offer pain relief but do not result in deformity correction. Thorough evaluation should be completed to rule out tight heel cords and decreased subtalar motion. UCBL heel cups are sometimes indicated for advanced cases with pain (symptomatic treatment only). Calcaneal lengthening osteotomy with or without medial soft tissue tightening may provide pain relief at the expense of inversion/eversion in adolescents with disabling pain refractory to every means of conservative treatment.

TABLE 3-21 RADIOLOGIC VIEWS FOR PES PLANUS

View	Assessment
Standing AP	Talar head coverage, talocalcaneal angle
Standing lateral	Calcaneal/talar equinus, talocalcaneal angle
Oblique	To rule out coalition

J. Habitual toe walker—Contracture of the Achilles tendon (often resolves with time). Usually responds to serial casting; sometimes requires Achilles tendon lengthening.

K. Accessory navicular—Normal variant seen in up to 12% of the population. Commonly associated with flat feet. The symptoms usually include medial arch pain with overuse; they usually resolve with activity restriction or immobilization. External oblique radiographic views are often helpful in the diagnosis. Most cases resolve spontaneously. Excision of the accessory bone is occasionally done, which can correct symptoms (but not flatfoot) in most patients.

L. Ball-and-socket ankle—Abnormal formation with a spherical talus (ball) and a cup-shaped tibiofibular articulation (socket). It usually requires no treatment but should be recognized because of its high association with tarsal coalition (50%), absent lateral rays (50%), fibular deficiency, and LLD.

M. Congenital toe disorders

1. Syndactyly—Fusion of the soft tissues (simple) and sometimes bone (complex) of the toes. Simple syndactyly usually does not require treatment; complex syndactyly is treated the same as it is in the hand.
2. Polydactyly (extra digits)—May be AD and usually involves the lateral ray in patients with a positive family history. Treatment includes ablation of the extra digit and any bony protrusion of the common metatarsal (the border digit is typically excised; not the best-formed digit). The procedure is usually done at age 9-12 months, but some rudimentary digits can be ligated in the newborn nursery.
3. Oligodactyly—Congenital absence of the toes. May be associated with more proximal agenesis (i.e., fibular hemimelia) and tarsal coalition. The disorder usually requires no treatment.
4. Atavistic great toe (congenital hallux varus)—Deformity involving great-toe adduction that is often associated with polydactyly. Must be differentiated from metatarsus adductus. The deformity usually occurs at the metatarsophalangeal joint and includes a short, thick first metatarsal and a firm band (abductor hallucis longus muscle) that may be responsible for the disorder. Surgery is sometimes required and includes release of the abductor hallucis longus muscle.
5. Overlapping toe—The fifth toe overlaps the fourth (usually bilaterally) and may cause

problems with footwear. Initial treatment includes passive stretching and "buddy" taping. Surgical options include tenotomy, dorsal capsulotomy, and syndactylization to the fourth toe (McFarland).

6. Underlapping toe (congenital curly toe)—Usually involves the lateral three toes and is rarely symptomatic. Surgery (flexor tenotomies) is occasionally indicated.

Selected Bibliography

BONE DYSPLASIAS (DWARFISM)

Ain MC, Browne JA: Spinal arthrodesis with instrumentation for thoracolumbar kyphosis in pediatric achondroplasia. Spine 29:2075–2080, 2004.

Bassett GS: Lower extremity abnormalities in dwarfing conditions. Instr Course Lect 39:389–397, 1991.

Bassett GS: Orthopedic aspects of skeletal dysplasias. Instr Course Lect 39:381–387, 1991.

Beals RK, Rolfe B: Current concepts review: Vater association: A unifying concept of multiple anomalies. J Bone Joint Surg [Am] 71:948–950, 1989.

Beals RK, Stanley G: Surgical correction of bowlegs in achondroplasia. J Pediatr Orthop 14(part B):245–249, 2005.

Bethem D, Winter RB, Lutter L, et al: Spinal disorders of dwarfism. J Bone Joint Surg [Am] 63:1412–1425, 1981.

Brook CG, de Vries BB: Skeletal dysplasias. Arch Dis Childhood 79:285–289, 1998.

Dawe C, Wynne-Davies R, Fulford GE: Clinical variation in dyschondrosteosis: A report on 13 individuals in 8 families. J Bone Joint Surg [Br] 64:377–381, 1982.

Dietz FR, Mathews KD: Update on the genetic bases of disorders with orthopaedic manifestations. J Bone Joint Surg [Am] 78:1583–1598, 1996.

Gluckman E: Bone marrow transplantation in children with hereditary disorders. Curr Opin Pediatr 8:42–44, 1996.

Kopits SE: Orthopedic complications of dwarfism. Clin Orthop 114:153–179, 1976.

McKusick VA: Heritable disorders of connective tissue, 4th ed. St. Louis, CV Mosby, 1972.

Rubin P: Dynamic classification of bone dysplasias. Chicago, Year Book Medical Publishers, 1964.

Stanscur V, Stanscur R, Maroteaux P: Pathogenic mechanisms in osteochondrodysplasias. J Bone Joint Surg [Am] 66:817–836, 1984.

Warman ML: Human genetic insights into skeletal development, growth, and homeostasis. Clin Orthop Relat Res Suppl 379:S40–S54, 2000.

CHROMOSOMAL AND TERATOLOGIC DISORDERS

Doyle JS, Lauerman WC, Wood KB, Krause DR: Complications and long-term outcome of upper cervical spine arthrodesis in patients with Down syndrome. Spine 21:1223–1231, 1996.

Huang TJ, Lubicky JP, Hammerberg KW: Scoliosis in Rhett syndrome. Orthop Rev 23:931–937, 1994.

Loder R, Lee C, Richards B: Orthopedic aspects of Rhett syndrome: A multicenter review. J Pediatr Orthop 9:557–562, 1989.

Milbrandt TA, Johnston CE II: Down syndrome and scoliosis: A review of a 50-year experience at one institution. Spine 30:2051–2055, 2005.

Rees D, Jones MW, Owen R, et al: Scoliosis surgery in the Prader-Willi syndrome. J Bone Joint Surg [Br] 71:685–688, 1989.

Segal LS, Drummond DS, Zanott RM, et al: Complications of posterior arthrodesis of the cervical spine in patients who have Down syndrome. J Bone Joint Surg [Am] 73:1547–1554, 1991.

Smith DW: Recognizable pattern of human malformation, 2nd ed. Philadelphia, WB Saunders, 1983.

Uno K, Kataoka O, Shiba R: Occipitoatlantal and occipitoaxial hypermobility in Down syndrome. Spine 21:1430–1434, 1996.

HEMATOPOIETIC DISORDERS

Diggs LW: Bone and joint lesions in sickle-cell disease. Clin Orthop 52:119–143, 1967.

Gill JC, Thometz JC, Scott JP. Musculoskeletal problems in hemophilia in the child and adult. New York, Raven Press, 1989.

Lofqvist T, Nilsson IM, Petersson C: Orthopaedic surgery in hemophilia: 20 years' experience in Sweden. Clin Orthop Relat Res 332:232–241, 1996.

Ribbans WJ, Giangrande P, Beeton K: Conservative treatment of hemarthrosis for prevention of hemophilic synovitis. Clin Orthop Relat Res 343:12–18, 1997.

Triantafylluo S, Hanks G, Handal JA, et al: Open and arthroscopic synovectomy in hemophilic arthropathy of the knee. Clin Orthop 283:196–204, 1992.

Thomas HB: Some orthopaedic findings in ninety-eight cases of hemophilia. Clin Orthop Relat Res 343:3–5, 1997.

METABOLIC DISEASE/ARTHRITIDES

Albright JA, Miller EA: Osteogenesis imperfecta [editorial comment]. Clin Orthop 159:2, 1981.

Birch JG, Herring JA: Spinal deformity in Marfan syndrome. J Pediatr Orthop 7:546–552, 1987.

Certner JM, Root L: Osteogenesis imperfecta. Orthop Clin North Am 21:151–162, 1990.

Cole WG: Advances in osteogenesis imperfecta. Clin Orthop Relat Res 401:6–16, 2002.

Gamble JG, Strudwick WJ, Rinsky LA, et al: Complications of intramedullary rods in osteogenesis imperfecta: Bailey-Dubow rods versus non-elongating rods. J Pediatr Orthop 8:645–649, 1989.

Hashkes PJ, Laxer RM: Medical treatment of juvenile idiopathic arthritis. JAMA 294:1671–1684, 2005.

Hensinger RN, DeVito PD, Ragsdale CG: Changes in the cervical spine in juvenile rheumatoid arthritis. J Bone Joint Surg [Am] 68:189–199, 1986.

Kulas DT, Schanberg L: Juvenile idiopathic arthritis. Curr Opin Rheumatol 13:392–398, 2001.

Mankin HJ: Rickets, osteomalacia and renal osteodystrophy: An update. Orthop Clin North Am 21:81–96, 1990.

Robelo I, Peredra DA, Silva L, et al: Effects of synthetic salmon calcitonin therapy in children with osteogenesis imperfecta. J Int Med Res 17:401–405, 1989.

Schaller JG: Chronic arthritis in children: Juvenile rheumatoid arthritis. Clin Orthop 182:79–89, 1984.

Shapiro F: Consequences of an osteogenesis imperfecta diagnosis for survival and ambulation. J Pediatr Orthop 5:456–462, 1985.

Sherry DD: What's new in the diagnosis and treatment of juvenile rheumatoid arthritis. J Pediatr Orthop 20:419–420, 2000.

Sillence DO: Osteogenesis imperfecta: An expanding panorama of variance. Clin Orthop 159:11, 1981.

Sofield HA, Miller EA: Fragmentation realignment and intramedullary rod fixation of deformities of the long bones in children. J Bone Joint Surg [Am] 41:1371, 1959.

Sponseller PD, Jones KB, Ahn NU, et al: Protrusio acetabuli in Marfan syndrome: Age-related prevalence and associated hip function. J Bone Joint Surg [Am] 88:486–495, 2006.

Tortolani PJ, McCarthy EF, Sponseller PD: Bone mineral density deficiency in children. J Am Acad Orthop Surgeons 10:57–66, 2002.

Wendt S, Mengel E, Beck M: Gaucher disease and miscellaneous. Acta Paediatr Suppl 95:139–144, 2006.

Zeitlin L, Fassier F, Glorieux FH: Modern approach to children with osteogenesis imperfecta. J Pediatr Orthop 12(part B):77–87, 2003.

BIRTH INJURIES

Bellew M, Kay SP, Webb F, Ward A: Developmental and behavioural outcome in obstetric brachial plexus palsy. J Hand Surg [Br] 25:49–51, 2000.

Canale ST, Griffin TW, Hubbard CN: Congenital muscular torticollis: A long-term follow-up. J Bone Joint Surg [Am] 64:810–816, 1982.

Davids JR, Wenger DR, Mubarak SJ: Congenital muscular torticollis: Sequelae of intrauterine or perinatal compartment syndrome. J Pediatr Orthop 13:141–147, 1993.

Gilbert A, Brockman R, Carlioz H: Surgical treatment of brachial plexus birth palsy. Clin Orthop 264:39–47, 1991.

Hentze VR, Meyer RD: Brachial plexus microsurgery in children. Microsurgery 12:175–185, 1991.

Jahnke AH, Bovill DF, McCarroll HR, et al: Persistent brachial plexus birth palsies. J Pediatr Orthop 11:533–537, 1991.

Moukoko D, Ezaki M, Wilkes D, Carter P: Posterior shoulder dislocation in infants with neonatal brachial plexus palsy. J Bone Joint Surg [Am] 86:787–793, 2004.

Smith NC, Rowan P, Benson LJ, et al: Neonatal brachial plexus palsy: Outcome of absent biceps function at three months of age. J Bone Joint Surg [Am] 86:2163–2170, 2004.

Quinlan WR, Brady PG, Regan BF: Congenital pseudarthrosis of the clavicle. Acta Orthop Scand 51:489–492, 1980.

Waters PM: Comparison of the natural history, the outcome of microsurgical repair, and the outcome of operative reconstruction in brachial plexus birth palsy. J Bone Joint Surg [Am] 81:649–659, 1999.

CEREBRAL PALSY

Albright AL, Barron WB, Fasick MP, et al: Continuous intrathecal baclofen infusion for spasticity of cerebral origin. JAMA 270:2475–2477, 1993.

Barnes MJ, Herring JA: Combined split anterior tibial-tendon transfer and intramuscular lengthening of the posterior tibial tendon. J Bone Joint Surg [Am] 73:734–738, 1991.

Bell KJ, Ounpuu S, DeLuca PA, Romness MJ: Natural progression of gait in children with cerebral palsy. J Pediatr Orthop 22:677–682, 2002.

Bleck EE: Current concepts review: Management of the lower extremities in children who have cerebral palsy. J Bone Joint Surg [Am] 72:140, 1990.

Bleck EE. Orthopedic management of cerebral palsy. Philadelphia, JB Lippincott, 1987.

Coleman SS, Chestnut WJ: A simple test for hindfoot flexibility in the cavovarus foot. Clin Orthop 123:60–62, 1977.

Dobson F, Boyd RN, Parrott J, et al: Hip surveillance in children with cerebral palsy: Impact on the surgical management of spastic hip disease. J Bone Joint Surg [Br] 84:720–726, 2002.

Elmer EB, Wenger DR, Mubarak SJ, et al: Proximal hamstring lengthening in the sitting cerebral palsy patient. J Pediatr Orthop 12:329–336, 1992.

Ferguson RL, Allen BL: Considerations in the treatment of cerebral palsy patients with spinal deformities. Orthop Clin North Am 19: 419–425, 1988.

Gage JR: Gait analysis: An essential tool in the treatment of cerebral palsy. Clin Orthop 288:126–134, 1993.

Gage JR: The clinical use of kinetics for evaluation of pathologic gait in cerebral palsy. J Bone Joint Surg [Am] 76:622–631, 1994.

Koman LA, Mooney JF, Goodman A: Management of valgus hindfoot deformity in pediatric cerebral palsy patients by medial displacement osteotomy. J Pediatr Orthop 13:180–183, 1993.

Koman LA, Mooney JF, Smith BP, et al: Management of spasticity in cerebral palsy with botulinum-A toxin: Report of preliminary, randomized, double-blind trial. J Pediatr Orthop 14:299–303, 1994.

Mubarak SJ, Valencia FG, Wenger DR: One stage correction of the spastic dislocated hip. J Bone Joint Surg [Am] 74:1347–1357, 1994.

Ounpuu S, Muik E, Davis RB, et al: Rectus femoris surgery in children with cerebral palsy. Part II: A comparison between the effect of transfer and release of the distal rectus femoris on knee motion. J Pediatr Orthop 13:331–335, 1993.

Rang M, Silver R, de la Garza JR, et al: Cerebral palsy. In Lovell R, Winter R, eds: Pediatric Orthopedics, 2nd ed. Philadelphia, JB Lippincott, 1986.

Rang M, Wright J: What have 30 years of medical progress done for cerebral palsy?. Clin Orthop 247:55–60, 1989.

Renshaw TS, Green NE, Griffin PP, Root L: Cerebral palsy: Orthopaedic management. Instr Course Lect 45:475–490, 1996.

Sutherland DH, Davids JR: Common gait abnormalities of the knee in cerebral palsy. Clin Orthop 288:139–147, 1993.

Thomas SS, Aiona MD, Buckon CE, Piatt JH Jr: Does gait continue to improve 2 years after selective dorsal rhizotomy?. J Pediatr Orthop 17:387–391, 1997.

NEUROMUSCULAR DISORDERS

Allen BL Jr, Ferguson RL: The Galveston technique of pelvic fixation with Luque-rod instrumentation of the spine. Spine 9:388–394, 1984.

Alman BA: Duchenne muscular dystrophy and steroids: Pharmacologic treatment in the absence of effective gene therapy. J Pediatr Orthop 25:554–556, 2005.

Babat LB, Ehrlich MG: A paradigm for the age-related treatment of knee dislocations in Larsen's syndrome. J Pediatr Orthop 20:396–401, 2000.

Banta JV, Drummond DS, Ferguson RL: The treatment of neuromuscular scoliosis. Instr Course Lect. 48:551–562, 1999.

Drennan JC: Foot deformities in myelomeningocele. Instr Course Lect 40:287–291, 1991.

Drennan JC: Current concepts in myelomeningocele. Instr Course Lect 48:543–550, 1999.

Drummond DS, Moreau M, Cruess RL: The results and complications of surgery for the paralytic hip and spine in myelomeningocele. J Bone Joint Surg [Br] 62:49–53, 1980.

Emans JB: Current concepts review: Allergy to latex in patients who have myelodysplasia. J Bone Joint Surg [Am] 74:1103–1109, 1992.

Evans GA, Drennan JC, Russman BS: Functional classification and orthopedic management of spinal muscular atrophy. J Bone Joint Surg [Br] 63:516–522, 1981.

Greene WB: Treatment of hip and knee problems in myelomeningocele. Instr Course Lect 48:563–574, 1999.

Hall JG: Arthrogryposis multiplex congenita: Etiology, genetics, classification, diagnostic approach, and general aspects. J Pediatr Orthop 6(part B):159–166, 1997.

Hoffer MM, Feiwell E, Perry R, et al: Functional ambulation in patients with myelomeningocele. J Bone Joint Surg [Am] 55:137–148, 1973.

Lindseth RE: Spine deformity in myelomeningocele. Instr Course Lect. 40:273–279, 1991.

Mazur JM, Shurtleff D, Menelaus M, et al: Orthopedic management of high-level spina bifida: Early walking compared with early use of a wheelchair. J Bone Joint Surg [Am] 71:56, 1989.

Mendell JR, Sahenk Z: Recent advances in diagnosis and classification of Charcot-Marie-Tooth disease. Curr Opin Orthop 4:39–45, 1993.

Shapiro F, Bresnan MJ: Orthopedic management of childhood neuromuscular disease. Part II: Peripheral neuropathies, Friedreich's ataxia, and arthrogryposis multiplex congenita. J Bone Joint Surg [Am] 64:949–953, 1982.

Shapiro F, Specht L: Current concepts review: The diagnosis and orthopedic management of inherited muscular disorders of childhood. J Bone Joint Surg [Am] 75:439–454, 1993.

Sodergard J, Ryoppy S: Foot deformities in arthrogryposis multiplex congenita. J Pediatr Orthop 14:768–772, 1994.

Sussman M: Duchenne muscular dystrophy. J Am Acad Orthop Surgeons 10:138–151, 2002.

PEDIATRIC SPINE

Bellah RD, Summerville DA, Treves ST, et al: Low-back pain in adolescent athletes: Detection of stress injury to the pars interarticularis with SPECT. Radiology 180:509–512, 1991.

Betz RR, Shufflebarger H: Anterior versus posterior instrumentation for the correction of thoracic idiopathic scoliosis. Spine 26:1095–1100, 2001.

Bollini G, Bergion M, Labriet C, et al: Hemivertebrae excision and fusion in children aged less than 5 years. J Pediatr Orthop 1(part B):95–101, 1993.

Bradford DS, Ahmed KB, Moe JH, et al: The surgical management of patients with Scheuermann's disease: A review of twenty-four cases managed by combined anterior and posterior spine fusion. J Bone Joint Surg [Am] 62:705–712, 1980.

Bradford DS, Hensinger RM, eds: The pediatric spine. New York, Thieme-Stratton, 1985.

Bradford DS, Lonstein JE, Ogilvie JB, et al, eds: Moe's textbook of scoliosis & other spinal deformities, 2nd ed. Philadelphia, WB Saunders, 1987.

Bridwell KH, McAllister JW, Betz RR, et al: Coronal decompensation produced by Cotrel-Dubousset "derotation" maneuver for idiopathic right thoracic scoliosis. Spine 16:769–777, 1991.

Carr WA, Moe JH, Winter RB, et al: Treatment of idiopathic scoliosis in the Milwaukee brace. J Bone Joint Surg [Am] 62:599–612, 1980.
Crawford AH, Schorry EK: Neurofibromatosis in children: The role of the orthopaedist. J Am Acad Orthop Surgeons 7:217–230, 1999.
Denis F: Cotrel-Dubousset instrumentation in the treatment of idiopathic scoliosis. Orthop Clin North Am 19:291–311, 1988.
Dobbs MB, Weinstein SL: Infantile and juvenile scoliosis. Orthop Clin North Am 30, vii, 331–341, 1999.
Dimeglio A: Growth of the spine before age 5 years. J Pediatr Orthop 1(part B):102–107, 1993.
Engler GL: Preoperative and intraoperative considerations in adolescent idiopathic scoliosis. Instr Course Lect. 38:137–141, 1989.
Evans SC, Edgar MA, Hall-Craggs MA, et al: MRI of "idiopathic" juvenile scoliosis: A prospective study. J Bone Joint Surg [Br] 78:314–317, 1996.
Fielding JW, Hawkins RJ: Atlantoaxial rotatory fixation. J Bone Joint Surg [Am] 59:37–44, 1977.
Fielding JW, Hensinger RN, Hawkins RJ: Os odontoideum. J Bone Joint Surg [Am] 62:376–383, 1980.
Fitch RD, Turi M, Bowman BE, et al: Comparison of Cotrel-Dubousset and Harrington rod instrumentation in idiopathic scoliosis. J Pediatr Orthop 10:44–47, 1990.
Karachalios T, Roidis N, Papagelopoulos PJ, Karachalios GG: The efficacy of school screening for scoliosis. Orthopedics 23:386–391, 2000.
King HA, Moe JH, Bradford DS, et al: The selection of fusion levels in thoracic idiopathic scoliosis. J Bone Joint Surg [Am] 65:1302–1313, 1983.
Koop SE, Winter RB, Lonstein JE: The surgical treatment of instability of the upper part of the cervical spine in children and adolescents. J Bone Joint Surg [Am] 66:403–411, 1984.
Lenke LG, Bridwell KH, Baldus C, et al: Cotrel-Dubousset instrumentation for idiopathic scoliosis. J Bone Joint Surg [Am] 74:1056–1068, 1992.
Lenke LG, Betz RR, Clements D, et al: Curve prevalence of a new classification of operative adolescent idiopathic scoliosis: Does classification correlate with treatment?. Spine 27:604–611, 2002.
Lenke LG: Lenke classification system of adolescent idiopathic scoliosis: Treatment recommendations. Instr Course Lect 54:537–542, 2005.
Lonstein JE, Carlson JM: The prediction of curve progression in untreated idiopathic scoliosis during growth. J Bone Joint Surg [Am] 66:1061–1071, 1984.
Lonstein JE: Congenital spine deformities: Scoliosis, kyphosis, and lordosis. Orthop Clin North Am 30:387–405, 1999.
Lowe TG: Current concepts review: Scheuermann's disease. J Bone Joint Surg [Am] 72:940–945, 1990.
Lowe TG, Edgar M, Margulies JY, et al: Etiology of idiopathic scoliosis: Current trends in research. J Bone Joint Surg [Am] 82:1157–1168, 2000.
Luque ER: Segmental spinal instrumentation for correction of scoliosis. Clin Orthop 163:192–198, 1982.
McMaster MJ, Ohtsuka K: The natural history of congenital scoliosis: A study of two hundred and fifty-one patients. J Bone Joint Surg [Am] 64:1128–1137, 1982.
Mehta MH: The rib-vertebra angle in the early diagnosis between resolving and progressive infantile scoliosis. J Bone Joint Surg [Br] 54:230–243, 1972.
Miller NH: Cause and natural history of adolescent idiopathic scoliosis. Orthop Clin North Am 30: vii,343–352, 1999.
Montgomery S, Hall J: Congenital kyphosis: Surgical treatment at Boston Children's Hospital. Orthop Trans 5:25, 1981.
Pang D, Wilberger JE Jr: Spinal cord injury without radiographic abnormalities in children. J Neuro Surg 57:114–129, 1982.
Picetti GD III, Ertl JP, Bueff HU: Anterior endoscopic correction of scoliosis. Orthop Clin North Am 33:421–429, 2002.
Ring D, Wenger DR: Magnetic resonance imaging scans in discitis: Sequential studies in a child who needed operative drainage: A case report. J Bone Joint Surg [Am] 76:596–601, 1994.
Schrock RD: Congenital abnormalities at the cervicothoracic level. Instr Course Lect 6, 1949.
Scoles PV, Quinn TP: Intervertebral discitis in children and adolescents. Clin Orthop 162:31–36, 1982.
Sorenson KH: Scheuermann's juvenile kyphosis. Copenhagen, Munksgaard, 1964.
Thompson GH, Akbarnia BA, Kostial P, et al: Comparison of single and dual growing rod techniques followed through definitive surgery: A preliminary study. Spine 30:2039–2044, 2005.
Tredwell SJ, Newman DE, Lockitch G: Instability of the upper cervical spine in Down syndrome. J Pediatr Orthop 10:602–606, 1990.
Tucker SK, Noordeen MH, Pitt MC: Spinal cord monitoring in neuromuscular scoliosis. J Pediatr Orthop 10(part B):1–5, 2001.
Weinstein SL, Ponseti IV: Curve progression in idiopathic scoliosis. J Bone Joint Surg [Am] 65:447–455, 1983.
Weinstein SL: Natural history. Spine 24:2592–2600, 1999.
Winter RB, Lonstein JE, Drogt J, et al: The effectiveness of bracing in the nonoperative treatment of idiopathic scoliosis. Spine 11:790–791, 1986.
Winter RB, Moe JH, Lonstein JE: The incidence of Klippel-Feil syndrome in patients with congenital scoliosis and kyphosis. Spine 9:363–366, 1984.
Winter RB, Moe JH, Lonstein JE: The surgical treatment of congenital kyphosis: A review of 94 patients age 5 years or older, with 2 years or more follow-up in 77 patients. Spine 10:224–231, 1985.

UPPER EXTREMITY PROBLEMS

Carson WG, Lovell WW, Whitesides TE Jr: Congenital elevation of the scapula: Surgical correction by the Woodward procedure. J Bone Joint Surg [Am] 62:1199–1207, 1981.
Liebovic SJ, Erlich MG, Zaleske DJ: Sprengel deformity. J Bone Joint Surg [Am] 72:192–197, 1990.
Woodward JW: Congenital elevation of the scapula: Correction by release and transplantation of muscle origins. J Bone Joint Surg [Am] 43:219–228, 1961.

LOWER EXTREMITY PROBLEMS

Berg EF: A reappraisal of metatarsus adductus and skewfoot. J Bone Joint Surg [Am] 68:1185–1196, 1986.
Bleck EE: Metatarsus adductus: Classification and relationship to outcomes of treatment. J Pediatr Orthop 3:2–9, 1983.
Crawford AH, Gabriel KR: Foot and ankle problems. Orthop Clin North Am 18:649–666, 1987.
Green WB: Metatarsus adductus and skewfoot. Instr Course Lect 43:161–178, 1994.
Kling TF, Hensinger RN: Angular and torsional deformities of the lower limbs in children. Clin Orthop 176:136–147, 1983.
Staheli LT, Clawson DK, Hubbard DD: Medial femoral torsion: Experience with operative treatment. Clin Orthop 146:222–225, 1980.
Staheli LT, Corbett M, Wyss C, et al: Lower extremity rotational problems in children: Normal values to guide management. J Bone Joint Surg [Am] 67:39–47, 1985.

HIP AND FEMUR

Blanco JS, Taylor B, Johnston CE II: Comparison of single pin vs. multiple pin fixation in treatment of slipped capital femoral epiphysis. J Pediatr Orthop 12:384–389, 1992.
Canale ST, Harkness RM, Thomas PA, et al: Does aspiration of bones and joints affect results of later bone scanning? J Pediatr Orthop 5:23–26, 1985.
Chiari K: Medial displacement osteotomy of the pelvis. Clin Orthop 98:55–71, 1974.
Christensen F, Soballe K, Ejsted R, et al: The Catterall classification of Perthes disease: An assessment of reliability. J Bone Joint Surg [Br] 68:614–615, 1986.
Daoud A, Saighi-Bouaouina A: Treatment of sequestra, pseudarthroses, and defects in the long bones of children who have chronic hematogenous osteomyelitis. J Bone Joint Surg [Am] 71:1448–1468, 1989.
Epps CH Jr: Current concepts review: Proximal femoral focal deficiency. J Bone Joint Surg [Am] 65:867–870, 1983.
Fabry F, Meire E: Septic arthritis of the hip in children: Poor results after late and inadequate treatment. J Pediatr Orthop 3:461–466, 1983.
Faciszewski T, Coleman SS, Biddolpf G: Triple innominate osteotomy for acetabular dysplasia. J Pediatr Orthop 13:426–430, 1993.
Faciszewski T, Keifer G, Coleman SS: Pemberton osteotomy for residual acetabular dysplasia in children who have congenital dislocation of the hip. J Bone Joint Surg [Am] 5:643–649, 1993.
Gage JR, Winter RB: Avascular necrosis of the capital femoral epiphysis as a complication of closed reduction of congenital dislocation of the hip: A critical review of twenty years' experience at Gillette Children's Hospital. J Bone Joint Surg [Am] 54:373–388, 1972.
Galpin RD, Roach JW, Wenger DR, et al: One-stage treatment of congenital dislocation of the hip in older children, including femoral shortening. J Bone Joint Surg [Am] 71:734–741, 1989.
Gillingham BL, Sanchez AA, Wenger DR: Pelvic osteotomies for the treatment of hip dysplasia in children and young adults. J Am Acad Orthop Surgeons 7:325–337, 1999.

Green NE, Edwards K: Bone and joint infections in children. Orthop Clin North Am 18:555–576, 1987.

Green SA: Patient management during limb lengthening. Instr Course Lect 46:547–554, 1997.

Guille JT, Pizzutillo PD, MacEwen GD: Developmental dysplasia of the hip from birth to six months. J Am Acad Orthop Surgeons 8:232–242, 2000.

Harke HT, Grissom LE: Performing dynamic ultrasonography of the infant hip. AJR Am J Roentgenol 155:837–844, 1990.

Haynes RJ: Developmental dysplasia of the hip: Etiology, pathogenesis, and examination and physical findings in the newborn. Inst. Course Lect 50:535–540, 2001.

Herndon WA, Knaur S, Sullivan JA, et al: Management of septic arthritis in children. J Pediatr Orthop 6:576–578, 1986.

Herring JA, Neustadt JB, Williams JJ, et al: The lateral pillar classification of Legg-Calvé-Perthes disease. J Pediatr Orthop 12:143–150, 1992.

Herring JA, Kim HT, Browne R: Legg-Calvé-Perthes disease. Part I: Classification of radiographs with use of the modified lateral pillar and Stulberg classifications. J Bone Joint Surg [Am] 86:2103–2120, 2004.

Herring JA, Kim HT, Browne R: Legg-Calvé-Perthes disease. Part II: Prospective multicenter study of the effect of treatment on outcome. J Bone Joint Surg [Am] 86:2121–2134, 2004.

Jackson MA, Nelson JD: Etiology and medical management of acute suppurative bone and joint infections in pediatric patients. J Pediatr Orthop 2:313–323, 1982.

Kocher MS, Zurakowski D, Kasser JR: Differentiating between septic arthritis and transient synovitis of the hip in children: An evidence-based clinical prediction algorithm. J Bone Joint Surg [Am] 81:1662–1670, 1999.

Loder RT, Aronsson DD, Dobbs MB, Weinstein SL: Slipped capital femoral epiphysis. Instr Course Lect 50:555–570, 2001.

Matan AJ, Smith JT: Pediatric septic arthritis. Orthopedics 20:630–635, 1997.

Mausen JPGM, Rozing PM, Obermann WR: Intertrochanteric corrective osteotomy in slipped capital femoral epiphysis: A long-term follow-up study of 26 patients. Clin Orthop 259:100–109, 1990.

Morrissey RT, ed: Lovell, & Winter's pediatric orthopedics, 3rd ed. Philadelphia, JB Lippincott, 2000.

Moseley CF: Assessment and prediction in leg length discrepancy. Instr Course Lect 38:325–330, 1989.

Moseley CF: Developmental hip dysplasia and dislocation: Management of the older child. Instr Course Lect 50:547–553, 2001.

Mubarak SJ, Beck LR, Sutherland DH: Home traction in the management of congenital dislocation of the hips. J Pediatr Orthop 6:721–723, 1986.

Mubarak SJ, Garfin S, Vance R, et al: Pitfalls in the use of the Pavlik harness for treatment of congenital dysplasia, subluxation, and dislocation of the hip. J Bone Joint Surg [Am] 63:1239–1248, 1981.

Norlin R, Hammerby S, Tkaczuk H: The natural history of Perthes disease. Int Orthop 15:13–16, 1991.

Paley D: Current techniques of limb lengthening. J Pediatr Orthop 8:73–92, 1988.

Price CT: Metaphyseal and physeal lengthening. Instr Course Lect 38:331–336, 1989.

Richardson EG, Rambach BE: Proximal femoral focal deficiency: A clinical appraisal. South Med J 72:166–173, 1979.

Ritterbusch JF, Shantharam SS, Gelinas C: Comparison of lateral pillar classification and Catterall classification of Legg-Calvé-Perthes disease. J Pediatr Orthop 13:200–202, 1993.

Salter RB, Hansson G, Thompson GH: Innominate osteotomy in the management of residual congenital subluxation of the hip in young adults. Clin Orthop 182:53–68, 1984.

Southwick WO: Compression fixation after biplane intertrochanteric osteotomy for slipped capital femoral epiphysis. J Bone Joint Surg [Am] 55:1218–1224, 1973.

Song J, Letts M, Monson R: Differentiation of psoas muscle abscess from septic arthritis of the hip in children. Clin Orthop Relat Res 391:258–265, 2001.

Staheli LT, Chew DE: Slotted acetabular augmentation in childhood and adolescence. J Pediatr Orthop 12:569–580, 1992.

Steele HH: Triple osteotomy of the innominate bone. J Bone Joint Surg [Am] 55:343–350, 1973.

Sutherland DH, Greenfield R: Double innominate osteotomy. J Bone Joint Surg [Am] 59:1082–1091, 1977.

Suzuki S, Yamamuro T: Avascular necrosis in patients treated with Pavlik harness for congenital dislocation of the hip. J Bone Joint Surg [Am] 72:1048–1055, 1990.

Tachdjian MO: Pediatric Orthopedics, 3rd ed. Philadelphia, WB Saunders, 2001.

Thompson GH, Price CT, Roy D, et al: Legg-Calvé-Perthes disease: Current concepts. Instr Course Lect 51:367–384, 2002.

Vitale MG, Skaggs DL: Developmental dysplasia of the hip from six months to four years of age. J Am Acad Orthop Surgeons 9:401–411, 2001.

Willis RB: Developmental dysplasia of the hip: Assessment and treatment before walking age. Instr. Course Lect 50:541–545, 2001.

KNEE AND LEG

Brown FW, Pohnert WH: Construction of a knee joint in meromelia tibia (congenital absence of the tibia): A 15-year follow-up study. J Bone Joint Surg [Am] 54:1333, 1972.

Cain EL, Clancy WG: Treatment algorithm for osteochondral injuries of the knee. Clin Sports Med 20:321–342, 2001.

Dickhaut SC, DeLee JC: The discoid lateral meniscus syndrome. J Bone Joint Surg [Am] 64:1068–1073, 1982.

Jacobsen ST, Crawford AH, Miller EA, et al: The Syme amputation in patients with congenital pseudarthrosis of the tibia. J Bone Joint Surg [Am] 65:533–537, 1983.

Johnston CE II: Congenital pseudarthrosis of the tibia: Results of technical variations in the Charnley-Williams procedure. J Bone Joint Surg [Am] 84:1799–1810, 2002.

Laville JM, Chau E, Willemen L, et al: Blount's disease: Classification and treatment. J Pediatr Orthop 8(part B):19–25, 1999.

Langenskiold A: Tibia vara: Osteochondrosis deformans tibiae: Blount's disease. Clin Orthop 158:77–82, 1981.

Letts M, Vincent N: Congenital longitudinal deficiency of the fibula (fibular hemimelia): Parental refusal of amputation. Clin Orthop 287:160–166, 1993.

Roach JW, Shindell R, Green NE: Late onset pseudarthrosis of the dysplastic tibia. J Bone Joint Surg [Am] 75:1593–1601, 1993.

FEET

Coleman SS. Complex foot deformities in children. Philadelphia, Lea & Febiger, 1983.

Crawford AH, Marxen JL, Osterfeld DL: The Cincinnati incision: A comprehensive approach for surgical procedures of the foot and ankle in childhood. J Bone Joint Surg [Am] 64:1355–1358, 1982.

Cummings RJ, Davidson RS, Armstrong PF, Lehman WB: Congenital clubfoot. Instr Course Lect 51:385–400, 2002.

Cummings RJ, Davidson RS, Armstrong PF, Lehman WB: Congenital clubfoot. J Bone Joint Surg [Am] 84:290–308, 2002.

Drennan JC: Congenital vertical talus. Instr Course Lect 45:315–322, 1996.

Drennan JC: Tarsal coalitions. Instr Course Lect 45:323–329, 1996.

Jacobs RF, Adelman L, Sack CM, et al: Management of Pseudomonas osteochondritis complicating puncture wounds of the foot. Pediatrics 69:432–435, 1982.

McHale KA, Lenhart MK: Treatment of residual clubfoot deformity, the "bean-shaped" foot, by opening wedge medial cuneiform osteotomy and closing wedge cuboid osteotomy: Clinical review and cadaver correlations. J Pediatr Orthop 11:374–381, 1991.

Morcuende JA, Abbasi D, Dolan LA, Ponseti IV: Results of an accelerated Ponseti protocol for clubfoot. J Pediatr Orthop 25:623–626, 2005.

Mosca VS: The cavus foot. J Pediatr Orthop 21:423–424, 2001.

Onley BW, Asher MA: Excision of symptomatic coalition of the middle facet of the talocalcaneal joint. J Bone Joint Surg [Am] 69:539–544, 1987.

Pentz AS, Weiner DS: Management of metatarsus adductovarus. Foot Ankle 14:241–246, 1993.

Peterson HA: Skewfoot (forefoot adduction with heel valgus). J Pediatr Orthop 6:24–30, 1986.

Piqueres X, de Zabala S, Torrens C, Marin M: Cubonavicular coalition: A case report and literature review. Clin Orthop Relat Res 396:112–114, 2002.

Simons GW: Analytical radiography of club feet. J Bone Joint Surg [Br] 59:485–489, 1974.

Sullivan JA: Pediatric flatfoot: Evaluation and management. J Am Acad Orthop Surgeons 7:44–53, 1999.

Turco VJ: Resistant congenital clubfoot: One-stage posteromedial release with internal fixation: A follow-up report of a 15 year experience. J Bone Joint Surg [Am] 61:805–814, 1979.

CHAPTER 4

Sports Medicine

Joshua A. Baumfeld, Jennifer A. Hart, and Mark D. Miller

CONTENTS

SECTION 1 Knee

I. Anatomy and Biomechanics

A. Anatomy—The knee is much more than a simple hinge joint because both gliding and rolling are essential to its kinematics. An understanding of the interactions of ligaments, menisci, capsular structures, and musculature is imperative. Although a thorough discussion of anatomy is included in Chapter 2, Anatomy, a brief review of knee anatomy is relevant.

1. Ligaments—Four major ligaments and several other supporting ligaments and structures provide stability to the knee joint.
   a. Despite being the subject of intensive research, the function and anatomy of the **anterior cruciate ligament** (ACL) are still debated. The tibial insertion is a broad, irregular, oval area just anterior to and between the intercondylar eminences of the tibia. The femoral attachment is a semicircular area on the posteromedial aspect of the lateral femoral condyle (Fig. 4–1). The ACL is approximately 33 mm long and 11 mm in diameter. The ACL is often said to be composed of two "bundles"—an anteromedial bundle that is tight in flexion and a posterolateral bundle that is tight in extension. The ACL is composed of 90% type I collagen and 10% type III collagen. The blood supply to both cruciate ligaments is via branches of the middle geniculate artery and the fat pad. Mechanoreceptor nerve fibers within the ACL have been found and may have a proprioceptive role.
   b. The **posterior cruciate ligament** (PCL) originates from a broad, crescent-shaped area anterolaterally on the medial femoral condyle and inserts into a tibial sulcus that is below the articular surface (see Fig. 4–1). It is also composed of two bundles—an anterolateral portion that is tight in flexion and a posteromedial portion that is tight in extension. The PCL is approximately 38 mm in length and 13 mm in diameter. Variable meniscofemoral ligaments (Humphry's [anterior]; Wrisberg's [posterior]) originate from the posterior horn of the lateral meniscus and insert into the substance of the PCL. The neurovascular supply of the PCL is similar to that of the ACL.
   c. The **medial collateral ligament** (MCL) is composed of superficial and deep fibers. The superficial MCL (tibial collateral ligament) lies deep to the gracilis and semitendinosus tendons; originates from the medial femoral epicondyle; and inserts onto the periosteum of the proximal tibia, deep to the pes anserinus. The anterior fibers of the superficial MCL tighten during the first 90 degrees of motion, while the posterior fibers tighten in extension. The deep portion of the ligament (medial capsular ligament) is a capsular thickening that blends with the superficial fibers and is intimately associated with the medial meniscus (coronary ligaments).
   d. The **lateral collateral ligament** (LCL), or fibular collateral ligament, is a cordlike structure that originates on the lateral femoral epicondyle posterior and superior to the insertion of the popliteus tendon and inserts on the lateral aspect of the fibular head. Because it is located behind the axis of knee rotation, the LCL is tight in extension and lax in flexion.
   e. The **posteromedial corner**, a structure deep and posterior to the superficial MCL and

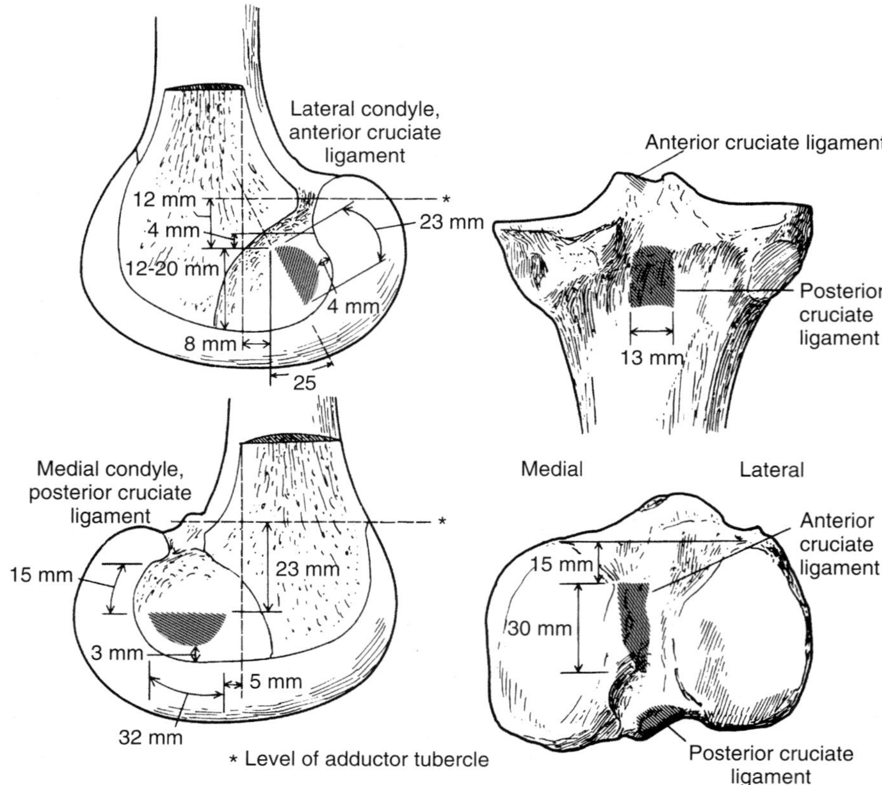

FIGURE 4–1 Origins and insertions of the anterior cruciate ligament and posterior cruciate ligament. (From Girgis FG, Marshall JL, Al Monajem ARS: The cruciate ligaments of the knee joint: Anatomical, functional, and experimental analysis. Clin Orthop 106:216-231, 1975.)

contiguous with the deep MCL, is important to rotary stability. The posteromedial corner consists of the capsular thickening of the multiple insertions of the semimembranosus; the posterior oblique ligament (POL), which originates on the adductor tubercle; and the oblique popliteal ligament, or thickening of the posterior capsule.

f. The **posterolateral corner** is becoming increasingly important in treating the multiple ligament–injured knee. It consists of the biceps, iliotibial band, and popliteus (which originates on the back of the tibia and inserts medial, anterior, and distal to the LCL); the popliteofibular ligament; the lateral capsule; the arcuate ligament (which is contiguous with the oblique popliteal ligament medially); and the fabellofibular ligament (the lateral two are really just thickenings of the joint capsule).

2. Medial structures of the knee—The medial structures of the knee are composed of three layers (Table 4–1) (Fig. 4–2).
3. Lateral structures of the knee—The lateral structures of the knee are also composed of three layers (Table 4–2) (see Fig. 4–2).
4. Menisci—The menisci are crescent-shaped, fibrocartilaginous structures that are triangular in cross section. They are composed predominantly of type 1 collagen. Only the peripheral 20-30% of the medial meniscus and 10-25% of the lateral meniscus are vascularized (medial and lateral genicular arteries, respectively). The medial meniscus is more C shaped, and the lateral meniscus is more circular in shape (see Fig. 4–1). These structures deepen the articular surfaces of the tibial plateau and have a role in stability, lubrication, and nutrition. They are connected anteriorly by the transverse (intermeniscal) ligament and are attached peripherally via the coronary ligaments.
5. Joint relationships—The anteroposterior dimensions of the lateral femoral condyle are greater than those of the medial condyle. The alignment of the condyles is also different; the lateral condyle is relatively straight, but the medial condyle is curved (allowing the medial tibial plateau to rotate externally in full extension—the "screw-home mechanism"). The lateral condyle can also be identified by its terminal sulcus and groove of the popliteus insertion (Fig. 4–3). The patellofemoral joint is composed of the patella (with variably sized medial and lateral facets) and the femoral trochlea. The patella is restrained in the trochlea by the valgus axis of the quadriceps mechanism (Q angle), the oblique fibers of the vastus medialis (VMO) and lateralis muscles (and their extensions—the patella retinaculum), and the patellofemoral ligaments. The articular surface of the patella is the thickest in the body; the patella can withstand forces several times those of body weight. The medial patellofemoral ligament (MPFL) is present in the second medial layer, originates just anterior and distal to the adductor tubercle or just superior to the origin of the superficial medial collateral ligament, and inserts into the medial border of the patella as well as the undersurface of the VMO. It has a major role in preventing lateral displacement of the patella, contributing more than 50% of the total medial restraint to lateral subluxation (Fig. 4–4).

TABLE 4-1 MEDIAL STRUCTURES OF THE KNEE

Layer	Components
I	Sartorius and fascia
II	Superficial MCL, posterior oblique ligament, semimembranosus
III	Deep MCL, capsule

Note: The gracilis, semitendinosus, and saphenous nerves run between layers I and II. MCL, medial collateral ligament.

B. Biomechanics

1. Ligamentous biomechanics—The role of the ligaments of the knee is to provide passive restraints to abnormal motion (Table 4–3).
2. Structural properties of ligaments—The tensile strength of a ligament, or maximal stress that a ligament can sustain before failure, has been characterized for all knee ligaments. However, it is important to consider age, orientation, preparation of the specimen, and other factors prior to determining which graft to use. The ACL's tensile strength is approximately 2200 N and up to 2500 N in young individuals. The tensile strength of a 10-mm patellar tendon graft (young specimen) is more than 2900 N and is about 30% stronger when it is rotated 90 degrees. However, this strength quickly diminishes in vivo. Studies suggest that the quadrupled hamstring graft is even greater but is dependent on graft fixation. The PCL is thought to have a higher tensile strength than the ACL (2500-3000 N), but its value is disputed. The MCL has approximately twice the stiffness and tensile strength as the ACL, whereas the strength of the LCL is approximately 750 N.
3. Kinematics—The motion of the knee joint and interplay of ligaments have been described as a four-bar cruciate linkage system (Fig. 4–5). As the knee flexes, the center of joint rotation (intersection of the cruciate ligaments) moves posteriorly, causing rolling and gliding at the articulating surfaces. The concept of ligament "isometry" remains controversial. Reconstructed ligaments should approximate normal anatomy and lie within the flexion axis in all positions of knee motion. Ligaments anterior to the flexion axis stretch, and ligaments posterior to the axis shorten as the joint flexes. Although many instruments have been designed to achieve isometry, other considerations, such as graft impingement and avoiding flexion contractures, may be more important factors to consider for ligament reconstructions.
4. Meniscal biomechanics—The collagen fibers of the menisci are arranged radially and longitudinally (Fig. 4–6). The longitudinal fibers help dissipate

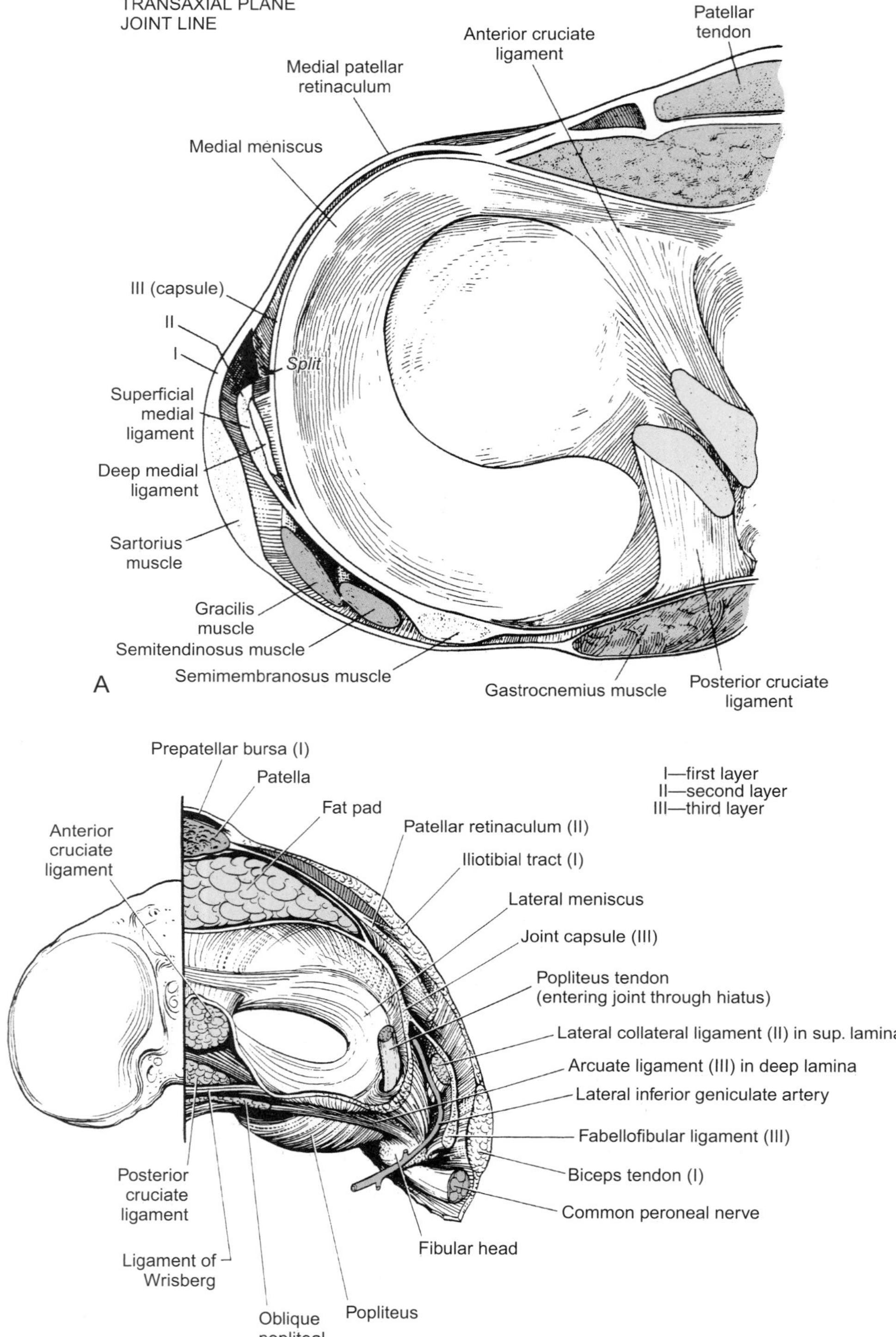

FIGURE 4–2 Medial and lateral supporting structures of the knee. **A**, Medial structures of the knee include the sartorius and its fascia and the patellar retinaculum (layer I), the hamstring tendons and superficial medial collateral ligament (MCL) (layer II), and the deep MCL (layer III). **B**, Lateral structures of the knee include the iliotibial tract and biceps (layer I), patellar retinaculum (layer II), and capsule and lateral collateral ligament (layer III). (**A** from Warren LF, Marshal JL: The supporting structures and layers of the medial side of the knee. J Bone Joint Surg [Am] 61:56-62, 1979. **B** from Seebacher JR, Ingilis AE, Marshall JL, et al: The structure of the posterolateral aspect of the knee. J Bone Joint Surg [Am] 64:536-541, 1982.)

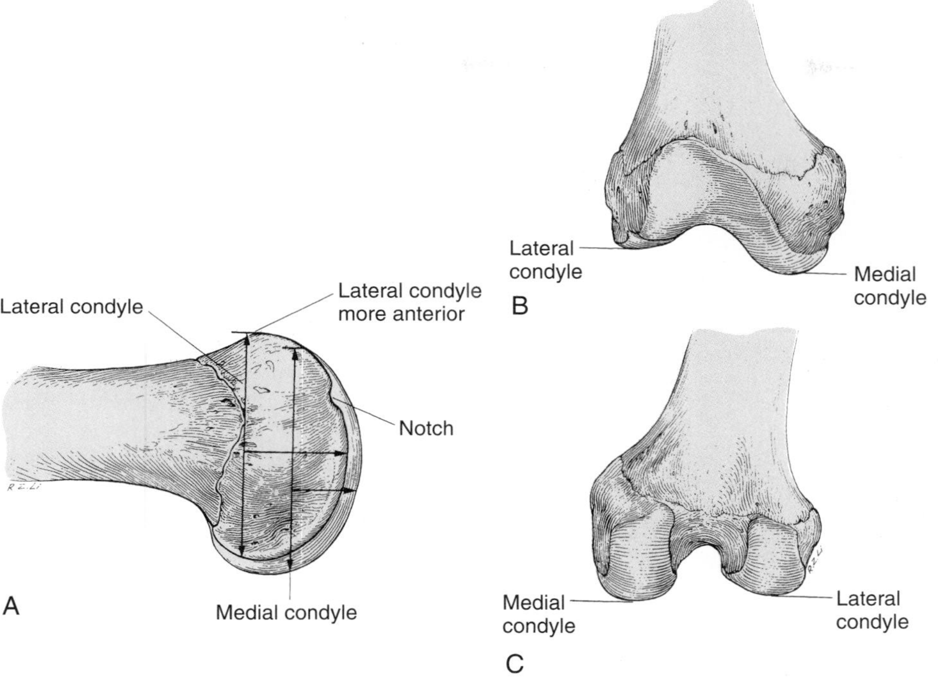

FIGURE 4–3 Relationships of the femoral condyles. **A**, On the lateral projection, the lateral condyle projects more anteriorly and is notched. Anterior (**B**) and posterior (**C**) views demonstrate the difference in size and curvature of the medial femoral condyle. (From Tria AJ, Klein KS: An Illustrated Guide to the Knee, p 5. New York, Churchill Livingstone, 1992.)

the hoop stresses in the menisci, and the combination of fibers allows the meniscus to expand under compressive forces and increase the contact area of the joint. The lateral meniscus has twice the excursion of the medial meniscus during knee range of motion (ROM) and rotation. Studies have shown that an ACL deficiency may result in abnormal meniscal strain, particularly in the posterior horn of the medial meniscus.

5. Patellofemoral joint—The patellofemoral joint must withstand forces that are more than three times those of body weight. The main restraint to lateral displacement of the patella is the MPFL, contributing more than 50% of the total restraining force.

TABLE 4-2 LATERAL STRUCTURES OF THE KNEE

Layer	Components
I	Iliotibial tract, biceps, fascia
II	Patellar retinaculum, patellofemoral ligament
III	Arcuate ligament, fabellofibular ligament, capsule, LCL

Note: The inferior lateral geniculate artery is deep to the LCL and is at risk with aggressive meniscal resection.

LCL, lateral collateral ligament.

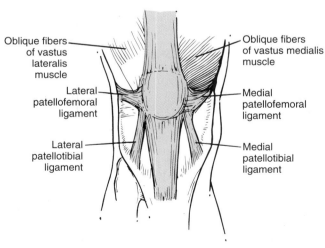

FIGURE 4–4 Patellar restraints include the patellofemoral and patellotibial ligaments as well as the oblique fibers of the vastus medialis and lateralis. (From Walsh WM: Patellofemoral joint. In DeLee JC, Drez D Jr, eds: Orthopaedic Sports Medicine: Principles and Practice. Philadelphia, WB Saunders, 1994, p 1168.)

TABLE 4-3 LIGAMENT BIOMECHANICS

Ligament	Restraint
ACL	Anterior translation of the tibia relative to the femur (85%)
PCL	Posterior tibial displacement (95%)
MCL	Valgus angulation
LCL	Varus angulation
MCL and LCL	Act in concert with posterior structures to control axial rotation of the tibia on the femur
PCL and posterolateral corner	Act synergistically to resist posterior translation and posterolateral rotary instability

ACL, anterior cruciate ligament; LCL, lateral collateral ligament; MCL, medial collateral ligament; PCL, posterior cruciate ligament.

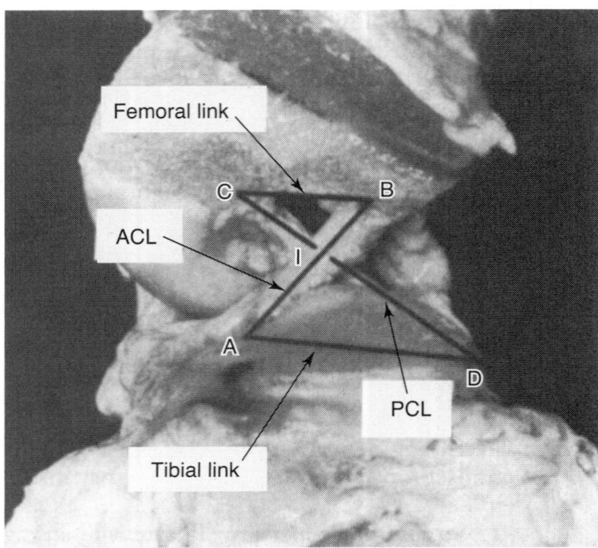

FIGURE 4–5 The four-bar linkage system consists of the anterior cruciate ligament (ACL) (AB), the posterior cruciate ligament (PCL) (CD), the femoral link (CB), and the tibial link (AD). I represents the intersection of the cruciate ligaments. (From O'Connor J, Shercliff T, Fitzpatrick D, et al: Geometry of the knee. In Daniels DM, Akeson WH, O'Connor JJ, eds: Knee Ligaments: Structure, Function, Injury, and Repair, pp 163-199. New York, Raven Press, 1990. Reprinted with permission from the Institution of Mechanical Engineers, London.)

II. Diagnostic Techniques

A. History—A complete history and clarification of the mechanism of injury is essential. The age of the patient is important because younger patients with traumatic injuries often have meniscal or ligamentous injuries, whereas older patients are more likely to have degenerative conditions. Several key historical points should be sought (Table 4–4).

B. Physical examination—Key examination points are shown in Table 4–5 (some may be best elicited with an examination under anesthesia).

C. Instrumented knee laxity measurement—KT-1000 and KT-2000 (MED-metric, San Diego) are the most commonly accepted devices for standardized laxity measurement. ACL laxity is measured with the knee in slight flexion (20-30 degrees) with the application of a standard force (30 pounds). Values are reported as millimeters of anterior displacement, with comparisons to the opposite (normal) side. More than 3 mm difference between sides is considered to be significant. PCL laxity can also be measured with this device, although it is less accurate.

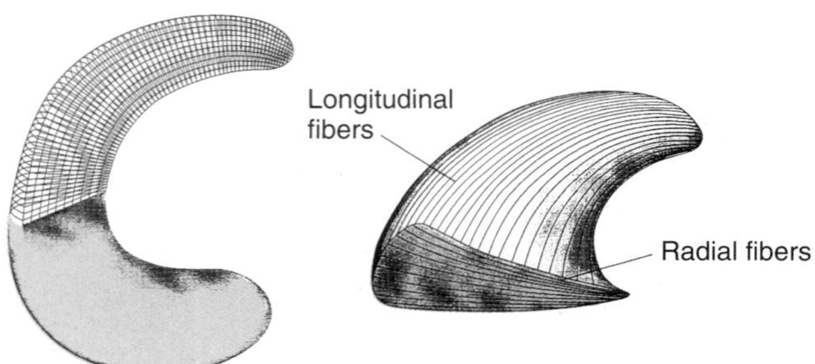

FIGURE 4–6 Longitudinal and radial fibers of the menisci. (From Tria AJ, Klein KS: An Illustrated Guide to the Knee, p 37. New York, Churchill Livingstone, 1992.)

D. Imaging the knee

1. Standard radiographs—Standard plain films include an anteroposterior (AP) view, a 45-degree posteroanterior (PA) weight-bearing view, a lateral view, and a Merchant or Laurin view of the patella. Additional views include long-cassette, lower extremity hip-to-ankle views; obliques; and stress radiographs. Several findings and their significance are listed in Table 4–6. Normal bony anatomy is demonstrated in Figure 4–7A. Many of these findings are illustrated in Figure 4–7B. Evaluation of patella height is accomplished by one of three commonly used methods (Fig. 4–7C).
2. Stress radiographs—These are useful for evaluating injuries to the femoral physis (to differentiate from MCL injury) and are becoming the gold standard in diagnosing and quantifying PCL injury.
3. Nuclear imaging—Technetium-99m bone scans are useful in diagnosing stress fractures, early degenerative joint disease (DJD), and complex regional pain syndrome (CRPS).
4. Magnetic resonance imaging (MRI)—This has become the imaging modality of choice for diagnosis of ligament injuries, meniscal pathology, avascular necrosis (AVN), spontaneous osteonecrosis of the knee (SONK), and articular cartilage defects and has replaced the use of arthrograms.
5. Magnetic resonance arthrogram—An intra-articular MR arthrogram is the most accurate imaging method for confirming the diagnosis of meniscal re-tears after repair.
6. Computed tomography (CT)—CT has been replaced largely by MRI, but it is still useful in the evaluation of bony tumors, patellar tilt, and fractures.
7. Arthrography—This technique was useful historically for the diagnosis of MCL tears and has been

TABLE 4-4 KEY HISTORICAL POINTS THAT INDICATE MECHANISM

History	Significance
Pain after sitting/climbing stairs	Patellofemoral etiology
Locking/pain with squatting	Meniscal tear
Non–contact injury with "pop"	ACL tear, patellar dislocation
Contact injury with "pop"	Collateral ligament, meniscus, fracture
Acute swelling	ACL, peripheral meniscal tear, osteochondral fracture, capsule tear
Knee "gives way"	Ligamentous laxity, patellar instability
Anterior force—**dorsiflexed foot**	Patellar injury
Anterior force—**plantar-flexed foot**	PCL injury
Dashboard injury	PCL or patellar injury
Hyperextension, varus, and tibial external rotation	Posterolateral corner injury

ACL, anterior cruciate ligament; PCL, posterior cruciate ligament.

TABLE 4-5 KEY EXAMINATION POINTS

Examination/Test	Method	Significance
Standing/gait	Observe gait	Based on pathology
Deformity	Observe patient standing	Based on pathology
Effusion	Patella: ballot/milk	Ligament/meniscus injury (acute), arthritis (chronic)
Point of maximum tenderness	Palpate for tenderness	Based on location (joint line tenderness = meniscal tear)
Range of motion (ROM)	Active and passive	Block = meniscus injury (bucket handle), loose body, ACL tear impinging
Patella crepitus	With passive ROM	Patellofemoral pathology
Patella grind	Push patella with quadriceps contraction	Patellofemoral pathology
Patella apprehension	Push patella laterally at 20-30 degrees of flexion	Patella subluxation/dislocation
Q angle	ASIS-patella-tibial tubercle	Increased with patella malalignment (normal < 15 degrees)
Flexion Q angle	ASIS-patella-tibial tubercle	Increased with patella malalignment
J sign	Lateral deviation of the patella in extension	Patella instability
Patella tilt	Tilt up laterally	>15 degrees = lax, <0 degrees = tight lateral constraint
Patella glide	Like apprehension	>50 degrees = increased medial constraint laxity
Active glide	Lateral excursion with quadriceps contraction	Lateral > proximate excursion = increased functional Q-angle quadriceps
Quadriceps circumference	10 cm (VMO), 15 cm (quadriceps)	Atrophy from inactivity
Symmetrical extension	Back of knee from ground or prone heel height difference	Contracture, displaced meniscal tear, or other mechanical block
Varus/valgus stress	30 degrees	MCL/LCL laxity (grade I: opening = 1-5 mm; grade II: opening = 6-10 mm; grade III [complete]: opening > 10 mm)
Varus/valgus stress	0 degrees	MCL/LCL and PCL
Apley's	Prone-flexion compression	DJD, meniscal pathology
Lachman	Tibia forward at 30 degrees of flexion	ACL injury (most sensitive)
Finacetto	Lachman with tibia subluxing beyond posterior horns of menisci	ACL injury (severe)
Anterior drawer	Tibia forward at 90 degrees of flexion	ACL injury
Internal-rotation drawer	Foot internally rotated with drawer	Tighter (normal), looser = ACL injury
External-rotation drawer	Foot externally rotated with drawer	Loose (normal), looser = ACL/MCL injury
McMurray	Varus/valgus stress and tibial rotation while extending knee	Meniscal pathology
Pivot shift	Flexion with internal rotation and valgus	ACL injury (EUA)
Pivot jerk	Extension with internal rotation and valgus	ACL injury (EUA)
Posterior drawer	Tibia backward at 90 degrees of flexion	PCL injury
Tibia sag	Flex 90 degrees, observe	PCL
90 degrees quadriceps active test	Extend flexed knee	PCL
Asymmetrical external rotation	"Dial" feet externally at 30 and 90 degrees of flexion	Asymmetrical increased external rotation >10 to 15 degrees = posterolateral corner (PLC) injury if asymmetrical at 30 degrees only; asymmetrical at both 30 and 90 degrees = PCL + PLC
External rotation recurvatum	Pick up great toes	PCL injury
Reversed pivot	Extension with external rotation and valgus	PCL injury
Posterolateral drawer	Posterior drawer, lateral > medial	PCL injury

ACL, anterior cruciate ligament; ASIS, anterior superior iliac spine; DJD, degenerative joint disease; EUA, exam under anesthesia; LCL, lateral collateral ligament; MCL, medial collateral ligament; PCL, posterior cruciate ligament; ROM; range of motion; VMO, vastus medialis obliquus.

supplanted by MRI. However, it can be useful when MRI is not available or tolerated by the patient, and it can be combined with CT.

8. Tomography—Tomograms are preferred to CT in the evaluation of tibial plateau fractures at some medical centers.
9. Ultrasonography—This technique is useful for soft tissue lesions about the knee, including patellar tendinitis, hematomas, and extensor mechanism ruptures, in some centers.

III. Knee Arthroscopy (see Color Plates)

A. Introduction—The gold standard for diagnosis of knee pathology. The benefits of arthroscopic versus open techniques include smaller incisions, less morbidity, improved visualization, and decreased recovery time.

B. Portals—Standard portals include superomedial and superolateral outflow portals (made with the knee in extension but may not be necessary with newer pump systems) and inferomedial and inferolateral portals (made with the knee in flexion) for

TABLE 4-6 RADIOGRAPHIC FINDINGS

View/Sign	Findings	Significance
Lateral-high patellar	Patella alta	Patellofemoral pathology
Congruence angle	$\mu = -6$ degrees; SD = 11 degrees	Patellofemoral pathology
Tooth sign	Irregular anterior patella	Patellofemoral chondrosis
Varus/valgus stress view	Opening	Collateral ligament injury; Salter-Harris fracture
Lateral capsule (Segund) sign	Small tibial avulsion off lateral tibia	ACL tear
Pellegrini-Stieda lesion	Avulsion of medial femoral condyle	Chronic MCL injury
Lateral-stress view—stress to anterior tibia with knee flexed 70 degrees	Asymmetrical posterior tibial displacement	PCL injury
Weight-bearing PA flexion		Early DJD, OCD, notch evaluation
Fairbank changes	Square condyle, peak eminences, ridging, narrowing	Early DJD (postmeniscectomy)
Square lateral condyle	Thickened joint space	Discoid meniscus

ACL, anterior cruciate ligament; DJD, degenerative joint disease; MCL, medial collateral ligament; OCD, osteochondral defect; PA, posteroanterior; PCL, posterior cruciate ligament; SD, standard deviation.

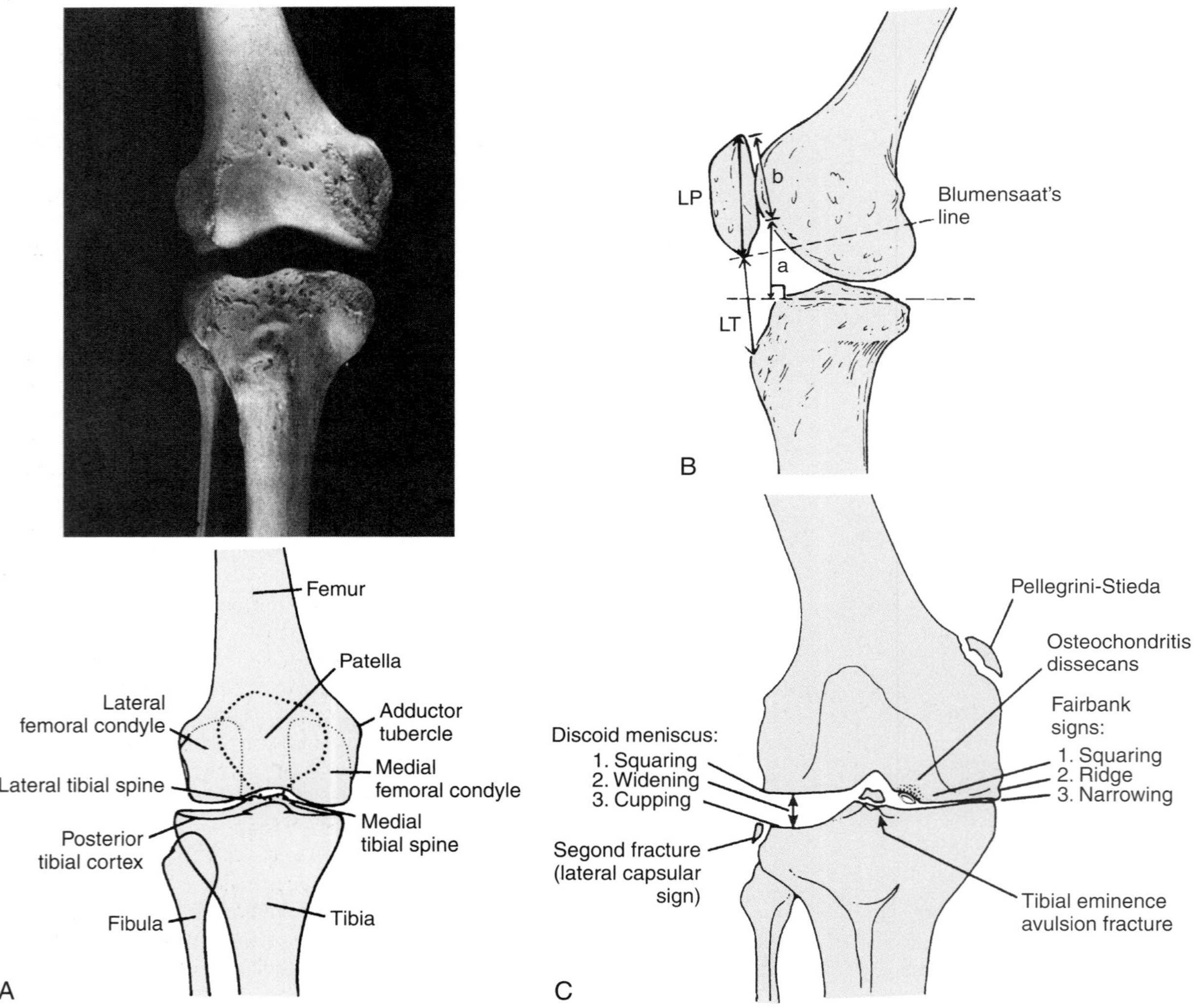

FIGURE 4–7 **A**, Anterior view and drawing demonstrating the bones of the knee. **B**, Three popular methods for evaluating patella alta and baja. (1) Blumensaat's line: With the knee flexed 30 degrees, the lower border of the patella should lie on a line extended from the intercondylar notch. (2) Insall-Salvati index: Ratio, or index, of patella tendon length (LT) to patella length (LP) should be 1.0. An index of 1.2 is alta and 0.8 is baja. (3) Blackburne-Peel index: Ratio of the distance from the tibial plateau to the inferior articular surface of the patella (a) to the length of the articular surface of the patella (b) should be 0.8. An index of 1.0 is alta. **C**, Common radiographic abnormalities. (**A** from Weissman BNW, Sledge CB: Orthopedic Radiology, p 498. Philadelphia, WB Saunders, 1986. **B** from Harner CD, Miller MD, Irrgang JJ: Management of the stiff knee after trauma and ligament reconstruction. In Siliski JM, ed: Traumatic Disorders of the Knee, p 364. New York, Springer-Verlag, 1994.)

instrument placement and the arthroscope, respectively (Fig. 4–8). Accessory portals, sometimes helpful for visualizing the posterior horns of the menisci and PCL, include the posteromedial portal (1 cm above the joint line behind the MCL [be careful to avoid saphenous nerve branches]) and the posterolateral portal (1 cm above the joint line between the LCL and biceps tendon [avoiding the common peroneal nerve]). The transpatellar portal (1 cm distal to the patella, splitting the patellar tendon fibers) can be used for central viewing or grabbing but should be avoided in patients requiring subsequent autogenous patellar tendon harvesting. Other, less commonly used portals include the medial and lateral midpatellar portals; the proximal superomedial and superolateral portals (4 cm proximal to the patella), which are used for patellofemoral compartment visualization; and the far medial and far lateral portals, which are used for accessory instrument placement (loose-body removal).

C. Technique—A systematic examination of the knee should include evaluation of the patellofemoral joint, medial and lateral gutters, medial and lateral compartments, and the intercondylar notch. The posteromedial corner can be best visualized with a 70-degree arthroscope placed through the notch (modified Gillquist's view) or a posteromedial portal. Each knee arthroscopy should include an evaluation of the suprapatellar pouch; patellofemoral joint and tracking; medial and lateral gutters; medial compartment, including the medial meniscus and the articular surface; the lateral compartment, including the lateral meniscus and the articular surface; and the intercondylar notch to visualize the ACL and PCL.

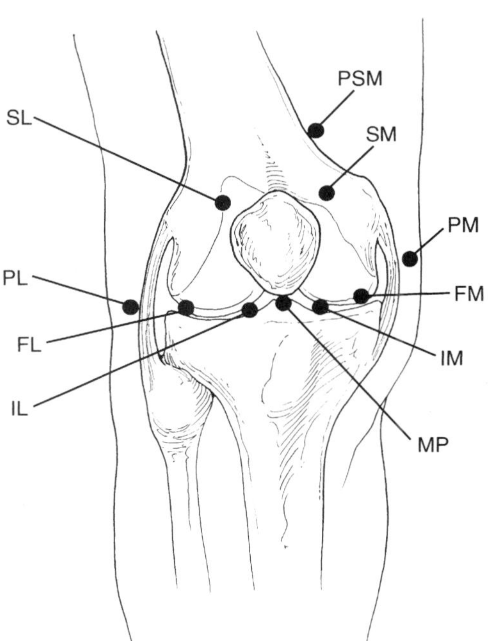

FIGURE 4–8 Arthroscopic portals. FL, far lateral; FM, far medial; IL, inferolateral; IM, inferomedial; MP, midpatellar; PL, posterolateral; PSM, proximal superomedial; SL, superolateral. (From Miller MD, Osborne JR, Warner JJP, et al: MRI-Arthroscopy Correlative Atlas, p 50. Philadelphia, WB Saunders, 1997.)

D. Arthroscopic complications—The most common arthroscopic complication is iatrogenic articular cartilage damage. Additional complications include instrument breakage, hemarthrosis, infection, and neurovascular injury.

IV. Meniscal Injuries

A. Meniscal tears

1. Overview—Meniscal tears are the most common injury to the knee that requires surgery. The medial meniscus is torn approximately three times more often than the lateral meniscus. Traumatic meniscal tears are common in young patients with sports-related injuries. Degenerative tears usually occur in older patients and can have an insidious onset. Meniscal tears can be classified based on their location in relation to the vascular supply (and healing potential), their position (anterior, middle, or posterior third), and their appearance and orientation (Fig. 4–9).
2. Treatment—In the absence of intermittent swelling, catching, locking, or giving way, meniscal tears, particularly those degenerative in nature, may be treated conservatively. Younger patients with acute tears, tears causing mechanical symptoms, and those that fail to improve with conservative measures may benefit from operative treatment.
   a. Partial meniscectomy—Tears that are not amenable to repair (i.e., peripheral, longitudinal tears), excluding those that do not require any treatment (i.e., partial-thickness tears, those >5 mm in length, and those that cannot be displaced >1-2 mm), are best treated by partial meniscectomy. In general, complex, degenerative, and central/radial tears are treated with resection of a minimal amount of normal meniscus. A motorized shaver is helpful for creating a smooth transition zone (Fig. 4–10). The role of lasers or other devices for this purpose is still under investigation. There is some concern about possible iatrogenic chondral injury caused by lasers and other thermal devices.
   b. Meniscal repair—Should be done for all peripheral longitudinal tears, especially in young patients and in conjunction with an ACL reconstruction. Augmentation techniques (fibrin clot, vascular access channels, synovial rasping) may extend the indications for repair. Four techniques are commonly used: open, "outside-in," "inside-out," and "all-inside" (Fig. 4–11). Newer techniques for all-inside repairs (arrows, darts, staples, screws, etc.) are popular because of their ease of use; however, they are probably not as reliable as vertical mattress sutures. The latest generation of "all-inside" devices

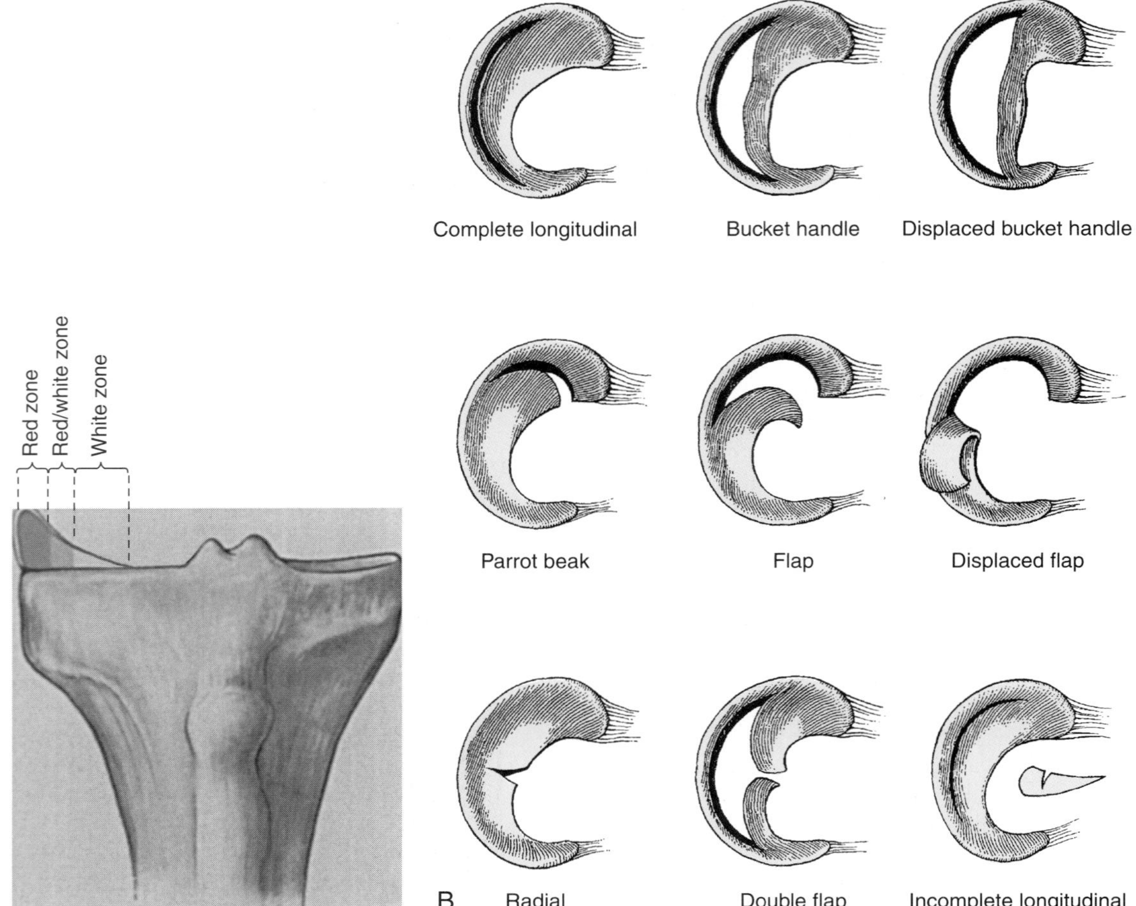

FIGURE 4–9 Classification of meniscal tears. **A**, Vascular zones. The red zone has the highest potential for meniscal healing, and the white zone has essentially no potential for healing without enhancement. **B**, Common meniscal tear appearance and orientation. (**A** modified from Miller MD, Warner JJP, Harner CD: Meniscal repair. In Fu FH, Harner CD, Vince KG, eds: Knee Surgery, p 616. Baltimore, Williams & Wilkins, 1994. **B** from Tria AJ, Klein KS: An Illustrated Guide to the Knee. New York, Churchill Livingstone, 1992.)

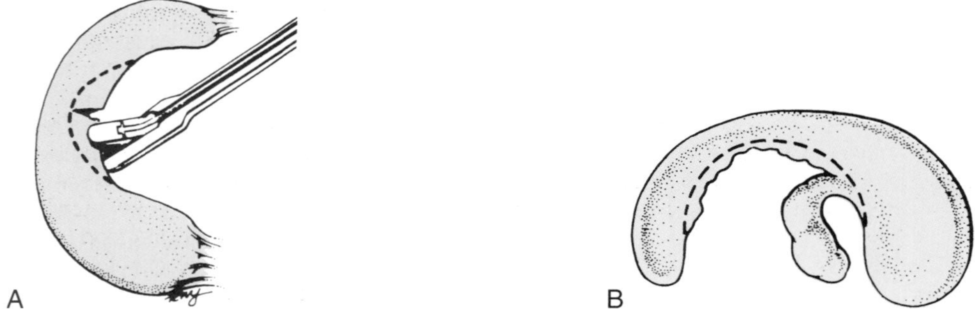

FIGURE 4–10 Outlines of partial meniscectomies necessary for a radial tear (**A**) and a degenerative flap tear (**B**). (From Ciccotti MG, Shields CL, El Attrache N: Meniscectomy. In Fu FH, Harner CD, Vince KG, eds: Knee Surgery. Baltimore, Williams & Wilkins, 1994.)

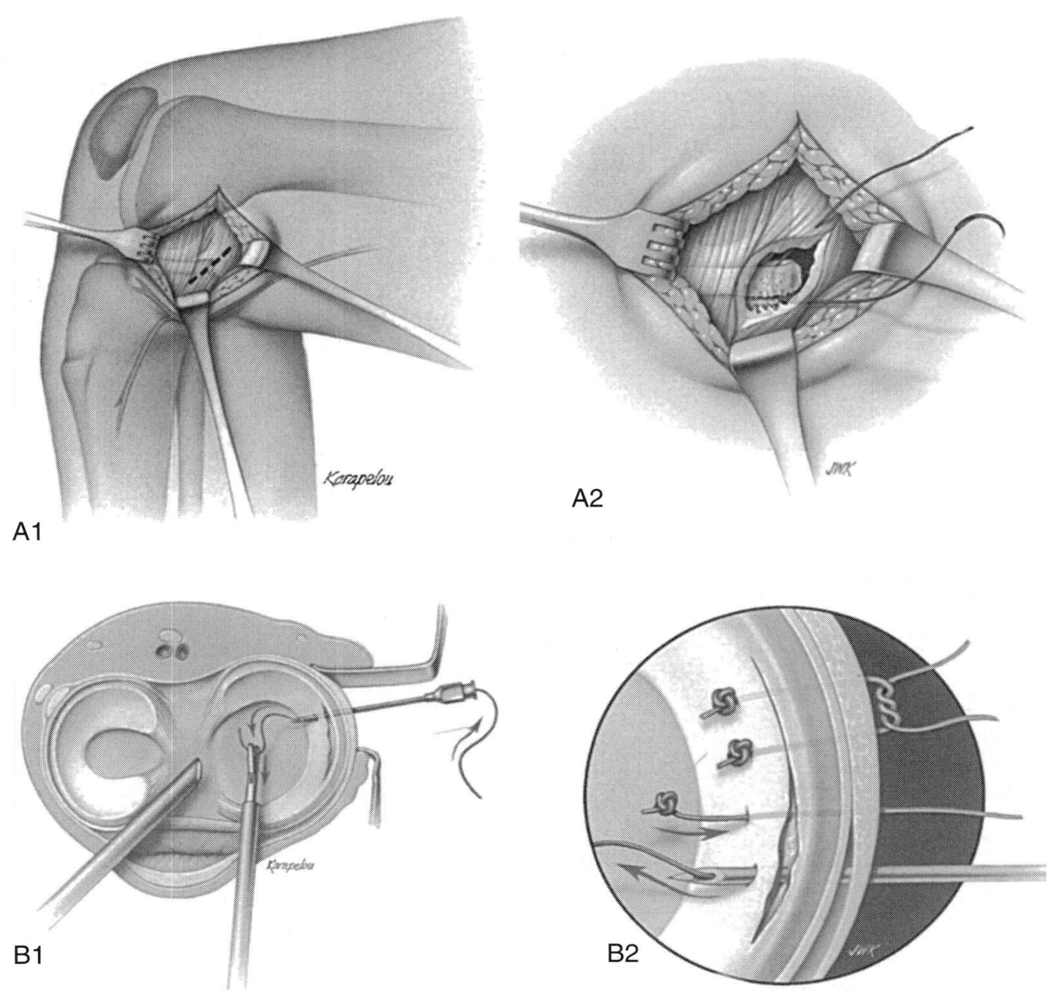

FIGURE 4–11 Meniscal repair techniques. **A**, Open repair of the medial meniscus (right knee). **B**, "Outside-in" repair of the medial meniscus (right knee).

Continued

allows tensioning of the construct. Nevertheless, the gold standard for meniscal repair remains the inside-out technique with vertical mattress sutures. Regardless of the technique used, it is essential to protect the saphenous nerve branches during medial repairs and the peroneal nerve during lateral repairs (Fig. 4–12).

c. Results of meniscal repair—Several studies report 80–90% success rates with meniscal repairs. However, this depends upon location, type of tear, and chronicity. It is generally accepted that the results of meniscal repair are best with acute peripheral tears in young patients with concurrent ACL reconstruction. Generally, a 90% success rate can be achieved with meniscal repair performed in conjunction with an ACL reconstruction, 60% success with a repair in which there is an intact ACL, and 30% with a repair in which there is an ACL-deficient knee.

B. Meniscal cysts—Occur primarily in conjunction with horizontal cleavage tears of the lateral meniscus (Fig. 4–13). Operative treatment consisting of arthroscopic partial meniscectomy and decompression through the tear (sometimes including "needling" of the cyst) has been shown to be effective. En bloc excision is no longer favored for most meniscal cysts. Popliteal (Baker's) cysts are commonly related to meniscal disorders and usually resolve with treatment of the primary disorder. They are usually located between the semimembranosus and medial head of the gastrocnemius.

C. Discoid menisci ("popping knee syndrome")—Can be classified as (1) incomplete, (2) complete, or (3) Wrisberg's variant (Fig. 4–14). Patients may develop mechanical symptoms, or "popping," with the knee in extension. Plain radiographs may demonstrate a widened joint space, squaring of the lateral femoral condyle, cupping of the lateral tibial plateau, and a hypoplastic lateral intercondylar spine. MRI (three consecutive sagittal images demonstrating a contiguous lateral meniscus) can be helpful and may also demonstrate associated tears. Treatment includes partial meniscectomy (saucerization) for tears, meniscal repair for peripheral detachments (Wrisberg's

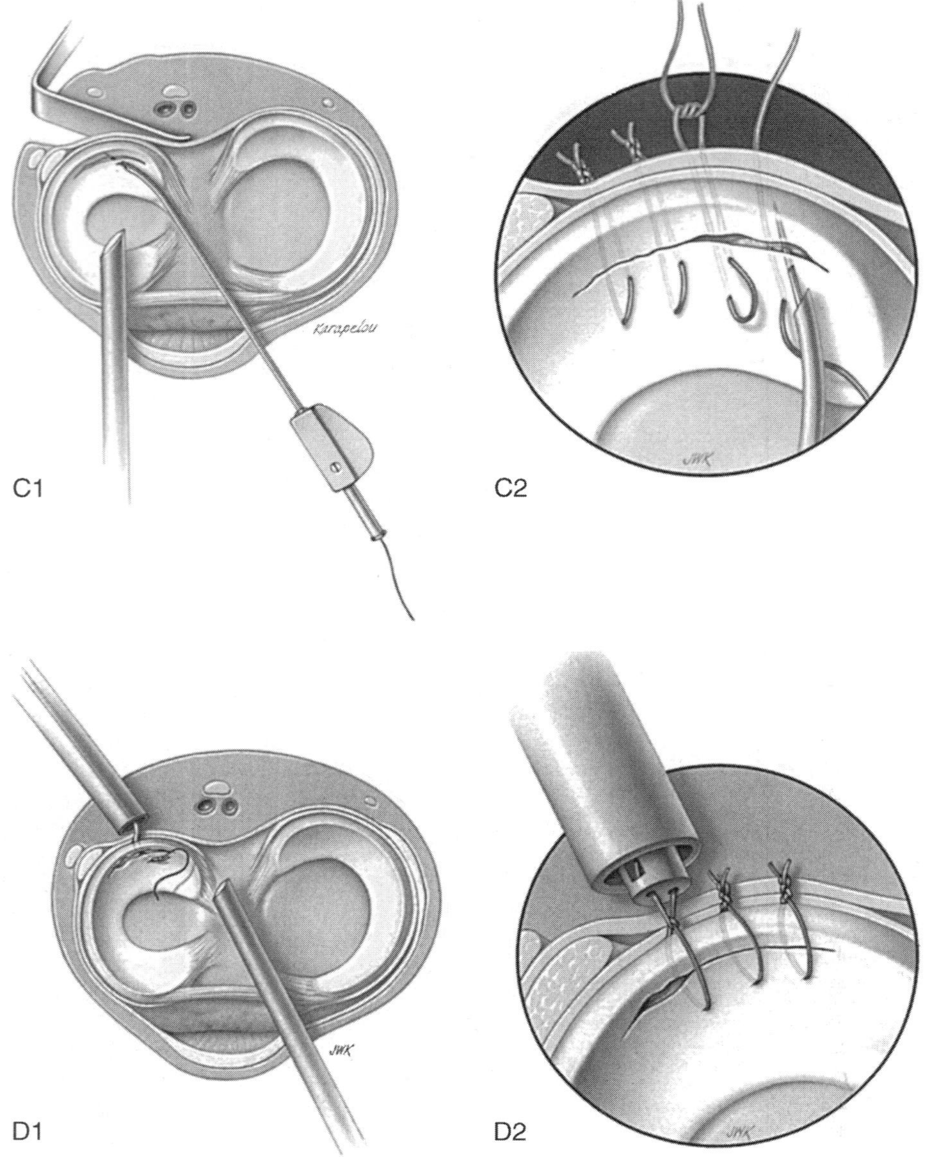

FIGURE 4–11, cont'd **C**, "Inside-out" repair of the lateral meniscus (right knee). **D**, "All-inside" repair of the lateral meniscus (right knee). (From Miller MD: Atlas of meniscal repair. Op Tech Orthop 5:70-71, 1995.)

FIGURE 4–12 Incisions for meniscal repair must be planned to allow for retraction and protection of the saphenous nerve branches during medial meniscal repairs (**A**) and the peroneal nerve during lateral meniscal repairs (**B**). MCL, medial cruciate ligament; ITT, iliotibial tract. (From Scott WN, ed: Arthroscopy of the Knee: Diagnosis and Treatment. Philadelphia, WB Saunders, 1990.)

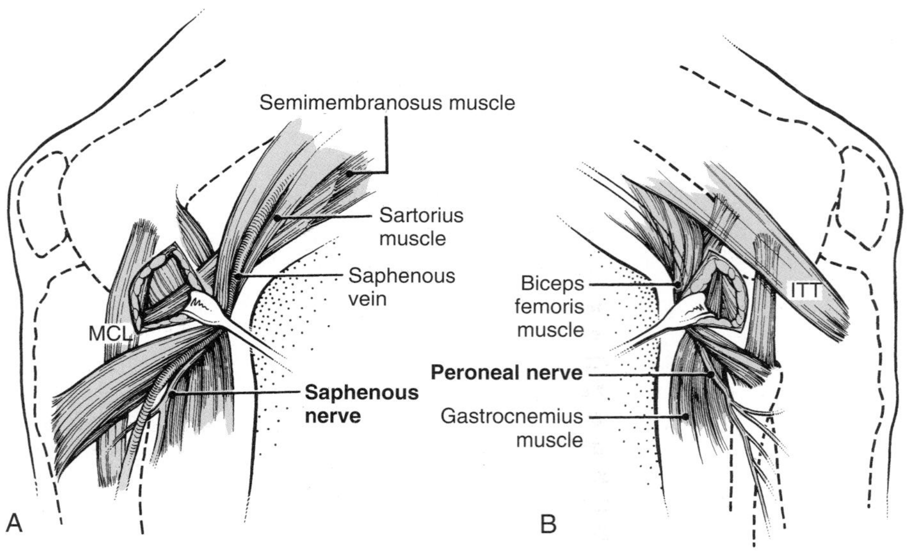

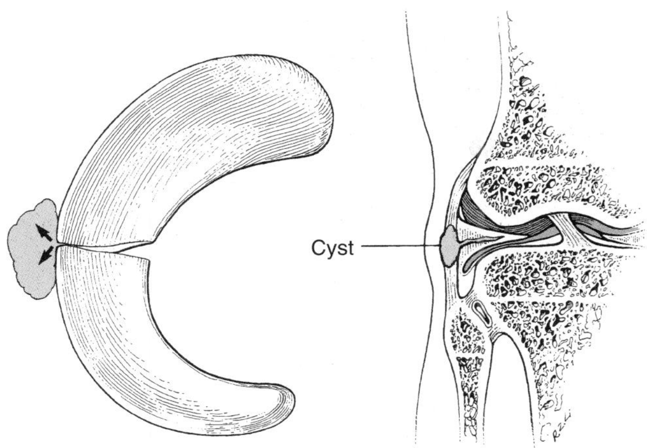

FIGURE 4–13 Meniscal cysts usually involve the lateral meniscus. (From Tria AJ, Klein KS: An Illustrated Guide to the Knee, p 101. New York, Churchill Livingstone, 1992.)

variant), and simple observation for discoid menisci without tears.

D. Meniscal transplantation—Remains controversial but may be indicated for young patients who have had near-total meniscectomy (especially lateral meniscectomy) and who have early symptomatic chondrosis. Relative contraindications include diffuse grades III-IV chondral lesions, kissing lesions (chondral lesions adjacent to each other on the femur and tibia), advanced patient age, and joint space narrowing. ACL deficiency as well as limb alignment needs to be addressed to increase the success rates of meniscal transplants. Pain relief is the most consistent benefit, with most studies having short- to mid-term (5-year) data available. Three-phase bone scans can be used diagnostically in patients who fit inclusion criteria to help determine if they are good surgical candidates. Allograft tissue needs to be appropriately sized and is typically harvested under a sterile technique, appropriately screened, and frozen. Techniques for implantation include the use of individual bone plugs for the anterior and posterior horns and the use of a bone bridge, especially laterally.

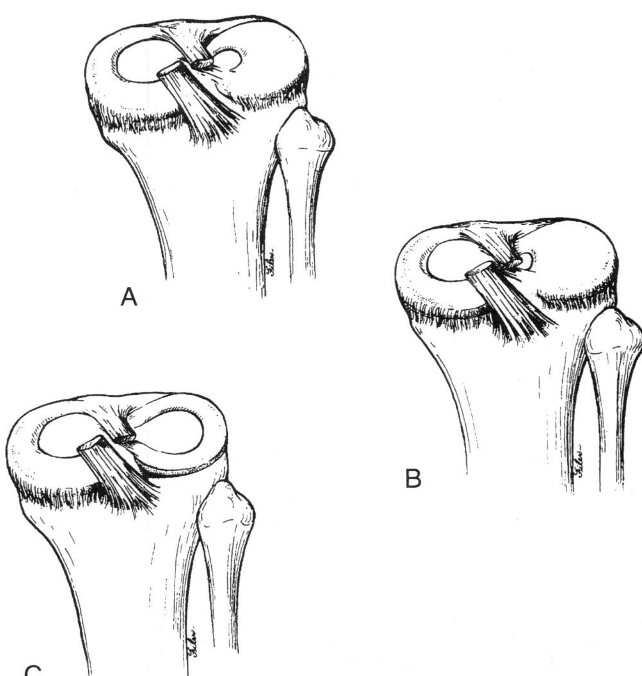

FIGURE 4–14 Classification of lateral discoid menisci. **A**, Incomplete. **B**, Complete. **C**, Variant of Wrisberg's ligament. (From Neuschwander DC: Discoid lateral meniscus. In Fu FH, Harner CD, Vince KG, eds: Knee Surgery, p 394. Baltimore, Williams & Wilkins, 1994.)

V. Ligament Injuries

A. ACL injury

1. Introduction—Controversy continues regarding the development of late arthritis in ACL-deficient versus reconstructed knees. Nevertheless, chronic ACL deficiency is associated with a higher incidence of complex meniscal tears not amenable to repair and chondral injury. It has been shown in several studies that there is a higher incidence of arthritis associated with the use of BPTB autograft than hamstring autograft at 5 to 7 years after ACL reconstruction. Bone bruises (trabecular microfractures) occur in more than half of acute ACL injuries and are typically located near the sulcus terminalis on the lateral femoral condyle and the posterolateral aspect of the tibia. Although the long-term significance of these injuries is unknown, they may be related to late cartilage degeneration. Treatment decisions should be individualized based on age, activity level, instability, associated injuries, and other factors (Fig. 4–15). The ACL injury rate is higher in female than male individuals and is thought to be due to smaller notches, smaller ligaments, and different landing biomechanics in this group. The in situ force of the ACL is highest at 30 degrees of flexion in response to anterior tibial load.
2. History and physical examination—ACL injuries are often the result of noncontact pivoting injuries and are commonly associated with an audible "pop" with an immediate hemarthrosis. Associated injuries, including meniscal tears (75%), are common. Lateral meniscal tears are more common than medial tears acutely, while medial tears occur more often in the chronic ACL-deficient knee. The Lachman test is the most sensitive examination for acute ACL injuries. The pivot shift or jerk is helpful in evaluating an ACL-deficient knee, especially with an examination under anesthesia. The KT-1000 and KT-2000 are useful in quantifying laxity. Plain radiographs are essential in evaluating ACL injuries, and MRI has become a useful tool to confirm the diagnosis.
3. Treatment—Intra-articular reconstruction is currently favored for patients who meet the criteria indicated in Figure 4–14. Graft selection depends on patient factors and surgeon preference and

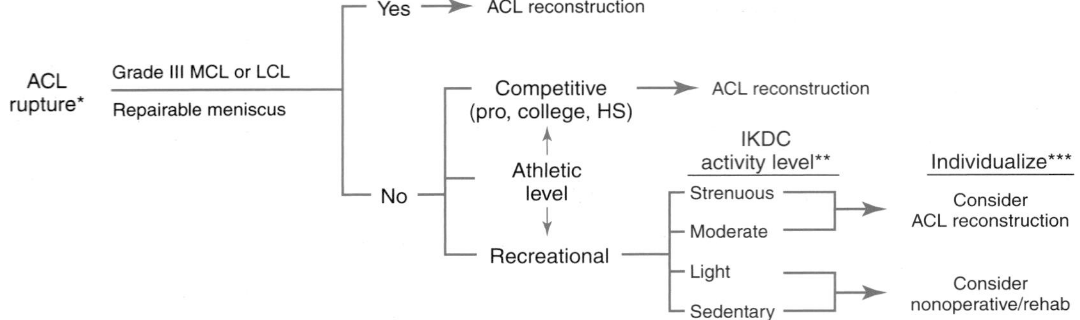

FIGURE 4–15 Algorithm for the treatment of ruptures of the anterior cruciate ligament. *Midsubstance tears. **Strenuous: jumping/pivoting sports; moderate: heavy manual work, skiing; light: manual work, running; and sedentary: activities of daily living. ***Individualize based on age, arthritis, occupation, activity modification, and/or other medical conditions. ACL, anterior cruciate ligament; IKDC, International Knee Documentation Committee; LCL, lateral collateral ligament; MCL, medial collateral ligament. (From Spindler KP, Walker RN: General approach to ligament surgery. In Fu FH, Harner CD, Vince KG, eds: Knee Surgery, p 652. Baltimore, Williams & Wilkins, 1994.)

usually includes (1) a bone-patella, tendon-bone autograft; (2) a four-strand hamstring autograft, (3) a quadriceps tendon autograft, and (4) an allograft. Primary repair of ACL tears is not currently recommended. Myofibroblasts "coat" the end of the ACL stumps, making primary healing impossible. Significant controversy exists regarding the double-bundle ACL reconstruction.

4. Partial ACL tears—The existence and treatment of "partial" ACL tears are controversial, although clinical examination and functional stability remain the most important factors for determining the need for reconstruction. One-bundle tears can occur and may be addressed with reconstruction of the injured bundle and preservation of the intact bundle.
5. Postoperative rehabilitation—Rehabilitation has evolved, and early motion (emphasis on extension) and weight bearing are encouraged in most protocols. Closed-chain rehabilitation has been emphasized because it allows physiologic co-contraction of the musculature around the knee. No difference has been found between accelerated and nonaccelerated rehabilitation programs. Postoperative bracing has not been proven to be beneficial after ACL reconstruction except in downhill skiers.
6. Complications—Complications in ACL surgery are usually a result of aberrant tunnel placement (often the femoral tunnel is placed too far anteriorly, limiting flexion) and early surgery (resulting in knee stiffness). Arthrofibrosis, which can occur often with acute ACL reconstruction, and aberrant hardware placement (interference screw divergence of >30 degrees [for endoscopic femoral tunnels] and >15 degrees [for tibial tunnels]) can also result in complications.

B. PCL injury

1. History—Injuries occur most commonly as a result of a direct blow to the anterior tibia with the knee flexed (the "dashboard injury"), hyperflexion, or hyperextension. A fall onto the ground with a plantar-flexed foot is also a mechanism of injury for PCL tears.
2. Physical examination and classification—The key examination is the posterior drawer test with an absent or posteriorly directed tibial "step-off." In grade I there is an isolated PCL injury in which the tibia remains anterior to the femoral condyles. In grade II there is usually an isolated, complete injury in which the anterior an tibia becomes flush with the femoral condyles. In grade III the tibia is posterior to the femoral condyles.
3. Treatment
   a. Nonoperative treatment is favored for most isolated grades I and II PCL injuries.
   b. Grade III injuries indicate a combined injury, usually to the posterolateral corner.
   c. Bony avulsion fractures can be repaired primarily with good results, although primary repair of midsubstance PCL (and ACL) injuries has not been successful.
   d. Chronic PCL deficiency can result in late chondrosis of the patellofemoral compartment and/or medial femoral condyle.
   e. PCL reconstruction is recommended for functionally unstable or combined injuries (Fig. 4–16). Generally, the results of PCL reconstruction are not as good as those of ACL reconstruction, and there is often some residual posterior laxity. For a successful reconstruction, concomitant ligament injuries must be addressed. There are many published techniques for PCL reconstruction, and they can generally be divided into tibial inlay versus transtibial, and single-bundle versus double-bundle. There are biomechanical advantages to the tibial inlay, such as a decrease in the "killer turn" and decreased attenuation of the graft. Double-bundle techniques may improve biomechanical function in both extension and flexion, but a clinical advantage to those techniques has not yet been shown. The anterolateral bundle is the most

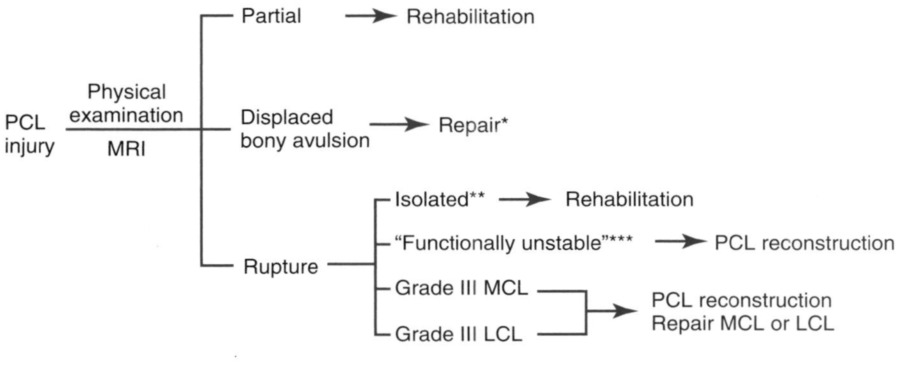

FIGURE 4–16 Algorithm for treatment of injuries to the posterior cruciate ligament. *With an intact ligament. **Without posterolateral injury or combined ligamentous injury. ***Failed rehabilitation or unstable/symptomatic in activities of daily living. LCL, lateral collateral ligament; MCL, medial collateral ligament; PCL, posterior cruciate ligament. (From Spindler KP, Walker RN: General approach to ligament surgery. In Fu FH, Harner CD, Vince KG, eds: Knee Surgery, p 655. Baltimore, Williams & Wilkins, 1994.)

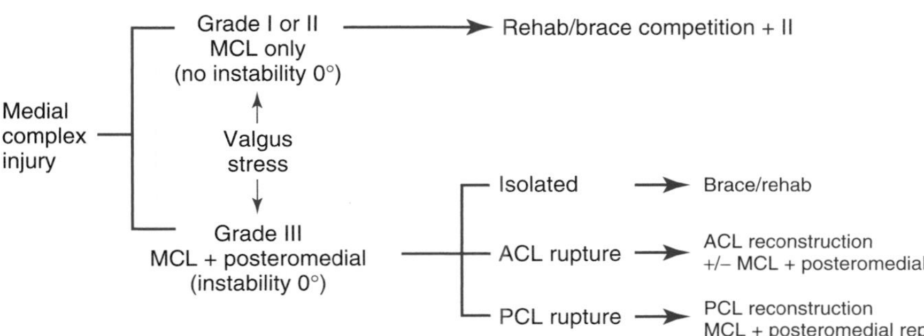

FIGURE 4–17 Algorithm for treatment of injuries to the medial collateral ligament (MCL). ACL, anterior cruciate ligament; PCL, posterior cruciate ligament. (From Spindler KP, Walker RN: General approach to ligament surgery. In Fu FH, Harner CD, Vince KG, eds: Knee Surgery. Baltimore, Williams & Wilkins, 1994.)

important for posterior stability at 90 degrees of flexion and should be tensioned in flexion, while the posteromedial bundle has a reciprocal function and should be tensioned in extension.

C. Collateral ligament injury

1. MCL injury

a. History and physical examination—Occurs as a result of valgus stress to the knee. Pain and instability with valgus stress testing at 30 degrees of flexion (and not in full extension) is diagnostic. Opening in full extension usually signifies other concurrent injuries (ACL and PCL). Injuries most commonly occur at the femoral insertion of the ligament.

b. Treatment—Nonoperative treatment (hinged knee brace) is highly successful for isolated MCL injuries. Prophylactic bracing may be helpful for football players, especially interior linemen. Advancement and reinforcement of the ligament are rarely necessary for chronic injuries that do not respond to conservative treatment (Fig. 4–17). Chronic injuries may have calcification at the medial femoral condyle insertion (Pellegrini-Stieda sign). Pellegrini-Stieda syndrome, which can occur with chronic MCL injury, usually responds to a brief period of immobilization followed by progressive motion.

2. LCL injury—Varus instability in 30 degrees of flexion is diagnostic only for an isolated LCL ligament injury. Isolated injuries to the LCL ligament are uncommon and should be managed nonoperatively if laxity is mild (Fig. 4–18).

D. Posterolateral corner injury

1. History—These injuries are rarely isolated but are usually associated with other ligamentous injuries (especially the PCL). Because of poor results with chronic reconstructions, acute repair combined with reconstruction is advocated. Examination for

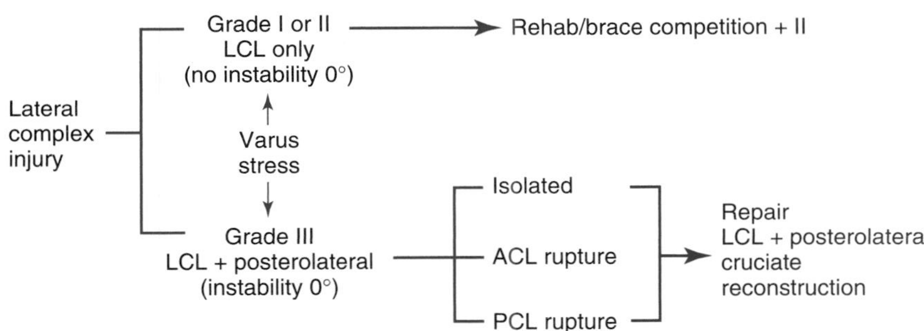

FIGURE 4–18 Algorithm for treatment of injuries to the lateral collateral ligament (LCL). ACL, anterior cruciate ligament; PCL, posterior cruciate ligament. (From Spindler KP, Walker RN: General approach to ligament surgery. In Fu FH, Harner CD, Vince KG, eds: Knee Surgery. Baltimore, Williams & Wilkins, 1994.)

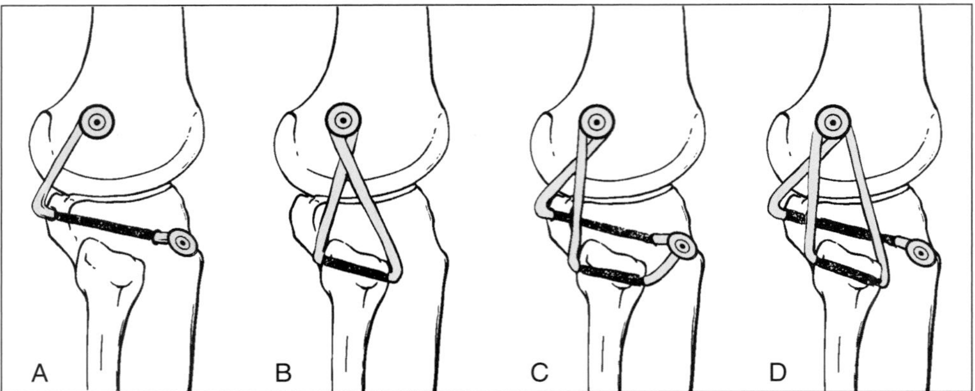

FIGURE 4–19 Techniques for posterolateral corner reconstruction. **A**, Popliteal bypass (Muller). **B**, Figure eight (Larsen). **C**, Two-tailed (Warren). **D**, Three-tailed (Warren/Miller). (From Miller MD, Cooper DE, Warner JJP: Review of Sports Medicine and Arthroscopy, 2nd ed. Philadelphia, WB Saunders, 2002.)

increased external rotation, the external rotation recurvatum test, the posterolateral drawer test, and the reverse pivot shift test are important.

2. Treatment—Early anatomic repair is often successful, but these injuries are frequently missed. Procedures recommended for chronic injuries include posterolateral corner advancement (only if structures are attenuated but intact); popliteal bypass (not currently favored); two- and three-tailed reconstruction; biceps tenodesis; and (more recently) "split" grafts and anatomic reconstructions, which are used to reconstruct both the LCL and the popliteal/posterolateral corner (Figs. 4–19 and 4–20).

E. Multiple-ligament injury

1. History and physical examination—Combined ligamentous injuries (especially ACL-PCL injuries) can be a result of a knee dislocation, and neurovascular injury must be suspected (Table 4–7). The incidence of vascular injury after anterior knee dislocation is 30-50%. Liberal use of vascular studies is recommended early (Fig. 4–21). In one study, serial examinations including ankle-brachial index (ABI) >90% over 48 hours were used to determine whether an arteriogram was necessary. The authors noted success with this technique and noted that a four-ligament injury was associated with a higher rate of vascular injury. Dislocations are classified based on the direction of tibial displacement (Fig. 4–22).

2. Treatment—Treatment is usually operative. Emergent surgical indications include popliteal artery injury, compartment syndrome, open dislocations, and irreducible dislocations. Most surgeons recommend delaying surgery 1-2 weeks to ensure that there is no vascular injury. The use of the arthroscope, especially with a pump, must be limited during these procedures because of the risk of fluid extravasation. Avulsion injuries can be repaired primarily; however, interstitial injuries must be reconstructed. Early motion is critical to avoid a stiff knee after these combined procedures, which has a high incidence.

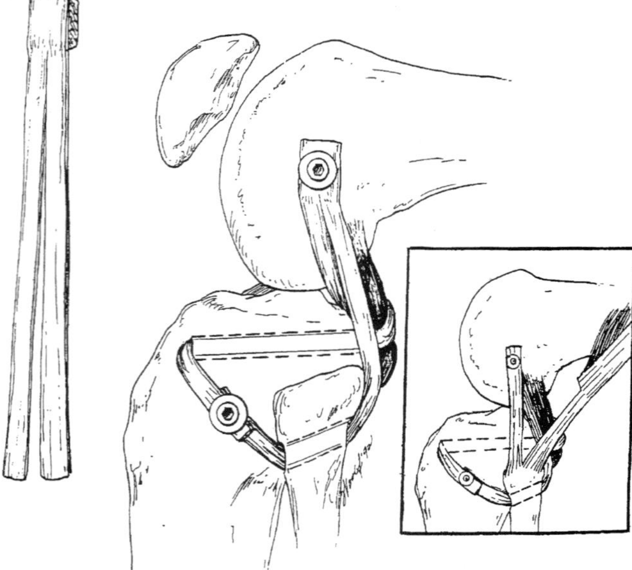

FIGURE 4–20 Split posterolateral corner graft. (From McKernan DJ, Paulos LE: Graft selection. In Fu FH, Harner CD, Vince KG, eds: Knee Surgery, p 669. Baltimore, Williams & Wilkins, 1994.)

VI. Osteochondral Lesions

A. Osteochondritis dissecans (OCD)

1. Introduction—Involves subchondral bone and overlying cartilage separation, most likely as a result of occult trauma. The lesion most often involves the lateral aspect of the medial femoral condyle. The lateral femoral condyle is involved in 15-20% of cases, and OCD is rarely seen in the patella. Spontaneous resolution is seen in the majority of the juvenile cases, in about 50% in the adolescent group, and rarely in the adult.

TABLE 4-7 SCHENCK CLASSIFICATION OF KNEE DISLOCATIONS*

Classification	Ligaments Affected
KDI	ACL + MCL or LCL
KDII	ACL + PCL
KDIII	ACL + PCL + one collateral ligament
KDIIIM	MCL
KDIIIL	LCL
KDIV	ACL + PCL + MCL + LCL

ACL, anterior cruciate ligament; KD, knee dislocation(s); LCL, lateral collateral ligament; MCL, medial collateral ligament; PCL, posterior cruciate ligament.

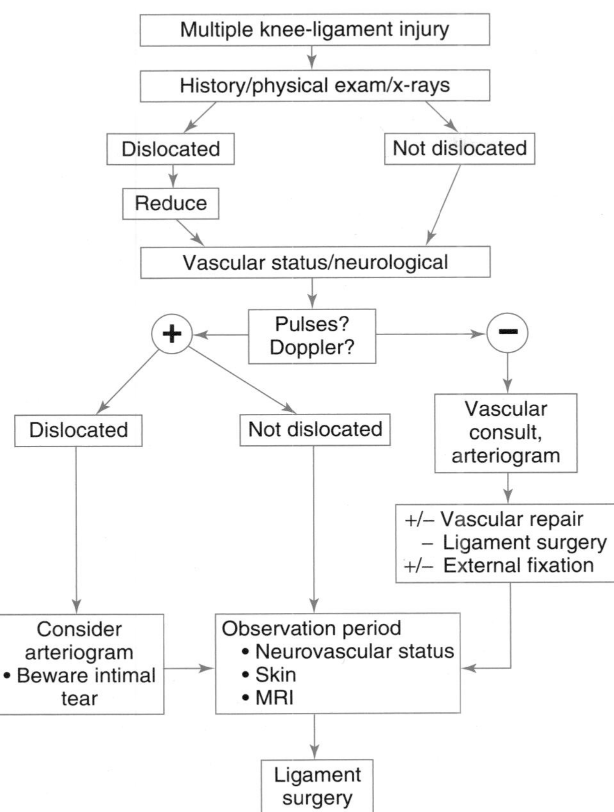

FIGURE 4–21 Algorithm for treatment of injuries to multiple knee ligaments. (From Marks PH, Harner CD: The anterior cruciate ligament in the multiple ligament-injured knee. Clin Sports Med 12:825-838, 1993.)

2. Diagnosis—Patients usually have poorly localized, vague complaints. Radiographs, nuclear imaging, and MRI can be helpful in determining the size, location, and characteristics of the lesion.
3. Treatment and prognosis—Children with open growth plates have the best prognosis, and often these lesions can be simply observed. In situ lesions can be treated with retrograde drilling. Detached lesions may require abrasion chondroplasty or newer, more aggressive techniques. OCD in adults is usually symptomatic and leads to arthritis if left untreated.

B. Articular cartilage injury
1. Overview—The distinction between articular cartilage injury and OCD is not often clear, but articular cartilage injury occurs as a result of rotational forces in direct trauma. It usually occurs on the medial femoral condyle. The lesions are classified according to their arthroscopic appearance.
2. Treatment—Débridement and chondroplasty are currently recommended for symptomatic lesions. Displaced osteochondral fragments can sometimes be replaced and secured with small, recessed screws or absorbable pins. Several treatment options for discrete, isolated, full-thickness cartilage injuries are in clinical use. These include microfracture, periosteal patches (chondrocyte implantation), and osteochondral transfer (plugs) (Fig. 4–23). Donor-site problems and the creation of true articular cartilage at the recipient site are still challenges. Age, lesion size, patient demand level, alignment, meniscal integrity, and ligamentous stability must all be taken into consideration when deciding on the appropriate treatment option. There is still debate regarding the best treatment options. An algorithm is presented in Figure 4–24.

C. DJD—Diffuse chondral damage is usually not considered "sports medicine," but treatment modalities include medications, nutritional supplements such as glucosamine with chondroitin sulfate, hyaluronic acid injections, arthroscopic débridement, osteotomies, and arthroplasty. These treatment modalities are addressed in detail in Chapter 5, Adult Reconstruction.

D. Osteonecrosis
1. Atraumatic osteonecrosis is similar to idiopathic osteonecrosis of the hip. Risk factors are similar to those of the hip and are common in elderly females.
2. Spontaneous osteonecrosis of the knee (SONK) is thought to represent a subchondral insufficiency fracture and is typically a self-limiting condition. SONK can follow knee arthroscopy in middle-aged females. It may be treated with limited weight bearing until it resolves.

VII. Synovial Lesions

A. Pigmented villonodular synovitis (PVNS)—Patients may present with pain and swelling and may have a palpable mass. There are nodular and diffuse types. The diffuse type has a higher recurrence rate. Synovectomy is effective, but there is a high recurrence rate. Arthroscopic techniques are as effective

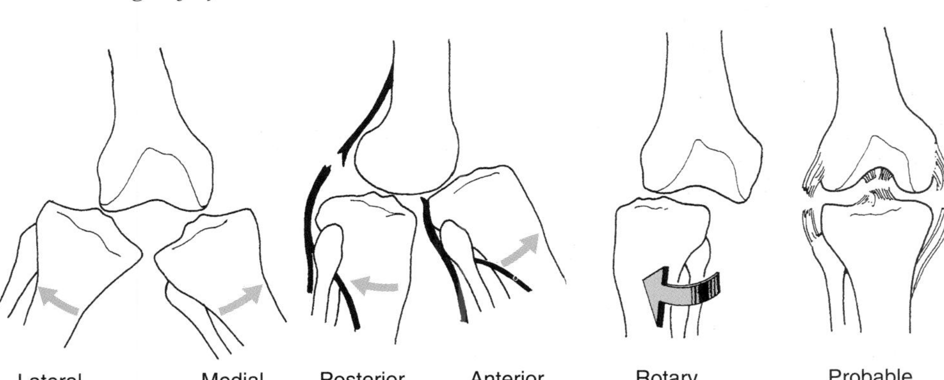

FIGURE 4–22 Classification of knee dislocations. (From Miller MD, Cooper DE, Warner JJP: Review of Sports Medicine and Arthroscopy, p 51. Philadelphia, WB Saunders, 1995.)

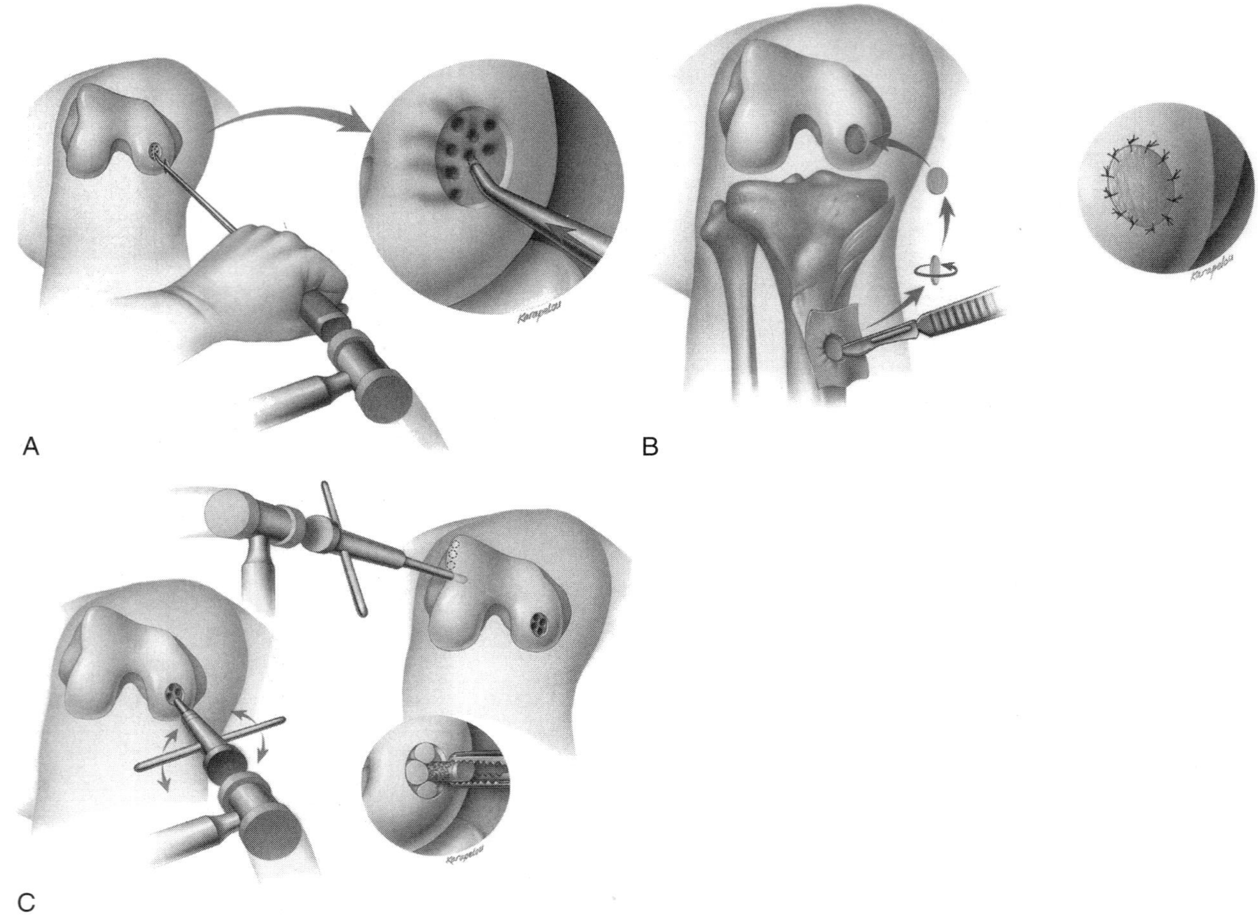

FIGURE 4–23 Treatment of chondral injuries. **A**, Microfracture. Awls, with various degrees of angulation, are introduced throughout the ipsilateral arthroscopic portal and used to penetrate the subchondral bone and encourage stem cell production of ''cartilage-like'' tissue. **B**, Periosteal graft. The periosteum is used as a ''patch.'' The inner cambium layer is rotated so that it is facing outward. The patch is carefully sewn in place, and ''cartilage'' may grow out from the undifferentiated cambium layer of the graft. **C**, Osteochondral plugs. Cylindrical ''plugs'' of exposed bone are removed from the defect. Plugs of normal, non-weight-bearing cartilage and bone are harvested and placed into the defect. (From Miller MD: Atlas of chondral injury treatment. Op Tech Orthop 7:289-294, 1997.)

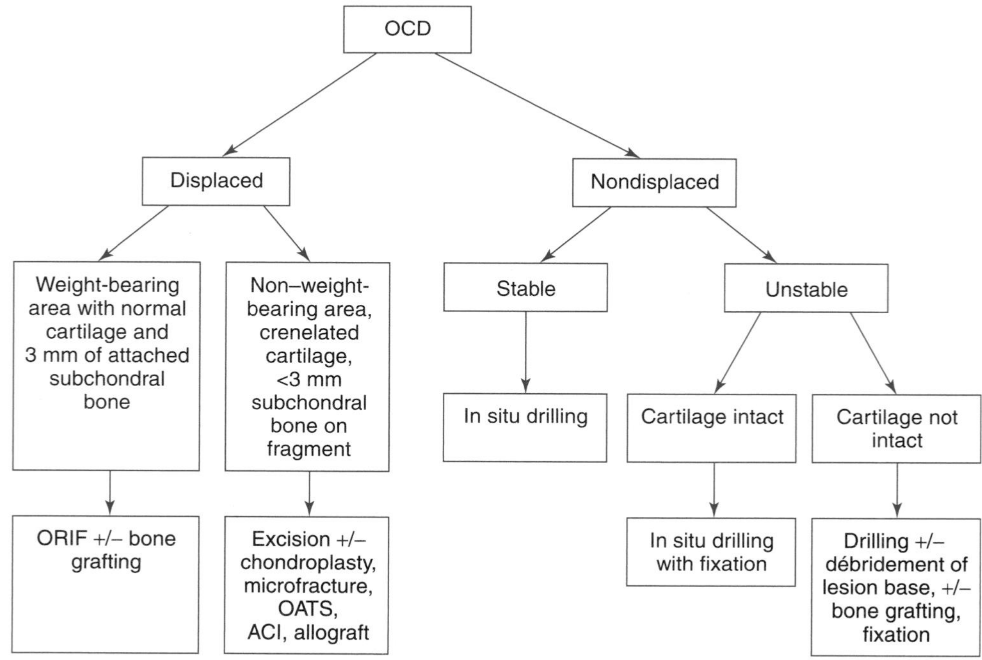

FIGURE 4–24 A treatment algorithm for stable and unstable osteochondritis dissecans lesions. ACI, autologous chondrocyte implantation; OATS, osteochondral autograft transplantation; ORIF, open reduction with internal fixation. (From Miller M, Cole B: Textbook of Arthroscopy. Philadelphia, WB Saunders, 2004.)

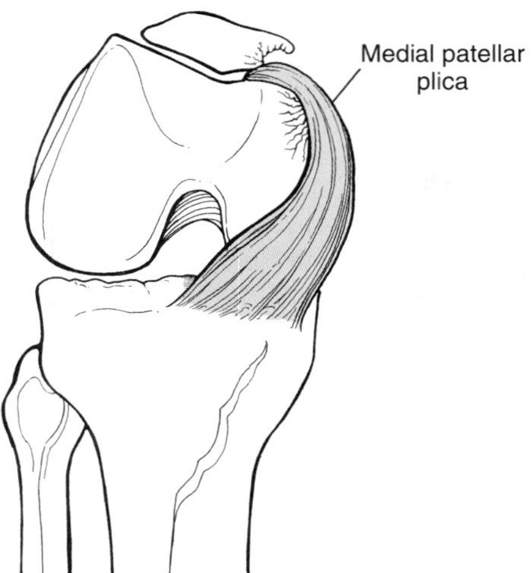

FIGURE 4–25 Medial patellar plica with associated chondromalacia of the medial femoral condyle and patella. (From Miller MD, Cooper DE, Warner JJP: Review of Sports Medicine and Arthroscopy, 2nd ed. Philadelphia, WB Saunders, 2002.)

as traditional open procedures if a complete synovectomy with multiple portals is done.

B. Synovial chondromatosis—This proliferative disease of the synovium is associated with cartilaginous metaplasia, resulting in multiple intra-articular loose bodies.

C. Other synovial lesions that respond to synovectomy include (osteo)chondromatosis, pauciarticular juvenile rheumatoid arthritis, and hemophilia. Additional arthroscopic portals are required for complete synovectomy.

D. Plicae—Synovial folds that are embryologic remnants. They are occasionally pathologic, particularly the medial patellar plica, which can cause abrasion of the medial femoral condyle and sometimes responds to arthroscopic excision (Fig. 4–25).

VIII. Patellofemoral Disorders

A. Introduction—Anterior knee pain is classified based on etiologic factors (Box 4–1). The term "chondromalacia" should be replaced with a specific diagnosis based on this classification.

B. Trauma—Includes fractures of the patella (discussed in Chapter 11, Trauma) and tendon injuries.

1. Tendon ruptures—Quadriceps tendon ruptures are more common than patellar tendon ruptures and occur most often in patients over 40 years old with indirect trauma. Patellar tendon ruptures occur in younger patients (<40 years) with direct or indirect trauma. Both types of tendon rupture are more common in patients with underlying disorders of the tendon. A palpable defect and the inability to extend the knee are diagnostic. Patella alta is consistent with patella tendon rupture. Primary repair with temporary stabilization (McLaughlin wire or suture) is indicated.

2. Repetitive trauma—Overuse injuries

a. Patellar tendinitis (jumper's knee)—This condition, perhaps better termed "tendinosis," is most common in athletes who participate in

Box 4–1 Classification of Patellofemoral Disorders

- I. Trauma (conditions caused by trauma in the otherwise normal knee)
  - A. Acute trauma
    - 1. Contusion (924.11)
    - 2. Fracture
      - a. Patella (822)
      - b. Femoral trochlea (821.2)
      - c. Proximal tibial epiphysis (tubercle) (823.0)
    - 3. Dislocation (rare in the normal knee) (836.3)
    - 4. Rupture
      - a. Quadriceps tendon (843.8)
      - b. Patellar tendon (844.8)
  - B. Repetitive trauma (overuse syndromes)
    - 1. Patellar tendinitis ("jumper's knee") (726.64)
    - 2. Quadriceps tendinitis (726.69)
    - 3. Peripatellar tendinitis (e.g., anterior knee pain of the adolescent due to hamstring contracture) (726.699)
    - 4. Prepatellar bursitis ("housemaid's knee") (726.65)
    - 5. Apophysitis
      - a. Osgood-Schlatter disease (732.43)
      - b. Sinding-Larsen-Johansson disease (732.42)
  - C. Late effects of trauma (905)
    - 1. Post-traumatic chondromalacia patellae
    - 2. Post-traumatic patellofemoral arthritis
    - 3. Anterior fat pad syndrome (post-traumatic fibrosis)
    - 4. Reflex sympathetic dystrophy of the patella
    - 5. Patellar osseous dystrophy
    - 6. Acquired patella infera (719.366)
    - 7. Acquired quadriceps fibrosis
- II. Patellofemoral dysplasia
  - A. Lateral patellar compression syndrome (LPCS) (718.365)
    - 1. Secondary chondromalacia patellae (717.7)
    - 2. Secondary patellofemoral arthritis (715.289)
  - B. Chronic subluxation of the patella (CSP) (718.364)
    - 1. Secondary chondromalacia patellae (717.7)
    - 2. Secondary patellofemoral arthritis (715.289)
  - C. Recurrent dislocation of the patella (RDP) (718.361)
    - 1. Associated fractures (822)
      - a. Osteochondral (intra-articular)
      - b. Avulsion (extra-articular)
    - 2. Secondary chondromalacia patellae (717.7)
    - 3. Secondary patellofemoral arthritis (715.289)
  - D. Chronic dislocation of the patella (718.362)
    - 1. Congenital
    - 2. Acquired
- III. Idiopathic chondromalacia patellae (717.7)
- IV. Osteochondritis dissecans
  - A. Patella (732.704)
  - B. Femoral trochlea (732.703)
- V. Synovial plicae (727.8916) (anatomic variant made symptomatic by acute or repetitive trauma)
  - A. Medial patellar ("shelf") (727.89161)
  - B. Suprapatellar (727.89163)
  - C. Lateral patellar (727.89165)

Note: Orthopaedic ICD-9-CM (International Classification of Diseases [of the World Health Organization]-9-Master in Surgery) Expanded Diagnostic Codes in parentheses.

From Merchant AC: Classification of patellofemoral disorders. Arthroscopy 4:235, 1988.

sports such as basketball and volleyball and is associated with pain and tenderness near the inferior border of the patella (worse in extension than flexion). Treatment includes nonsteroidal anti-inflammatory drugs (NSAIDs), physical therapy (strengthening and ultrasound), and orthoses (patella tendon strap). Surgery involving excision of necrotic tendon fibers is rarely indicated.

b. Quadriceps tendinitis—Less common than tendinosis but just as painful. Patients may note painful clicking and localized pain at the superior border of the patella. Operative treatment is occasionally necessary.

c. Prepatellar bursitis (housemaid's knee)— The most common form of bursitis of the knee and associated with a history of prolonged kneeling. Supportive treatment (knee pads, occasional steroid injections) and (rarely) bursal excision are recommended. Aspiration is advocated in wrestlers because of the kneeling on the flexed knee required for this sport.

d. Iliotibial band friction syndrome—Can occur in runners (especially those running hills) and cyclists and is a result of abrasion between the iliotibial band and the lateral femoral condyle. Localized tenderness, worse with the knee flexed 30 degrees, is common. The Ober test (patient lies in a lateral decubitus position with hyperextension of the hip; the leg can be brought from abduction to adduction to demonstrate tightness of the iliotibial band) is helpful in making the diagnosis. Rehabilitation is usually successful. Surgical excision of an ellipse of the iliotibial band is occasionally necessary.

e. Semimembranosus tendinitis—Most common in male athletes in their early thirties, this condition can be diagnosed with MRI or nuclear imaging and often responds to stretching and strengthening. A steroid injection may be added if no improvement is seen.

f. Pes anserinus bursitis—This is characterized by localized pain, tenderness, and swelling over the proximal anteromedial tibia at the insertion site of the sartorius, gracilis, and semitendinosus (approximately 6 cm inferior to the joint line). It is treated conservatively with oral anti-inflammatory medication, localized injections, and activity modification.

C. Late effects of trauma

1. Patellofemoral arthritis—Injury and malalignment can contribute to patellar DJD. Lateral release may be beneficial early only if there is objective evidence of patellar tilting; however, other procedures may be required for advanced patellar arthritis. Options include anterior (Maquet) or anteromedial (Fulkerson) transfer of the tibial tubercle or patellectomy for severe cases. Patellofemoral arthroplasty has been introduced as another treatment option but remains controversial.

2. Anterior fat pad syndrome (Hoffa's disease)—Trauma to the anterior fat pad can lead to fibrous changes and pinching of the fat pad, especially in patients with genu recurvatum. Activity modification, ice, knee padding, and injection can be helpful. Arthroscopic excision is occasionally beneficial.

3. **Complex regional pain syndrome** (CRPD) (formerly known as reflex sympathetic dystrophy)—Characterized by pain out of proportion to physical findings, this condition is an exaggerated response to injury. Three stages, progressing from swelling, warmth, and hyperhidrosis to brawny edema and trophic changes and finally to glossy, cool, dry skin and stiffness, are typical. Patellar osteopenia and a "flamingo gait" are also common. Treatment includes nerve stimulation, NSAIDs, and sympathetic or epidural blocks, which can be both diagnostic and therapeutic.

D. Patellofemoral dysplasia

1. Lateral patellar facet compression syndrome—This problem is associated with a tight lateral retinaculum and excessive lateral tilt without excessive patellar mobility. Treatment includes activity modification, NSAIDs, and VMO strengthening. Arthroscopy and lateral release are occasionally required but indicated only in the setting of objective evidence of lateral tilt that has not responded to extensive nonoperative management. The best candidates have a neutral or negative tilt with a medial patellar glide of less than one quadrant and a lateral patellar glide of less than three quadrants. Arthroscopic visualization through a superior portal demonstrates that the patella does not articulate medially with 40 degrees of knee flexion.

2. Patellar instability

a. Recurrent subluxation/dislocation of the patella can be characterized by lateral displacement of the patella, a shallow intercondylar sulcus, or patellar incongruence. When it is associated with femoral anteversion, genu valgum, and pronated feet, the symptoms can be exacerbated, especially in adolescents ("miserable malalignment syndrome"). Extensive rehabilitation is often curative. Females with previous instability are at increased risk. Several radiographic findings are somewhat helpful in diagnosing patellar malalignment (Fig. 4–26). Surgical procedures include proximal and/or distal

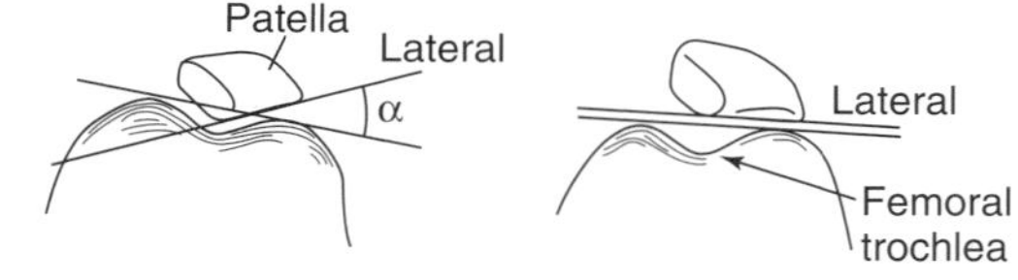

FIGURE 4–26 The measurement of the lateral patellofemoral angle. One line is drawn across the slope of the femoral condyles. A second line is drawn across the slope of the lateral patellar facet. A normal angle (shown on the left) opens laterally.

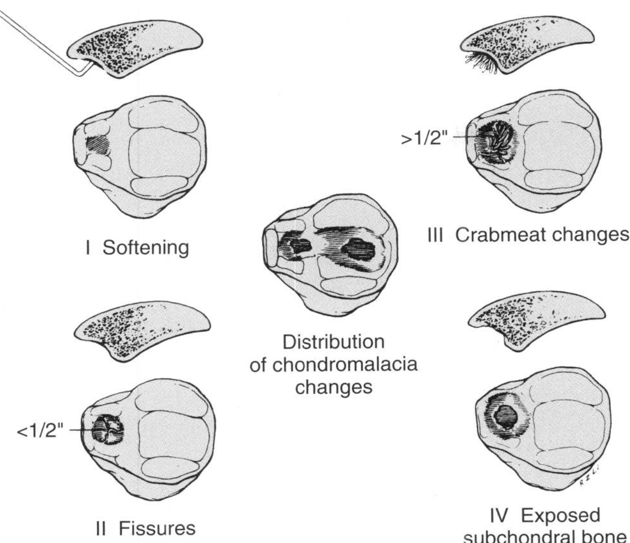

FIGURE 4–27 Outerbridge classification of chondromalacia. (From Tria AJ, Klein KS: An Illustrated Guide to the Knee. New York, Churchill Livingstone, 1992.)

realignment. Acute, first-time patella dislocations may be best treated with arthroscopic evaluation/débridement and acute repair of the medial patellofemoral ligament (usually at the medial epicondyle). This is still somewhat controversial. These patients should be evaluated with radiographs for fractures and loose bodies. If a loose body is suspected, an MRI can help make the diagnosis. The articular cartilage of the medial patellar facet is the most common donor site.

b. Abnormalities of patellar height—Patella alta (high-riding patella) and patella baja (low-riding patella) are determined based on various measurements made on lateral radiographs of the knee (see Fig. 4–7). Patella alta can be associated with patellar instability because the patella may not articulate with the sulcus, which normally constrains the patella. Patella baja is often the result of fat pad and tendon fibrosis and may require proximal transfer of the tubercle in refractory cases.

E. Idiopathic chondromalacia patellae—Although this term has fallen into disfavor, articular damage and changes to the patella are common. Treatment is usually symptomatic and has a heavy emphasis on physical therapy. Débridement procedures are of questionable benefit. The Outerbridge classification system is still in common use today (Fig. 4–27).

IX. Pediatric Knee Disorders

A. Physeal injuries—Most often involve Salter-Harris II fractures of the distal femoral physis. Pain, swelling, and an inability to ambulate are common. Stress radiographs and/or MRI may be necessary to make the diagnosis. Open reduction and internal fixation are indicated for Salter-Harris III and IV fractures and Salter-Harris I and II fractures that cannot be adequately reduced. It is important to counsel the parents that knee physeal injuries may have a worse prognosis than other physeal fractures.

B. Ligament injuries

1. Classification—Avulsion fractures of the intercondylar eminence of the tibia are described as types I through IV.
   a. Type I—<3 mm displacement
   b. Type II—Avulsion and elevation of the anterior ⅓-½
   c. Type III—Displacement of entire fragment
   d. Type IV—Comminuted
2. Treatment—Most ligament injuries are treated like those in adults.
   a. Midsubstance ACL injuries in skeletally immature individuals remain a subject of considerable debate. Procedures that do not violate the growth plate, especially on the femoral side, are usually recommended for young patients with wide, open physes. Delay in treatment is associated with medial meniscal tears. Several studies report no angular deformities or bony bridges in Tanner 2-4 children after ACL reconstruction despite the use of multiple grafts and different techniques.
   b. Types I and II avulsion fractures can usually undergo closed treatment. Types III and IV and types I and II that fail closed treatment can undergo open or arthroscopic reduction and fixation of the fragment. The lateral meniscus may become trapped beneath the bony fragment and thus prevent reduction if not addressed.

C. Traction apophysitis—This includes Osgood-Schlatter disease and Sinding-Larsen-Johansson disease. It is usually treated symptomatically, with immobilization as needed. Procedures such as ossicle excision are occasionally indicated for refractory cases (Fig. 4–28).

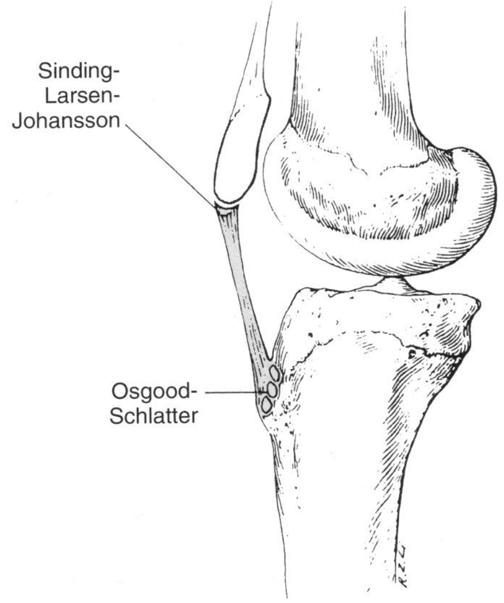

FIGURE 4–28 Two types of traction apophysitis affecting adolescent knees. (From Tria AJ, Klein KS: An Illustrated Guide to the Knee. New York, Churchill Livingstone, 1992, p 140.)

SECTION 2 Thigh, Hip, and Pelvis

I. Contusions

A. Iliac crest contusions ("hip pointer")—Direct trauma to this area can occur in contact sports. An avulsion of the iliac apophysis should be ruled out in adolescent athletes. Treatment consists of ice, compression, pain control, and placing the affected leg on maximum stretch. Corticosteroid injections have occasionally been advocated. Additional padding is indicated after the acute phase.

B. Groin contusions—An avulsion fracture of the lesser trochanter, traumatic phlebitis, thrombosis, or femoral neuropathy must be ruled out before supportive treatment is initiated.

C. Quadriceps contusions—This can result in hemorrhage and late myositis ossificans. Acute management includes cold compression and immobilization in flexion. Close monitoring for compartment syndrome is indicated in the acute phase.

II. Muscle Injuries

A. Hamstring strain—This common injury is often the result of sudden stretch on the musculotendinous junction during sprinting. These injuries can occur anywhere in the posterior thigh. Treatment is supportive, followed by stretching and strengthening. To prevent recurrence, return to play should be delayed until strength is approximately 90% that of the opposite side.

B. Athletic pubalgia/"sports hernia"—Common in sports such as soccer, these injuries must be differentiated from subtle hernias. Injury to the muscles of the abdominal wall or adductor longus produce anterior pelvis and/or groin pain without the classic physical findings of a true inguinal hernia. This injury can result from acute trauma or microtrauma associated with overuse of the affected muscle. Rule out other causes of pain with an x-ray, bone scan, and/or MRI. Treat nonoperatively for 6-8 weeks with rest and therapy. Repair or reinforcement of the anterior abdominal wall is indicated after failed conservative measures and after other causes have been excluded.

C. Rectus femoris strain—Acute injuries are usually located more distally on the thigh, but chronic injuries are usually nearer the muscle origin. Pain is elicited with resisted hip flexion or extension. Treatment includes ice and stretching/strengthening.

III. Bursitis

A. Trochanteric bursitis—Occurs frequently in female runners and is associated with training on banked surfaces. Treatment includes oral anti-inflammatory drugs, stretching, and rest. Corticosteroid injections are occasionally advocated.

B. Iliopsoas bursitis—A cause of anterior hip pain in athletes and often associated with mechanical irritation of the iliopsoas tendon.

C. Ischial bursitis—Caused by direct trauma or prolonged sitting and hard to distinguish from hamstring injuries.

IV. Nerve Entrapment Syndromes

A. Ilioinguinal nerve entrapment—This nerve can be constricted by hypertrophied abdominal muscles as a result of intensive training. Hyperextension of the hip may exacerbate the pain that patients experience, and hyperesthesia symptoms are common. Surgical release is occasionally necessary.

B. Obturator nerve entrapment—Can lead to chronic medial thigh pain, especially in athletes with well-developed hip adductor muscles (e.g., skaters). Nerve conduction studies are helpful for establishing the diagnosis. Treatment is usually supportive.

C. Lateral femoral cutaneous nerve entrapment—Can lead to a painful condition known as meralgia paresthetica. Tight belts and prolonged hip flexion may exacerbate symptoms. Release of compressive devices, postural exercises, and NSAIDs are usually curative.

D. Sciatic nerve entrapment—Can occur anywhere along the course of the nerve, but the two most common locations are at the level of the ischial tuberosity and by the piriformis muscle, known as "piriformis syndrome."

V. Bone Disorders

A. Stress fractures—A history of overuse, an insidious onset of pain, and localized tenderness and swelling are typical. A bone scan can be diagnostic, even with normal plain radiographs. MRI is the most specific test for detecting stress fractures. Treatment includes protected weight bearing, rest, cross-training, analgesics, and therapeutic modalities. There are several especially problematic stress fractures.

1. Femoral neck stress fractures—Tension (transverse) fractures are more serious than compression fractures (on the medial side of the neck) and may require operative stabilization.
2. Femoral shaft stress fractures—Usually respond to protected weight bearing but can progress to complete fractures if unrecognized. The "fulcrum" test may be helpful in making this diagnosis.
3. Pelvic stress fractures—Stress fractures to the sacrum and pubis are rare but can occur.

B. Proximal femoral fractures—Can occur in athletes, especially cross-country skiers (skier's hip). Release bindings have reduced the incidence of these injuries.

C. AVN—Traumatic hip subluxation can disrupt the arterial blood supply to the hip and result in avascular necrosis. Early recognition of these injuries, which are seen in football players, is essential. With posterior subluxation or dislocation, one study found a 25% incidence of AVN. Obtaining obturator oblique films to determine the presence of an avulsion injury and an MRI are recommended. This should be followed by aspiration of the hip if a large hemarthrosis is present, 6 weeks of minimal weight bearing, and a repeat MRI. A search for other causative factors (alcohol, catabolic

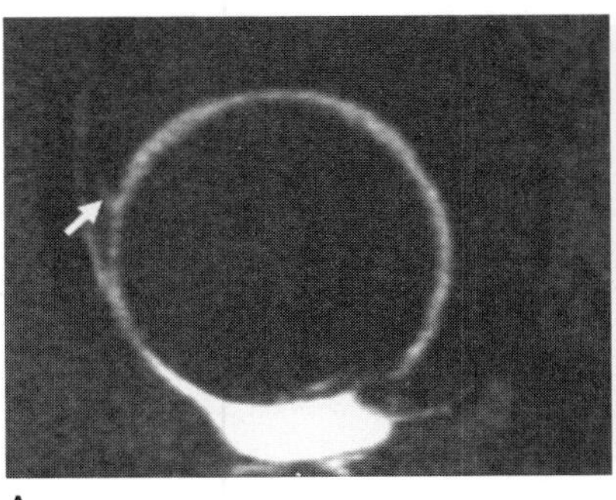

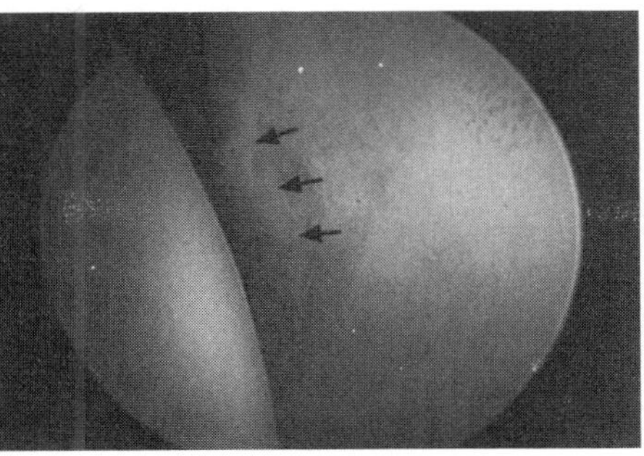

A B

FIGURE 4–29 A 27-year-old with mechanical symptoms in the left hip. **A**, Sagittal MRI with gadolinium arthrography reveals a tear of the anterior labrum *(arrow)*. **B**, Arthroscopic picture showing the anterior labral tear. (From Miller MD, Cooper DE, Warner JJP: Review of Sports Medicine and Arthroscopy, 2nd ed. Philadelphia, WB Saunders, 2002.)

steroids, and decompression sickness) should be made in the atraumatic population.

D. Osteitis pubis—Repetitive trauma can cause an inflammation of the symphysis. It occurs frequently in soccer players, hockey players, and runners. Conservative management is usually curative.

E. Tumors—Because more than 10% of all musculoskeletal tumors occur in the hip and pelvis, they must be suspected in cases of unexplained pain.

VI. Intra-articular Disorders

A. Loose bodies—These often result from trauma or diseases such as synovial chondromatosis. They must be removed, either open or arthroscopically, to prevent third-body wear.

B. Labral tears—Often a cause of mechanical hip pain presenting with vague symptoms. An MR arthrogram has a greater than 90% sensitivity and is often used for diagnosis, but arthroscopy is the gold standard (Fig. 4–29). The highest incidence of labral tears is present in patients with acetabular dysplasia. Underlying hip pathology should be addressed in addition to the labral tear for the best results. Arthroscopic labral débridement has shown good short- and mid-term results. New techniques and data that suggest that labral repair may yield better results than débridement are beginning to emerge.

C. Chondral injuries—Articular surface injury is often a cause of mechanical hip pain. Microfracture is effective in the treatment of focal lesions.

D. Ruptured ligamentum teres—Associated with mechanical hip pain as the ruptured ligament catches within the joint after a hip dislocation. Débridement is often necessary. The viability of the femoral head is not in jeopardy with a ruptured ligamentum teres.

E. Femoroacetabular impingement (FAI)—A frequent initiator of arthritis in the nondysplastic hip. Impingement may be caused by acetabular retroversion; an old slipped capital femoral epiphysis (SCFE); a nonspherical head; decreased femoral offset or decreased head-to-neck ratio (the Cam effect); overhang of the anterosuperior acetabular rim (pincer mechanism); protrusio; and a retroverted femoral neck (postfracture). Treatment options include open or arthroscopic procedures to trim the femoral head/neck or acetabular rim, periacetabular osteotomy, femoral osteotomy, combinations of the above with labral débridement, and repair. Total hip arthroplasty (THA) is reserved for those with significant arthritic changes.

VII. Other Hip Disorders

A. Snapping hip—Condition in which the iliotibial band abruptly catches on the greater trochanter or the iliopsoas impinges on the hip capsule. The iliotibial condition (*external snapping hip*) is more common in females with wide pelvises and prominent trochanters and can be exacerbated by running on banked surfaces. The snapping may be reproduced with passive hip flexion from an adducted position. Stretching/strengthening, modalities such as ultrasonography, and occasionally surgical release may relieve the snapping. This condition must be differentiated from the less common snapping iliopsoas tendon (*internal snapping hip*), which can be diagnosed with extension and internal rotation of the hip from a flexed and externally rotated position. Arthrography and/or bursography may also be helpful in making the diagnosis.

VIII. Hip Arthroscopy (see Color Plates)

A. Indications—As techniques improve, so do the indications. Hip arthroscopy is currently effective for the treatment of loose bodies, labral tears, chondral injuries, AVN, synovial disease, ruptured ligamentum teres, impinging osteophytes, and unexplained mechanical symptoms.

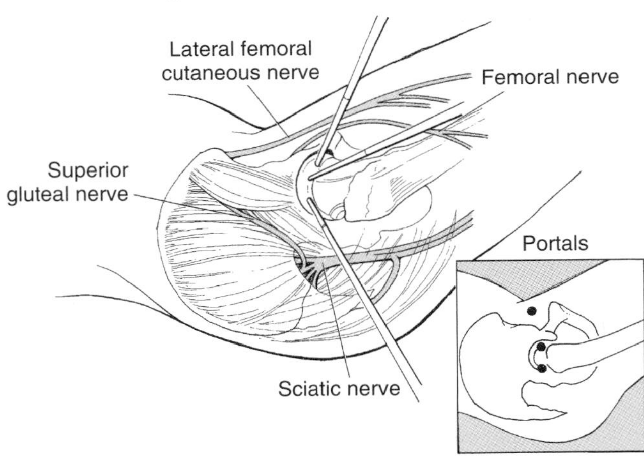

FIGURE 4–30 Portals for hip arthroscopy include the anterior portal and two portals adjacent to the greater trochanter. (From Miller MD, Cooper DE, Warner JJP: Review of Sports Medicine and Arthroscopy, p 107. Philadelphia, WB Saunders, 1995.)

B. Setup—Typically performed in the supine or lateral position with approximately 50 lb of traction and a well-padded perineal post.
C. Portals—Three portals are commonly used for instrumentation—one on each side of the greater trochanter and an additional anterior portal (Fig. 4–30).
D. Complications—Complications are rare but are associated with traction injuries, iatrogenic chondral injuries, and neurovascular injury due to aberrant portal placement. The anterolateral portal is associated with injury to the superior gluteal nerve. The anterior portal puts the lateral femoral cutaneous nerve, the ascending branch of the lateral femoral circumflex artery, and the femoral neurovascular bundle at risk.

SECTION 3 Leg, Foot, and Ankle

I. Nerve Entrapment Syndromes

A. Saphenous nerve entrapment—When compressed at Hunter's canal or in the proximal leg, the saphenous nerve can cause painful symptoms inferior and medial to the knee.
B. Peroneal nerve entrapment—The common peroneal nerve can be compressed behind the fibula or injured by a direct blow to this area. The superficial peroneal nerve can be entrapped about 12 cm proximal to the tip of the lateral malleolus, where it exits the fascia of the anterolateral leg, as a result of inversion injuries. Fascial defects can be present as well, contributing to the problem. Compartment release is sometimes indicated. The deep peroneal nerve can be compressed by the inferior extensor retinaculum, leading to anterior tarsal tunnel syndrome and sometimes necessitating release of this structure.
C. Tibial nerve entrapment—When the tibial nerve is compressed under the flexor retinaculum behind the medial malleolus, it may result in tarsal tunnel syndrome. Electromyography/nerve conduction evaluation is helpful, and surgical release is sometimes indicated. Distal entrapment of the first branch of the lateral plantar nerve (to the adductor digiti quinti), between the fascia of the abductor hallucis longus and the medial side of the quadratus plantae, has also been described.
D. Medial plantar nerve entrapment—Occurs at the point where the flexor digitorum longus and flexor hallucis longus cross (knot of Henry) and is most commonly caused by external compression from orthoses. Commonly called jogger's foot, this condition usually responds to conservative measures.
E. Sural nerve entrapment—Can occur anywhere along its course but is most vulnerable 12-15 mm distal to the tip of the fibula as the foot rests in equinus. Surgical release is usually effective.
F. Interdigital nerve—Commonly called Morton's neuroma, entrapment can occur during the push-off phase while running in athletes and with the demi-pointe position in dancers. It usually occurs between the third and fourth metatarsals plantar to the transverse metatarsal ligament and responds to surgical resection if conservative measures fail.

II. Muscle Injuries

A. Gastrocnemius-soleus strain—Nicknamed tennis leg because of its common association with tennis, this injury is probably much more common than rupture of the plantaris tendon. Supportive treatment is indicated.

III. Tendon Injuries

A. Peroneal tendon injuries
   1. Subluxation/dislocation—Violent dorsiflexion of the inverted foot can result in injury of the fibro-osseous peroneal tendon sheath. Diagnosis is confirmed by observing the subluxation or dislocation by means of eversion and dorsiflexion of the foot. Plain radiographs may demonstrate a rim fracture of the lateral aspect of the distal fibula. Treatment of acute injuries includes restoration of the normal anatomy (Fig. 4–31). Chronic reconstruction involves direct repair, groove-deepening procedures, tissue transfers, or bone block techniques.
   2. Tenosynovitis—These injuries are being recognized more frequently with MRI and often lead to tears of the peroneal tendons.
   3. Longitudinal tears of the peroneal tendons (especially the peroneus brevis tendon)—These injuries are now recognized with increasing frequency. Repair and decompression are generally recommended.
B. Posterior tibialis tendon injury—This injury can occur in older athletes. Patients complain of midarch foot pain, with difficulty pushing off. Débridement of partial ruptures and flexor digitorum longus transfer for chronic injuries are recommended.
C. Anterior tibialis tendon injury—Rupture is uncommon but has been reported in elderly athletes. Repair is recommended.
D. Achilles tendon injuries
   1. Tendinitis/tendinosis—Overuse injury to the Achilles tendon usually responds to rest and physical therapy, with an eccentric loading program and local modalities. Progression to partial rupture may necessitate surgical excision of scar and granulation tissue.
   2. Rupture—Complete rupture of the tendon is caused by maximum plantar flexion with the foot planted. Patients may relate that they felt as if they were "shot." The Thompson test (squeezing the calf results in normal plantar flexion of the foot) is helpful for confirming the diagnosis. Treatment remains controversial; however,

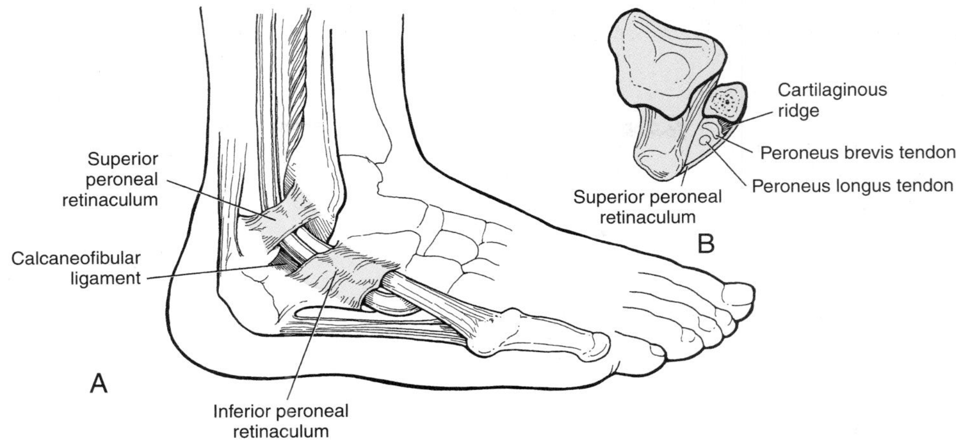

FIGURE 4–31 Normal relationship of the peroneal tendons. Note the superior and inferior retinacula and the cartilaginous ridge on the posterolateral fibula. **A**, Lateral view. **B**, Superior view. (From Miller MD, Cooper DE, Warner JJP: Review of Sports Medicine and Arthroscopy, p 82. Philadelphia, WB Saunders, 1995.)

recurrence rates are reduced with primary repair, while other complications (i.e., wound problems) are increased with surgical repair.

IV. Chronic Exertional Compartment Syndrome

Although it is more commonly encountered with trauma, sports-related compartment syndrome is becoming more frequently diagnosed. Athletes (especially runners and cyclists) may note pain that has a gradual onset during exercise, ultimately restricting their performance. Compartment pressures taken before, during, and after exercise (pressures >20 mm Hg 5 minutes after exercise or absolute values above 15 mm Hg while resting or above 30 mm Hg 1 minute after exercise) can help establish the diagnosis. The anterior compartment of the leg is the most frequently involved. Fasciotomy is sometimes indicated for refractory cases (Fig. 4–32).

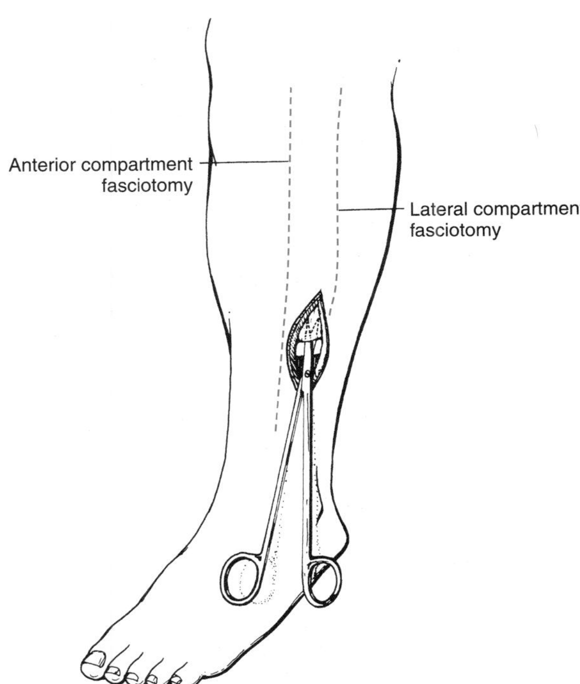

FIGURE 4–32 Anterior and lateral compartment release. (From DeLee JC, Drez D Jr: Orthopaedic Sports Medicine: Principles and Practice, p 1618. Philadelphia, WB Saunders, 1994.)

V. Fractures

A. Stress fractures—Common in athletes who have undergone a change in their training routines and in female endurance athletes (must ask about a menstrual history). Usually responds to rest and activity modification. Recalcitrant fractures may need operative fixation.

1. Tibial shaft fractures—This is a complication of unrecognized tibial stress fractures and can be a difficult problem. Persistence of the "dreaded black line" (Fig. 4–33) for more than 6 months, especially

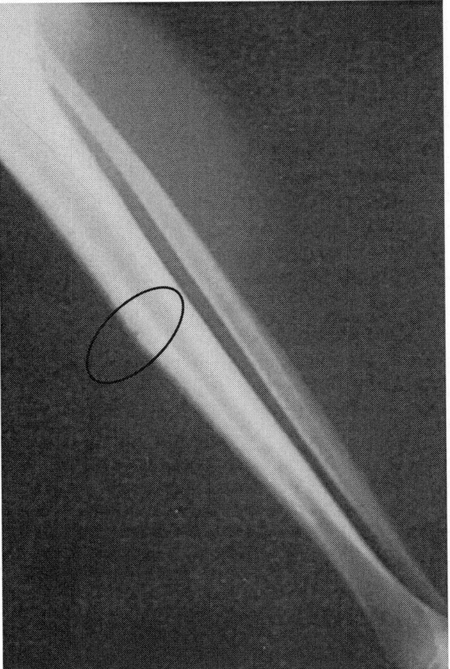

FIGURE 4–33 Radiograph demonstrating the "dreaded black line" *(circled area)* associated with an impending complete fracture of the tibial shaft. (From Miller MD, Cooper DE, Warner JJP: Review of Sports Medicine and Arthroscopy, p 81. Philadelphia, WB Saunders, 1995.)

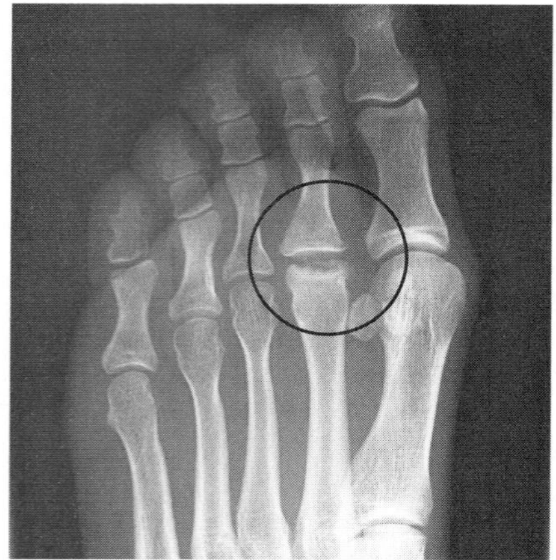

FIGURE 4–34 Radiographic appearance of Freiberg infarction *(circled area)*.

with a positive bone scan, can be an indication for bone grafting and/or intramedullary nailing.

2. Tarsal navicular fractures—This injury is often found in basketball players. Immobilization and non–weight bearing are important during the early management of these stress fractures. Open reduction with internal fixation is occasionally indicated with linear fractures (as seen on CT).
3. Freiberg infarction—Flattening of the second metatarsal head, usually due to stress overloading in a child's foot. Conservative management is indicated unless the patient is having mechanical symptoms (Fig. 4–34).

B. Jones fractures—Fractures at the metaphyseal-diaphyseal junction of the fifth metatarsal in an athlete can be treated more aggressively with early intramedullary screw fixation to allow earlier healing and an earlier return to conditioning activities. A screw with a minimum diameter of 4 mm should be used (Fig. 4–35).

VI. Other Foot and Ankle Disorders

A. Plantar fasciitis—Inflammation of the plantar fascia, usually in the central to medial subcalcaneal region, is common in runners. Rest, orthoses, stretching, NSAIDs, and local steroid injections are helpful. Partial plantar fasciotomy is occasionally necessary, but recovery can be protracted. Refractory cases may be treated with extracorporeal shock wave therapy.

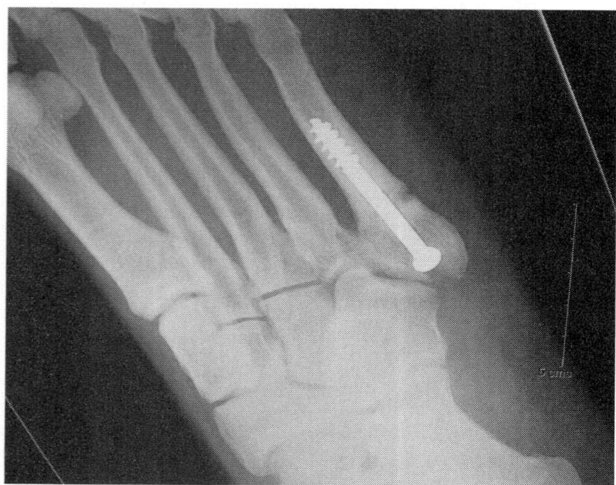

FIGURE 4–35 Radiographic appearance of Jones fracture after open reduction with internal fixation with a 6.5 screw.

B. Os trigonum (posterior impingement) syndrome—An os trigonum can cause impingement with plantar flexion of the foot, especially in ballet dancers. Treatment may include local anesthetic injection and other supportive measures. Surgical excision of the offending bone with or without release of the **flexor hallucis longus** (FHL) is occasionally necessary, and arthroscopic techniques have been described.

C. Ankle sprains and instability—These injuries are common in athletes and most often involve the anterior talofibular ligament (ATFL) and occasionally the calcaneofibular ligament (CFL). The posterior talofibular ligament (PTFL) is rarely involved. The Ottawa ankle rules indicate that radiographs are required only in patients with distal (especially posterior) tibia or fibula tenderness, tenderness at the base of the fifth metatarsal or navicular, and an inability to bear weight. Surgical treatment is reserved for recurrent, symptomatic ankle instability with excessive tilt and a positive anterior drawer on examination/stress radiographs that have not responded to orthoses and peroneal strengthening/proprioceptive exercises over an extended period. Anatomic procedures (modified Brostrom) are usually successful. Involvement of the subtalar joint requires tendon rerouting procedures that include this joint. Patients with "high" ankle sprains involving the syndesmosis require recovery periods of almost twice those for patients with common ankle sprains.

D. Turf toe—Severe dorsiflexion of the metatarsophalangeal (MTP) joint of the great toe (injuring the plantar plate) can result in a tender, stiff, swollen toe. Treatment includes motion, ice, and taping in plantar flexion. If symptoms persist, a stress fracture of the proximal phalanx should be ruled out with a bone scan or MRI.

E. Snowboarder's foot and ankle—Fracture of the lateral process of the talus (Fig. 4–36). The injury involves the leading leg on the board. A CT scan can help confirm the diagnosis. A fracture with small fragments (<2 mm) can be treated in a short leg cast for 6 weeks, whereas a fracture with large fragments should undergo open reduction with internal fixation.

VII. Ankle Arthroscopy (see Color Plates)

A. Indications—Include treatment of osteochondral injuries of the talus, débridement of post-traumatic synovitis, anterolateral impingement secondary to chronic pain from an ankle sprain, removal of anterior tibiotalar spurring, os trigonum excision, and cartilage débridement in conjunction with ankle fusions.

1. Osteochondral injuries of the talus—Treatment includes drilling of the base of these lesions and fixation of replaceable lesions. Lateral lesions are

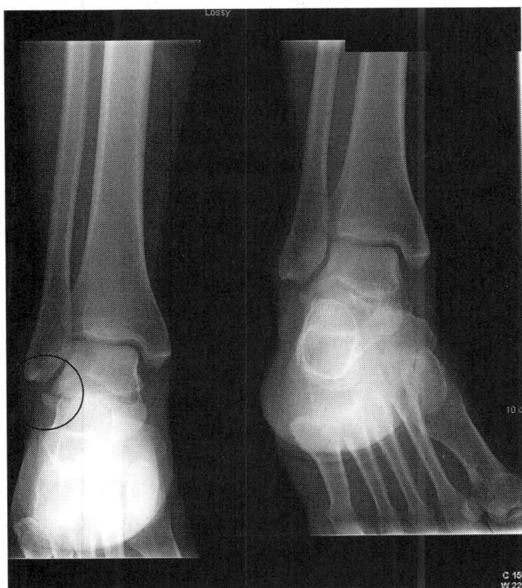

FIGURE 4–36 Radiographic appearance of snowboarder's ankle *(circled area)*.

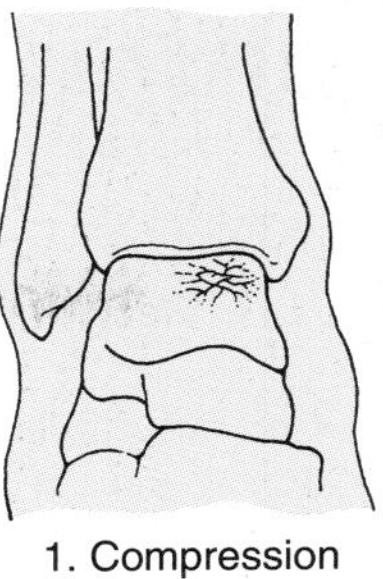

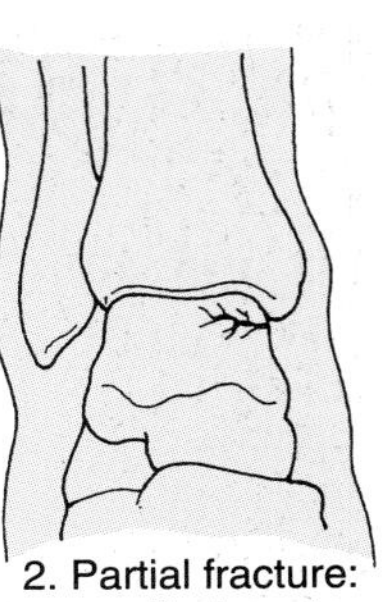

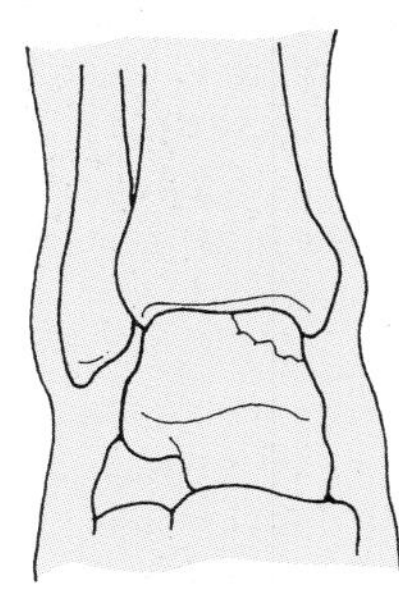

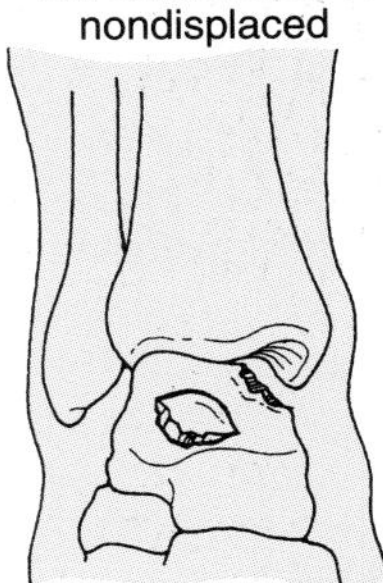

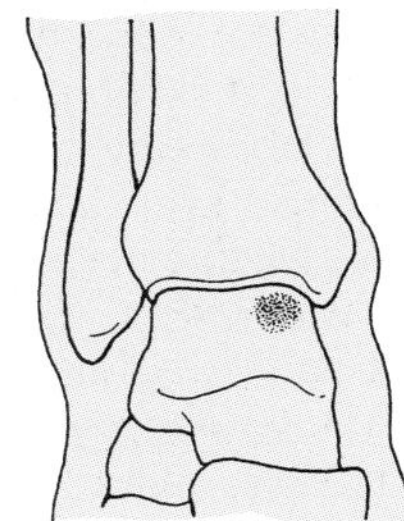

FIGURE 4–37 Loomer and coworkers' modification to the Berndt and Harty classification of osteochondral lesions of the talus. (From Miller MD, Cooper DE, Warner JJP: Review of Sports Medicine and Arthroscopy, p 95. Philadelphia, WB Saunders, 1995.)

usually traumatic, shallow, and anterior, while medial lesions are atraumatic, deeper, and posterior. The modification to the Berndt and Harty classification scheme (Fig. 4–37) by Loomer and coworkers is helpful in the management of these osteochondral lesions of the talus.

B. Technique—Supine positioning with the leg over a well-padded bolster and an external traction device are currently popular. Five portals have been suggested (Fig. 4–38), but most surgeons avoid the posteromedial portal because of the risk to the posterior tibial artery and tibial nerve and avoid the anterocentral portal because of the risk to the dorsalis pedis and deep peroneal nerve. The "nick and spread" method is advocated for the anterolateral portal (superficial peroneal nerve) and the anteromedial portal (saphenous vein).

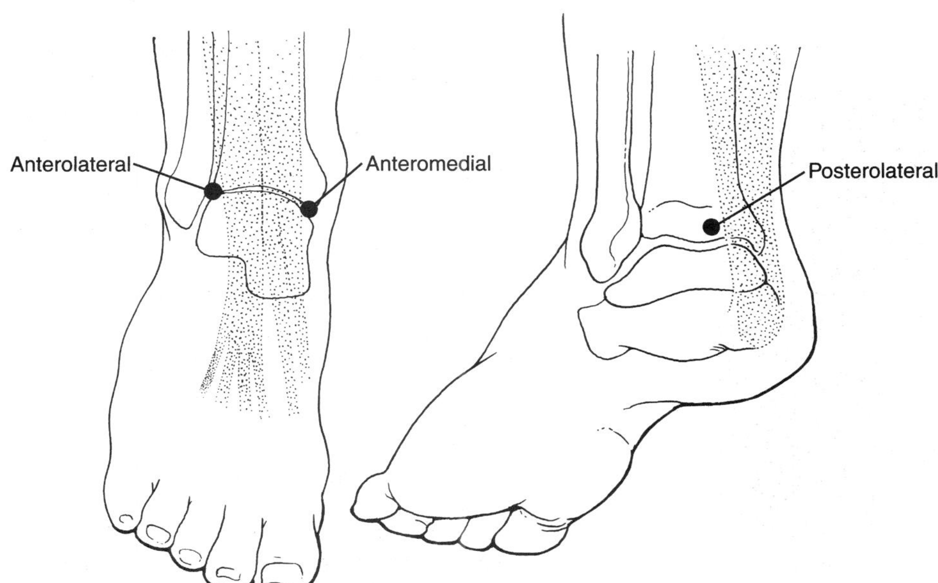

FIGURE 4–38 Portals for ankle arthroscopy are the anteromedial, anterolateral, and posterolateral. (From Miller MD, Osborne JR, Warner JJP, et al: MRI-Arthroscopy Correlative Atlas, p 134. Philadelphia, WB Saunders, 1997.)

SECTION 4 Shoulder

I. Anatomy and Biomechanics*

The shoulder consists of three bones and four joints.

A. Osteology

1. Clavicle—An S-shaped bone, it is the last to ossify (the medial growth plate fuses in the early twenties).
2. Scapula—Serves as the insertion site for 17 muscles. It has two important prominences: the coracoid process and the acromion. Os acromiale, an unfused secondary ossification center, occurs with a 3% incidence and 60% bilaterality. The most common location is at the junction of the meso-acromion and meta-acromion.
3. Humeral head—It is approximately spheroidal in 90% of individuals and has an average diameter of 43 mm. It is normally retroverted an average of 30 degrees to the transepicondylar axis of the distal humerus, with its articular surface inclined an average of 130 degrees superiorly relative to the shaft.
4. Glenoid—The shoulder "socket," or glenoid cavity, is a lateral projection of the scapula. Its rim is surrounded by fibrocartilaginous thickening known as the labrum, which serves to both deepen the socket (acting as a chock block) and anchor the inferior glenohumeral ligament complex. Its surface is pear shaped, with an average upward tilt of 5 degrees and an average range of 7 degrees of retroversion to 10 degrees of anteversion.

B. Articulations—The shoulder consists of four joints: the glenohumeral (GH), sternoclavicular (SC), acromioclavicular (AC), and scapulothoracic (ST).

1. GH joint—A spheroidal (ball-and-socket) joint, it is the principal articulation of the shoulder and is stabilized by both static and dynamic restraints (see the following discussion on biomechanics). Part of the static restraints, the glenohumeral ligaments are discrete capsular thickenings that act as a kind of checkrein to limit excessive humeral head rotation or translation. The capsuloligamentous structures include the superior glenohumeral ligament (SGHL), coracohumeral ligament (CHL), middle glenohumeral ligament (MGHL), and inferior glenohumeral ligament complex (IGHLC) (Fig. 4–39). Additional capsular elements include the posterior capsule, which is the thinnest portion (<1 mm) of the shoulder capsule, and the rotator interval. This interval includes the capsule and CHL that bridge the gap between the supraspinatus and the subscapularis. It is bounded medially by the lateral coracoid base, superiorly by the anterior edge of the supraspinatus (biceps tendon), and inferiorly by the superior border of the subscapularis. The transverse humeral ligament forms its apex laterally.
2. SC joint—This is a gliding joint with a disc that serves to anchor the shoulder girdle to the chest wall. Elevation of the arm from 0-90 degrees produces clavicular rotation about its longitudinal axis and elevation at the SC joint of 0-40 degrees. The posterior capsule is the primary restraint of excessive anterior and posterior translation.
3. AC joint—The articulation of the scapula with the clavicle occurs through a diarthrodial joint containing an incomplete intra-articular disc. It is stabilized by the AC ligaments, which primarily resist anteroposterior translation, and the coracoclavicular (CC) ligaments, which prevent inferior translation of the coracoid and acromion from the clavicle (Fig. 4–40).
4. ST joint—The medial border of the scapula articulates with the posterior aspect of the second to seventh ribs. It is angled 30 degrees anteriorly and has a 3 degree upward tilt. There are two major ST

*See Chapter 2, Anatomy, for a more detailed description of shoulder anatomy.

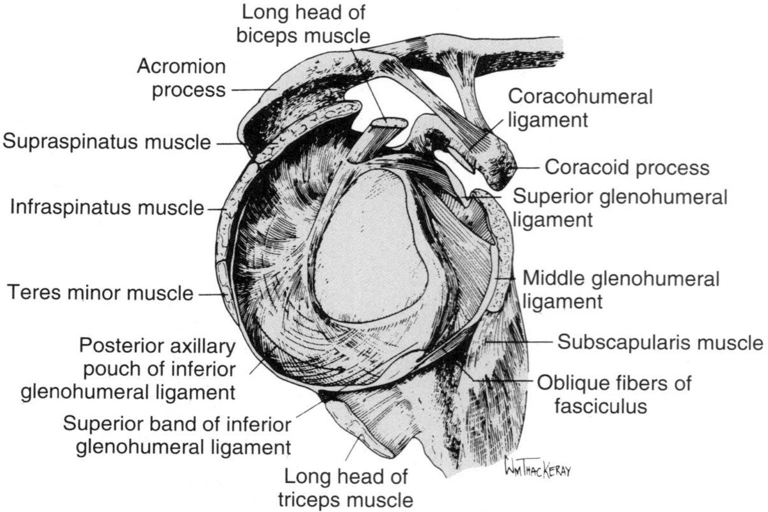

FIGURE 4–39 Important ligaments of the shoulder. (From Turkel SJ, Panio MW, Marshall JL, et al: Stabilizing mechanisms preventing anterior dislocation of the glenohumeral joint. J Bone Joint Surg [Am] 63:1209, 1981.)

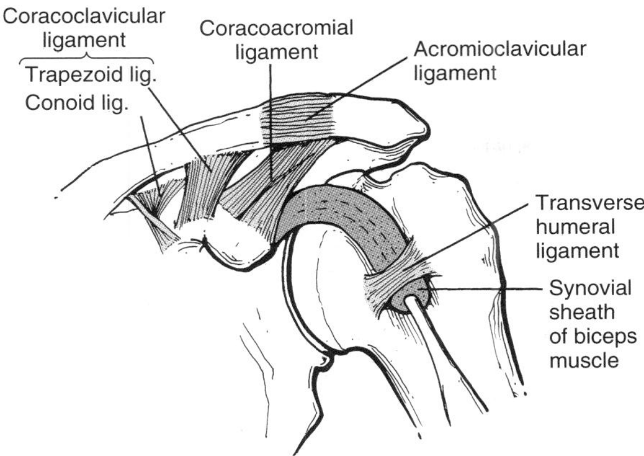

FIGURE 4–40 Acromioclavicular joint anatomy. (From Tibone J, Patek R, Jobe FW, et al: Functional anatomy, biomechanics, and kinesiology: The shoulder. In DeLee JC, Drez D Jr, eds: Orthopaedic Sports Medicine: Principles and Practice, p 465. Philadelphia, WB Saunders, 1994.)

bursae. The ratio of GH to ST motion during shoulder abduction is approximately 2:1.

C. Supporting structures—It is helpful to consider the shoulder in layers (Fig. 4–41).

D. Biomechanics—The shoulder is stabilized by both static and dynamic restraints.

1. Static restraints—These include the glenoid labrum, articular version, articular conformity, negative intra-articular pressure, capsule (posterior capsule and rotator interval), and capsuloligamentous structures. Imbrication of the rotator interval decreases inferior and posterior translation, while its release produces increased forward flexion and external rotation. The SGHL and CHL are reinforcing structures of the rotator interval, limiting inferior translation and external rotation when the arm is adducted and posterior translation when the arm is flexed forward, adducted, and internally rotated. The MGHL limits external rotation of the adducted humerus, inferior translation of the adducted and externally rotated humerus, and anterior and posterior translation of the partly abducted (45 degrees) and externally rotated arm. The IGHLC serves as the primary restraint to anterior, posterior, and inferior GH translation at 45-90 degrees of GH elevation (Table 4–8).

2. Dynamic restraints—These include joint concavity compression produced by synchronized contraction of the rotator cuff (RTC), acting to stabilize the humeral head within the glenoid; increased capsular tension produced by direct attachments of the RTC to the capsule; the scapular stabilizers that act to maintain a stable glenoid platform ("ball on a seal's nose"); and proprioception.

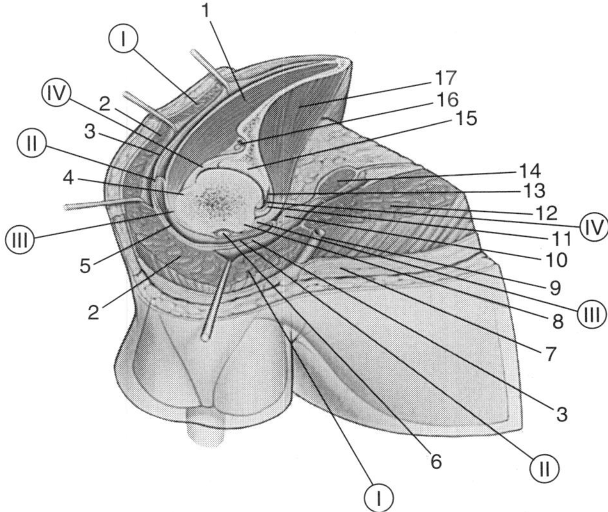

FIGURE 4–41 Cross-sectional view of the right shoulder at the level of the lesser tuberosity. Note the four layers of the shoulder and their components: I—deltoid (2), pectoralis major (12), cephalic vein (9); II—conjoined tendon (10), pectoralis minor (14), clavipectoral fascia (7); III—subdeltoid bursa (5), rotator cuff muscles (1, 17), glenohumeral capsule (11), greater tuberosity (4), long head of biceps (6), lesser tuberosity (8), fascia (3), synovium (13), glenoid (15). (From Cooper DE, O'Brien SJ, Warren RF: Supporting layers of the glenohumeral joint: An anatomic study. Clin Orthop 289:151, 1993.)

E. Throwing—Significant forces are generated when throwing and can result in injury. The five phases of throwing are shown in Figure 4–42. Maximum torque is generated during two actions—maximum external rotation (late cocking) and just after ball release (deceleration).

II. Diagnostic Techniques

A. History—Age and chief complaint are two important considerations. Instability, AC injuries, and distal clavicle osteolysis are more common in young patients. RTC tears, arthritis, and proximal humeral fractures are more common in older patients. Direct blows are usually responsible for AC separations. Instability occurs with injury to the abducted, externally rotated arm. Chronic overhead pain and night pain are associated with RTC tears.

B. Physical examination—Observation, palpation, and strength testing can provide important diagnostic clues. Examination includes range and quality of motion (forward flexion of 150-180 degrees, external rotation with the arm adducted 30-60 degrees, and internal rotation reaching T4-T8 are considered normal) as well as specific muscle testing (Table 4–9; Figs. 4–43 and 4–44). Note that the scapula

TABLE 4-8 GLENOHUMERAL LIGAMENTS

Structure	Arm Position	Resists
SGHL/CHL	Adduction	Inferior translation/ER
	FF/abduction/IR	Posterior translation
MGHL	ADD/ER	ER
	45-degree ABD/ER	Anterior/posterior translation
IGHL	45-90–degree GH elevation	Primary restraint to anterior/posterior/inferior GH translation

ABD/ER, abduction/external rotation; ADD/ER, adduction/external rotation; CHL, coracohumeral ligament; FF, forward flexion; GH, glenohumeral; IGHL, inferior glenohumeral ligament; IR, internal rotation; MGHL, middle glenohumeral ligament; SGHL, superior glenohumeral ligament.

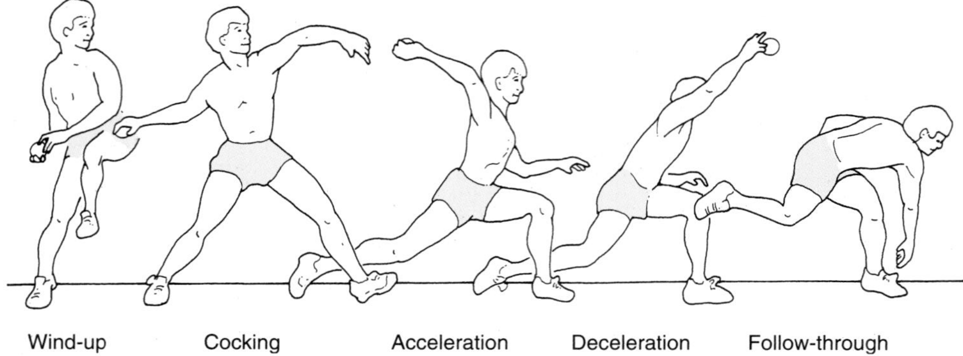

FIGURE 4–42 The five phases of throwing. (From Miller MD, Cooper DE, Warner JJP: Review of Sports Medicine and Arthroscopy, p 123. Philadelphia, WB Saunders, 1995.)

must be stabilized to evaluate true ROM of the glenohumeral joint.

C. Imaging the shoulder
   1. Trauma series—The trauma series of radiographs includes a "true" anteroposterior view (plate is placed parallel to the scapula, about 45 degrees from the plane of the thorax) and an axillary lateral view.
   2. Other views—Other views that are sometimes helpful include a scapular Y or trans-scapular

TABLE 4-9 MUSCLE TESTING FOR SHOULDER INJURIES

Examination	Technique	Significance
Impingement/RTC		
Impingement sign	Passive FF >90 degrees	Pain = impingement syndrome
Impingement test	Same after subacromial injection	Relief of pain = impingement syndrome
Hawkins test	Passive FF 90 degrees and IR	Pain = impingement syndrome
Jobe test	Resisted pronation/FF 90 degrees	Pain = supraspinatus lesion
Drop-arm test	Maintain FF in plane of scapula	Inability = supraspinatus lesion
Hornblower sign	Resisted maximum ER/abd 90 degrees	Pain = infraspinatus/(post)supraspinatus lesion
Rubber band sign	Resisted maximum ER/slight abd	Pain = infraspinatus lesion
Liftoff test	Arm IR behind back	Inability to elevate from back = subscapularis lesion
Modified liftoff test	Resisted arm held off back	Inability to keep elevated off back = subscapularis lesion
Belly-push test	Elbow held anterior with abd pressure	Inability to hold elbow forward = subscapularis lesion
Instability		
Apprehension test	Supine abd 90 degrees and ER	Apprehension = anterior instability
Relocation test (see Fig. 4–43)	Apprehension with posterior force	Relief of apprehension = anterior instability
Load-and-shift test	Anterior/posterior force on humeral head	Degree of translation = laxity vs. instability (see grading)
Modified load-and-shift test	Supine load/shift with elbow bending	Degree of translation = laxity vs. instability (see grading)
Jerk test	Post force with arm add and FF	"Clunk" = posterior subluxation
Sulcus sign	Inferior force with arm at side	Increased acromiohumeral interval = inferior laxity vs. instability (see sulcus grading)
Labrum/Biceps		
Active compression test	10 degrees add, 90 degrees FF, maximum pronation	Pain with resistance = SLAP lesion
Anterior slide test	Hand on hip, joint loading	Pain with resistance = SLAP lesion
Crank test	Full abd, humeral loading, rotation	Pain = SLAP lesion
Speed test	Resisted FF in scapular plane	pain = bicipital tendinitis
Yerguson test	Resisted supination	pain = bicipital tendinitis
Miscellaneous		
Spurling maneuver (see Fig. 4–44)	Lateral flexion, rotation, cervical loading	Cervical spine pathology
Wright's test	Ext-abd-ER of arm with neck rotated away	Loss of pulse and reproduction of symptom(s) = thoracic outlet syndrome

abd, Abduction; add, adduction; ER, external rotation; ext, extension; FF, forward flexion; IR, internal rotation; RTC, rotator cuff; SLAP, superior labrum from anterior to posterior.

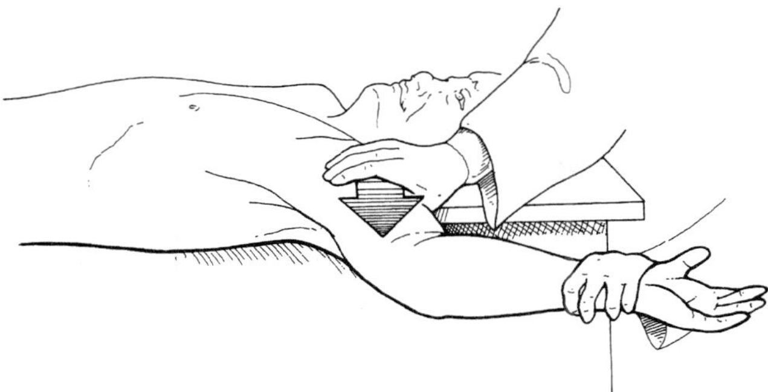

FIGURE 4–43 Relocation test. Anterior pressure on the proximal arm relocates the humerus and causes relief of apprehension. (From Miller MD, Cooper DE, Warner JJP: Review of Sports Medicine and Arthroscopy, p 128. Philadelphia, WB Saunders, 1995.)

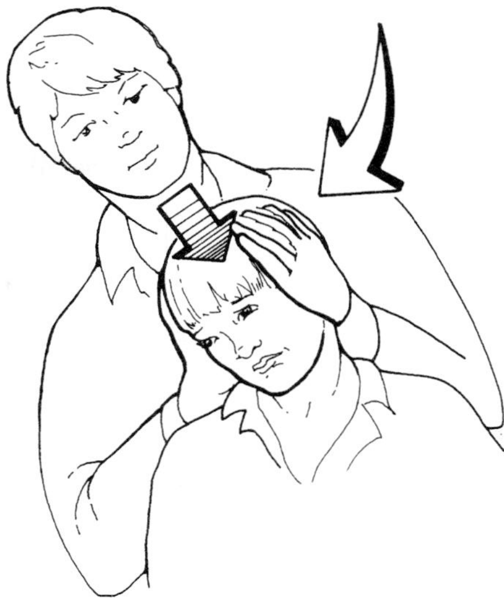

FIGURE 4–44 Spurling's test. Lateral flexion and rotation with some compression may cause nerve root encroachment and pain on the ipsilateral side in patients with impingement of the cervical nerve root. (From Miller MD, Cooper DE, Warner JJP: Review of Sports Medicine and Arthroscopy, p 129. Philadelphia, WB Saunders, 1995.)

view and anteroposterior radiographs in internal and external rotation. Special radiographic views have also been developed for certain other abnormalities. For example, the supraspinatus outlet view is helpful in the evaluation of impingement (Fig. 4–45; Table 4–10).

III. Shoulder Arthroscopy (see Color Plates)

A. Portals
   1. Standard portals
      a. Posterior portal (2 cm distal and medial to the posterolateral border of the acromion, primarily used for viewing)
      b. Anterior portal (just anterior to the AC joint)
      c. Lateral portal (1-2 cm distal to the lateral acromial edge)
   2. Additional portals
      a. Supraspinatus (Neviaser) portal for anterior glenoid visualization (through the supraspinatus fossa)
      b. Anterolateral and posterolateral portals (Port of Wilmington, just anterior to the posterolateral corner of the acromion), which are useful for labral tears or superior labrum from anterior to posterior (SLAP) tears and RTC repair
      c. Anteroinferior (5 o'clock position) portal for Bankart repair and stabilization procedures
      d. Posteroinferior (7 o'clock position) portal for stabilization procedures (Fig. 4–46)

B. Technique—Systematic evaluation of intra-articular structures should be performed. As the number and variety of arthroscopic procedures grow, so does the opportunity for iatrogenic injury. Maintaining adequate visualization through hemostasis, avoiding chondral abrasion, maintaining adequate flow with thermal devices, and preventing fluid extravasation by preserving muscle fascial layers will help minimize the risk.

IV. Shoulder Instability

A. Diagnosis—Due to the shoulder's extensive ROM, it is at risk for developing instability and is the most commonly dislocated joint in the body. Instability is a pathologic condition manifesting as pain due to

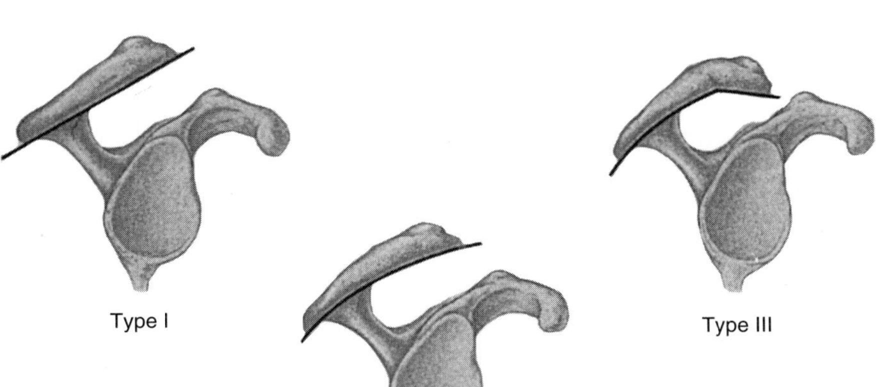

FIGURE 4–45 Acromion morphology is classified on the basis of the supraspinatus outlet view as originally described by Bigliani. (From Esch JC: Shoulder arthroscopy in the older age group. Op Tech Orthop 1:200, 1991.)

TABLE 4–10 RADIOGRAPHIC VIEWS

View/Sign	Findings	Significance
View of supraspinatus outlet	Acromial morphology (types I-III)	Type III acromion associated with impingement
View of 30-degree caudal tilt	Subacromial spurring	Area below level of clavicle = impingement area
Zanca 10-degree cephalic tilt	AC joint pathology	AC DJD, distal clavicle osteolysis
West Point	AI glenoid evaluation	Bony Bankart lesion seen with instability
Garth view	AI glenoid evaluation	Bony Bankart lesion seen with instability
Stryker notch	Humeral head evaluation	Hill-Sachs impression fracture
Anteroposterior internal rotation	Humeral head evaluation	Hill-Sachs defect
Hobbs view	SC injury	AP dislocations
Serendipity view	SC injury	AP dislocations
45-degree abduction, true AP	Glenohumeral space	Subtle DJD
Arthrography	Rotator cuff injuries	Dye above cuff = tear
CT	Fractures	Classification easier
MRI ± arthrography	Soft tissue evaluation	Labral, cuff, muscle tears

AC, acromioclavicular; AI, anteroinferior; AP, anteroposterior; CT, computed tomography; DJD, degenerative joint disease; MRI, magnetic resonance imaging; SC, sternoclavicular.

excessive translation of the humeral head on the glenoid during active shoulder motion, representing a spectrum of injury to the shoulder stabilizers. Diagnosis is based on history, physical examination, and imaging. Clinical evidence of instability includes positive load-and-shift, modified load-and-shift, and apprehension-relocation testing as well as a sulcus sign (see Table 4–9). Grading of instability is shown in Table 4–11.

1. TUBS syndrome—*T*raumatic *u*nilateral dislocations with a *B*ankart lesion often require *s*urgery because they typically occur in young patients and have recurrence rates of up to 80-90% with nonoperative management.
2. AMBRI syndrome—*A*traumatic *m*ultidirectional *b*ilateral shoulder dislocation/subluxation often responds to *r*ehabilitation, and sometimes an *i*nferior capsular shift or plication is required.

B. Treatment—Several open and arthroscopic techniques have been developed to address instability (Table 4–12). These procedures have been broadened to address both capsuloligamentous laxity (e.g., capsular plication, rotator interval closure) and labral pathology via a variety of instruments, suture passage and knot-tying techniques, and fixation devices (both absorbable and nonabsorbable).

1. First-time dislocations—Debate still exists regarding the treatment of first-time dislocations. External rotation bracing for 3-6 weeks has been effective in decreasing the short-term rates of recurrent dislocation, at least in an Asian population. The lowest rates of recurrent dislocation (generally <10%) are seen after operative treatment, either open or arthroscopic. The newest data show that arthroscopic anterior stabilization is equivalent to open repairs. Some have advocated repair of first-time dislocations because of

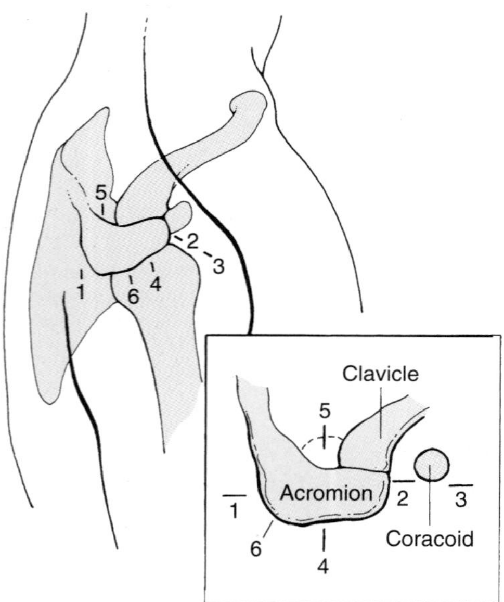

FIGURE 4–46 Arthroscopic portals of the shoulder. 1, posterior; 2, anterosuperior; 3, anteroinferior; 4, lateral; 5, supraspinatus (Neviaser); 6, port of Wilmington. (From Miller MD, Cooper DE, Warner JJP: Review of Sports Medicine and Arthroscopy, p 135. Philadelphia, WB Saunders, 1995.)

TABLE 4–11 GRADES OF INSTABILITY

Grade	Anteroposterior Grading Scheme*	Sulcus Grading Scheme†
Grade 0	Normal small amount of humeral head translation	n/a
Grade 1	Humeral head translation to but not over the glenoid rim	Acromiohumeral interval <1 cm
Grade 2	Humeral head translation over the glenoid rim with spontaneous reduction when the applied force is withdrawn	Acromiohumeral interval 1-2 cm
Grade 3	Humeral head translation with locking over the glenoid rim	Acromiohumeral interval >2 cm

**Abnormal (vs. contralateral shoulder): anterior instability is ≥ grade 1; posterior instability is ≥ grade 3.*
†Abnormal (vs. contralateral shoulder): ≥ grade 2.

TABLE 4-12 TREATMENT OF SHOULDER INSTABILITY

Procedure	Essential Features	Comments/Complications
Bankart	Reattachment of labrum (and IGHLC) to glenoid	Gold standard
Staple capsulorrhaphy	Capsular reattachment and tightening	Staple migration/articular injury
Putti-Platt	Subscapularis advancement capsular coverage	Decreased external rotation, DJD
Magnuson-Stack	Subscapularis transfer to greater tuberosity	Decreased external rotation
Boyd-Sisk	Transfer of biceps laterally and posteriorly	Nonanatomic, recurrence
Bristow/Laterjet	Coracoid transfer to inferior glenoid	Nonunion, migration, labral tears
Bone block osteotomy	Anterior bone block	Nonunion, migration, articular injury
Capsular shift	Inferior capsule shifted superiorly—"pants over vest"	Overtightening, gold standard for MDI

DJD, degenerative joint disease; IGHLC, inferior glenohumeral ligament complex; MDI, multidirectional instability.

the decreased rate of dislocation 6 years after repair and the higher quality of life associated with operative treatment; however, this is still controversial.

2. Complications of open procedures—Complications of open procedures include subscapularis overtightening (Z-lengthening required) or rupture (repair or pectoralis transfer required) and hardware problems.
3. Instability—Although the role for the arthroscopic treatment of instability is being broadened, clinical studies have not yet established a clear role for the treatment of instability in the contact athlete.
4. Thermal capsular shrinkage—The role of thermal capsular shrinkage has yet to be clearly elucidated. Good short-term results have been reported, but newer long-term results have demonstrated worsening outcomes. Poor tissue quality and chondral damage at the time of revision have been noted after thermal shrinkage. Despite this, there may still be a role for thermal shrinkage as an adjunct to capsulolabral repair.

C. Posterior instability—Patients may exhibit positive load-and-shift and jerk testing. When they are recognized, posterior dislocations respond well to acute reduction and immobilization. Patients may present with their arms internally rotated, with observable coracoid and posterior prominence. An axillary lateral radiograph is extremely helpful in making the diagnosis. Rehabilitation focuses on RTC and deltoid strengthening, with surgical management (arthroscopic or open posterior Bankart repair with or without capsular shift) reserved for refractory cases.

D. Kim lesion—This is an incomplete and concealed avulsion of the posteroinferior labrum. It may be associated with posterior and multidirectional instability. The jerk (posterior lesion) and Kim (posteroinferior lesion) tests have been shown to be highly sensitive and specific. An MR arthrogram can be helpful in making the diagnosis. However, the findings may be subtle or falsely negative. After failure of conservative treatment, arthroscopic labroplasty (with a posterior capsular shift in primary posterior instability) or posterior labroplasty (with an inferior capsular shift and rotator interval closure when associated with multidirectional instability) has been effective.

V. Impingement Syndrome/Rotator Cuff Disease

A. Overview—RTC disease is a continuum beginning with mild impingement and progressing toward partial RTC tear, full-thickness RTC tear, massive tear, and finally RTC arthropathy. Tears associated with chronic impingement syndrome typically begin on the bursal surface or within the tendon substance, in contrast to those that occur on the articular surface because of tension failure in younger overhead athletes (Table 4–13).

B. Epidemiology of RTC tear—Millions of Americans have some aspect of RTC disease. Twenty-eight percent of those over 60 years of age have a full-thickness tear, while 65% of patients older than 70 years have a full-thickness tear. There is a 50% risk of having bilateral tears in those over 60 years old with a tear. In those with a unilateral, painful, full-thickness tear, there is a 56% chance of having an asymptomatic, contralateral, full- or partial-thickness tear. Fifty percent of those with an asymptomatic tear will develop symptoms at 3 years, and 40% of these patients may have progression of the tear.

C. Diagnosis

1. Physical examination—Patients typically present with an insidious onset of pain exacerbated by overhead activities. Complaints of night discomfort, pain in the deltoid region, muscular weakness, and differences in active versus passive ROM are common, with more significant weakness and loss of motion indicating a higher degree of cuff involvement. Acute pain and weakness may be seen after traumatic RTC rupture. In young athletes, it is critical to exclude GH instability that causes a secondary impingement (nonoutlet impingement) from primary

TABLE 4-13 ROTATOR CUFF TEARS

Stage	Age (yr)	Pathology	Clinical Course	Treatment
I	<25	Edema and hemorrhage	Reversible	Conservative
II	25-40	Fibrosis and tendinitis	Activity-related pain	Therapy/operative
III	>40	AC spur and cuff tear	Progressive disability	Acromioplasty/repair

impingement syndrome (pathology within the subacromial space). For specific testing, refer to Table 4–9.

2. Radiographs—May demonstrate classic changes within the acromion or coracoacromial ligament (spurring and calcification) in addition to cystic changes within the greater tuberosity. With chronic RTC pathology, superior migration of the humeral head with extensive degenerative change may be present.

D. Treatment

1. Nonoperative treatment—Initially indicated for impingement syndrome, chronic atraumatic cuff tears, noncompliant patients, medical contraindications to surgery, RTC arthropathy, and athletes with a combined picture of instability or cuff tearing resulting from articular-side, partial thickness failure. Activity modification, avoiding repeated forward flexion beyond 90 degrees, and an aggressive RTC and scapular-stabilizer strengthening program are initiated. Additionally, oral anti-inflammatory medications, therapeutic modalities, and judicious use of subacromial steroid injections may be implemented.

2. Chronic impingement syndrome—Symptoms that are refractory to a minimum of 4-6 months of nonoperative treatment may respond favorably to subacromial decompression. Similarly, patients indicated for RTC repair will often require concomitant subacromial decompression at the time of repair. Exceptions include massive, irreparable RTC tears that may benefit from débridement with preservation of the coracoacromial arch to prevent anterosuperior humeral migration. Additional exceptions include the acute, traumatic RTC tear or the overhead-movement athlete who may benefit from limited acromial smoothing and bursectomy, which is required for visualization and limiting postoperative irritation of the repair site.

3. RTC surgery—Surgery reliably decreases pain and improves motion and function. The operative approach has evolved from a classic open approach, to a "mini-open" or deltoid-sparing approach, to an all-arthroscopic technique. Independent of the technique, the rate-limiting step for recovery is the biologic healing of the RTC tendon to the humerus, estimated to require a minimum of 8-12 weeks.

   a. Acute RTC tears—Should have early repair, as the disease process is accelerated in this setting.

   b. Articular-side, partial-thickness tears—Treatment with débridement versus repair remains controversial. Considerations include the depth of the tear, the pattern of the tear (avulsion versus degeneration), the amount of footprint uncovered, and the activity level of the patient.

   c. Patients with a preponderance of impingement findings and a tear of less than 50% thickness may benefit from débridement and subacromial decompression. Despite the excellent results reported with RTC repair, a high percentage of repairs either do not heal or re-tear. Despite this outcome, functional and subjective results remain high. A correlation appears to exist between younger age and repair success.

E. Subscapularis tears—May occur after anterior dislocation and anterior shoulder surgery (e.g., shoulder arthroplasty). Symptoms include increased external rotation and the presence of a liftoff, modified liftoff, or belly-press sign. Surgical treatment, either open or arthroscopic, is generally indicated, with chronic cases occasionally requiring a pectoralis transfer.

F. RTC arthropathy—Defined as a massive RTC tear combined with fixed superior migration of the humeral head and severe GH arthrosis, presumably due to chronic loss of the concavity-compression effect. Hemiarthroplasty may be helpful if the anterior deltoid is preserved. This is a good option for patients with pain as the predominant symptom. The use of a reverse shoulder prosthesis remains controversial. It requires a competent deltoid and good glenoid bone stock. It is recommended only for older patients (typically over the age of 70 years) with low functional demands. More predictable functional results are seen with the reverse prosthesis than hemiarthroplasty, but a high rate of complications (40%) has been reported with its use.

G. Subcoracoid impingement—Patients with long or excessively laterally placed coracoid processes may have impingement of this process on the proximal humerus with forward flexion (120-130 degrees) and internal rotation of the arm. This condition may occur after surgery that causes posterior capsular tightness and loss of internal rotation. Local anesthetic injection should relieve these symptoms. A CT scan performed with the arms crossed on the chest is helpful to evaluate this problem. Less than 7 mm between the humerus and coracoid process is considered to be abnormal. Treatment of chronic symptoms involves resection of the lateral aspect of the coracoid process and reattachment of the conjoined tendon to the remaining coracoid. Arthroscopic coracoplasty has also been successful in treating this condition without detachment of the conjoined muscle group.

H. Internal impingement

1. Impingement of the posterior labrum and cuff can occur in a throwing-motion or overhead-movement athletes with external rotation and anterior translation (secondary impingement). A Bennett lesion (glenoid exostosis) may occasionally be seen on radiographs. It is often associated with **glenohumeral internal rotation deficit** (GIRD) secondary to a tight posterior capsule. Glenohumeral kinematics is altered, leading to a posterosuperior shift of the humeral head, with abduction and external rotation of the arm leading to the internal impingement. This may lead to pain associated with SLAP/biceps

anchor pathology a well as undersurface RTC tears of the posterior aspect of the supraspinatus and infraspinatus tendons. A "peel-back" phenomenon of the superior labrum can be appreciated intraoperatively with abduction and external rotation of the arm.

2. Treatment—Primary treatment should include physical therapy and avoidance of aggravating activities. Patients with GIRD may benefit from posterior capsular stretching exercises such as the sleeper stretch. Diagnosis can be aided with an MR arthrogram. An ABER view can at times show the internal impingement and associated lesions. Operative treatment includes arthroscopic débridement or repair of the labrum, with débridement of the undersurface RTC lesion. Some suggest repairing the RTC if it is significantly thinned either by using a trans-cuff technique or by taking down the remaining thinned cuff and advancing the unaffected normal tendon. A posterior capsular release can be considered in those that have GIRD and have failed to improve with nonoperative stretching.

VI. Superior Labral and Biceps Tendon Injuries

A. Superior labrum lesions—SLAP lesions have been classified into many varieties (Fig. 4–47), with specific types associated with instability and RTC disease. In addition to biceps tenderness patients may exhibit a positive active compression (O'Brien's) test, anterior slide, or crank test. The dynamic labral shear test has recently been described, with a sensitivity of 86% and specificity of 100% in diagnosing a SLAP tear (Table 4–14). Treatment involves débridement (types I and III) with or without stabilization of the biceps anchor (types II and IV).

B. Biceps tendinitis—Often associated with impingement, RTC tears (subscapularis and leading-edge supraspinatus tears), and stenosis of the bicipital groove. Like most other cases of "tendinitis," this is probably best considered to be a "tendinosis." Diagnosis is made by direct palpation, with the arm internally rotated 10 degrees, and confirmed with Speed and Yergason tests. Initial management includes strengthening and local injection (around but not into the tendon). Surgical release (with or without tenodesis) is usually reserved for refractory cases.

C. Biceps tendon subluxation—This is most commonly associated with a subscapularis tear. A tear of the CHL or transverse humeral ligament may produce tendon subluxation as well. Arm abduction and external rotation may produce a palpable click with palpation as the tendon subluxates or dislocates outside of the groove. Nonoperative treatment is similar to that for tendinitis, whereas operative treatment includes repair of the subscapularis and supporting structures of the bicipital groove but more often involves tenotomy or tenodesis.

VII. Acromioclavicular and Sternoclavicular Injuries

A. AC separation

1. Overview—These injuries are typically caused by a direct blow to the shoulder, are common athletic injuries, and can be classified into six types (Fig. 4–48).
2. Treatment of type III injuries—Management of type III injuries is somewhat controversial, with most advocating conservative treatment and some advocating surgical reduction and repair or reconstruction. The literature suggests that those treated acutely with surgery have a higher rate of reoperation than that of primary surgery for those who are initially treated nonoperatively.
3. Management of types IV through VI injuries—These are typically treated surgically. Note that a type V injury is defined by a coracoclavicular distance that is greater than 100% of the opposite side (bilateral AC views are required), and a type IV injury can only be diagnosed on an axillary lateral view.
4. Surgical treatment of failed, conservatively treated injuries or acute treatment—Involves reduction of the AC joint by various methods. Coracoclavicular (CC) ligament reconstruction with a free soft tissue graft is now becoming popular to allow for an anatomic reconstruction. The distal clavicle is often resected in the chronic situation, and the CA ligament may then be transferred to the distal clavicle (modified Weaver-Dunn). Backup CC stabilization is usually required for a successful outcome. Free tendon grafts have recently been advocated for anatomic CC reconstructions.

B. AC DJD—Due to the transmission of large loads through a small surface area, the AC joint may begin to degenerate as early as the second decade. Additionally, direct blows or low-grade AC separation may cause post-traumatic arthritis. The condition is diagnosed by direct palpation, pain elicited by crossed-chest adduction, radiographic evidence of osteophytes and joint-space narrowing, and pain relief with selective AC joint injection. Treatment includes both open and arthroscopic distal clavicle resections (Mumford procedure).

C. Distal clavicle osteolysis—Common in weightlifters and those with a history of traumatic injury. Radiographs of the distal clavicle reveal osteopenia, osteolysis, tapering, and cystic changes. After failure of selective corticosteroid injection, NSAIDs, and activity modification, this condition responds favorably to distal clavicle excision.

D. SC subluxation/dislocation—Often caused by motor vehicle accidents or direct trauma, this injury can be best diagnosed by CT. Plain imaging includes the Hobbs and Serendipity views. Closed reduction is often successful. The posterior capsule is the most important for anteroposterior

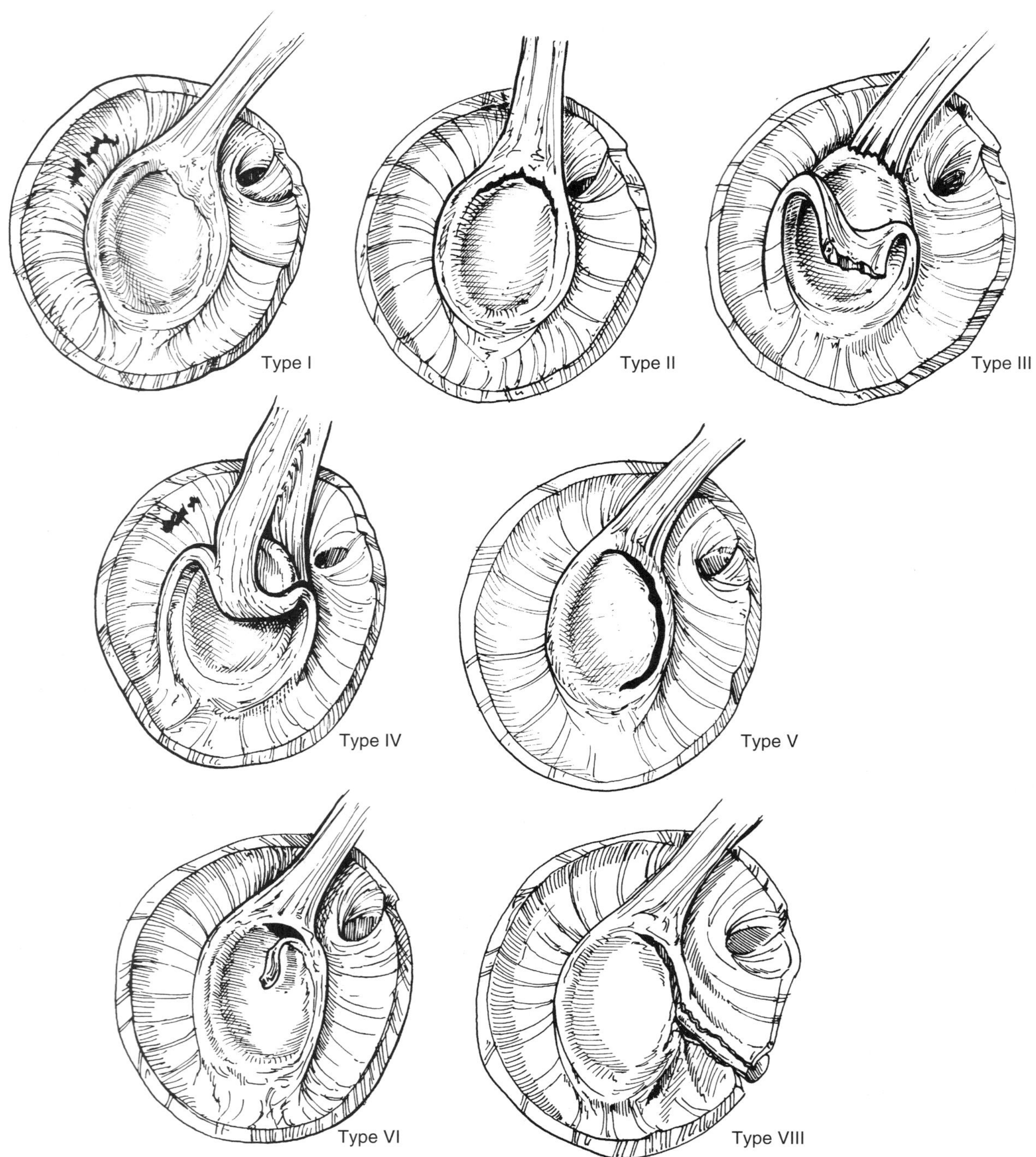

FIGURE 4–47 Anterior and posterior lesion types I-IV and V-VII of the superior labrum. (From Miller MD, Osborne JR, Warner JJP, et al: MRI-Arthroscopy Correlative Atlas, p 157. Philadelphia, WB Saunders, 1997.)

translation. Anterior dislocation should be first treated with acute, closed reduction. Failed attempts and chronic dislocations are treated conservatively. Posterior dislocation should undergo closed reduction and open reduction if necessary, particularly with compression of the posterior structures. Consultation with a cardiothoracic surgeon may be appropriate. The use of hardware should be avoided whenever possible.

VIII. Muscle Ruptures

A. Pectoralis major—Injury to this muscle is caused by excessive tension on a maximally eccentrically contracted muscle, often found in weightlifters. Localized swelling and ecchymosis, a palpable defect, and weakness with adduction and internal rotation are characteristic findings. Surgical repair to bone is usually necessary. Pectoralis major ruptures have not been reported in females.

TABLE 4-14 SUPERIOR LABRAL AND BICEPS TENDON INJURIES

Type	Description	Treatment
I	Biceps fraying, intact anchor on superior labrum	Arthroscopic débridement
II	Detachment of biceps anchor	Reattachment/stabilization
III	Bucket-handle superior labral tear; biceps intact	Arthroscopic débridement
IV	Bucket-handle tear of superior labrum into biceps	Repair or tenodesis of tendon based on symptoms and condition of remaining tendon
V	Labral tear + SLAP	Stabilize both
VI	Superior flap tear	Débride
VII	Capsular injury + SLAP	Repair and stabilize

SLAP, superior labrum from anterior to posterior.

B. Deltoid—Complete rupture of this muscle is unusual, and injuries are most often strains or partial tears. Repair to bone is required for complete ruptures. Iatrogenic injury may occasionally occur during open RTC repair, with some cases requiring deltoidplasty, which consists of mobilization and anterior transfer of the middle third of the deltoid. Unfortunately, this procedure is not always possible or successful.

C. Triceps—Ruptures of the triceps is most often associated with systemic illness (e.g., renal osteodystrophy) or steroid use. Primary repair of avulsions is indicated.

D. Latissimus dorsi rupture—This is a very rare condition exhibiting local tenderness and pain with shoulder adduction and internal rotation. Although nonoperative treatment may allow resumption of activities, operative repair has been described for the high-demand athlete.

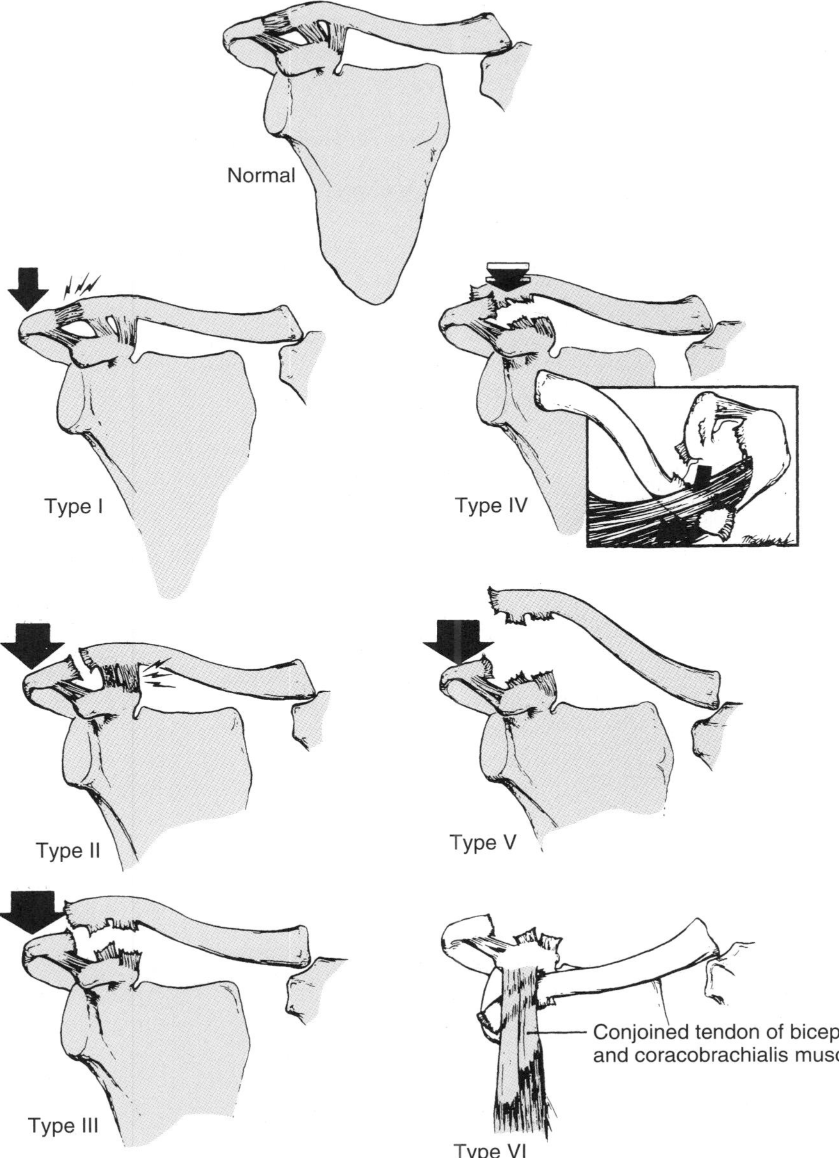

FIGURE 4–48 Classification of acromioclavicular (AC) separations. Type I injuries involve only an AC sprain. Type II injuries are characterized by a complete AC tear but intact coracoclavicular (CC) ligaments. Type III injuries involve both the AC and CC ligaments, with a CC distance of up to 100% of that of the opposite shoulder. Type IV injuries are associated with posterior displacement of the clavicle through the trapezius muscle. Type V injuries involve superior displacement, with a CC distance of more than twice that of the opposite side. This injury is usually associated with rupture of the deltotrapezial fascia, leaving the distal end of the clavicle subcutaneous. Type VI injuries are rare and defined on the basis of inferior displacement of the clavicle below the coracoid. (From Rockwood CA Jr, Young DC: Disorders of the acromioclavicular joint. In Rockwood CA Jr, Matsen FA III, eds: The Shoulder, 2nd ed, p 495. Philadelphia, WB Saunders, 1998.)

IX. Calcifying Tendinitis and Shoulder Stiffness

A. Calcifying tendinitis—A self-limiting condition of unknown etiology that affects predominantly the supraspinatus tendon and occurs slightly more frequently in women. Radiographs demonstrate characteristic calcification within the tendon. Three stages have been elucidated: precalcific, calcific, and postcalcific. Nonoperative treatment is the rule, consisting of physical therapy, modalities, and injections. "Needling" of the lesion under image guidance has been described and is often successful. Arthroscopic or open removal of the deposit is occasionally necessary. The rotator cuff should be repaired if it is significantly involved.

B. Shoulder stiffness

1. Adhesive capsulitis—This disorder (also known as "frozen shoulder") is characterized by pain and restricted GH joint motion. Factors associated with the development of adhesive capsulitis include trauma after chest or breast surgery, prolonged immobilization, diabetes, thyroid disease (etiology probably autoimmune), and other medical conditions. The essential lesion involves the CHL and the rotator interval capsule. Arthrography may demonstrate a loss of the normal axillary recess, revealing contracture of the joint capsule. Three clinical and four arthroscopic stages have been defined (Table 4–15).
2. Post-traumatic shoulder stiffness—This is an asymmetrical loss of GH motion secondary to a post-traumatic or postsurgical complication due to excessive scar formation. Motion loss is related to the area of surgery or trauma and may involve the humeroscapular motion interface between the proximal humerus and overlying deltoid and conjoined tendon as well as contracture of the RTC and capsule.
3. Treatment—For idiopathic adhesive capsulitis, a supervised physical therapy program combined with anti-inflammatory medications and/or glenohumeral steroid injections will successfully treat the majority of patients within 12 weeks. Prolonged post-traumatic shoulder stiffness is unlikely to respond to nonsurgical treatment. If no improvement is seen after 12-16 weeks of nonsurgical treatment, operative intervention consisting of open or arthroscopic lysis of adhesions and manipulation under anesthesia is recommended.

TABLE 4–15 STAGES OF SHOULDER STIFFNESS

Stage	Characteristics
Clinical	
Painful	Gradual onset of diffuse pain
Stiff	Decreased ROM; affects activities of daily living
Thawing	Gradual return of motion
Arthroscopic	
1	Patchy, fibrinous synovitis
2	Capsular contraction, fibrinous adhesions, synovitis
3	Increased contraction, resolving synovitis
4	Severe contraction

ROM, range of motion.

X. Nerve Disorders

A. Brachial plexus injury—Minor traction and compression injuries, commonly known by football players as "burners" or "stingers," can be serious if they are recurrent or persist for more than a short time. Injury results from compression of the plexus between the shoulder pad and the superior medial scapula when the pad is compressed into Erb's point superior to the clavicle. Complete resolution of symptoms is required before return to play. If burners occur more than one time, the player should be removed from competition until cervical spine radiographs can be obtained. Three grades of nerve injury are commonly recognized (Table 4–16).

B. Thoracic outlet syndrome—Compression of the nerves and vessels that pass through the scalene muscles and first rib can result in this disorder. This condition can be associated with cervical rib, scapular ptosis, or scalene muscle abnormalities. Patients may note pain and ulnar paresthesias. Wright's test (see Table 4–9) and neurological evaluation can be diagnostic. First-rib resection is occasionally required.

C. Long thoracic nerve palsy—Injury to this nerve can result in medial scapular winging secondary to serratus anterior dysfunction. This condition can be caused by a compression injury (such as that occurring in backpackers) or traction injury (as seen in weightlifters). Simple observation is usually called for because many of these injuries spontaneously resolve within 18 months. Treatment with a modified thoracolumbar brace may be beneficial, and (rarely) pectoralis major transfer may be required for chronic palsies that do not recover.

D. Suprascapular nerve compression—This nerve may become compressed by various structures, including a ganglion in the spinoglenoid notch or suprascapular notch or fracture callus in the area of the transverse scapular ligament. Weakness and atrophy of the supraspinatus (proximal lesions) and infraspinatus are present along with pain over the dorsal aspect of the shoulder. Cysts within the spinoglenoid notch affect only the infraspinatus. Electrodiagnostic studies and MRI may confirm and elucidate the nature of the nerve compression. Compression due to a cyst associated with a SLAP lesion may respond to arthroscopic decompression and labral repair. In the absence of a

TABLE 4–16 GRADES OF NERVE INJURY

Grade	Description	Pathophysiology
1	Neurapraxia	Selective demyelination of the axon sheath
2	Axonotmesis	Disruption of axon and myelin sheath
3	Neurotmesis	Disruption of epineurium and endoneurium

structural lesion, release of the transverse scapular ligament may provide relief.

E. Quadrilateral space syndrome—This condition is defined as axillary nerve compression within the quadrilateral space and is characterized by pain and paresthesias with overhead activity. This is most often seen in throwing athletes and is associated with late cocking and acceleration with the abducted, extended, and externally rotated arm. Diagnosis is confirmed by compression of the posterior humeral circumflex artery on arteriogram.

F. Other nerve injuries—Other injuries, including those of the axillary nerve, the spinal accessory nerve (lateral scapular winging), and the musculocutaneous nerve, are usually the result of surgical injury to these structures. Several months of observation is appropriate before considering exploration and repair of the affected nerve.

XI. Other Shoulder Disorders

A. GH DJD—Although it is more common in older patients, athletes who engage in throwing may develop arthritis at a younger age than usual. Arthritis may also be associated with other shoulder disorders, including instability and RTC disease. Certain iatrogenic factors may also contribute to the development of osteoarthritis of the shoulder, including the use of hardware in and around the shoulder and overtightening of the shoulder capsule during shoulder reconstruction. Radiographs, including a true anteroposterior view taken in abduction, can be helpful in characterizing the amount of arthritis. In some cases, arthroscopic débridement may be a temporizing measure before considering joint arthroplasty. Progressive pain, decreased ROM, and the inability to perform activities of daily living are reasonable indications for considering prosthetic replacement.

B. Scapulothoracic crepitus—This condition is also known as "snapping scapula syndrome." The presentation is that of painful scapulothoracic crepitus associated with elevation of the arm. Scapulothoracic dyskinesis may be present, and the pain is generally relieved with manual stabilization of the scapula. Many possible causes of symptomatic crepitus exist. Patients may respond to scapular strengthening exercises, local injections, or anti-inflammatory medications. The differential diagnosis includes osteochondroma and elastofibroma dorsi. For more refractory cases, open or arthroscopic bursectomy and sometimes resection of the superomedial scapular border are necessary.

C. Scapular winging—Can occur as a result of a nerve injury, bony abnormality, muscle contracture, intra-articular pathology, or voluntarily. The description of the direction of the winging is based on the movement of the inferior border of the scapula. Nerve injuries include injury to the spinal accessory nerve (trapezius palsy, lateral winging), the long thoracic nerve (serratus anterior palsy, medial winging), and the dorsal scapular nerve (rhomboid palsy). Osseous causes include osteochondromas and fracture malunions. Selective muscle strengthening may improve winging. Surgical treatment includes lateral transfer of the levator scapulae and rhomboids (Eden-Lange procedure) for lateral winging and pectoralis major transfer for medial winging.

D. Complex regional pain syndrome (formerly known as "reflex sympathetic dystrophy")—As in the knee, this condition is fraught with a poor response to both conservative and surgical treatments and, in a litigious medicolegal environment, is often associated with malingering and issues of secondary gain. Diagnosis may be confirmed with a three-phase bone scan. Treatment options are numerous and may include sympathetic nerve block.

E. Little Leaguer's shoulder—This disorder commonly occurs in young baseball players and is actually a Salter-Harris type I fracture of the proximal humerus. Overuse of the shoulder as a result of failure to limit pitch count and provide periods of adequate rest are the key factors implicated in the development of this condition. It has also been suggested that breaking pitches not be thrown until after skeletal maturity is reached. Radiographs may demonstrate widening of the proximal humeral physis. MRI can assist with the diagnosis if it is in question. The condition responds to rest and activity modification, with return to play allowed when symptoms have resolved completely. Recommendations regarding age and pitch counts have been made (Table 4–17).

TABLE 4–17 PITCH COUNT RECOMMENDATIONS FOR YOUTH BASEBALL

	Pitch Count			
Age	*Per Game*	*Per Week*	*Per Season*	*Per Year*
9-10	50	75	1000	2000
11-12	75	100	1000	3000
13-14	75	125	1000	3000

SECTION 5 Elbow

I. Tendon Injuries

A. Lateral epicondylitis (tennis elbow)

1. Causes and diagnosis—Commonly occurs with activities that involve repetitive pronation and supination of the forearm with the elbow in near extension (backhand in tennis). The injury is initiated as a microtear at the origin of the extensor carpi radialis brevis (ECRB) but may also involve the

origin of the extensor carpi radialis longus (ECRL) and extensor carpi ulnaris (ECU). Microscopic evaluation of this tissue shows angiofibroblastic hyperplasia. Diagnosis is clinical, with reproducible, localized tenderness at the extensor origin and reproduction of symptoms with resisted wrist extension.

2. Treatment—Treatment is predominantly nonoperative, with activity modification (slower playing surfaces, more flexible racquet, lower string tension, larger grip), physical therapy (stretching, ultrasound), anti-inflammatory medications, counterforce bracing, and up to three corticosteroid injections at the site of maximum tenderness, all achieving up to 95% success. Recalcitrant cases require open or arthroscopic débridement of the ECRB origin (Fig. 4–49). Excessive resection can jeopardize the LCL and should be avoided.

B. Medial epicondylitis (golfer's elbow)—This condition is classified as an overuse syndrome of the flexor/pronator mass. It is much less common and more difficult to treat than tennis elbow. Resisted forearm pronation and wrist flexion worsen the pain. Treatment is similar to that for lateral epicondylitis. Multiple corticosteroid injections and medial epicondylectomy should be avoided.

C. Distal biceps tendon rupture—Occurs almost exclusively in men after forceful, eccentric overload of the partially flexed elbow. Up to 50% loss of supination power has been documented after rupture. Intraosseous tendon reattachment with the two-incision (Boyd-Anderson) technique has been traditionally favored. A one-incision technique is coming back into favor with some by using a single-incision repair with an endobutton, suture anchors, or an interference screw. In a cadaveric model, the endobutton had the greatest load to failure when compared with the standard suture technique, suture anchors, and interference screw fixation. Cyclic loading did not show any statistically significant differences in gap formation among the fixation techniques. Care must be taken not to disrupt the syndesmosis. Complications include neurovascular injury, loss of motion, and heterotopic ossification.

D. Distal triceps tendon avulsion—This extremely uncommon injury results from a deceleration force to the outstretched elbow and is associated with multiple corticosteroid injections or chronic olecranon bursitis. Repair with transosseous tunnels is mandatory for the restoration of extension power.

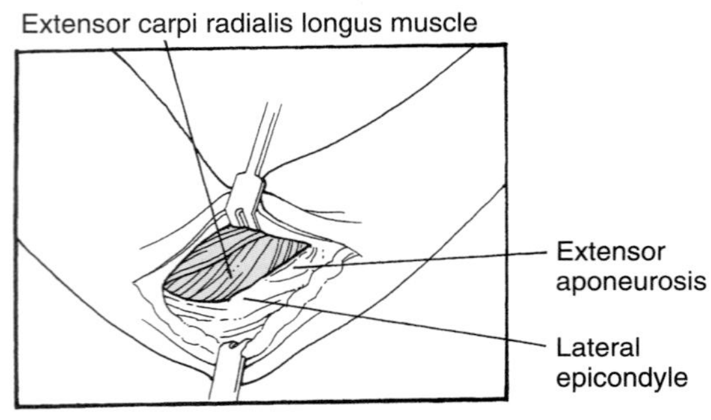

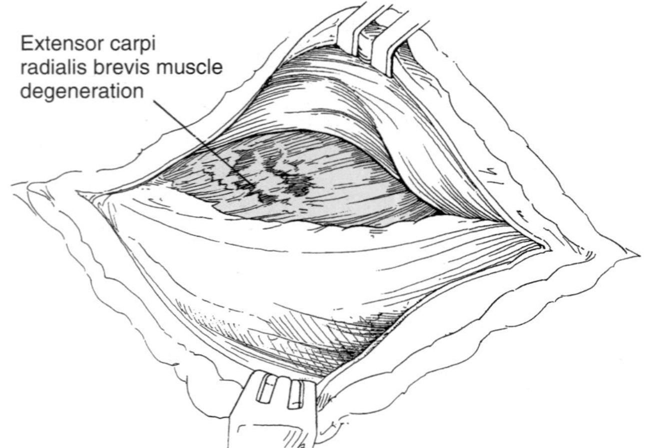

FIGURE 4–49 Operative exposure for lateral epicondylitis. (From Miller MD, Cooper DE, Warner JJP: Review of Sports Medicine and Arthroscopy, p 178. Philadelphia, WB Saunders, 1995.)

II. Ligament Injuries

A. Ulnar collateral ligament (UCL) injury

1. Causes and diagnosis—Repetitive, high-velocity valgus stress to the medial aspect of the elbow results in attenuation or rupture of the anterior band of the UCL. The late-cocking and acceleration phases of throwing are periods of high stress generation. Patients present with acute or chronic medial elbow tenderness and (frequently) associated ulnar nerve symptoms. The pain is localized to the course of the ligament from the medial epicondyle to the sublime tubercle. Valgus instability is demonstrable in only 50% of patients because it is usually a dynamic phenomenon (Fig. 4–50). The "moving valgus stress test" of O'Driscoll has been shown to have a high sensitivity and specificity in detecting UCL injury. An MR arthrogram is useful for confirmation of the diagnosis.

2. Treatment—Initial treatment is with rest, physical therapy, and maintenance of joint motion. Surgery is required only in high-level athletes who desire a return to sports. Ligament reconstruction is favored over direct repair, and treatment of chronic injuries has demonstrated better results than those of acute injuries. The ligament is reconstructed with a palmaris tendon graft woven in a figure-eight fashion (Tommy John procedure) (Fig. 4–51). Nearly 75-80% of patients return to sports at the same or better level 1 year after reconstruction. Complications include loss of motion, graft site morbidity, and neurologic injury.

B. LCL injury—Typically the first ligament disrupted in elbow dislocation. Patients with LCL insufficiency may complain of clicking or locking with elbow extension and often demonstrate posterolateral rotatory instability (Fig. 4–52). Surgical reconstruction with a palmaris longus autograft and capsular

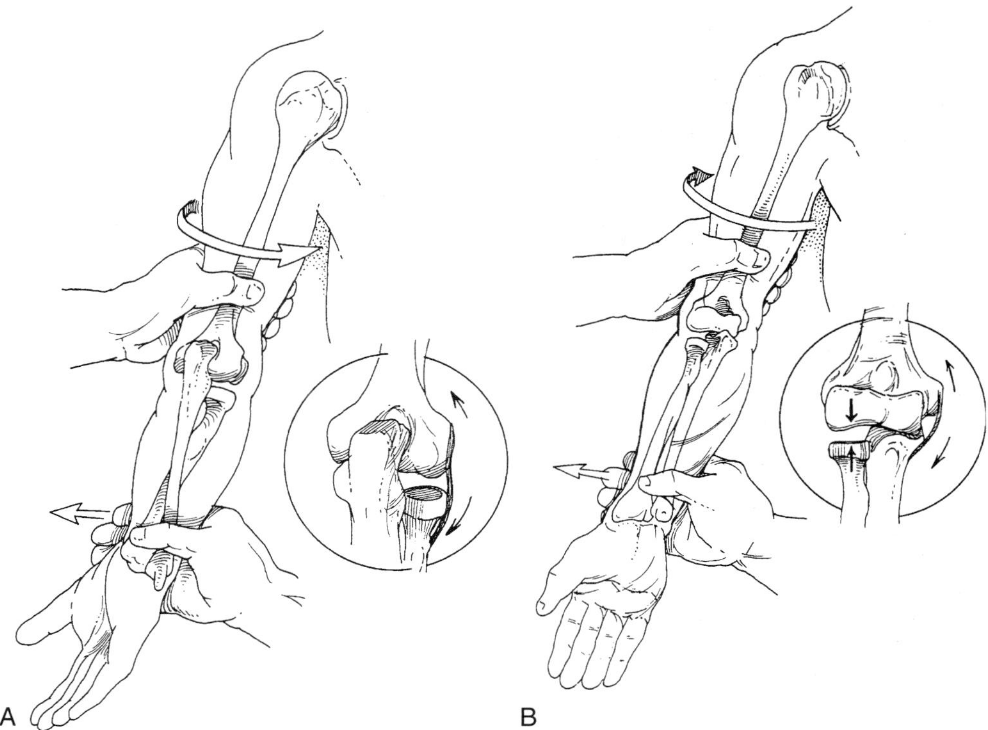

FIGURE 4–50 Varus (**A**) and valgus (**B**) instability testing of the elbow. Note the position and rotation of the arm. (From Morrey BF: The Elbow and Its Disorders, 2nd ed, p 83. Philadelphia, WB Saunders, 1994.)

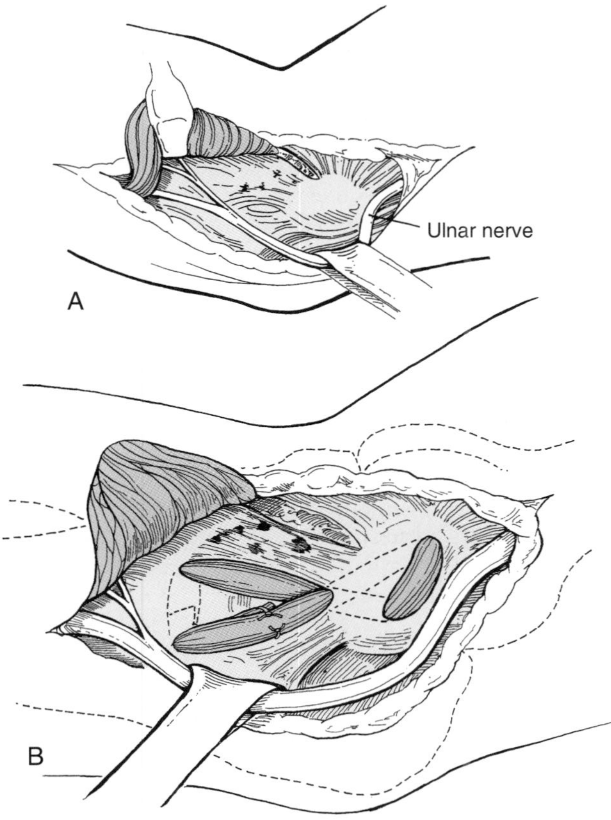

FIGURE 4–51 Reconstruction of the (medial) ulnar collateral ligament. **A**, Exposure with protection of the ulnar nerve. **B**, Figure 8 palmaris graft (Tommy John procedure). (From Miller MD, Cooper DE, Warner JJP: Review of Sports Medicine and Arthroscopy. Philadelphia, WB Saunders, 1995, p 179.)

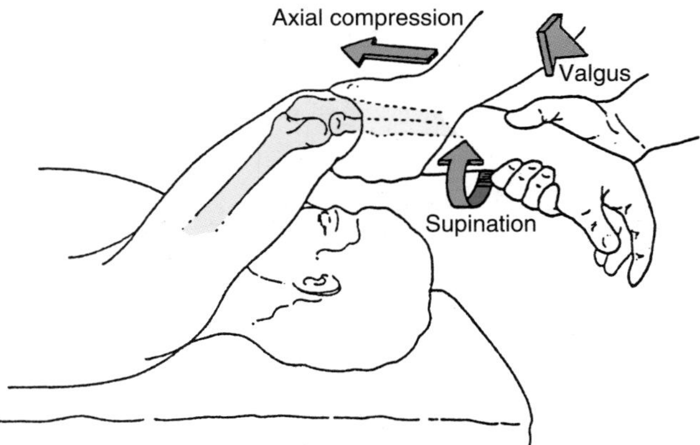

FIGURE 4–52 Lateral pivot shift test of the elbow for posterolateral rotatory instability. (Redrawn from O'Driscoll SW, Bell DF, Morrey BF: Posterolateral instability of the elbow. J Bone Joint Surg [Am] 73:404-446, 1991.)

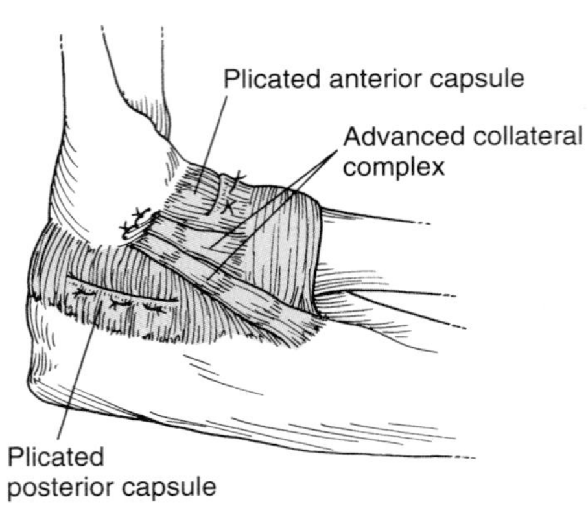

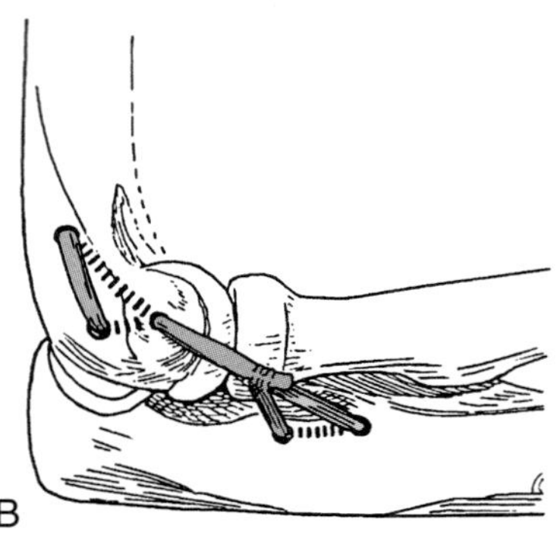

FIGURE 4–53 **A**, Imbrication and advancement of the ulnar band and radial part of the radial collateral ligament, respectively. **B**, Palmaris longus tendon through the ulnar and humeral tunnels and tied to itself. (From Canale ST, ed: Campbell's Operative Orthopaedics, 9th ed, p 1397. St. Louis, CV Mosby, 1998.)

plication is indicated for patients with recurrent instability, pain, or mechanical symptoms (Fig. 4–53).

III. Articular Injuries

A. Osteochondritis dissecans—Typically occurs in the capitellum of the adolescent athlete engaged in repetitive overhead or upper extremity weight-bearing activities. The cause is thought to be related to vascular insufficiency and repetitive microtrauma. Plain radiographs and improvement with activity modification confirm the diagnosis. If the fragment is stable, this condition can be treated with activity modification and supportive methods. Separated fragments may be arthroscopically reduced and stabilized or excised and the defects drilled. Osteochondrosis of the capitellum is seen in younger patients (Panner's disease) and is associated with a more benign course.

B. Little Leaguer's elbow—This condition is defined as a stress fracture of the medial epicondyle in adolescents due to repetitive valgus loading with throwing. Rest and limitation of the number of innings pitched per week help to reduce the incidence of complete fracture (see Table 4–17).

C. Pitcher's elbow—Involves medial tension, lateral compression, and posterior extension overload. Adaptive changes common to this condition include increased valgus, pronator mass hypertrophy, and loss of extension. Radiographic changes include posteromedial olecranon osteophytes and chondromalacia of the medial wall of the olecranon fossa.

D. Osteoarthritis—Primary elbow osteoarthritis disproportionately affects football linemen, participants in racquet sports, and throwers. These patients present with a decreased arc of motion and pain at the extremes of motion. Plain radiographs demonstrating joint space narrowing and osteophytic spurring confirm the diagnosis. Surgical treatment consists of arthroscopic débridement, soft tissue release, and loose-body removal. Persistent symptoms are treated with distraction/interposition arthroplasty, ulnohumeral arthroplasty, or total elbow arthroplasty.

IV. Elbow Stiffness

A. The loss of motion and function results from capsular contracture; olecranon, coronoid, and radial fossa overgrowth; or heterotopic ossification about the elbow after a single acute injury or because of degenerative disease. Treatment involves open surgical débridement by means of a collateral ligament–sparing approach (Hastings-Cohen), olecranon fossa fenestration and débridement (Outerbridge-Kashiwagi procedure) (Fig. 4–54), or arthroscopic osteocapsular arthroplasty with resection of bone osteophytes and resection of the capsule. Success is largely dependent on a motivated patient. Loss of terminal extension is common after elbow dislocation and is usually managed with simple observation.

V. Elbow Arthroscopy (see Color Plates)

A. Indications—This procedure is typically indicated for diagnostic confirmation of suspected elbow pathology; removal of loose bodies; treatment of osteochondritis dissecans of the capitellum;

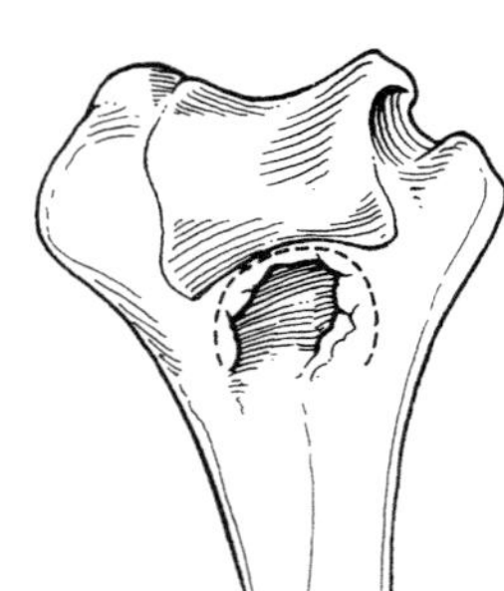

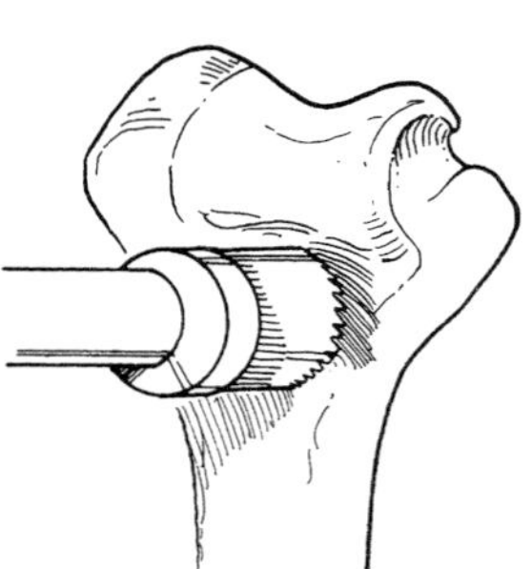

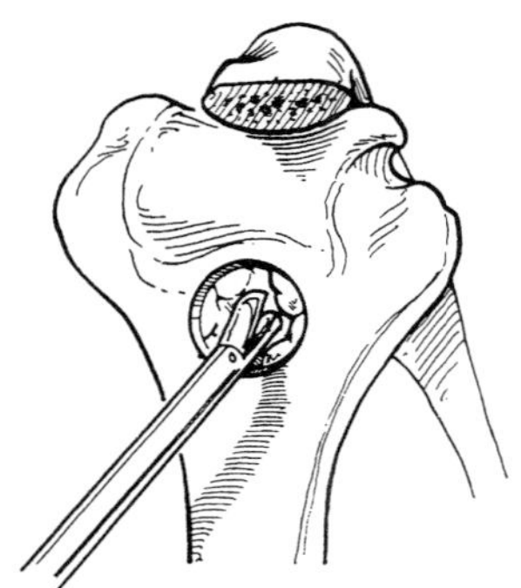

FIGURE 4–54 Outerbridge-Kashiwagi arthroplasty performed through a triceps-splitting approach. The coronoid is approached through a Cloward drill hole in the olecranon fossa. The olecranon can also be débrided with this approach. (From Miller MD, Cooper DE, Warner JJP: Review of Sports Medicine and Arthroscopy, p 180. Philadelphia, WB Saunders, 1995.)

osteophyte débridement (as seen with chronic valgus overload in pitchers); capsular release and débridement of the olecranon, radial, and coronoid fossa in the stiff elbow; and synovectomy. Successful arthroscopic intervention depends on technical expertise in elbow arthroscopy and thorough anatomic familiarity because vital neurovascular structures are proximal to the intra-articular space and are thus prone to injury, particularly with overexuberant débridement.

B. Risks—The "nick and spread" method of portal placement is used to minimize inadvertent neurovascular injury. The use of far-proximal portals may decrease these risks. Other risks include injury to the ulnar nerve (proximal medial portal) and brachial artery injury with loose-body removal (anteriorly).

C. Portals—The following represent the common portals (Fig. 4–55).

1. Anterolateral portal—Placed after joint distention 1 cm distal and 1 cm anterior to the lateral epicondyle. The lateral antebrachial cutaneous and radial nerves are at risk.
2. Anteromedial portal—Placed under direct visualization 2 cm distal and 2 cm anterior to the medial epicondyle. The medial antebrachial cutaneous and median nerves are at risk.
3. Posterolateral portal—Placed 2 cm proximal to the olecranon and just lateral to the triceps tendon.

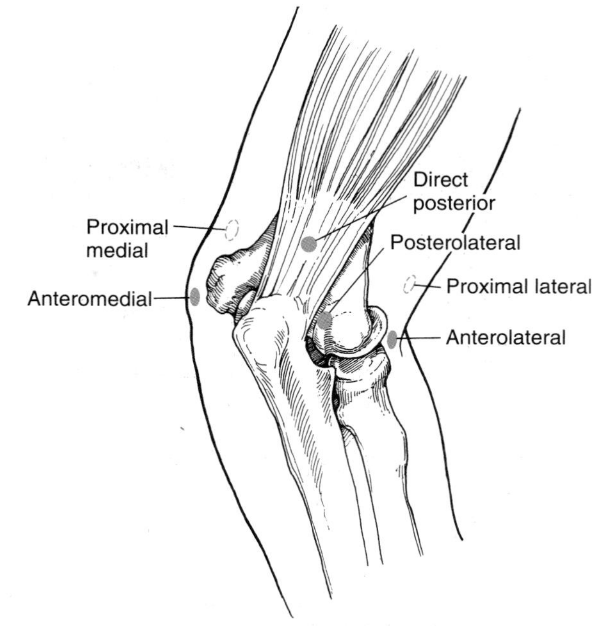

FIGURE 4–55 Arthroscopic portals for elbow arthroscopy. (From Miller MD, Osborne JR, Warner JJP, et al: MRI-Arthroscopy Correlative Atlas, p 197. Philadelphia, WB Saunders, 1997.)

SECTION 6 Hand and Wrist

I. Tendon Injuries (Fig. 4–56)

A. De Quervain disease—Refers to stenosing tenosynovitis of the first dorsal wrist compartment (abductor pollicis longus [APL] and extensor pollicis brevis [EPB]) and typically occurs in racquet sports and in golfers. Ulnar deviation of the wrist with the thumb in the palm (Finkelstein's test) generally reproduces patient symptoms. Treatment includes activity modification, splinting, local corticosteroid injection, and occasionally surgical release (Fig. 4–57). The APL and EPB may lie in separate subsheaths in the first dorsal compartment, and care must be taken to release both of them.

B. Flexor carpi radialis/flexor carpi ulnaris tendinitis—Wrist flexor tendinitis is common and is associated with overuse, especially in golfers and in players of racquet sports. Ulnar deviation and supination lead to dislocation. Activity modification, splinting, and NSAIDs are generally effective. Surgical tenolysis is rarely necessary.

C. Extensor carpi ulnaris tendinitis—Tendinitis or subluxation of the sixth dorsal compartment frequently occurs in tennis and hockey players. Patients experience painful snapping with forearm supination (tendon subluxates) and pronation (tendon reduces). This condition must be distinguished from other ulnar wrist disorders. Long-arm cast immobilization in

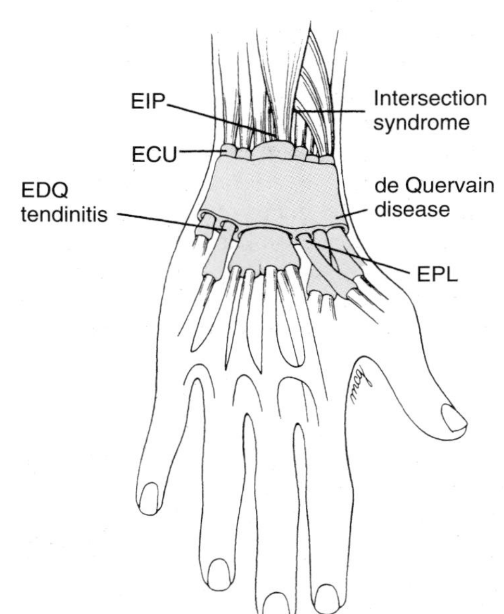

FIGURE 4–56 Location of common sites of tendinitis about the wrist. ECU, extensor carpi ulnaris; EDQ, extensor digiti quinti; EIP, extensor indicis proprius; EPL, extensor pollicis longus. (From Kiefhaber TR, Stern PJ: Upper extremity tendinitis and overuse syndromes in the athlete. Clin Sports Med 11:43, 1992.)

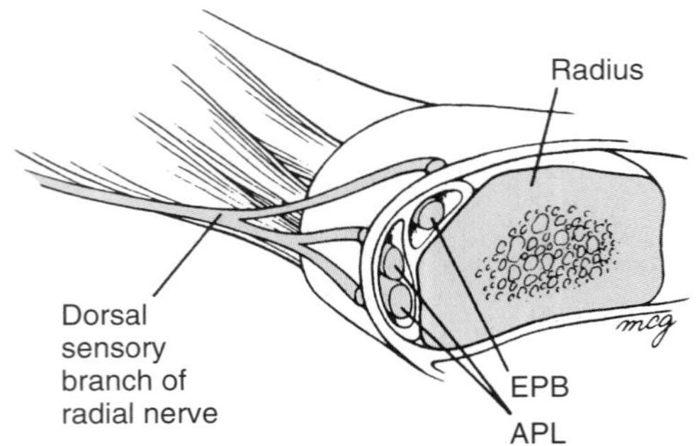

FIGURE 4–57 Surgical release of the first compartment for refractory de Quervain's syndrome should include preservation of the dorsal sensory branch of the radial nerve. APL, abductor pollicis longus; EPB, extensor pollicis brevis. (From Kiefhaber TR, Stern PJ: Upper extremity tendinitis and overuse syndromes in the athlete. Clin Sports Med 11:44, 1992.)

pronation may allow healing. Surgical débridement of the sixth dorsal compartment and reconstruction of the fibro-osseous tunnel with a slip of extensor retinaculum are occasionally necessary (Fig. 4–58).

D. Intersection syndrome—Involves painful crepitus at the dorsal forearm due to irritation and inflammation of the crossing point of the first (APL and EPB) with the second (ECRL and ECRB) dorsal compartments and is typically seen in rowers and weightlifters. Splinting and local injections are typically effective for this self-limiting condition. Surgical decompression of the crossing point is rarely necessary.

E. Other extensor tendon tendinitis—May affect the extensor pollicis longus (EPL), extensor indicis proprius (EIP), or extensor digiti quinti (EDQ) and is usually responsive to local measures and surgical release, if indicated.

F. "Jersey finger"—Refers to an avulsion injury of the flexor digitorum profundus tendon from its insertion at the base of the proximal interphalangeal joint (PIP), with the ring finger being the most commonly affected. The avulsion occurs with sudden hyperextension during finger flexion and may be seen on plain x-ray. The Leddy classification describes three types: type I, retraction of tendon into palm; type II, retraction to PIP; and type III; associated with a large, bony articular fragment, usually without significant retraction due to the A4 pulley. These injuries require retrieval of the retracted tendon and reattachment to the base of the PIP. Type I injuries must be repaired early (within 1 week) because of loss of blood supply to the tendon. Arthrodesis is generally favored over late (>3 months) repair due to finger stiffness after tendon grafting.

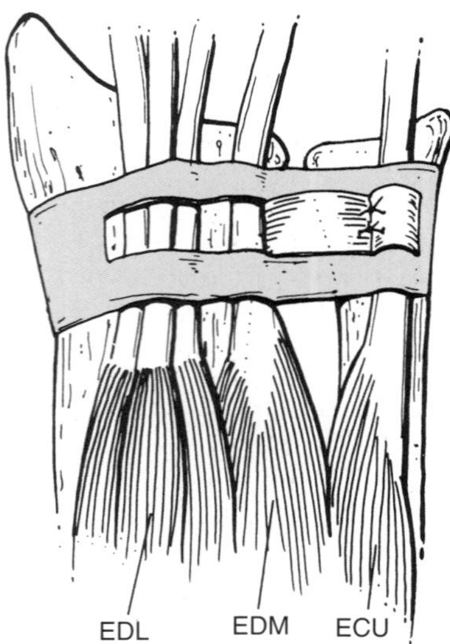

FIGURE 4–58 Stabilization of the extensor carpi ulnaris (ECU) with a flap of the extensor retinaculum. EDL, extensor digitorum longus; EDM, extensor digiti minimi. (From Spinner M, Kaplan EB: Extensor carpi ulnaris. Clin Orthop 68:124-129, 1970.)

G. "Mallet finger"—Refers to an avulsion of the terminal extensor tendon. X-ray is used to rule out fracture. These injuries are typically treated with prolonged (>6 weeks) extension splinting. Results are almost uniformly good. Chronic injuries may result in significant swan-neck deformities due to chronic overpull of the extensor tendon at the PIP with flexion of the distal interphalangeal joint (DIP). Chronic deformities in young patients with preserved passive finger motion may be corrected by restoring the balance between extensors and flexors.

H. Sagittal band rupture ("boxer's knuckle")—Typically occurs in pugilists due to forceful subluxation of the extensor tendon. This condition usually involves the index and long fingers in professionals and the ring and small fingers in amateurs. Acute injuries are treated with extension splinting for 4 weeks. Chronic injury will lead to persistent extensor tendon subluxation and should be repaired or reconstructed with a slip of extensor tendon looped around the collateral ligament.

II. Ligament Injuries

A. Scapholunate (SL) ligament injury

1. Diagnosis—The most common wrist ligament injury. Patients experience snuffbox tenderness after hyperextension of a pronated wrist, such as that occurring after a fall. Radial deviation of the hand with volar stabilization of the scaphoid (Watson test) may reproduce pain. Radiographic hallmarks include an increased SL interval (>3 mm), a cortical ring sign (proximal and distal poles of scaphoid overlap on posteroanterior projection), and an increased SL angle (>70 degrees) on lateral projection. Persistent SL dissociation with attenuation of extrinsic structures leads to an extended posture of the lunate (dorsal intercalated segment instability [DISI]) (Fig. 4–59) that unloads its articulation with the radius and increases contact forces at the radioscaphoid articulation, leading to progressive arthrosis. Diagnosis may be made with an MR arthrogram, which may help to increase the sensitivity and specificity.
2. Treatment—Treatment involves either closed reduction and percutaneous pinning of the SL joint for 8-10 weeks or open reduction and internal fixation of the articulation combined with a capsulodesis. Partial tears can be treated with débridement or thermal modulation.

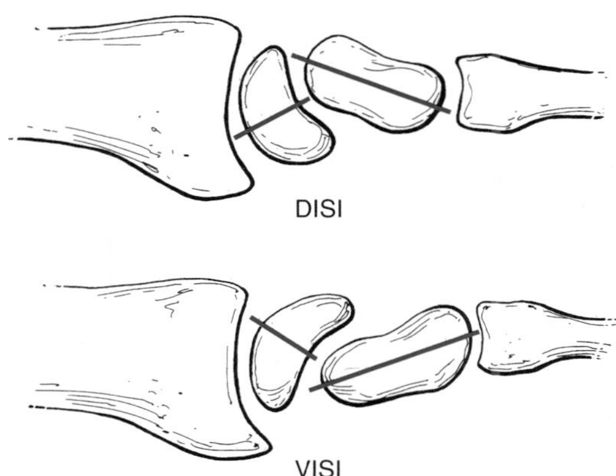

FIGURE 4–59 Scapholunate instability is associated with a dorsal intercalated instability pattern (dorsal intercalated segmental instability [DISI]). Triquetrum-lunate instability may have a volar intercalated instability pattern (volar intercalated segmental instability [VISI]). Note the increased scapholunate angle (> 60 degrees) with the DISI pattern (normal, 30 degrees). (From McCue FC, Bruce JF: The wrist. In DeLee JC, Drez D Jr, eds: Orthopaedic Sports Medicine: Principles and Practice, p 918. Philadelphia, WB Saunders, 1994.)

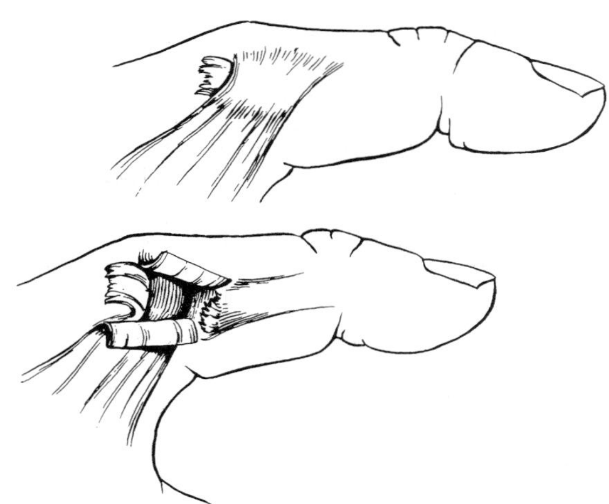

FIGURE 4–60 Stener's lesion. The adductor aponeurosis separates the two ends of the ulnar collateral ligament, and the aponeurosis must be incised to repair the ligament. (From Green DP, Strickland JW: The hand. In DeLee JC, Drez D Jr, eds: Orthopaedic Sports Medicine: Principles and Practice, p 976. Philadelphia, WB Saunders, 1994.)

B. **Lunotriquetral** (LT) ligament injury—LT ligament injury is less common than SL ligament injury. Patients describe ulnar-sided wrist pain after a fall that is worse with pronation and ulnar deviation (power grip). Examination seeks to distinguish LT injuries from the spectrum of injuries that usually accompany them (chondral lesions, triangular fibrocartilage complex [TFCC] tears). Pain is reproduced with ballottement or shuck of the LT articulation. Radiographic hallmarks include widening of the LT interval, volar flexion of the lunate, an increase in the capitolunate angle, and a decrease in the SL angle. An MR arthrogram may help to confirm the diagnosis. Treatment after failure of conservative care is through débridement of the LT ligament with or without ulnar shortening. Arthrodesis is useful for refractory cases.

C. Hand ligament injury
   1. Digital collateral ligament injury—Often the result of a "jammed finger." Simple tears are managed with buddy taping for 3 weeks, whereas complete tears should be buddy taped for 6 weeks. Radial collateral ligament injury of the index finger PIP should be surgically repaired because of the need for pinch stability of this joint.
   2. PIP dislocation—Typically occurs in a dorsal direction and results in a volar plate injury. Reduction is usually accomplished by the athlete, and incomplete reduction may be due to volar plate interposition. After reduction, the finger is buddy taped to the adjacent digit for 3-6 weeks. ROM should begin early. A flexion contracture of the PIP joint (pseudo-boutonnière) may develop late but generally resolves with therapy and appropriate splinting. Volar PIP dislocation (central slip injury) is unusual and generally results in a tear of the central slip insertion. Treatment includes 6-8 weeks of immobilization with the PIP joint in extension.
   3. Collateral ligament injury of the thumb—Includes radial and ulnar collateral ligament injuries; "gamekeeper's or skier's thumb." Instability should be examined in extension and at 30 degrees. X-rays are helpful to rule out fracture, with stress x-rays and MRI also playing a role in confirming the diagnosis. Nondisplaced, bony avulsions should not undergo stress radiography because of the risk of displacement. Incomplete ulnar injuries may be immobilized. Injuries with greater than 15 degrees of side-to-side difference or greater than 45 degrees of opening require operative intervention because the aponeurosis of the adductor becomes interposed between the ends of the torn ligament (Stener's lesion) (Fig. 4–60). Aponeurotic interposition does not occur on the radial side. These rare injuries are often treated closed.

III. Fractures

A. Scaphoid fracture—Fractures here occur frequently in contact sports. Because the vascular supply enters distally, proximal fractures have a high rate of nonunion and avascular necrosis. Acute and subacute, nondisplaced fractures less than 8 weeks old may be treated in a thumb-spica cast. Percutaneous fixation of nondisplaced fractures leads to earlier union, ROM, return to work, and possibly return to play. Displaced fractures should be managed operatively with either percutaneous or limited open fixation. Nonunion may be managed with a local vascularized bone graft and internal fixation. A CT scan can be used to assess displacement, while MRI is helpful to rule out occult fracture and assess vascularity.

B. Hamate fracture—Hook-of-hamate fractures typically occur in a golfer or baseball batter after repeated direct contact. Diagnosis is confirmed by a carpal tunnel view or CT scan. Treatment is either cast immobilization or excision of the hook. The latter allows more rapid return to play.

C. Metacarpal and phalanx fractures—Many of these fractures heal with closed reduction and immobilization. Fourth and fifth metacarpal fractures can accept greater angulation than the index and long finger. Displaced fractures, those involving the joints, and those resulting in rotational malalignment should be treated surgically. Early motion is the key to successful rehabilitation. Fractures involving the base of the thumb carpometacarpal (CMC) joint (Bennett's fracture, Rolando's fracture) often require operative reduction and stabilization.

IV. Ulnar Wrist Pain

A. Differential diagnosis—The differential diagnosis of ulnar-sided wrist pain in athletes includes TFCC tear, pisotriquetral arthritis, fracture (ulnar styloid, hook-of-hamate), LT ligament injury, ECU subluxation or tendinitis, ulnar nerve entrapment at Guyon's canal, ulnar artery thrombosis (hypothenar hammer syndrome), chondral lesions, and wrist ganglia.

B. TFCC/DRUJ (distal radioulnar joint)—Patients seek treatment after a fall onto a pronated, extended wrist or after a traction injury to the ulnar aspect of the wrist. Point tenderness is present at the base of the "ulnar snuffbox," which is between the triquetrum and ulnar styloid. Symptoms are reproduced with ulnar deviation (compresses TFCC) or radial deviation (applies tension to peripheral tear). Diagnosis can also be made clinically, with pain associated with wrist extension and applied axial load with resisted pronosupination. Arthrography and MRI may help diagnosis a tear, but both are highly user dependent and have a high rate of false-positive results (Table 4–18). Arthroscopy is the diagnostic gold standard. Treatment is based on tear type, the presence of DRUJ instability/arthritis, and ulnar variance. See Figure 4–61 for the treatment algorithm.

C. Ulnocarpal abutment syndrome—Typically occurs in patients with ulnar-positive variance. Pain is exacerbated with rotation or ulnar loading of the wrist. Sclerotic and cystic changes may be seen in the lunate and distal ulna. If supportive measures fail, ulnar shortening (wafer procedure, ulnar-shortening osteotomy) provides predictable pain relief. Ulnar head resection (Darrach), hemiresection with interpositional arthroplasty, the Suave-Kapandji

TABLE 4–18 CLASSIFICATION OF INJURIES TO THE TRIANGULAR FIBROCARTILAGE COMPLEX

Class	Description	Treatment
1A	Horizontal tear adjacent to sigmoid notch	Débridement
1B	Avulsion from ulna ± ulnar styloid fracture	Suture repair
1C	Avulsion from carpus; exposes pisiform	Débridement
1D	Avulsion from sigmoid notch	Débridement
2A	Thinning of triangular fibrocartilage complex without perforation	Débridement
2B	Thinning of disc with chondromalacia	Débridement
2C	Perforation of disc with chondromalacia	Débridement
2D	Perforation of disc, chondromalacia, partial tear of lunotriquetral ligament	Débridement
2E	Perforation of disc, chondromalacia, complete tear of lunotriquetral ligament, ulnocarpal degenerative joint disease	Débridement

Note: Type 1, traumatic lesions; type 2, degenerative lesions. Treatment for degenerative lesions includes débridement of loose, degenerated discs; intra-articular resection of the ulnar head; and débridement of lunotriquetral ligament tears with percutaneous pinning of the lunotriquetral joint based on the pathology present.

From Miller MD, Cooper DE, Warner JJP, et al: Review of Sports Medicine and Arthroscopy, p 188. Philadelphia, WB Saunders, 1995.

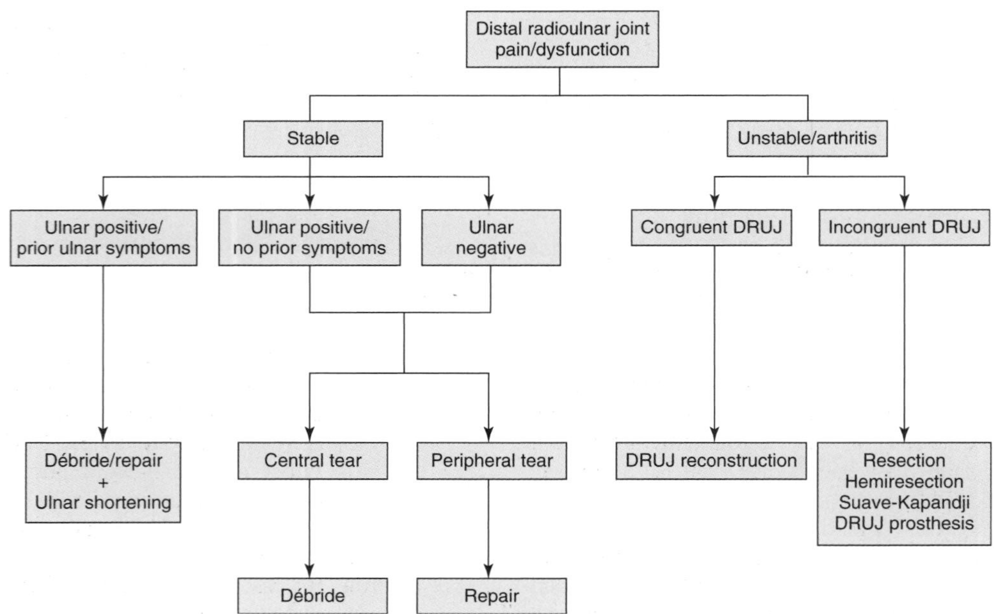

FIGURE 4–61 Algorithmic approach to treatment of injuries to the triangular fibrocartilage complex. DRUJ, distal radioulnar joint.

procedure, and prosthetic ulnar head replacement are useful if significant arthritis is present.

D. Hypothenar hammer syndrome—Involves ulnar artery constriction, which can occur in baseball pitchers. Allen's test will show decreased ulnar filling. Doppler evaluation and vascular referral may be necessary.

E. Guyon's canal syndrome (handlebar palsy)—This condition is characterized by pain and ulnar paresthesias, with weakness of the intrinsic hand muscles. Treatment includes modification of the cyclist's grip and occasionally ulnar nerve decompression.

V. Post-traumatic Dysfunction of the Wrist and Hand

A. Scaphoid avascular necrosis—A common complication due to the tenuous blood supply of this bone. Bone grafting and internal fixation are usually curative. Unrecognized injuries may lead to the development of scaphoid nonunion–advanced collapse (SNAC), which in turn requires radial styloid excision, scaphoid excision and partial wrist arthrodesis (four-corner fusion), proximal row carpectomy, and/or total wrist fusion.

B. Osteochondrosis of the capitate—Most often found in gymnasts and may respond to débridement or limited wrist fusions.

C. Kienbock's disease—Avascular necrosis and collapse of the lunate is probably related to overuse and ulnar negative wrist variance. Early in the disease process, ulnar lengthening or radial shortening may be helpful in arresting progression to collapse. Limited wrist fusions may be necessary for cases of advanced collapse.

VI. Wrist Arthroscopy

A. Introduction—This procedure serves as a useful diagnostic and staging adjunct and as an alternative to arthrotomy for the manipulation of intra-articular structures. It is indicated for the establishment of a diagnosis for unexplained wrist pain, treatment of mechanical symptoms secondary to interosseous ligament injuries or TFCC tears, assistance in the anatomic reduction and fixation of intra-articular fractures, débridement of chondral lesions, removal of loose bodies, and synovectomy.

B. Technique—The wrist is placed in a traction apparatus, and a 2.5- or 3.0-mm scope is used. Portals are named in relation to the dorsal wrist compartments (Fig. 4–62). The 3-4 portal is established first and the 4-5 portal is used for instrumentation. The 6R portal serves as a useful adjunct for visualization and instrumentation. The midcarpal portals are necessary for complete carpal visualization, and the radiocarpal portals often allow confirmation of pathology. The scaphotrapeziotrapezoid (STT) portal is typically used by advanced arthroscopists to evaluate localized pathology.

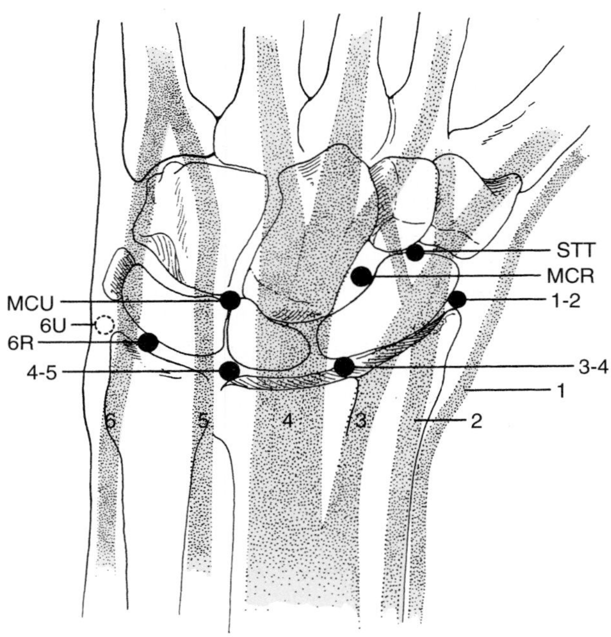

FIGURE 4–62 Arthroscopic wrist portals. Numbers indicate wrist extensor compartments and associated portals. MCR, midcarpal radial; MCU, midcarpal ulnar; R, radial; STT, scaphotrapeziotrapezoid; U, ulnar. (From Miller MD, Osborne JR, Warner JJP, et al: MRI-Arthroscopy Correlative Atlas, p 220. Philadelphia, WB Saunders, 1997.)

SECTION 7 Head and Spine

I. Head Injuries

A. Diffuse brain injuries—Include mild and "classic" cerebral concussions and diffuse axonal injury. Mild concussions occur without loss of consciousness and can be subdivided into three grades, which are shown in Table 4–19.

B. Postconcussion syndrome

1. Presentation—Characterized by persistent headaches, irritability, confusion, and difficulty concentrating and can occur with grades 2 and 3 mild concussions. Classic concussion includes a period of loss of consciousness. If it lasts more than 5 minutes, head CT should be obtained.
2. Evaluations—Can be made with the **standard assessment of concussion** (SAC), neuropsychological testing, memory testing, and the **balance error scoring system** (BESS).
3. Return to play—The athlete can return to play 1 week to 1 month after the first episode; after a second episode, the athlete should be out for the entire season. Diffuse axonal injury occurs with loss of consciousness lasting over

TABLE 4–19 GRADES OF MILD CONCUSSIONS

Grade	Symptoms	Duration	Recommended RTP
1	Confusion, no amnesia	Minutes	When symptoms resolve
2	Retrograde amnesia	Hours to days	1 wk
3	Amnesia after impact	Days	1 mo

RTP, return to play.

6 hours; athletes who suffer this injury should consider total avoidance of future contact sports. Return to play should be prohibited if there is loss of consciousness, symptoms lasting more than 15 minutes, recurrence of symptoms with exertion, amnesia, and a history of prior concussion.

C. Second-impact syndrome—May occur with a second minor blow before initial symptoms have resolved. Leads to loss of autoregulation of the brain's blood supply and potential herniation. Second-impact syndrome is associated with a 50% mortality rate.

D. Focal brain syndromes—Include contusions, intracranial hematomas, epidural hematomas, and subdural hematomas. CT scanning is helpful for distinguishing these entities (Fig. 4–63). Although epidural hematomas are classically said to be characterized by a period of lucidity followed by loss of consciousness, this sequence may not occur. Neurosurgical consultation and monitoring in an intensive care unit are necessary. Surgical treatment of intracranial hematomas may be indicated and are followed by seizure prophylaxis.

E. Prevention—Head protection, especially in contact sports, equestrian events, hockey, boxing, skating, and skiing, should be encouraged. Strict adherence to guidelines for return to play for these injuries can minimize the risk of second-impact syndrome.

II. Cervical Spine Injuries

A. Introduction—Catastrophic injury to the cervical spine is unfortunately all too common in contact sports (especially football and rugby). Soft tissue injuries of the cervical spine, as well as fractures and dislocations in athletes, are treated in the same manner as that used to treat other traumatic injuries to the spine (see Chapter 8, Spine). Underlying cervical stenosis, or narrowing of the **anteroposterior diameter of the spine (<13 mm)**, can make these injuries worse (Fig. 4–64). Recommendations for return to play for athletes with cervical stenosis with transient symptoms are controversial (see below). Congenital conditions of the odontoid are usually contraindications to participation in contact sports. Football players who repeatedly use poor tackling techniques can develop a condition known as "spear tackler's spine," which includes developmental cervical stenosis, loss of lordosis, and other radiographic abnormalities. The return to contact sports should be avoided. Spinal cord injury may lead to thermoregulatory problems.

B. On-field management—As with any trauma victim, careful handling of the patient and immobilization are critical. The mechanism of injury usually involves an axial load with flexion and compression of the spine. In football, the helmet and shoulder pads should not be removed. However, the facemask should be removed in the event that an emergent airway is needed. The sequence for proper cervical spine stabilization includes the following:
   1. Stabilize the head
   2. Log-roll the individual to the supine position
   3. Take off the facemask (**not** helmet)
   4. Administer cardiopulmonary resuscitation (CPR) if necessary
   5. Apply a backboard
   6. Transport the individual

C. No return to play—Criteria include transient quadriplegia with severe stenosis; cervical neurapraxia with ligamentous instability; congenital anomalies, with failure of fusion (os odontoideum, odontoid agenesis, odontoid hypoplasia); and spear tackler's spine.

III. Thoracic and Lumbar Spine Injuries*

A. Overview—Injuries commonly associated with sports include muscle injury, fractures, disc disease, and spondylolysis/spondylolisthesis.

*See Chapter 8, Spine, for a more complete description of these injuries.

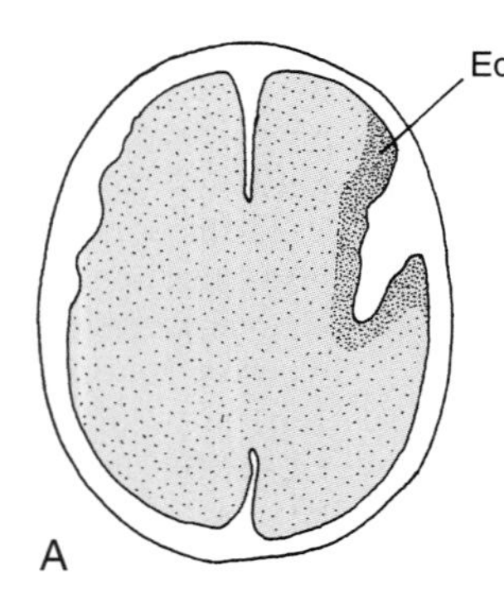

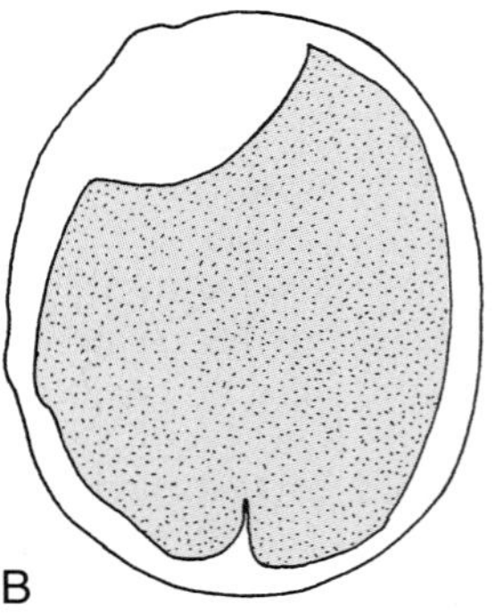

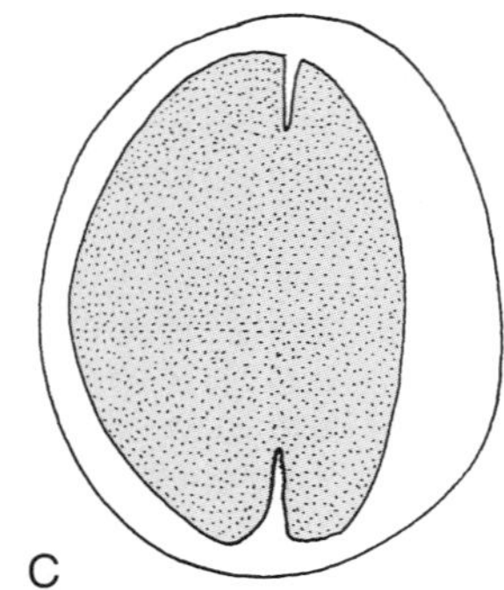

FIGURE 4–63 Computed tomographic findings. **A**, Contusion includes a hemorrhagic area and surrounding edema. **B**, Epidural hematomas typically have a biconvex appearance. **C**, Subdural hematomas have a concave or crescentic appearance. (From Miller MD, Cooper DE, Warner JJP: Review of Sports Medicine and Arthroscopy, p 204. Philadelphia, WB Saunders, 1995.)

B. Spondylolysis/spondylolisthesis
1. Diagnosis—This condition is common in football interior line positions and gymnasts owing to the repetitive hyperextension of the spine involved in these sports. Oblique radiographs (only 32% sensitive), bone scanning with **single-photon emission computed tomography** (SPECT) (the most sensitive and effective in the acute setting), and CT (useful in assessing healing) are all helpful for establishing the diagnosis.
2. Treatment—Treatment includes activity modification, bracing, and fusion for high-grade slips. Individuals with grade I or II injuries may play if they are asymptomatic. For those with grades III, IV, or V injuries who are experiencing intractable pain and/or a progressive slip, a posterolateral fusion should be considered.

C. **Herniated nucleus pulposus** (HNP)—Adolescent athletes may have a variety of findings that contribute to this diagnosis. Typical among these are pain that is worse in flexion, sitting intolerance, the presence of radicular symptoms, and testing for a positive **straight-leg raise** (SLR). Treatment depends on the degree of herniation and may range from core muscle strengthening and injections to surgical decompression with or without fusion.

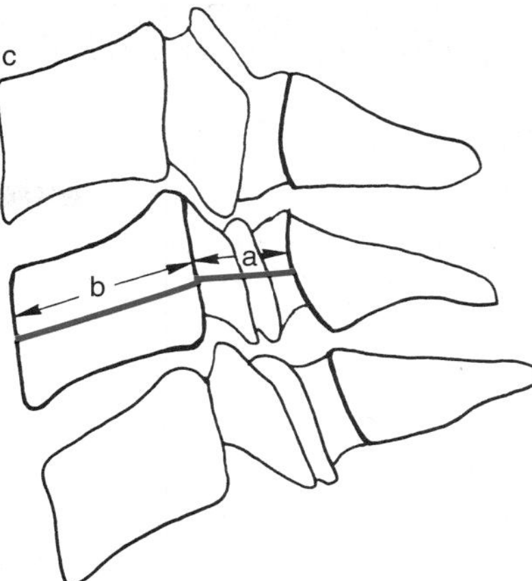

FIGURE 4–64 Pavlov's ratio (a/b) of 0.8 is consistent with cervical stenosis. (Note that this ratio may not apply to larger individuals.) (From Pavlov H, Porter IS: Criteria for cervical instability and stenosis. Op Tech Sports Med 1:170, 1993.)

SECTION 8 Medical Aspects of Sports Medicine

I. Preparticipation Physical Examination

The orthopaedic history questionnaire is the most helpful for identifying musculoskeletal problems. A family history of sudden cardiac death or any personal history of exertional chest pain or dyspnea requires further evaluation and cardiac workup.

II. Muscle Physiology

There are three types of muscle: I, IIA, and IIB. Muscle of type I is slow twitching/aerobic and is helpful in endurance sports. Training can increase the number of mitochondria and increase capillary density. Muscle of types IIA and IIB is fast twitching/anaerobic and is helpful for sprinters. These muscles have high contraction speeds, quick relaxation, and low triglycerine stores. The mode of energy utilization differentiates type IIA from type IIB muscle: IIA has both aerobic and anaerobic capabilities, whereas IIB is primarily anaerobic. Immobilization of muscle results in a shorter position with a decreased ability to generate tension.

III. Exercise

A. Benefits—Done on a regular basis, exercise can decrease heart rate and blood pressure (hypertension), decrease insulin requirements in diabetics, decrease cardiovascular risk, and increase lean body mass. It has also been shown to reduce cancer risk, osteoporosis, and hypercholesterolemia.

B. Aerobic threshold and conditioning—The aerobic threshold can be determined by measuring oxygen consumption and is useful for evaluating endurance athletes. Sports-specific conditioning involves aerobic and anaerobic conditioning in different proportions, based on the season and the sport. In the off-season, long-distance runs can enable sprinters to increase aerobic recovery capability after sprints. Several exercise categories have been described. Stretching has also been shown to have a beneficial effect (Table 4–20).

IV. Delayed-Onset Muscle Soreness

This condition often follows unaccustomed eccentric exercise, usually appearing 24-48 hours after the activity. The etiology involves inflammation and edema of the connective tissue, with elevated creatine kinase levels.

V. Cardiac Abnormalities in Athletes

A. Sudden cardiac death—Usually related to an underlying heart condition, especially hypertrophic cardiomyopathy in young athletes and coronary artery disease in older athletes. Screening that includes electrocardiography can identify this problem early.

B. Commotio cordis—Cardiac contusion from a direct blow to the chest (e.g., in Little League baseball) has a poor prognosis, even when immediately recognized and treated.

C. Hypertrophic cardiomyopathy and cardiac murmurs—Diastolic murmurs found on routine examination warrant further cardiac evaluation. Murmurs that

TABLE 4-20 EXERCISE TYPES

Exercise	Description	Benefit
Isometric	Muscle tension without change in unit length	Muscle hypertrophy; not endurance
Isotonic	Weight training with a constant resistance through arc of motion	Improved motor performance
Isokinetic	Weight training with a constant velocity, variable resistance	Increase strength; less time consuming but more expensive
Plyometric	Rapid shortening	Power generation
Functional	Aerobic fitness	Easily performed

increase in intensity with Valsalva maneuvers are consistent with hypertrophic cardiomyopathy. Sports participation is contraindicated in cases of outflow obstruction.

VI. Metabolic Issues in Athletes

A. Dehydration—Fluid and electrolyte loss can lead to decreased cardiovascular function and work capacity. Absorption is increased with solutions of low osmolarity (<10%).

B. Nutritional supplements—Continue to be a source of controversy. Creatine, one of the more popular supplements, increases the water retention in cells. In-season use can increase the incidence of dehydration and cramps. The use of glucosamine with chondroitin sulfate has yielded improvement over placebo in some studies of knee arthritis.

VII. Ergogenic Drugs

A. Anabolic steroids—Derivatives of testosterone are abused by athletes attempting to increase muscle mass and strength and increase erythropoiesis. Adverse effects include liver dysfunction, hypercholesterolemia, cardiomyopathy, testicular atrophy, gynecomastia, and irreversible alopecia. Urine sampling has been the standard for evaluation by the International Olympic Committee.

B. **Human growth hormone** (HGH)—Made from recombinant DNA; illegal use of this drug is common. Athletes attempting to increase muscle size and weight abuse this drug, which has side effects similar to those of steroids as well as hypertension and gigantism. **Insulin-like growth factor-1** (IGF-1) has effects similar to HGHs.

C. Prohormones—Derivatives of testosterone, **dehydroepiandrosterone** (DHEA) and androstenedione, have been used as anabolic agents. However, their effects are controversial.

D. Other commonly abused drugs—Include amphetamines, blood doping, diuretics, and laxatives

VIII. Female Athlete–Related Issues

A. Physiologic differences—Women are typically smaller and lighter and have higher body fat. Lower maximum oxygen consumption (max $\dot{V}O_2$), cardiac output, hemoglobin, and muscular mass/strength are also important considerations. Other differences contribute to the increased incidence of patellofemoral disorders, stress fractures, and knee ACL injuries in females (especially in basketball, soccer, and rugby).

B. Amenorrhea—This problem may be related to a low percentage of body fat and/or stress. The incidence approaches 50% in elite runners and is related to stress fractures (osteopenia) and eating disorders (female athlete triad). Dietary management and birth control pills are helpful in treating this problem.

IX. Other Sports-Related Injuries/Issues

A. Blunt trauma—Can cause injury to solid organs. These injuries may be subtle and require a high index of suspicion. The kidney is the most commonly injured organ (especially in boxing), followed by the spleen (injured in football).

B. Chest injuries—Can be serious and require immediate on-field action. Decreased breath sounds and hypotension may signify a tension pneumothorax. Treatment entails placing a 14-gauge intravenous needle in the second intercostal space at the midclavicular line, followed by the placement of a chest tube. Airway obstructions must also be anticipated and treated. Rib fractures may also occur in contact sports. The player usually has "had the air knocked out" of him or her, which is usually related to a problem with the diaphragm.

C. Eye injuries—These injuries are best avoided with proper protection. A hyphema (blood in the eye) is associated with a vitreous or retinal injury in more than 50% of cases.

D. Ear injuries—Auricular hematomas ("cauliflower ear"), common in wrestlers, should be treated with aspiration and wrapping.

E. Tooth injuries—The tooth or teeth should be replaced immediately but may be temporarily placed in the buccal fold or in milk if necessary.

F. Heat illness—Heat stroke, common during the football preseason, is characterized by collapse, with neurologic deficits, tachycardia, tachypnea, hypotension, and anhidrosis. Treatment involves rapidly cooling the body's core temperature. Heat stroke is the second leading cause of death in football players.

G. Cold injury—Rewarm in 110-112°F warm-water bath.

H. Exercise-induced bronchospasm—This condition involves transient airway obstruction resulting from exertion. Symptoms include the triad of coughing, shortness of breath, and wheezing. It commonly occurs in cold-weather sports, and the diagnosis is confirmed by a low forced expiratory volume. Inhaled β_2 agonists are the first-line treatment.

I. Pneumothorax—A chest tube or large-bore angiocatheter must be inserted at the second intercostal space for tension pneumothorax.

J. **Deep vein thrombosis** (DVT) after knee arthroscopy—A 10% incidence of DVT after knee arthroscopy, with 2% being proximal without prophylaxis. It is prudent to treat high-risk patients (older patient age, personal or family history of DVT, concomitant medical illness) with prophylaxis against DVT.

K. On-field bleeding—The affected player must be immediately removed from play and may not return until the bleeding has stopped and the wound has been covered with an occlusive dressing.

L. Infectious disease in athletes

1. **Methicillin-resistant *Staphylococcus aureus*** (MRSA)—Can be a training room disaster because it is spread by direct physical contact and sharing of equipment. It typically occurs around the area of previous skin trauma and is characterized by pustules on an erythematous base. It is treated with trimethoprim-sulfamethoxazole (Bactrim) and rifampin.
2. **Human immunodeficiency virus** (HIV)—An athlete's HIV status is confidential and by itself is insufficient reason to restrict athletic participation. Wound care in this population is the same as that for all athletes, with the use of universal precautions, application of compressive dressing, and waiting until the bleeding has stopped before a return to play.
3. Infectious mononucleosis—The primary concern for athletic participation in athletes that have been diagnosed with this condition is the risk of spleen rupture associated with it. Participation in contact sports should be restricted for 3-5 weeks, and splenomegaly must have resolved before a return to play.
4. Meningitis—A concern in athletes because of the ease of spread from the "close quarters" environment of the training room. Symptoms include fever, headache, and nuchal rigidity. The evaluation of **cerebrospinal fluid** (CSF) is important to identify cases of bacterial meningitis.
5. Other skin infections—Conditions such as tinea corporis ("ringworm"), herpes simplex, herpes gladiatorum, and impetigo are common in sports such as wrestling that involve close contact among athletes. Treatment is administered with antifungal and antiviral medications, as appropriate. Athletic participation should be restricted until all skin lesions have resolved.

M. Special athletes—Special considerations may be necessary for patients with congenital heart disease and Down syndrome. Patients with Down syndrome may have congenital cervical instability, which should be assessed radiographically before sports participation. More than 9 mm atlanto–dens interval (ADI) with flexion and extension views is an indication for surgical fusion.

Selected Bibliography

GENERAL

Buckwalter JA, Einhorn TA, Simon SR, eds: Orthopaedic Basic Science: Biology and Biomechanics of the Musculoskeletal System, 2nd ed. Rosemont, IL, American Academy of Orthopaedic Surgeons, 2000.

Koval KJ, ed: Orthopaedic Knowledge Update 7 American Academy of Orthopaedic Surgeons.

KNEE

Anatomy and Biomechanics

Arnoczky SP: Anatomy of the anterior cruciate ligament. Clin Orthop 172:19–25, 1983.

Arnoczky SP, Warren RF: Microvasculature of the human meniscus. Am J Sports Med 10:90–95, 1982.

Chhabra A, Elliot C, Miller MD: Normal anatomy and biomechanics of the knee. Sports Med Arthrosc Rev 9:166–177, 2002.

Cooper DE, Deng XH, Burnstein AL, et al: The strength of the central third patellar tendon graft: A biomechanical study. Am J Sports Med 21:818–824, 1993.

Daniel DM, Akeson WH, O'Connor JJ, eds: Knee Ligaments: Structure, Function, Injury, and Repair. New York, Raven Press, 1990.

Fu FH, Harner CD, Johnson DL, et al: Biomechanics of knee ligaments: Basic concepts and clinical application. J Bone Joint Surg 75:1716–1725, 1993.

Giffin JR, Vogrin TM, Zantop T, et al: Effects of increasing tibial slope on the biomechanics of the knee. Am J Sports Med 32:376–382, 2004.

Girgis FG, Marshall JL, Al Monajem ARS: The cruciate ligaments of the knee joint: Anatomical, functional and experimental analysis. Clin Orthop 106:216–231, 1975.

Jackson DW, Evans NA, Thomas BM: Accuracy of needle placement into the intra-articular space of the knee. J Bone Joint Surg [Am] 84:1522–1527, 2002.

Noyes FR, Butler DL, Grood ES, et al: Biomechanical analysis of human ligament grafts used in knee-ligament repairs and reconstructions. J Bone Joint Surg [Am] 66:344–352, 1984.

Seebacher JR, Inglis AE, Marshall JL, et al: The structure of the posterolateral aspect of the knee. J Bone Joint Surg [Am] 64:536–541, 1982.

Thompson WO, Theate FL, Fu FH, et al: Tibial meniscal dynamics using three-dimensional reconstruction of magnetic resonance images. Am J Sports Med 19:210–216, 1991.

Warren LF, Marshall JL: The supporting structures and layers of the medial side of the knee. J Bone Joint Surg [Am] 61:56–62, 1979.

Warren R, Arnoczky SP, Wickiewicz TL: Anatomy of the knee. In Nicholas JA, Hershman EB, eds: The Lower Extremity and Spine in Sports Medicine, pp 657–694. St. Louis, CV Mosby, 1986.

History and Physical Examination

Fetto JF, Marshall JL: Injury to the anterior cruciate ligament producing the pivot shift sign. J Bone Joint Surg [Am] 61:710–714, 1979.

Fulkerson JP, Kalenak A, Rosenberg TD, et al: Patellofemoral pain. Instr Course Lect 41:57–71, 1992.

Galway RD, Beaupre A, MacIntosh DL: Pivot shift. J Bone Joint Surg [Br] 54:763, 1972.

Hosea TM, Tria AJ: Physical examination of the knee: Clinical. In Scott WN, ed: Ligament and Extensor Mechanism Injuries of the Knee: Diagnosis and Treatment. St. Louis, CV Mosby, 1991.

Ritchie JR, Miller MD, Harner CD: History and physical examination of the knee. In Fu FH, Harner CD, Vince KG, eds: Knee Surgery. Baltimore, Williams & Wilkins, 1994.

Slocum DB, Larson RL: Rotatory instability of the knee. J Bone Joint Surg [Am] 50:211–225, 1968.

Imaging

Blackburne JS, Peel TE: A new method of measuring patellar height. J Bone Joint Surg [Br] 59:241–242, 1977.

Blumensaat C: Die lageabweichunger und verrenkungen der kniescheibe. Ergeb Chir Orthop 31:149–223, 1938.

Insall J, Salvati E: Patella position in the normal knee joint. Radiology 101:101–104, 1971.

Jackson DW, Jennings LD, Maywood RM, et al: Magnetic resonance imaging of the knee. Am J Sports Med 16:29–38, 1988.

Jackson RW: The painful knee: Arthroscopy or MR imaging. J Am Acad Orthop Surg 4:93–99, 1996.

Merchant AC, Mercer RL, Jacobsen RH, et al: Roentgenographic analysis of patellofemoral congruence. J Bone Joint Surg [Am] 56:1391–1396, 1974.

Moseley JB, O'Malley K, Petersen NJ, et al: A controlled trial of arthroscopic surgery for osteoarthritis of the knee. N Engl J Med 347:81–88, 2002.

Newhouse KE, Rosenberg TD: Basic radiographic examination of the knee. In Fu FH, Harner CD, Vince KG, eds: Knee Surgery, pp 313–324. Baltimore, Williams & Wilkins, 1994.

Rosenberg TD, Paulos LE, Parker RD, et al: The forty-five degree posteroanterior flexion weight-bearing radiograph of the knee. J Bone Joint Surg [Am] 70:1479–1483, 1988.

Thaete FL, Britton CA: Magnetic resonance imaging. In Fu FH, Harner CD, Vince KG, eds: Knee Surgery. Baltimore, Williams & Wilkins, 1994.

Vives MJ, Homesley D, Ciccotti MG, Schweitzer ME: Evaluation of recurring meniscal tears with gadolinium-enhanced magnetic resonance imaging: A randomized, prospective study. Am J Sports Med 31:868–873, 2003.

Knee Arthroscopy

DeLee JC: Complications of arthroscopy and arthroscopic surgery: Results of a national survey. Arthroscopy 4:214–220, 1988.

DiGiovine NM, Bradley JP: Arthroscopic equipment and set-up. In Fu FH, Harner CD, Vince KG, eds: Knee Surgery. Baltimore, Williams & Wilkins, 1994.

Gillquist J: Arthroscopy of the posterior compartments of the knee. Contemp Orthop 10:39–45, 1985.

Ilahi OA, Reddy J, Ahmad I: Deep venous thrombosis after knee arthroscopy: A meta-analysis. Arthroscopy 21:727–730, 2005.

Johnson LL: Arthroscopic Surgery: Principles and Practice, 3rd ed. St. Louis, CV Mosby, 1986.

O'Connor RL: Arthroscopy in the diagnosis and treatment of acute ligament injuries of the knee. J Bone Joint Surg [Am] 56:333–337, 1974.

Rosenberg TD, Paulos LE, Parker RD, et al: Arthroscopic surgery of the knee. In Chapman MW, ed: Operative Orthopaedics, pp 1585–1604. Philadelphia, JB Lippincott, 1988.

Small NC: Complications in arthroscopy: The knee and other joints. Arthroscopy 2:253–258, 1986.

Watanabe M, Takeda S: The number 21 arthroscope. J Jpn Orthop Assoc 34:1041, 1960.

Meniscus

Arnoczky SP, Warren RF, Spivak JM: Meniscal repair using an exogenous fibrin clot—an experimental study in dogs. J Bone Joint Surg [Am] 70:1209–1220, 1988.

Baratz ME, Fu FH, Mengato R: Meniscal tears: The effect of meniscectomy and of repair on intra-articular contact areas and stresses in the human knee. Am J Sports Med 14:270–275, 1986.

Belzer JP, Cannon WD: Meniscus tears: Treatment in the stable and unstable knee. J Am Acad Orthop Surg 1:41–47, 1993.

Boenisch UW, Faber KJ, Ciarelli M, et al: Pull out strength and stiffness of meniscal repair using absorbable arrows or Ti-Cron vertical and horizontal loop sutures. Am J Sports Med 27:626–631, 1999.

Carter TR: Meniscal allograft transplantation. Sports Med Arthrosc Rev 7:51–62, 1999.

Cannon WD, Vittori JM: The incidence of healing in arthroscopic meniscal repairs in anterior cruciate ligament reconstructed knees versus stable knees. Am J Sports Med 20:176–181, 1992.

DeHaven KE, Black KP, Griffiths HJ: Open meniscus repair: Technique and two to nine year results. Am J Sports Med 17:788–795, 1989.

DeHaven KE: Meniscus repair. Am J Sports Med 27:242–250, 1999.

Dickhaut SC, DeLee JC: The discoid lateral meniscus syndrome. J Bone Joint Surg [Am] 64:1068–1073, 1982.

Fairbank TJ: Knee joint changes after meniscectomy. J Bone Joint Surg [Br] 30:664–670, 1948.

Henning CE, Lynch MA, Yearout KM, et al: Arthroscopic meniscal repair using an exogenous fibrin clot. Clin Orthop Relat Res 252:64–72, 1990.

Jordan MR: Lateral meniscal variants: Evaluation and treatment. J Am Acad Orthop Surg 4:191–200, 1996.

Miller MD, Ritchie JR, Royster RM, et al: Meniscal repair: An experimental study in the goat. Am J Sports Med 23:124–128, 1995.

Miller MD, Warner JJP, Harner CD: Mensical repair. In Fu FH, Harner CD, Vince KG, eds: Knee Surgery. Baltimore, Williams & Wilkins, 1994.

Neuschwander DC, Drez D, Finney TP: Lateral meniscal variant with absence of the posterior coronary ligament. J Bone Joint Surg [Am] 74:1186–1190, 1992.

Noyes FR, Barber-Westin SD, Rankin M: Meniscal transplantation in symptomatic patients less than fifty years old. J Bone Joint Surg [Am] 86:1392–1404, 2004.

Parisien JS: Arthroscopic treatment of cysts of the menisci: A preliminary report. Clin Orthop 257:154–158, 1990.

Sekiya JK, Giffin JR, Irrgang JJ, et al: Clinical outcomes after combined meniscal allograft transplantation and anterior cruciate ligament reconstruction. Am J Sports Med 31:896–906, 2003.

Warren RF: Meniscectomy and repair in the anterior cruciate ligament–deficient patient. Clin Orthop 252:55–63, 1990.

Osteochondral Lesions

Bauer M, Jackson RW: Chondral lesions of the femoral condyles: A system of arthroscopic classification. Arthroscopy 4:97–102, 1988.

Buckwalter JA: Restoration of injured or degenerated articular cartilage. J Am Acad Orthop Surg 2:192–201, 1994.

Buckwalter JA, Mankin HJ: Articular cartilage (Parts I and II): Instructional course lectures. J Bone Joint Surg [Am] 79:600–632, 1997.

Bugbee WD, Convery FR: Osteochondral allograft transplantation. Clin Sports Med 18:67–75, 1999.

Cahill BR: Osteochondritis dissecans of the knee: Treatment of juvenile and adult forms. J Am Acad Orthop Surg 3:237–247, 1995.

Ecker ML, Lotke PA: Spontaneous osteonecrosis of the knee. J Am Acad Orthop Surg 2:173–178, 1994.

Horas U, Pelinkovic D, Herr G, et al: Autologous chondrocyte implantation and osteochondral cylinder transplantation in cartilage repair of the knee joint: A prospective, comparative trial. J Bone Joint Surg [Am] 85:185–192, 2003.

Guhl J: Arthroscopic treatment of osteochondritis dissecans. Clin Orthop 167:65–74, 1982.

Knutsen G, Engebretsen L, Ludvigsen TC, et al: Autologous chondrocyte implantation compared with microfracture in the knee: A randomized trial. J Bone Joint Surg [Am] 86:455–464, 2004.

Mandelbaum BR, Browne JE, Fu FH, et al: Articular cartilage lesions of the knee: Current concepts. Am J Sports Med 26:853–861, 1998.

Menche DS, Vangsness CT, Pitman M, et al: The treatment of isolated articular cartilage lesions in the young individual. AAOS Instr Course Lect 47:505–515, 1998.

Murray PB, Rand JA: Symptomatic valgus knee: The surgical options. J Am Acad Orthop Surg 1:1–9, 1993.

Newman AP: Articular cartilage repair: Current concepts. Am J Sports Med 26:309–324, 1998.

O'Driscoll SW: Current concepts review: The healing and regeneration of articular cartilage. J Bone Joint Surg [Am] 80:1795–1812, 1998.

Schenck RC, Goodnight JM: Current concepts review: Osteochondritis dissecans. J Bone Joint Surg [Am] 78:439–456, 1996.

Synovial Lesions

Curl WW: Popliteal cysts: Historical background and current knowledge. J Am Acad Orthop Surg 4:129–133, 1996.

Ewing JW: Plica: Pathologic or not?. J Am Acad Orthop Surg 1:117–121, 1993.

Flandry F, Hughston JC: Current concepts review: Pigmented villonodular synovitis. J Bone Joint Surg [Am] 69:942–949, 1987.

Knee Ligament Injuries

Almekinders LC, Dedmond BT: Outcomes of operatively treated knee dislocations. Clin Sports Med 19:503–518, 2000.

Albright JP, Brown AW: Management of chronic posterolateral rotatory instability of the knee: Surgical technique for the posterolateral corner sling procedure. AAOS Instr Course Lect 47:369–378, 1998.

Bergfeld JA, Graham SM, Parker RD, et al: A biomechanical comparison of posterior cruciate ligament reconstructions using single- and double-bundle tibial inlay techniques. Am J Sports Med 33:976–981, 2005.

Carson EW, Simonian PT, Wickiewicz TL, et al: Revision anterior cruciate ligament reconstruction. AAOS Instr Course Lect 47:361–368, 1998.

Chen FS, Rokito AS, Piutman MI: Acute and chronic posterolateral rotary instability of the knee. J Am Acad Orthop Surg 8:97–110, 2000.

Clancy WG, Ray JM, Zoltan DJ: Acute tears of the anterior cruciate ligament: Surgical versus conservative treatment. J Bone Joint Surg [Am] 70:1483–1488, 1988.

Cooper DE, Warren RF, Warner JJP: The posterior cruciate ligament and posterolateral structures of the knee: Anatomy, function, and patterns of injury. Instr Course Lect 40:249–270, 1991.

Dye SF, Wojtys EM, Fu FH, et al: Factors contributing to function of the knee joint after injury or reconstruction of the anterior cruciate ligament. J Bone Joint Surg [Am] 80:1380–1393, 1998.

Fowler PJ, Messieh SS: Isolated posterior cruciate ligament injuries in athletes. Am J Sports Med 15:553–557, 1987.

France EP, Paulos LE: Knee bracing. J Am Acad Orthop Surg 2:281–287, 1994.

Frank CB: Ligament healing: Current knowledge and clinical applications. J Am Acad Orthop Surg 4:74–83, 1996.

Frank CB, Jackson DW: Current concepts review: The science of reconstruction of the anterior cruciate ligament. J Bone Joint Surg [Am] 79:1556–1576, 1997.

Frassica FJ, Sim FH, Staeheli JW, et al: Dislocation of the knee. Clin Orthop 263:200–205, 1991.

Fu FH, Bennett CH, Lattermann C, Ma CB: Current trends in anterior cruciate ligament reconstruction, Part I. Am J Sports Med 27:821–830, 1999.

Fu FH, Bennett CH, Ma CB, Menetrey J, Lattermann C: Current trends in anterior cruciate ligament reconstruction, Part II. Am J Sports Med 28:124–130, 2000.

Good L, Johnson RJ: The dislocated knee. J Am Acad Orthop Surg 3:284–292, 1995.

Harner CD, Hoher J: Evaluation and treatment of posterior cruciate ligament injuries: Current concepts. Am J Sports Med 26:471–482, 1998.

Harner CD, Irrgang JJ, Paul J, et al: Loss of motion following anterior cruciate ligament reconstruction. Am J Sports Med 20:507–515, 1992.

Howell SM, Taylor MA: Failure of reconstruction of the anterior cruciate ligament due to impingement by the intercondylar roof. J Bone Joint Surg [Am] 75:1044–1055, 1993.

Indelicato PA: Isolated medial collateral ligament injuries in the knee. J Am Acad Orthop Surg 3:9–14, 1995.

Indelicato PA, Hermansdorfer J, Huegel M: Nonoperative management of complete tears of the medial collateral ligament of the knee in intercollegiate football players. Clin Orthop 256:174–177, 1990.

Larson RL, Taillon M: Anterior cruciate ligament insufficiency: Principles of treatment. J Am Acad Orthop Surg 2:26–35, 1994.

Lopez MJ, Markel MD: Anterior cruciate ligament rupture after thermal treatment in a canine model. Am J Sports Med 31:164–167, 2003.

Margheritini F, Mauro CS, Rihn JA, et al: Biomechanical comparison of tibial inlay versus transtibial techniques for posterior cruciate ligament reconstruction: Analysis of knee kinematics and graft in situ forces. Am J Sports Med 32:587–593, 2004.

Miller MD, Bergfeld JA, et al: The posterior cruciate ligament injured knee: Principles of evaluation and treatment. AAOS Instr Course Lect 48:199–207, 1999.

Miller MD, Osborne JR, Gordon WT, et al: The natural histories of bone bruises. Am J Sports Med 26:15–19, 1998.

Myers MH, Harvey JP: Traumatic dislocation of the knee joint. J Bone Joint Surg [Am] 53:16–29, 1971.

Noyes FR, Barber-Westin SD, Butler DL, et al: The role of allografts in repair and reconstruction of knee joint ligaments and menisci. AAOS Instr Course Lect 47:379–396, 1998.

O'Brien SJ, Warren RF, Pavlov H, et al: Reconstruction of the chronically insufficient anterior cruciate ligament with the central third of the patellar ligament. J Bone Joint Surg [Am] 73:278–286, 1991.

Paulos LE, Rosenberg TD, Drawbert J, et al: Infrapatellar contracture syndrome: An unrecognized cause of knee stiffness with patellar entrapment and patella infra. Am J Sports Med 15:331–341, 1987.

Shelbourne KD, Nitz P: Accelerated rehabilitation after anterior cruciate ligament reconstruction. Am J Sports Med 18:292–299, 1990.

Shelbourne KD, Muthukaruppan Y: Subjective results of nonoperatively treated, acute, isolated posterior cruciate ligament injuries. Arthroscopy 21:457–461, 2005.

Shelton WR, Treacy SH, Dukes AD, et al: Use of allografts in knee reconstruction. J Am Acad Orthop Surg 6:165–175, 1998.

Sisto DJ, Warren RF: Complete knee dislocation: A follow-up study of operative treatment. Clin Orthop 198:94–101, 1985.

Sitler M, Ryan J, Hopkinson W, et al: The efficacy of a prophylactic knee brace to reduce knee injuries in football: A prospective, randomized study at West Point. Am J Sports Med 18:310–315, 1990.

Stannard JP, Sheils TM, Lopez-Ben RR, et al: Vascular injuries in knee dislocations: The role of physical examination in determining the need for arteriography. J Bone Joint Surg [Am] 86:910–915, 2004.

Veltri DM, Warren RF: Isolated and combined posterior cruciate ligament injuries. J Am Acad Orthop Surg 1:67–75, 1993.

Yamamoto Y, Hsu WH, Woo SL, et al: Knee stability and graft function after anterior cruciate ligament reconstruction: A comparison of a lateral and an anatomical femoral tunnel placement. Am J Sports Med 32:1825–1832, 2004.

Anterior Knee Pain

Boden BP, Pearsall AW, Garrett WE, et al: Patellofemoral instability: Evaluation and management. J Am Acad Orthop Surg 5:47–57, 1997.

Cooper DE, DeLee JC: Reflex sympathetic dystrophy of the knee. J Am Acad Orthop Surg 2:79–86, 1994.

Cramer KE, Moed BR: Patellar fractures: Contemporary approach to treatment. J Am Acad Orthop Surg 5:323–331, 1997.

Fulkerson JP: Anteromedialization of the tibial tuberosity for patellofemoral malalignment. Clin Orthop 177:176–181, 1983.

Fulkerson JP: Patellofemoral pain disorders: Evaluation and management. J Am Acad Orthop Surg 2:124–132, 1994.

Fulkerson JP, Shea KP: Disorders of patellofemoral alignment: Current concepts review. J Bone Joint Surg [Am] 72:1424–1429, 1990.

Gambardella RA: Technical pitfalls of patellofemoral surgery. Clin Sports Med 18:897–903, 1999.

James SL: Running injuries to the knee. J Am Acad Orthop Surg 3:309–318, 1995.

Kelly MA: Algorithm for anterior knee pain. AAOS Instr Course Lect 47:339–343, 1998.

Kilowich P, Paulos L, Rosenberg T, et al: Lateral release of the patella: Indications and contraindications. Am J Sports Med 18:361, 1990.

Larson RL, Cabaud HE, Slocum DB, et al: The patellar compression syndrome: Surgical treatment by lateral retinacular release. Clin Orthop 134:158–167, 1978.

Matava MJ: Patellar tendon ruptures. J Am Acad Orthop Surg 4:287–296, 1996.

Merchant A: Classification of patellofemoral disorders. Arthroscopy 4:235–240, 1988.

Merchant AC, Mercer RL, Jacobsen RJ, et al: Roentgenographic analysis of patellofemoral congruence. J Bone Joint Surg [Am] 56:1391–1396, 1974.

Post WR: Clinical evaluation of patients with patellofemoral disorders. Arthroscopy 15:841–851, 1999.

Wang CT, Lin J, Chang CJ, et al: Therapeutic effects of hyaluronic acid on osteoarthritis of the knee: A meta-analysis of randomized controlled trials. J Bone Joint Surg [Am] 86:538–545, 2004.

Childhood and Adolescent Knee Disorders

Andrish JT: Meniscal injuries in children and adolescents: Diagnosis and management. J Am Acad Orthop Surg 5:231–237, 1996.

Aronowitz ER, Ganley TJ, Goode JR, et al: Anterior cruciate ligament reconstruction in adolescents with open physes. Am J Sports Med 28:168–175, 2000.

Baxter MP, Wiley JJ: Fractures of the tibial spine in children: An evaluation of knee stability. J Bone Joint Surg [Br] 70:228–230, 1988.

Edwards PH, Grana WA: Physical fractures about the knee. J Am Acad Orthop Surg 3:63–69, 1995.

Lo IKY, Bell DM, Fowler PJ: Anterior cruciate ligament injuries in the skeletally immature patient. AAOS Instr Course Lect 47:351–359, 1998.

Lowe J, Chaimsky G, Freedman A, et al: The anatomy of tibial eminence fractures: Arthroscopic observations following failed closed reduction. J Bone Joint Surg [Am] 84:1933–1938, 2002.

McCarroll JR, Rettig AC, Shelbourne KD: Anterior cruciate ligament injuries in the young athlete with open physes. Am J Sports Med 16:44–47, 1988.
Meyers MH, McKeever FM: Fractures of the intercondylar eminence of the tibia. J Bone Joint Surg [Am] 41:209–222, 1959.
Micheli LJ, Foster TE: Acute knee injuries in the immature athlete. Instr Course Lect 42:473–481, 1993.
Millett PJ, Willis AA, Warren RF: Associated injuries in pediatric and adolescent anterior cruciate ligament tears: Does a delay in treatment increase the risk of meniscal tear?. Arthroscopy 18:955–959, 2002.
Ogden JA, Tross RB, Murphy MJ: Fractures of the tibial tuberosity in adolescents. J Bone Joint Surg [Am] 62:205–215, 1980.
Parker AW, Drez D, Cooper JL: Anterior cruciate ligament injuries in patients with open physes. Am J Sports Med 22:44–47, 1994.
Riseborough EJ, Barrett IR, Shapiro F: Growth disturbances following distal femoral physeal fracture-separations. J Bone Joint Surg [Am] 65:885–893, 1983.
Shelbourne KD, Gray T, Wiley BV: Results of transphyseal anterior cruciate ligament reconstruction using patellar tendon autograft in Tanner stage 3 or 4 adolescents with clearly open growth plates. Am J Sports Med 32:1218–1222, 2004.
Stanitski CL: Anterior cruciate ligament injury in the skeletally immature patient: Diagnosis and treatment. J Am Acad Orthop Surg 3:146–158, 1995.
Stanitski CL: Patellar instability in the school age athlete. AAOS Instr Course Lect 47:345–350, 1998.

OTHER PROBLEMS IN LOWER EXTREMITY SPORTS MEDICINE

Nerve Entrapment Syndromes

Baxter DE: Functional nerve disorders in the athlete's foot, ankle, and leg. AAOS Instr Course Lect 42:185–194, 1993.
Beskin JL: Nerve entrapments of the foot and ankle. J Am Acad Orthop Surg 5:261–269, 1997.
Styf J: Entrapment of the superficial peroneal nerve: Diagnosis and results of decompression. J Bone Joint Surg [Br], 71:131–135, 1989.

Contusions

Jackson DW, Feagin JA: Quadriceps contusions in young athletes. J Bone Joint Surg [Am] 55:95–105, 1973.
Renstrom PAHF: Tendon and muscle injuries in the groin area. Clin Sports Med 11:815–831, 1992.
Ryan JB, Wheeler JH, Hopkinson WJ, et al: Quadriceps contusions: West Point update. Am J Sports Med 19:299–304, 1991.

Muscle Injury

Garrett WE: Muscle strain injuries. Am J Sports Med 24:S2–S8, 1996.
Zarins B, Ciullo JV: Acute muscle and tendon injuries in athletes. Clin Sports Med 2:167–182, 1983.

Tendon Injuries

Almekinders LC: Tendinitis and other chronic tendinopathies. J Am Acad Orthop Surg 6:157–164, 1998.
Bassett FH, Speer KP: Longitudinal rupture of the peroneal tendons. Am J Sports Med 21:354–357, 1993.
Biedert R: Dislocation of the tibialis posterior tendon. Am J Sports Med 20:775–776, 1992.
Brage ME, Hansen ST: Traumatic subluxation/dislocation of the peroneal tendons. Foot Ankle 13:423–430, 1992.
Jones DC: Tendon disorders of the foot and ankle. J Am Acad Orthop Surg 1:87–94, 1993.
Millar AP: Strains of the posterior calf musculature ("tennis leg"). Am J Sports Med 7:172–174, 1979.
Myerson MS, McGarvey W: Disorders of the insertion of the Achilles tendon and Achilles tendinitis. J Bone Joint Surg [Am] 80:1814–1824, 1998.
Ouzounian TJ, Myerson MS: Dislocation of the posterior tibial tendon. Foot Ankle 13:215–219, 1992.
Saltzman CL, Tearse DS: Achilles tendon injuries. J Am Acad Orthop Surg 6:316–325, 1998.
Sobel M, Geppert MJ, Olson EJ, et al: The dynamics of peroneus brevis tendon splits: A proposed mechanism, technique of diagnosis, and classification of injury. Foot Ankle 13:413–421, 1992.
Teitz CC, Garrett WE Jr, Miniaci A, et al: Tendon problems in athletic individuals. AAOS Instr Course Lect 46:569–582, 1997.
Williams JGP: Achilles tendon lesions in sport. Sports Med 3:114–135, 1986.

Compartment Syndrome

Beckham SG, Grana WA, Buckley P, et al: A comparison of anterior compartment pressures in competitive runners and cyclists. Am J Sports Med 21:36–40, 1993.
Eisele SA, Sammarco GJ: Chronic exertional compartment syndrome. AAOS Instr Course Lect 42:213–217, 1993.
Pedowitz RA, Horgens AR, Mubarak SJ, et al: Modified criteria for the objective diagnosis of compartment syndrome of the leg. Am J Sports Med 18:35–40, 1990.
Rorabeck CH, Bourne RB, Fowler PJ: The surgical treatment of exertional compartment syndromes in athletes. J Bone Joint Surg [Am] 65:1245–1251, 1983.
Rorabeck CH, Fowler PJ, Nitt L: The results of fasciotomy in the management of chronic exertional compartment syndrome. Am J Sports Med 16:224–227, 1986.

Stress Fractures

Anderson EG: Fatigue fractures of the foot. Injury 21:274–279, 1990.
Blickenstaff LD, Morris JM: Fatigue fracture of the femoral neck. J Bone Joint Surg [Am] 48:1031–1047, 1966.
Green NE, Rogers RA, Lipscomb AB: Nonunions of stress fractures of the tibia. Am J Sports Med 13:171–176, 1985.
Khan KM, Fuller PJ, Brukner PD, et al: Outcome of conservative and surgical management of navicular stress fracture in athletes: Eighty-six cases proven with computerized tomography. Am J Sports Med 20:657–661, 1992.
McBryde AM: Stress fractures in athletes. J Sports Med 3:212, 1973.
Rettig AC, Shelbourne KD, McCarroll JR, et al: The natural history and treatment of delayed union stress fractures of the anterior cortex of the tibia. Am J Sports Med 16:250–255, 1988.
Shin AY, Gillingham BL: Fatigue fractures of the femoral neck in athletes. J Am Acad Orthop Surg 5:293–302, 1997.

Other Hip Disorders

Allen WC, Cope R: Coxa saltans: The snapping hip revisited. J Am Acad Orthop Surg 3:303–308, 1995.
Buckwalter JA, Lane NE: Athletics and osteoarthritis. Am J Sports Med 25:873–881, 1997.
Clanton TO, Coupe KJ: Hamstring strains in athletes: Diagnosis and treatment. J Am Acad Orthop Surg 6:237–248, 1998.
Cooper DE, Warren RF, Barnes R: Traumatic subluxation of the hip resulting in aseptic necrosis and chondrolysis in a professional football player. Am J Sports Med 19:322–324, 1991.
Holmes JC, Pruitt AL, Whalen NJ: Iliotibial band syndrome in cyclists. Am J Sports Med 21:419–424, 1993.
Mardones RM, Gonzalez C, Chen Q, et al: Surgical treatment of femoroacetabular impingement: Evaluation of the effect of the size of the resection. Surgical technique. J Bone Joint Surg [Am] 88(Suppl 1, Part 1):84–91, 2006.
Martens M, Libbrecht P, Burssens A: Surgical treatment of the iliotibial band friction syndrome. Am J Sports Med 17:651–654, 1989.
Moorman CT III, Warren RF, Hershman EB, et al: Traumatic posterior hip subluxation in American football. J Bone Joint Surg [Am] 85:1190–1196, 2003.

Other Foot and Ankle Disorders

Baxter DE, Zingas C: The foot in running. J Am Acad Orthop Surg 3:136–145, 1995.
Churchill JA, Mazur JM: Ankle pain in children: Diagnostic evaluation and clinical decision-making. J Am Acad Orthop Surg 3:183–193, 1995.
Colville MR: Surgical treatment of the unstable ankle. J Am Acad Orthop Surg 6:368–377, 1998.
Donahue SW, Sharkey NA: Strains in the metatarsals during the stance phase of gait: Implications for stress fractures. J Bone Joint Surg [Am] 81:1236–1244, 1999.
Garrick JG, Requa RK: The epidemiology of foot and ankle injuries in sports. Clin Sports Med 7:29–36, 1988.

Gill LH: Plantar fasciitis: Diagnosis and conservative management. J Am Acad Orthop Surg 5:109–117, 1997.
Hamilton WG, Thompson FM, Snow SW: The modified Brostrom procedure for lateral ankle instability. Foot Ankle 14:1–7, 1993.
Hopkinson WJ, St. Pierre P, Ryan JB, et al: Syndesmosis sprains of the ankle. Foot Ankle 10:325–330, 1990.
Lynch S, Renstrom P: Treatment of acute lateral ankle ligament rupture in the athlete: Conservative vs. surgical treatment. Sports Med 27:61–71, 1999.
Marotta JJ, Micheli LJ: Os trigonum impingement in dancers. Am J Sports Med 20:533–536, 1992.
Miller CM, Winter WG, Bucknell AL, et al: Injuries to the midtarsal joint and lesser tarsal bones. J Am Acad Orthop Surg 6:249–258, 1998.
Mizel MS, Yodlowski ML: Disorders of the lesser metatarsophalangeal joints. J Am Acad Orthop Surg 3:166–173, 1995.
Mologne TS, Lundeen JM, Clapper MF, O'Brien TJ: Early screw fixation versus casting in the treatment of acute Jones fractures. Am J Sports Med 33:970–975, 2005.
Porter DA, Duncan M, Meyer SJ: Fifth metatarsal Jones fracture fixation with a 4.5-mm cannulated stainless steel screw in the competitive and recreational athlete: a clinical and radiographic evaluation. Am J Sports Med 33:726–733, 2005.
Reese K, Litsky A, Kaeding C, et al: Cannulated screw fixation of Jones fractures: A clinical and biomechanical study. Am J Sports Med 32:1736–1742, 2004.
Renstrom PAFH: Persistently painful sprained ankle. J Am Acad Orthop Surg 2:270–280, 1994.
Rodeo SA, O'Brien S, Warren RF, et al: Turf toe: An analysis of metatarsal phalangeal joint pain in professional football players. Am J Sports Med 18:280–285, 1990.
Thacker S, Stroup D, Branche CM, et al: The prevention of ankle sprains in sports: A systematic review of the literature. Am J Sports Med 27:753–760, 1999.
Valderrabano V, Perren T, Ryf C, et al: Snowboarder's talus fracture: Treatment outcome of 20 cases after 3.5 years. Am J Sports Med 33:871–880, 2005.
Wuest TK: Injuries to the distal lower extremity syndesmosis. J Am Acad Orthop Surg 5:172–181, 1997.

Hip and Ankle Arthroscopy

Angermann P, Jensen P: Osteochondritis dissecans of the talus: Long-term results of surgical treatment. Foot Ankle 10:161–163, 1989.
Basset FH, Billy JB, Gates HS: A simple surgical approach to the posteromedial ankle. Am J Sports Med 21:144–146, 1993.
Ferkel RD, Scranton PE: Current concepts review: Arthroscopy of the ankle and foot. J Bone Joint Surg [Am] 75:1233–1243, 1993.
Glick JM, Sampson TG, Gordon RB, et al: Hip arthroscopy by the lateral approach. Arthroscopy 3:4–12, 1987.
Loomer R, Fisher C, Lloyd-Smith R, et al: Osteochondral lesions of the talus. Am J Sports Med 21:13–19, 1993.
McCarroll JR, Schrader JW, Shelbourne KD, et al: Meniscoid lesions of the ankle in soccer players. Am J Sports Med 15:257, 1987.
McCarthy JC, Day B, Busconi B: Hip arthroscopy: Applications and technique. J Am Acad Orthop Surg 3:115–122, 1995.
Meislin RJ, Rose DJ, Parisien S, et al: Arthroscopic treatment of synovial impingement of the ankle. Am J Sports Med 21:186–189, 1993.
Ogilvie-Harris DJ, Lieverman I, Fitsalos D: Arthroscopically assisted arthrodesis for osteoarthritic ankles. J Bone Joint Surg [Am] 75:1167–1174, 1993.
Stetson WB, Ferkel RD: Ankle arthroscopy. J Am Acad Orthop Surg 4:17–34, 1996.
Stone JW: Osteochondral lesions of the talar dome. J Am Acad Orthop Surg 4:63–73, 1996.
Thein R, Eichenblat M: Arthroscopic treatment of sports-related synovitis of the ankle. Am J Sports Med 20:496–499, 1992.

SHOULDER

Anatomy and Biomechanics

Cooper DE, Arnoczsky SP, O'Brien SJ, et al: Anatomy, histology, and vascularity of the glenoid labrum. J Bone Joint Surg [Am] 74:46–52, 1992.
Cooper DE, O'Brien SJ, Warren RF: Supporting layers of the glenohumeral joint: An anatomic study. Clin Orthop 289:144–155, 1993.
Ferrari DA: Capsular ligaments of the shoulder: Anatomical and functional study of the anterior superior capsule. Am J Sports Med 18:20–24, 1990.
Flatow EL: The biomechanics of the acromioclavicular, sternoclavicular, and scapulothoracic joints. AAOS Instr Course Lect 42:237–245, 1993.
Harryman DT, Sidles JA, Harris SL, Matsen FA: The role of the rotator interval capsule in passive motion and stability of the shoulder. J Bone Joint Surg [Am] 74:53–66, 1992.
Harryman DT II: Common surgical approaches to the shoulder. AAOS Instr Course Lect 41:3–11, 1992.
Iannotti JP, Gabriel JP, Schneck SL, et al: The normal glenohumeral relationships: An anatomical study of one hundred and forty shoulders. J Bone Joint Surg [Am] 74:491–500, 1992.
Kibler WB: The role of the scapula in athletic shoulder function: Current concepts. Am J Sports Med 26:325–337, 1998.
O'Brien SJ, Neves MC, Rozbruck SR, et al: The anatomy and histology of the inferior glenohumeral ligament complex of the shoulder. Am J Sports Med 18:449–456, 1990.
O'Connell PW, Nuber GW, Mileski RA, et al: The contribution of the glenohumeral ligaments to anterior stability of the shoulder joint. Am J Sports Med 18:579–584, 1990.
Sher JS: Anatomy, biomechanics, and pathophysiology of rotator cuff disease. In Iannotti JP, Williams GR, eds: Disorders of the Shoulder. Lippincott, Williams & Wilkins, 1999.
Speer KP: Anatomy and pathomechanics of shoulder instability. Clin Sports Med 14:751–760, 1995.
Warner JJP, Deng XH, Warren RF, et al: Static capsuloligamentous restraints to superior-inferior translation of the glenohumeral joint. Am J Sports Med 20:675–685, 1992.
Warner JJP, Deng XH, Warren RF, et al: Superior-inferior translation in the intact and vented glenohumeral joint. J Shoulder Elbow Surg 2:99–105, 1993.

History and Physical Examination

Altchek DW, Dines DM: Shoulder injuries in the throwing athlete. J Am Acad Orthop Surg 3:159–165, 1995.
Gerber C, Ganz R: Clinical assessment of instability of the shoulder with special reference to anterior and posterior drawer tests. J Bone Joint Surg [Br] 66:551–556, 1984.
Hawkins RJ, Hobeika P: Physical exam of the shoulder. Orthopaedics 6:1270–1278, 1983.
Neer CS, Welsh RP: The shoulder in sports. Orthop Clin North Am 8:583–591, 1977.

Imaging of the Shoulder

Beltran J: The use of magnetic resonance imaging about the shoulder. J Shoulder Elbow Surg 1:287–295, 1992.
Bigliani LU, Morrison D, April EW: The morphology of the acromion and its relationship to rotator cuff tears. Orthop Trans 10:228, 1986.
Garth WP Jr, Slappey CE, Ochs CW: Roentgenographic demonstration of instability of the shoulder: The apical oblique projection—a technical note. J Bone Joint Surg [Am] 66:1450–1453, 1984.
Herzog RJ: Magnetic resonance imaging of the shoulder. J Bone Joint Surg [Am] 79:934–953, 1997.
Hill HA, Sachs MD: The grooved defect of the humeral head: A frequently unrecognized complication of dislocations of the shoulder joint. Radiology 35:690–700, 1940.
Hobbs DW: Sternoclavicular joint: A new axial radiographic view. Radiology 90:801–802, 1968.
Kozo O, Yamamuro T, Rockwood CA: Use of a thirty-degree caudal tilt radiograph in the shoulder impingement syndrome. J Shoulder Elbow Surg 1:246–252, 1992.
Zanca P: Shoulder pain: Involvement of the acromioclavicular joint: Analysis of 1000 cases. AJR Am J Roentgenol 112:493–506, 1971.

Arthroscopy of the Shoulder

Altchek DW, Carson EW: Arthroscopic acromioplasty: Indications and technique. AAOS Instr Course Lect 47:21–28, 1998.
Bell RH: Arthroscopic distal clavicle resection. AAOS Instr Course Lect 47:35–41, 1998.
Caborn DM, Fu FH: Arthroscopic approach and anatomy of the shoulder. Op Tech Orthop 1:126–133, 1991.

Lintner SA, Speer KP: Traumatic anterior glenohumeral instability: The role of arthroscopy. J Am Acad Orthop Surg 5:233–239, 1997.

Nisbet JK, Paulos LE: Subacromial bursoscopy. Op Tech Orthop 1:221–228, 1991.

Skyhar MJ, Altchek DW, Warren RF, et al: Shoulder arthroscopy with the patient in the beach chair position. Arthroscopy 4:256–259, 1988.

Wolf EM: Anterior portals in shoulder arthroscopy. Arthroscopy 5:201–208, 1989.

Shoulder Instability

Altchek DW, Warren RF, Skyhar MJ, et al: T-plasty modification of the Bankart procedure for multidirectional instability of the anterior and inferior types. J Bone Joint Surg [Am] 73:105–112, 1991.

Arciero RA, Wheeler JH III, Ryan JB, et al: Arthroscopic Bankart repair for acute, initial anterior shoulder dislocations. Am J Sports Med 22:589–594, 1994.

Black KP, Schneider DJ, Yu JR, Jacobs CR: Biomechanics of a Bankart repair: Relationship between glenohumeral translation and labral fixation site. Am J Sports Med 27:339–344, 1999.

Bottoni CR, Franks BR, Moore JH, et al: Operative stabilization of posterior shoulder instability. Am J Sports Med 33:996–1002, 2005.

Cole BJ, Warner JJP: Arthroscopic vs. open Bankart repair for traumatic anterior shoulder instability: Decision making and results. Clin Sports Med 19:19–47, 2000.

Cole BJ, Romeo AA, Warner JJP: The use of bioabsorbable implants to treat shoulder instability. Tech Sports Med 8:197–205, 2000.

Cooper RA, Brems JJ: The inferior capsular shift procedure for multidirectional instability of the shoulder. J Bone Joint Surg [Am] 74:1516–1521, 1992.

Grana WA, Buckley PD, Yates CK: Arthroscopic Bankart suture repair. Am J Sports Med 21:348–353, 1993.

Harryman DT II, Sidles JA, Harris SL, et al: Laxity of the normal glenohumeral joint. J Shoulder Elbow Surg 1:66–76, 1992.

Kim SH, Ha KI, Park JH, et al: Arthroscopic posterior labral repair and capsular shift for traumatic unidirectional recurrent posterior subluxation of the shoulder. J Bone Joint Surg [Am] 85:1479–1487, 2003.

Kim SH, Ha KI, Yoo JC, Noh KC: Kim's lesion: An incomplete and concealed avulsion of the posteroinferior labrum in posterior or multidirectional posteroinferior instability of the shoulder. Arthroscopy 20:712–720, 2004.

Kim SH, Park JC, Park JS, Oh I: Painful jerk test: A predictor of success in nonoperative treatment of posteroinferior instability of the shoulder. Am J Sports Med 32:1849–1855, 2004.

Kirkley A, Werstine R, Ratjek A, Griffin S: Prospective randomized clinical trial comparing the effectiveness of immediate arthroscopic stabilization versus immobilization and rehabilitation in first traumatic anterior dislocations of the shoulder. Arthroscopy 21:55–63, 2005.

Lippit S, Matsen FA III: Mechanisms of glenohumeral joint stability. Clin Orthop 291:20–28, 1993.

Mazzocca AD, Brown FM Jr, Carreira DS, et al: Arthroscopic anterior shoulder stabilization of collision and contact athletes. Am J Sports Med 33:52–60, 2005.

Mohtadi NG, Bitar IJ, Sasyniuk TM, et al: Arthroscopic versus open repair for traumatic anterior shoulder instability: A meta-analysis. Arthroscopy 21:652–658, 2005.

Morgan CD, Bodenstab AB: Arthroscopic Bankart suture repair: Techniques and early results. Arthroscopy 3:111–112, 1982.

Neer CS II, Foster CR: Inferior capsular shift for involuntary inferior and multidirectional instability of the shoulder: A preliminary report. J Bone Joint Surg [Am] 62:897–908, 1980.

Pollock RG, Bigliani LU: Glenohumeral instability: Evaluation and treatment. J Am Acad Orthop Surg 1:24–32, 1993.

Rowe CR, Patel D, Southmayd WW: The Bankart procedure: A long-term end-result study. J Bone Joint Surg [Am] 55:445–460, 1973.

Schenk TJ, Brems JJ: Multidirectional instability of the shoulder: Pathophysiology, diagnosis, and management. J Am Acad Orthop Surg 6:65–72, 1998.

Turkel SJ, Panio MW, Marshall JL, et al: Stabilizing mechanisms preventing anterior dislocation of the glenohumeral joint. J Bone Joint Surg [Am] 63:1208–1217, 1981.

Zuckerman JD, Matsen FA III: Complications about the glenohumeral joint related to the use of screws and staples. J Bone Joint Surg [Am] 66:175–180, 1984.

Impingement Syndrome/Rotator Cuff

Bigliani LU, Cordasco FA, McIlveen SJ, et al: Operative treatment of failed repairs of the rotator cuff. J Bone Joint Surg [Am] 74:1505–1515, 1992.

Bigliani LU, Levine WN: Current concepts review: Subacromial impingement syndrome. J Bone Joint Surg [Am] 79:1854–1868, 1997.

Budoff JE, Nirschl RP, Guidi EJ: Current concepts review: Débridement of partial-thickness tears of the rotator cuff without acromioplasty. J Bone Joint Surg [Am] 80:733–748, 1998.

Caspari RB, Thal R: A technique for arthroscopic subacromial decompression. Arthroscopy 8:23–30, 1992.

Cordasco FA, Bigliani LU: The treatment of failed rotator cuff repairs. AAOS Instr Course Lect 47:77–86, 1998.

Ellman H, Kay SP, Worth M: Arthroscopic treatment of full-thickness rotator cuff tears: Two to seven year follow-up study. Arthroscopy 9:301–314, 1993.

Flatow EL, Warner JJP: Instability of the shoulder: Complex problems and failed repairs (Part I). J Bone Joint Surg [Am] 80:122–140, 1998.

Flatow EL, Miniaci A, Evans PJ, et al: Instability of the shoulder: Complex problems and failed repairs (Part II). J Bone Joint Surg [Am] 80:284–298, 1998.

Galatz LM, Ball CM, Teefey SA, et al: The outcome and repair integrity of completely arthroscopically repaired large and massive rotator cuff tears. J Bone Joint Surg [Am] 86:219–224, 2004.

Gartsman GM: Arthroscopic management of rotator cuff disease. J Am Acad Orthop Surg 6:259–266, 1998.

Gerber C, Terrier F, Ganz R: The role of the coracoid process in the chronic impingement syndrome. J Bone Joint Surg [Br] 67:703–708, 1985.

Holsbeeck E: Subacromial impingement: Open versus arthroscopic decompression. Arthroscopy 8:173–178, 1992.

Ianotti JP: Full-thickness rotator cuff tears: Factors affecting surgical outcome. J Am Acad Orthop Surg 2:87–95, 1994.

McConville OR, Iannotti JP: Partial-thickness tears of the rotator cuff: Evaluation and management. J Am Acad Orthop Surg 7:32–43, 1999.

Neer CS II: Anterior acromioplasty for the chronic impingement syndrome in the shoulder. J Bone Joint Surg [Am] 54:41–50, 1972.

Norberg FB, Field LD, Savoie FH III: Repair of the rotator cuff: Mini open and arthroscopic repairs. Clin Sports Med 19:77–99, 2000.

Rockwood CA Jr, Lyons FR: Shoulder impingement syndrome: Diagnosis, radiographic evaluation, and treatment with a modified Neer acromioplasty. J Bone Joint Surg [Am] 75:409–424, 1993.

Speer KP, Lohnes J, Garrett WC: Arthroscopic subacromial decompression: Results in advanced impingement syndrome. Arthroscopy 7:291–296, 1991.

Williams GR: Painful shoulder after surgery for rotator cuff disease. J Am Acad Orthop Surg 5:97–108, 1997.

Zeman CA, Arcand MA, Cantrell JS, et al: The rotator cuff-deficient arthritic shoulder: Diagnosis and surgical management. J Am Acad Orthop Surg 6:337–348, 1998.

Biceps Injuries

Andrews J, Carson W, McLeod W: Glenoid labrum tears related to the long head of the biceps. Am J Sports Med 13:337–341, 1985.

Froimson AI, Oh I: Keyhole tenodesis of biceps origin at the shoulder. Clin Orthop 112:245–249, 1974.

Gartsman GM, Hammerman SM: Superior labrum, anterior and posterior lesions. Clin Sports Med 19:115–124, 2000.

Mileski RA, Snyder SJ: Superior labral lesions in the shoulder: Pathoanatomy and surgical management. J Am Acad Orthop Surg 6:121–131, 1998.

Resch H, Golser K, Thoeni H, et al: Arthroscopic repair of superior glenoid labral detachment (the SLAP lesion). J Shoulder Elbow Surg 2:147–155, 1993.

Snyder SJ, Wuh HCK: Arthroscopic evaluation and treatment of the rotator cuff and superior labrum anterior posterior lesion. Op Tech Orthop 1:207–220, 1991.

Tennent TD, Beach WR, Meyers JF: Clinical sports medicine update. Am J Sports Med 31:301–307, 2003.

Acromioclavicular and Sternoclavicular Injuries

Cahill BR: Osteolysis of the distal part of the clavicle in male athletes. J Bone Joint Surg [Am] 64:1053–1058, 1982.

Gartsman GM: Arthroscopic resection of the acromioclavicular joint. Am J Sports Med 21:71–77, 1993.

Lemos MJ: The evaluation and treatment of the injured acromioclavicular joint in athletes: Current concepts. Am J Sports Med 26:137–144, 1998.
Nuber GW, Bowen MK: Acromioclavicular joint injuries and distal clavicle fractures. J Am Acad Orthop Surg 5:11–18, 1997.
Richards RR: Acromioclavicular joint injuries. AAOS Instr Course Lect 42:259–269, 1993.
Rockwood CA Jr, Young DC: Disorders of the acromioclavicular joint. In Rockwood CA Jr, Matsen FA III, eds: The Shoulder, pp 413–476. Philadelphia, WB Saunders, 1990.
Scavenius M, Iverson BF: Nontraumatic clavicular osteolysis in weight lifters. Am J Sports Med 20:463–467, 1992.
Wirth MA, Rockwood CA Jr: Acute and chronic traumatic injuries of the sternoclavicular joint. J Am Acad Orthop Surg 4:268–278, 1996.

Muscle Ruptures

Caughey MA, Welsh P: Muscle ruptures affecting the shoulder girdle. In Rockwood CA Jr, Matsen FA III, eds: The Shoulder, pp 863–873. Philadelphia, WB Saunders, 1991.
Gerber C, Krushell RJ: Isolated rupture of the tendon of the subscapularis muscle. J Bone Joint Surg [Br] 73:389–394, 1991.
Kretzler HH Jr, Richardson AB: Rupture of the pectoralis major muscle. Am J Sports Med 17:453–458, 1989.
Miller MD, Johnson DL, Fu FH, et al: Rupture of the pectoralis major muscle in a collegiate football player. Am J Sports Med 21:475–477, 1993.
Wolfe SW, Wickiewicz TL, Cavanaugh JT: Ruptures of the pectoralis major muscle: An anatomic and clinical analysis. Am J Sports Med 20:587–593, 1992.

Calcific Tendinitis and Adhesive Capsulitis

Ark JW, Flock TJ, Flatow EL, et al: Arthroscopic treatment of calcific tendinitis of the shoulder. Arthroscopy 8:183–188, 1992.
Coventry MB: Problem of the painful shoulder. JAMA 151:177–185, 1953.
Faure G, Daculsi G: Calcified tendinitis: A review. Ann Rheum. Dis 42(Suppl):49–53, 1983.
Grey RG: The natural history of "idiopathic" frozen shoulder. J Bone Joint Surg [Am] 60:564, 1978.
Harmon HP: Methods and results in the treatment of 2580 painful shoulders: With special reference to calcific tendinitis and the frozen shoulder. Am J Surg 95:527–544, 1958.
Harryman DT II: Shoulders: Frozen and stiff. AAOS Instr Course Lect 42:247–257, 1993.
Leffert RE: The frozen shoulder. AAOS Instr Course Lect 34:199–203, 1985.
Miller MD, Wirth MA, Rockwood CA Jr: Thawing the frozen shoulder: The "patient" patient. Orthopedics 19:849–853, 1996.
Murnaghan JP: Adhesive capsulitis of the shoulder: Current concepts and treatment. Orthopaedics 2:153–158, 1988.
Murnaghan JP: Frozen shoulder. In Rockwood CA Jr, Matsen FA III, eds: The Shoulder. Philadelphia, WB Saunders, 1990.
Neviaser JS: Adhesive capsulitis and the stiff and painful shoulder. Orthop Clin North Am 2:327–331, 1980.
Neviaser TJ: Adhesive capsulitis. In McGinty JB, ed: Operative Arthroscopy, pp 561–566. New York, Raven Press, 1991.
Neviaser RJ, Neviaser TJ: The frozen shoulder: Diagnosis and management. Clin Orthop 223:59–64, 1987.
Shaffer B, Tibone JE, Kerlan RK: Frozen shoulder: A long-term follow-up. J Bone Joint Surg [Am] 74:738–746, 1992.
Uthoff HK, Loehr JW: Calcific tendinopathy of the rotator cuff: Pathogenesis, diagnosis, and management. J Am Acad Orthop Surg 5:183–191, 1997.
Warner JJP: Frozen shoulder: Diagnosis and management. J Am Acad Orthop Surg 5:130–140, 1997.
Warner JJP, Greis PE: The treatment of stiffness of the shoulder after repair of the rotator cuff. J Bone Joint Surg [Am] 79:1260–1269, 1997.

Nerve Disorders

Black KP, Lombardo JA: Suprascapular nerve injuries with isolated paralysis of the infraspinatus. Am J Sports Med 18:225–228, 1990.
Burkhead WZ, Scheinberg RR, Box G: Surgical anatomy of the axillary nerve. J Shoulder Elbow Surg 1:31–36, 1992.
Drez D: Suprascapular neuropathy in the differential diagnosis of rotator cuff injuries. Am J Sports Med 4:443, 1976.
Fechter JD, Kuschner SH: The thoracic outlet syndrome. Orthopedics 16:1243–1254, 1993.
Kauppila LI: The long thoracic nerve: Possible mechanisms of injury based on autopsy study. J Shoulder Elbow Surg 2:244–248, 1993.
Leffert RD: Neurological problems. In Rockwood CA Jr, Matsen FA III, eds: The Shoulder, pp 750–773. Philadelphia, WB Saunders, 1990.
Leffert RD: Thoracic outlet syndrome. J Am Acad Orthop Surg 2:317–325, 1994.
Markey KL, DiBenedito M, Curl WW: Upper trunk brachial plexopathy: The stinger syndrome. Am J Sports Med 23:650–655, 1993.
Marmor L, Bechtal CO: Paralysis of the serratus anterior due to electric shock relieved by transplantation of the pectoralis major muscle. J Bone Joint Surg [Am] 45:156–160, 1983.
Post M, Grinblat E: Suprascapular nerve entrapment: Diagnosis and results of treatment. J Shoulder Elbow Surg 2:190–197, 1993.
Vastamaki M, Kauppila LI: Etiologic factors in isolated paralysis of the serratus anterior muscle: A report of 197 cases. J Shoulder Elbow Surg 2:244–248, 1993.
Warner JJP, Krushell RJ, Masquelet A, et al: Anatomy and relationships of the suprascapular nerve: Anatomical constraints to mobilization of the supraspinatus and infraspinatus muscles in the management of massive rotator cuff tears. J Bone Joint Surg [Am] 74:36–45, 1992.

Other Shoulder Disorders

Burkhart SS, Morgan CD, Kibler WB: The disabled throwing shoulder: Spectrum of pathology, Part I: Pathoanatomy and biomechanics. Arthroscopy 19:404–420, 2003.
Carson WG, Gasser SI: Little Leaguer's elbow: A report of 23 cases. Am J Sports Med 26:575–580, 1998.
Fees M, Decker T, Snyder-Mackler L, et al: Upper extremity weight-training modifications for the injured athlete: Current concepts. Am J Sports Med 26:732–742, 1998.
Goss TP: Scapular fractures and dislocations: Diagnosis and treatment. J Am Acad Orthop Surg 3:22–33, 1995.
Green A: Current concepts of shoulder arthroplasty. AAOS Instr Course Lect 47:127–133, 1998.
Kuhn JE, Plancher KD, Hawkins RJ: Scapular winging. J Am Acad Orthop Surg 3:319–325, 1995.
Kuhn JE, Plancher KD, Hawkins RJ: Symptomatic scapulothoracic crepitus and bursitis. J Am Acad Orthop Surg 6:267–273, 1998.
Matthews LS, Wolock BS, Martin DF: Arthroscopic management of degenerative arthritis of the shoulder. In McGinty JB, ed: Operative Arthroscopy, pp 567–572. New York, Raven Press, 1991.
Miller, MD, and Warner, JJP: The abduction (weight bearing) radiograph of the shoulder (poster). American Academy of Orthopaedic Surgeons 61st Annual Meeting, New Orleans, 1994.
Olsen SJ II, Fleisig GS, Dun S, et al: Risk factors for shoulder and elbow injuries in adolescent baseball pitchers. Am J Sports Med 34:905–912, 2006.
Schlegel TF, Hawkins RJ: Displaced proximal humeral fractures: Evaluation and treatment. J Am Acad Orthop Surg 2:54–66, 1994.
Simpson NS, Jupiter JB: Clavicular nonunion and malunion: Evaluation and surgical management. J Am Acad Orthop Surg 4:1–8, 1996.

ELBOW AND WRIST

General Elbow

Ball CM, Galatz LM;, Yamaguchi K: Elbow instability: Treatment strategies and emerging concepts. AAOS Instr Course Lect 51:53–61, 2002.
Bradley JP, Petrie RS: Osteochondritis dissecans of the humeral capitellum: Diagnosis and treatment. Clin Sports Med 20:565–590, 2001.
Burra G, Andrews JR: Acute shoulder and elbow dislocations in the athlete. Orthop Clin North Am 33:479–495, 2002.
Ciccotti MG: Epicondylitis in the athlete. AAOS Instr Course Lect 48:375–381, 1999.
Ciccotti MG, Jobe FW: Medial collateral ligament instability and ulnar neuritis in the athlete's elbow. AAOS Instr Course Lect 48:383–391, 1999.
Field LD, Savoie FH: Common elbow injuries in sport. Sports Med 26:193–205, 1998.
Grana W: Medial epicondylitis and cubital tunnel syndrome in the throwing athlete. Clin Sports Med 20:541–548, 2001.
Haake M, Konig IR, Decker T, et al: Extracorporeal shock wave therapy in the treatment of lateral epicondylitis: A randomized multicenter trial. J Bone Joint Surg [Am] 84:1982–1991, 2002.
Izzi J, Dennison D, Noerdlinger M, et al: Nerve injuries of the elbow, wrist, and hand in athletes. Clin Sports Med 20:203–217, 2001.

Kelly EW, Morrey BF, O'Driscoll SW: Complications of elbow arthroscopy. J Bone Joint Surg [Am] 83:25–34, 2001.

Lee DH: Posttraumatic elbow arthritis and arthroplasty. Orthop Clin North Am 30:141–162, 1999.

Maloney MD, Mohr KJ, el Attrache NS: Elbow injuries in the throwing athlete: Difficult diagnoses and surgical complications. Clin Sports Med 18:795–809, 1999.

Moskal MJ: Arthroscopic treatment of posterior impingement of the elbow in athletes. Clin Sports Med 20:11–24, 2001.

Norberg FB, Savoie FH III, Field LD: Arthroscopic treatment of arthritis of the elbow. AAOS Instr Course Lect 49:247–253, 2000.

Oka Y: Débridement arthroplasty for osteoarthrosis of the elbow: 50 patients followed mean 5 years. Acta Orthop Scand 71:185–190, 2000.

Petty DH, Andrews JR, Fleisig GS, Cain EL: Ulnar collateral ligament reconstruction in high school baseball players: Clinical results and injury risk factors. Am J Sports Med 32:1158–1164, 2004.

Ramsey ML: Elbow arthroscopy: Basic setup and treatment of arthritis. AAOS Instr Course Lect 51:69–72, 2002.

Reddy AS, Kvitne RS, Yocum LA, el Attrache NS, et al: Arthroscopy of the elbow: A long-term clinical review. Arthroscopy 16:588–594, 2000.

Rettig AC: Traumatic elbow injuries in the athlete. Orthop Clin North Am 33:509–522, 2002.

Rettig AC, Sherrill C, Snead DS, Mendler JC, et al: Nonoperative treatment of ulnar collateral ligament injuries in throwing athletes. Am J Sports Med 29:15–17, 2001.

Rizio L, Uribe JW: Overuse injuries of the upper extremity in baseball. Clin Sports Med 20:453–468, 2001.

Savoie FH III, Nunley PD, Field LD: Arthroscopic management of the arthritic elbow: Indications, technique, and results. J Shoulder Elbow Surg 8:214–219, 1999.

Schickendantz MS: Diagnosis and treatment of elbow disorders in the overhead athlete. Hand Clin 18:65–75, 2002.

Sevier TL, Wilson JK: Treating lateral epicondylitis. Sports Med 28:375–380, 1999.

Sofka CM, Potter HG: Imaging of elbow injuries in the child and adult athlete. Radiol Clin North Am 40:251–265, 2002.

Stubbs MJ, Field LD, Savoie FH III: Osteochondritis dissecans of the elbow. Clin Sports Med 20:1–9, 2001.

General Wrist

Bond CD, Shin AY, McBride MT, Dao KD: Percutaneous screw fixation or cast immobilization for nondisplaced scaphoid fractures. J Bone Joint Surg [Am] 83:483–488, 2001.

Berger RA: Arthroscopic anatomy of the wrist and distal radioulnar joint. Hand Clin 15:393–413, 1999.

Chou CH, Lee TS: Peripheral tears of triangular fibrocartilage complex: Results of primary repair. Int Orthop 25:392–395, 2001.

Cober SR, Trumble TE: Arthroscopic repair of triangular fibrocartilage complex injuries. Orthop Clin North Am 32:279–294, 2001.

Dailey SW, Palmer AK: The role of arthroscopy in the evaluation and treatment of triangular fibrocartilage complex injuries in athletes. Hand Clin 16:461–476, 2000.

De Smet L: Ulnar variance and its relationship to ligament injuries of the wrist. Acta Orthop Belg 65:416–417, 1999.

Geissler WB: Carpal fractures in athletes. Clin Sports Med 20:167–188, 2001.

Grechenig W, Peicha G, Fellinger M, et al: Anatomical and safety considerations in establishing portals used for wrist arthroscopy. Clin Anat 12:179–185, 1999.

Haims AH, Schweitzer ME, Morrison WB, et al: Limitations of MR imaging in the diagnosis of peripheral tears of the triangular fibrocartilage of the wrist. AJR Am J Roentgenol 178:419–422, 2002.

Hanker GJ: Radius fractures in the athlete. Clin Sports Med 20:189–201, 2001.

Hester PW, Blazar PE: Complications of hand and wrist surgery in the athlete. Clin Sports Med 18:811–829, 1999.

Izzi J, Dennison D, Noerdlinger M, et al: Nerve injuries of the elbow, wrist, and hand in athletes. Clin Sports Med 20:203–217, 2001.

Kocher MS, Waters PM, Micheli LJ: Upper extremity injuries in the paediatric athlete. Sports Med 30:117–135, 2000.

Le TB, Hentz VR: Hand and wrist injuries in young athletes. Hand Clin 16:597–607, 2000.

Mastey RD, Weiss AP, Akelman E: Primary care of hand and wrist athletic injuries. Clin Sports Med 16:705–724, 1997.

Morgan WJ, Slowman LS: Acute hand and wrist injuries in athletes: Evaluation and management. J Am Acad Orthop Surg 9:389–400, 2001.

Morley J, Bidwell J, Bransby-Zachary M: A comparison of the findings of wrist arthroscopy and magnetic resonance imaging in the investigation of wrist pain. J Hand Surg [Br] 26:544–546, 2001.

Nakamura T, Takayama S, Horiuchi Y, Yabe Y: Origins and insertions of the triangular fibrocartilage complex: A histological study. J Hand Surg [Br] 26:446–454, 2001.

Potter HG, Weiland AJ: Magnetic resonance imaging of triangular fibrocartilage complex lesions. J Hand Surg [Am] 27:363–364, author reply [364], 2002.

Shih JT, Lee HM, Tan CM: Early isolated triangular fibrocartilage complex tears: Management by arthroscopic repair. J Trauma 53:922–927, 2002.

Stamos BD, Leddy JP: Closed flexor tendon disruption in athletes. Hand Clin 16:359–365, 2000.

Strickland JW: Considerations for the treatment of the injured athlete. Clin Sports Med 17:397–400, 1998.

Tomaino MM, Weiser RW: Combined arthroscopic TFCC débridement and wafer resection of the distal ulna in wrists with triangular fibrocartilage complex tears and positive ulnar variance. J Hand Surg [Am] 26:1047–1052, 2001.

Treihaft MM: Neurologic injuries in baseball players. Semin Neurol 20:187–193, 2000.

Westkaemper JG, Mitsionis G, Giannakopoulos PN, Sotereanos DG: Wrist arthroscopy for the treatment of ligament and triangular fibrocartilage complex injuries. Arthroscopy 14:479–483, 1998.

Tendon Injuries of the Elbow and Wrist

Boyd HB, Anderson LD: A method for reinsertion of the distal biceps brachii tendon. J Bone Joint Surg [Am] 43:1041–1043, 1961.

Boyd HB, McLeod AC: Tennis elbow. J Bone Joint Surg [Am] 55:1183–1187, 1973.

Burhkhart SS, Wood MB, Linscheid RL: Posttraumatic recurrent subluxation of the extensor carpi ulnaris tendon. J Hand Surg 7:1, 1982.

Conrad RW: Tennis elbow. AAOS Instr Course Lect 35:94–101, 1986.

D'Alessandro DF, Shields CL, Tibone JE, et al: Repair of distal biceps tendon ruptures in athletes. Am J Sports Med 21:114–119, 1993.

Froimson AI: Treatment of tennis elbow with forearm support band. J Bone Joint Surg [Am] 53:183–184, 1971.

Gabel GT, Morrey BF: Tennis elbow. AAOS Instr Course Lect 47:165–172, 1998.

Green DP, Strickland JW: The hand. In DeLee JC, Drez D Jr, eds: Orthopaedic Sports Medicine, pp 945–1017. Philadelphia, WB Saunders, 1993.

Ilfeld FW: Can stroke modification relieve tennis elbow?. Clin Orthop 276:182–185, 1992.

Jobe FW, Ciccotti MG: Lateral and medial epicondylitis of the elbow. J Am Acad Orthop Surg 2:1–8, 1994.

Kiefhaber TR, Stern PJ: Upper extremity tendinitis and overuse syndromes in the athlete. Clin Sports Med 11:39–55, 1992.

Leddy JP: Soft tissue injuries of the hand in the athlete. AAOS Instr Course Lect 47:181–186, 1998.

Leddy JP, Packer JW: Avulsion of the profundus tendon insertion in athletes. J Hand Surg 2:66–69, 1977.

Morrey BF: Reoperation of failed surgical treatment of refractory lateral epicondylitis. J Shoulder Elbow Surg 1:47–55, 1992.

Moss JG, Steingold RF: The long-term results of mallet finger injury: A retrospective study of one hundred cases. Hand 15:151–154, 1983.

Nirschl RP: Sports and overuse injuries to the elbow. In Morrey BF, ed: The Elbow and Its Disorders, 2nd ed, pp 537–552. Philadelphia, WB Saunders, 1993.

Nirschl RP, Pettrone F: Tennis elbow: The surgical treatment of lateral epicondylitis. J Bone Joint Surg [Am] 61:832–839, 1979.

Regan W, Wold LE, Conrad R, Morrey BF: Microscopic histopathology of chronic refractory lateral epicondylitis. Am J Sports Med 20:746–749, 1992.

Rettig AC: Closed tendon injuries of the hand and wrist in the athlete. Clin Sports Med 11:77–99, 1992.

Strickland JW: Management of acute flexor tendon injuries. Orthop Clin North Am 14:827–849, 1983.

Tarsney FF: Rupture and avulsion of the triceps. Clin Orthop 83:177–183, 1972.

Wood MB, Dobyns JH: Sports-related extraarticular wrist syndromes. Clin Orthop 202:93–102, 1986.

Ligamentous Injuries of the Elbow and Wrist

Alexander CE, Lichtman DM: Ulnar carpal instabilities. Orthop Clin North Am 15:307–320, 1984.

Bednar JM, Osterman AL: Carpal instability: Evaluation and treatment. J Am Acad Orthop Surg 1:10–17, 1993.

Bennett JB, Green MS, Tullos HS: Surgical management of chronic medial elbow instability. Clin Orthop 278:62–68, 1992.

Berger RA: Radial-sided carpal instability. AAOS Instr Course Lect 47:219–228, 1998.

Betz RR, Browne EZ, Perry GB, et al: The complex volar metacarpophalangeal joint dislocation. J Bone Joint Surg [Am] 64:1374–1375, 1982.

Campbell CS: Gamekeeper's thumb. J Bone Joint Surg [Br] 37:148–149, 1955.

Conway JE, Jobe FW, Glousman RE, et al: Medial instability of the elbow in throwing athletes: Surgical treatment by ulnar collateral ligament repair or reconstruction. J Bone Joint Surg [Am] 74:67–83, 1992.

Cooney WP III, Linscheid RL, Dobyns JH: Carpal instability: Treatment of ligament injuries of the wrist. AAOS Instr Course Lect 41:33–44, 1992.

Eaton RG, Malerich MM: Volar plate arthroplasty of the proximal interphalangeal joint: A review of ten years' experience. J Hand Surg 5:260–268, 1980.

Green DP, Strickland JW: The hand. In DeLee JC, Drez D Jr, eds: Orthopaedic Sports Medicine, pp 945–1017. Philadelphia, WB Saunders, 1993.

Habernek H, Ortner F: The influence of anatomic factors in elbow joint dislocation. Clin Orthop 274:226–230, 1992.

Heyman P: Injuries to the ulnar collateral ligament of the thumb metacarpophalangeal joint. J Am Acad Orthop Surg 5:224–229, 1997.

Hinterman B, Holzach PJ, Schultz M, et al: Skier's thumb: The significance of bony injuries. Am J Sports Med 21:800–804, 1993.

Isani A, Melone CP Jr: Ligamentous injuries of the hand in athletes. Clin Sports Med 5:757–772, 1986.

Jobe FW, Kvitne RS: Elbow instability in the athlete. AAOS Instr Course Lect 40:17, 1991.

Kaplan EB: Dorsal dislocation of the metacarpophalangeal joint of the index finger. J Bone Joint Surg [Am] 39:1081–1086, 1957.

Kozin SH: Perilunate injuries: Diagnosis and treatment. J Am Acad Orthop Surg 6:114–120, 1998.

Light TR: Buttress pinning techniques. Orthop Rev 10:49–55, 1981.

Lubahn JD, Cermak MB: Uncommon nerve compression syndromes of the upper extremity. J Am Acad Orthop Surg 6:378–386, 1998.

McCue FC, Bruce JF: The wrist. In DeLee JC, Drez D Jr, eds: Orthopaedic Sports Medicine, pp 913–944. Philadelphia, WB Saunders, 1993.

McElfresh EC, Dobyns JH, O'Brien ET: Management of fracture-dislocation of the proximal interphalangeal joints by extension-block splinting. J Bone Joint Surg [Am] 54:1705–1711, 1972.

McLaughlin HL: Complex "locked" dislocation of the metacarpal phalangeal joints. J Trauma 5:683–688, 1965.

Miller CD, Savoie FH III: Valgus extension injuries of the elbow in the throwing athlete. J Am Acad Orthop Surg 2:261–269, 1994.

Morrey BF: Acute and chronic instability of the elbow. J Am Acad Orthop Surg 4:117–128, 1996.

Morrey BF: Complex instability of the elbow. J Bone Joint Surg [Am] 79:460–469, 1997.

O'Driscoll SW, Morrey BF: Arthroscopy of the elbow: Diagnostic and therapeutic benefits and hazards. J Bone Joint Surg [Am] 74:84–94, 1992.

O'Driscoll SW, Morrey BF, Korinek S, et al: Elbow subluxation and dislocation: A spectrum of instability. Clin Orthop 280:17–28, 1992.

O'Driscoll SW, Lawton RL, Smith AM: The "moving valgus stress test" for medial collateral ligament tears of the elbow. Am J Sports Med 33:231–239, 2005.

Palmer AK, Louis DS: Assessing ulnar instability of the metacarpophalangeal joint of the thumb. J Hand Surg 3:542–546, 1978.

Redler I, Williams JT: Rupture of a collateral ligament of the proximal interphalangeal joint of the fingers: Analysis of eighteen cases. J Bone Joint Surg [Am] 49:322–326, 1967.

Short WH: Wrist instability. AAOS Instr Course Lect 47:203–208, 1998.

Stener B: Displacement of the ruptured collateral ligament of the metacarpophalangeal joint of the thumb: A clinical and anatomical study. J Bone Joint Surg [Br] 44:869–879, 1962.

Viegas SF: Ulnar-sided wrist pain and instability. AAOS Instr Course Lect 47:215–218, 1998.

Watson HK, Ballet FL: The SLAC wrist: Scapholunate advanced collapse pattern of degenerative arthritis. J Hand Surg [Am] 9:358–365, 1984.

Wilson FD, Andrews JR, Blackburn TA, et al: Valgus extension overload in the pitching elbow. Am J Sports Med 11:83–88, 1983.

Articular Injuries of the Elbow and Wrist

Armstead RB, Linscheid RL, Dobyns JH, et al: Ulnar lengthening in the treatment of Kienbock's disease. J Bone Joint Surg [Am] 64:170–178, 1982.

Aulicino PL, Siegel L: Acute injuries of the distal radioulnar joint. Hand Clin 7:283–293, 1991.

Bauer M, Jonsson K, Josefsson PO, Linden B: Osteochondritis dissecans of the elbow: A long-term follow-up study. Clin Orthop 284:156–160, 1992.

Bennett JB: Articular injuries in the athlete. In Morrey BF, ed: The Elbow and Its Disorders, 2nd ed, pp 581–595. Philadelphia, WB Saunders, 1993.

DeHaven KE, Evarts CM: Throwing injuries of the elbow in athletes. Orthop Clin North Am 1:801, 1973.

Dell PC: Traumatic disorders of the distal radioulnar joint. Clin Sports Med 11:141–159, 1991.

Gelberman RH, Salamon PB, Jurist JM, et al: Ulnar variance in Kienbock's disease. J Bone Joint Surg [Am] 57:674–676, 1975.

Morrey BF: Primary arthritis of the elbow treated by ulno-humeral arthroplasty. J Bone Joint Surg [Br] 74:409–413, 1992.

Murakami S, Nakajima H: Aseptic necrosis of the capitate bone. Am J Sports Med 12:170–173, 1984.

Nalebuff EA, Poehling GG, Siegel DB, et al: Wrist and hand: Reconstruction. In Frymoyer JW, ed: Orthopaedic Knowledge Update 4. Home Study Syllabus, pp 389–402. Rosemont, IL, American Academy of Orthopaedic Surgeons, 1993.

Osterman AL: Arthroscopic débridement of triangular fibrocartilage complex tears. Arthroscopy 6:120–124, 1990.

Palmer AK: Triangular fibrocartilage disorders: Injury patterns and treatment. Arthroscopy 6:125–132, 1990.

Singer KM, Roy SP: Osteochondrosis of the humeral capitellum. Am J Sports Med 12:351–360, 1984.

Watson HK, Ryu J, DiBella WS: An approach to Kienbock's disease: Triscaphoarthrodesis. J Hand Surg [Am] 10:179–187, 1985.

Woodward AH, Bianco AJ: Osteochondritis dissecans of the elbow. Clin Orthop Relat Res 110:35–41, 1975.

Arthroscopy of the Elbow and Wrist

Adams BD: Endoscopic carpal tunnel release. J Am Acad Orthop Surg 2:179–184, 1994.

Andrews JR, Carson WG: Arthroscopy of the elbow. Arthroscopy 1:97–107, 1985.

Boe S: Arthroscopy of the elbow: Diagnosis and extraction of loose bodies. Acta Orthop Scand 57:52–53, 1986.

Carson W: Arthroscopy of the elbow. AAOS Instr Course Lect 37:195, 1988.

Chidgey LK: The distal radioulnar joint: Problems and solutions. J Am Acad Orthop Surg 3:95–108, 1995.

Cooney WP, Dobyns JH, Linscheid RL: Arthroscopy of the wrist: Anatomy and classification of carpal instability. Arthroscopy 6:133–140, 1990.

Guhl J: Arthroscopy and arthroscopic surgery of the elbow. Orthopedics 8:1290–1296, 1985.

Lindenfeld TN: Medial approach in elbow arthroscopy. Am J Sports Med 18:413–417, 1990.

Lynch G, Meyers J, Whipple T, et al: Neurovascular anatomy and elbow arthroscopy: Inherent risks. Arthroscopy 2:191, 1986.

Osterman AL: Arthroscopic débridement of triangular fibrocartilage complex tears. Arthroscopy 6:120–124, 1990.

Poehling GG, Siegel DB, Koman LA, et al: Arthroscopy of the wrist and elbow. In DeLee JC, Drez D Jr, eds: Orthopaedic Sports Medicine, pp 189–214. Philadelphia, WB Saunders, 1993.

Roth JH, Poehling GG, Whipple TL: Arthroscopic surgery of the wrist. AAOS Instr Course Lect 37:183–194, 1988.

Whipple TL: Diagnostic and surgical arthroscopy of the wrist. In Nichols JA, Hershman EB, eds: The Upper Extremity in Sports Medicine, pp 399–418. St. Louis, CV Mosby, 1990.

Other Upper Extremity Problems

O'Driscoll SW: Elbow arthritis: Treatment options. J Am Acad Orthop Surg 2:106–116, 1993.

Rettig AC: Fractures in the hand in athletes. AAOS Instr Course Lect 47:187–190, 1998.

Simonian PT, Trumble TE: Scaphoid nonunion. J Am Acad Orthop Surg 2:185–191, 1994.

Szabo RM, Steinberg DR: Nerve entrapment syndromes in the wrist. J Am Acad Orthop Surg 2:115–123, 1994.

HEAD AND SPINE INJURIES

Head Injuries

Bruno LA: Focal intracranial hematoma. In Torg JS, ed: Athletic Injuries to the Head, Neck and Face, 2nd ed. St. Louis, Mosby–Year Book, 1991.

Cantu RC: Criteria for return to competition after a closed head injury. In Torg JS, ed: Athletic Injuries to the Head, Neck and Face, 2nd ed. St. Louis, Mosby–Year Book, 1991.

Cantu RC: Guidelines to return to sports after cerebral concussion. Phys Sports Med 14:76, 1986.

Cantu RC: Return to play guidelines after a head injury. Clin Sports Med 17:45–60, 1998.

Gennarelli TA: Head injury mechanisms and cerebral concussion and diffuse brain injuries. In Torg JS, ed: Athletic Injuries to the Head, Neck and Face, 2nd ed. St. Louis, Mosby–Year Book, 1991.

Jordan BD, Tsairis P, Warren RF: Sports Neurology. Rockville, MD, Aspen Press, 1989.

Lindsay KW, McLatchie G, Jennett B: Serious head injuries in sports. BMJ 281:789–791, 1980.

Wojtys EM, Hovda D, Landry G, et al: Current concepts: Concussion in sports. Am J Sports Med 27:676–687, 1999.

Cervical Spine Injuries

Albright JP, Moses JM, Feldich HG, et al: Non-fatal cervical spine injuries in interscholastic football. JAMA 236:1243–1245, 1976.

Ghiselli G, Schaadt G, McAllister DR: On-the-field evaluation of an athlete with a head or neck injury. Clin Sports Med 22:445–465, 2003.

Bracken MD, Shepard MJ, Collins WF, et al: A randomized, controlled trial of methylprednisolone or naloxone in the treatment of acute spinal cord injury. N Engl J Med 322:1405–1411, 1990.

Pavlov H, Torg JS, Robie B, et al: Cervical spinal stenosis: Determination with vertebral body ratio method. Radiology 164:771–775, 1987.

Thompson RC: Current concepts in management of cervical spine fractures and dislocations. Am J Sports Med 3:159, 1975.

Torg JS, Gennarelli TA: Head and cervical spine injuries. In DeLee JC, Drez D Jr, eds: Orthopaedic Sports Medicine: Principles and Practice, pp 417–462. Philadelphia, WB Saunders, 1994.

Torg JS, Pavlov H, Genuario SE, et al: Neuropraxia of the cervical spinal cord with transient quadriplegia. J Bone Joint Surg [Am] 68:1354–1370, 1986.

Torg JS, Sennett B, Pavlov H, et al: Spear tackler's spine: An entity precluding participation in tackle football and collision activities that expose the cervical spine to axial energy inputs. Am J Sports Med 21:640–649, 1993.

Torg JS, Sennett B, Vegso JJ, et al: Axial loading injuries to the middle cervical spine segment: An analysis and classification of twenty-five cases. Am J Sports Med 19:6–20, 1991.

Torg JS, Vegso JJ, O'Neill J, et al: The epidemiologic, pathologic, biomechanical and cinematographic analysis of football-induced cervical spine trauma. Am J Sports Med 18:50–57, 1990.

Waninger K: On field management of potential cervical spine injury in helmeted football players. Clin J Sports Med 8:124–129, 1998.

White AA, Johnson RM, Panjabi MM: Biomechanical analysis of clinical stability in the cervical spine. Clin Orthop 109:85–93, 1975.

Thoracic and Lumbar Spine Injuries

Bradford DS, Boachie-Adjei O: Treatment of severe spondylolisthesis by anterior and posterior reduction and stabilization: A long-term follow-up study. J Bone Joint Surg [Am] 72:1060–1066, 1990.

Eismont FJ, Currier B: Surgical management of lumbar intervertebral disc disease. J Bone Joint Surg [Am] 71:1266–1271, 1989.

Eismont FJ, Kitchel SH: Thoracolumbar spine. In DeLee JC, Drez D Jr, eds: Orthopaedic Sports Medicine, pp 1018–1062. Philadelphia, WB Saunders, 1994.

Jackson D, Wiltse L, Dingeman R, et al: Stress reactions involving the pars interarticularis in young athletes. Am J Sports Med 9:305, 1981.

Keene JS, Albert MJ, Springer SL, et al: Back injuries in college athletes. J Spinal Disord 2:190–195, 1989.

Mundt DJ, Kelsey JL, Golden AL, et al: An epidemiological study of sports and weightlifting as possible risk factors for herniated lumbar and cervical discs. Am J Sports Med 21:854–860, 1993.

MEDICAL ASPECTS

Drugs

Beiner JM, Jokl P, Cholewicki J, et al: The effect of anabolic steroids and corticosteroids on healing of muscle contusion injury. Am J Sports Med 27:2–9, 1999.

Berger RG: Nonsteroidal anti-inflammatory drugs: Making the right choices. J Am Acad Orthop Surg 2:255–260, 1994.

Fadale PD, Wiggins ME: Corticosteroid injections: Their use and abuse. J Am Acad Orthop Surg 2:133–140, 1994.

Ergogenic Drugs

Aronson V: Protein and miscellaneous ergogenic aids. Physician Sports Med 14:209–212, 1986.

Brien AJ, Simon TL: The effects of red blood cell infusion on 10-km race time. JAMA 257:2761–2765, 1987.

Cowart VS: Human growth hormone: The latest ergogenic aid. Physician Sports Med 16:175, 1988.

Haupt HA: Anabolic steroids and growth hormone: Current concepts. Am J Sports Med 21:468–474, 1993.

Perlmutter G, Lowenthal DT: Use of anabolic steroids by athletes. Am Fam Physician 32:208–210, 1985.

Pope HG, Katz DL, Champoux R: Anabolic-androgenic steroid use among 1,010 college men. Physician Sports Med 16:75, 1988.

Robinson JB: Ergogenic drugs in sports. In DeLee JC, Drez D Jr, eds: Orthopaedic Sports Medicine, pp 294–306. Philadelphia, WB Saunders, 1994.

Cardiovascular

Abraham P, Chevalier J-M, Leftheriotis G, et al: Lower extremity arterial disease in sports. Am J Sports Med 25:581–584, 1997.

Alpert SA, et al: Athletic heart syndrome. Physician Sports Med 12:103–107, 1989.

Basilico FC: Cardiovascular disease in athletes: Current concepts. Am J Sports Med 27:108–121, 1999.

Braden DS, Strong WB: Preparticipation screening for sudden cardiac death in high school and college athletes. Physician Sports Med 16:128–140, 1988.

Finney TP, D'Ambrosia RD: Sudden cardiac death in an athlete. In DeLee JC, Drez D Jr, eds: Orthopaedic Sports Medicine, pp 404–416. Philadelphia, WB Saunders, 1994.

James TN, Froggatt P, Marshall TK: Sudden death in young athletes. Ann Intern Med 67:1013–1021, 1967.

Maron BJ, Epstein SE, Roberts WC: Causes of sudden death in competitive athletes. J Am Coll. Cardiol 7:204–214, 1986.

Maron BJ, Roberts WC, McAllister HA, et al: Sudden death in young athletes. Circulation 62:218–229, 1980.

Van Camp SP: Exercise-related sudden deaths: Risks and causes. Physician Sports Med 16:97–112, 1988.

Exercise Physiology

Almekinders LC, Oman J: Isokinetic muscle testing: Is it clinically useful?. J Am Acad Orthop Surg 2:221–225, 1994.

Cahill BR, Misner JE, Boileau RA: The clinical importance of the anaerobic energy system and its assessment in human performance: Current concepts. Am J Sports Med 25:863–872, 1997.

Fleck SJ, Schutt RC: Types of strength training. Clin Sports Med 4:159–168, 1985.

Galloway M, Jikl P: Aging successfully: The importance of physical activity in maintaining health and function. J Am Acad Orthop Surg 8:37–44, 2000.

Katch FI, Drumm SS: Effects of different modes of strength training on body composition and arthropometry. Clin Sports Med 5:413–459, 1986.

Kirkendall DT, Garrett WE Jr: The effects of aging and training on skeletal muscle: Current concepts. Am J Sports Med 26:598–602, 1998.

Latzka W, Montain S: Water and electrolyte requirements for exercise. Clin Sports Med 18:513–524, 1999.

Lephart SM, Pincivero DM, Giraldo JL, et al: The role of proprioception in the management and rehabilitation of athletic injuries. Am J Sports Med 25:130–137, 1997.

Paulos LE, Grauer JD: Exercise. In DeLee JC, Drez D Jr, eds: Orthopaedic Sports Medicine: Principles and Practice, pp 228–243. Philadelphia, WB Saunders, 1994.

Pipes TV: Isokinetic vs isotonic strength training in adult men. Med Sci Sports 7:262–274, 1975.

Taylor DC, Dalton JD, Seaber AV, et al: Viscoelastic properties of muscle-tendon units: The biomechanical effects of stretching. Am J Sports Med 18:300–309, 1990.

Yamamoto SK, Hartman CW, Feagin JA, et al: Functional rehabilitation of the knee: A preliminary study. J Sports Med 3:228–291, 1976.

Female Athletes

Barrow G, Saha S: Menstrual irregularity and stress fractures in collegiate female distance runners. Am J Sports Med 16:209–215, 1988.

Eisenberg T, Allen W: Injuries in a women's varsity athletic program. Physician Sports Med 6:112–116, 1978.

Hunter L, Andrews J, Clancy W, et al: Common orthopaedic problems of the female athlete. AAOS Instr Course Lect 31:126–152, 1982.

Otis C, Drinkwater B, et al: American College of Sports Medicine position stand: The female athlete triad. Med Sci Sports Exerc 29:1–9, 1997.

Powers J: Characteristic features of injuries in the knee in women. Clin Orthop 143:120–124, 1979.

Protzman R: Physiologic performance of women compared to men: Observations of cadets at the United States Military Academy. Am J Sports Med 7:191–194, 1979.

Tietz CC, Hu SS, Arendt EA: The female athlete: Evaluation and treatment of sports-related problems. J Am Acad Orthop Surg 5:87–96, 1997.

Voss LA, Fadale PD, Hulstyn MJ: Exercise-induced loss of bone density in athletes. J Am Acad Orthop Surg 6:349–357, 1998.

Whiteside P: Men's and women's injuries in comparable sports. Physician Sports Med 8:130–140, 1980.

CHAPTER 5

Adult Reconstruction

Edward J. McPherson

CONTENTS

SECTION 1 Technical Considerations

I. The Prosthetic Articular Bearing

A. Hard-on-soft hip and shoulder replacement bearings
   1. Coupling—In hip and shoulder replacement surgery, the traditional bearing has been a "hard-on-soft" couple. Hard-on-soft bearing couples include metallic heads (Co-Cr alloy or Ti alloy) mated to a polyethylene (PE) cup. The other hard-on-soft couple is a ceramic head (alumina ceramic or zirconia ceramic) mated to a PE cup.
      a. Metallic heads—Of the metallic-head options, the Co-Cr–PE couple is considered the best. For hip and shoulder replacement, Ti alloy heads should be avoided. This metallic bearing is susceptible to scratching from third-body debris. A rough, scratched surface will cause rapid wear of the PE surface.
      b. Ceramic heads—It is now generally accepted that Zirconia femoral heads should not be used with PE. Zirconia ceramic is a metastable substance. It is manufactured and inserted in a stabilized tetragonal crystal phase. In vivo, Zirconia can undergo phase transformation into a monoclinic crystal state, which adversely affects surface roughness and can lead to accelerated PE wear.
   2. Optimum wear—For both Co-Cr–PE and ceramic-PE couples, optimum wear is related to the **roughness** of the head surface and its **sphericity.** In Co-Cr heads, residual roughness is a result of carbide asperites that stick up from the surface after polishing. For ceramic heads, residual pits within the surface cause it to be rough.
   3. Hip lubrication—The lubrication regimen for a hard-on-soft bearing in the hip is always **boundary lubrication.** In this regimen, the lubricant (i.e., synovial fluid) is not thick enough to prevent contact between the asperites (i.e., high points on the bearing surface) of the two opposing surfaces. However, the synovial fluid, with its long-chain protein molecules, can separate the two surfaces enough to prevent severe wear.

B. Hard-on-soft knee replacement bearings
   1. Metallic components—For knee replacement surgery the vast majority of prosthetic components manufactured employ a Co-Cr alloy femoral surface

mated to a PE tibial surface. Similar to the recommendation for the hip and shoulder, Ti alloy is not used, because this metal alloy is susceptible to scratching from third-body debris. The rare exception for using a Ti alloy femoral component would be a patient with a documented nickel allergy. The Co-Cr alloys used for prosthetic implants contain a small percentage of nickel.

2. Ceramic components—Ceramic femoral components for TKR are much less commonly used. Ceramic femoral components have the advantage of greater scratch resistance than Co-Cr alloy but the disadvantage of being more brittle, which may potentially lead to prosthetic breakage. The biggest disadvantage of a ceramic implant employed in any joint replacement scenario is its low toughness (defined as resistance to fracture).
3. Polyethylene—The type of PE used for hard-on-soft bearing couples is ultra–high-molecular-weight polyethylene (UHMWPE). The wear of PE is the major factor in causing osteolysis and prosthetic failure in all hard-on-soft bearing couples. PE wear is related to three factors: PE manufacturing, sterilization after processing, and shelf life (i.e., how long the PE product has remained on the shelf unused).
   a. Manufacturing techniques—UHMWPE for prosthetic devices in general is made by four different manufacturing techniques. They are (1) ram bar extrusion with secondary machining into the desired product (Fig. 5–1), (2) hot isostatic pressing into bars with secondary machining into the desired product, (3) compression molding into bars with secondary machining into the desired product, and (4) direct compression molding from PE powder to the desired product. Better wear of UHMWPE has been consistently achieved with the **direct compression molding** process.
   b. Calcium stearate—Calcium stearate should not be added in the production of PE. Calcium stearate prevents PE from caking onto processing equipment and acts as a corrosion inhibitor that protects processing equipment. Studies have shown that calcium stearate added to PE adversely affects PE consolidation by creating areas with unfused PE particles **(fusion defects).** These areas of fusion defect significantly diminish the mechanical properties of finished PE implants.
   c. Techniques and effects of sterilization—The sterilization of PE after processing significantly affects PE performance and wear characteristics. PE sterilization techniques involve either nonenergetic (i.e., no irradiation) or energetic (i.e., radiation) processes. The techniques in which no irradiation is used are gas plasma sterilization and ethylene oxide sterilization. Irradiation of UHMWPE for sterilization is performed at two different levels: the traditional low dose (2.5-4.5 Mrad) and the newer high dose (5-15 Mrad).
   d. PE cross-linking—UHMWPE treated with low-dose irradiation in an inert environment *without* oxygen favors cross-linking of PE.
      (1) Advantages—Cross-linking of UHMWPE improves resistance to adhesive and abrasive wear. In addition, cross-linked PE improves bearing wear rates. The newer techniques of high-dose irradiation further increase cross-linking of PE to further improve PE wear rates. UHMWPE treated with high-dose irradiation is called **highly cross-linked PE (HCLPE).** Remember that irradiation of UHMWPE in an oxygen environment promotes oxidation of PE, and this is detrimental. Oxidation of PE causes molecular chain scission, which in turn causes accelerated PE wear and failure. The techniques of gas plasma and ethylene oxide sterilization have no effect on the cross-linking of UHMWPE. When these techniques are used alone, the wear rates of UHMWPE are generally higher than those for cross-linked PE.
      (2) Methods—There are at least four different methods to produce HCLPE with high-dose irradiation. The key factor in all of these techniques is maintaining optimum **crystallinity** of the PE. The PE in a manufactured implant exists in two different phases: crystalline and amorphous (Fig. 5–2). With irradiation after processing, only the amorphous areas cross-link. The crystallinity of PE that is over 70% is associated with higher PE failure rates. When high-dose irradiation techniques are used, the manufacturing techniques must keep the crystalline phase to 50-56%.
      (3) Disadvantages of cross-linked PE—It is important to remember that HCLPE has disadvantages. Increasing cross-linking *diminishes* the mechanical properties of

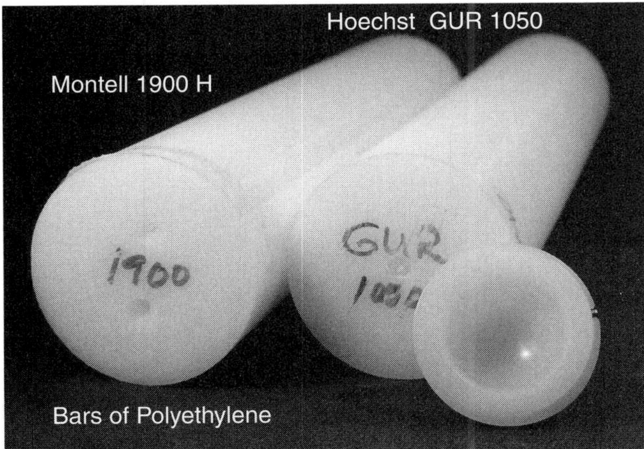

FIGURE 5–1 Ram bar-extruded polyethylene. Samples are from Hoechst GUR 1050 and Montell 1900 H. Hip and knee polyethylene products are cut and machined from these bars.

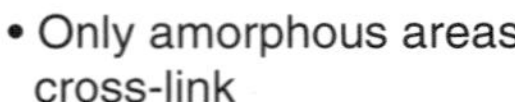
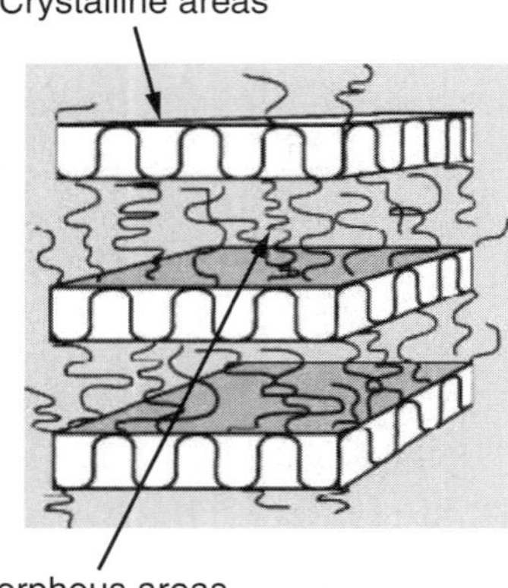
Crystalline areas
• Polyethylene has two different phases: Crystalline and amorphous
• Only amorphous areas cross-link
Amorphous areas

FIGURE 5–2 The molecular structure of ultra-high-molecular-weight polyethylene. There are two distinct phases. One is the crystalline phase, which coexists with the adjacent amorphous regions. It is the amorphous regions that are cross-linked with irradiation treatment.

the PE. With HCLPE, there is decreased tensile strength (pulling force to break), decreased fatigue strength (maximum cyclic stress the material can withstand), decreased fracture toughness (force to propagate a crack), and decreased ductility (elongation without fracture). The decreased mechanical properties may have deleterious clinical effects when the PE is edge loaded. In the hip, edge loading can occur when the prosthetic femoral neck impinges on the edge of the acetabular insert of the HCLPE, which may cause localized fracture. Furthermore, HCLPE may not be desirable in the knee because the diminished mechanical properties may lead to macroscopic failure of the PE if high stresses are applied. An example of this situation in the knee would be edge loading of the femoral component onto the PE. HCLPE has not yet been shown to reduce osteolysis and improve implant survival because there are no long-term outcome studies with these devices. Finally, when compared with conventional PE, the particles generated by HCLPE during bearing wear have a *decreased* average particle size.

e. Heat annealing—The secondary processes involved in high-dose irradiation of PE generally involve the heating of PE to remove the remaining free radicals. **Heat annealing** is the process of heating PE close to the melting point to remove free radicals. If the heating is kept below the melting point, there is little reordering of the PE structure. If the heating is taken above the melting point, there is structural reordering of the PE chains, which can increase the crystallinity of PE with certain techniques.

f. PE degradation from storage and packaging—PE performance can be adversely affected by its **shelf storage time** (the time the PE product sits on the shelf before implantation). The extent of PE degradation while it remains on the shelf depends on two major factors: the extent of radiation treatment and the type of packaging.

(1) Oxidation of PE products—Irradiation of PE produces free radicals. If PE products are packaged and irradiated in an oxygen-free environment, oxidation of PE is minimized. However, if PE products are allowed to sit on the shelf and age, oxygen diffusion into the PE can occur, resulting in oxidation.

(2) Packaging—The extent of oxygen diffusion into PE depends on the type of packaging. In experimental studies, free radicals are known to survive within PE for as long as 2-3 years. The higher the radiation dose, the more free radicals produced. Therefore, a long shelf life can adversely affect PE performance via **on-the-shelf** oxidation. A PE product that has been on the shelf a long time may have already developed significant oxidative structural changes before implantation. The worst-case scenario is irradiated PE packaged in air (i.e., oxygen) and allowed to sit for years on the shelf. This occurs with odd lot sizes (i.e., very small or very large product sizes that are infrequently used). If these odd-lot parts are implanted, PE wear rates may be severe. It is recommended that irradiated PE products sit on the shelf no longer than several years. Nonirradiated PE products are not affected significantly by shelf storage time.

C. Hard-on-hard hip replacement bearings

1. Advantages—The "hard-on-hard" bearing couple has been reintroduced as an alternative bearing for THR. The main impetus for employing the hard-on-hard bearing surface is the associated structural bone damage and prosthetic failure incurred from PE particulate–induced osteolysis with hard-on-soft couples. The particle size range of 0.2-7 μm has been demonstrated to trigger the immune response, which leads to the osteolytic reaction. For hard-on-hard bearings, the particulate debris generated is much smaller in size (range, 0.015-0.12 μm). It is believed that these smaller-sized particles induce a much less intense osteolytic reaction. Ironically, even though hard-on-hard bearings show very low **linear wear rates** and low wear volumes, the number of particles generated is still *greater* than hard-on-soft bearing couples. The reason is that the particles are so much smaller compared with PE particles that the calculated total particle aggregate is greater.

2. Clearance of debris/cancer risk—The very small particle sizes generated with hard-on-hard bearing couples change the physiologic clearance of debris. These very small particles are absorbed regionally and are disseminated throughout the body via

lymphatic channels. This is a concern with metal-on-metal (i.e., Co-Cr alloy) bearings, with which increased cobalt and chromium ion levels in the blood and urine have been documented. At present, the primary concern of long-term induction of neoplasia is unfounded. Long-term studies have shown no increase in cancer levels associated with metal-on-metal hip bearings. Ceramic particles within the body are essentially inert, and the cancer risk with ceramic-on-ceramic bearings is not an issue.

3. Lubrication—The lubrication regimen for a hard-on-hard bearing is **mixed lubrication,** which means that part of the time the lubrication regimen is **boundary** and part of the time **hydrodynamic** (also known as fluid film lubrication).
   a. Hydrodynamic lubrication—With hydrodynamic lubrication, the two opposing bearing surfaces are completely separated by the lubricant. Hydrodynamic lubrication with a hard-on-hard bearing is governed by the **lambda ratio,** a complicated formula that takes into consideration bearing surface roughness, head size, fluid viscosity (constant with synovial fluid), and angular velocity. A lambda ratio greater than 3 indicates fluid film mechanics. An extremely smooth bearing surface is more likely to achieve hydrodynamic lubrication, which is directly related to the head radius. A head size of 38 mm or greater is more likely to achieve hydrodynamic lubrication during walking. Finally, it is important to remember that the fluid film state *requires* angular velocity; the joint must be in motion. Therefore, for any hard-on-hard bearing construct used, hydrodynamic lubrication does not occur while the patient is at rest or when head motion is slow. It is thought that a bearing that is lubricated part-time by hydrodynamic lubrications has longer bearing wear than one that is lubricated completely by boundary lubrication.
4. Other factors—The success of hard-on-hard bearing couples depends on several important factors: **surface roughness, sphericity**, and **radial clearance.**
   a. Surface roughness—For optimum lubrication, a hard-on-hard bearing surface must be very smooth. The rougher the surface, the more difficult it is to separate with lubricant. Metal (i.e., Co-Cr alloy) surfaces have a surface roughness (R_a) of 0.05 μm. Ceramic surfaces have an R_a of 0.02 μm. In comparison, machined UHMWPE has a roughness of several hundred micrometers.
   b. Sphericity—Also affects bearing lubrication. It should be kept below 10 μm. Variation in sphericity creates small, high points on the surface, which causes localized stress points that can adversely affect lubrication and increase wear.
   c. Radial clearance—Defined as the difference in radius of the head and cup. If the radius of the head is larger than the cup, bearing contact is **equatorial.** An equatorial bearing has high frictional torque because there is no space for lubricant ingress and egress. If the diameter of the head is smaller than the cup, bearing contact is **polar.** Polar contact with low conformity (i.e., high radial clearance) also causes high friction and wear. The small bearing contact area causes high stress, resulting in poor lubrication. The *optimum* design is polar contact with high bearing conformity (Fig. 5–3). In this situation, the radial clearance is small (typically <150 μm). The low radial clearance is still enough to allow ingress and egress of the lubricant into the bearing.

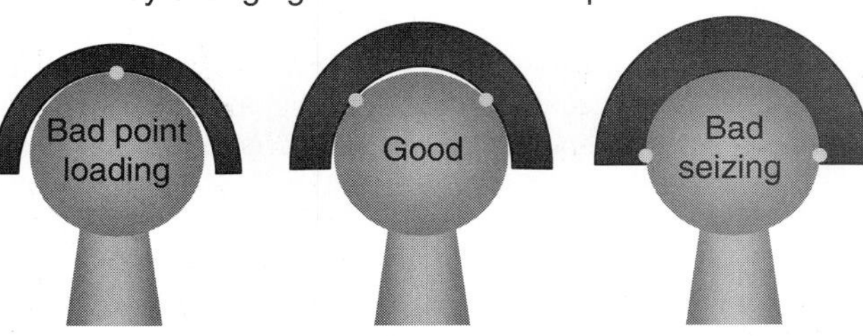

FIGURE 5–3 The three different areas of bearing contact that can be employed for a hard-on-hard bearing couple for hip replacement. Polar contact allows fluid lubrication, but contact stress at the pole is high, causing high friction and wear. Midpolar contact is the best because contact loads are optimized and there is good bearing lubrication. Equatorial contact prevents fluid lubrication and can cause high friction and wear.

5. Wear on bearings—Hard-on-hard bearings have a phenomenon of **"run-in" wear.** There is typically a higher wear rate within the first 1 million cycles of wear that diminishes to a lower steady-state wear rate after the run-in period. It is thought that during the run-in period, high stress points (i.e., sphericity discrepancies) and the larger surface asperites are polished out of the bearing couple.
   a. Stripe wear—A common pattern of wear seen with a hard-on-hard bearing is *stripe* wear. Initially described with alumina-on-alumina hip bearings, stripe wear can potentially occur with any hard-on-hard bearing surface combination. A stripe line is a crescent-shaped line that forms on a femoral head (Fig. 5–4). A corresponding stripe line forms on the acetabular component, which is always near the edge. Depending on component orientation and patient position during heavy hip loads, the stripe line on the acetabulum can be seen in various locations about the acetabular edge.
   b. Stripe line/surface wear—The stripe line microscopically represents an area of surface wear (1-60 μm deep). With a ceramic surface, grain pullout is the mechanism of wear. With a metal surface, abrasive wear is the mechanism. Pathomechanically, stripe wear occurs

when the femoral head loads near the edge of the acetabular cup. When edge loading occurs, surface contact loads within the "stripe zone" are significantly increased, which causes increased wear in this region. Stripe wear is seen more frequently in acetabular cups that are more vertically oriented (i.e., high theta angle orientation).

6. Hip edge loading—This action can occur in several scenarios, but the common theme is that the axial hip load passes through the femoral head and then onto the acetabular cup near the edge. If the axial hip load passes through the pole of the acetabular cup, the contact area is maximized and contact loads are relatively low. In contrast, if the axial hip load passes near the edge of the acetabular cup, the contact area is reduced and contact loads are significantly increased. Therefore, to reduce stripe wear clinically, acetabular and femoral stem orientations must be carefully checked to maximize polar cup loading in the positions of high hip loads. High hip-loading positions occur at heel strike during walking, stair climbing, and rising from a chair.

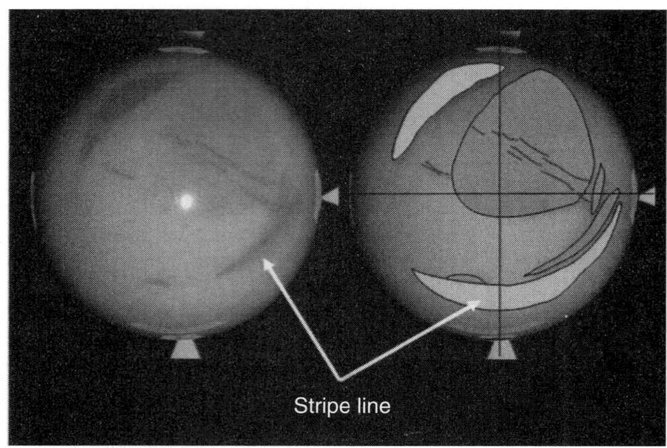

FIGURE 5–4 A retrieved ceramic head showing wear indicated by a stripe line. The picture on the left shows a crescent-shaped stripe line that is covered with debris particles. The picture on the right shows overlay diagrams on the head where the stripe line extends when viewed microscopically. (Courtesy of Ian Clarke, PhD, Peterson Tribology Research Center.)

SECTION 2 Joint Replacements and Procedures

I. Hip Replacement Surgery

A. Fixation in **total hip replacement** (THR)—Long-term fixation of component parts for prosthetic joint replacement is accomplished with cement or biologic interdigitation of bone to the prosthetic interface.

1. Choice of fixation technique—The recommended fixation for primary hip arthroplasty remains controversial. The **National Institutes of Health** (NIH) consensus statement for total hip arthroplasty recommends that a cemented femoral component with the use of a modern cementing technique, paired with a porous-coated hemispherical acetabular component, can give excellent long-term results. This recommendation is based on data showing a higher loosening rate with cemented acetabular sockets than that with porous-coated, noncemented sockets. On the other hand, there are so many different noncemented femoral stem designs and variations of coatings that there is no identified superiority of noncemented femoral stem over cemented femoral stem fixation. However, the general tendency is to use noncemented femoral stems in younger, more active patients, in which cemented stems have a reportedly higher loosening rate in long-term follow-up. It is thought that the increased cycles (one step equals one hip cycle) and higher stresses applied to the hip joint in young, more active patients lead to a more rapid failure of cemented components. Cemented fixation provides a static mechanical interlocking of methylmethacrylate to the interstices of bone. If microfractures occur with continued cyclic loading, the cement cannot remodel and will ultimately loosen. In contrast, with noncemented components there is dynamic biologic fixation to the prosthesis. If microfractures occur with cyclic loading in this system, there is the potential for bone remodeling, which produces a potentially lifelong bond. Furthermore, removing cement from the system provides one less interface that can fail.
2. Cemented fixation—Cement fixation for hip replacement surgery requires a good technique to provide optimum interdigitation of cement to bone. Paradoxically, with increasing severity of osteoporosis, the mechanical integrity of cement implant fixation increases as a result of the greater bone porosity.
   a. Cement preparation—The technique for cement preparation has undergone several generations of development and is summarized in Table 5–1.
   b. Size of cement mantle—The size of the cement mantle surrounding the femoral stem is controversial. It is suggested that a minimum of 2 mm of cement thickness be allowed between the prosthesis and bone, which would be impractical in narrow canals, where a very small stem diameter would be required. A more practical approach is the

TABLE 5-1 CEMENT PREPARATION TECHNIQUE FOR TOTAL HIP REPLACEMENT

First Generation	Second Generation (began in 1975)	Third Generation (began in 1982)
Finger packing	Cement gun (began 1971)	Porosity reduction (vacuum)
No canal preparation	Pulsatile lavage	Pressurization cement
No cement plug	Canal preparation (brush and dry)	Precoat stem
No cement gun	Cement restrictor	Rough surface finish on stem
No pressurization	Super alloy stem (forged)	Stem centralizer
Cast stem	Broad and round medial border	
Narrow medial border on stem	Collar on stem	
Sharp edges on stem		

two-thirds rule, in which two thirds of the canal is displaced by the femoral stem and the other third by cement. Cement *mantle defects* should be avoided. A mantle defect in which the prosthesis touches bone creates an area of concentrated stress and is associated with a higher loosening rate (Fig. 5–5).

c. Femoral stem
   (1) Design—The design of the femoral stem affects cemented stem performance. A stiffer material (i.e., increased Young's modulus) is preferred. A more flexible material and stem design can put bending and torsional forces onto the cement mantle, creating cracks. Similarly, to reduce the stress points on the cement mantle, the stem should have no sharp corners. Precoating a stem with **polymethylmethacrylate** (PMMA) and adding a medial calcar flange to contact the medial calcar bone do not improve performance. With cemented THR, it is usually the acetabular socket that fails first from loosening. Ranawat states that if the subgroups of patients with rheumatoid arthritis (or other similar inflammatory conditions), protrusio deformity, hip dysplasia, and excessive bleeding are excluded, the long-term results of cemented sockets are comparable to those of noncemented sockets.
   (2) Alternative cemented technique—For femoral stem implantation, an alternative cemented technique is to use a highly polished, tapered stem with square edges and no centralizer (Ling's technique). With this procedure, careful studies have documented that the stem settles within the cement mantle and over time finds a stable mechanical state. It is thought that this technique reduces mechanical stresses on the cement–bone mantle, which may reduce the long-term rates of stem loosening.

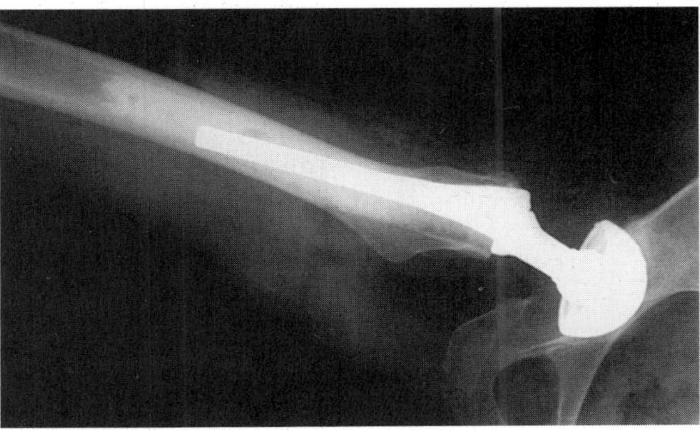

FIGURE 5–5 Lateral radiograph of a cemented femoral stem with a mantle defect. Note the distal stem tip that touches bone.

3. Noncemented (biologic) fixation—Biologic fixation is done using either a porous-coated metallic surface that provides bone **ingrowth** fixation or a grit-blasted metallic surface that provides bone **on-growth** fixation. Biologic fixation by host bone requires viable bone. Prior irradiation to the pelvis and hip predictably increases the risk of aseptic failure due to lack of adequate prosthesis–bone ingrowth or on-growth.
   a. Surfaces
      (1) Porous coating—With a porous-coated surface, pores into which the bone can grow and secure the prosthesis to host bone are created on the metallic surface. Successful bone ingrowth requires an optimum pore size of 50-350 μm (preferably 50-150 μm). The **porosity** of the porous-coated surface, which should be 40-50%, is important for allowing bone to fill in a significant area of the prosthesis. Greater porosity than this is detrimental because the porous-coated surface would be at risk of shearing off. In addition, **pore depth** is a factor in the strength of the prosthesis–bone interlock. A deeper pore depth into the prosthesis provides greater interface shear strength with loading. Finally, **gaps** between the prosthesis and bone must be less than 50 μm.
      (2) Grit blasting—With a grit-blasted surface, a metallic surface is roughened with an abrasive spray of particles that pits the metallic surface. The resulting peaks and valleys in the surface provide areas for bone to interdigitate and develop a stable construct. With this method, the success of the bone on-growth fixation is related to **surface roughness**, which is defined as the average distance from the peak to the valley on the roughened surface. An increase in surface roughness is directly related to an increase in interface shear strength. The drawback to a grit-blasted surface is that bone fixation occurs only on the surface and therefore requires a more extensive area of coating

to secure the prosthesis. The entire prosthesis typically needs to be grit blasted to ensure adequate fixation.

b. Requirements of biologic (noncemented) fixation
   (1) Rigid fixation—Successful bone ingrowth or on-growth requires initial rigid fixation. Micromotion of the prosthesis must be kept below 150 μm (preferably 50-100 μm) or the prosthesis will be secured only by fibrous tissue (fibrous ingrowth), which will allow continued prosthetic micromotion and pain. If gross motion is allowed, the prosthesis will be encapsulated with fibrous tissue rather than fibrous ingrowth, which will cause the prosthesis to settle and remain mechanically unstable. Therefore, the technique for insertion of noncemented components is very important.
      (a) Press-fit technique—Initial rigid fixation of porous-coated implants is usually accomplished by the **press-fit technique,** in which the bone prepared for the acetabular cup or the femoral stem is sized slightly smaller in diameter (usually 1-2 mm undersized). When the component is inserted, the bone expands around the prosthesis, generating **hoop stresses** that keep the prosthesis in position and minimize micromotion.
      (b) Line-to-line fit—The other technique is a **line-to-line fit,** in which the bone is fitted to the same size as the implant and secured with additional measures. In the cup, a line-to-line technique requires screws for additional fixation. For the femoral stem, an extensive porous coating along the entire stem is required to obtain an interference fit, which provides a rough surface over a large area and prevents excessive motion.
   (2) Cortical bone seating—Another important factor for stable bone ingrowth is to have the implant seated against cortical bone rather than cancellous bone. Although cancellous bone will provide bone ingrowth, it is now known that the mechanical strength of an implant seated onto cortical bone is much higher. Therefore, in the acetabulum it is important to achieve a good fit of the acetabular cup to the cortical rim. On the femoral side, it is important that the implant design and surgical preparation allow for cortical contact with the porous-coated or grit-blasted surface.
   (3) Surface coating—**Hydroxyapatite** (HA) [$Ca_{10}(PO_4)_6(OH)_2$] is used as an adjuvant surface coating on porous-coated and grit-blasted surfaces. HA is an *osteoconductive* agent that allows for more rapid closure of gaps. Its surface readily receives osteoblasts and thus provides a bidirectional closure of gaps (i.e., bone to prosthesis and prosthesis to bone), which clinically shortens the time to biologic fixation. HA has been reported to delaminate off the prosthetic interface, and its use may be better suited to porous coated surfaces, with which the bone–HA bond is not the sole means of fixation. The successful use of HA as an adjuvant surface coating requires high crystallinity and optimum thickness (approximately 50 μm).
   (4) Porous coating—The recommended amount of porous coating on a femoral stem is controversial. With proximal porous coating, the porous surface is kept in the metaphyseal and upper metadiaphyseal regions of the femur. With this design concept, proximal bone ingrowth allows proximal bone loading and less stress shielding (Fig. 5–6). Conversely, an extensively coated stem has a porous coating over its entire surface. Most bone ingrowth occurs in the diaphysis, and the weight-bearing forces bypass the proximal femur. The classic radiographic finding of a well-fixed, extensively porous-coated stem is the *spot weld;* increased bone density is seen *surrounding* the distal extent of the porous coating but not inside the medullary canal, which would be seen in a loose stem with a bony intramedullary pedestal.

4. Complications in fixation
   a. Stress shielding—Stress shielding in THR describes the phenomenon of proximal femoral *bone density loss* observed over time in the presence of a solidly fixed implant. In the hip, stress shielding typically occurs with noncemented implants. However, stress shielding can occur in cemented implants and can be seen in other areas where a stem is implanted into bone (i.e., shoulder stem or long-stem tibial implant in **total knee replacement** [TKR]). Dual-energy x-ray absorption studies have confirmed proximal bone density loss with extensively coated, noncemented femoral stems and cemented femoral stems.
      (1) Causes of stress shielding—**Stem stiffness** is the primary factor causing stress shielding. Biomechanically, there is a decrease in the physiologic stress to bone caused by the stiffer structure that shares its load. The extent of porous coating has some effect on stress shielding but is less important than stem stiffness.
      (2) Factors affecting stem stiffness—Stem size, metal choice, stem geometry. (a) Stem stiffness increases exponentially in relation to stem size. Specifically, stem stiffness increases in proportion to the **fourth power of the stem radius** (r^4). (b) A stiffer metal also increases stem

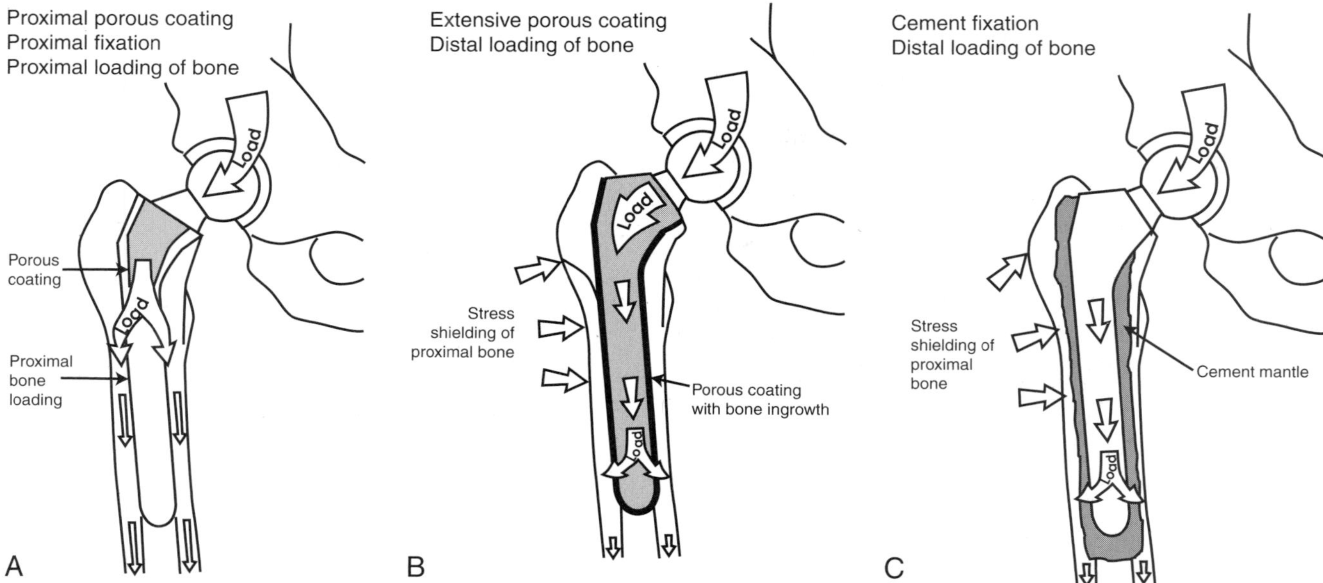

FIGURE 5–6 Bone loading in relation to femoral stem fixation. **A**, Proximal porous coating, no cement. **B**, Extensive porous coating, no cemented fixation. **C**, Cemented fixation.

stiffness. Cobalt chrome (Co-Cr) alloy has a higher modulus of elasticity (Young's modulus) than titanium alloy and therefore is stiffer. (c) Stem geometry can significantly influence its stiffness. Stems that are solid and round are stiffer. Stem geometry that is less stiff includes stems that are hollow or tapered and stems that have slots or flutes. The archetypal scenario of stress shielding in THR is a large-diameter stem (>16 mm) that is made of Co-Cr alloy; has a round, solid cylindrical shaft; and has an extensive porous coating. Although a well-fixed stem with stress shielding appears not to affect implant survival, revision of a stem with significant stress shielding is difficult. Because of stress shielding, femoral cortical bone is thin and more prone to damage during the revision procedure.

b. Fat embolus syndrome—In hip replacement, **fat embolus syndrome** is most often associated with cementing of the femoral stem in an elderly patient. In knee replacement, fat embolism syndrome is more commonly associated with the use of intramedullary guide rods during preparation for bone cuts. The risk increases in direct relation to the number of intramedullary guide rods used (four is the maximum with bilateral TKR).

(1) In hip replacement, fat embolus syndrome is described as a rapid onset of hypotension and hypoxia soon after insertion of a cemented implant. The pressure generated within the intramedullary canal forces fat out of the bone and into the venous system. Microscopic fat emboli then travel to the lungs, where their effects are most dramatic. They lodge in lung capillary parenchymal tissues, preventing oxygenation. A secondary response occurs, creating systemic vasodilatation and hypotension.

(2) Elderly patients are affected more for two main reasons. First, it is more common for elderly patients to have osteoporotic bone that allows cement to squeeze out more fat and marrow elements. Second, it is more common for elderly patients to have coexisting cardiopulmonary disease, making them less able to compensate for the embolic fat showering the lungs. Treatment is supportive, with fluid and pressure support, mechanical ventilation, and oxygenation.

B. Hip stability—Primary and revision surgery

1. Dislocation of THR—The etiology of dislocated THR is complex and often multifactorial. An understanding of the factors involved in the unstable total hip can provide value to the surgeon in both primary and revision arthroplasty. The dislocation incidence after primary THR is on average 1-2%, but it has been reported to be as high as 9.5%. Dislocation after revision is higher and reported as high as 26% in cases of multiple revisions. The highest incidence of dislocation in primary hip arthroplasty is in the subgroup of elderly patients (>80 years old) whose repair was converted to THR after failed osteosynthesis for femoral neck fracture. In this subgroup, the dislocation incidence in one European study was 82%.
2. Assessment of hip stability—The assessment of hip stability involves four major areas: component design, component alignment, soft tissue tensioning, and soft tissue function.
   a. Component design—In the area of component design, the ball-cup articulation is most important.

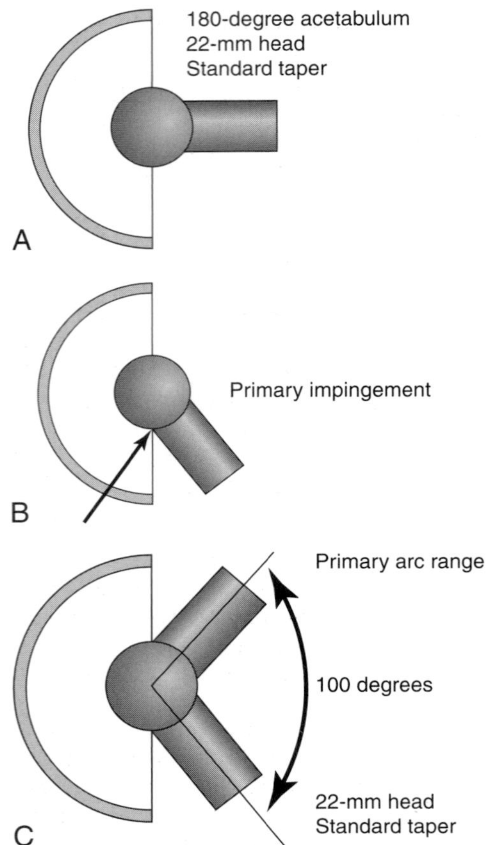

FIGURE 5–7 The articulation of total hip replacement demonstrating primary arc range. **A**, a 22-mm head articulating with 180-degree acetabulum. **B**, At the end of the range, primary impingement occurs. **C**, Primary arc range is the arc of motion allowed between the two ends of primary impingement.

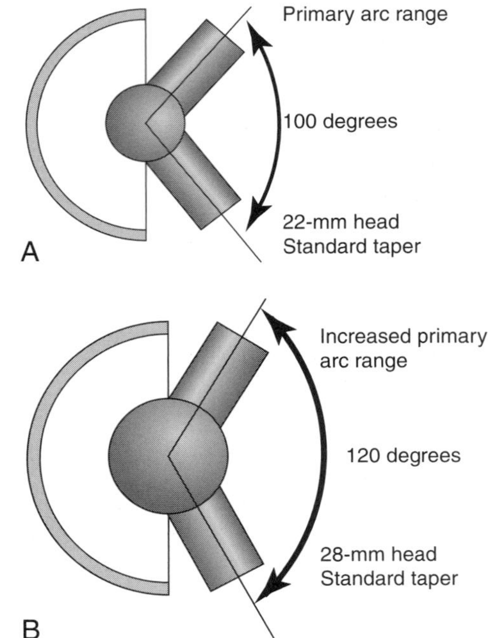

FIGURE 5–8 Comparison of primary arc range between 22-mm head and 28-mm head. **A**, Primary arc range with 22-mm head. **B**, Primary arc range with 28-mm head. The only change in this illustration is the head size, which increases the head-to-neck ratio, in turn allowing for an increased arc range.

(1) **Primary arc range**—Defines the arc this articulation moves before impinging and levering out (Fig. 5–7). The major determinant of primary arc range is the **head-neck ratio,** which is defined as the ratio of the femoral head diameter to the femoral neck diameter. A larger head-neck ratio allows greater arc of motion before primary impingement (Fig. 5–8).

(2) **Excursion distance**—At the point of primary impingement, the head will begin to lever out of the cup. The distance a head must travel to dislocate is defined as excursion. The greater the excursion distance a ball must travel to dislocate when levered out, the more stable the hip. The excursion distance is usually one half the diameter of the femoral head. Comparing a 32-mm head with a 22-mm head shows that the excursion distance is 16 mm in the first compared with 11 mm in the second. In addition, a 32-mm head is more stable because of a more favorable head-neck ratio. Taken to the extreme, a hemiarthroplasty head is the most inherently stable because of a very favorable head-neck ratio femoral prosthetic neck.

(3) Size of the taper—Influences stability by affecting the head-neck ratio. Narrow neck tapers provide more stability via a more favorable head-neck ratio. Conversely, the addition of a collar on a modular femoral head (seen in long neck lengths) increases neck diameter and adversely affects the head-neck ratio.

(4) Acetabular augmentation—Augmented acetabular liners (i.e., hoods) decrease the primary arc range because the arc of the opening is decreased (i.e., less than the standard opening of 180 degrees) (Fig. 5–9). The larger the hood, the more likely there will be impingement and excursion. Large hoods should be avoided.

(5) Head-neck ratio—An optimal head-neck ratio also helps prevent prosthetic neck–cup impingement. Repetitive neck–cup impingement can cause localized damage to prosthetic components, which is especially salient with a ceramic-on-ceramic bearing, where edge impingement can cause ceramic fracture.

(6) Constrained liner—A **constrained liner** that covers almost the entire femoral head provides inherent stability but at a cost. The primary arc range is *dramatically reduced* (Fig. 5–10). If the patient consistently exceeds this primary arc range, the acetabulum can undergo early mechanical failure. The repetitive impingement imparts a levering force on the acetabular component, leading to early loosening.

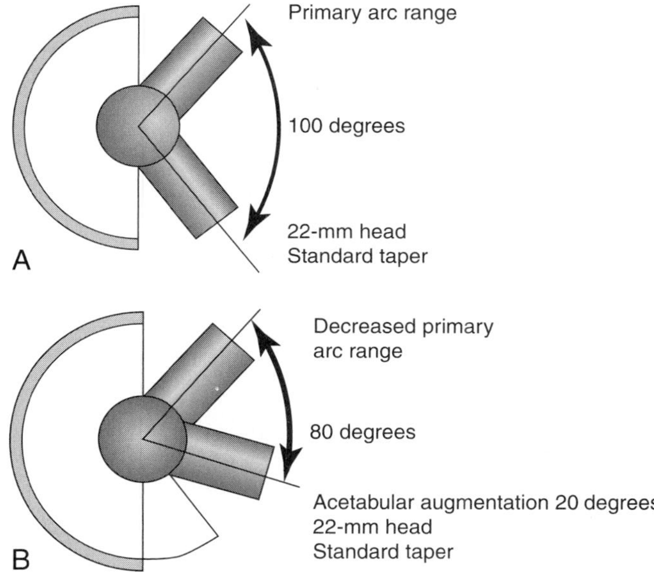

FIGURE 5–9 Comparison of primary arc range between nonhooded and hooded acetabular liners. **A**, Primary arc range with 22-mm head. **B**, Primary arc range with augmented acetabular liner (i.e., hood). Primary arc range is reduced as a result of the augmented liner.

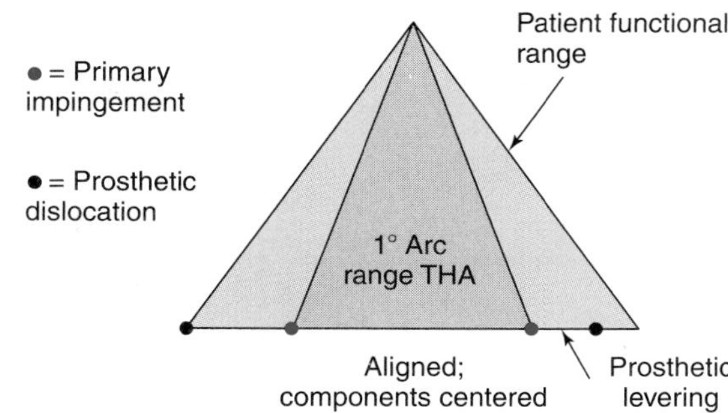

FIGURE 5–11 The difference in the patient's functional hip range of motion compared with the prosthetic range. Because smaller heads are used in prosthetic hip replacement, prosthetic arc range is smaller than native hip range. Prosthetic arc range should be centered within the patient's functional range to minimize dislocation. THA, total hip arthroplasty.

b. Component alignment—This consideration is another important factor in hip stability. Because the patient's native femoral head is much larger than a prosthetic THR head, it is more stable and has a larger primary arc range than a prosthetic replacement. Therefore, when inserting acetabular and femoral components, the goal is to center the prosthetic primary arc range in the middle of the patient's functional range (Fig. 5–11). By doing so, there is still some stability with the prosthetic excursion distance if the primary arc range is exceeded. Poorly aligned components do not decrease the primary arc range; rather, the arc range is not centered in the patient's functional range. As a result, on one side of the arc range the head will suffer excessive excursion and hip dislocation (Fig. 5–12). Because surgeon preference and training vary, there is no one correct answer for the proper component position. On the acetabulum, anteversion should be 15-30 degrees, and the theta angle (i.e., coronal tilt), 35-45 degrees (Fig. 5–13). Intraoperative trials are important to ensure that component placement is optimal. The hip must be taken through all extremes of end range to ensure stability.

c. Soft tissue tensioning—This factor also plays a critical role in hip stability. Components that are properly placed may still dislocate if there is inadequate soft tissue tension to hold the components in place.

(1) Offset—The major key to hip stability is the **abductor complex**, which consists primarily of the gluteus medius and minimus. Maintaining the correct tension in this complex will provide optimum stability. **Preoperative templating** should assess **head offset** and **neck length** such that when the prosthetic stem is inserted, the appropriate neck length and offset are restored (Fig. 5–14). Restored hip

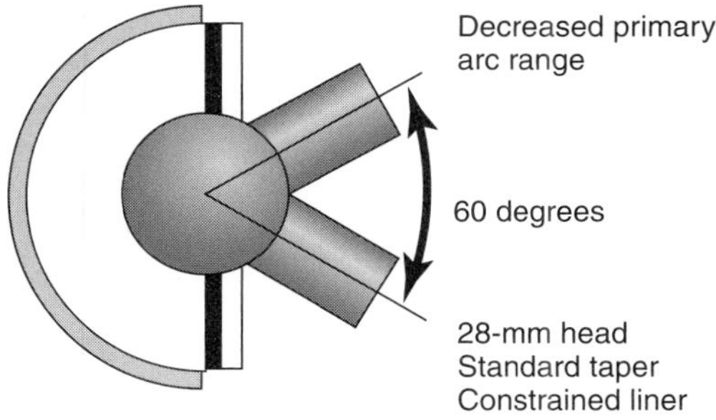

FIGURE 5–10 A constrained acetabular liner. A constrained liner covers the femoral head past its equator, which keeps the ball from coming out of its socket. This action has the adverse effect of severely restricting primary arc range.

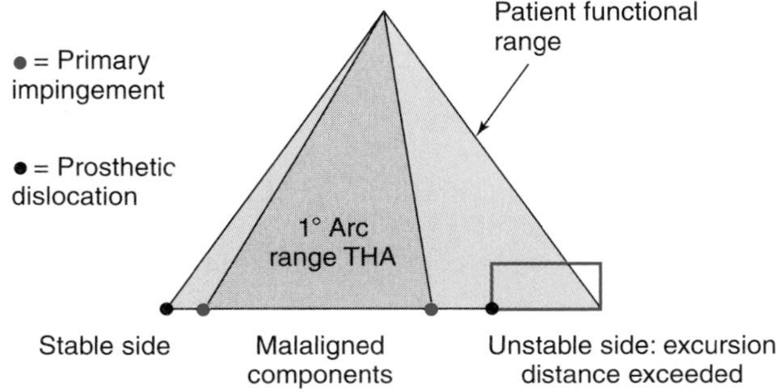

FIGURE 5–12 Prosthetic malalignment. In this example, prosthetic arc range is positioned to one side of the patient's functional range. On one side, the hip will be very stable. However, on the other side, the hip is at risk for dislocation. Specifically, the patient's arc range will exceed prosthetic arc range. Primary impingement will occur, followed by head levering, head excursion, and then dislocation. If the patient is unwilling to accept the limited functional range, recurrent dislocation will result. THA, total hip arthroplasty.

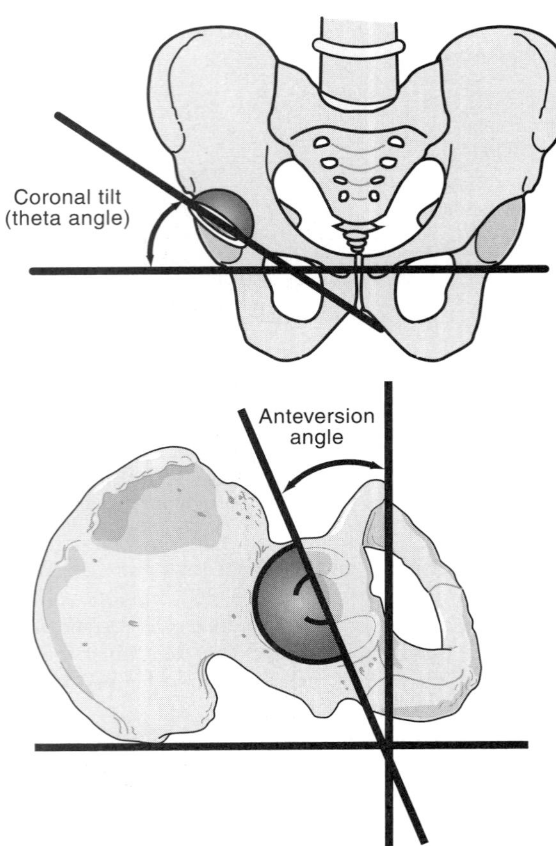

FIGURE 5–13 The acetabular cup position in coronal and sagittal planes. Coronal tilt (also known as theta angle) should be 35-45 degrees. In the sagittal plane, cup anteversion should be 15-30 degrees.

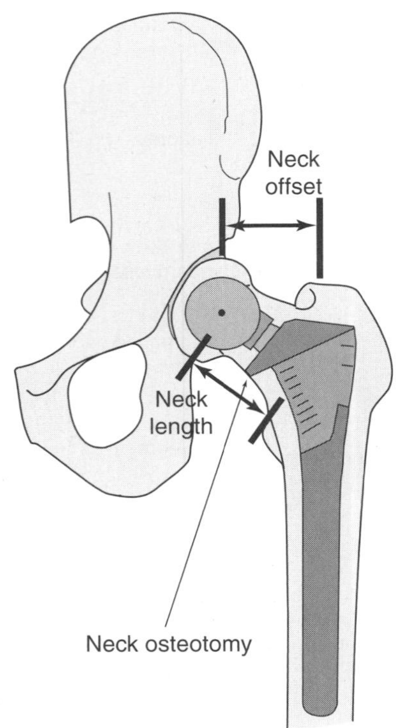

FIGURE 5–14 Preoperative templating for proper femoral stem positioning. The prosthetic stem should be positioned such that femoral stem offset (center of head to greater trochanter) matches the native hip. Also, femoral neck length must be restored. Restoring head offset and neck length optimizes abductor tension, providing stability.

mechanics confers hip stability via optimized abductor tension. Conversely, reduced hip length and offset can lead to instability. A THR short in neck length results in a lax abductor complex and may not generate the force required to keep the hip in place. Additionally, a short neck length can cause trochanteric impingement with abduction and rotation, causing the hip to lever out of the socket. Hip stability can also be affected by a decreased offset. With a **narrow offset** the greater trochanter can impinge, allowing the hip to lever out of the socket. The worst-case scenario would be a THR with a shortened neck length and a narrow offset. It is very important to template x-rays preoperatively to see if neck length and offset can be adequately restored. If not, a different prosthetic system may be required.

(2) Greater trochanter deficiency or trochanteric escape (seen after trochanteric osteotomy)—This often leads to hip instability. With the loss of the greater trochanter attachment to the femur, there is a loss of abductor power and hip compressive forces. In addition, with the loss of the greater trochanter, the hip is allowed a greater range of motion, leading to prosthetic neck impingement, head excursion, and dislocation.

d. Soft tissue function—The abductor complex and surrounding soft tissues of the hip are controlled by the synchronized neurologic firing from the brain delivered through the peripheral nervous system. Any disruption in this system can adversely affect function and hip stability. Soft tissue function can be broken into two main issues: central and peripheral. **Central issues** involve the brain, brainstem, and spinal cord. Problems in this area can include stroke, cerebellar dysfunction, Parkinson's disease, multiple sclerosis, dementia, cervical stenosis/myelopathy, and psychiatric disorders. The issue common to all of these is the coordinated firing of muscles to keep the hip stable. The problem could be from paralysis, spasticity, or loss of coordinated movements of the surrounding hip musculature. **Peripheral issues** involve the area of the peripheral nerves and muscles that support the hip. The peripheral issues that can affect hip stability include lumbar stenosis, peripheral neuropathy, myopathy, localized soft tissue trauma, and radiation therapy. The cause of poor soft tissue function may be multifactorial in the elderly patient. Sometimes it is difficult to preoperatively ascertain the extent of soft tissue dysfunction, and it is only after multiple dislocations that one appreciates the significance of these deficits.

3. Management of the dislocated THR—Treatment of the dislocated THR depends on the reason for dislocation.
   a. Indications—During closed reduction, it is important to take the hip through the full range of positions and assess those that make the hip dislocate. If the dislocating positions noted are near the extremes of the end range, the prognosis for long-term stability is good. On the other hand, if the hip dislocates easily within the patient's functional range, revision surgery is probably necessary. As a general rule, if the hip dislocates more than two times, recurrent dislocation is likely and the hip should be revised to enhance stability.
   b. Closed reduction and immobilization—Approximately two thirds of patients with a dislocated THR can be treated successfully with closed reduction and a period of hip immobilization. Immobilization can be effected by means of either a spica cast or brace. A knee immobilizer is effective as well; it keeps the patient from putting the hip in a compromised position. However, immobilization in a hip brace or cast affords a better chance for soft tissues to heal in a more contracted position.
   c. Surgical options—The surgical options for recurrent dislocation depend on its cause. Although in many circumstances the cause of recurrent dislocation is multifactorial, there is usually one main area that stands out.
      (1) THR revision—If the THR components are poorly aligned, they should be revised, even if they are well fixed. The choice of implants for revision surgery should take into account factors that restore normal hip offset and neck length and provide an optimum arc range. Optimizing the head-neck ratio with a larger head should take priority over **polyethylene** (PE) thickness if this provides the stability needed for a successful outcome. In some situations in which the component parts of the hip are reasonably aligned, trochanteric osteotomy with distal advancement is a good option (Fig. 5–15). Distal advancement places the abductor complex under tension, providing more hip compressive force. Trochanteric advancement, if performed, is usually accompanied by postoperative immobilization in a spica cast or brace. In the scenario in which a prior trochanteric osteotomy has detached and migrated proximally, reattaching the greater trochanter is not very successful. In the abductor-deficient patient, hip stability may be achieved only by using a larger femoral head and/or a constrained PE liner.

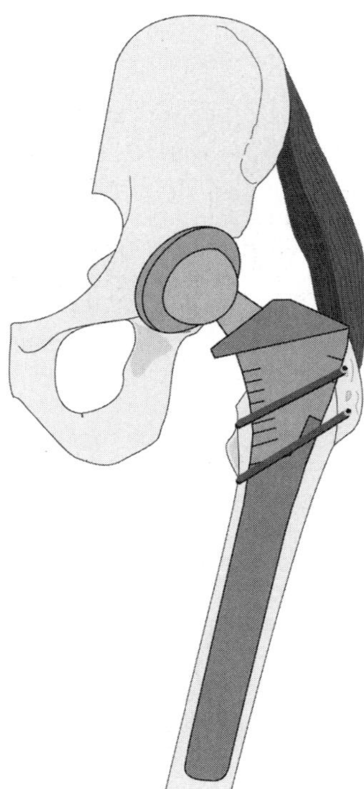

FIGURE 5–15 Trochanteric advancement. Distal advancement tightens the hip abductor complex, restoring compressive force to the hip joint.

      (2) THR conversion to a hemiarthroplasty with a large femoral head.
         (a) Indications—Used only when there is soft tissue deficiency or dysfunction. If the hemiarthroplasty can be seated firmly on the bony acetabular rim and there is acceptable remaining bone stock, conversion to a hemiarthroplasty is an option.
         (b) Contraindications—Conversion to a monopolar or bipolar head cannot be used in situations in which the acetabular bone is compromised (i.e., segmental deficiencies). If acetabular wall deficiencies are present, there is a high likelihood of intrapelvic migration.
      (3) Conversion to a constrained PE liner—Used when soft tissue deficiency and dysfunction are the main problems. The advantage of a constrained liner is that it can be used in the reconstructed acetabulum, where there is acetabular deficiency. The main problem with a constrained liner is the very limited range of motion it provides. If a patient is not compliant with the limited range, the acetabular cup may rapidly become mechanically loose from levering forces. Conversion to a constrained liner

should not be the first surgical option if other procedures will take care of the problem.

(4) Resection arthroplasty—Used when other options have been exhausted. Resection arthroplasty is usually used in the patient with significant soft tissue deficiency along with significant bone loss who has undergone multiple revisions. This procedure is also used for the psychiatric patient who purposely dislocates the hip for secondary gratification (e.g., narcotics, hospitalization).

C. Leg length discrepancy—Postoperative leg length discrepancy is divided into true versus apparent leg length discrepancy. A common method to discern between apparent and true leg length discrepancy is to draw the transverse ischial line on the anteroposterior radiograph of the pelvis (Fig. 5–16).

1. Apparent leg length discrepancy—In patients in whom the hip mechanics are accurately restored and true leg lengths are equal, the transverse ischial line will pass through the same region of the lesser trochanter. An apparent leg discrepancy usually results from contracture of the hip abductor complex or scoliosis, with resulting pelvic obliquity. In the case of a postoperative abduction contracture, the apparent leg length discrepancy will resolve, typically over a period of 3-6 months. In the scenario of long-standing scoliosis with pelvic obliquity, the apparent leg length discrepancy will remain. When scoliosis and pelvic obliquity are present, the patient should be counseled preoperatively about the possibility of residual postoperative leg length discrepancy.
2. True leg length discrepancy—If the leg is lengthened as a result of the total hip procedure, the transverse ischial line will show a discrepancy. With a lengthened leg, the lesser trochanter will usually be in a caudal position relative to the contralateral lesser trochanter, which was not operated on.

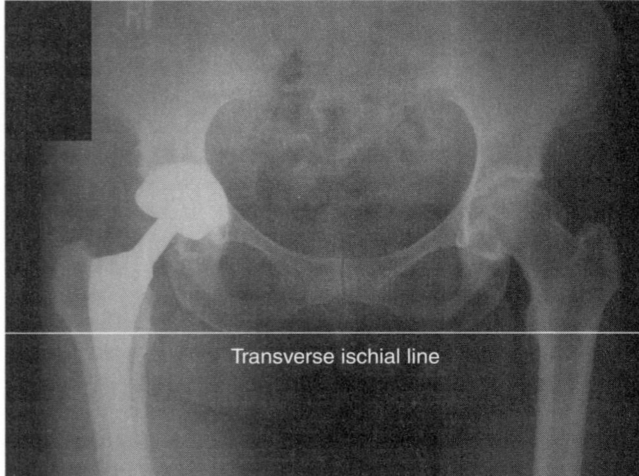

FIGURE 5–16 Anteroposterior pelvic radiograph demonstrating the transverse ischial line. The lesser tuberosity on the right hip is lower than the corresponding region on the left hip. In this case, the right leg has been anatomically lengthened, and there is a "true" leg-length discrepancy. If the lesser tuberosities are at the same level, the anatomic leg lengths are equal.

D. Hip loosening

1. Indications for revision surgery—Aseptic femoral and acetabular loosening are the most common indications for revision surgery. In cemented hip replacement, the most common reason for revision is failure of the cemented acetabular component. In noncemented THR, the most common reason for revision is failure of the femoral component (usually from osteolysis).
2. Radiographic evaluation—Standard radiographs taken in the same rotational position are required to assess interval changes.
   a. Radiographic zones—Radiographic analysis is based on dividing the acetabular and femoral components into radiographic zones. The acetabulum is divided into three zones, as described by DeLee and Charnley. The femoral component is divided into seven zones, as described by Gruen (Fig. 5–17). The development of radiolucent lines around these zones (with either cemented or noncemented implants) in a progressive fashion suggests loosening.
   b. Differentiating age-related changes from interval changes—It is important to distinguish progressive radiolucent lines in the femur from the typical age-related expansion of the femoral canal and cortical thinning, which may give the appearance of progressively widening radiolucency. Age-related radiolucent zones generally do not have the associated sclerotic line seen about loose femoral stems. In addition, radiolucent lines associated with osteolysis tend to be more irregular, with variable areas of cortical thinning and ectasia.
   c. Modes of failure—With cemented femoral implants, Gruen describes four modes of failure, which are defined in Table 5–2. The acetabular cup is considered loose if there is radiolucency greater than 2 mm in all three zones, there are progressive radiolucent lines in zones 1 and 2, or there is a change in component position.

E. Resurfacing hip arthroplasty

1. Disadvantages—**Total articular resurfacing** (TAR) arthroplasty of the hip has been used infrequently in the past because of the high failure rate from PE osteolysis. The large-diameter head articulates with a relatively thin PE insert. Volumetric wear is great, and the amount of PE debris generated is markedly greater than that with a traditional THR head of 28-32 mm.
2. New developments—With the advent of alternative bearing constructs, metal-on-metal TAR has seen a resurgence. Early- and intermediate-term survival of metal-on-metal TAR is comparable to traditional THR. Patient selection and surgical

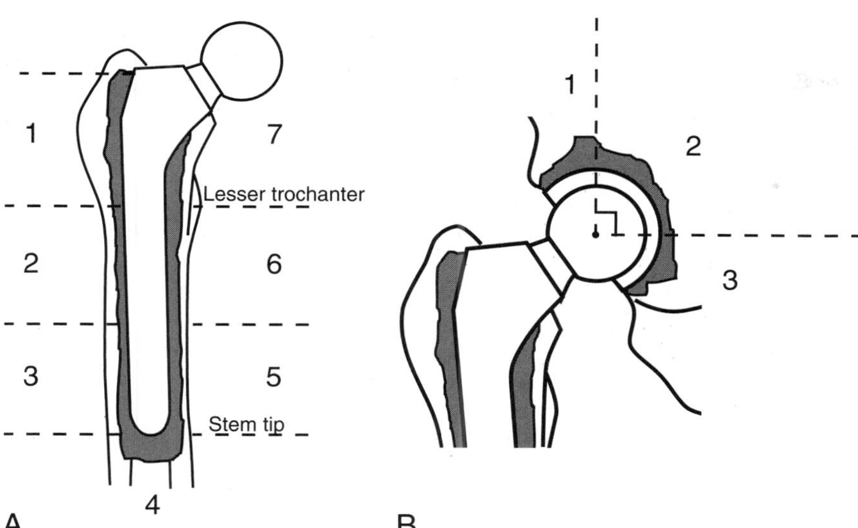

FIGURE 5–17 Seven Gruen zones for femoral stem (**A**) and three DeLee-Charnley zones for acetabular cup (**B**).

technique are important for success. In general, normal acetabular and femoral anatomy is required for TAR because it prevents abnormal neck impingement and failure.

3. Complications—The most common complication of current TAR is periprosthetic fracture at the femoral head. Fracture risk is increased when (1) a notch is made in the superior femoral neck during bone preparation, (2) there is significant osteoporosis, (3) the femoral head has a moderate to large area of osteonecrosis, and/or (4) there is a misplaced acetabular cup causing neck impingement.

F. Revision THR

1. Problems—Revision hip surgery is often difficult and complex. The results are less satisfactory than those from primary hip replacement. Postoperative complications of infection, dislocation, nerve palsy, cortical perforation, fracture, and deep vein thrombosis are higher than those found in primary hip replacement.
2. Goals—The surgical goals in revision hip replacement are (1) removal of loose components without significant destruction of host bone and tissue, (2) reconstruction of bone defects with bone graft and/or metal augmentation, (3) stable revision implants, and (4) restoration of a normal hip center of rotation.
3. Acetabular defects
   a. Reconstruction of acetabulum—Acetabular reconstruction first requires defining the extent of bone loss. Acetabular defects are classified as follows: (1) **segmental** (type I)—loss of part of the acetabular rim or medial wall; (2) **cavitary** (type II)—volumetric loss in the bony substance of the acetabular cavity; (3) **combined deficiency** (type III)—combination of segmental bone loss and cavitary deficiency; (4) **pelvic discontinuity** (type IV)—complete separation between the superior and inferior acetabulum, usually due to combined deficiencies and fracture; and (5) **arthrodesis** (type V)—obliteration of the acetabulum due to arthrodesis.
   b. Revision of acetabulum—In acetabular revision, a porous-coated hemisphere cup secured with superior screws is the preferred choice, provided that the rim is intact.

TABLE 5-2 MODES OF CEMENTED FEMORAL STEM FAILURE

Mode	Mechanism	Causes	Findings
IA	Pistoning behavior	Subsidence of stem within cement	RLLs between stem and cement in zones 1 and 2 Distal cement fracture Stem displaced distally in cement
IB	Pistoning behavior	Subsidence of cement mantle and stem within bone	RLLs in all 7 zones
II	Medial stem pivot	Lack of superomedial and inferolateral cement support	Medial migration proximal stem Lateral migration distal tip Cement fracture zones 2 and 6
III	Calcar pivot	Medial and lateral toggles of distal stem "Hang up" of stem collar on medial cortex "Windshield wiper" reaction at distal stem	Sclerosis and thickening of bone at stem tip RLL zones 4 and 5
IV	Cantilever bending	Loss of proximal cement support, leaving distal stem still fixed; allows for proximal cantilever bending	Stem crack or fracture RLL zones 1 and 2, 6 and 7

RLL(s), radiolucent line(s).

A porous-coated hemisphere cup can be used even with segmental deficiency of the acetabular rim. As a general rule, a hemisphere cup can be used if at least *two thirds* of the rim remains and there is still a good "rim fit." The cup must be secured with screws. Cavitary deficiencies with an intact rim are filled with particulate graft, and the acetabular cup will hold the graft in place. The acetabular rim provides stability for the acetabular cup when the cup is inserted with a press-fit technique. Because acetabular bone stock is weakened in revision surgery, superior screws should be placed to augment stability. The correct placement of acetabular screws is important. Figure 5–18 diagrams the safe zones for correct screw placement. Incorrect placement can lead to catastrophic vascular injury or neurologic damage.

c. Reconstruction of acetabular bone deficiency

(1) Structural allograft—Acetabular deficiencies that are rim deficient and/or have large cavitary deficiencies will require a structural and/or particulate allograft. A structural allograft (as opposed to a particulate graft) is a large, solid piece of bone that supports weight-bearing stress. The failure rate is high if a cup is placed into a large structural allograft. Failure is usually due to graft resorption and subsequent component migration. The failure rate of noncemented components with a large structural allograft is 40-60%. The failure rate with a cemented socket is 40%.

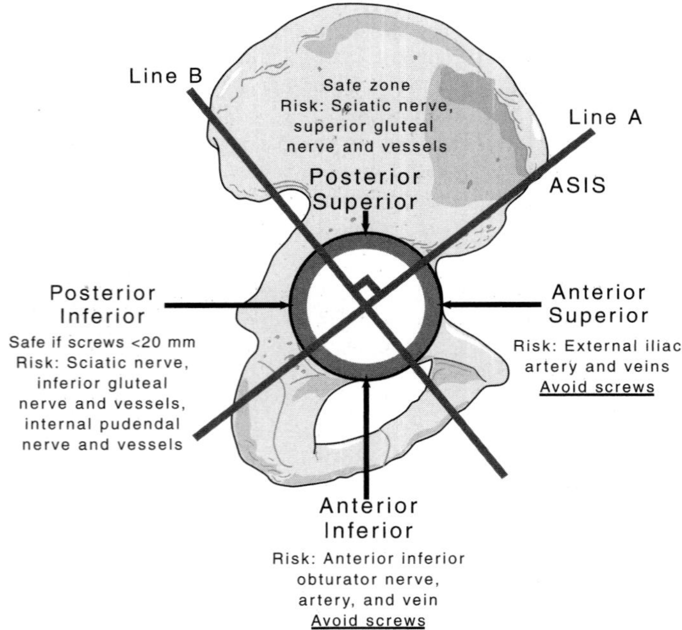

FIGURE 5–18 Acetabular zones for screw insertion. Line A is formed by drawing a line from the anterior superior iliac spine (ASIS) to the center of the acetabular socket. Line B is then drawn perpendicular to line A, also passing through center of socket. The posterior superior quadrant is the preferred zone for screw insertion.

(2) Reconstruction cage—A much higher success rate is achieved when the structural deficiencies are reinforced by a reconstruction cage (Fig. 5–19). For segmental deficiencies of the acetabulum, a reconstruction cage with morcellized bone graft is a preferred revision construct. Placement of a structural allograft behind the cage is an acceptable alternative. If a reconstruction cage is used, typically an all-PE acetabular component is usually cemented into the cage. More recently, all-metal cups (metal-metal bearing) have been cemented into the reconstruction cage. With this technique, the reconstruction cage must have inherent stability with the native pelvis. This stability is achieved by placing long screws through the cage and allograft into the ilium (posterosuperior safe zone) and providing solid flange fixation onto the pelvis. The most common mechanism of failure of a reconstruction cage is **abduction pullout** (Fig. 5–20). Failure occurs because the bulk allograft does not heal to host bone. When a bulk allograft is not used, cage failure occurs due to loss of fixation to the pelvis.

4. Femoral bone defects

a. Classification—Femoral bone defects, like acetabular defects, are primarily either segmental or cavitary. The complete classification of femoral bone deficiencies is as follows: (1) **segmental** (type I)—any loss of bone of the supporting shell of the femur; (2) **cavitary** (type II)—loss of endosteal bone but an intact cortical shell; (3) **combined deficiency** (type III)—combined segmental and cavitary defects; (4) **malalignment** (type IV)—loss of normal femoral geometry due to prior surgery, trauma, or disease; (5) **stenosis** (type V)—occlusion of the canal from trauma, fixation devices, or bony hypertrophy; and (6) **femoral discontinuity** (type VI)—loss of femoral integrity from fracture or nonunion.

b. Revision of femoral stem—With femoral stem revision, the most commonly used technique is a noncemented, extensively porous-coated (or porous coating/grit-blast combination), long-stem prosthesis. The revision stem should pass 2-3 cm below the original stem in order to bypass stress risers that may occur from stem extraction or osteolysis. If there is a femoral cortical violation (i.e., hole in bone), the revision stem should pass at least **two shaft diameters** below the defect. Ectatic, cavitary lesions can be grafted with particulate graft. Segmental deficiencies are usually reconstructed with cortical onlay struts secured with cerclage wires or multifilament cables (Fig. 5–21).

c. Impaction bone grafting (Ling's technique) —This procedure can be used for some

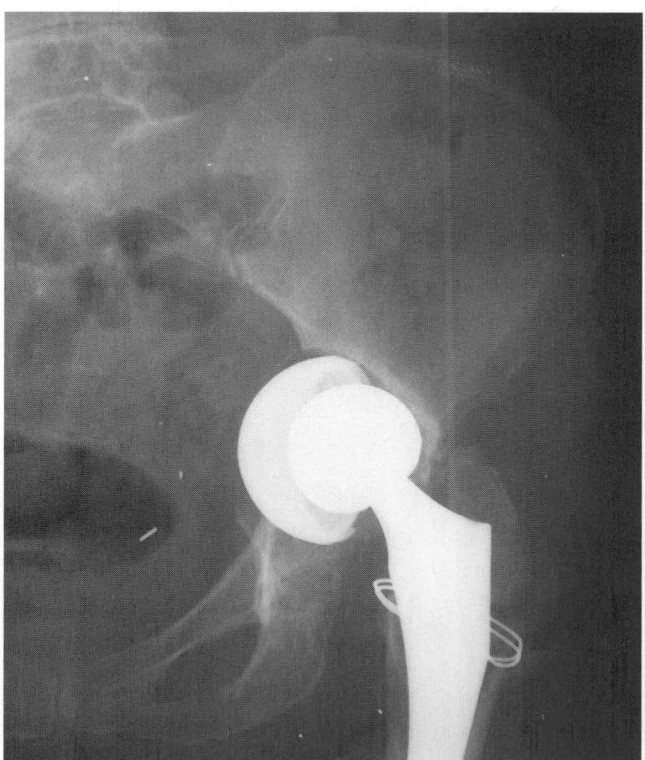

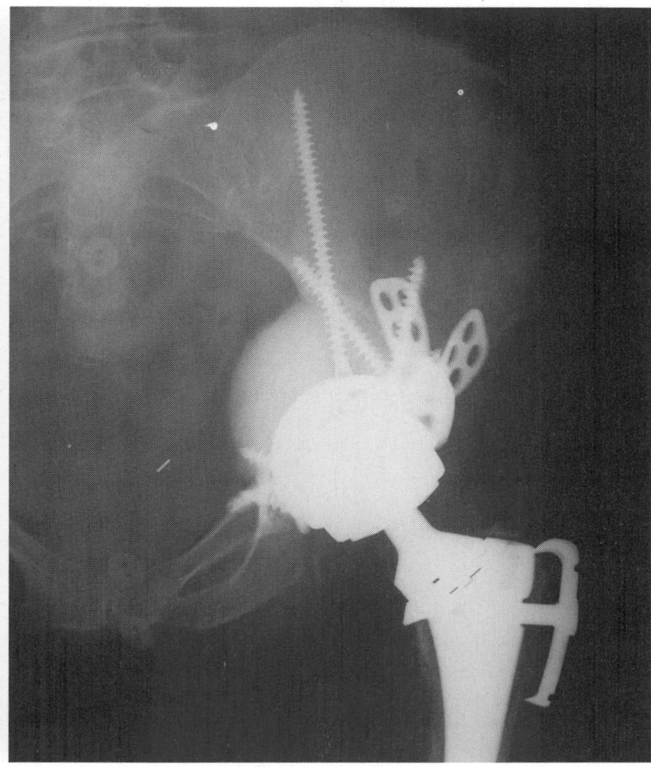

A B

FIGURE 5–19 Pelvic and acetabular reconstruction employing reconstruction cage. **A**, Preoperative radiograph showing significant destruction of the acetabulum. At the time of surgery, complete pelvic discontinuity was evident. Notice that the hip center is markedly elevated, indicating significant segmental iliac bone loss. **B**, One-year postoperative X-ray showing pelvic reconstruction employing a triflange reconstruction cage and allograft. The cage is secured with screws into the ilium, ischium, and superior ramus. Allograft is placed behind the cage. An all-metal acetabular cup is cemented into the cage. The large-ball construct enhances stability. This construct allows weight-bearing forces to be distributed from the cage to the pelvis, allowing the allograft to remodel and incorporate to host bone.

revisions in which there is a large ectatic canal and narrow, thin cortices (destroyed by osteolysis). This technique uses morcellized, fresh-frozen allograft packed tightly into the ectatic proximal femur. A smooth, tapered stem is cemented into the allograft. This technique requires an intact cortical tube, although small segmental defects can be patched with a wire mesh. The most common complication of this technique is stem settling.

G. Periprosthetic fracture—The management of periprosthetic fractures of the femur depends on the location of the fracture and whether the stem is well-fixed or loose.

1. Locations, causes, and timing of fractures—Femurs with bone ingrowth prostheses tend to fracture within the first 6 months after implantation. The most likely reason is the development of stress risers created by reaming and broaching of the femoral canal. With proximal porous-coated noncemented stems, the femur tends to fracture in the proximal metaphysis/diaphysis. The proximal portion of these stems is usually wedged in very tightly during insertion. Any small, undetected cracks at the time of insertion are prone to fracture. With fully porous stems, the femur tends to fracture distally. These stems are usually straight and impacted to achieve an interference fit throughout the length of the stem. During insertion, the stem can abut the anterior femoral cortex and create a crack. Cemented implants tend to fracture late (5 years on average). Fractures in cemented implants occur most often about the stem tip or distal to the prosthesis. In revision THR, fractures tend to occur at the sites of cortical defects from previous operations. Fractures also occur when the new stem does not bypass a cortical defect by greater than **two cortical diameters.**

2. Treatment of fractures with a loose prosthesis—Fractures that occur where there is a loose prosthesis (cemented or noncemented) should be revised with a noncemented bone ingrowth, long-stem prosthesis that bypasses the last cortical defect by two diameters of the femoral shaft. In addition, if a hemiarthroplasty is in place at the time of revision and the patient has significant groin pain, the acetabulum should be resurfaced concomitantly. If an existing acetabular component is loose, the acetabular cup should be revised along with the femoral stem. When significant osteolysis is present and the acetabular PE liner is worn, the modular acetabular liner should be exchanged during stem revision if the cup is deemed stable.

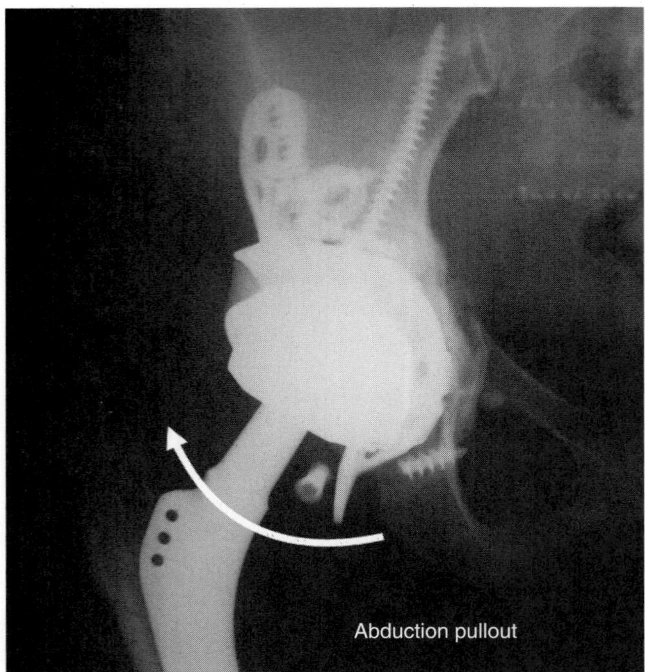

FIGURE 5–20 Five year x-ray demonstrating abduction pullout of acetabular reconstruction cage. The acetabulum was reconstructed with triflange cage and particulate allograft placed behind the cup. Reconstruction cages do not have porous coating behind them; thus, they are susceptible to cyclic failure, which occurred in this active 54-year-old female.

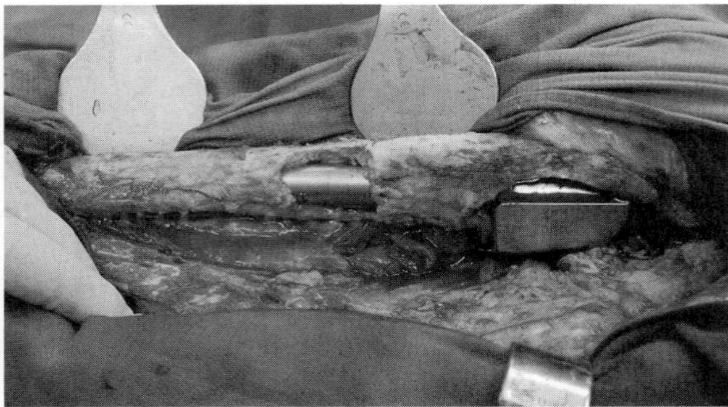

A

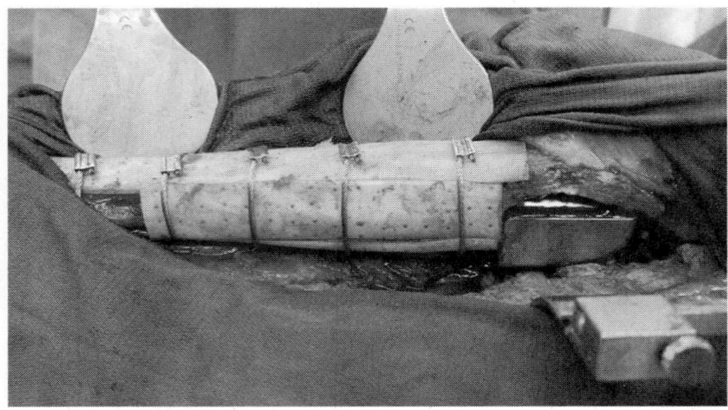

B

FIGURE 5–21 Application of cortical onlay struts to cover segmental deficiencies. Hip revision was performed for mechanical loosening and osteolysis of cemented total hip replacement in an active 40 year-old female with juvenile rheumatoid arthritis. **A**, Photograph showing segmental deficiency of proximal femoral diaphysis. **B**, Note the longer lateral strut to cover a more distal defect. The allograft struts used were demineralized, which provides some pliability to mold around the femur.

3. Treatment of fractures with an intact prosthesis—The treatment of fractures with an intact prosthetic interface depends on the site of the fracture and the extent of its involvement. A fracture classification (Beals and Tower) with recommended treatment alternatives is reviewed in Table 5–3.

H. Heterotopic ossification—**Heterotopic ossification** (HO) after hip replacement surgery most frequently affects males. Predisposing risk factors include hypertrophic osteoarthritis, ankylosing spondylitis, **diffuse idiopathic skeletal hyperostosis** (DISH), post-traumatic arthritis, prior hip arthrodesis, and a history of previous development of HO. HO is seen more often with the direct lateral approach to the hip (Harding approach). If HO is seen in the contralateral hip, its incidence in the ipsilateral hip is high.

1. Diagnosis/prognosis—When it is pronounced, HO limits hip motion but does not usually cause pain or muscle weakness. Reoperation to remove HO is not recommended unless there is severe restriction of hip range or severe pain from impingement. Recurrence is likely unless prophylactic measures are taken. Once HO is seen radiographically, there is no treatment to prevent further progression. Instead, treatment for HO is directed toward identifying those patients at high risk for developing HO and treating this subgroup prophylactically.
2. Treatment—Prophylactic treatment with low-dose radiation or certain **nonsteroidal anti-inflammatory drugs** (NSAIDs) is an effective measure to prevent HO. A single dose of 600-750 cGy (rad) is considered the lowest effective dose for HO. Treatment must be delivered within 72 hours of surgery (preferably within the first 48 hours) to be effective. If noncemented prosthetic components are used, these areas should be shielded from the radiation beam to avoid reducing bone ingrowth potential. Indomethacin is the most commonly used NSAID for heterotopic ossification. Other NSAIDs have also shown effectiveness. The recommended indomethacin dose is 75 mg per day for 6 weeks. The efficacy of indomethacin in preventing recurrent HO after excision is not well documented.

I. Nerve injury—Nerve injury during THR involves the sciatic nerve 80% and the femoral nerve 20% of the time. When the sciatic nerve is injured, it is usually the peroneal division that is involved. The peroneal division is closer to the acetabulum than the tibial division is. The sciatic nerve passes closest to the acetabulum at the level of the *ischium*. The most common reason for sciatic nerve injury is errant retractor placement in this region. Compression of the nerve is the most common pathologic mechanism

TABLE 5-3 CLASSIFICATION AND TREATMENT OF PERIPROSTHETIC FEMORAL FRACTURE

Fracture Locations and Descriptions	Recommended Treatments
Greater trochanter	Nonoperative
Proximal metaphysis	1. Nonoperative 2. Cerclage fixation
Diaphysis—stem tip Cemented stem <25% disruption of cement mantle	1. ORIF—lateral plate and screws ± cerclage cables 2. ORIF—cortical allograft struts with cerclage cables 3. Long-stem, cementless revision + ORIF
Diaphysis—stem tip Cemented stem >25% disruption of cement mantle	Long-stem, cementless revision + ORIF
Diaphysis—stem tip Cementless stem Implant still well fixed	1. ORIF—lateral plate and screws ± cerclage cables 2. ORIF—cortical allograft struts with cerclage cables 3. Long-stem, cementless revision + ORIF
Supracondylar fracture distant to stem tip	1. Nonoperative if stable 2. ORIF—lateral supracondylar plate and screws
Supracondylar fracture at the tip of a long-stem prosthesis	1. Nonoperative if stable 2. ORIF—lateral plate and screws ± cerclage cables

ORIF, open reduction with internal fixation.

of injury. Hip hematoma from anticoagulation can cause sciatic nerve palsy from compression. Treatment is initiated by prompt surgical evacuation. Associated risk factors for nerve injury include female sex, revision surgery, and DDH. In the case of DDH, the risk of nerve palsy increases with leg lengthening of more then 3.5 cm.

II. Knee Replacement Surgery

A. Preoperative examination and radiographs—Among the preoperative plans are a good clinical examination of the knee and preoperative radiographs, which are used to identify corrections needed in alignment and defects in bone that will require bone grafting or augmentation. Box 5–1 lists the recommended series of preoperative radiographs. Consistent clinical results are predicated on good preoperative planning.

B. Goals—The technical goals of knee replacement surgery are (1) restoring mechanical alignment, (2) preserving (or restoring) of the joint line, (3) balancing ligaments, and (4) maintaining or restoring a normal Q angle.

1. Restoring mechanical alignment—Restoring neutral mechanical alignment ensures that the forces through the leg pass through the center of the hip, knee, and ankle. Restoring this alignment in knee replacement surgery allows an optimum load share through the medial and lateral sides of the prosthetic components. In a knee replacement in which mechanical alignment is not restored, a net varus or valgus moment is created, placing excessive stress on one side of the knee and leading to excessive wear and early failure.
2. Location of the anatomic and mechanical axes—Identifying the anatomic and mechanical axes on preoperative radiographs and with intraoperative instrumentation is essential. Figure 5–22 defines the anatomic and mechanical axes of the femur and tibia.
   a. **Femoral anatomic axis**—In the femur, the anatomic axis is defined by the medullary canal and most often exits in the intercondylar notch region. The exit of the anatomic axis at the distal end of the femur defines the medullary entry point for the intramedullary rod of the femoral jigs used to prepare the femur. In some cases, the anatomic axis may be located just medial or lateral to the intercondylar notch due to distal femoral bowing deformities. A preoperative standing, full-length radiograph can be used to identify the anatomic axis and femoral entry point.
   b. **Femoral mechanical axis**—The femoral mechanical axis starts from the center of the femoral head and ends at the point of intersection with the femoral anatomic axis at the intercondylar notch.
   c. **Valgus cut angle**—The angle measured between the femoral anatomic axis and mechanical axis is called the valgus cut angle. This angle can be measured in each case using a standing anteroposterior full-length radiograph of the leg; in most cases it measures 5-7 degrees. The goal is to cut the distal femur at an angle perpendicular to the *mechanical* axis. With the distal femur cut at the valgus cut angle, the femoral prosthesis will point toward the center of the femoral head and be in a mechanically neutral position. Cases in which the valgus cut angle should be measured with a full-length radiograph are patients who are very tall or short, those who have post-traumatic deformities of the femur, and those who have congenital femoral bowing deformities. Patients who are very tall will often have a valgus cut angle of less than 5 degrees, whereas those who are very short may have a valgus cut angle of more than 7 degrees.
   d. **Tibial anatomic and mechanical axes**—The anatomic axis of the tibia is the line

Box 5–1 Recommended Preoperative Radiographs in Knee Replacement Surgery

- Standing full-length anteroposterior radiograph from hip to ankle (when angular deformity is present)
- Standing anteroposterior of knees on large cassette (14″ × 17″)
- Standing extension lateral on large cassette
- Flexion lateral (90-100 degrees) on large cassette
- Merchant's view

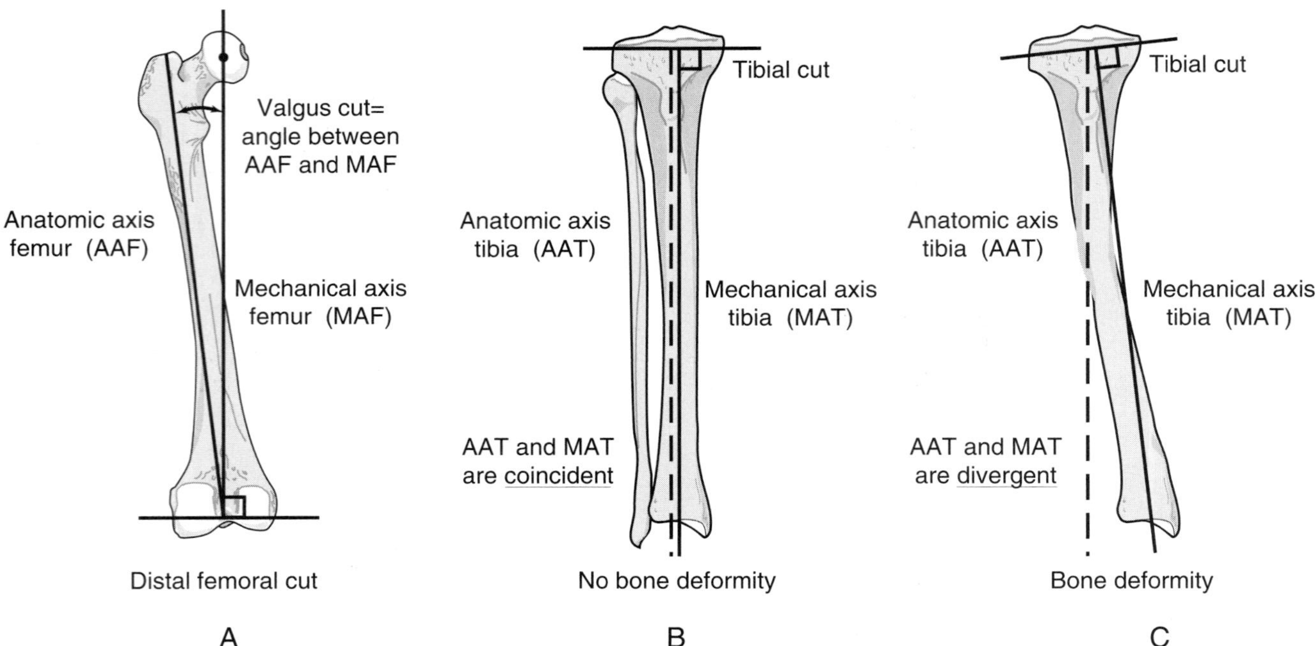

FIGURE 5–22 The mechanical and anatomic axes of the leg. **A**, In the femur, the anatomic axis follows the femoral shaft, whereas the mechanical axis lies along the line from the hip center to the knee center (mechanical and anatomic axes intersect at knee). **B**, In the tibia, the anatomic axis follows the tibial shaft. The mechanical axis runs from knee center to the ankle joint center. When deformities are absent, the tibial anatomic axis and mechanical axis are usually coincident. **C**, When deformities are present, these axes are divergent.

defining the medullary canal, and in the majority of cases it is coincident with the mechanical axis. The cases in which the tibial anatomic and mechanical axes are disparate are in post-traumatic and congenital bowing deformities. The goal in either case is to cut the tibial surface perpendicular to the mechanical axis such that leg stresses are passed evenly through the medial and lateral sides of the prosthetic tibial surface. When the anatomic and mechanical tibial axes are coincident, an intramedullary rod will readily assist in determining the correct cut. However, in a post-traumatic tibial deformity the medullary rod may not pass. In this instance, an extramedullary guide device placed over the center of the ankle up to the center of the tibia or center of the tibial tubercle will be necessary.

2. Restoring the joint line—The next technical aspect in knee replacement surgery is to remove a sufficient amount of bone so that the prosthesis, when placed, will re-create the original thickness of cartilage and bone. This ensures that the *joint line is re-created*, which is important because knee ligaments play a vital role in prosthetic knee kinematics. Knee function is optimized when the joint line is preserved.
   a. Usual technique—Current total knee instrumentation is capable of providing precise bone cuts, but the surgeon should never be lulled into a sense of complacency. Cutting jigs can be pinned improperly or may shift as sawing occurs, causing inaccurate cuts. The surgeon should always double-check cuts and alignment during the trialing process. Furthermore, during the bone cut and trialing process, bone defects should be identified and restored. If not, malalignment may occur. If bone defects are small (<1 cm deep), they can be filled with cement. Larger defects may require bone grafts or, more commonly, metallic augmentation, which is provided with many modular knee replacement systems.
   b. Modified technique—An extra-articular angular deformity of the femur as a result of prior fracture requires modification of the surgical technique. Specifically, an extra-articular deformity in the supracondylar region requires a simultaneous distal femoral osteotomy and TKR when the deformity is greater than 10 degrees in the coronal plane or 20 degrees in the sagittal plane. The osteotomy site is usually stabilized with a laterally placed supracondylar plate and screws.
3. Ligament balancing—Knee ligament balancing is another important aspect for successful knee replacement. In the degenerative process, ligaments may become scarred and contracted, or they may become stretched from excessive bowing deformities. Ligaments must be balanced to provide optimum function and wear for the prosthesis. Balancing must be accomplished in both the coronal and sagittal planes.
   a. Coronal plane—In the coronal plane, the two deformities are varus and valgus.

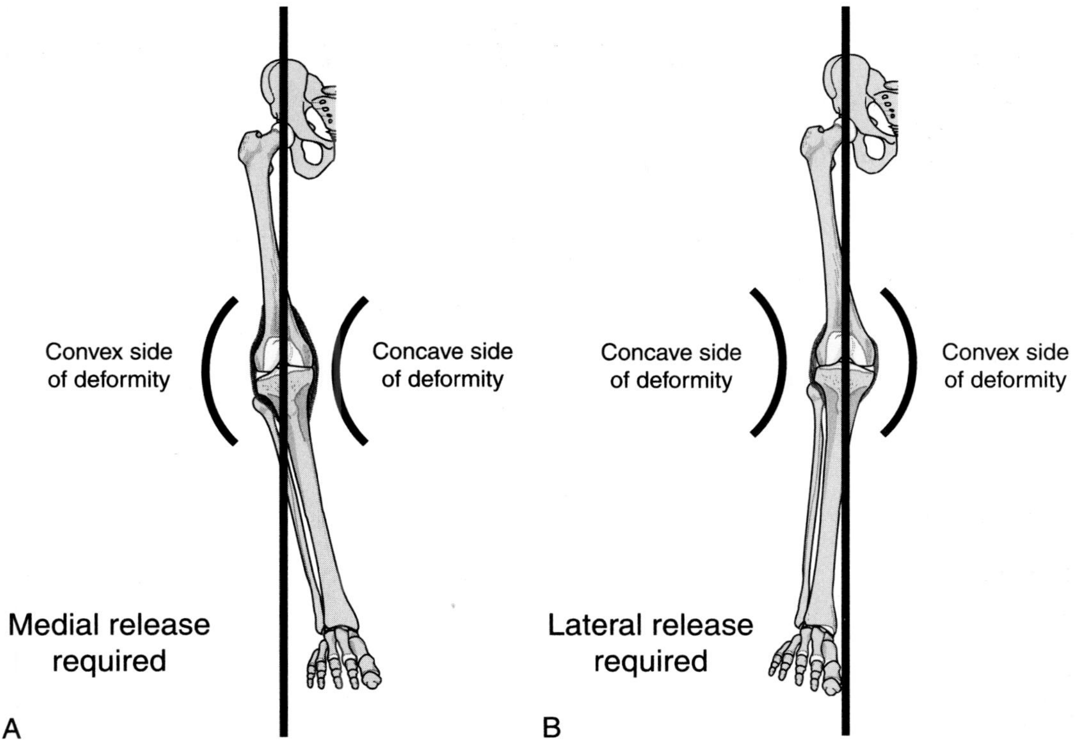

FIGURE 5–23 Principle of releases for coronal plane deformities in the knee. **A**, Varus deformity. **B**, Valgus deformity.

The basic principle in coronal plane balancing is to **release on the concave side** of the deformity and **fill up the convex side** until the ligament is taut. Figure 5–23 illustrates the principle for varus and valgus deformities. Table 5–4 lists the structures to be released for varus and valgus deformities.

(1) Varus deformities—Typically for varus deformities, the release of osteophytes and the deep medial collateral ligament (MCL) is all that is required to make the medial and lateral compartments symmetrical. More significant deformities require the release of the posteromedial corner along with the attachment of the semimembranosus muscle. For more significant deformities, sequential subperiosteal elevation of the superficial MCL (at the pes anserinus region) is required. The ligament cannot be fully released or it will become incompetent. If over-release occurs, a constrained knee device is required. In rare instances, the posterior cruciate ligament (PCL) may be a deforming factor in significant varus deformities, and one should consider release of the PCL if other releases fail to achieve proper balance.

(2) Valgus deformities—For valgus deformities, there should be an initial release of osteophytes and the lateral capsule off the tibia. If the lateral compartment remains tight in extension, release of the iliotibial band (with either a Z-type release of the tendon or a release off Gerdy's tubercle) is recommended. If the lateral compartment is tight in flexion, release of the popliteus tendon is recommended. In many situations in which the valgus deformity is large (>15 degrees), both the iliotibial band and popliteal tendon need to be released. For severe valgus deformities, balancing may require the release of the lateral collateral ligament. If this is done, then one should strongly consider the use of a constrained-type prosthetic design.

TABLE 5-4 CORONAL PLANE KNEE LIGAMENT BALANCING

Problem	Solution	Structures to be Released
Varus deformity	Medial release	Osteophytes Deep medial collateral ligament (meniscotibial ligament) Posteromedial corner with semimembranosus Superficial medial collateral ligament and pes anserinus complex Posterior cruciate ligament (rare occasions)
Valgus deformity	Lateral release	Osteophytes Lateral capsule Iliotibial band if tight in extension Popliteus if tight in flexion Lateral collateral ligament

TABLE 5-5 SAGITTAL PLANE BALANCING IN TOTAL KNEE REPLACEMENT

Scenarios	Problem	Solutions
Tight in extension (contracture) Tight in flexion (will not bend fully)	*Symmetrical* gap Did not cut enough tibial bone	Cut more proximal tibia
Loose in extension (recurvatum) Loose in flexion (large-drawer test)	*Symmetrical* gap Cut too much tibia	Use thicker polyethylene insert Perform metallic tibial augmentation
Extension good Flexion loose (large-drawer test)	*Asymmetrical* gap Cut too much posterior femur	1. Increase size of femoral component from anterior to posterior (i.e., go up to next size) Fill up posterior gap with either cement or metal augmentation 2. Use thicker polyethylene insert and readdress as tight extension gap
Extension tight (contracture) Flexion good	*Asymmetrical* gap Did not cut enough distal femur or release enough posterior capsule	Release posterior capsule Take off more distal femur bone (1-2 mm at a time)
Extension good Flexion tight (will not bend fully)	*Asymmetrical* gap Did not cut enough posterior bone or PCL scarred and too tight (assuming use of a PCL-retaining knee system) No posterior slope in tibial bone cut (i.e., anterior slope)	1. Decrease size of femoral component from anterior to posterior (i.e., recut to next smaller size) 2. Recess PCL 3. Check posterior slope of tibia and recut if anterior slope is present
Extension loose (recurvatum) Flexion good	*Asymmetrical* gap Cut too much distal femur or anteroposterior size too big	1. Perform distal femoral augmentation with metal augments 2. Use smaller femur (anteroposterior) and readdress as symmetrical gap problem 3. Use thicker tibial polyethylene inset and readdress as tight flexion gap

Correction of significant valgus deformity places the peroneal nerve on stretch.

(3) Combined deformities—The deformity *most often* associated with peroneal nerve palsy is combined valgus deformity with flexion contracture. Correction of both deformities places the nerve on significant stretch. If postoperative peroneal nerve palsy is noted, initial treatment should be the release of all compressive dressings and flexion of the knee. If the peroneal nerve function does not return after 3 months, exploration of the nerve via a posterolateral knee incision is recommended. Not infrequently, fascial constriction of the nerve is seen. The release of constrictions will frequently allow the return of nerve function.

b. Sagittal plane—In this plane, balancing becomes more sophisticated. In the sagittal plane, the knee has two radii of curvatures; one for the patellofemoral articulation and one for the remaining weight-bearing portion of the knee. The knee, like the hand metacarpal, acts as a modified cam. Stability in extension and flexion is provided by different parts of the collateral ligament structures. Balancing in the sagittal plane may require soft tissue releases but may also require additional bone resection to achieve the correct balance. The goal in sagittal plane balancing is to obtain a gap in extension equal to the gap in flexion. By achieving this goal, the tibial insert will be stable throughout the arc of motion. The general rule to follow when balancing the knee in the sagittal plane is as follows: If the gap problem is symmetrical (i.e., same problem in flexion and extension), adjust the tibia; if the gap problem is asymmetrical (i.e., different problem in flexion and extension), adjust the femur. The six scenarios for knee balancing are illustrated in Table 5–5.

4. Maintaining the Q angle—The final important factor in knee replacement surgery is avoiding techniques that result in an increased Q angle. The most common complications in TKR involve the patellofemoral articulation. An increased Q angle leads to increased lateral subluxation forces, which can adversely affect patellofemoral tracking. The subsequent discussion of patellofemoral articulation addresses the technical factors in avoiding patellofemoral maltracking.

C. Primary TKR

1. Prosthesis design—Current total knee prosthesis designs are of three types: unconstrained, constrained-nonhinged, and constrained-hinged. The unconstrained designs are used in almost all primary total knee replacements. Constrained-nonhinged and constrained-hinged are used in revision knee replacement (see Revision TKR).

a. Unconstrained design—There are two design types in the unconstrained category: the posterior cruciate–retaining and posterior

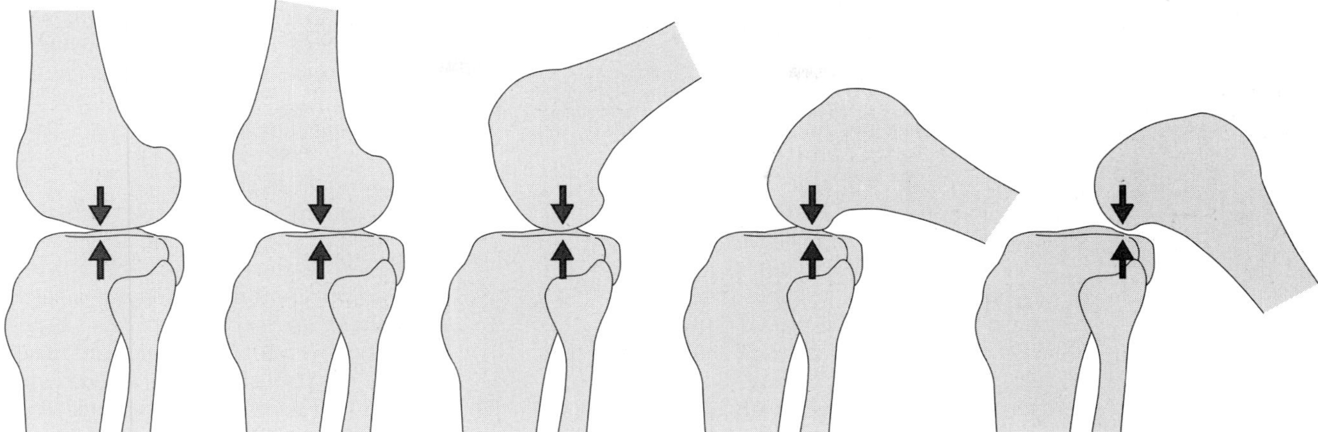

FIGURE 5–24 Femoral rollback is a posterior shift of the femoral-tibial contact point as the knee flexes. Rollback allows the femur to clear the tibia to provide further flexion.

cruciate–substituting (often referred to as posterior stabilized) implants. Initial unconstrained total knee resurfacing designs sacrificed both the anterior cruciate ligament (ACL) and the PCL. The drawback of such designs was limited knee flexion (in the range of 95 degrees) and flexion instability. With knee flexion, the femur could subluxate or dislocate anterior to the tibia.

(1) PCL-retaining prosthesis
   (a) Mechanism—By preserving the PCL, flexion instability is mitigated as the PCL becomes taut with knee flexion and prevents anterior dislocation of the femur on the tibia (provided that adequate knee balancing has been performed). In addition, by preserving the PCL, **femoral rollback** is produced. This term refers to the posterior shift in the femoral-tibial contact point in the sagittal plane as the knee flexes (Fig. 5–24). The posterior shift in the femoral-tibial contact point allows the posterior femur to flex further without impinging on the posterior tibia. Femoral rollback is controlled by both the ACL and PCL working in concert, but it can still occur without the ACL to an extent. Total knee prosthetic designs that preserve the PCL do achieve better knee flexion by allowing femoral rollback.
   (b) Disadvantage—The disadvantage of this design is that femoral rollback occurs without the aid of the ACL, and the consequent rollback is a combination of roll and slide. For rollback to occur, the tibial PE needs to be relatively flat, but this shape has the detrimental effect of creating high-contact stresses. The combination of sliding wear and high-contact stresses on the PE can lead to rapid PE wear and failure (see the later section on catastrophic wear). To combat this problem, recent PCL-retaining designs contain a more congruent PE insert that allows for less rollback. A more congruent articulation reduces the contact stresses on the PE, but it relegates the PCL to function as a static stabilizer to prevent anterior dislocation of the femur on the tibia. Increased knee flexion is achieved with a posterior offset center of rotation (usually 4-6 mm) and re-creation of the normal posterior tibial slope.

(2) PCL-substituting implants—These employ the use of a tibial PE post in the middle of the knee along with a cam situated between the femoral condyles (Fig. 5–25).

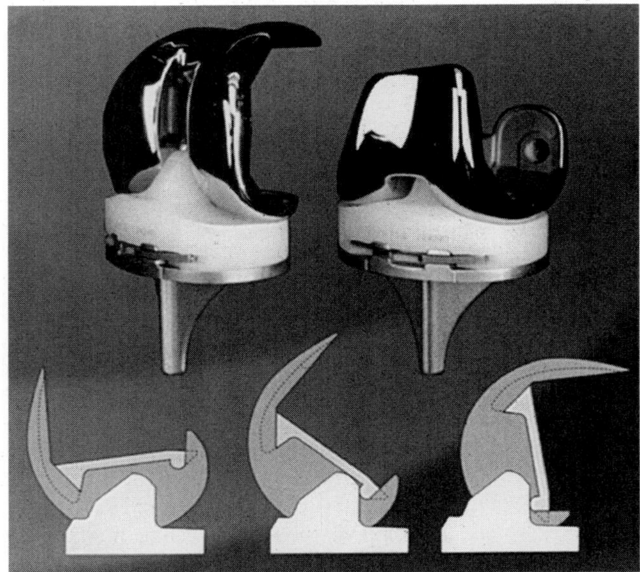

FIGURE 5–25 Posterior cruciate-substituting (also known as posterior stabilized) knee. Note the central polyethylene post and femoral cam device on femur when the knee flexes.

(a) Mechanism—Depending on the design parameters, the femoral cam will engage against the tibial post at a designated flexion point. At that point the femur is unable to translate anteriorly, and with further flexion it will mechanically reproduce the roll-back. With the knee in the flexed position, the tibial post will prevent the cam from translating anteriorly, thus providing stability. PCL-substituting designs achieve improved knee flexion and allow for mechanical roll-back. Because rollback is controlled mechanically, a congruent articulation surface can be used, which reduces contact stresses on the tibial PE.

(b) Advantages—A cruciate-substituting design is favored over a cruciate-retaining design in several situations. First, patients with a previous patellectomy should have a cruciate-substituting prosthesis because the weakened extensor force allows for easier anterior femoral dislocation even if the PCL is retained. Second, patients with *inflammatory arthritis* can have continued inflammatory changes that will cause late PCL ruptures in total knees that retain the PCL. Third, patients with prior trauma to the PCL with rupture or attenuation should have a posterior stabilized implant. The fourth indication for a cruciate-substituting device is over-release of the PCL during knee ligament balancing. If the tibial articular profile is flat, the knee can translate anteriorly and become unstable. In this situation, conversion to a cruciate-substituting device is preferred.

(c) Disadvantage—The disadvantage of the cruciate-substituting design is that knee balancing must be carefully addressed. If the flexion gap is loose, the femur can jump over the tibial post and dislocate (Fig. 5–26). If dislocation occurs, reduction requires sedation or general anesthetic. The reduction maneuver consists of knee flexion (at 90 degrees), distraction, and an anterior drawer maneuver. A cam jump can occur with hyperflexion even if the knee is well balanced. With a hyperflexed knee, the femur will impinge on the tibia and lever the femur over the tibial post. Therefore, if knee motion after knee replacement surgery is expected to be beyond 130 degrees, a cruciate-retaining design should be considered.

b. Rotating tibial platform—Another design modification for primary TKR implants is the rotating tibial platform, also known as the **mobile-bearing tibia** (MBT). In this design the tibial PE rotates on a polished metal tibial baseplate. The theoretical advantage to this design is better femoral-tibial conformity through the entire knee range.

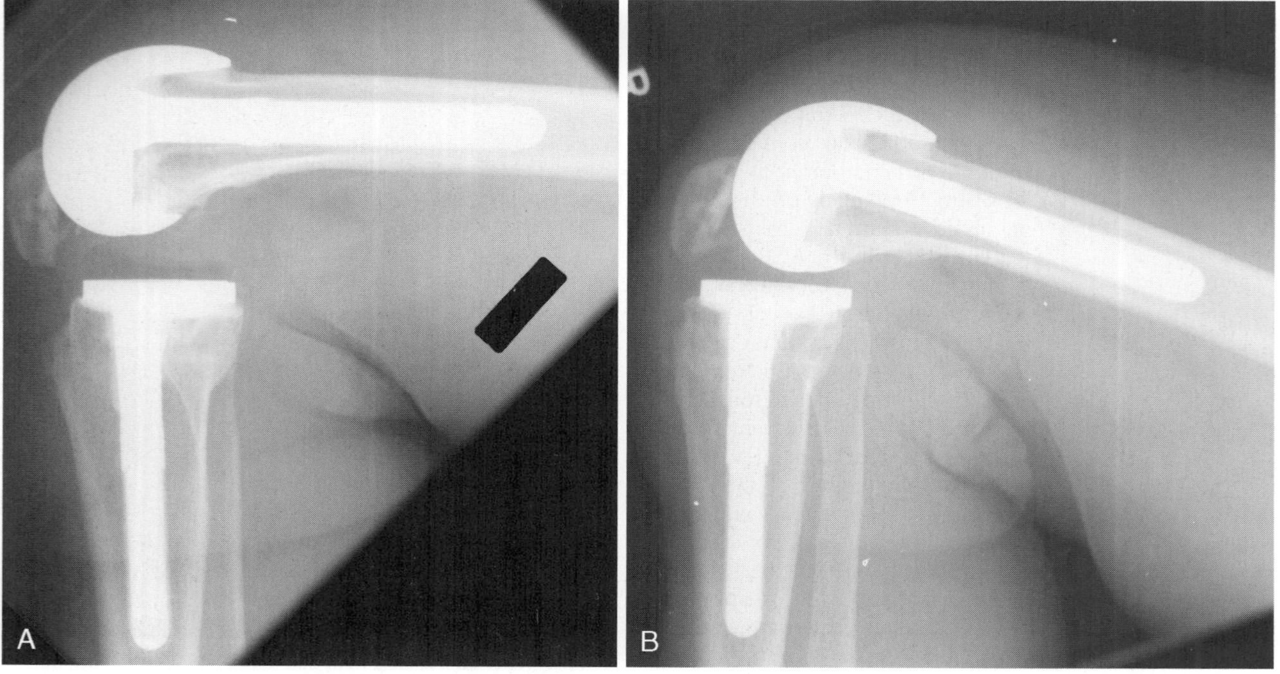

FIGURE 5–26 **A**, Lateral radiograph of the femoral cam jump. The femur has hyperflexed, allowing the cam to rise above the tibial post and dislocate anteriorly. Once in this position, it is very difficult to reduce unless an anesthetic is administered. **B**, Postreduction radiograph of the same knee.

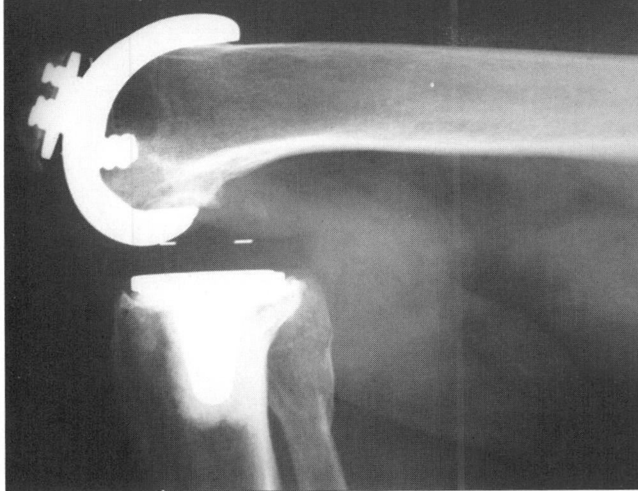

A

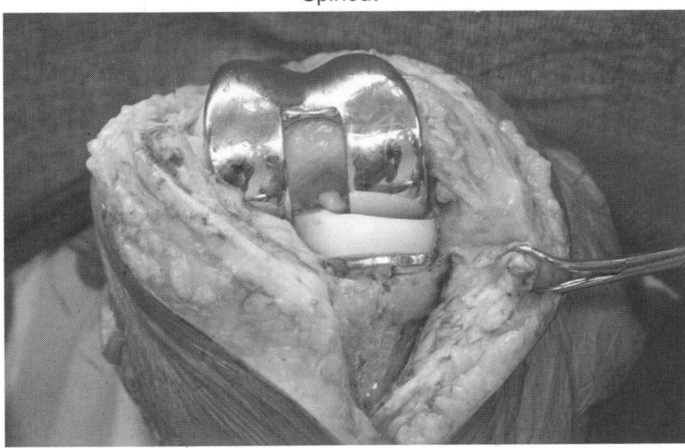

B

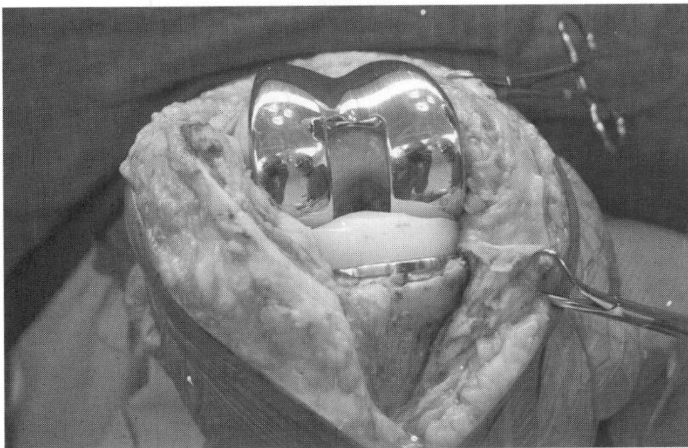

C

FIGURE 5–27 Radiographic and intraoperative pictures demonstrating bearing spinout. **A**, Lateral radiograph showing the anteroposterior profile of the tibial polyethylene bearing. **B**, Intraoperative finding where the lateral portion of the tibial bearing is dislocated posterior to the prosthetic lateral femoral condyle. **C**, The reduced position of the mobile-bearing tibial.

Better overall conformity is thought to reduce PE wear. The MBT shows survivorship equivalent to fixed-bearing designs at long-term follow-up, but the results are not superior. The unique problem with the MBT design is *bearing spinout* (Fig. 5–27). Bearing spinout occurs when the knee flexion gap is loose. The loose flexion gap allows the tibial bearing to rotate beyond the normal constraints of the knee, which clinically presents as knee locking and perching. Bearing spinout requires knee revision and correction of the loose flexion gap.

2. Patellofemoral articulation—The most common complications in TKR involve abnormal patellar tracking. Avoiding patellar problems in knee replacement is essentially an exercise in Q angle management and understanding the technical aspects that alter the knee joint line. The Q angle is an angle formed by the intersection of the extensor mechanism axis above the patella with the axis of the patellar tendon. The significance of the Q angle in knee replacement surgery is that an increased Q angle is associated with increased lateral patellar subluxation forces. Additionally, most patellofemoral prosthetic designs are not as constraining as the native knee. Thus, an increased Q angle can frequently cause the patella to track laterally. The goal in TKR is to maintain a normal Q angle with techniques that *do not compromise* mechanical alignment or ligament stability. Several technical rules in TKR should be followed to prevent abnormal patellar tracking, summarized in Table 5–6. The evaluation of component rotation in the scenario of patellofemoral instability is best performed with a CT scan to identify the epicondylar axis and compare it with the posterior condylar line of the femoral prosthesis. On the tibial side, tibial component rotation can be compared with its position with the tibial tubercle.
   a. Femoral component—Femoral component position, if it can be adjusted, should be either centered or lateralized. A medialized femoral component places the trochlear groove in a more medial position, which increases the Q angle. Thus, this position should be avoided. Internal rotation of the femoral component must be avoided because it causes lateral patellar tilt and a net increase in the Q angle (Fig. 5–28). An internally rotated femoral component also creates an asymmetrical flexion gap, which can present clinically as a stiff, painful TKR with an overly tight medial flexion gap. The other clinical presentation with an internally rotated femoral component is flexion instability with an overly loose lateral flexion gap. The preferred rotational alignment of the femur is slight external rotation to the neutral axis. Normally, the proximal tibia is in slight varus (3 degrees) (Fig. 5–29). In TKR, the

TABLE 5-6 PREVENTION OF ABNORMAL PATELLOFEMORAL TRACKING

Technical Issue	Guidelines	Problems	Preferred Solutions
Femoral component rotation	Do not internally rotate femoral component past neutral axis	Internal rotation of femoral component results in net lateral patellar tilt and increased lateral subluxation Internal rotation forces patella medially, which increases Q angle	Slight external rotation of femoral component
Femoral component position	Do not medialize femoral component	Increases Q angle	Either central or lateral position of femoral component
Tibial component rotation	Do not internally rotate tibial component past medial side of tibial tubercle	Internal rotation of tibial component results in net external rotation of tibial tubercle and increases Q angle	Tibial component centered in area between medial border of tibial tubercle and middle of tibial tubercle
Mechanical alignment of leg	Do not leave leg with net valgus mechanical alignment (i.e., avoid excess valgus)	Excessive valgus alignment increases Q angle	Femoral and tibial bone cuts that restore a *neutral* mechanical alignment of leg
Patellar component position	Avoid lateralization of patellar component on patella	Lateralization of patellar component increases Q angle (patella is pushed medially)	Patellar component placed in center of patella or in medial position
	Avoid inferior position of patellar component on patella	Inferior positioning can result in relative patella baja, causing loss of knee flexion	Patellar component placed in center of patella or in superior position
Joint line position	Avoid bone cuts that raise the joint line.	Creates or enhances patella baja—causes loss of knee flexion	Maintain joint line, and lower joint line if possible when baja deformity is present.

tibia is cut at 90 degrees (i.e., perpendicular to the mechanical axis). In order to maintain a symmetrical flexion gap, the femoral component must be externally rotated by the same amount to create a symmetrical flexion gap. This allows for balanced ligaments in flexion. Identifying the neutral rotational axis for the femur is not always easy. Occasionally, landmarks can be damaged during the degenerative process. Three generally accepted femoral landmarks can be used to define the neutral femoral rotational axis. They are the anteroposterior axis of the femur, the epicondylar axis, and the posterior condylar axis (Fig. 5–30).

(1) The **anteroposterior axis** of the femur is defined as a line running from the center of the trochlear groove to the top of the

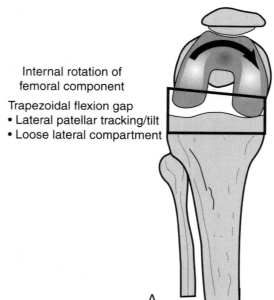

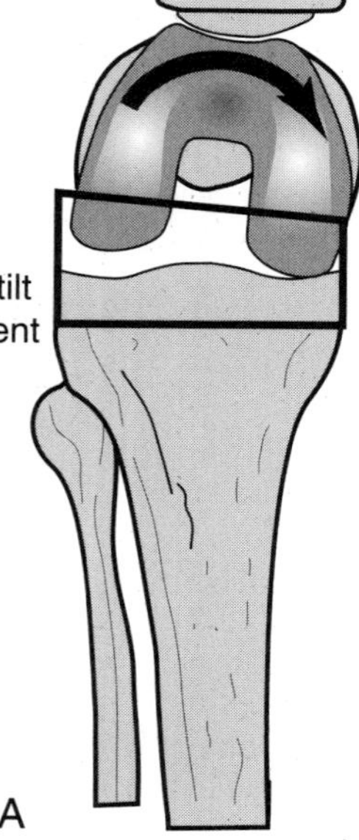

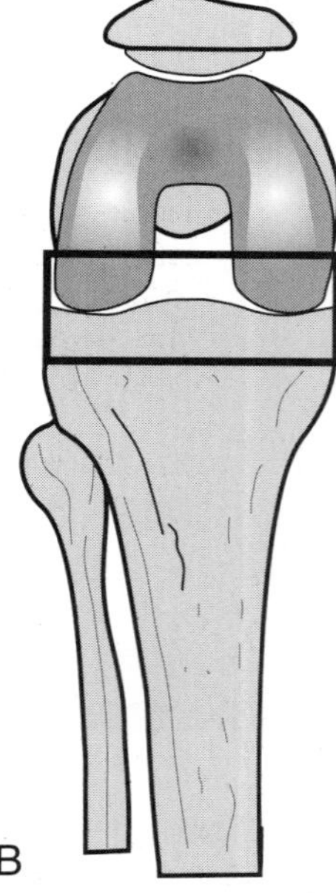

FIGURE 5–28 Femoral component rotation in coronal plane. **A**, Illustration of a femoral component that is placed in internal rotation. Internal rotation of femoral component causes the lateral flange of the femoral component to push the patella medially. The result is an increased Q angle. Although the patella is neutrally positioned, internal rotation of the femoral component gives the effect of a lateral patellar tilt. In addition, internal rotation of the femoral component creates an asymmetrical flexion gap, making it more difficult to balance the knee. **B**, Femoral component in slight external rotation (ER). This action creates symmetrical flexion gap, and the trochlear groove matches the patella. The knee is balanced.

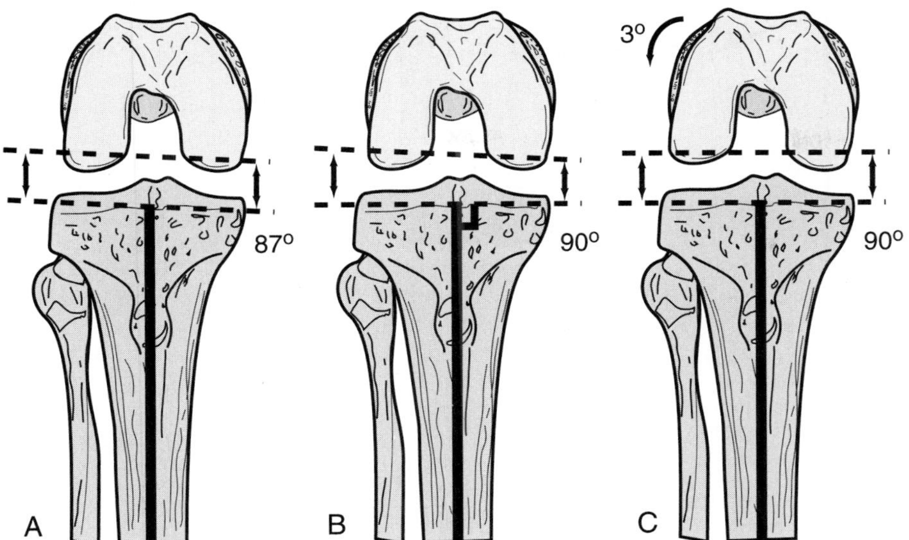

FIGURE 5–29 Rotational alignment of knee in coronal plane in flexion. **A**, Tibia on average has 3 degrees varus tilt. To match this tilt, the medial femoral condyle is slightly bigger than the lateral femoral condyle. **B**, The proximal tibia is cut at 90 degrees, perpendicular to the mechanical axis of the tibia. In flexion, this creates an asymmetrical flexion gap when the femur is cut parallel to the posterior femoral condyles. **C**, Anteroposterior (AP) cut of the femur made in slight external rotation. The AP cut matches the tibial cut in flexion, creating a symmetrical flexion gap. The flexion gap is now balanced.

intercondylar notch. A line perpendicular to this defines the neutral rotational axis. When patellofemoral dysplasia is present, it is difficult to accurately define the anteroposterior axis, which should not be used in this situation.

(2) The **epicondylar axis** is a line that is drawn between the center of the medial and lateral epicondyles. The epicondylar axis is generally parallel to the neutral rotational axis. Sometimes, because of anatomic variance, the epicondyles are shallow and round, making accurate pinpointing of the centers difficult. In this scenario, another axis line should help corroborate the neutral rotational axis.

(3) The **posterior condylar axis** is a line drawn between the bottom of the medial and lateral femoral condyles with the knee at 90 degrees of flexion. A line made 3-5 degrees in external rotation to this line defines the neutral rotational axis. The posterior condylar axis is inaccurate when there is lateral femoral condylar hypoplasia. When the lateral femoral condyle is hypoplastic, the posterior condylar axis will be in significant internal rotation. If the standard 3-5 degrees of external rotation is chosen to define the neutral rotational axis, the femoral component will be misplaced into internal rotation.

b. Tibial component—Internal rotation of the tibial component must be avoided because it effectively results in relative external rotation of the tibial tubercle. This action increases the Q angle (Fig. 5–31).

c. Mechanical alignment—Anatomic valgus deformities must be corrected to a normal range (5-7 degrees preferred). The actual goal in TKR is to restore a neutral mechanical alignment. Distal femoral and proximal bone cuts should be made to achieve this goal. If excessive valgus remains, there will be an increased Q angle.

d. Patellar component—When resurfacing the patella, the desired position of the patellar component is central or medialized. A medialized patellar component reduces the Q angle, but it requires the use of a smaller patellar dome (Fig. 5–32). The need for lateral release is less when a small patellar dome is used in a medialized position. Placing a small patellar component in a lateralized position increases the Q angle and lateral subluxation forces.

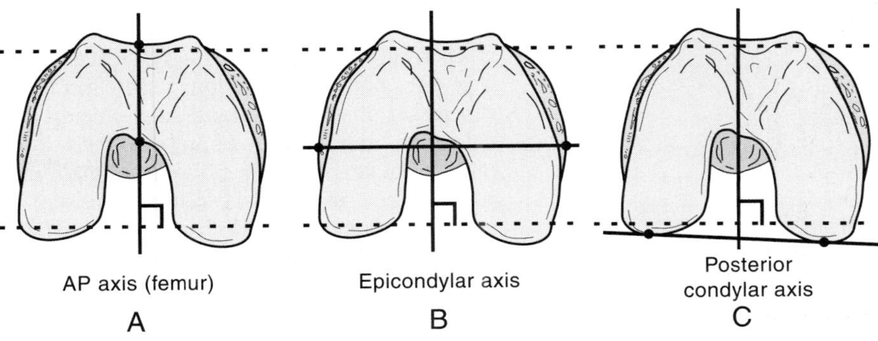

FIGURE 5–30 Determination of the femoral component of external rotation. **A**, Anteroposterior (AP) axis: defined by the center of the trochlear groove and intercondylar notch (dots). The AP cut is made perpendicular to this axis. **B**, Epicondylar axis: defined by a line connecting the centers of medial and lateral epicondylar condyles *(dots)*. The AP cut is made parallel to this axis. **C**, Posterior condylar axis: defined by a line connecting the bottom of the medial and lateral posterior condyles. The AP cut is made in 3 degrees of external rotation to this axis line.

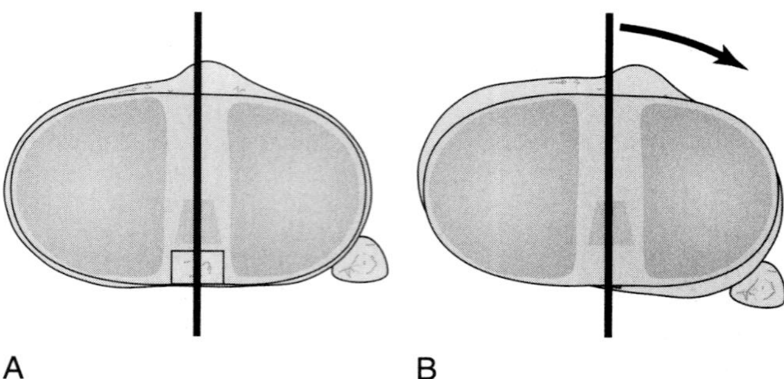

FIGURE 5–31 Demonstration of the tibial component of internal rotation. **A**, The tibial component centered over the medial third of the tibial tubercle. This is generally considered the preferred position. **B**, Internal rotation of tibial component. This action causes a net effect of externally rotating the tibial tubercle to the lateral side, which increases the Q angle.

e. Patella baja—Patella baja (or patella infera) is not an infrequent problem encountered in TKR. Patella baja is a condition manifested by a shortened patellar tendon. With patella baja, *knee flexion is limited* due to patellar impingement on the tibia as the knee flexes. Patella baja is most frequently seen in patients who have had a proximal tibial osteotomy, tibial tubercle shift or transfer, or prior fracture to the proximal tibia. Patella baja is encountered in various degrees. The solutions are limited. First, when performing a TKR, avoid bone cuts that *raise the joint line*. Raising the joint line will effectively increase the baja deformity. Conversely, lowering the joint line will decrease the deformity. Lowering the joint line can be achieved by using distal femoral metallic augmentation and cutting off more proximal tibia (Fig. 5–33). Lowering the joint line does not get rid of the deformity entirely, but it does help to provide increased knee flexion. Resurfacing the patella with a small patellar dome placed superiorly can effectively increase patellar tendon length. Inferior bone can be trimmed to prevent impingement. Another useful technique is trimming the anterior tibial PE and patellar PE at the impingement points (Fig. 5–34), which is achieved sharply with a scalpel. It will provide some improved flexion. Shave only the PE that does not compromise component stability or patellar tracking. If the baja deformity is severe, one last option is to cut the patella but not resurface. This creates less patellar impingement, allowing for more knee flexion. Lastly, for severe baja impingement, a complete patellectomy may be required.

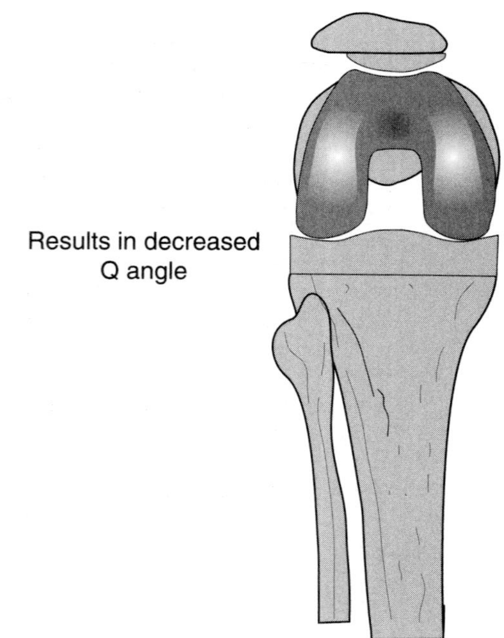

FIGURE 5–32 Medialization of the patellar component. With this technique, a small patellar dome is placed on the medial side of the cut patella (usually centered over the trochlear ridge). Because the entire patella does not need to be centered in the trochlea, the center of the patellar bone is in a lateralized position that reduces the Q angle. In addition, the lateral retinaculum is more relaxed, with the patella in the lateral position.

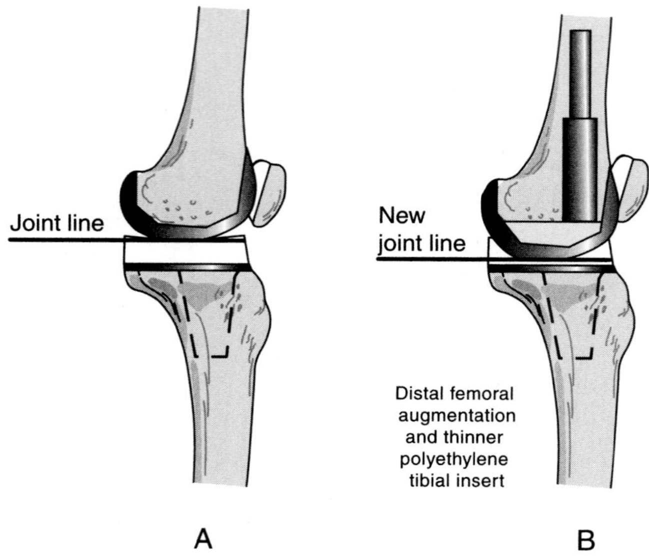

FIGURE 5–33 The effect of lowering the joint line with distal femoral augmentation to improve baja deformity. **A**, Total knee with baja deformity. **B**, Distal femoral augmentation (augments behind the femoral component) moves the joint line inferiorly. Less tibial polyethylene thickness is required. Baja deformity is improved.

3. Catastrophic wear—Catastrophic wear in knee replacement surgery refers to the premature failure of prosthetic implants due to excessive loading, *macroscopic* failure of PE, and subsequent mechanical loosening (Fig. 5–35). Catastrophic wear does not refer to the long-term effect of the generation of submicron and small-micron particle debris and associated bony osteolysis. It is a problem of large-scale PE failure resulting from a combination of several factors involved in implant design and biomechanics. The problem is seen primarily in TKR, but depending on the situation and conditions it can also be seen in prosthetic hip and shoulder replacement. The main issues involved in the phenomenon of

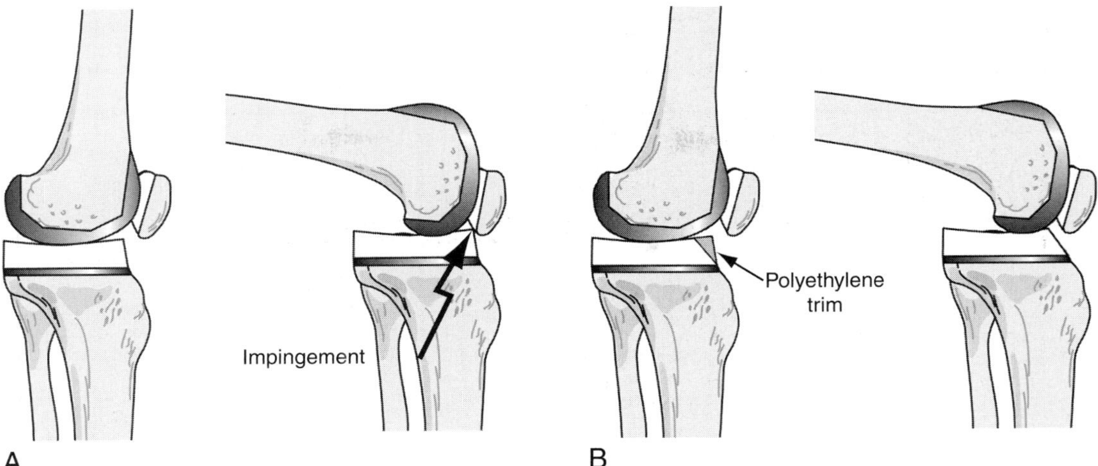

FIGURE 5–34 Technique of trimming polyethylene at the impingement points in patella baja. **A**, Total knee replacement with baja deformity. Note impingement of the inferior pole of the patella component with anterior tibial polyethylene. **B**, Trimming of polyethylene to decrease impingement. Trimming is performed with a scalpel and should not compromise the articulating surfaces or stability. Trimming provides some improvement (usually up to 10 degrees) in flexion range.

catastrophic wear are (1) PE thickness, (2) articular geometry, (3) sagittal plane knee kinematics, (4) PE sterilization, and (5) PE machining. The problem of catastrophic wear is multidimensional. The factors involved and the problems encountered are summarized in Table 5–7. The elimination of only one of the problems will not solve the situation; it will only serve to temporarily mitigate or slow the eventual result. Only with an understanding of all the factors involved can there be an effective change in component design and manufacturing to prevent this problem from occurring.

a. PE thickness—PE thickness is of critical importance in the process of catastrophic wear. To keep joint contact stresses below the yield strength of UHMWPE, PE thickness must be at least 8 mm. Thinner sections transmit joint stresses to a localized area only, resulting in microscopic and macroscopic PE failure. It is important to understand that when a tibial PE insert is placed into a metal tray, the PE thickness reported represents the total thickness of the metal tray (usually 2-3 mm) plus the PE. Therefore, in many instances in which 8-10–mm PE inserts are used with a metal base tray, the actual PE thickness at the nadir of the concavity on the articular surface may be as thin as 4-5 mm. Consequently, in many cases in which thin PE inserts are used, the yield strength of UHMWPE is exceeded. This result is seen most often when thin bone–cut resections are used in younger patients to preserve bone stock for future revision. In this scenario, the young, active patient will cycle the prosthetic joint at a much higher rate, leading to rapid failure (4-5 years in some instances).

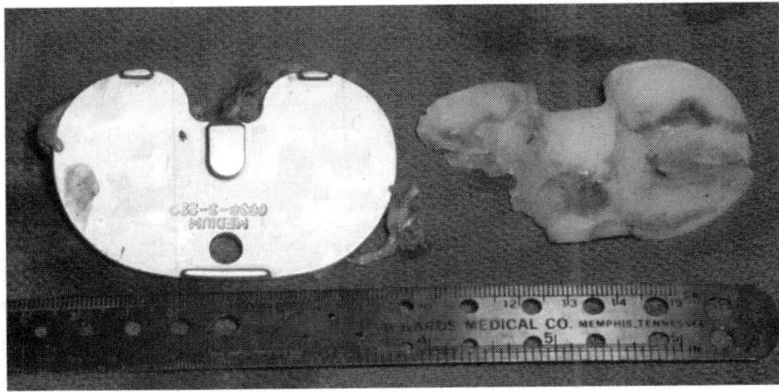

FIGURE 5–35 Catastrophic wear of polyethylene in a total knee replacement. Note gross fragmentation of tibial polyethylene.

b. Articular geometry—Another important factor leading to catastrophic failure is articular geometry. A majority of the prosthetic knee implants associated with catastrophic wear have a relatively flat PE articular surface. A flat articular design is disadvantageous in terms of biomechanical loading. With such a design, prosthetic contact areas between the femur and the tibia are low, and contact loads are high. Instead, the goal in prosthetic knee design is to **minimize contact loads**, which is achieved **by maximizing the surface contact area.** Newer-generation prosthetic knee designs have improved contact areas by increasing articular congruency, which is achieved by increasing congruency in the coronal and sagittal planes. As a result, instead of using a flat PE insert, newer components tend to be more "dished" in both the coronal and sagittal planes.

c. Sagittal plane knee kinematics—Sagittal plane kinematics played an important role in the design choice of flat PE inserts. In an effort to improve knee flexion, prosthetic designs used the PCL to provide femoral rollback, which is the posterior shift of the

TABLE 5-7 CATASTROPHIC WEAR IN TOTAL KNEE REPLACEMENT

Factors Involved	Problem	Solutions
PE thickness	PE < 8 mm thickness will exceed yield strength when loaded	Keep thinnest portion of PE above 8 mm • Thicker tibial cut • All-PE tibia (needs to be congruent articulation)
Articular surface design	Flat tibia PE • Low-contact surface area • High-contact stress load	Use congruent articular surface design • High-contact surface area • Low-contact stress load
Kinematics	Femoral rollback with only PCL (no ACL) • Dyskinetic motion in sagittal plane • Sliding wear	1. Minimize rollback with PCL-retained implant design. • Posterior offset center of rotation for flexion • Posterior slope to improve flexion 2. Use PCL-substituting implant • Posterior stabilized knee • Anterior stabilized knee (i.e., extended anterior PE lip)
PE sterilization	Irradiation in air • PE oxidation • Diminished mechanical properties of PE • Subsurface delamination, pitting, and fatigue cracking	1. Irradiation in inert gas or vacuum • Facilitate polyethylene cross-linking • Improved wear resistance of PE 2. Use alternative bearing surface • Ceramic-to-ceramic (future prospect)
PE machining	Machining stretches PE chains in subsurface region of 1-2 mm • This area more at risk to oxidation • Causes subsurface delamination, pitting, and fatigue cracking	Use direct-compression molding of PE with no machining of articular surface

ACL, anterior cruciate ligament; PCL, posterior cruciate ligament; PE, polyethylene.

femoral-tibial contact as the knee flexes. Femoral rollback allows the femur to clear the posterior tibia and bend further. In the native knee, femoral rollback is controlled by both the ACL and PCL. It can still occur without an ACL, but fluoroscopic studies observing rollback in PCL-retained TKRs show that the posterior rollback is kinetically displeasing. Instead of a smooth, gradual roll, there is a combination of forward sliding, backward sliding, and posterior rolling. In addition, to allow the knee to roll back, a flat PE insert is required. The dyskinetic sagittal plane movements seen with PCL-retained implants that have flat PE inserts contribute to the catastrophic wear process. Laboratory studies do show that sliding movements (i.e., femoral component translation on the tibia) result in surface and subsurface cracking and significant wear. In contrast, pure rolling movements generated minimum cracking and wear. Therefore, newer prosthetic knee designs incorporate less femoral rollback and provide a more congruent articular PE surface. Knee flexion is achieved with other design techniques, such as using a posterior center of rotation, using a posterior slope, or using a PCL-substituting knee design.

d. PE sterilization—The next major factor in catastrophic wear involves the sterilization of PE. As discussed in the section on osteolysis and PE wear, PE components irradiated in an oxygen environment suffer from PE oxidation. Oxidized PE is mechanically weaker, and the threshold for catastrophic wear is lowered. Excessive loading of oxidized PE can result in rapid PE failure.

e. PE machining—More recent studies have implicated the **machining process** of PE as a factor leading to PE breakdown. During the machining of PE, cutting tools (lathing or burring tools) create shear forces at the cutting interface that microscopically stretch the PE chains (Fig. 5–36). This effect is most pronounced in the subsurface region of 1-2 mm. In the "sensitized" subsurface region, the PE molecule chains (specifically those in the amorphous regions) are microscopically stretched and are at an increased energy state. Therefore, any oxidation will be more apt to affect this region. As a result, oxidative changes within the machined PE tibial component will show a classic **white band** of oxidation in the subsurface region, which also explains why wear patterns in total-knee tibial bearings consist of subsurface delamination and the associated patterns of pitting and fatigue cracking (Fig. 5–37). The lack of this sensitized region in direct compression–molded components may be the reason that delamination and subsurface oxidation are rarely observed in this process.

4. Knee flexion range—The single most important factor governing the ultimate flexion range after TKR is preoperative flexion range. As a general rule, postoperative flexion range is equal to preoperative flexion range ±10 degrees. Preoperative flexion contractures must be corrected at

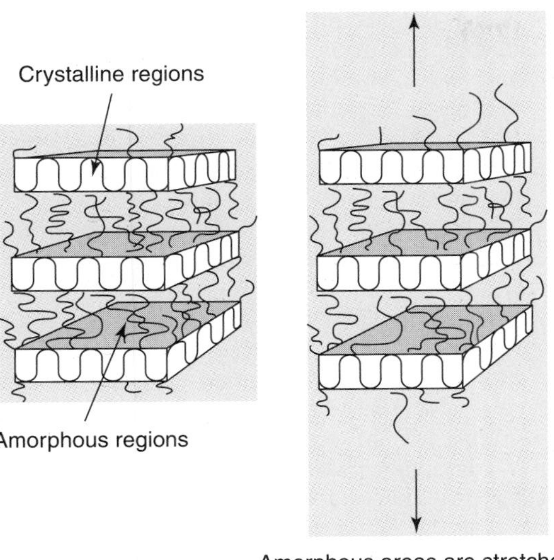

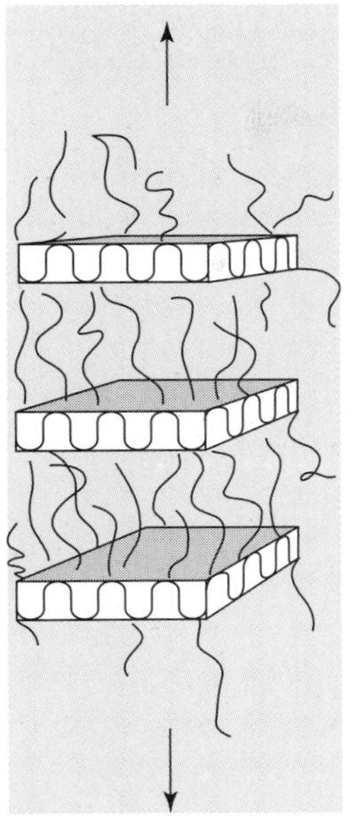

FIGURE 5–36 The effect of machining on polyethylene. **A**, Polyethylene in its two forms in situ in a molded tibial insert. Gamma irradiation affects the amorphous areas of the polyethylene (either oxidation or cross-linking). **B** and **C**, Machining stretches the amorphous areas, mostly 1-2 mm below the polyethylene surface. Gamma irradiation to this *sensitized* region will have greater oxidation effect.

the time of surgery because fixed contractures usually do not stretch out. On the other hand, the flexion contracture seen postoperatively after intraoperative correction of a knee contracture is usually due to hamstring tightness and spasm. After an anterior arthrotomy, the quadriceps musculature is not firing vigorously, so there is a relative overpull by the hamstring complex. As knee swelling abates, the quadriceps becomes more active and will counter hamstring overpull. Almost all postoperative knee flexion contractures due to hamstring overpull will stretch out by 6 months. The few that exist after this time may still stretch out by 1 year. It is important for patients to be diligent with extension and flexion range exercises up to 3 months postoperatively.

a. Flexion closure—Recent studies have also examined flexion closure of total knee wounds as a means of obviating the need for postoperative **continuous passive motion** (CPM) devices. Knees closed in flexion tend to recover quicker in the perioperative period and do not need concomitant use of CPM machines.
b. TKR and arthrofibrosis—Manipulation of TKR for arthrofibrosis should be carried out in the range of 4-6 weeks postoperatively. The risk of waiting too long for manipulation is that one increases the chance of causing a

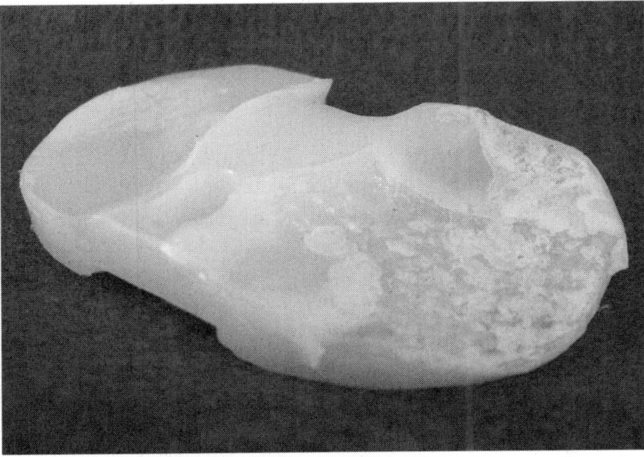

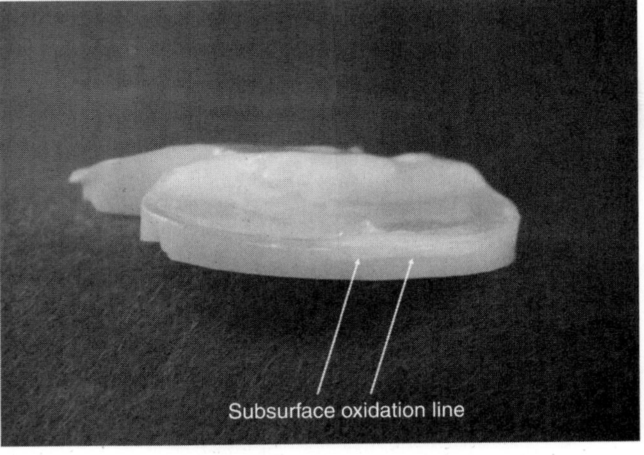

FIGURE 5–37 Pattern of catastrophic polyethylene wear in a modular polyethylene tibial insert. **A**, The typical wear pattern of subsurface delamination, fatigue cracking, and pitting. **B**, The lateral edge of the insert, where one can see the white band of oxidation, starting 1-2 mm below the articular surface.

supracondylar femur fracture. Adhesions in the medial and lateral gutter areas of the knee are the main cause in limiting knee range when arthrofibrosis does occur. Furthermore, one must be aware of a femoral notch when considering knee manipulation. A femoral notch is a small violation of the anterior femoral cortex when the anterior femoral cut is made during TKR. A femoral notch has a mild detrimental effect on the torsional strength of the femur. However, an anterior notch significantly reduces *bending* strength. In the presence of a femoral notch, a knee manipulation is more likely to cause a supracondylar fracture. In the case of a significant cortical notch, a knee manipulation should be avoided if at all possible.

5. Patellar clunk syndrome—Patellar clunk syndrome is seen with posterior stabilized total-knee implants. A fibrous lump of tissue forms on the posterior surface of the quadriceps tendon just above the superior pole of the patella. This nodule of tissue causes symptoms when it gets caught in the box of the posterior stabilized femoral component as the knee comes from flexion into extension, which usually occurs as the knee reaches 30-45 degrees of flexion range. As the knee extends further, tension is applied to the entrapped nodule, which subsequently pops out of the box with a palpable and often auditory clunk. The reason for the scar formation is not clear. It may occur from a stimulated healing response from cutting the patella and abrading the adjacent quadriceps tissue. Another proposed reason is the use of a small patellar component that fails to lift the quadriceps tendon away from the anterior edge of the intercondylar notch. Recommended treatment is arthroscopic or open débridement of the nodule (Fig. 5–38).

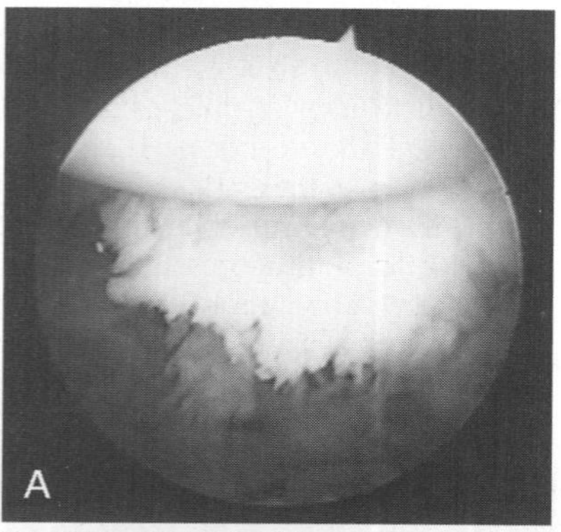

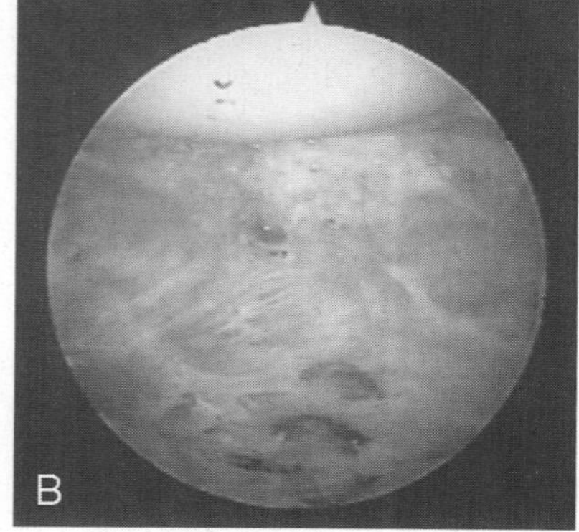

FIGURE 5–38 Arthroscopic photographs of patient with patellar clunk syndrome. **A**, Cephalic view of the patella, showing nodule of fibrous tissue hanging down in front of the patella. It is this tissue that gets caught in the central box region of the posterior stabilized femoral component. **B**, The same cephalic view after arthroscopic débridement of fibrous nodule. Patellar clunk syndrome resolved postoperatively.

D. Less invasive surgical technique—A less invasive surgical technique for TKR has recently been emphasized. The main benefit of this technique is reduced hospital stay and faster early rehabilitation. The less invasive technique is accomplished via the use of smaller-sized knee-cutting jigs and preparation jigs. The size of the femoral component generally determines the minimum length of incision required. Complication rates are higher than those in a standard, full, open procedure. Difficulty in exposure often causes tissue trauma and tearing. If the patellar tendon peels off the tibial tubercle or other soft tissue tearing occurs, the incision should be fully extended. In the case in which the patellar tendon peels off the tibial tubercle, two thirds of the patellar tendon is usually allowed to peel before a formal extensor reconstruction is required.

E. Revision TKR—Aseptic failure of a TKR is caused by several factors, which include component loosening, PE wear (catastrophic wear and osteolysis), ligament instability, and patellofemoral maltracking. Tibial component loosening is more common than femoral component loosening.
   1. Goals of revision—The major goals of revision knee surgery are (1) extraction of knee components, with minimal bone and soft tissue destruction; (2) restoration of cavitary and segmental bone defects; (3) restoration of the original joint line as efficaciously as possible; (4) balanced knee ligaments; and (5) stable knee components.
   2. Surgical exposure—The surgical exposure for revision TKR should be extensile. In the case where knee stiffness and arthrofibrosis is present, a **rectus snip** may be required to expose the knee joint and evert the patella. In a rectus snip, an oblique transverse cut is made across the upper portion of the quadriceps tendon from medial to lateral. The common complication with this technique is diastasis of the repair, causing an extensor lag.
   3. Implant choice
      a. Unconstrained prosthesis—If the PCL is attenuated and/or the joint line remains significantly altered, a posterior stabilized implant (PCL-substituting implant) is recommended. A posterior stabilized implant is *not* a constrained design and does not assist at all in varus/valgus stability of the knee (Fig. 5–39). If a PCL-retaining system is used instead, the option of a posterior stabilized implant should be available at the time of surgery. The integrity of the PCL at the time of revision is often unpredictable.

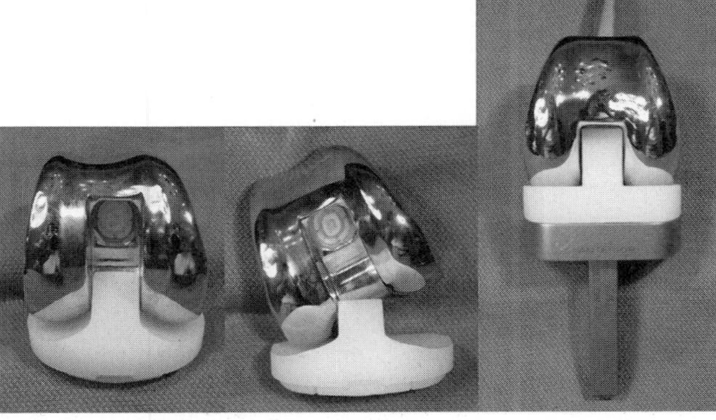

FIGURE 5–39 Photographs comparing a posterior stabilized knee implant with a high-post constrained implant. A constrained implant (nonhinged) has a high central post that will not allow the knee to open to varus or valgus stress. Note how the smaller posterior stabilized post will allow the knee to completely open to varus or valgus stress.

b. Constrained-nonhinged prosthesis—The next choice in revision TKR implants is the constrained-nonhinged prosthesis, which is an implant that has a large central post that *substitutes* for MCL or lateral collateral ligament (LCL) function. The central post is wider and taller than the posterior stabilized design. The high central post restricts opening of the knee to varus/valgus stress and restricts rotation. The indications for use of a constrained-nonhinged TKR are MCL attenuation, LCL attenuation or deficiency, and flexion gap laxity. A knee with a loose flexion gap can be made stable with a tall post. The use of a constrained-nonhinged TKR for complete MCL deficiency is controversial. With complete MCL deficiency, all varus loading forces are placed upon the PE post. Consequently, PE post breakage can occur even with normal (nonexcessive) activity.

c. Constrained-hinged knee implant—The most constrained revision TKR implant currently used is a hinged knee with a rotating platform (Fig. 5–40). In this design, the femur and tibia are mechanically linked with a connecting bar and bearing. The tibial component is allowed to rotate within a yoke, which allows internal and external rotation during the gait cycle. The rotating platform is needed to reduce the rotational forces that would otherwise be placed upon the prosthesis–bone interface. Historically, hinged-knee designs that did not have a rotating platform had a very high loosening rate. A constrained-hinged knee with a rotating platform should be used only when absolutely necessary. The indications for use of this device are global ligament deficiency (usually post-trauma or the multiply revised TKR), hyperextension instability seen with polio, and resection of the knee for tumor or infection. Relative indications include

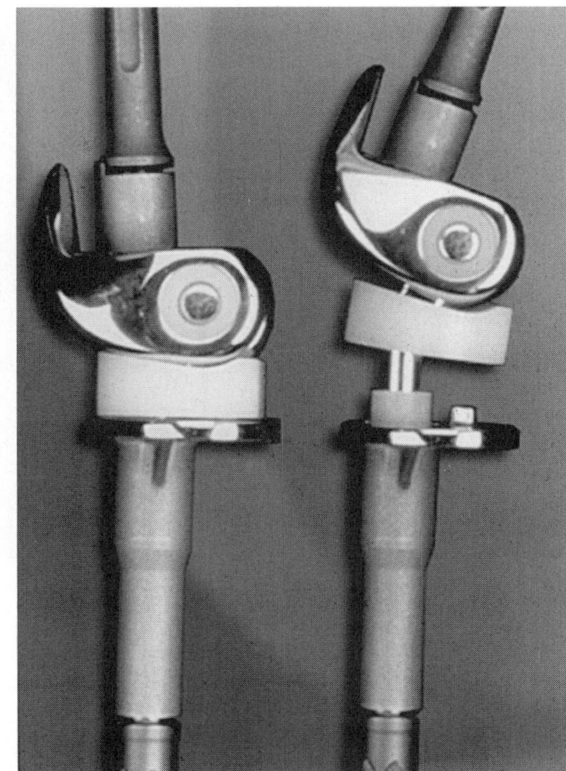

FIGURE 5–40 A constrained hinged knee with a rotating tibial platform. The tibial polyethylene bearing is mechanically linked to the femur via a large connecting pin. The tibial polyethylene has a distal extension (called a yoke) that goes into the metal tibial tray to allow for some internal and external rotation during the knee gait cycle. This action relieves some of the rotational forces that would otherwise be placed on the prosthesis-bone interface.

Charcot arthropathy and complete MCL deficiency (controversial). When a constrained device for revision TKR (either nonhinged or hinged) is chosen, medullary stems in the femur and tibia *must* always be used. With the use of constrained implants, the forces at the prosthesis–bone interface are increased. These increased interface forces can be partially ameliorated by the use of diaphyseal stems that can share the load in the revision construct.

4. Metaphyseal bone damage—In many circumstances, the metaphyseal bone in the knee is damaged from mechanical abrasion, osteolysis, or an extraction technique. When these deficiencies are encountered, the affected areas should be supported with medullary stem extensions, which assist with load sharing. Cavitary defects can be filled with either particulate bone graft or cement. Generally, contained defects 1 cm deep or less can be filled with cement. Segmental deficiencies can be reconstructed with metal augmentation devices (wedges or blocks) and/or structural bone grafts. Large segmental deficiencies may require bulk-support allografts or modular endoprosthetic devices (Fig. 5–41). Almost all revision TKRs are cemented at the metaphyseal interfaces. In most cases, stem extensions are

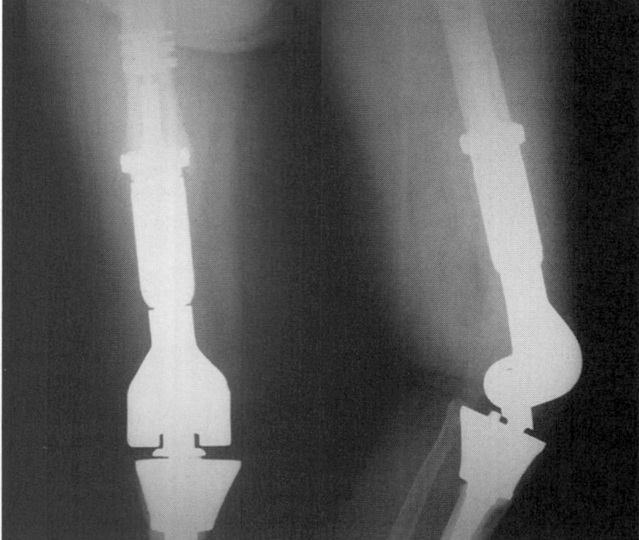

FIGURE 5–41 Radiograph of salvage knee reimplantation at 2.5 years. This 86-year-old female presented with massive infection of a revision total knee arthroplasty. A significant bone resection was required due to infection. A femoral endoprosthesis is secured with biologic fixation to the end of femoral diaphysis using a femoral compress device. The extensor tendon is still intact, with a clinical lag of 30 degrees.

noncemented and inserted with a press-fit technique. Cementing medullary stems is acceptable.

5. Knee reconstruction after component removal—Reconstruction of the knee after component removal should proceed first with the tibial side, which allows the joint line to be established. A useful guideline in determining the normal joint line is to identify the proximal tip of the fibular head. The joint line is usually about 1.5-2 cm above the fibular head. If the contralateral knee is not replaced, a radiograph of the native knee can be used to determine more accurately the distance from the fibular head to the joint line. Once the joint line has been established, the femur is reconstructed to match the tibia. Balancing is then performed to equalize flexion and extension gaps and balance medial and lateral spaces. If reconstruction proceeds in this manner, the patellofemoral articulation is usually situated in the appropriate position. If patella baja occurs, it should be addressed accordingly (see discussion of patellofemoral tracking).

J. Periprosthetic fracture
   1. Supracondylar fracture—Supracondylar fractures of the femur occur infrequently (less than 1%). The scenario most likely to cause supracondylar fracture is anterior femoral notching in a patient with weak bone (especially from rheumatoid arthritis). Supracondylar fracture can also occur as a result of overexuberant manipulation of the total knee under anesthesia.
      a. Nondisplaced—Nondisplaced fractures are treated with nonoperative management (cast or cast brace). However, if the prosthesis is mechanically loose, revision with a long-stem prosthesis is required.
      b. Displaced—For fractures that are displaced, there is no one recommended treatment. Open treatment, no matter what method is chosen, is often difficult and demanding. If the total-knee implant is mechanically loose or the fracture disrupts the prosthetic interface, revision with a long-stem prosthesis is required. If the implant is solidly fixed, an attempt should be made to reduce the fracture and restore anatomic alignment. If the fracture is stable, then treatment with a cast or cast brace is preferred. If the fracture is unstable, the three options for open fixation include (1) a supracondylar plate/screw system, (2) a supracondylar nail with proximal and distal fixation, and (3) revision TKR with a long medullary stem. Fractures that extend distal to the supracondylar prosthetic flange leave little bone for fixation with either a plate or nail construct. In this situation, revision TKR with a long medullary stem is recommended. Some total-knee designs and sizes may not allow passage of a supracondylar nail because either an intercondylar box is closed (seen in posterior stabilized knee designs) or the intercondylar dimensions of the available bone are too small for passage of the nail. Comminuted fractures with osteopenic bone (i.e., elderly patients with thin bone) do not respond well to plating or nailing. Revision TKR with a long medullary stem is preferred.
   2. Tibial fracture—Tibial fractures below a total-knee implant are uncommon. Nondisplaced fractures are best treated by immobilization and restricted weight bearing. Displaced fractures are best treated with a long-stem revision prosthesis.

K. Wound necrosis—Wound necrosis after TKR usually occurs after a difficult/complex surgical reconstruction. Major complications occur more frequently in the following groups: (1) an anterior knee with multiple parallel incisions that create skin bridges, (2) prior knee trauma with localized soft tissue loss, (3) significant knee stiffness that requires significant dissection, and (4) chronic infection with associated soft tissue loss. In the above conditions, knee closure under tension should be avoided. When an open wound develops and a tension-free closure is not possible, the recommended treatment requires the rotation of a **medial gastrocnemius muscle flap** to the anterior knee. This flap has good excursion and can be rotated even to the lateral side of the knee (Fig. 5–42). The blood supply to the medial gastrocnemius muscle is through the medial sural artery. In contrast, the lateral gastrocnemius muscle has little excursion. Its role should be limited to covering isolated lateral knee wounds. The lateral gastrocnemius muscle is pulled over the peroneal nerve when the muscle is rotated to the knee region. Therefore, the common complication with a rotation of the lateral

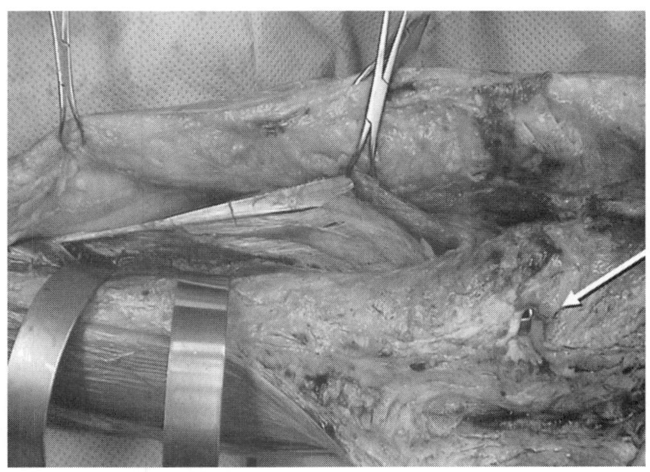

A

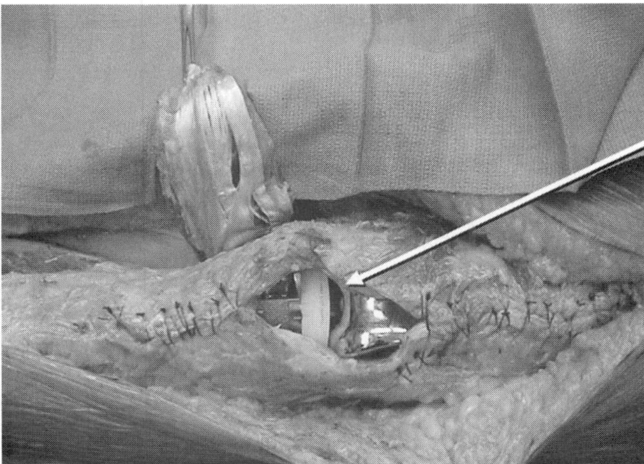

B

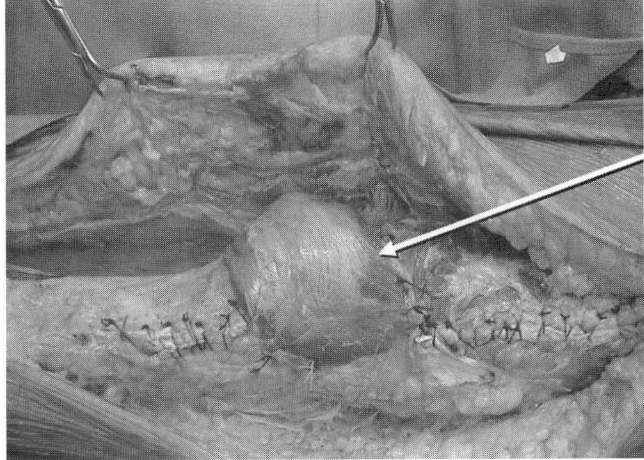

C

FIGURE 5–42 Intraoperative photographs showing an open anterior knee wound and a medial gastrocnemius rotational flap. **A**, Harvesting of medial gastrocnemius muscle. Note that the anterior knee wound must be opened, débrided, and lavaged. **B**, The medial gastrocnemius muscle is completely detached except for its proximal origin. Note also the anterior knee wound reapproximated with tension-free closure. **C**, Note how the medial gastrocnemius muscle can be mobilized to cover the anterolateral aspect of the knee.

gastrocnemius muscle is peroneal nerve palsy from flap traction on the nerve.

L. **Unicompartmental knee arthroplasty** (UKA)—Unicompartmental knee arthroplasty is considered an alternative to knee osteotomy and TKR when degenerative arthritis involves only one compartment. In UKA, only one of the three compartments of the knee is replaced. The most common UKA performed is clearly a medial UKA (i.e., resurfacing of medial femoral condyle and medial tibial condyle). The greatest documented advantage of medial UKA over TKR is faster early recovery and rehabilitation. In addition, there are generally fewer short-term complications, and the incision is smaller than that made for TKR. There is a high rate of short- to mid-term satisfaction, but long-term survivorship is not comparable to TKR when revision rates are compared.

1. Patient selection criteria—Careful patient selection is critical for the success of a UKA. Arthritic pain must be localized to the affected compartment. In general, isolated medial compartment arthritis produces more degeneration in extension. The wear pattern shows eburnated bone on the distal end of the medial femoral condyle (i.e., not posterior) and the anterior portion of the medial tibial condyle. The pain presenting with this condition is anteromedial. In contrast, isolated patellofemoral arthritis presents with pain that is retropatellar, superomedial, and superolateral. Pain not infrequently can radiate distally toward the ankle. Isolated arthritis of the lateral compartment presents with anterolateral pain. Isolated patellofemoral arthritis usually results from preexisting maltracking and dysplasia. With isolated patellofemoral replacement, concomitant proximal extensor realignment is often needed.
2. Contraindications—Contraindications for a medial UKA (concepts also apply to lateral UKA) are (1) ACL deficiency, (2) fixed varus deformity that cannot be corrected on clinical examination, (3) previous meniscectomy in the opposite compartment, (4) knee flexion contracture, (5) lack of knee flexion (>90 degrees required), (6) inflammatory arthritis, and (7) significant tricompartmental disease. When the ACL is deficient, knee flexion kinematics is significantly altered, creating increased sliding translation in the medial compartment. This action increases prosthetic wear, leading to early failure. A fixed varus or valgus deformity preoperatively indicates a rigid deformity that cannot be balanced adequately with a unicompartmental technique. Finally, a UKA should not be used in a highly active patient or laborer because the UKA PE tibial insert is usually thin and can fail early with increased wear.
3. Overcorrection and undercorrection—For medial UKA, varus deformity should be corrected only to 1-5 degrees of anatomic valgus. Overcorrection leads to accelerated disease progression in the lateral compartment. Undercorrection results in implant overload, with subsequent failure of the implant or underlying bone (i.e., a subsiding implant). Fixed-bearing implants usually fail due to mechanical loosening, whereas mobile-bearing implants fail because of disease progression in the unresurfaced compartments.

III. Shoulder Replacement Surgery

A. Contraindications—Shoulder arthroplasty is *contraindicated* in the following conditions: (1) when both the deltoid and the rotator cuff are not functional, (2) when active infection is present, (3) with neuropathic arthropathy, (4) with intractable instability, and (5) with a noncompliant patient.

B. Approach—The most common approach for shoulder arthroplasty is deltopectoral. In this procedure, the subscapularis muscle and anterior capsule are released off the humeral head. The shoulder is dislocated anteriorly. The most common complication with this approach is damage to the axillary nerve. Rehabilitation after shoulder arthroplasty should include avoiding excessive *passive* external rotation exercises in order to avoid pull-off of the subscapularis muscle.

C. Total shoulder replacement (TSR) versus hemiarthroplasty

1. TSR is the preferred procedure for patients with either glenohumeral osteoarthritis or inflammatory arthritis. Superior pain relief is noted with TSR compared with humeral hemiarthroplasty in long-term follow-up. Loosening of the glenoid component is the most common reason for revision TSR.
2. The best indication for humeral hemiarthroplasty is osteonecrosis of the humeral head in a young patient with normal glenoid articular cartilage. A successful hemiarthroplasty requires normal glenoid bone and anatomy. Late glenoid pain is a problem in hemiarthroplasty. Furthermore, late conversion to TSR is not always successful. Problems include significant glenoid bone loss from mechanical wear, unpredictable glenoid pain relief, and limited postoperative motion.

D. Total shoulder replacement

1. Technical demands—Although it has similarities to THR, TSR has technical demands that set it apart. First, the range of motion in the shoulder far surpasses the range in either the hip or the knee. The success of shoulder replacement surgery is far more dependent on the proper functioning of the soft tissues. Second, the glenoid is far less constrained than the acetabulum, and the shear forces on the glenoid are significant, which make the glenoid more prone to mechanical loosening and PE wear. The two most important factors to take into consideration in TSR are the condition of the rotator cuff and the amount of glenoid bone stock available for resurfacing.
   a. Rotator cuff condition—The biomechanics of active shoulder elevation is complex. The rotator cuff provides a compressive force for the humeral head against the glenoid. This action keeps the humeral head center of rotation in a relatively fixed position against the glenoid, which allows the deltoid and other shoulder elevators to lift the arm over a fixed, efficient fulcrum. When the rotator cuff is deficient, the compressive force for the humeral head against the glenoid is lost. Deltoid tensioning pulls the arm and humeral head cephalad against the acromion. The humeral head center of rotation is superior and eccentric in relation to the glenoid socket. Active shoulder elevation is lost due to the loss of the fixed fulcrum around the glenoid.

b. Glenoid stock integrity—The other critical factor when considering shoulder replacement surgery is the integrity of the glenoid. The glenoid fossa is relatively small and shallow. Mechanical abrasion by the degenerative process may leave little bone and little chance for glenoid resurfacing.
   (1) Preoperative evaluation—A preoperative axillary lateral x-ray is an essential part of preoperative evaluation. If there is any question about the integrity of the glenoid bone stock, a CT scan should be obtained. If the glenoid is eroded down to the coracoid process, glenoid resurfacing is *contraindicated*. There should be enough glenoid bone to ensure adequate glenoid orientation and solid fixation for long-term implant survival. It is also important to assess glenoid version preoperatively. Some suggest using a limited preoperative CT anteversion study to evaluate glenoid version (Fig. 5–43).
   (2) Intraoperative correction—Patients with osteoarthritis tend to have posterior glenoid erosion and a relative retroversion of the glenoid. This retroversion needs to be corrected intraoperatively to a neutral version. This is most often accomplished with anterior reaming or (less often) with posterior bone graft augmentation.
   (3) Choice of components—It is now generally accepted that an all-PE glenoid component be used if glenoid resurfacing is undertaken. Because the glenoid is relatively small and shallow, taking away bone during resurfacing arthroplasty is avoided. Preparation for resurfacing usually entails reaming the remaining cartilage and some subchondral bone while glenoid depth is preserved. Keel holes or peg holes are made through the subchondral bone to anchor the prosthesis. As a result, the thickness of the glenoid component used for resurfacing is small (generally 4-6 mm). If a porous-ingrowth, metal-backed component is used, PE thickness will be reduced, which may decrease prosthetic longevity.

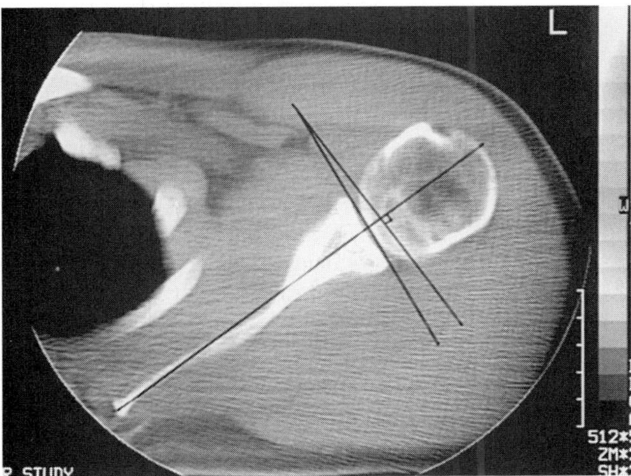

FIGURE 5–43 Anteversion study by CT. A limited scan is performed, providing a transverse computed tomographic image of the shoulder. A line is then drawn from medial tip of the scapula to the midpoint of the glenoid fossa. A line perpendicular to this defines neutral version. A line drawn from the anterior glenoid to the posterior glenoid defines the patient's glenoid version, which is then compared with neutral version line. In this example, the glenoid has 7 degrees of retroversion.

2. Fixation of humeral stem—The choice of humeral stem fixation is similar to that of hip fixation. Successful long-term results can be achieved with cemented stems by using a modern cement technique (see hip section) or with noncemented, porous-coated implants. Noncemented, porous-coated stems have a design rationale similar to that of the hip: a proximal porous coating to preserve proximal bone stock, as opposed to an extensive porous coating that has the potential for stress shielding in the proximal humerus. When considering the choice of humeral implant and fixation, one should take into consideration that the humeral shaft is not as thick and sturdy as the femoral shaft. If revision surgery is required, the humeral shaft is more likely to succumb to the effects of osteolysis and mechanical extraction techniques. Therefore, a proximal porous stem is favored in this respect. The positioning of the humeral stem should be in retroversion, generally 20-30 degrees. Its position should allow mating with the glenoid. In the difficult situation in which glenoid retroversion is accepted, less humeral retroversion is required to avoid posterior dislocation of the humeral head.
3. Complications—The most common pattern of instability after TSR is anterior instability as a result of subscapularis pull-off. If this pattern occurs, early exploration and repair are recommended. A test for subscapularis muscle pull-off is the "arm-to-chest" test (also known as the belly press test). If the subscapularis muscle is detached, the patient cannot internally rotate the shoulder and therefore cannot press the arm against the chest. Furthermore, the patient is unable to put the hand into the back pocket or tuck the shirt behind the back.

E. Treatment of specific conditions
   1. Four-part fractures—The treatment of four-part fractures of the shoulder with hemiarthroplasty is challenging. Anatomic repositioning of the greater and lesser tuberosities is the key to successful function. To maintain stability and function, the greater tuberosity with the superior rotator cuff and the lesser tuberosity with the subscapularis muscle must be positioned and heal anatomically. Nonunion of the greater tuberosity renders the shoulder rotator cuff deficient, and loss of active shoulder elevation results. Nonunion of the lesser tuberosity renders the

shoulder subscapularis deficient, and loss of active internal rotation results. Furthermore, if the lesser tuberosity is brought too far toward the greater tuberosity, the subscapularis will be stretched, and the patient will not be able to externally rotate the shoulder. Lastly, nonunion of the lesser tuberosity may cause the shoulder to become anteriorly unstable.

2. Rotator cuff deficiency—**Rotator cuff arthropathy** (RTA) refers to the condition of a shoulder that is completely devoid of the superior rotator cuff mechanism (i.e., supraspinatus and infraspinatus tendons). In this condition there is superior migration of the humeral head, with articulation of the head on the bony acromion, creating mechanical bone pain. Because of the abnormal biomechanics, secondary glenohumeral arthritis develops. The RTA shoulder is recognized on anteroposterior shoulder radiographs (Fig. 5–44). In the rotator cuff–deficient shoulder, glenoid resurfacing is *contraindicated*. Resurfacing of the glenoid in this circumstance will place excessive shear stress on the superior glenoid and will lead to rapid mechanical loosening and failure.
   a. Treatment with humeral hemiarthroplasty—In the situation of a rotator cuff–deficient shoulder with degenerative arthritis, several variations of humeral hemiarthroplasty are considered.
      (1) The most common is humeral hemiarthroplasty with a large head that will stay located within the confines of the glenoid and subacromial space. A variant of this technique is a bipolar arthroplasty. This procedure provides no additional benefit to active range or function. In either situation, active motion will be very limited, usually to 40-70 degrees of elevation.
      (2) A less frequent option is a modified reconstruction of the remaining rotator cuff by superior advancement of the subscapularis and teres minor, with closure of the superior rotator cuff defect. This procedure is combined with humeral head resurfacing with the use of a humeral head, generally of a smaller size, to allow closure of the superior defect. In some circumstances, this technique may provide improved active range of motion.
      (3) In all variations of the hemiarthroplasty procedure, it is critically important to **preserve the coracoacromial ligament.** Release of the coracoacromial ligament in the rotator cuff–deficient shoulder will result in superoanterior subluxation of the humeral head. Not infrequently, the humeral head can migrate into the superior subcutaneous tissue (Fig. 5–45).
   b. Treatment with reverse total shoulder—A newer alternative for treatment for rotator cuff arthropathy with associated glenohumeral arthritis is the use of a **reverse total shoulder**. With this method, a hemisphere ball is placed onto the bony glenoid surface, and an articulating cup is placed into the humerus (Fig. 5–46). With this construct, a stable glenohumeral fulcrum is created, which allows the deltoid and other shoulder elevators to lift the arm with increased (but not normal) efficiency. Patients with rotator cuff arthropathy and glenohumeral arthritis who are being considered for reverse total shoulder must meet the following criteria: (1) have intact glenoid bone stock, (2) have intact axillary nerve and functioning deltoid muscle, (3) accept a low level of physical activity (i.e., do not participate in sports or do medium/heavy physical labor), and (4) be free of active infection. A relative contraindication is significant glenoid osteoporosis. The most common mechanism of failure is glenoid prosthetic loosening. The results at this time are only short to intermediate term.

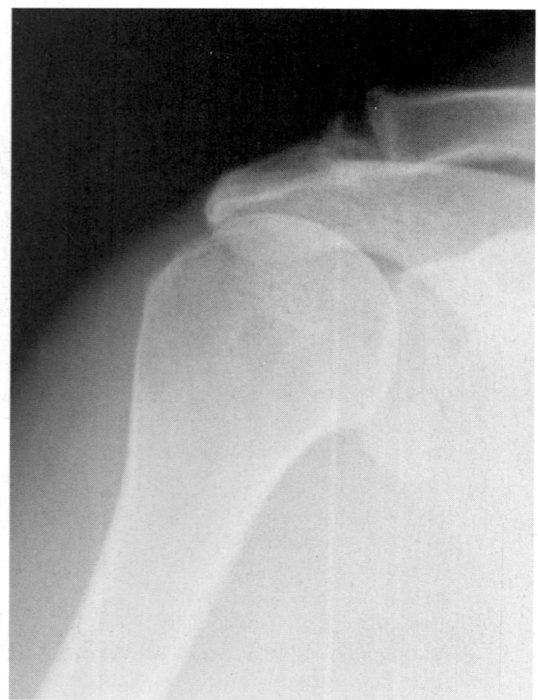

FIGURE 5–44 Radiograph of a shoulder with chronic rotator cuff deficiency. With absence of the rotator cuff, the humeral head articulates with the undersurface of acromion. The head does not remain centralized with the glenoid fossa.

IV. Osteotomy

A. Hip osteotomy
   1. Introduction—Hip osteotomy is used to treat hip dysplasia. Hip dysplasia, as opposed to primary osteoarthritis, is increasingly considered to be a cause of noninflammatory coxarthrosis of the hip. In fact, the incidence of hip dysplasia is reported to be as high as 43% in the United States and 80% in Japan. Untreated dysplasia leads to degenerative arthritis in approximately 50% of patients by

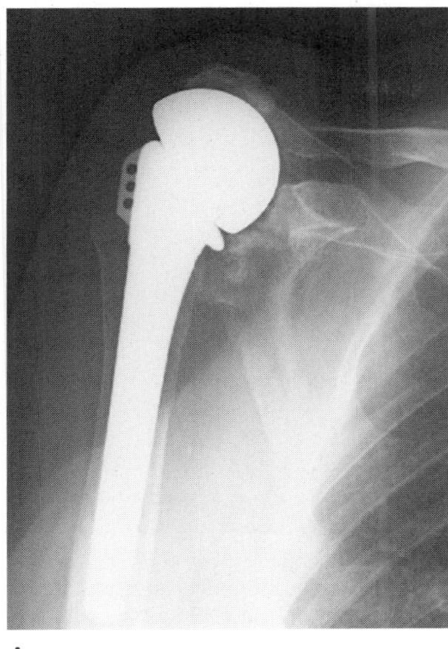
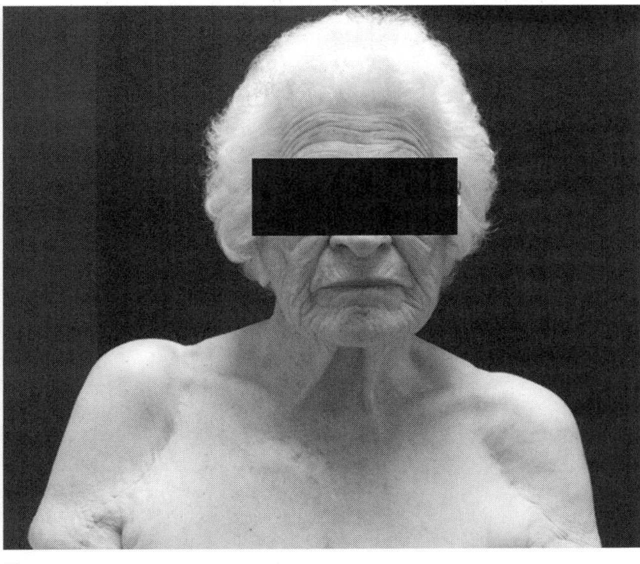

A B

FIGURE 5–45 Example of a rotator cuff-deficient shoulder with superior subcutaneous dislocation. In this case, the coracoacromial ligament was released. **A**, Radiograph of superoanterior subluxation. **B**, Clinical photograph of the superior subcutaneous dislocation of the humeral hemiarthroplasty with attempt at shoulder elevation.

age 50. Adult hip dysplasia is now recognized as a spectrum ranging from subtle to severe.

2. Forms of hip dysplasia—The classic definitions of hip dysplasia are reviewed in Box 5–2 and are illustrated in Figure 5–47. The newer-described forms of hip dysplasia are acetabular retroversion, acetabular overcoverage, and proximal femoral head-neck dysplasia with reduced head-neck offset.
   a. Acetabular retroversion, as the name implies, describes a condition in which the acetabular socket faces backward. There is excessive anterior wall coverage over the femoral head and deficient posterior wall coverage. On an anteroposterior pelvic radiograph, the **crossover sign** (i.e., Reynold's sign) is pathognomonic. In addition to the crossover sign, the ischial spine is seen prominently (Fig. 5–48).
   b. With acetabular overcoverage, the acetabular socket extends beyond a hemisphere, mechanically decreasing the range of motion of the femoral head. Acetabular overcoverage can be manifested as excessive anterior rim coverage, excessive lateral rim coverage, or a combination of both (Fig. 5–49).

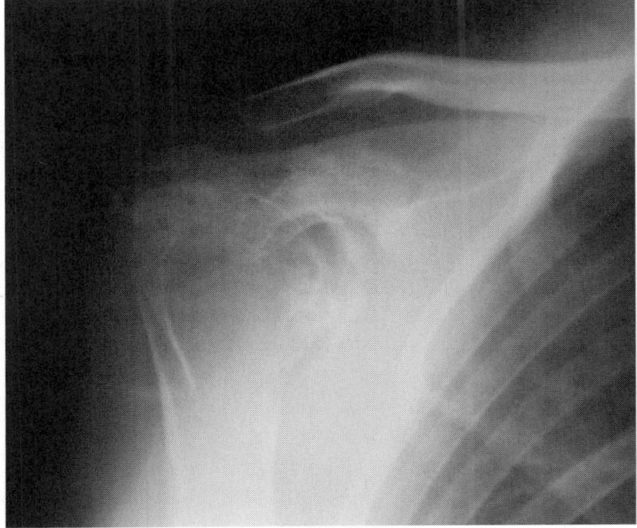
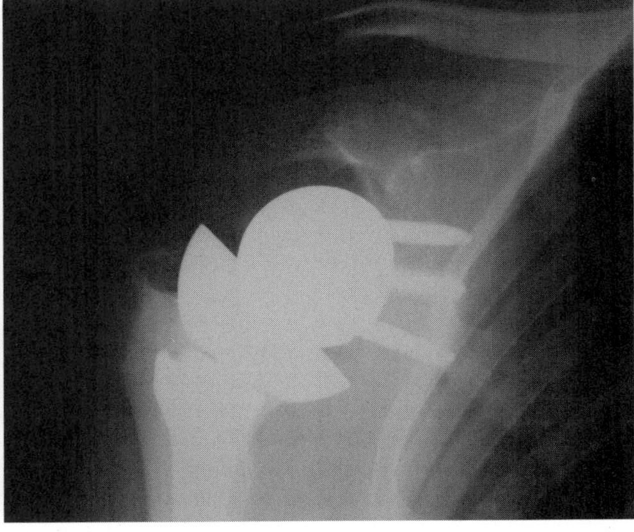

A B

FIGURE 5–46 Radiographs showing rotator cuff arthropathy and reconstruction with a reverse total shoulder. **A**, Anteroposterior (AP) radiograph showing loss of the glenohumeral joint space and irregularity. The superior head articulates with the acromion. The irreparable rotator cuff deficiency was confirmed by MRI. **B**, AP radiograph demonstrating reverse total shoulder replacement. Glenoid baseplate is secured with biologic, porous ingrowth with screws. The ball is then attached to a metallic baseplate. The humeral socket sits under the ball. Superior migration is minimized with this design.

Box 5–2 Hip Dysplasia—Classic Definition

Lateral center edge angle (CEA): <20 degrees
- Also known as Wiberg angle
- Lateral CEA measured on AP radiograph of pelvis

Anterior center edge angle: <20 degrees
- Also known as Lequesne angle
- Anterior CEA measured on modified lateral radiograph of hip

Acetabular index (AI): >5 degrees
- Also known as Tönnis angle
- AI measured on AP radiograph of pelvis

c. In proximal femoral dysplasia there is a decrease in the normal offset between the femoral head and femoral neck. The offset between the femoral head and neck is required for functional hip range (Fig. 5–50). In proximal femoral dysplasia the normal head-neck offset is lost, resulting in early bony impingement (Fig. 5–51).

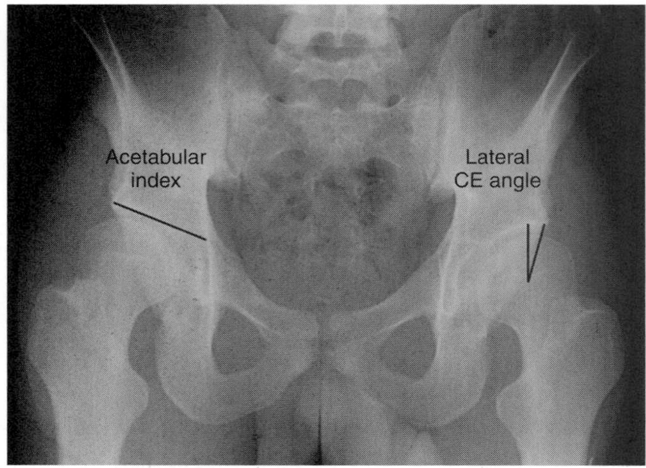

FIGURE 5–47 Radiograph of anteroposterior pelvis demonstrating measurement methods to assess the extent of acetabular dysplasia. The right hip shows the acetabular index line, which defines the slope of the superior acetabular rim (also known as acetabular sourcil). The index should be zero (i.e., horizontal). The left hip demonstrates a center edge (CE) angle. The CE angle should measure greater than 25 degrees (a larger number means a deeper socket).

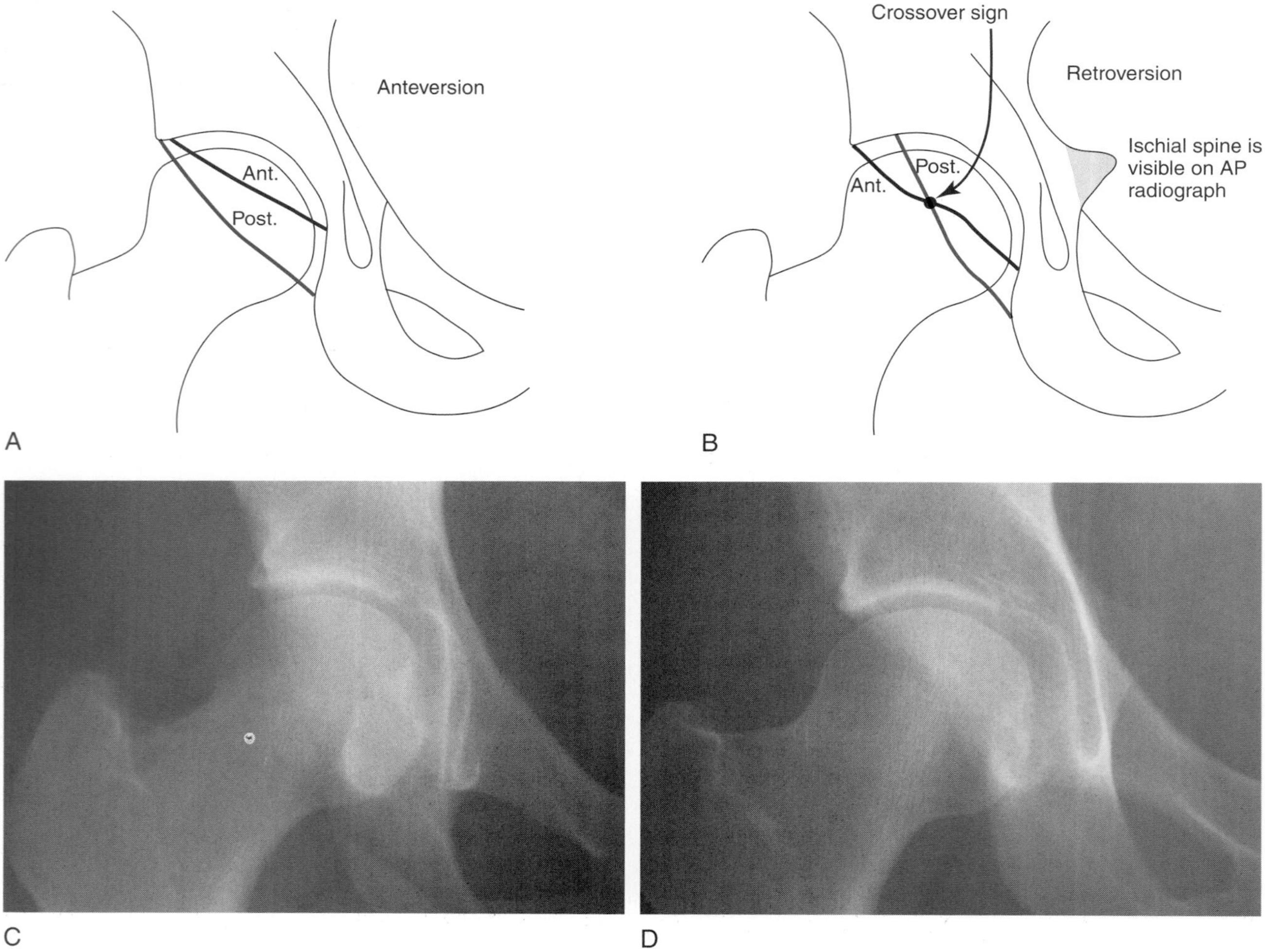

FIGURE 5–48 **A**, Diagram of a normal acetabulum on AP view. Anterior and posterior acetabular rims are marked. Note that the anterior rim is anterior to the posterior rim. **B**, Diagram of a retroverted acetabulum on AP view. The anterior rim is now farther down, and the anterior rim line crosses over the posterior rim line, which creates a **crossover sign.** Note also the prominent ischial spine. (Courtesy of Chris Peters, MD.) **C**, Radiograph of a normal acetabular version. **D**, Radiograph of a retroverted acetabulum.

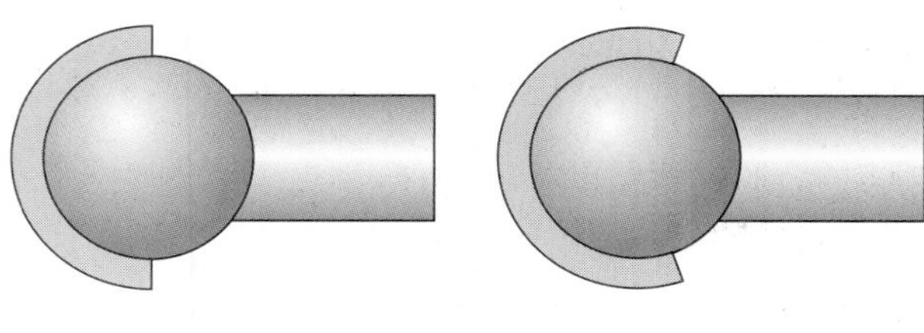

FIGURE 5–49 The normal acetabulum generally circumscribes a hemisphere over the femoral head. In acetabular overcoverage, the acetabulum covers more than a hemisphere, which causes early impingement with hip flexion.

3. Acetabular impingement—**Femoral acetabular impingement** (FAI) is a newly described entity that is associated with mild forms of adult dysplasia. In FAI, there is abnormal impingement between the femoral neck and anterior acetabular rim. The impingement zone is in the anterosuperior zone of the acetabulum. Supraphysiologic demand in a young patient may precipitate symptoms. Repetitive impingement causes labral degeneration, resulting in tears. Later, chondral degeneration occurs in the impingement zone, leading to chondral flap tears. Degenerative joint disease is the end result. Hip arthroscopy with isolated labral débridement will not solve the problem. The anatomic deformities causing impingement require surgical correction.
4. Treatment—Treatment of symptomatic adult hip dysplasia follows three primary avenues: joint replacement, joint preservation, and surgical hip decompression.
   a. Joint replacement—Regardless of age, if end-stage arthritis is present, THR is the preferred procedure. Hip arthrodesis is relegated to use in the young, active male laborer with isolated unilateral hip arthritis. In severe forms of acetabular dysplasia, additional measures are required for acetabular cup placement. A medial ream technique through the medial wall is an accepted method of deepening the acetabular socket. A modified porous hemisphere cup with metallic augmentation and additional screws may be required to achieve initial rigid fixation. If a pseudoacetabulum is present, the recommended placement of the cup is back into the native acetabulum. Placement of the cup into the

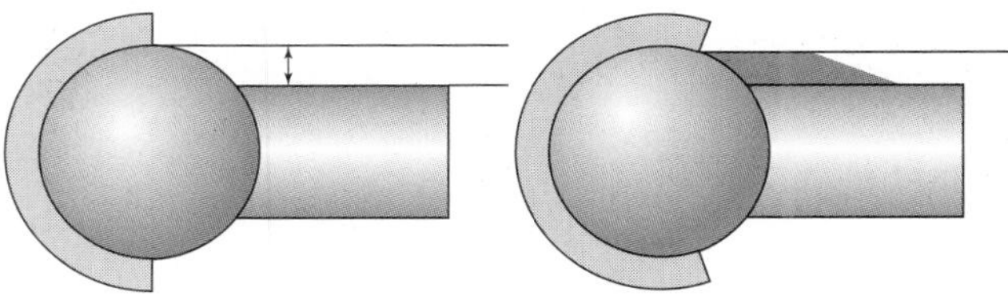

FIGURE 5–50 Proximal femoral dysplasia. On the left side, normal head-neck offset allows adequate range of motion. On the right side, the head-to-neck offset is significantly reduced. Therefore, the relatively large neck impinges on the acetabulum in early flexion.

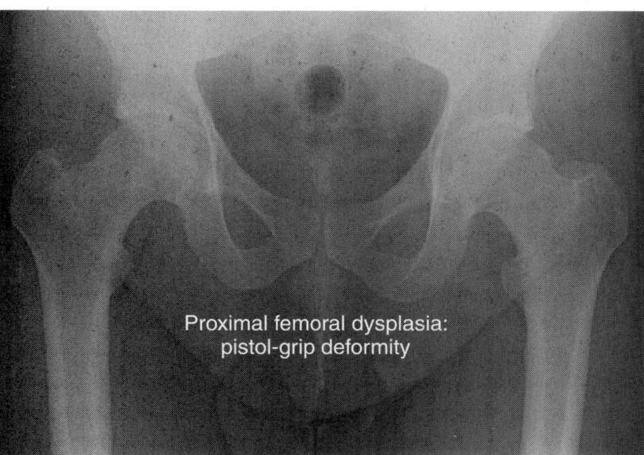

FIGURE 5–51 Anteroposterior radiograph demonstrating proximal femoral dysplasia with reduced head-neck offset. In this radiograph, the distance between the edge of the femoral head and neck is short. Native head-neck ratio is diminished, which leads to early impingement in flexion. The classic description of this condition is the pistol-grip deformity.

normal acetabulum re-creates the normal hip center of rotation and thus lowers joint reaction forces. On the femoral side, if significant leg shortening is associated with a dislocated femoral head, a proximal diaphyseal subtrochanteric osteotomy is required to remove a segment of bone. This procedure allows the hip to be reduced into the native acetabulum. It also reduces neurovascular stretch. Sciatic nerve palsy increases with lengthening over 3.5 cm, so lengthening greater than this amount should be avoided.
   b. Joint preservation—There are two joint preservation techniques used to treat symptomatic hip dysplasia.
      (1) Ganz **periacetabular osteotomy** (PAO)—When the primary deformity involves the acetabulum, the treatment is a PAO (Fig. 5–52). The PAO has four advantages over other salvage osteotomies: (1) it allows for multiplanar correction of the deformity; (2) it is versatile enough to allow large, angular corrections; (3) it provides joint medialization; and (4) it has relatively inherent stability (posterior column is preserved). In the coronal plane (i.e., anteroposterior pelvic view), the acetabulum can be rotated enough to bring acetabular cartilage to cover the superior and anterior femoral head. The goal is to correct the acetabular index to zero. In the sagittal plane, acetabular retroversion can be corrected to reduce FAI. In addition, by virtue of rotating the acetabulum to a normal theta angle (i.e., abduction angle), the acetabular center of rotation is medialized, which reduces joint reaction forces at the hip. Finally, with the PAO, the posterior column is preserved, providing inherent pelvic stability. The PAO requires only 3 or 4 long screws for

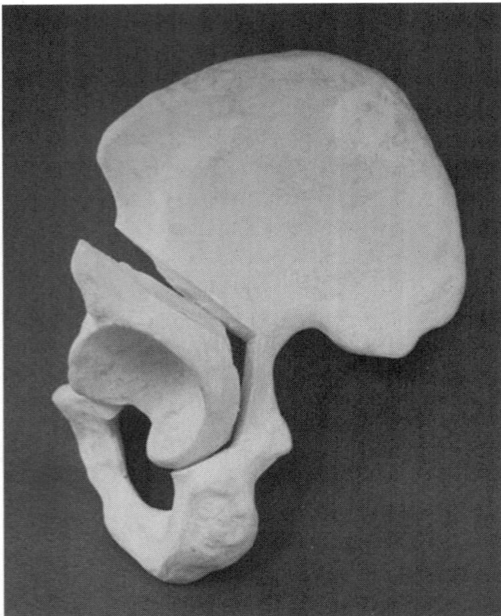

FIGURE 5–52 Model of Ganz periacetabular osteotomy. In this osteotomy, the posterior column is preserved, which provides pelvic stability. The osteotomy cuts are close to the acetabulum, which allows significant rotational and angular corrections.

fixation. The osteotomy is also performed via an anterior approach, so the hip abductors are not disturbed.

(2) Subtrochanteric osteotomy—Correction of severe coxa valga is currently the main use for proximal femoral subtrochanteric osteotomy. Excess femoral head anteversion is associated with the coxa valga deformity. Thus, a varus-producing **derotational** osteotomy is needed to fully correct the deformity. The osteotomy site is usually secured with a lateral hip plate and screws. The disadvantage of proximal femoral osteotomy is the potentially more difficult stem insertion when converting to THR. The osteotomy affects the displacement, rotation, and angulation of the proximal femur. Careful preoperative planning is necessary to ensure that the chosen osteotomy will not greatly interfere with future hip replacement surgery. Of particular note, flexion osteotomy (see under Osteonecrosis) should not be performed with anterior closing wedges. Such wedges are predisposed to significant displacement of the distal fragment and compromise future femoral stem insertion. Instead, gaps created by the osteotomy can be easily filled with bone graft and heal with predictable success.

c. Surgical hip decompression (SHD)—Used for mild forms of hip dysplasia that present with femoral acetabular impingement. In this procedure, the hip is dislocated anteriorly (head and neck vascularity are carefully preserved). The femoral neck and anterior acetabulum are trimmed of excess bone (Fig. 5–53). On the femoral side, neck offset is improved. On the acetabular side, the frequently damaged acetabular labrum is repaired. In mild forms of acetabular retroversion, the anterior acetabular rim can be removed and the labrum reattached.

B. Knee osteotomy—Varus or valgus deformities common in degenerative arthritis of the knee cause an abnormal distribution of weight-bearing stresses through the joint. These deformities concentrate stress either medially or laterally, accelerating the degenerative changes in that compartment.

1. Indications—The best indication for osteotomy about the knee is in the young, active patient (<50 years old) in whom arthroplasty would fail due to excessive wear. Osteotomy is most

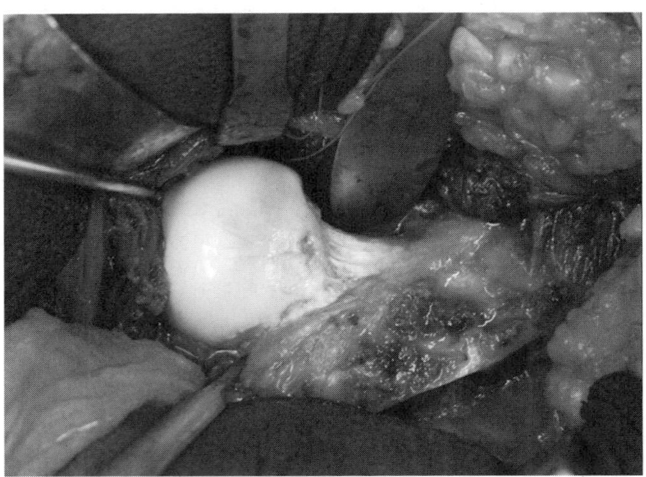

A

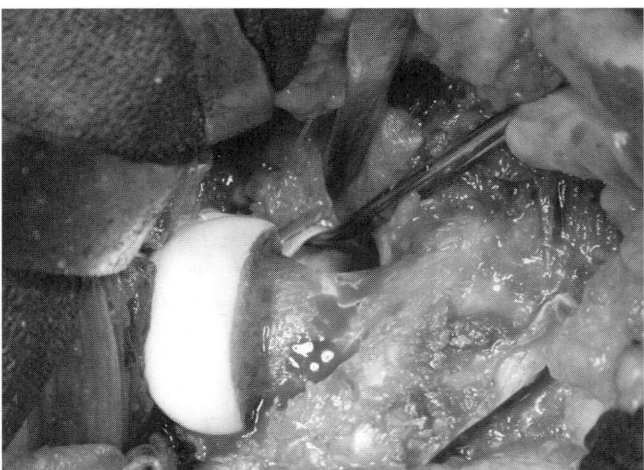

B

FIGURE 5–53 Intraoperative photographs showing surgical decompression of the right hip in a 35-year-old female tennis player. **A**, The hip is approached via a lateral incision with an anterior trochanteric slide maneuver. The hip is dislocated anteriorly. Note the excess bone on the anterior femoral neck. **B**, The femoral neck bone has been removed up to the subcapital line of the femoral head, restoring the head-neck offset. Note the hemostat under the detached labrum, which occurred from repetitive impingement. The labrum was reattached to the bone with four suture anchors.

likely to succeed when the arthritic disease affects predominantly *one* compartment.

1. Choice of osteotomy—The type of osteotomy chosen depends on the anatomic deformity and mechanical malalignment. In any osteotomy chosen, the goals are to (1) unload the involved joint compartment by correcting the malalignment and (2) maintain the joint line perpendicular to the mechanical axis of the leg. In the knee joint, varus deformity with medial compartment degenerative arthritis is generally treated with a valgus-producing proximal tibial osteotomy. This option is chosen because the knee deformity is typically caused by relative proximal tibia vara. A valgus deformity with lateral compartment degenerative arthritis is treated with a varus-producing distal femoral supracondylar osteotomy. This option is chosen because the knee deformity is typically caused by relative lateral femoral condylar hypoplasia.
2. Indications for *proximal tibial valgus–producing osteotomy* are (1) pain and disability resulting from degenerative arthritis that significantly interfere with work and recreation, (2) evidence on weight-bearing radiographs of degenerative arthritis confined to one compartment, (3) the ability of the patient to be compliant postoperatively with partial weight bearing and the motivation to carry out a rehabilitation program, and (4) good vascular status without serious arterial insufficiency.
3. Contraindications—Contraindications to proximal tibial valgus osteotomy are (1) narrowing of lateral compartment cartilage space with stress radiographs, (2) lateral tibial subluxation of more than 1 cm, (3) medial compartment bone loss of more than 2-3 mm, (4) flexion contracture of more than 10 degrees, (5) knee flexion of less than 90 degrees, (6) varus deformity >10 degrees, and (7) inflammatory arthritis (e.g., rheumatoid arthritis). In addition, a relative contraindication is a knee that shows a varus thrust. The best results are achieved when overcorrection to a valgus alignment of 8-10 degrees is achieved and the patient is not overweight. Patients with both risk factors—undercorrection and overweight—had a 60% failure rate after 3 years.
4. Techniques—The surgical technique should avoid significant translation of osteotomy fragments in order to prevent further complications during subsequent TKR. In addition, the surgical technique should maintain a normal posterior slope of the knee.
   a. **Proximal tibial valgus–producing osteotomy**
      (1) Lateral closing wedge procedure—The more common technique for proximal tibial valgus–producing osteotomy is a lateral closing wedge. In this technique, a wedge of bone is removed from the tibia via an anterolateral approach. The osteotomy is usually held closed with laterally placed internal fixation. The main complications of this technique include recurrence of the deformity, loss of native posterior tibial slope, and patella baja deformity. Patella baja is thought to form as a result of retropatellar scarring with tendon contracture. When patella baja occurs, knee flexion is limited due to bony impingement of the patella on the tibia.
      (2) Open wedge procedure—Another technique for proximal tibial valgus–producing osteotomy is a medial open wedge. In this procedure, a transverse bone cut is made in the proximal tibia, and the tibia is wedged open from the medial side. The wedge can be held open with internal fixation or placement of an external fixation device. Bone graft is placed into the open gap. This technique has the advantage of more effectively maintaining native tibial posterior slope as well as minimizing patella baja. The main complications with this technique include nonunion and loss of valgus correction (i.e., collapse of the open wedge).
   b. **Distal femoral varus–producing osteotomy**—The goal of this technique is to produce a horizontal joint line and a tibiofemoral angle of 0 degrees (i.e., anatomic alignment of 0 degrees). The single most common complication in converting to a TKR after supracondylar osteotomy is the inability to restore the desired anatomic valgus alignment.
   c. **Proximal tibial varus–producing osteotomy**—This technique can be done if there is a tibial valgus deformity. The deformity should be less than 12 degrees. However, when the valgus deformity is more than 12 degrees, the plane of the joint line deviates significantly from horizontal, and a distal femoral osteotomy is preferred.

V. Arthrodesis

A. Hip arthrodesis

1. Indications—Arthrodesis of the hip is generally reserved for young, active patients who are, or plan to be, in a heavy-labor occupation and have advanced isolated *unilateral* hip arthritis. Hip replacement surgery in these patients would fail rapidly owing to excessive stresses placed on the total hip construct. Arthrodesis of the hip should be considered an alternative treatment to joint replacement in patients younger than 35 years of age with severe, usually posttraumatic arthritis.
2. Contraindications and cautions—The absolute contraindication to hip arthrodesis is active infection of the joint. Relative contraindications include degenerative changes in the lumbosacral spine, contralateral hip, and ipsilateral knee. Another relative contraindication is poor bone stock from either severe osteoporosis or loss of bone stock. Careful patient selection is

important. Hip arthrodesis increases stresses in the lumbar spine, contralateral hip, and ipsilateral knee, and it requires approximately 30% more energy expenditure for ambulation. Therefore, hip arthrodesis should be performed only in young, healthy patients. Degenerative changes develop in adjacent joints 15-25 years after surgery. The most commonly affected joints involved, in decreasing order, are lumbar spine (55-100%), ipsilateral knee and contralateral knee (45-68%), and contralateral hip (25-63%).

3. Position— Regardless of the technique, the hip should be fused in approximately 20-25 degrees of flexion, zero degrees of adduction, and 0-15 degrees of external rotation. Abduction is to be *avoided* because it creates pelvic obliquity and increases the incidence of back pain. Internal rotation should also be avoided.
4. Technique—The choice of surgical technique for hip arthrodesis is important if later conversion to THR is desired.
   a. If lateral plating of the hip and ileum using a cobra plate is chosen, one should strongly consider a trochanteric osteotomy and elevation of the abductor mechanism to protect it for later use. Once the cobra plate is placed, the trochanter can be placed back down and secured. This technique ensures optimum preservation of the abductors for future use in hip replacement surgery.
   b. The other technique for hip fusion is anterior plating of the femur, with the fusion plate taken into the pelvis, across the anterior column of the pelvis, and superiorly toward the sacroiliac joint. The surgical approach for this technique is the extended Smith-Peterson method. Through this anterior approach, the femoral head and acetabulum can still be prepared for hip arthrodesis without violating the abductor mechanism.
5. Conversion to THR—Conversion of a hip arthrodesis to a THR is difficult and is associated with a high complication rate. The main indications for conversion are severe, persistent low back pain or painful pseudarthrosis after unsuccessful fusion. Another less compelling indication is ipsilateral knee pain. If hip replacement is to be considered, it is important to know whether abductor function is present. This determination can be made with electromyogram and nerve conduction velocity testing of the gluteus medius. Absent abductor function is a contraindication for conversion. The failure rate of THR converted from hip arthrodesis is high: 33% at 10 years. The reasons for failure include loosening, infection, and recurrent dislocation.

B. Knee arthrodesis
   1. Indications—The indications for knee arthrodesis are similar to those for hip arthrodesis. Other indications for primary arthrodesis include (1) painful ankylosis after infection, tuberculosis, or trauma; (2) neuropathic arthropathy; and (3) resection of malignant lesions about the knee. The most frequent indication for knee arthrodesis is currently salvage of a failed TKR.
   2. Position— For primary arthrodesis, the desired position is 5-8 degrees of valgus, 0-10 degrees of external rotation (to match the other foot), and 0-15 degrees of flexion.
   3. Technique—Intramedullary nailing is the preferred technique for arthrodesis when extensive bone loss (seen after failed total knee or tumor resection) does not allow compression to be exerted across broad areas of cancellous bone. Union rates in this scenario are much higher (up to 100%) with medullary rod fixation than with external fixation (38%). Bone graft can be used to augment arthrodesis when bone loss is encountered.

C. Shoulder arthrodesis
   1. Indications—Specific indications for shoulder arthrodesis are (1) painful ankylosis after infection; (2) stabilization in paralytic disorders; (3) post-traumatic brachial plexus palsy; (4) stabilization after massive, unreconstructible rotator cuff tears with arthropathy; (5) salvage of failed shoulder replacement; (6) degenerative arthritis in patients not suited for shoulder replacement; (7) stabilization after resection of neoplastic lesions; and (8) recurrent shoulder dislocations.
   2. Contraindications— Shoulder fusion is contraindicated in a patient with an ipsilateral elbow fusion.
   3. Position—The recommended position of shoulder arthrodesis is 30-30-30: 20-30 degrees of abduction, 20-30 degrees of flexion, and 20-30 degrees of internal rotation. The position of *rotation* is the most critical factor in obtaining optimum function.

SECTION 3 Complications

I. Osteolysis and Wear in Prosthetic Joint Replacement

A. Osteolysis—Osteolysis remains the most vexing problem in total joint arthroplasty.
   1. Cause—In its most basic form, osteolysis represents a histiocytic response to wear debris, primarily PE. PE debris formation and osteolysis are problems of bearing wear. Clinically, young patients are more likely to develop osteolysis for two reasons. First, they are much more active

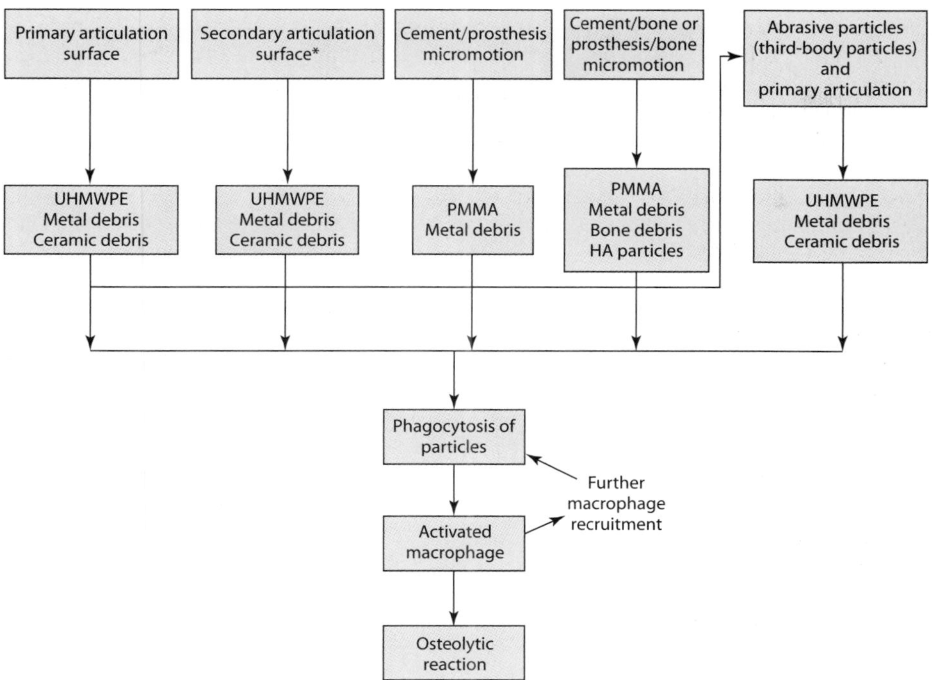

FIGURE 5–54 Wear sources in total joint replacement. HA, hydroxyapatite; PMMA, polymethylmethacrylate; UHMWPE, ultra-high-molecular-weight polyethylene.

and thus cycle their prosthetic joints more frequently than elderly patients. Second, a young, active patient will place higher hip loads on the bearing, thus increasing bearing wear.

2. Sources of wear—The osteolysis process begins with **wear sources** that generate particulate debris, which initiate the osteolytic reaction. The potential sources of wear are listed in Figure 5–54. Although any particle can serve as a source of wear debris and cause osteolysis, debris that is known to elicit an enhanced histiocytic response includes **ultra–high-molecular-weight polyethylene** (UHMWPE), PMMA, Co-Cr, and titanium (Ti). Because PE is relatively softer than other materials used in joint replacement surgery, it is considered the major source of the osteolytic process by virtue of the volume of PE generated compared with other sources.
3. Osteolytic process—As a result of particle ingestion by the macrophages, the *activated macrophage* liberates osteolytic factors, including **tumor necrosis factor** (TNF)-α, interleukin-1β, interleukin-6, prostaglandins, oxide radicals, hydrogen peroxide, and acid phosphatase. These factors activate the osteoclast system and together assist in the dissolution of bone. Osteoclastic resorption of bone around the prosthesis allows prosthetic micromotion to occur. This leads to further generation of wear debris. Additional lysis of bone allows for prosthetic macromotion, loosening, and pain.

B. Effective joint space
1. Definition—The effective joint space is the potential space where joint fluid can be pumped and thereby allow particle debris to travel (Fig. 5–55). The effective joint space comprises the joint itself and the surfaces where the prosthesis (or cement) contacts host bone. Once particulate debris is generated and the osteolytic process begins, the inflammatory response generated within the joint produces increased hydrostatic pressure, which allows for dissemination of particulate debris within the effective joint space. Osteolysis can occur anywhere within the effective joint space.
2. Pattern of osteolysis and fracture—The observed pattern of osteolysis is design dependent but can be predicted by remembering one basic rule: fluid (and therefore PE particles) will flow along the **path of least resistance**. If the femoral implant is not cemented and contains noncircumferential proximal porous coating, fluid can be pumped to the distal stem. Osteolysis is therefore more prevalent in this region. When the femoral implant contains proximal circumferential porous coating, the canal is sealed off. Osteolysis will then be seen predominantly in the greater trochanter. In this scenario, a fracture of the greater trochanter can occur due to the significant loss of bone. On the acetabular side, fluid can be pumped between porous patches, creating significant

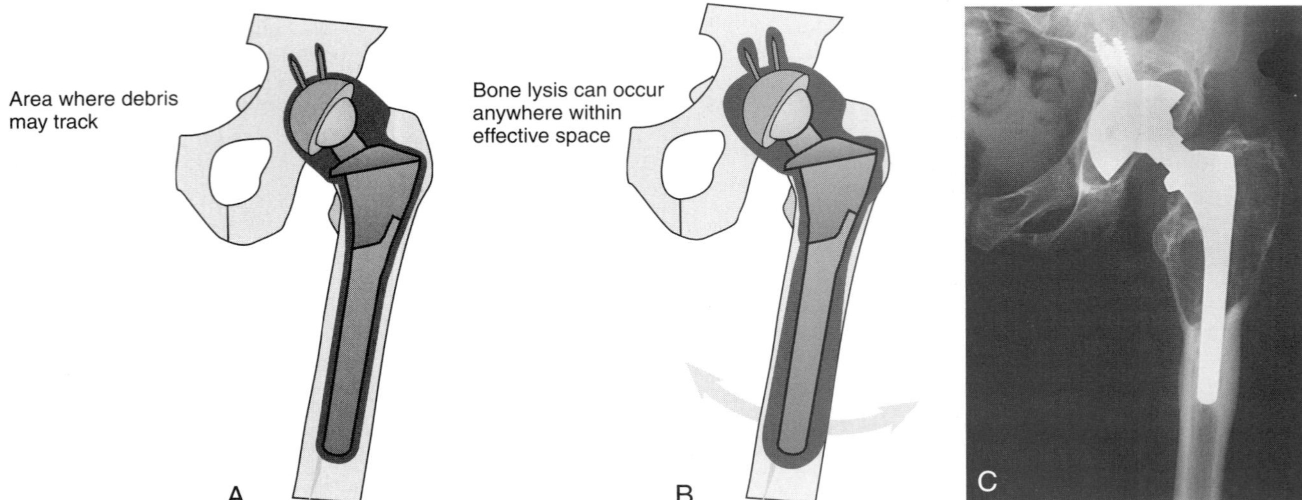

FIGURE 5–55 Effective joint space. **A**, Area of effective joint space, which includes any area around prosthetic construct, including screws. **B**, Osteolysis can occur in any region of the effective joint space. Particles are pumped via the path of least resistance. **C**, X-ray film example of massive osteolysis. Note the eccentric position of femoral head, indicating polyethylene wear.

osteolytic lesions in the ilium or ischium. When the acetabular cup is fully porous coated, fluid can still be pumped behind the cup through screw channels. Mechanically, the fluid travels between the PE insert and the metal acetabular cup. The fluid then continues along the acetabular screw (or open screw hole), where PE particles can be deposited.

3. Treatment—When an osteolytic screw lesion is seen and the porous acetabular cup is well fixed, it is not recommended to remove the cup. Instead, the modular PE insert is exchanged, and the osteolytic lesion is débrided. Bone graft is placed through the acetabular screw holes. Bone grafting of the lesions via a small, open trap door on the ilium is an accepted alternative technique.

C. Particle size—The size of the particles implicated in osteolysis is very small. The particles are in the micron or submicron range (0.2-7 μm). The main culprit in osteolysis is the submicron shedding of PE particles as a result of **adhesive** wear occurring on the primary articular surface.

D. Mechanisms of particle wear—Wear particles within the total joint construct are generated by three mechanisms—abrasion, third-body wear, and adhesion. In **abrasive** wear, particles are generated by rough articular surfaces (e.g., scratches, carbide asperites) either at the primary articulation or at other secondary surfaces (backside of PE insert with metal-backed shell). **Third-body particles** (see Fig. 5–54) can generate debris through an abrasive process when they insert in between the two articular surfaces. The loss of PE at the primary articulation occurs via a process of **adhesive wear.** Remember, PE is produced by the heating of small PE beads into a congealed mass. On the femoral head surface, the small submicron beads can be pulled off by the passing of the adjacent articulation surface. The generation of these small particles is significant (Fig. 5–56). The combination of adhesive and abrasive wear can generate many billions of particles that are then disseminated throughout the effective joint space. Efforts to minimize osteolysis in total joint replacement are primarily focused on minimizing adhesive wear at the primary articulation and also abrasive wear within the total joint construct.

E. Size of femoral head—Head size affects the rate of acetabular PE wear and osteolysis. Biomechanically, a large femoral head has a larger surface contact area than a small head and therefore a larger wear surface. However, because of the larger contact area, a large femoral head has *decreased* contact stress (hip loading force remains unchanged). With a traditional

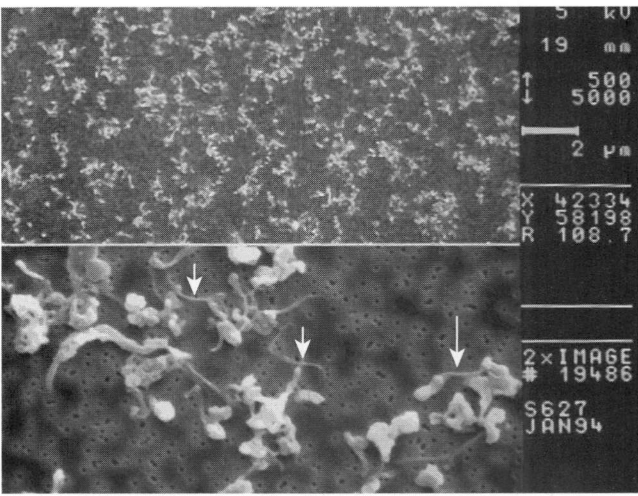

FIGURE 5–56 Scanning electron micrograph of polyethylene (PE) beads at the bottom of a wear simulator. The top photograph shows a 2-μm guide to the right. Note that most of the PE particles are submicron size. In the bottom photograph, *arrows* point to "tails" on the PE beads, indicating that these PE heads are being pulled off the surface via adhesive wear. (Courtesy of Harry McKellop, PhD.)

metal head and PE cup, a large femoral head will produce a greater amount of PE particles but have less linear wear. In contrast, a small femoral head has a smaller surface contact area and therefore a smaller wear surface. However, because of the *decreased* contact area, a small femoral head has increased contact stress (hip loading force remains unchanged). With a traditional metal head and PE cup, a small femoral head will produce a smaller amount of PE particles but have higher linear wear.

F. PE sterilization—The sterilization process of PE has been implicated as a factor causing high wear rates and rapid PE failure. PE components sterilized via radiation and stored in an oxygen environment generate oxidized PE that, under repetitive cyclic loading, can excessively wear, delaminate, and crack, leading to PE failure. The pathways of irradiated PE are outlined in Figure 5–57. Irradiated PE undergoes an intermediate step of free radical formation. At this point there are four pathways that can be taken: **recombination, nonsaturation, chain scission**, and **cross-linking.** The two important pathways concerning PE wear are chain scission and cross-linking. In the presence of an oxygen environment, oxidized PE is favored. In an environment without oxygen, *cross-linking* is favored. Cross-linked PE has *improved* resistance to adhesive and abrasive wear and improves wear rates in simulated data. The disadvantage of cross-linking PE is diminished mechanical properties. Therefore, cross-linked PE may fail catastrophically if excessive stresses are applied. Conversely, oxidized PE causes subsurface delamination and cracking, leading to accelerated PE failure. Oxidized PE should be avoided. If PE is irradiated, modern techniques involve packing in an environment free of oxygen. This task is achieved via argon, nitrogen, or vacuum packaging. Two other methods of sterilization are ethylene oxide gas sterilization and peroxide gas plasma sterilization. The disadvantage of ethylene oxide gas sterilization is that residues left by the gas sterilization process may have deleterious effects on the surrounding human tissues.

II. Prosthetic Joint Infection

A. Categories of infections—Prosthetic joint infection is one of the most devastating complications that can occur in joint replacement surgery. Studies as to the correct treatment abound; general guidelines are reviewed here. Prosthetic joint infection can be divided into three main categories: (1) early postoperative infection, (2) hematogenous infection, and (3) chronic infection. Table 5–8 describes the three categories and recommended treatment options.

1. Early postoperative infection—With early postoperative infection, the infection is identified within 3 weeks of the joint replacement surgery. In this setting, the infection is usually confined to the joint space and has not had sufficient time to invade the prosthesis–bone interface and persist.
    a. Laboratory tests—The recommended studies to evaluate a patient for an acute periprosthetic infection include serum **C-reactive protein** (CRP), **Westergren sedimentation rate** (WSR), **complete blood count** (CBC) with differential, and

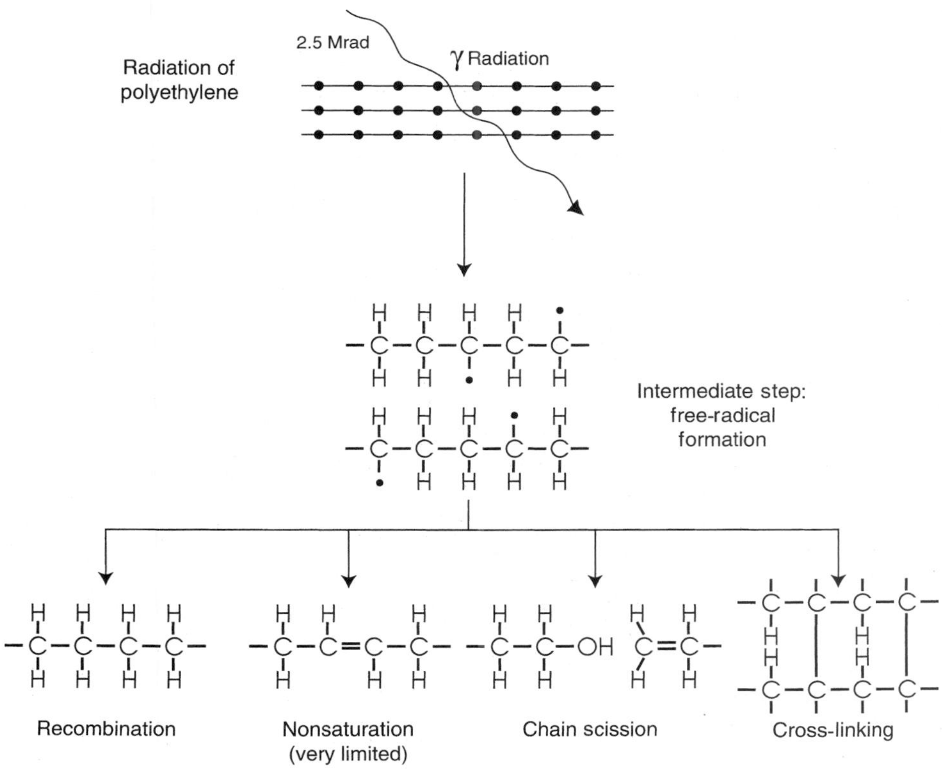

FIGURE 5–57 Potential pathways of gamma radiation on polyethylene.

TABLE 5-8 CLASSIFICATION AND MANAGEMENT OF PROSTHETIC JOINT INFECTION

Infection Type	Duration	Treatment
Early postoperative infection	Under 3 wk from initial joint replacement	1. I&D with retention of components Exchange of modular polyethylene parts Postoperative IV antibiotics (6 wk) 2. Resection of components if I&D fails
Hematogenous infection	Under 3 wk from initial hematogenous seeding	1. I&D with retention of components Exchange of modular polyethylene parts Postoperative IV antibiotics (6 wk) 2. Resection of components if I&D fails
Chronic infection	>3 wk from initial joint replacement >3 wk from initial hematogenous seeding	1. Two-stage reimplantation with an interval period of IV antibiotics Interpositional high-dose antibiotic PMMA spacer in joint Reimplantation in 3 months if free of infection 2. Two-stage arthrodesis with an interval period of IV antibiotics 3. Permanent resection arthroplasty with IV antibiotics postoperatively 4. Amputation

I&D, irrigation and débridement; IV, intravenous; PMMA, polymethylmethacrylate

joint aspiration analysis. In an acute periprosthetic infection, CRP and WSR are always elevated. The CBC with its differential can be normal early in acute infection. Joint fluid analysis will show an elevated **white blood cell** (WBC) count (<500 WBC/mL^3 is normal), and the differential will show a preponderance of neutrophils. Gram stain is not always predictable and not infrequently is negative.

b. Surgical intervention—If periprosthetic infection is suspected and laboratory data corroborate, immediate surgical intervention is recommended. One should not wait for the results of aspiration culture. Surgical débridement with component retention is recommended. The prognosis for infection-free recovery is good (usually 90% or greater). Modular parts must be removed to débride the fibrin layer that develops between metal and plastic parts. This fibrin layer can harbor organisms causing persistent infection. Postoperative intravenous antibiotics are recommended, usually for a minimum of 4-6 weeks. If reinfection occurs, the prosthetic components must be resected.

2. Hematogenous infection—In hematogenous infection, the prosthetic joint has been in place for years. An infection that develops at another body site (e.g., necrotic gallbladder, sternal wound infection) results in hematogenous seeding of the prosthesis. The affected joint usually becomes painful and swollen soon after the hematogenous event, but the pain and swelling may be masked by other medical treatments, such as antibiotics and steroids. The treatment for an acute hematogenous infection is the same as that for an early postoperative infection. Recurrent infection requires surgical extirpation of the prosthetic components if débridement fails.

3. Chronic infection—In a chronic infection, infection has been present for more than 3 weeks. The bacteria most frequently encountered in chronic prosthetic infection are the coagulase-negative *Staphylococcus* species. The persistent infection has had time to enter the bone–prosthesis interface and persist. Furthermore, the bacteria form a biofilm on the implant. (A biofilm is a bacteria-developed polysaccharide layer that allows bacteria to adhere to prosthetic implants and seals off some of the bacteria colony from immune system attack.) All organisms seen with chronic prosthetic infection develop a biofilm. Although some of the biofilm can be scrubbed off mechanically, there is no chemical that can be used to safely remove it completely. Therefore, once an infection is allowed to take hold by existing in the prosthesis–bone interface and forming a biofilm, eradication of the infection requires prosthesis removal along with débridement of infected bone and soft tissue.

B. Reconstruction of infected joint—Once the prosthetic implant has been removed, treatment continues with intravenous antibiotics for 4-6 weeks. Reconstruction of the infected joint is predicated on a benign clinical examination, a normal serum laboratory analysis (normal WSR and CRP), and aspiration cultures showing no growth.

1. Parameters for choice of reconstructive process—The type of reconstructive process (see Table 5–8) depends on the patient's overall medical and immune system condition and the condition of the local wound. Amputation is reserved for patients who are very ill or who have severe soft tissue destruction in which neither arthrodesis nor reconstructive salvage will help.

a. Medical condition—A patient who is ill with multiple medical problems and a compromised immune system will have a higher likelihood for perioperative complications and reinfection. In this situation, leaving the patient with a resection arthroplasty may be the best solution. If the patient's medical/immune condition is good, the choice for the reconstruction depends on the condition of the local wound.

b. Wound condition—The condition of the local wound is the most important factor in determining the type of reconstruction after removal of an infected total joint. The destructive inflammatory process of chronic infection causes bone defects, ligament/tendon loss or attenuation, and muscle loss and/or scarring. If significant soft tissue destruction has occurred and the anticipated function of the joint is going to be poor, joint arthrodesis may be a better reconstructive solution.

2. Techniques for preservation of joint function
   a. Reimplantation arthroplasty—Used if joint function can be adequately preserved.
   b. Local muscle transfer—If soft tissue deficits are present, a local muscle transfer can be rotated to cover the defect and allow for a tension-free closure.
   c. Modular revision implants—Bony defects can be accommodated with modular-revision implants or (in some cases) modular oncologic implants.
   d. Bulk-support allograft—A bulk-support allograft is an acceptable alternative for large bony defects. The disadvantage of using an allograft for reconstruction is that the surrounding tissues (damaged by the infection) may have an attenuated blood supply and the graft may not heal and be incorporated. Furthermore, if the allograft is placed in a superficial position (e.g., proximal tibia), it can become easily infected from minor wound dehiscence or prolonged drainage. Once the allograft is colonized, eradication of the infection is nearly impossible because the allograft is a dead, porous structure in which bacteria can easily hide.
   e. Metallic augmentation—Deficits filled by metallic augmentation have only an outer surface for bacteria to adhere to. If colonization does occur, it can be treated successfully with early irrigation and débridement before a biofilm is allowed to form.

3. Antibiotics for preservation of soft tissue—Antibiotic-loaded cement (PMMA) spacers for prosthetic joint infection are used to preserve the soft-tissue envelope during the period between resection and reimplantation of the prosthetic joint. The elution of antibiotics from methylmethacrylate depends on the porosity of the cement, surface area, and antibiotic concentration. Increased porosity allows for better elution of antibiotics. Some PMMA powders have larger monomer beads and are more porous in solid form. The addition of large quantities of antibiotics increases porosity even further. Antibiotic beads have a larger surface area than a block and elute more antibiotic but do not provide mechanical joint stability. Higher doses of antibiotics in the cement allow for higher antibiotic elution and longer elution time. Antibiotics that are to be used in PMMA must be heat stable because the curing process of PMMA generates temperatures high enough to deactivate antibiotics. The common antibiotics used with PMMA for prosthetic joint infection are vancomycin, tobramycin, and gentamicin.

C. Dental prophylaxis—It is recommended that all patients who have undergone joint replacement surgery receive prophylactic antibiotic coverage for dental procedures during the first 2 years after surgery. Patients who are immunocompromised or immunosuppressed should receive lifetime prophylactic antibiotics. Examples of immunocompromised conditions include inflammatory arthropathies (rheumatoid arthritis, systemic lupus erythematosus) and medication-induced immunosuppression. Patients with comorbidities that alter immune system function should also receive lifetime dental prophylaxis. Examples include previous prosthetic joint infection, malnutrition, hemophilia, HIV infection, diabetes, and malignancy. Table 5–9 outlines the recommended prophylactic antibiotic coverage.

TABLE 5-9 DENTAL PROPHYLAXIS FOR PROSTHETIC JOINT REPLACEMENT PATIENTS

Patient Status	Recommended Antibiotic	Regimen
Patients not allergic to penicillin	Cephalexin, cephradine, or amoxicillin	2 g orally 1 hr before dental procedure
Patients not allergic to penicillin and unable to take oral medications	Cefazolin or ampicillin	Cefazolin 1 g or ampicillin 2 g intramuscularly or intravenously 1 hr before the dental procedure
Patients allergic to penicillin	Clindamycin	600 mg orally 1 hr before the dental procedure
Patients allergic to penicillin and unable to take oral medications	Clindamycin	600 mg intravenously 1 hr before the dental procedure

Box 5–3 Risk Factors for Osteonecrosis

Alcoholism
Antiphospholipid antibody syndrome
Dysbaric disorders
Endotoxic (Shwartzman) reactions
  Systemic bacterial infections
Gaucher's disease
Hemoglobinopathy
  Sickle cell disease
Hypercoagulable states
Hypercortisolism
  Endogenous (Cushing syndrome)
  Exogenous
Hyperlipidemic disorders
  Types II and IV hyperlipidemia
Hypersensitivity reactions
  Allograft organ rejection
  Anaphylactic shock
Inflammatory conditions
  Systemic lupus erythematosus
  Inflammatory bowel disease
  Gout
Malignancy
  Acute promyelocytic or lymphoid leukemia
  Metastatic carcinoma
Pregnancy
Radiation therapy
Transplant
  Bone marrow
  Renal
Traumatic
  Femoral head dislocation
  Intracapsular hip fracture
Viral infections
  Cytomegalovirus
  Hepatitis
  Human immunodeficiency virus
  Rubella
  Rubeola
  Varicella

TABLE 5–10 HEMATOLOGIC FACTORS INVOLVED IN HYPERCOAGULABLE STATES

Factor	Problem
Protein C	Deficiency
Protein S	Deficiency
Antithrombin III	Deficiency
Lupus anticoagulant	Presence
Factor V Leiden	Presence
Activated protein C resistance (APCR)	Presence
Prothrombin G-20210A mutation	Presence
Homocysteine	Excess
Lipoprotein (a)	Excess
Anticardiolipin antibody	Excess
Factor VIII, IX, or XI	Excess
Clonal increase in platelet count seen in myeloproliferative disorders	Excess

III. Osteonecrosis

A. Hip osteonecrosis—Osteonecrosis (ON) can occur in many sites, but it has received the most attention in the hip.
   1. Etiology—The final common pathway involved in ON is intravascular coagulation. The coagulopathy involves intraosseous microcirculation coagulation, leading to generalized venous thrombosis and retrograde arterial occlusion. A list of risk factors for ON is shown in Box 5–3. It is now believed that patients with idiopathic ON may have a hypercoagulability disorder and should undergo a hematologic evaluation. A list of factors that have recently been implicated in hypercoagulable states is shown in Table 5–10.
   2. Evaluation/classification—The accepted evaluation and rating system for ON of the hip is the Steinberg classification, which is modified from Ficat. The classification is listed in Table 5–11. Six stages are defined, and each stage is modified based on the quantity of head involvement. The head involvement is calculated by multiplying the percentage of head involvement on the coronal anteroposterior view by the percentage of head involvement on the sagittal lateral view. For example, a patient with 25% volume involvement has 50% head involvement on the anteroposterior view and 50% head involvement on the lateral view (i.e., $0.50 \times 0.50 = 0.25$).
   3. Treatment options—The treatment options for ON include observation, core decompression, femoral head rotational osteotomy, vascularized fibular strut grafting, and hip arthroplasty.
      a. Core decompression—This is generally reserved for the early stages of ON, *before* subchondral collapse is seen. Core decompression is effective in relieving *intraosseous hypertension*, which is seen in all stages of ON. Reducing intraosseous hypertension has the clinical effect of reducing pain. Additionally, a core decompression creates an intraosseous wound that stimulates vascular neogenesis and may allow healing of the infarcted area. Core decompression, even in the early stages, still may not prevent subsequent collapse. Generally poor results are seen with core decompression in steroid-induced ON.
      b. Rotational osteotomy—This has a role in relatively small lesions whereby the infarcted region can be rotated out of the main weight-bearing region of the hip. Defining the extent of the necrotic sector is the dominant variable in predicting the outcome for osteotomy. Success is *inversely* related to the size of the necrotic sector. From numerous studies, it is clear that intertrochanteric rotational osteotomy will fail if more than 50% of

TABLE 5-11 STAGING SYSTEM FOR OSTEONECROSIS OF THE HIP

Stage	Grade	Criteria
0		Normal x-ray, MRI, and bone scan
I		Normal x-ray Abnormal MRI and/or bone scan
II		Abnormal x-ray showing cystic or sclerotic changes in femoral head
III		Subchondral collapse producing *crescent* sign
IV		Flattening of femoral head
V		Joint narrowing with or without acetabular involvement
VI		Advanced degenerative changes
		Head involvement—quantification of extent
I and II	A	<15% volume head involvement on x-ray or MRI
	B	15-30%
	C	>30%
III	A	Crescent beneath <15% of articular surface
	B	Crescent beneath 15-30%
	C	Crescent beneath >30%
IV	A	<15% head surface collapse *and* < 2-mm depression
	B	15-30% head surface collapse or 2-5–mm depression
	C	>30% head surface collapse or >4-mm depression
V	A	Mild joint narrowing and/or acetabular changes
	B	Moderate
	C	Severe

MRI, magnetic resonance imaging.

the femoral head is involved at the time of surgery. The type of intertrochanteric rotational osteotomy depends on the location of the necrotic lesion within the femoral head. The principle is to rotate the femoral head such that there is viable bone and cartilage articulating with the superior weight-bearing portion of the acetabulum. Therefore, an intact lateral portion of the femoral head is a prerequisite for varus osteotomy. Conversely, an intact medial femoral head is required for valgus osteotomy. A flexion osteotomy is used in patients with anterior involvement in the sagittal plane. Conversely, an extension osteotomy can be used in patients with posterior involvement in the sagittal plane. Biplanar corrections are often required (e.g., flexion-valgus intertrochanteric osteotomy). Hungerford recommends that osteotomy be considered only when the arc of involvement is less than 50%. Larger lesions generally have poor results.

c. Vascularized fibular strut grafting—This procedure represents a relatively new concept in treating ON, which has been championed most recently by Urbanik. What is heard most about the procedure is the core decompression and insertion of the vascularized fibular strut grafting, but these two procedural steps constitute only one component. A very important part of the procedure involves the surgical extirpation of the necrotic bone through a large central core hole, followed by autogenous bone grafting (usually taken from the greater trochanter) of the necrotic segment. Curettage of the necrotic segment is taken all the way to subchondral bone. The fibular strut is placed up against subchondral bone, which then heals. This process prevents subchondral collapse as the rest of the autogenous bone graft heals. Vascularized fibular strut grafting is usually recommended for earlier stages of ON, but it has been shown to be effective even if some subchondral collapse has occurred. Sometimes the subchondral bone can even be tapped up to a more congruent position. Vascularized fibular strut grafting is contraindicated when there is "whole head" involvement.

d. Hip arthroplasty—This procedure is recommended in the advanced stages of ON, when degenerative arthritis is present, or when collapse of the femoral head is advanced. The choice of hemiarthroplasty versus THR depends on the patient's activity level, physiologic age, compliance, and preexisting arthritis. Young, active patients tend to do less well with hemiarthroplasty because of rapid wear of the acetabular articular cartilage and the development of pain, particularly in the groin. In contrast, an elderly patient whose ON is due to chronic alcohol use and who would be poorly compliant with total-hip precautions may be best suited for hemiarthroplasty. Patients with radiographic evidence of acetabular degenerative changes should have a THR.

e. Hip arthrodesis—This should be considered in the very young patient who is (or plans to be) in a heavy-labor occupation. Additional autogenous bone grafting is often required because the necrotic femoral head is collapsed. The results of hip fusion for ON are less favorable than those of hip fusion for degenerative arthritis without ON.

Selected Bibliography

American Dental Association, American Academy of Orthopedic Surgeons: Advisory Statement: Antibiotic prophylaxis for dental patients with total joint replacements. J Am Dent Assoc 134:895–899, 2003.

Anaissie E, Samonis G, Kontoyiannis D, et al: Role of catheter colonization and infrequent hematogenous seeding in catheter-related infections. Eur J Clin Microbiol Infect Dis 14:134, 1995.

Arima J, Whiteside LA, McCarthy DS, et al: Femoral rotational alignment, based on the anteroposterior axis, in total knee arthroplasty in a valgus knee. J Bone Joint Surg [Am] 77:1331, 1995.

Barrack RL, Mulroy RD, Harris WWH: Improved cementing techniques and femoral component loosening in young patients with hip arthroplasty: A 12-year radiographic review. J Bone Joint Surg [Br] 74:385, 1992.

Beals RK, Tower SS: Periprosthetic fractures of the femur. Clin Orthop 327:238, 1996.

Bloebaum RD, Rubman MH, Hofmann AA: Bone ingrowth into porous-coated tibial components implanted with autograft bone chips: Analysis of ten consecutively retrieved implants. J Arthroplasty 7:483, 1992.

Blunn GW, Joshi AB, Walker PS, et al: Wear in retrieved condylar knee arthroplasties: A comparison of wear in different designs of 280 retrieved condylar knee prostheses. J Arthroplasty 12:281–290, 1997.

Bobyn JD, Pilliar RM, Cameron HU, et al: The effect of porous surface configuration on the tensile strength of fixation of implants by bone ingrowth. Clin Orthop 149:291, 1980.

Bono JV, Sanford L, Toussaint JT: Severe polyethylene wear in total hip arthroplasty: Observations from retrieved AML PLUS hip implants with an ACS polyethylene liner. J Arthroplasty 9:119, 1994.

Brooker AF, Bowerman JW, Robinson RH, et al: Ectopic ossification following total hip replacement: Incidence and a method of classification. J Bone Joint Surg [Am] 55:1629, 1973.

Burke DW, Gates EI, Harris WH: Centrifugation as a method of improving tensile and fatigue properties of acrylic bone cement. J Bone Joint Surg [Am] 66:1265, 1984.

Canale ST: Campbell's Operative Orthopaedics, 9th ed. St. Louis, CV Mosby, 1998.

Cappello WN: Femoral component fixation in the 1990s: Hydroxyapatite in total hip arthroplasty: Five-year clinical experience. Orthopedics 17:781, 1994.

Cella JP, Salvati EA, Sculco TP: Indomethacin for the prevention of heterotopic ossification following total hip arthroplasty: Effectiveness, contraindications and adverse effects. J Arthroplasty 3:229, 1988.

Chandler HP, Reineck FT, Wixson RL, et al: Total hip replacement in patients younger than thirty years old: A five-year follow-up study. J Bone Joint Surg [Am] 63:1426, 1981.

Chen F, Mont MA, Bachner RS: Management of ipsilateral supracondylar femur fractures following total knee arthroplasty. J Arthroplasty 9:521, 1994.

Clarke IC, Manaka M, Green DD, et al: Current status of zirconia used in total hip implants. J Bone Joint Surg [Am] 85:73–84, 2003.

Cofield RH, Briggs BT: Glenohumeral arthrodesis: Operative and long-term functional results. J Bone Joint Surg [Am] 61:668, 1979.

Collier J, Mayor MB, McNamara JL, et al: Analysis of the failure of 122 polyethylene inserts from uncemented tibial knee components. Clin Orthop 273:232, 1991.

Cook SD, Barrack RL, Thomas KA, et al: Quantitative analysis of tissue growth into human porous total hip components. J Arthroplasty 3:249, 1988.

Dall DM, Miles AW: Reattachment of the greater trochanter: The use of the trochanter cable-grip system. J Bone Joint Surg [Br] 65:55, 1983.

D'Antonio J, McCarthy JC, Bargar WL, et al: Classification of femoral abnormalities in total hip arthroplasty. Clin Orthop 296:133, 1993.

David A, Eitemuller J, Muhr G, et al: Mechanical and histological evaluation of hydroxyapatite-coated, titanium-coated, and grit-blasted surfaces under weight-bearing conditions. Arch Orthop Trauma Surg 114:112, 1995.

Delaunay S, Dussault RG, Kaplan PA, et al: Radiographic measurements of dysplastic adult hips. Skel Radiol 26:75, 1997.

DeLee JG, Charnley J: Radiologic demarcation of cemented sockets in total hip replacement. Clin Orthop 121:20, 1976.

Ebramzadeh E, Sarmiento A, McKellop H, et al: The cement mantle in total hip arthroplasty: Analysis of long-term radiographic results. J Bone Joint Surg [Am] 76:77, 1994.

Emerson RH, Head WC, Peters PC: Soft-tissue balance and alignment in medial unicompartmental knee arthroplasty. J Bone Joint Surg [Br] 74:807, 1992.

Emerson RH, Malinin TI, Cuellar AD, et al: Cortical allografts in the reconstruction of the femur in revision total hip arthroplasty: A basic science and clinical study. Clin Orthop 285:35, 1992.

Engh CA, Bobyn JD: The influence of stem size and extent of porous coating on femoral bone resorption after primary cementless hip arthroplasty. Clin Orthop 231:7, 1988.

Engh CA, Bobyn JD, Glassman AH: Porous-coated hip replacement: The factors governing bone ingrowth, stress shielding, and clinical results. J Bone Joint Surg [Br] 69:45, 1987.

Engh CA, Glassman AH, Suthers KE: The case for porous-coated hip implants. Clin Orthop 261:63, 1990.

Engh CA, Glassman AH, Griffin WL, et al: Results of cementless revision for failed cemented total hip arthroplasty. Clin Orthop 235:91, 1988.

Estok DM, Harris WH: Long-term results of cemented femoral revision surgery using second-generation techniques: An average 11.7 year follow-up evaluation. Clin Orthop 299:190, 1994.

Eyerer P, Ellwanger R, Madler H, et al: Polyethylene. In Williams D, ed: Concise Encyclopedia of Medical and Dental Biomaterials, 1st ed, pp 271–279. Oxford, Pergamon Press, 1990.

Faris PM, Herbst SA, Ritter MA, et al: The effect of preoperative knee deformity on the initial results of cruciate-retaining total knee arthroplasty. J Arthroplasty 7:527, 1992.

Feighan JE, Goldberg VM, Davy D, et al: The influence of surface blasting on the incorporation of titanium-alloy implants in a rabbit intramedullary model. J Bone Joint Surg [Am] 77:1380, 1995.

Foglar C, Lindsey RW: C-reactive protein in orthopaedics. Orthopedics 21:687, 1998.

Frankle M, Siegal S, Pupello D, et al: The reverse shoulder prosthesis for glenohumeral arthritis associated with severe rotator cuff deficiency: A minimum two-year follow-up study of sixty patients. J Bone Joint Surg [Am] 87:1697, 2005.

Fredricks DN: Microbial etiology of human skin in health and disease. J Invest Dermatol Symp Proc 6:167, 2001.

Furman BD, Awad JN, Li S, et al: Material and Performance Differences Between Retrieved Machined and Molded Insall/Burstein Type Total Knee Arthroplasties, 43rd Annual ORS, Feb 9–13, 1997, San Francisco, Paper 643.

Furman BD, Ritter MA, Li S, et al: Effect of Resin Type and Manufacturing Method on UHMWPE Oxidation and Quality at Long Aging and Implant Times, 43rd Annual ORS, Feb 9–13, 1997, San Francisco, Paper 92.

Ganz R, Klaue K, Vinh TS, et al: A new periacetabular osteotomy for the treatment of hip dysplasias. Clin Orthop 232:26, 1988.

Georgopoulos D, Bouros D: Fat embolism syndrome. Chest 123:982, 2003.

Gillis A, Furman B, Li S, et al: Oxidation of In Vivo vs Shelf Aged Gamma Sterilized Total Knee Replacements, Society for Biomaterials 23rd Annual Meeting, April 30–May 4, 1997, New Orleans, Paper 73.

Greene N, Holtom PD, Warren CA, et al: In vitro elution of tobramycin and vancomycin polymethylmethacrylate beads and spacers from Simplex and Palacos. Am J Orthop 27:201, 1998.

Gristina AG, Costerton JW: Bacterial adherence to biomaterials and tissue: The significance of its role in clinical sepsis. J Bone Joint Surg [Am] 67:264, 1985.

Gruen TA, McNeice GM, Amstutz HC: "Modes of failure" of cemented stem-type femoral components: A radiographic analysis of loosening. Clin Orthop 141:17, 1979.

Gsell R, Johnson T, Taylor G, et al: Zimmer Polyethylene Overview, Zimmer Technical Report, Zimmer, Warsaw, IN, 1997.

Hawkins RJ, Neer CS II: A functional analysis of shoulder fusions. Clin Orthop 223:65, 1987.

Healy WL, Lo TCM, DeSimone AA, et al: Single-dose irradiation for the prevention of heterotopic ossification after total hip arthroplasty. J Bone Joint Surg [Am] 77:590, 1995.

Hedley AK, Mead LP, Hendren DH: The prevention of heterotopic bone formation following total hip arthroplasty using 600 rad in a single dose. J Arthroplasty 4:319, 1989.

Higgins JC, Roesener DR: Evaluation of Free Radical Reduction Treatments for UHMWPE, 42nd Annual Meeting of the ORS, Feb. 19–22, 1996, Atlanta, Paper 485.

Hofmann AA, Bloebaum RD, Rubman JH, et al: Microscopic analysis of autograft bone applied at the interface of porous-coated devices in human cancellous bone. Int Orthop 16:349, 1992.

Holtom PD, Warren CA, Green NW, et al: Relation of surface area to in vitro elution characteristics of vancomycin-impregnated polymethylmethacrylate spacers. Am J Orthop 27:207, 1998.

Hozack WJ, Rothman RH, Booth RE Jr, et al: The patellar clunk syndrome: A complication of posterior stabilized total knee arthroplasty. Clin Orthop 241:203, 1989.

Hubbard NT: The Effects of Manufacturing Techniques and Calcium Stearate on the Oxidation of UHMWPE, Perplas Medical Technical Report, Warsaw, IN, 1997.

Huiskes R: Biomechanical aspects of hydroxyapatite coatings on femoral hip prosthesis. In Manley MT, ed: Hydroxyapatite Coatings in Orthopaedic Surgery. New York, Raven Press, Ltd, 1993.

Jones JP, Steinberg ME, Hungerford DS, et al: Avascular necrosis: Pathogenesis, diagnosis, and treatment. AAOS Instr Course Lect 115:309–322, 1997.

Jonsson E, Lidgren L, Rydholm U: Position of shoulder arthrodesis measured with moiré photography. Clin Orthop 238:117, 1989.

Kaplan SJ, Thomas WH, Poss R: Trochanteric advancement for recurrent dislocation after total hip arthroplasty. J Arthroplasty 2:119–124, 1987.

Kjaersgaard-Andersen P, Ritter MA: Short-term treatment with non-steroidal anti-inflammatory medications to prevent heterotopic bone formation after total hip arthroplasty: A preliminary report. Clin Orthop 279:157, 1992.

Klapperich C, Komvopoulos K, Pruitt L: Tribological properties and molecular evolution of UHMWPE. Trans ASME J Tribol 12:394–402, 1999.

Koessler MJ, Pitto RP: Fat and bone marrow embolism in total hip arthroplasty. Acta Orthop Belg 67:97, 2001.

Kumar PJ, McPherson EJ, Dorr LD, et al: Rehabilitation after total knee arthroplasty: A comparison of two rehabilitation techniques. Clin Orthop 331:93, 1996.

Landy MM, Walker PS: Wear of Ultra-high-molecular-weight polyethylene components of 90 retrieved knee prostheses. J Arthroplasty (3 Suppl):S73–S85, 1988.

Laskin RS, Rieger M, Schob C, et al: The posterior stabilized total knee prosthesis in the knee with severe fixed deformity. J Knee Surg 1:199, 1988.

Lewonowski K, Dorr LD, McPherson EJ, et al: Medialization of the patella in total knee arthroplasty. J Arthroplasty 12:161, 1997.

Li S, Chang JD, Salvati E, et al: Nonconsolidated Polyethylene Particles and Oxidation in Charnley Acetabular Cups, CORR, No. 319, pp. 54–63, 1995.

Livermore J, Ilstrup D, Morrey B: Effect of femoral head size on wear of the polyethylene acetabular component. J Bone Joint Surg [Am] 72:518, 1990.

Lombardi AV, Mallory TH, Vaughan BK, Drouillard P: Aseptic loosening in total hip arthroplasty secondary to osteolysis induced by wear debris from titanium-alloy modular femoral heads. J Bone Joint Surg [Am] 71:1337, 1989.

Lombardi AV, Mallory TH, Vaughn BK, et al: Dislocation following primary posterior-stabilized total knee arthroplasty. J Arthroplasty 8:633, 1993.

Lonner JH, Siliski JM, Lotke PA: Simultaneous femoral osteotomy and total knee arthroplasty for treatment of osteoarthritis associated with severe extra-articular deformity. J Bone Joint Surg [Am] 82:342, 2000.

Manaka M, Clarke IC, Yamamoto K, et al: Stripe wear rates in alumina THR: Comparison of microseparation simulator study with retrieved implants. J Biomed Mater Res (Part B): Appl Biomater 69:149, 2004.

Mantas JP, Bloebaum RD, Skedros JG, et al: Implications of reference axes used for rotational alignment of the femoral component in primary and revision knee arthroplasty. J Arthroplasty 7:531, 1992.

McKellop HA, Shen FW, Campbell P, et al: Effect of Sterilization Method and Other Modifications on the Wear Resistance of UHMWPE Acetabular Cups, Polyethylene Wear in Orthopaedic Implants Workshop, Society for Biomaterials 23rd Annual Meeting, April 30–May 4, 1997, New Orleans.

McPherson EJ, Patzakis MJ, Gross JE, et al: Infected total knee arthroplasty: Two-stage reimplantation with a gastrocnemius rotational flap. Clin Orthop 341:73, 1997.

McPherson EJ, Tontz W, Patzakis MJ, et al: Outcome of infected total knee utilizing a staging system for prosthetic joint infection. Am J Orthop 28:161, 1999.

Mont MA, Dellon AL, Chen F, et al: The operative treatment of peroneal nerve palsy. J Bone Joint Surg [Am] 78:863, 1996.

Montes LF, Wilborn WH: Location of bacterial skin flora. Br J Dermatol 81:23, 1969.

Nashed RS, Becker DA, Gustilo RB: Are cementless acetabular components the cause of excess wear and osteolysis in total hip arthroplasty?. Clin Orthop 317:19, 1995.

National Institute of Arthritis and Musculoskeletal and Skin Diseases (NIAMS): Questions and answers about osteonecrosis. NIH Publication No. 06-4857. January 2001. Revised March 2006.

National Institutes of Health: Total hip replacement. NIH Consensus Conference, Sept. 2–14, 1994, Vol 12, p 1.

National Institutes of Health: Total hip replacement: NIH Consensus Conference. JAMA 273:1950, 1995.

Nelissen RGHH, Bauer TW, Weidenhielm RA, et al: Revision hip arthroplasty with the use of cement and impaction grafting. J Bone Joint Surg [Am] 77:412, 1995.

Nevelos JE, Ingham E, Doyle C, et al: Analysis of retrieved alumina ceramic components from Mittelmeier total hip prostheses. Biomaterials 20:1833, 1999.

Oh I, Bourne RB, Harris WH: The femoral cement compactor: An improvement in cementing technique in total hip replacement. J Bone Joint Surg [Am] 65:1335, 1983.

Otani T, Whiteside LA, White SE: The effect of axial and torsional loading on strain distribution in the proximal femur as related to cementless total hip arthroplasty. Clin Orthop 292:376, 1993.

Padgett DE, Kull L, Rosenberg A, et al: Revision of the acetabular component without cement after total hip arthroplasty. J Bone Joint Surg [Am] 75:663, 1993.

Pak JH, Paprosky WG, Jablonsky WS, et al: Femoral strut allografts in cementless revision total hip arthroplasty. Clin Orthop 295:172, 1993.

Paprosky WG, Perona PG, Lawrence JM: Acetabular defect classification on surgical reconstruction in revision arthroplasty. J Arthroplasty 9:33, 1994.

Passerini L, Lam K, Costerton JW, et al: Biofilms on indwelling vascular catheters. Crit Care Med 20:665, 1992.

Peters CL, Rivero DP, Kull LR, et al: Revision total hip arthroplasty without cement: Subsidence of proximally porous-coated femoral components. J Bone Joint Surg [Am] 77:1217, 1995.

Plitz W, Griss P: Clinical, histomorphological, and material related observations on removed alumina-ceramic hip joint components. In Weinstein A, Gibbons D, Brown S, Ruff W, eds: Implant Retrieval: Material and Biological Analysis. Washington, DC, National Bureau of Standards, 1981.

Poggie RA, Takeuchi MT, Averill R: Effects of Resin Type, Consolidation Method, and Sterilization on UHMWPE, Society for Biomaterials 23rd Annual Meeting, April 30–May 4, 1997, New Orleans, p 216.

Poilvache PL, Insall JN, Scuderi GR, et al: Rotational landmarks and sizing of the distal femur in total knee arthroplasty. Clin Orthop 331:35, 1996.

Possai KW, Dorr LD, McPherson EJ: Metal rings for deficient acetabular bone in total hip replacement. Instr Course Lect 45:161, 1996.

Raad I, Costerton W, Sabharwal U, et al: Ultrastructural analysis of indwelling vascular catheters: A quantitative relationship between luminal colonization and duration of placement. J Infect Dis 168:400, 1993.

Ranard G, Higgins J, Schroeder D: Density and Thermal Analysis of Molded and Machined UHMWPE Tibial Bearings, Transactions of the 24th Annual Meeting of the Society for Biomaterials, April 22–26, 1998, San Diego, Paper 497.

Ranawat CS, Peters LE, Umlas ME: Fixation of the acetabular component. Clin Orthop 334:207, 1997.

Ries MD, Lynch F, Rauscher LA, et al: Pulmonary function during and after total hip replacement. J Bone Joint Surg [Am] 75:581, 1993.

Ritter MA, Faris PM, Keating EM: Posterior cruciate ligament balancing during total knee arthroplasty. J Arthroplasty 3:323, 1988.

Ritter MA, Worland R, Meding JB, et al: Flat-on-Flat, Nonconstrained Compression Molded Polyethylene Total Knee Replacement, CORR, No. 321, December 1995, p. 79–85.

Ronk R, Higgins J, Kinsel A: Method For Detecting Non-consolidation in UHMWPE, Transactions of the 10th Annual ISTA Meeting, Sept. 25–27, 1997, San Diego, p. 64–65.

Rowe CR: Arthrodesis of the shoulder used in treating painful conditions. Clin Orthop 173:92, 1983.

Santore RF, Murphy SB: Osteotomies about the hip for the prevention and treatment of osteoarthrosis. AAOS Instr. Course Lect 115:98-116, 1997.

Schmalzried TP, Jasty M, Harris WH: Periprosthetic bone loss in total hip arthroplasty: Polyethylene wear debris and the concept of the effective joint space. J Bone Joint Surg [Am] 74:849, 1992.

Schroeder DW, Pozorski KM: Hip Simulator Wear Testing of Isostatically Molded UHMWPE: Effect of ETO and Gamma Irradiation, 42nd Annual Meeting of the ORS, Feb. 19–22, 1996, Atlanta.

Schulte KR, Callaghaan JJ, Kelley SS, et al: The outcome of Charnley total hip arthroplasty with cement after a minimum of twenty year follow-up. J Bone Joint Surg [Am] 75:961, 1993.

Scott RD, Cobb AG, McQueary FG, et al: Unicompartmental knee arthroplasty: 8 to 12 year follow-up with survivorship analysis. Clin Orthop 271:96, 1991.

Scully SP, Aaron RK, Urbaniak JR: Survival analysis of hips treated with core decompression or vascularized fibular grafting because of avascular necrosis. J Bone Joint Surg [Am] 80:1270, 1998.

Serekian P: Process application of hydroxyapatite coatings. In Manley MT, ed: Hydroxyapatite Coatings in Orthopaedic Surgery. New York, Raven Press, Ltd., 1993.

Shishido T, Clarke IC, Williams P, et al: Clinical and simulator wear study of alumina ceramic THR to 17 years and beyond. J Biomed Mater Res (Part B): Appl Biomater 67:638, 2003.

Sommerich R, Flynn T, Zalenski E, et al: The Effects of Sterilization on Contact Area and Wear Rate of UHMWPE, 42nd Annual Meeting of the ORS, Feb 19–22, 1996, Atlanta.

St. John KR, Takeichi MJ, Poggie RA: Effects of Radiation Dose and Packaging Condition on the Oxidation of UHMWPE, Society for Biomaterials 23rd Annual Meeting, April 30–May 4, 1997, New Orleans, Paper 46.

Steinberg ME, Hayken GD, Steinberg DR: A quantitative system for staging avascular necrosis. J Bone Joint Surg [Br] 77:34, 1995.

Stern SH, Becker MW, Insall JN: Unicondylar knee arthroplasty: An evaluation of selection criteria. Clin Orthop 286:143, 1993.

Stewart TD, Tipper JL, Insley G, et al: Long term wear of ceramic matrix composite materials for hip prostheses under severe swing phase microseparation. J Biomed Mater Res (Part B): Appl Biomater 66:567, 2003.

Stiehl JB, Komistek RD, Dennis DA, et al: Fluoroscopic analysis of kinematics after posterior cruciate–retaining knee arthroplasty. J Bone Joint Surg [Br] 77:884, 1995.

Streicher RM, Schaffner S: Significance of the Sterilization Method and Long-Term Aging on the In Vivo Wear Rate of UHMWPE, 42nd Annual Meeting of the ORS, Feb. 19–22, 1996, Atlanta.

Sun DC, Wang A, Dumbleton JH, et al: Development of Stabilized UHMWPE Implants with Improved Oxidation Resistance via Crosslinking, Scientific Exhibition, 63rd Annual AAOS, Feb. 22–26, 1996, Atlanta.

Tanner MG, Hoernschemeyer DG, Whiteside LA: Polyethylene Quality Variations in Currently Available Bar Stock, 64th Annual Meeting of the AAOS, Feb 13–17, 1997.

Tanzer M, Miller J, Richards GK: Preoperative assessment of skin colonization and antibiotic effectiveness in total knee arthroplasty. Clin Orthop Rel Res 299:163, 1994.

Tsukayama DT, Estrada R, Gustilo RB: Infection after total hip arthroplasty. J Bone Joint Surg [Am] 78:512, 1996.

Vince KG, McPherson EJ: The patella in total knee arthroplasty. Orthop Clin North Am 23:675, 1992.

Walter WL, Insley GM, Walter WK, et al: Edge loading in third generation alumina ceramic-on-ceramic bearings. J Arthroplasty 19:402, 2004.

Wang A, Essner A, Dumbleton JH, et al: Wear Mechanisms and Wear Testing of Ultra-High Molecular Weight Polyethylene in Total Joint Arthroplasty, Polyethylene Wear in Orthopaedic Implants Workshop, Society for Biomaterials 23rd Annual Meeting, April 30–May 4, 1997, New Orleans.

Wasielewski RC, Cooperstein LA, Kruger MP, et al: Acetabular anatomy and the transacetabular fixation of screws in total hip arthroplasty. J Bone Joint Surg [Am] 72:501, 1990.

Wilson PD Jr, Gordon SL, eds: NIH Consensus Development Conference: Total hip joint replacement. Bethesda, MD, March 1982. J Orthop Res 1:189, 1983.

Wong M, Eulenberger J, Schenk R, et al: Effect of surface topology on the osteointegration of implant materials in trabecular bone. J Bio Mat Res 29:1567, 1995.

Wroblewski BM, Siney PD: Charnley low-friction arthroplasty of the hip: Long-term results. Clin Orthop 292:191, 1993.

Wroblewski BM, Lynch M, Atkinson JR, et al: External wear of the polyethylene socket in cemented total hip arthroplasty. J Bone Joint Surg [Br] 69:61, 1987.

CHAPTER 6

Disorders of the Foot and Ankle

Gregory J. Roehrig, Judith Baumhauer, Brian D. Giordano, AND E. Greer Richardson

CONTENTS

This chapter provides a review of adult foot and ankle disorders and deformities. Pediatric and congenital deformities are covered in Chapter 3, Pediatric Orthopaedics.

I. Biomechanics of the Foot and Ankle

The foot and ankle are made up of 28 bones and approximately 44 joint articulations that are closely related in form and function. The primary functions of the foot and ankle are to provide support and forward ambulation. Through rhythmic and alternating limb and trunk movements, the body is propelled forward in an energy-efficient fashion. Shock absorption and adaptation to uneven ground lessen energy expenditure and oxygen demand during gait.

A. Parts of the foot

1. Forefoot—The bony forefoot comprises the metatarsals and phalanges. The first metatarsal is the widest and shortest; the second metatarsal is usually the longest and experiences more stress than the other lesser metatarsals. The lesser toes are controlled by a balance among the extrinsic muscles (**extensor digitorum longus** [EDL], **flexor digitorum longus** [FDL]), the intrinsic muscles (interossei, lumbricals), and passive restraints (plantar plate, extensor hood, joint capsule, collateral ligaments). The intrinsic tendons pass plantar (providing a flexion force) to the metatarsal–phalangeal joint axis proximally and pass dorsal to the axis distally (providing an extension force) (Fig. 6–1).
2. Midfoot—The midfoot comprises two rows of tarsal bones that articulate with the forefoot at the Lisfranc joint and with the hindfoot at the Chopart joint. The cuneiforms are wedge-shaped, narrowing inferiorly, and serve as cornerstones for the transverse arch. The second metatarsal is set into the distal tarsal row, further adding to the stability of the arch and the Lisfranc articulation. The plantar intermetatarsal ligaments are stronger than the dorsal ligaments. The Lisfranc ligament extends from the inferior aspect of the medial cuneiform to the base of the second metatarsal and is the strongest.
3. Hindfoot—The talus and calcaneus and their ligamentous attachments form the hindfoot. The spring ligament (inferior calcaneonavicular and superomedial calcaneonavicular ligaments) helps to support the longitudinal arch.

B. Foot positions versus foot motions—The nomenclature for motion about the foot and ankle can be confusing because the terms are often used variably and interchangeably, especially for motion in the Z-axis.

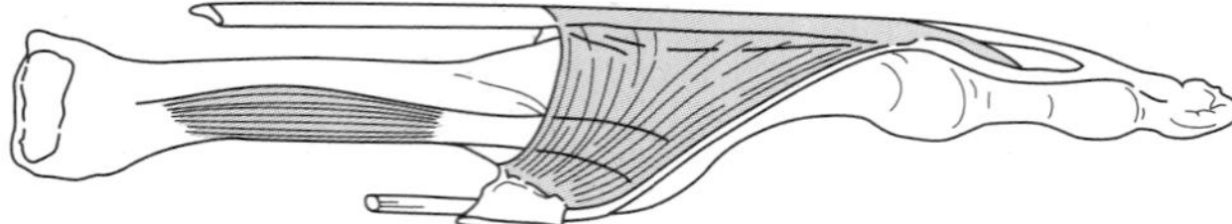

FIGURE 6–1 Anatomy of the intrinsic and extrinsic musculotendinous attachments of the lesser toes. (From Myerson MS: Foot and Ankle Disorders. Philadelphia, WB Saunders, 2000.)

Foot positions are defined in a manner different from that of foot motions. The foot positions are varus/valgus, abduction/adduction, and equinus/calcaneus. Foot motions in the three axes of rotation are illustrated in Figure 6–2 and summarized in Table 6–1. The critical assessment is to determine the relationship of the forefoot to the hindfoot. If the heel is in a neutral position (subtalar neutral), the forefoot should be parallel with the floor to meet the ground flush (plantigrade). If the first ray is elevated, the forefoot is in varus position. If the first ray is flexed, the forefoot is in valgus position (Fig. 6–3).

TABLE 6-1 MOTIONS OF THE FOOT AND ANKLE

Plane of Motion	Motion
Sagittal (X-axis)	Dorsiflexion Plantar flexion
Frontal (Coronal) (Z-axis)	Inversion Eversion
Transverse (Y-axis)	Forefoot/midfoot Adduction Abduction Ankle/hindfoot Internal rotation External rotation
Triplanar motion	Supination Adduction Inversion Plantar flexion Pronation Abduction Eversion Dorsiflexion

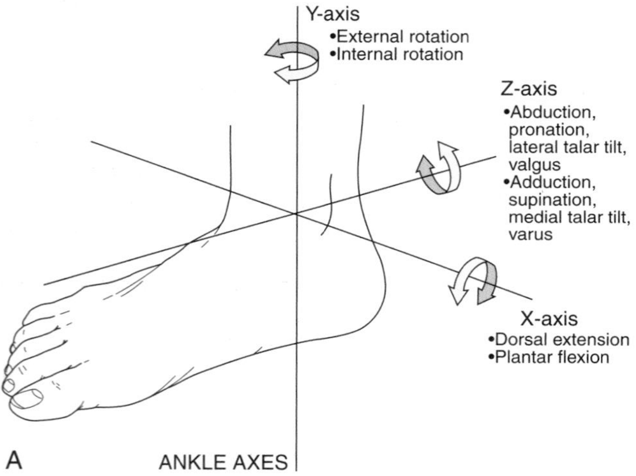

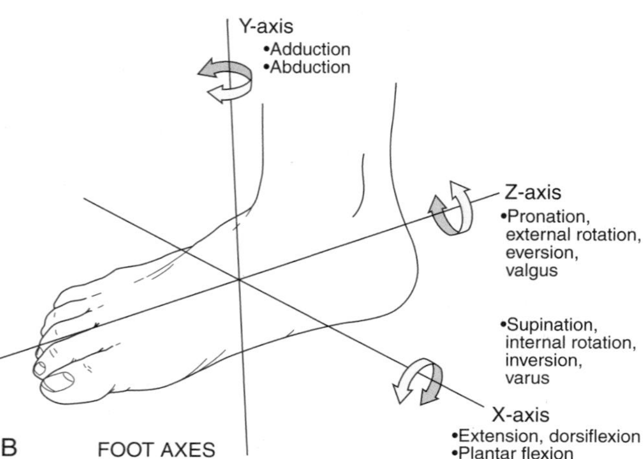

FIGURE 6–2 Axes of rotation of the ankle (**A**) and foot (**B**). (From Myerson MS: Foot and Ankle Disorders. Philadelphia, WB Saunders, 2000.)

C. Joints

1. Transverse tarsal joint—The calcaneocuboid and talonavicular joints make up the transverse tarsal joint. This joint is important for providing stability of the hindfoot and midfoot to produce a rigid lever at heel-rise for toe-off. When the foot is pronated (hindfoot valgus, forefoot abduction, and dorsiflexion of the ankle), the transverse tarsal joints are parallel and supple, adapting to the uneven ground. When the foot supinates (hindfoot varus, forefoot adduction, and plantar flexion of the ankle), these joints become divergent and lock, providing stiffness to the foot for forward propulsion (Fig. 6–4).

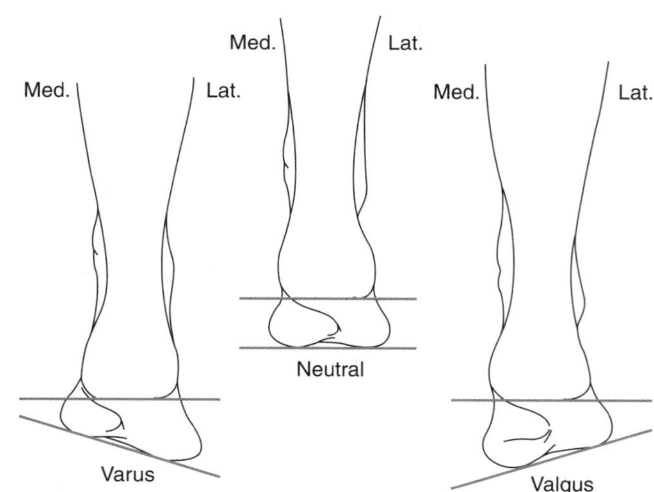

FIGURE 6–3 Varus, neutral, and valgus forefoot positions. Med., medial; Lat., lateral. (From Alexander IJ: The Foot: Examination and Diagnosis, 2nd ed. New York, Churchill Livingstone, 1997.)

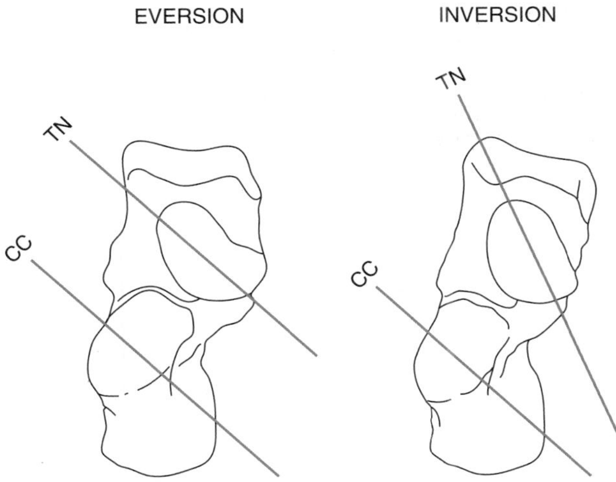

FIGURE 6–4 Function of the transverse tarsal joint. When the heel is everted, the transverse tarsal joints are parallel and unlocked, allowing the foot to be supple and pronate and accommodate to the floor. When the heel is inverted (varus), the transverse tarsal joint is divergent and locked, allowing for a stable hindfoot/midfoot complex for toe-off. CC, calcaneocuboid; TN, talonavicular.

2. Ankle joint—There is no single ankle axis of rotation. Instead, the topography of the tibiotalar articular surfaces results in a continually changing center of rotation with joint position. A simplified model of the ankle joint has a horizontal axis from anteromedial to posterolateral and a coronal axis from medial cephalic to lateral caudal (between the malleoli) (Fig. 6–5).

D. The gait cycle—One full gait cycle, from heel-strike to heel-strike, is termed a "stride." Each stride is composed of a stance phase (heel-strike to toe-off, 62% of the cycle) and a swing phase (toe-off to heel-strike, 38% of the cycle) (Fig. 6–6). During gait, the rotational displacement of the body ranges from 12-25 degrees. Vertical and lateral body displacements are both approximately 4-5 cm (Fig. 6–7). Ground reaction forces are approximately 1.5 times body weight during walking and 3-4 times body weight during running. This difference is due to the increased load after the float phase of running, in which there is no foot in contact with the ground. As the speed of gait increases, the stance phase decreases.

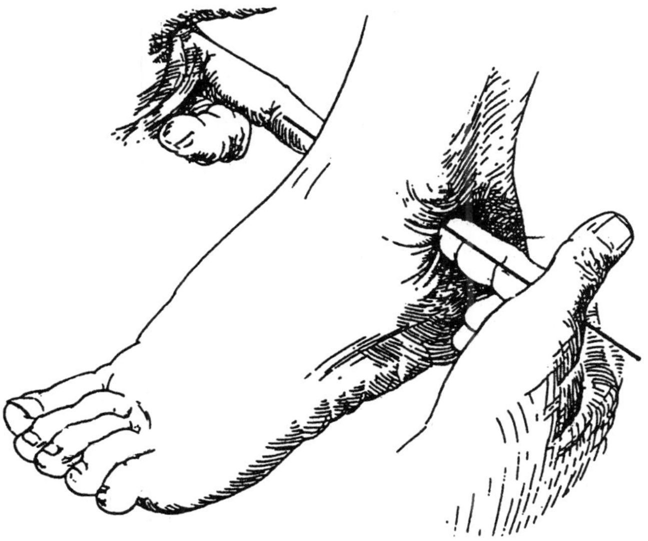

FIGURE 6–5 The ankle axis of movement can be clinically estimated by palpating the tips of the medial and lateral malleoli. (From Mann RA: Biomechanics of the foot and ankle. In Mann RA, Coughlin MJ, eds: Surgery of the Foot and Ankle, 6th ed. St. Louis, CV Mosby, 1993, p 17.)

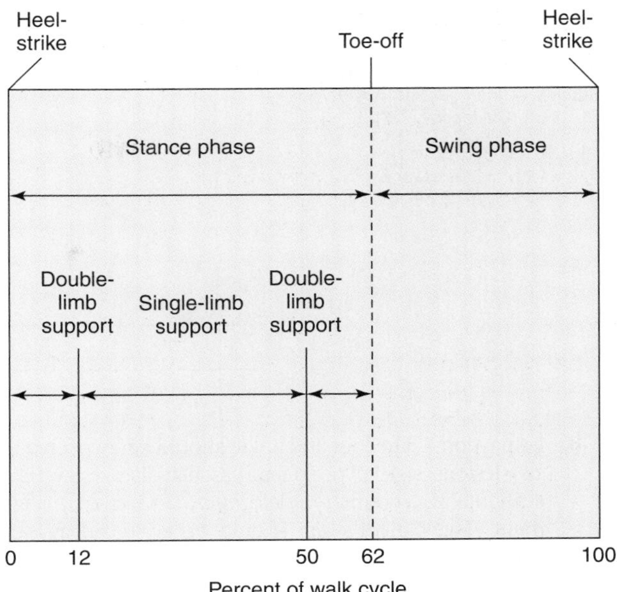

FIGURE 6–6 Phases of the walking cycle. Stance phase constitutes approximately 62% of the cycle, and swing phase 38%. Stance phase is further divided into two periods of double-limb support and one period of single-limb support. (From Coughlin MJ, Mann RA: Surgery of the Foot and Ankle. St. Louis, CV Mosby, 1999.)

E. Soft-tissue contributions to gait mechanics—During the swing phase the tibialis anterior muscle contracts concentrically, and after heel-strike it contracts eccentrically and lengthens until the foot-flat phase. At this point, the gastrocnemius-soleus complex contracts eccentrically and then concentrically as heel-rise/toe-off is occurring. In addition, as the foot progresses from heel-strike to toe-off, the following changes allow the foot to convert from a flexible shock absorber to a rigid propellant: (1) the plantar fascia, which attaches to the plantar medial heel and runs the length of the arch to the bases of each proximal phalanx, is tightened as the metatarsophalangeal (MTP) joints extend; (2) the longitudinal arch is accentuated; (3) the hindfoot supinates, with firing of the posterior tibial tendon; and (4) the transverse tarsal joint locks and provides a rigid lever arm for toe-off. This is called the windlass mechanism (Fig. 6–8). The opposite (eversion of the subtalar joint, unlocking of the transverse tarsal joints, internal rotation of the tibia) occurs from heel-strike to foot-flat.

II. Physical Examination of the Foot and Ankle

A. Overview—Symmetry of motion, strength, gait, and appearance between the feet and ankles should be assessed. The knee, hip, and back can influence the sensory, motor, and gait examination for the foot and ankle and need to be integrated into this assessment.

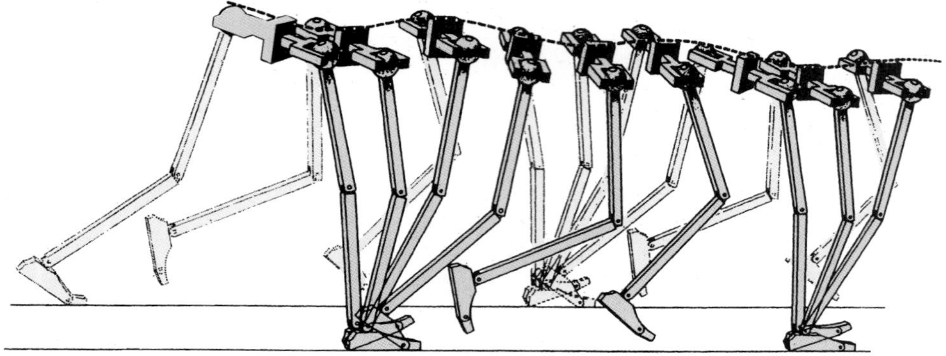

FIGURE 6–7 Vertical body displacement is about 4-5 cm. (From Coughlin MJ, Mann RA: Surgery of the Foot and Ankle. St. Louis, CV Mosby, 1999.)

B. Inspection—The foot and ankle should be inspected for skin lesions, signs of peripheral vascular disease, swelling, ecchymosis, symmetry, deformity, and overall alignment. The patient's gait should be evaluated as well. When pain is part of the presentation, it is helpful to ask the patient to locate the primary focus with one finger.

C. Neurovascular examination—Every physical examination of the foot and ankle should include a neurovascular assessment. Palpate the dorsalis pedis and posterior tibial pulses. If they are not present, consider Doppler signals, ankle-brachial indices, and toe pressures and/or arterial waveforms, especially if surgical intervention is planned. The sensory examination should assess the following five cutaneous nerves that supply the feet (Figs. 6–9 to 6–11).
   - Sural—Lateral border of the foot
   - Saphenous—Medial eminence region of the great toe
   - Superficial peroneal
     - Medial dorsal cutaneous—Dorsomedial foot
     - Intermediate dorsal cutaneous—Dorsolateral foot
   - Deep peroneal—First dorsal web space
   - Posterior tibial—Plantar foot

If sensory neuropathy is suspected, testing with Semmes-Weinstein monofilaments can be helpful. When assessing strength, keep in mind the relation the tendon has to the axis of the ankle. For example, if it passes medially and posteriorly, the function of that structure will be to provide plantar flexion and inversion (tibialis posterior). The tibialis anterior passes anterior and medial to the ankle and therefore accomplishes dorsiflexion and inversion. To isolate the posterior tibialis muscle, the ankle needs to be in plantar flexion to eliminate the contributions of the tibialis anterior muscle to inversion (Fig. 6–12). When assessing motor function of the foot and ankle, the following muscles should be tested:
   - Tibialis anterior—Ankle dorsiflexion, L3-4
   - Extensor hallucis longus—Great-toe extension, L4-5
   - Peroneus longus and brevis—Hindfoot eversion, L5-S1
   - Posterior tibialis—Hindfoot inversion, L4-5
   - Gastrocnemius complex—Ankle plantar flexion, S1

It is important to remember that neurologic deficits can be secondary to more proximal pathology

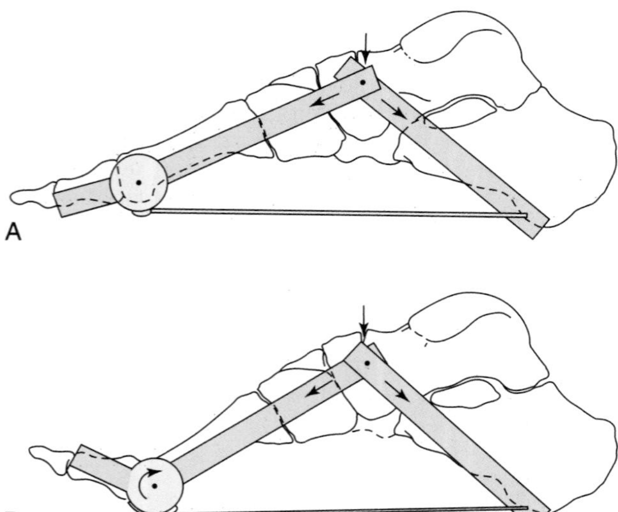

FIGURE 6–8 The windlass mechanism. As the foot progresses to the toe-off phase of the gait cycle, metatarsal phalangeal extension tightens the plantar fascia, the arch of the foot is accentuated, and the transverse tarsal joint locks, providing a stable lever for push-off. (From Myerson MS: Foot and Ankle Disorders. Philadelphia, WB Saunders, 2000.)

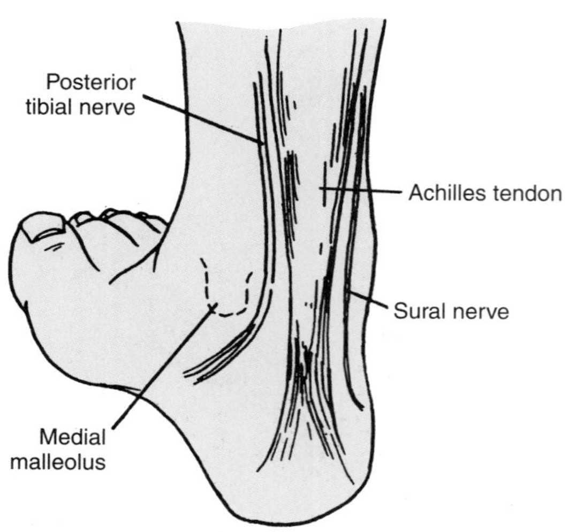

FIGURE 6–9 The location of the sural nerve and posterior tibial nerve in relation to the medial malleolus and Achilles tendon. (From Coughlin MJ, Mann RA: Surgery of the Foot and Ankle. St. Louis, CV Mosby, 1999.)

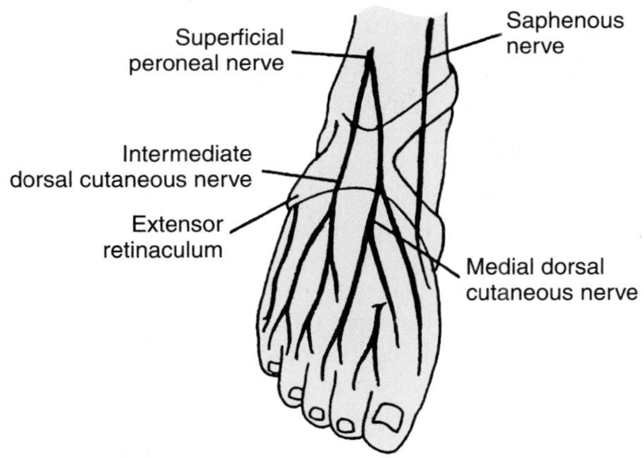

FIGURE 6–10 Locations of the cutaneous nerves of the foot. (From Coughlin MJ, Mann RA: Surgery of the Foot and Ankle. St. Louis, CV Mosby, 1999.)

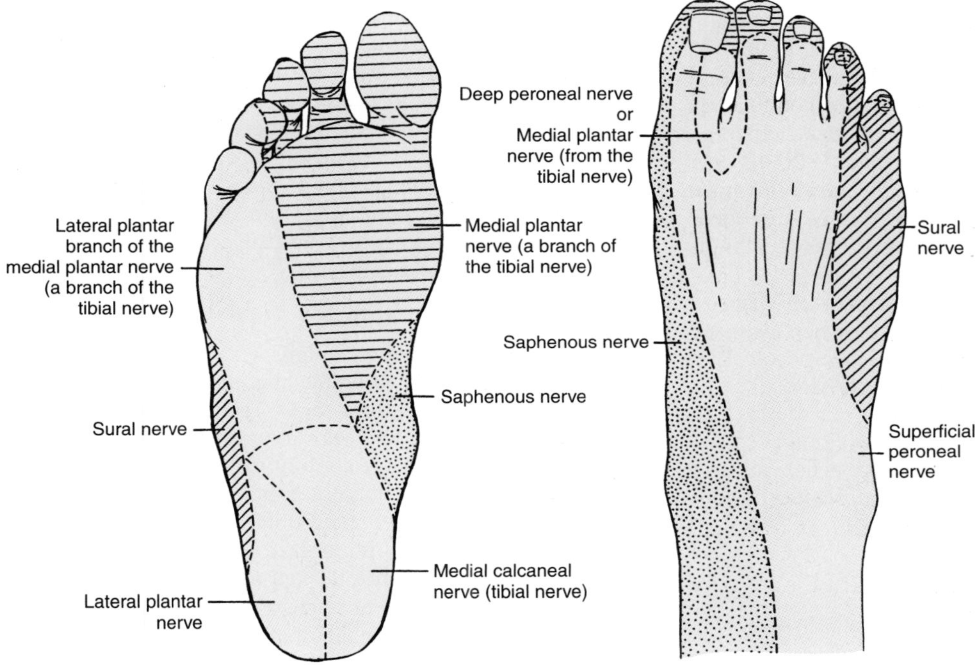

FIGURE 6–11 Sensory innervation of the foot. (From Myerson MS: Foot and Ankle Disorders. Philadelphia, WB Saunders, 2000.)

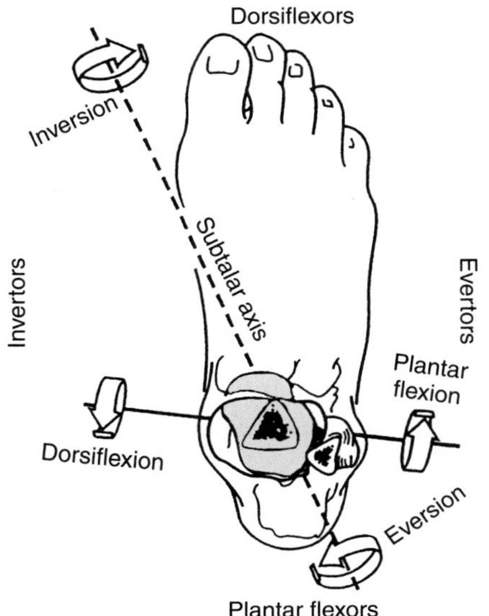

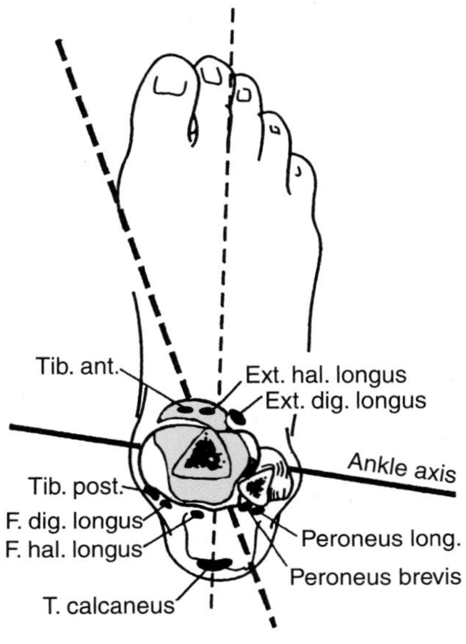

FIGURE 6–12 The relationships of the tendons to the axes of rotation of the ankle and subtalar joints. (From Mann RA: In American Academy of Orthopaedics Surgeons: Atlas of Orthotics, 3rd ed. St. Louis, CV Mosby, 1997.)

(central nervous system [CNS], spinal cord, nerve root, etc.).

D. Palpation and stability—Palpation of bony prominences such as the lateral malleolus, medial malleolus, fifth metatarsal base, metatarsal shafts, and first MTP joint can be revealing. The lateral and medial ankle ligaments should be palpated after trauma. The courses of all tendons are checked both at rest and during contraction for swelling, nodules, and subluxation. A Tinel sign should be sought for the posterior tibial nerve at the tarsal tunnel and for the **superficial peroneal nerve** (SPN) and **deep peroneal nerve** (DPN). The web space can be palpated for evidence of interdigital neuromas (Morton). Stability of the lateral ankle ligaments can be assessed with an anterior drawer test (isolates the anterior talofibular ligament when done in plantar flexion) and inversion of the ankle in dorsiflexion (to evaluate the calcaneofibular ligament).

E. Range of motion—Both passive and active range of motion should be compared with the contralateral side for the following structures and characteristics:
1. Ankle dorsiflexion/plantar flexion—20-40 degrees; the Silfverskiöld test (difference in ankle dorsiflexion with knee flexed versus extended) can help differentiate between gastrocnemius and Achilles tightness (Fig. 6–13)
2. Subtalar joint eversion/inversion—5-20 degrees; take care to eliminate tibiotalar tilt when assessing subtalar joint motion
3. Transverse tarsal joint—Abduction/adduction
4. First MTP—Flexion/extension
5. Coupled triplanar motions
6. Pronation—Abduction/eversion/dorsiflexion
7. Supination—Adduction/inversion/plantar flexion

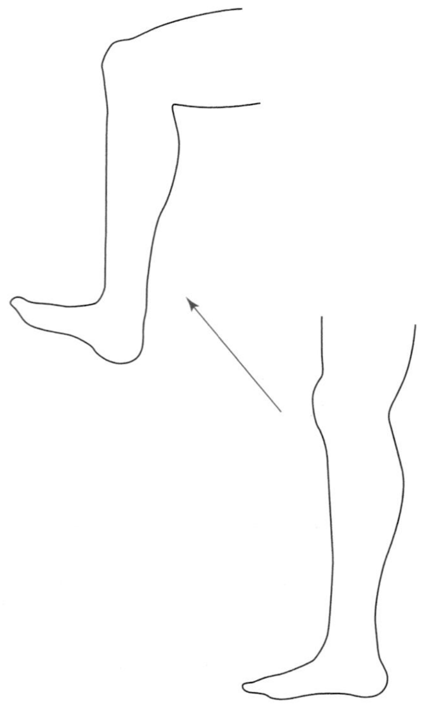

FIGURE 6–13 Silfverskiöld test to differentiate gastrocnemius tightness from Achilles tendon contracture.

III. Radiographic Evaluation of the Foot and Ankle

A. Views—Plain radiographs are instrumental in the initial evaluation of foot and ankle disorders. Weight-bearing views should be obtained when possible. The standard views of the ankle are anteroposterior, lateral, and mortise (a view of 15 degrees of internal rotation along the transmalleolar axis). Views of external rotation stress can be obtained to check the integrity of the syndesmosis. Anterior drawer and talar tilt views are helpful in cases of suspected ankle instability. The standard views of the foot should include anteroposterior, lateral, and oblique (Fig. 6–14). Special views are provided when the clinical presentation warrants it (Table 6–2). Comparison views of the contralateral foot or ankle are not routinely ordered but can be helpful in difficult cases.

B. Imaging procedures—**Computed tomography** (CT) of the foot and ankle is especially useful for complex fractures (pilon, calcaneus, talus, midfoot, Lisfranc) and tarsal coalition. **Magnetic resonance imaging** (MRI) aids the evaluation of osteochondral defects, osteonecrosis, neoplasm, and other soft tissue pathologies. Bone scans can detect stress fractures, and indium-tagged white blood cell (WBC) scans can detect osteomyelitis.

IV. Adult Hallux Valgus

A. Overview—**Hallux valgus** is a lateral deviation of the great toe. Although the etiology for bunions is multifactorial (Box 6–1), genetics and pointed, high-heeled shoes with a narrow toe box are felt to be the primary contributors to this deformity. Asymptomatic bunions are treated with patient education and observation only. If the patient is symptomatic, initial nonoperative measures should be tried, which include appropriately fitting shoes. More than 60% of women wear shoes that are one half to one size smaller than their measured foot size. The shoe should be wider and low-heeled with a soft upper part to accommodate the prominent medial eminence and decrease forefoot loading. A ring-and-ball stretcher can enlarge the area of the shoe over the eminence to avoid rubbing. An orthotic device can be used to support the arch and decrease pronation.

B. Pathophysiology (Figs. 6–15 and 6–16)
1. Medial capsular attenuation
2. Proximal phalanx drifts laterally, leading to the following conditions:
   a. Plantar-lateral migration of abductor hallucis
   b. Stretching of the extensor hood of the extensor hallucis longus
   c. Lateral deviation of the extensor hallucis longus and flexor hallucis longus, causing a muscular imbalance and deforming force for valgus progression
3. First metatarsal head moves medially off the sesamoids, increasing the intermetatarsal angle
4. Secondary contracture of the lateral capsule, adductor hallucis, lateral metatarsal-sesamoid ligament, and intermetatarsal ligament

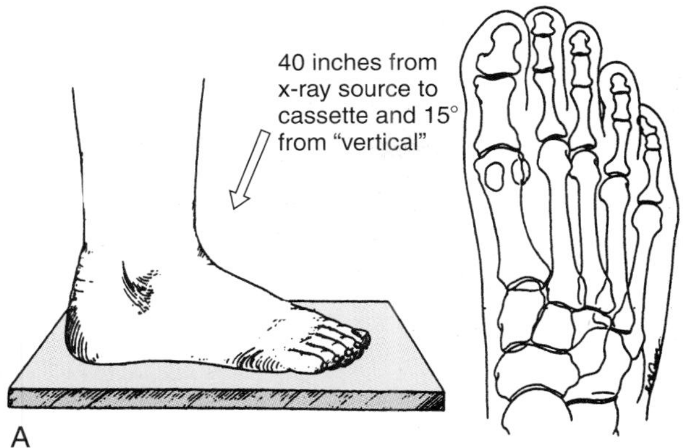

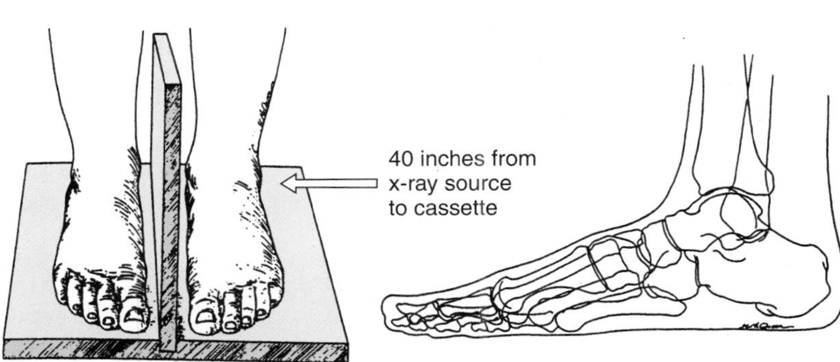

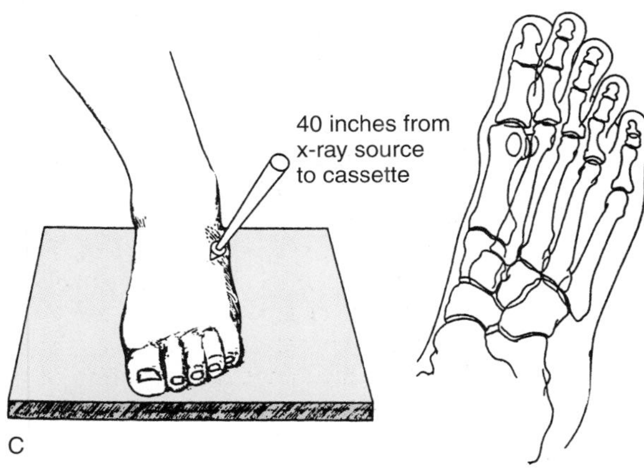

FIGURE 6–14 Radiographic views of the foot: anteroposterior (**A**), lateral (**B**), and non-weight-bearing lateral oblique (**C**). (From Richardson EG: Disorders of the hallux. In Canale ST, ed: Campbell's Operative Orthopaedics, 10th ed. St. Louis, CV Mosby, 2003.)

C. Assessment of hallux valgus severity—Measurement of various angles, joint congruity, sesamoid position, stability of the first tarsometatarsal (TMT) joint, and the presence or absence of arthritis have guided the operative intervention for hallux valgus.
   1. Angles (Fig. 6–17, Table 6–3)
   2. First TMT stability—Dorsal translation of first metatarsal base or plantar widening (Fig. 6–18)
   3. Sesamoid position—Normally centered under the first metatarsal head, the sesamoids stay in place and the first metatarsal head migrates medially off the sesamoids.
   4. First MTP arthritis

D. Surgical procedures (Fig. 6–19)

E. Bunion surgical complications
   1. Any osteotomy
      a. Nonunion
      b. Dorsal malunion and resulting transfer metatarsalgia
      c. Undercorrection (hallux valgus recurrence)—More common with distal (underpowered) osteotomies or isolated soft tissue procedures
      d. Overcorrection (hallux varus)—More common with proximal osteotomies
      e. First MTP arthritis or loss of motion—More common with proximal osteotomies
   2. Chevron (distal osteotomy) bunionectomy
      a. Avascular necrosis with or without segmental collapse—Once thought to be due to a concurrent release of first web space. This is currently being questioned.

TABLE 6-2 SPECIAL RADIOGRAPHIC VIEWS OF THE FOOT AND ANKLE

View	Specific Purpose
Canale view—15 degree internal rotation for foot	Talar neck view for fracture
Harris view—Axial heel view	Calcaneus fractures
Sesamoid view—Axial sesamoid view	Sesamoid fracture or arthritis
Broden's view—Tibiocalcaneal (subtalar) medial oblique views at 10 degree variations	Posterior, medial, and anterior facets of subtalar joint for fracture or arthritis
Anteroposterior view	Evaluation of tibiotalar joint, distal tibia and fibula, peripheral borders of tarsals, and talar dome
Lateral view	Assessment of effusion, talocalcaneal relationships, tibiofibular integrity, and tibiotalar joint congruity
Oblique views Internal—Plantar flexion plus 45 degrees internal rotation External—Plantar flexion plus 45 degrees external rotation	Additional information about ankle mortise, talar dome, and malleoli
Mortise view	Best information about mortise integrity and talar dome

Box 6–1 Etiologic Factors in Hallux Valgus Deformity

High-heeled shoes with a narrow toe box
Genetics
Trauma
Neuromuscular disorders with soft tissue imbalance
Pes planus foot
Connective tissue disorders with ligamentous laxity
Instability of the first tarsometatarsal joint
Inflammatory arthropathies (rheumatoid arthritis)

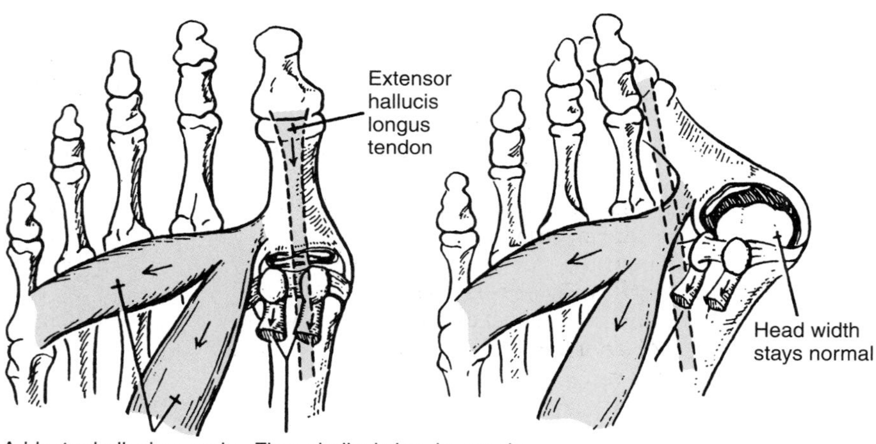

FIGURE 6–15 Pathophysiology of hallux valgus deformity. (From Coughlin MJ, Mann RA: Surgery of the Foot and Ankle. St. Louis, CV Mosby, 1999.)

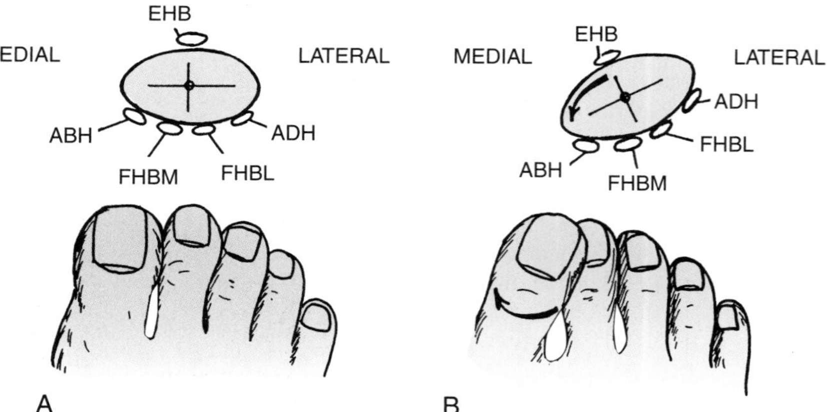

FIGURE 6–16 Schematic representation of tendons around first metatarsal head. **A**, Normal articulation in a balanced state. **B**, Relationship of tendons in hallux valgus deformity. ABH, abductor hallucis; ADH, adductor hallucis; EHB, extensor hallucis brevis; FHBL, flexor hallucis brevis lateral head; FHBM, flexor hallucis brevis medial head. (From Coughlin MJ, Mann RA: Surgery of the Foot and Ankle. St. Louis, CV Mosby, 1999.)

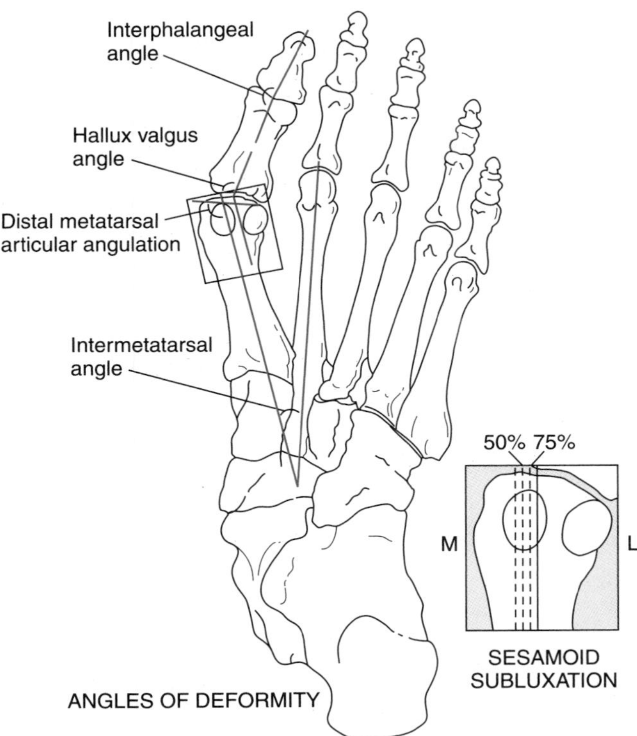

FIGURE 6–17 Radiographic angles of the first ray in hallux valgus.

3. Keller resection arthroplasty
   a. Transfer metatarsalgia
   b. Loss of toe weight-bearing function
   c. Cock-up toe deformity
   d. Salvage—First MTP arthrodesis with or without interpositional graft for length
4. Isolated distal soft tissue release and resection of medial eminence (Silver bunionectomy)
   a. Recurrence
   b. Original McBride with resection of lateral sesamoid lead to hallux varus deformity
5. First TMT arthrodesis (Lapidus)
   a. Dorsal malunion
   b. Nonunion (10-20%)

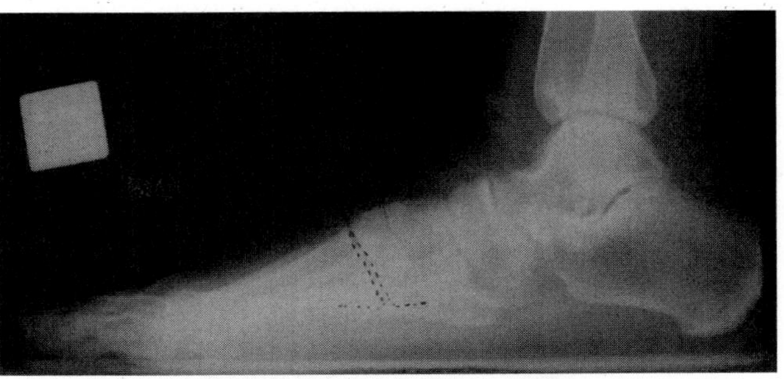

FIGURE 6–18 First tarsometatarsal joint instability with plantar widening.

6. First MTP arthrodesis
   a. Nonunion (5%)
   b. Malunion
      (1) 110 degrees dorsiflexion relative to the floor or 25 degrees dorsiflexion relative to the first metatarsal shaft
      (2) Neutral rotation
      (3) 10-15 degrees valgus
7. Proximal osteotomies
   a. Crescentic
      (1) Dorsal malunion
      (2) Hallux varus
   b. Scarf
      (1) "Troughing"—Malrotation deformity due to osteotomy cuts

V. Juvenile and Adolescent Hallux Valgus

A. Factors—Several factors separate these patients from adult patients with hallux valgus deformity.
   1. Pain, either at the MTP joint or beneath the lesser metatarsal heads, may not be the primary complaint.
   2. A bunion secondary to medial eminence and bursal hypertrophy may be a minor part of the deformity.
   3. Varus of the first metatarsal with a widened intermetatarsal angle (IMA) is almost always present. The distal metatarsal articular angle (DMAA) is increased.

TABLE 6-3 IMPORTANT RADIOGRAPHIC ANGLES IN THE EVALUATION OF HALLUX VALGUS

Angle	Location	Importance	Normal
Hallux valgus interphalangeus	Between long axes of first proximal phalanx and first distal phalanx, bisecting their diaphyses	Identifies degree of deformity at the IP joint	<8 degrees
Hallux valgus	Between long axes of first proximal phalanx and first metatarsal, bisecting their diaphyses	Identifies degree of deformity at the MTP joint	<15 degrees
Metatarsus primus varus	Between long axes of first metatarsal and first cuneiform	Identifies obliquity versus subluxation of MTC joint	<25 degrees
First intermetatarsal (Hardy and Clapham)	Between long axes of first and second metatarsals, bisecting shafts of first and second metatarsals	Not influenced by over-resection of medial eminence. Not accurate for postoperative evaluation of distal osteotomies	<10 degrees
Distal metatarsal articular	Angle of line bisecting MT shaft with line through base of distal articular cartilage cap	Offset of angle is predisposing factor in development of hallux valgus	<15 degrees
Phalangeal articular	Articular angle of base of proximal phalanx in relation to longitudinal axis	Offset of angle is predisposing factor in development of hallux valgus	7-10 degrees

IP, interphalangeal; MT, metatarsal; MTC, metatarsocuneiform; MTP, metatarsophalangeal.

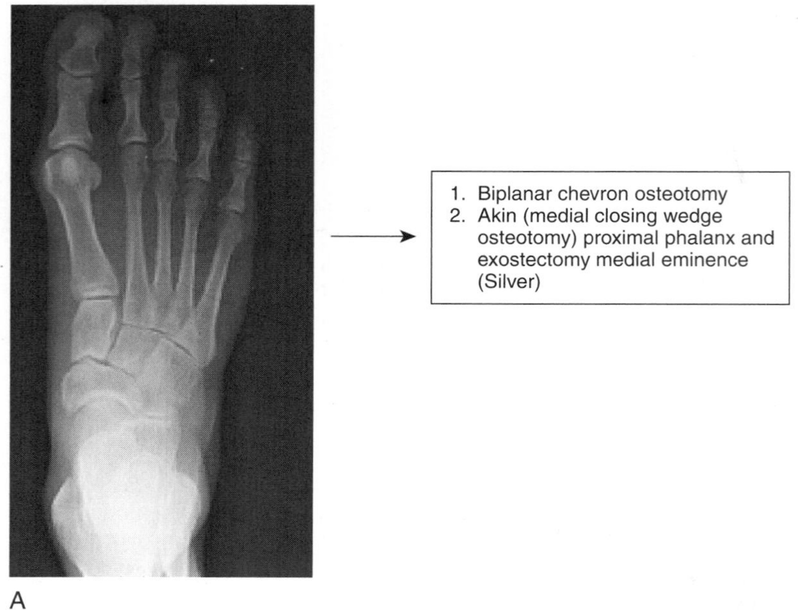

Congruent bunion:
DMAA < 10°
1. Biplanar chevron osteotomy
2. Akin (medial closing wedge osteotomy) proximal phalanx and exostectomy medial eminence (Silver)
A

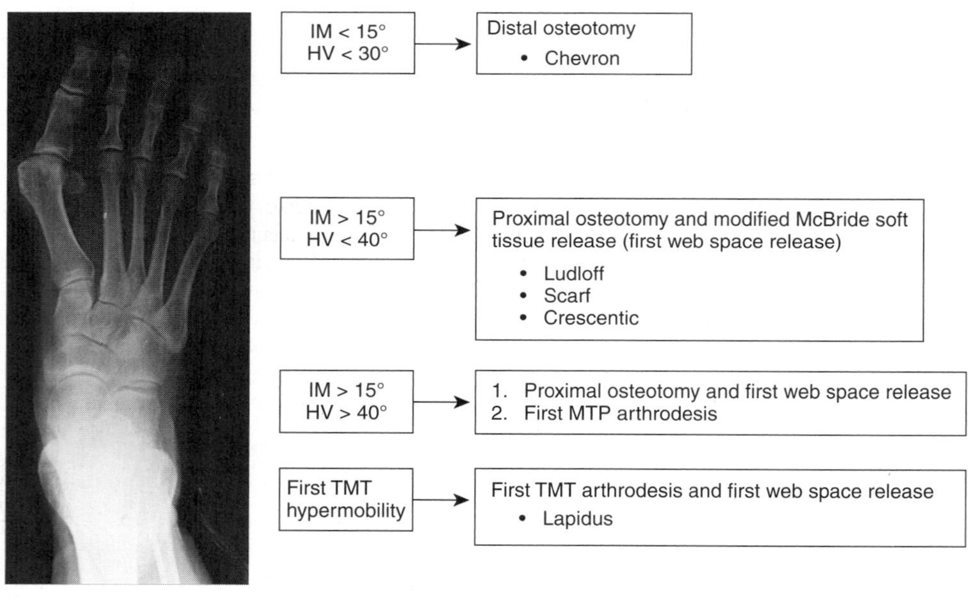

FIGURE 6–19 Treatment algorithm for hallux valgus. **A**, Congruent bunion. **B**, Incongruent bunion. HV, hallux valgus angle; IM, intermetatarsal angle.

4. Hypermobile flatfoot with pronation of the foot during weight bearing is frequently associated with the deformity (Coughlin's data do not support this).
5. Recurrence of the hallux valgus deformity is more frequent, especially with flatfoot deformity.
6. Hallux valgus interphalangeus may be prominent yet easily overlooked and may cause unsatisfactory correction of the deformity.
7. The family history is frequently positive for hallux valgus.
8. Soft tissue procedures alone are unlikely to result in permanent correction.
9. Osteotomy, single or double, of the first metatarsal is almost always necessary to obtain and maintain correction.

VI. Hallux Varus

A. Cause—Medial deviation of the great toe is most often an iatrogenic deformity secondary to overcorrection of hallux valgus.

Arthritic bunion, unreliable soft tissue balancing, or bunion recurrence

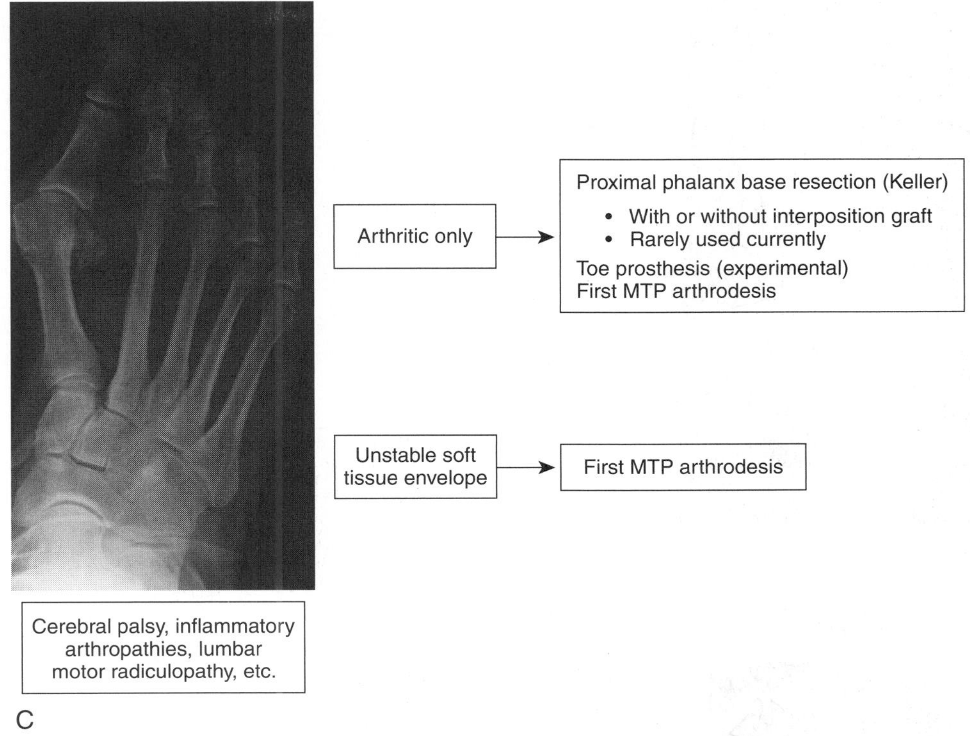

FIGURE 6–19, cont'd C, Arthritic bunion, unreliable soft tissue balancing, or bunion recurrence.

B. Treatment
   1. Nonoperative treatment—Nonoperative treatment is limited to accommodation of the deformity with shoe modifications (curved-last shoe) and shoe stretching.
   2. Operative treatment—Operative treatment of a flexible deformity can be addressed with the release of the abductor hallucis muscle and fascia and transfer of a portion of the extensor hallucis longus (EHL) or brevis tendon under the transverse intermetatarsal (IM) ligament to the proximal phalanx (Fig. 6–20). This acts as a "check ring" to limit adduction of the proximal phalanx. A fixed deformity or a deformity with limited first MTP motion is treated with a first MTP arthrodesis.

Medial capsular lengthening

Split EHL rerouting under IM ligament

FIGURE 6–20 Correction of flexible hallux varus deformity.

VII. Lesser-Toe Deformities

A. Anatomic considerations (Fig. 6–21)—The EDL forms three tendinous slips on the dorsum of each toe; the first inserts into the middle phalanx, and the remaining two merge and insert on the distal phalanx. In concert, the EDL and **extensor digitorum brevis** (EDB) extend the MTP, **proximal interphalangeal** (PIP), and **distal interphalangeal** (DIP) joints through their pull on the extensor hood. The FDL courses deep to the **flexor digitorum brevis** (FDB) on the plantar surface of the toe and acts as a powerful flexor at the DIP joint. The PIP and MTP joints are flexed through the combined action of the FDL and FDB tendons as well as the lumbrical

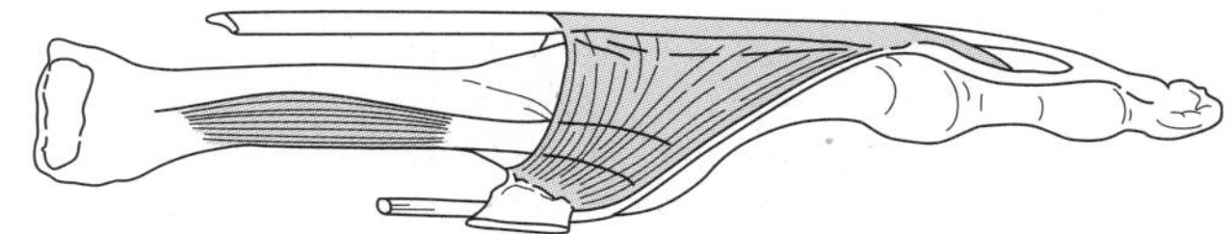

FIGURE 6–21 Anatomy of the intrinsic and extrinsic musculature in the normal MTP joint. (From Myerson MS: Foot and Ankle Disorders. Philadelphia, WB Saunders, 2000.)

and interosseous muscles. The intrinsics first pass plantar to the axis of MTP joint rotation and then dorsal to the axis of motion of the PIP and DIP joints. This anatomic relationship allows the intrinsics to act as flexors at the MTP joint and extensors at the PIP and DIP joints. Disruption of this delicate balance can lead to problematic disequilibrium between the intrinsics and extrinsics, which in turn can result in characteristic lesser-toe deformities and associated pressure phenomena.

B. Deformities—Of the three most common lesser-toe deformities (hammer toe, claw-toe, and mallet-toe), the hammer-toe deformity is the most common. The various anatomic properties that define each deformity are shown in Table 6–4 and Figure 6–22.

1. Hammer-toe deformity
   a. Diagnosis—The characteristic *hammer-toe* deformity is caused by an overpull of the EDL and imbalance of the intrinsics. Hammer-toe deformity occurs mostly in older women and may be isolated (usually the second toe) or multiple, flexible, or rigid. Symptoms usually occur as the result of painful corns that arise at the dorsal PIP joint. Manual manipulation or use of the "push-up test" (Fig. 6–23) should be performed to determine whether a flexible or rigid deformity exists. This distinction greatly influences the choice of surgical procedure.
   b. Treatment—In patients with flexible and mild deformities, accommodative footwear and protective padding are often successful in alleviating symptoms. On the other hand, patients with flexible deformities who fail nonoperative treatment may benefit from a flexor-to-extensor tendon transfer of the FDL. In a fixed deformity, surgical options include resection arthroplasty of the head and neck of the proximal phalanx or PIP arthrodesis.
2. Mallet-toe deformity
   a. Diagnosis—A *mallet toe* may consist of an isolated flexion deformity at the DIP joint or may exist in conjunction with a claw-toe deformity. This deformity usually occurs as the result of a contracted or spastic FDL in association with attenuation of the terminal extensor tendons. Although the condition is normally idiopathic, 75% of patients with mallet-toe deformity have elongation of the affected digit.
   b. Treatment—Conservative treatment modalities are similar to those used in treating patients with hammer-toe and claw-toe deformities. A flexible mallet toe can be corrected with percutaneous FDL tenotomy, whereas surgical alternatives for treating a rigid deformity include excisional arthroplasty of the DIP joint, middle phalangeal condylectomy, and terminal Syme's amputation (when underlying infection exists). Concurrent repair of the extensor tendon and percutaneous K-wire pinning should also be performed for added stabilization.
3. Claw-toe deformity
   a. Diagnosis—A *claw-toe* deformity rarely occurs in isolation. There is often clawing of all five toes, in which case an underlying neuromuscular condition is usually present and should be strongly considered. However, if present only in the second toe or occasionally the second and third toes, a

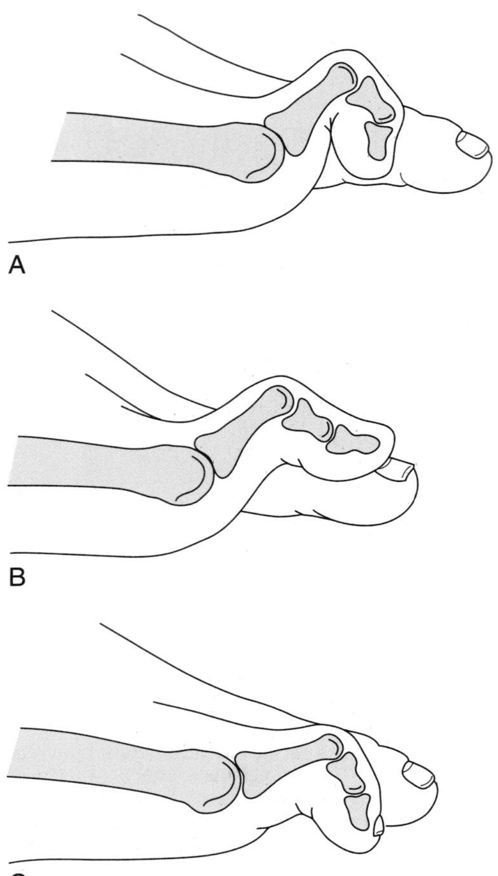

FIGURE 6–22 Examples of sagittal plane deformities. **A**, Hammer toe. Notice the proximal interphalangeal (PIP) joint flexion. **B**, Mild claw-toe deformity. Notice the flexion at the PIP joint and extension at the metatarsophalangeal joint. **C**, Advanced claw-toe deformity. Notice the flexion at the PIP and distal interphalangeal joints from flexor digitorum longus pull. (From Myerson MS: Foot and Ankle Disorders. Philadelphia, WB Saunders, 2000.)

TABLE 6–4 LESSER-TOE DEFORMITIES AND THEIR RELATIVE ANATOMIC RELATIONSHIPS

Lesser-Toe Deformity	Position		
	MTP Position	*PIP Position*	*DIP Position*
Hammer toe	Dorsiflexed	Flexed	Neutral/hyperextended
Claw toe	Dorsiflexed	Flexed	Flexed
Mallet toe	Neutral	Neutral	Flexed

DIP, distal interphalangeal; MTP, metatarsophalangeal; PIP, proximal interphalangeal.

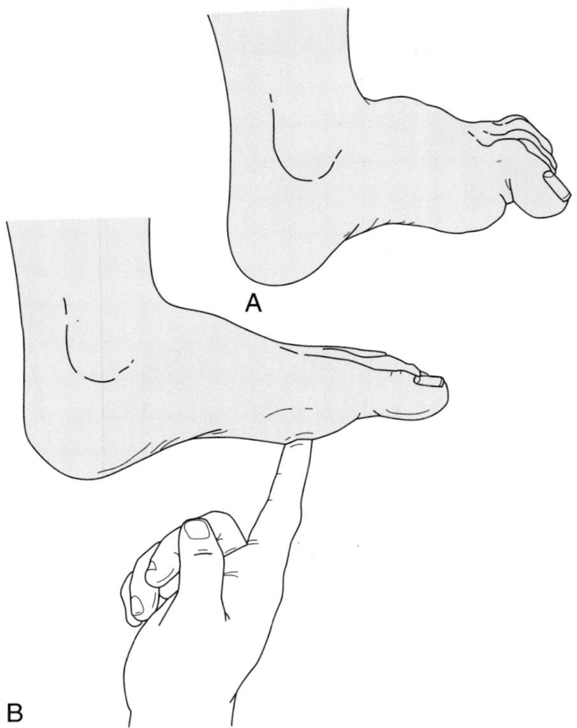

FIGURE 6–23 The push-up test is used to assess the flexibility of a lesser-toe deformity. **A**, Active dorsiflexion with extrinsic-overpowering intrinsics creates an intrinisic-minus deformity. **B**, The passive push-up test demonstrates an intrinsic-plus toe pattern after the overactive extrinsics are removed. (From Myerson MS: Foot and Ankle Disorders. Philadelphia, WB Saunders, 2000.)

neuromuscular cause is less likely. MTP joint hyperextension represents the primary pathology in claw-toe deformity (Fig. 6–24). Painful dorsal and terminal end corns are often created by the extended posture of the MTP joint and associated PIP and DIP flexion. Key components of the physical examination include assessment of the MTP joint for instability, evaluation of the extent of deformity, and documentation of the degree of flexibility.

b. Treatment—Nonsurgical treatment options are identical to those used for hammer toes and mallet toes but can also be expanded to include the use of semirigid orthotic devices with metatarsal padding for patients with claw toes and associated metatarsalgia. In patients with flexible deformity, a flexor-to-extensor transfer enables the FDL to assume the function of the intrinsics and maintain correction (Table 6–5). EDB tenotomy and EDL lengthening should also be performed to aid in soft tissue balancing. Patients with fixed deformities may benefit from a complete MTP capsulotomy and resection arthroplasty of the proximal phalanx or PIP arthrodesis. A Weil osteotomy (oblique-shortening metatarsal (MT) osteotomy, usually of the second metatarsal) is occasionally added for greater correction.

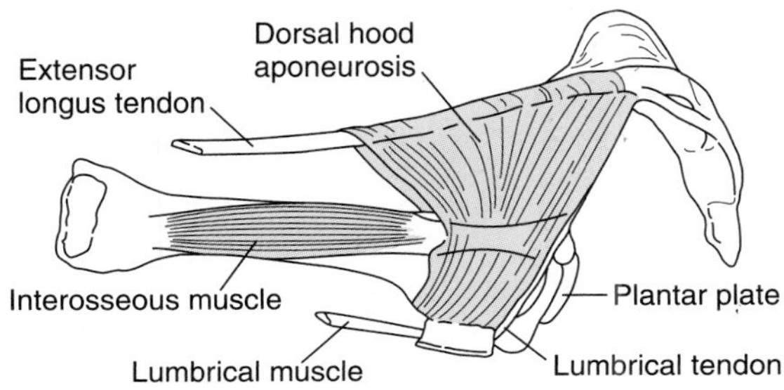

FIGURE 6–24 Anatomy of the intrinsic and extrinsic musculature in claw-toe deformity. (From Myerson MS: Foot and Ankle Disorders. Philadelphia, WB Saunders, 2000.)

4. Crossover second toe
   a. Diagnosis—Multiplanar instability of the second toe may cause the toe to lie dorsomedially relative to the hallux (Fig. 6–25). Commonly referred to as *crossover second toe*, this deformity occurs from attritional rupture of the lateral cruciate ligament (LCL) and lateral capsule in addition to attenuation or rupture of the first dorsal interosseous tendon and fibrocartilaginous plantar plate. Medial structures such as the lumbrical and interosseous tendons, medial cruciate ligament (MCL), and medial capsule become tight and contracted, thus creating an unopposed adduction moment at the MTP joint. This imbalance results in medial deviation of the second toe, which is often progressive.
   b. Treatment—Nonoperative measures, though historically unreliable, attempt to limit the degree of second MTP joint synovitis, which can lead to increased laxity at the MTP and eventually instability. In patients with mild disease, soft tissue release of the extensor tendon, dorsal and medial capsule, and MCL may help to correct the deformity and alleviate symptoms. However, if symptoms persist or instability is not fully addressed, flexor-to-extensor tendon transfer can be performed to further stabilize the deformity. EDB tendon transfer may also be used as a dynamic stabilizer of incompetent lateral structures. In patients with severe subluxation, bony procedures such as resection arthroplasty of the proximal phalanx or a distal MT shortening osteotomy (Weil osteotomy) may be needed to achieve a satisfactory degree of correction.
5. Fifth toe deformities
   a. Diagnosis—Several types of deformity exist, including underlapping, overlapping, rotatory, and cock-up fifth toe (Fig. 6–26). Subluxation at the fifth MTP results in weakened push-off during ambulation, a loss of coverage of the fifth metatarsal head, and subsequent callus formation under the dorsolateral aspect of the fifth toe.
   b. Treatment—Stretching or taping may be helpful with an overlapping fifth toe;

TABLE 6-5 SURGICAL TREATMENT OF LESSER-TOE DEFORMITIES

Deformity	Surgical Options	Comments
Hammer toe		
Flexible	FDL flexor-to-extensor tendon transfer	Add EDL lengthening or tenotomy if active flexion < 10-15 degrees
Fixed	Resection arthroplasty of head and neck of proximal phalanx with EDB tenotomy and EDL lengthening PIP arthrodesis	
Mallet toe		
Flexible	Percutaneous FDL tenotomy	
Fixed	Excisional arthroplasty of the DIP joint Middle phalangeal condylectomy Terminal Syme's amputation	Extensor tendon repair and percutaneous pinning should be performed for added stabilization Reserved as salvage procedure for infection
Claw toe		
Flexible	FDL flexor-to-extensor tendon transfer with EDB tenotomy and EDL lengthening	Look for underlying neuromuscular etiology when > 2 toes are involved
Fixed	Complete MTP capsulotomy and resection arthroplasty of the proximal phalanx with EDB tenotomy and EDL lengthening PIP arthrodesis	Weil osteotomy (oblique-shortening MT osteotomy with internal fixation, usually of 2nd MT) can be performed for added correction
All 4 lesser toes	Resection of PIP joint with MTP joint capsulotomy and tendon release/lengthening Distal MT shortening osteotomy (Weil)	Occasionally partial MT head resection arthroplasty and MT plantar condylectomy
Crossover 2nd toe	Soft tissue release of extensor tendon, dorsal and medial MTP joint capsule, and MCL	Lateral capsular imbrication can be performed for additional correction
Overlapping 5th toe	Release of dorsomedial MTP capsule, Z-plasty of contracted dorsal skin, lengthening of contracted EDL, dermodesis, and lateral imbrication EDL tendon transfer into the lateral capsule or abductor digiti minimi is another option	Bony resection or osteotomy can be added to soft tissue procedures for further correction Salvage options include syndactylization of the 5th toe or a Ruiz-Mora procedure Results are often disappointing
Underlapping 5th toe	Tenotomy of FDL and FDB in children (flexible deformities) Flexor-to-extensor tendon transfer, syndactylization, bony resection, and derotational soft tissue procedures in adults	
Hard corns (helomata durum)	Decompression of bony prominences at the lateral IP joint Partial cheilectomy Resection of the lateral proximal 5th phalanx or MT head Hemiphalangectomy of the proximal phalanx	
Soft corns (helomata molle)	Excision of offending bony prominences as well as adjacent skin lesions Basilar hemiphalangectomy with lateral condyle excision of the MT head for proximal lesions	Avoid web space incisions to minimize the risk of infection
Intractable plantar keratosis		
Discrete form	Partial plantar exostosectomy of the medial sesamoid or prominent plantar MT condyle (mild disease) Complete excision of the medial sesamoid (advanced disease)	Patients with IPK due to a plantar-flexed 1st ray may benefit from a dorsiflexion osteotomy of that ray
Diffuse form	Shortening or dorsiflexion osteotomy Duvries arthroplasty	Transfer metatarsalgia can develop excessive MT head resection Transfer lesions may also develop regardless of the success of the procedure
Bunionette (tailor's bunion)	Plantar/lateral MT head condylectomy (type I) Diaphyseal osteotomy (types II and III) MT head resection (salvage)	Three types: Type I: enlarged 5th MT head Type II: abnormally widened 4th to 5th IM angle Type III: lateral bowing of the 5th MT diaphysis Avoid proximal osteotomies due to the tenuous blood supply

DIP, distal interphalangeal; EDB, extensor digitorum longus; EDB, extensor digitorum brevis; EDL, extensor digitorum longus; FDB, flexor digitorum brevis; FDL, flexor digitorum longus; IM, intermetatarsal; IP, interphalangeal; IPK, intractable plantar keratosis; MCL, medial collateral ligament; MT, metatarsal; MTP, metatarsophalangeal; PIP, proximal interphalangeal.

however, if conservative measures fail, release of the dorsomedial capsule, Z-plasty of contracted dorsal skin, lengthening of contracted EDL, strategic dermodesis, and lateral imbrication may all be indicated. Surgical treatment for patients with cock-up toe deformity is similar. EDL tendon transfer into the lateral capsule or abductor digiti minimi has also met with success. Bony resection or osteotomy can be added to soft tissue procedures to achieve further correction. A salvage option is syndactylization

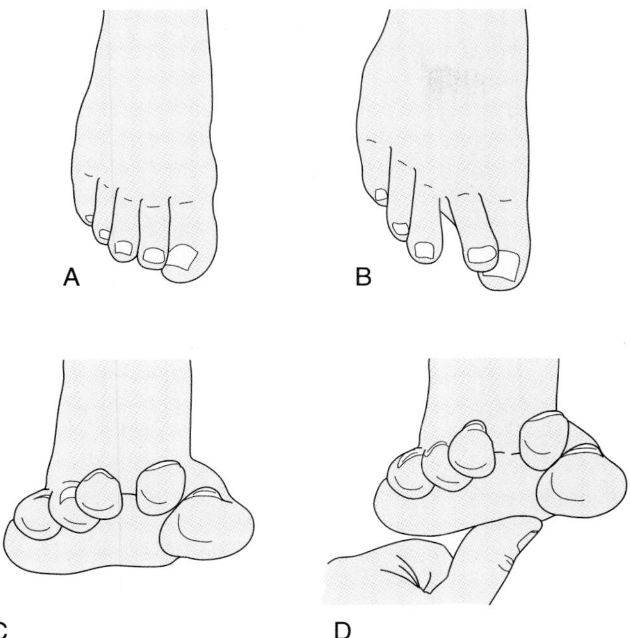

FIGURE 6–25 Crossover second-toe deformity, weight-bearing (**B** and **D**) and non-weight-bearing (**A** and **C**) views. (From Myerson MS: Foot and Ankle Disorders. Philadelphia, WB Saunders, 2000.)

of the fifth toe. An underlapping fifth toe (congenital curly toe) usually demonstrates attenuation of the dorsal capsule and EDL in addition to contracture of the plantar metaphalangeal joint capsule and FDL. Tenotomy of FDL and FDB has been recommended in children with flexible deformities. Flexor-to-extensor tendon transfer, syndactylization, bony resection, and derotational soft tissue procedures all have been proposed in isolation or in combination to correct the underlying deformity.

VIII. Hyperkeratotic Pathologies

A. Hard corns (helomata durum)

1. Diagnosis—Hard corns commonly occur over the fibular aspect of the fifth metaphalangeal or interphalangeal joints in response to frictional irritation or from pressure over bony prominences. Examination reveals epidermal hyperplasia with a conical central area.
2. Treatment—Conservative management consists of shaving or paring the corn with a pumice stone, followed by removal of the central inverted "seed" of the corn. Modification of shoe wear and protective padding can be employed to reduce extrinsic pressure. Surgical treatment, reserved for refractory cases that fail with conservative management, consists mainly of decompression of bony prominences at the fibular aspect of the interphalangeal joint. Partial cheilectomy, resection of the lateral proximal fifth phalanx or metatarsal head, and hemiphalangectomy of the proximal phalanx also represent effective surgical options.

B. Soft corns (helomata molle)

1. Diagnosis—Soft corns are characterized by hyperkeratoses that develop as the result of moisture between two adjacent toes as well as pressure from neighboring phalangeal condyles. There are two main types. In the first, a prominent medial condyle of the fifth proximal phalanx contacts the lateral base of the fourth proximal phalanx or metatarsal head. In the second, a distal phalangeal exostosis abuts its neighboring toe at various locations. On examination, the skin overlying the affected toe may be macerated and friable, with thickened callus and mediolateral squeezing causing significant pain.
2. Treatment—Conservative treatment includes absorptive padding and accommodative shoe wear that decreases contact pressure between the fourth and fifth toes and wicks excess moisture. Surgical measures include excision of offending bony prominences as well as adjacent skin lesions. Web space incisions should be avoided to minimize the risk of infection. Proximal lesions may be treated with basilar hemiphalangectomy with lateral condyle excision of the MT head.

C. Intractable plantar keratosis—**Intractable plantar keratosis** (IPK) develops on the plantar aspect of a

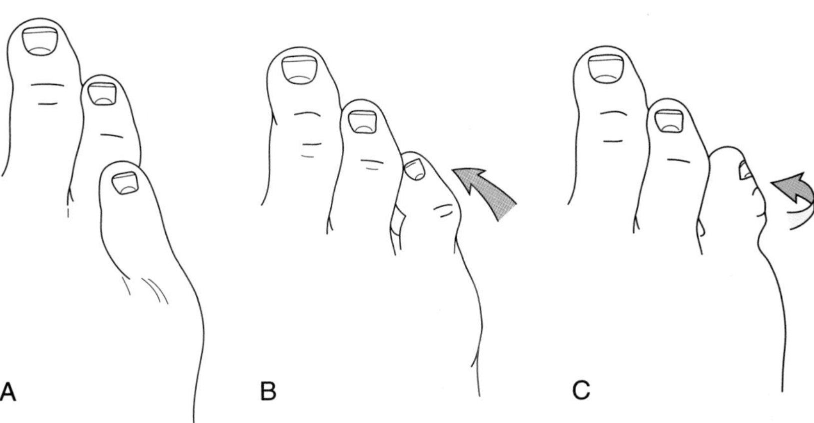

FIGURE 6–26 Rotational and angular deformities of the fifth toe. **A**, Congenital overlapping fifth toe. **B**, Congenital underlapping fifth toe. **C**, Primary rotatory deformity of the fifth toe. (From Myerson MS: Foot and Ankle Disorders. Philadelphia, WB Saunders, 2000.)

weight-bearing surface of the foot owing to excess pressure from a metatarsal head on the plantar fat pad. IPK is commonly associated with a prominent tibial sesamoid. Predisposing factors include fat pad atrophy, a plantar-flexed first ray, intrinsic-minus toe contracture, and hypertrophy of the sesamoid.

1. Discrete form—The discrete form of IPK is caused by shear forces and is associated with systemic diseases, biomechanical foot deformities, and fat pad atrophy. Initial treatment includes paring down the callus and encouraging the use of flat, soft-soled, strategically cushioned footwear. A total-contact orthosis or an extended steel shank can be considered for patients with significant fat pad atrophy. In patients with mild disease, partial plantar exostosectomy of the medial sesamoid or prominent plantar metatarsal condyle may provide symptomatic relief. In more advanced cases, complete excision of the medial sesamoid may be indicated. Patients with a plantar-flexed first ray may benefit from a dorsiflexion osteotomy.
2. Diffuse form—The diffuse form of IPK is characterized by a pressure phenomenon from the entire metatarsal head rather than from a prominent plantar condyle. It is commonly associated with an elongated first metatarsal or an excessively plantar-flexed first metatarsal. Conservative management is similar to that used with the discrete form of IPK. In patients for whom nonoperative management is unsuccessful, shortening or dorsiflexion osteotomy as well as Duvries arthroplasty may be effective. Transfer metatarsalgia can result from excessive metatarsal head resection, and transfer lesions may also develop regardless of the success of the procedure.

D. Bunionette deformity (tailor's bunion)

1. Diagnosis—A bunionette is a prominence over the distal aspect of the fifth metatarsal head and is commonly associated with pain over the lateral or plantar aspect of the MTP joint, particularly with compressive shoe wear. When a bunionette deformity occurs in conjunction with ipsilateral hallux valgus and metatarsus primus varus, the deformity is termed "splayfoot." Three distinct types have been described based on the anatomic location of the deformity along the fifth metatarsal (Fig. 6–27).
   a. Type I deformity—Distinguished by the presence of an enlarged fifth metatarsal head
   b. Type II deformity—Demonstrates lateral bowing of the fifth metatarsal diaphysis
   c. Type III deformity—Demonstrates an abnormally widened 4-5 metatarsal angle (intermetatarsal angle > 8 degrees)
2. Treatment—Initial treatment is conservative and usually effective. It consists of paring down or shaving the symptomatic callus in conjunction with shoe-wear modification and strategic padding. If coexisting pes planus is present or hyperkeratosis is plantar, a metatarsal pad or custom orthotic device may improve symptoms. Surgical treatments include lateral metatarsal head condylectomy, diaphyseal osteotomy, and metatarsal head resection. Proximal osteotomy should be avoided owing to the tenuous blood supply at the proximal metadiaphyseal junction of the fifth metatarsal (see Table 6–5).

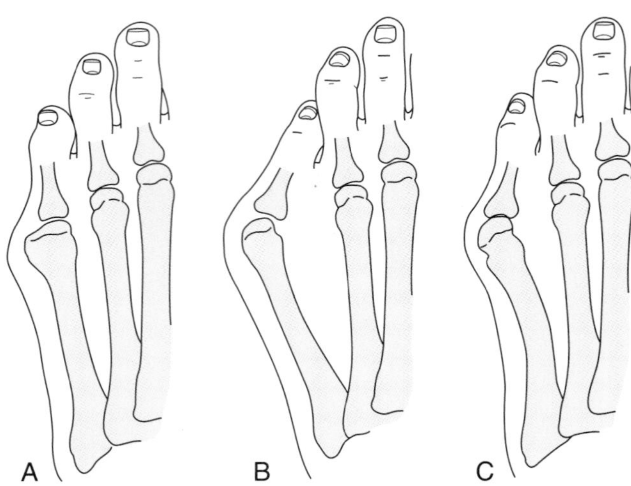

FIGURE 6–27 Types of bunionette deformities. **A**, Type I is associated with an enlarged head. **B**, Type II is associated with an increase in the 4-5 intermetatarsal angle. **C**, Type III is associated with lateral bowing of the metatarsal diaphysis. (From Myerson MS: Foot and Ankle Disorders. Philadelphia, WB Saunders, 2000.)

IX. Sesamoids

A. Anatomy—The medial and lateral hallucal sesamoids are part of the strong sesamoid capsuloligamentous complex that includes attachments from the flexor hallucis longus (FHL), flexor hallucis brevis (FHB), and metatarsosesamoid and intersesamoid ligaments. This complex may be analogous to the patella, as a mechanism to increase the mechanical advantage of the pulley function of the intrinsics (FHB). In addition, it protects the FHL and disperses the forces beneath the first metatarsal head.

B. Deformities—Sesamoid disorders can include acute injury (fracture, dislocation, sprain/"turf toe"), sesamoiditis, stress fracture, arthrosis, avascular necrosis, and IPK (Box 6–2).

1. Diagnosis—Patients usually present with pain under the first metatarsal head. Tenderness can

Box 6–2 Conditions Affecting the Hallucal Sesamoids

Fracture (acute, stress)
Dislocation
Inflammation (sesamoiditis)
- Traumatic
- Infectious
- Arthritic

Chondromalacia
Flexor hallucis brevis tendinitis
Osteochondritis dissecans

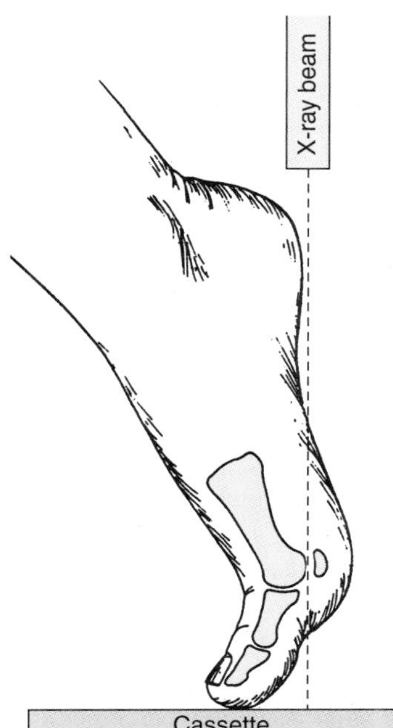

FIGURE 6–28 Axial sesamoid view obtained with a patient up on the toes. (From Richardson EG: Disorders of hallux. In Canale ST, ed: Campbell's Operative Orthopaedics, 10th ed. St. Louis, CV Mosby, 2003, p 4007.)

usually be elicited over the involved sesamoid. The most common mechanism of injury is that of forced dorsiflexion of the first MTP joint. This can result in avulsion of the plantar plate off the base of the phalanx and subsequent proximal migration of the sesamoids, seen on radiographs. The tibial sesamoid is more frequently involved in trauma but also more likely to be bipartite or multipartite. Special radiographic views include sesamoid anteroposterior, lateral, non–weight-bearing and weight-bearing axial, and oblique views to isolate the tibial or fibular sesamoid (Fig. 6–28).

2. Treatment—Treatment of sesamoid fractures should involve immobilization in a walking boot, short-leg cast, stiffened shoe, or postoperative shoe. Sesamoiditis can be treated with anti-inflammatory medications, rest, ice, and activity and shoe-wear modification. Symptomatic nonunions or cases that prove refractory to conservative care can be treated surgically with bone grafting or with partial or complete sesamoidectomy. The results of sesamoidectomy are unpredictable. The most common complications of medial and lateral sesamoidectomy are hallux valgus and varus, respectively. Cock-up deformity is possible if both sesamoids are excised, and with any sesamoid surgery, care should be taken to avoid loss of flexor function, especially in the high-performance athlete.

X. Accessory Bones (Fig. 6–29)

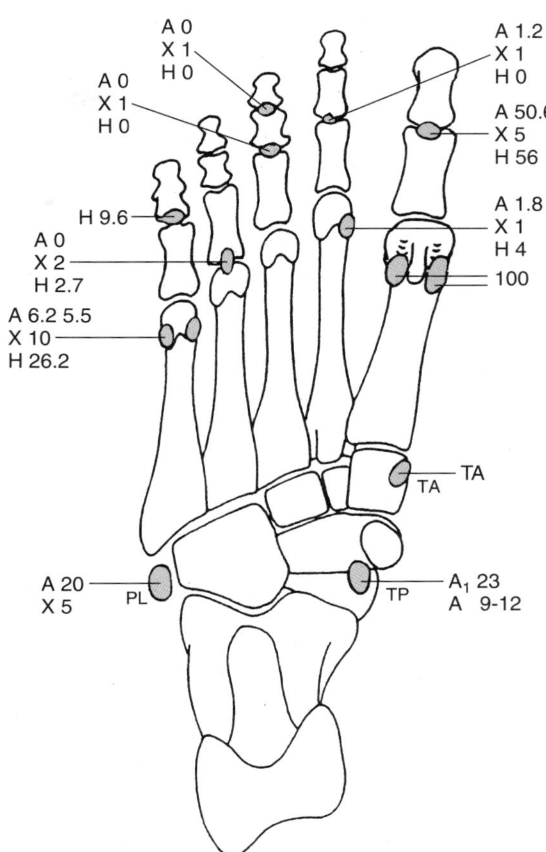

FIGURE 6–29 Sesamoids of the foot. Frequency of occurrence is based on anatomic evaluation (A), histoembryologic investigation (H), and radiographic investigation (X). TA, tibialis anterior; TP, tibialis posterior; PL, peroneus longus. (From Mann RA, Coughlin MJ, eds: Surgery of the Foot and Ankle, 6th ed, vol 1, p 500. St. Louis, CV Mosby, 1993.)

XI. Neurologic Disorders

A. **Interdigital neuritis (Morton neuroma)**—This is a compressive neuropathy of the interdigital nerve, usually between the third and fourth metatarsals (Fig. 6–30). The pathophysiology of this condition is still poorly understood but may involve compression/tension around the intermetatarsal ligament, repetitive microtrauma, vascular changes, excessive bursal tissue, endoneural edema, and eventual neural fibrosis.

1. Diagnosis—Patients (females more than males) complain of burning pain and paresthesia in the involved toes. These symptoms are exacerbated by footwear with narrow toe boxes and high heels. Palpation between and just distal to the metatarsal heads elicits plantar tenderness. Compressing all of the metatarsals while palpating the web space structures can provoke symptoms and occasionally a bursal "click" (Mulder click). Plain films should be performed to rule out bony masses or deformity. MRI has been used to diagnose the condition but is not used universally. Ultrasound may represent a more economical alternative, but a high-resolution device is required.
2. Treatment—Conservative care can include nonsteroidal anti-inflammatory drugs (NSAIDs) and injections, but the most important and effective intervention is modification of shoe wear. Patients should be instructed to avoid high heels and

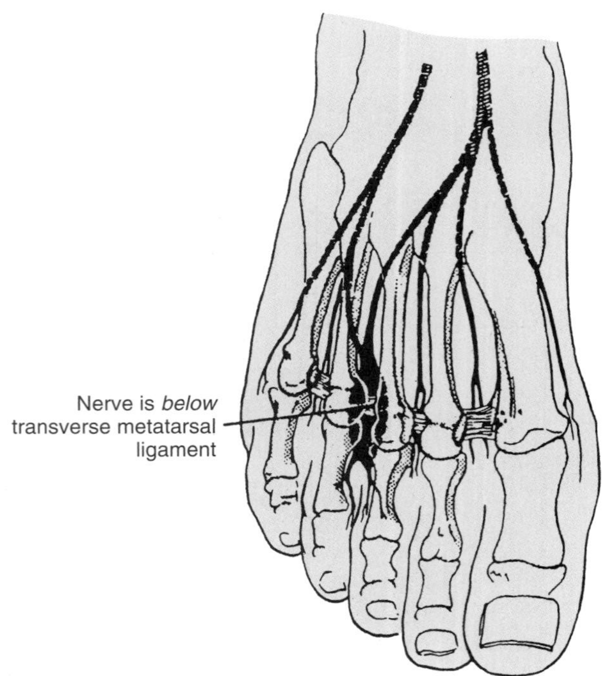

FIGURE 6–30 Third branch of the medial plantar nerve. Note that it courses in a plantar direction under the transverse metatarsal ligament. (From Mann RA, Coughlin MJ, eds: Surgery of the Foot and Ankle, 6th ed, vol 1, p 546. St. Louis, CV Mosby, 1993.)

narrow toe boxes. Metatarsal pads placed proximal to the focus of pain can prevent direct pressure and widen the intermetatarsal space during weight bearing, thereby indirectly decompressing the nerve. Success with surgical intervention is estimated to be 80-85%, so patients must understand that complete relief cannot be guaranteed with neurectomy. A dorsal approach is more common than a volar approach. The transverse intermetatarsal ligament is incised, the common digital nerve and its branches are dissected, and the nerve is resected 2-3 cm proximal to the intermetatarsal ligament, which is proximal to the small plantar branches (Fig. 6–31). This provides the best chance for the proximal stump to retract and minimizes formation of stump neuroma, the most common complication.

B. Recurrent neuroma—This is a secondary glioma or bulbous enlargement of the neural stump that is usually caused by inadequate proximal resection or failure of the nerve to retract.
   1. Diagnosis—In this clinical setting, careful palpation of the posterior tibial nerve and its branches distal to the flexor retinaculum is essential. These symptoms may represent an "irritable" posterior tibial nerve, and no diagnosis beyond this can be found in spite of an extensive workup. However, if the recurrent symptoms are very localized and reproducible and all nonoperative treatment has failed to relieve the patient's localized symptoms, a traction neuritis resulting from neural stump adherence to adjacent bony and soft tissue can be assumed.

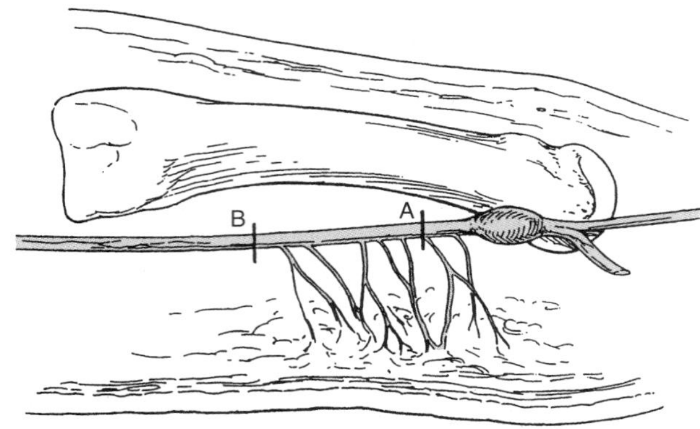

FIGURE 6–31 Treatment of Morton neuroma. Resection should be proximal to the plantar branches of the digital nerve (B). If resection is distal to the plantar branches (A), the nerve stump may not retract. (From Myerson MS: Foot and Ankle Disorders. Philadelphia, WB Saunders, 2000.)

   2. Treatment—This stump neuroma can be excised through another dorsal incision or through a plantar incision placed between the appropriate metatarsal heads. A plantar incision allows access to a very proximal location in which to place the resected neuroma stump. However, the dorsal incision also allows adequate resection if it is extended into the proximal aspect of the intermetatarsal space and the metatarsals are spread well apart during the dissection. The success rate after excision of a recurrent or stump neuroma is 65-75%, compared with the 80-85% success rate after initial excision.

C. **Tarsal tunnel syndrome**—This syndrome manifests compressive neuropathy of the posterior tibial nerve within the fibro-osseous tunnel posterior and inferior to the medial malleolus. The tunnel is bounded by the flexor retinaculum (lancinating ligament) superficially; the medial talus, medial calcaneus, and sustentaculum tali deep; and the abductor hallucis inferiorly. The other structures in the tarsal tunnel include the tendons of the FHL, FDL, and tibialis posterior; the posterior tibial artery; the venae comitantes; and the numerous septa that subdivide the tunnel. There are many reported causes of tarsal tunnel syndrome: tenosynovitis, engorged or varicose vessels, synovial or ganglion cysts, pigmented villonodular synovitis, nerve sheath tumors, lipomas, fracture of the sustentaculum tali or medial tubercle of the posterior process of the talus, middle facet tarsal coalition, and accessory muscles (accessory FDL, tibiocalcaneus internus). Systemic diseases such as diabetes mellitus, rheumatoid arthritis (RA), and ankylosing spondylitis may have an indirect effect by causing inflammatory edema.
   1. Clinical diagnosis—The symptoms of tarsal tunnel syndrome may be vague and misleading, but patients often have a burning sensation on the plantar surface of the foot and occasional sharp pains or paresthesias. Some will demonstrate a Tinel sign, symptoms with continuous deep compression over the nerve, or diminished two-point discrimination. Prolonged standing,

walking, or running can exacerbate the symptoms. All patients being evaluated for tarsal tunnel syndrome should be assessed for pes planus because this is felt to cause increased tension on the nerve. The medial plantar nerve can be entrapped in the master knot of Henry, and the first branch of the lateral plantar nerve (to the abductor digiti quinti muscle) can be entrapped while passing the abductor hallucis. Given the location of these symptoms, proximal plantar fasciitis should always be part of the differential diagnosis.

2. Diagnostic tests—The utility and interpretation of electrodiagnostic studies are still controversial. Motor conduction tests for detecting tarsal tunnel syndrome have demonstrated mixed results in the literature. It is felt that the motor axons are affected later in the disease process. Sensory conduction abnormality seems to occur earlier and is a more sensitive test. Mixed nerve conduction studies can therefore be a helpful diagnostic tool in the setting of a thorough patient history and clinical examination. MRI can direct the surgeon to the specific anatomic structure or abnormality that is causing the tibial nerve compression.
3. Treatment
   a. Conservative treatment—Management should begin with conservative measures unless there is a suspicious mass or suspected malignancy. NSAIDs, ice, elevation, and corticosteroid/lidocaine injections are the mainstays of nonoperative care. Physical therapy may include stretching, massage, desensitization, and iontophoresis. Orthoses to correct hindfoot valgus (medial sole and heel wedge) play an important role as well. In cases of acute inflammation or severe limitation because of pain, a brief course in short-leg casting can be helpful.
   b. Surgical treatment—After 3-6 months of unsuccessful conservative management, surgical release can be performed. A longitudinal incision is made over the course of the tibial nerve that curves distally behind the medial malleolus to the abductor musculature (Fig. 6–32). The nerve is identified proximally, and the proximal investing fascia and flexor retinaculum are released. Care should be taken to release any septa in the tunnel as well as the superficial and deep fascia of the abductor hallucis muscle (Fig. 6–33). Endoscopic tarsal tunnel release has been performed but is not the favored procedure (the other structures of the tarsal tunnel are placed at greater risk, and large-mass lesions cannot be addressed). Recurrence of tarsal tunnel syndrome is a challenging problem. Incomplete release is the most common etiology, and revision release is generally not recommended because the results are often poor.

D. Anterior tarsal tunnel syndrome—This syndrome manifests a compressive neuropathy of the DPN in the fibro-osseous tunnel formed by the Y-shaped inferior extensor retinaculum (Fig. 6–34). The nerve divides into the lateral motor and the medial sensory branches within the tunnel and is accompanied by the dorsalis pedis artery. The common causes of compression include tightly laced shoes; anterior osteophytes at the tibiotalar and talonavicular articulations; a bony prominence associated with pes cavus deformity or fracture; ganglion cysts; and tendinitis of the EDL, EHL, and tibialis anterior (Fig. 6–35).

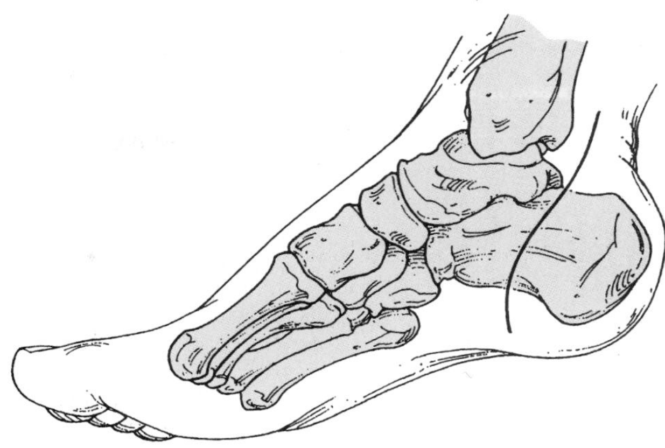

FIGURE 6–32 Incision for tarsal tunnel release. (From DiGiovanni BF, Gould JS: Tarsal tunnel syndrome and related entities. Foot Ankle Clin 3:405-426. 1998.)

1. Diagnosis—Patients present with burning pain and paresthesias along the medial second toe, lateral hallux, and first web space or even vague dorsal foot pain. Symptoms are often worse at night as the ankle assumes a plantar-flexed posture. On examination, decreased two-point discrimination and a Tinel sign can be elicited. The nerve is under greater stretch with the ankle plantar flexed and the toes dorsiflexed, making wearing high-heeled, narrow-toed shoes problematic.
2. Treatment—Night splints, NSAIDs, diagnostic/therapeutic injections, shoe tongue padding, and footwear with loose lacing are the conservative approaches. Surgical release involves incising the inferior extensor retinaculum, releasing both branches of the nerve, excising bone spurs, and carefully repairing the bony capsule to avoid exposing the nerve to bleeding bone while protecting the dorsalis pedis artery. Patients should understand that relief of the paresthesias and dysesthesias may take weeks or months.

E. Sequelae of upper motor neuron disorders—The most common CNS disorders that result in these problems include traumatic brain injury, stroke, and spinal cord injury.

1. Pathology—Disruption of the upper motor neuron pathways can lead to paralysis, muscular imbalance, acquired spasticity, and deformity of the foot and ankle. Secondary problems include fixed contractures, calluses, pressure sores, hygiene issues, joint subluxation, shoe-wear

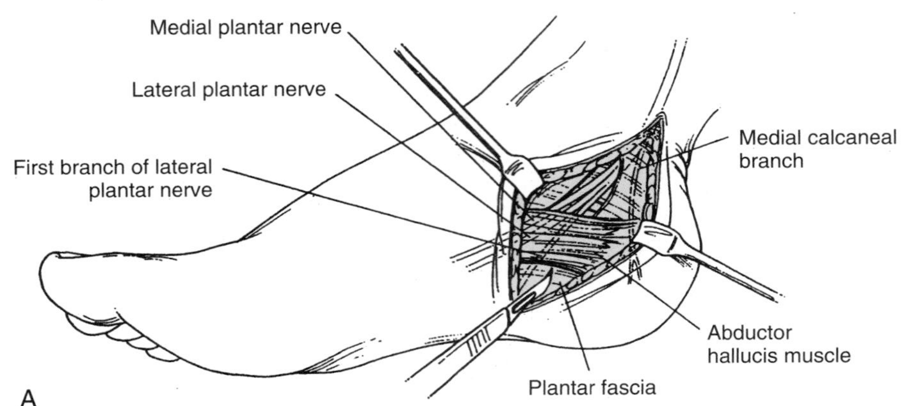

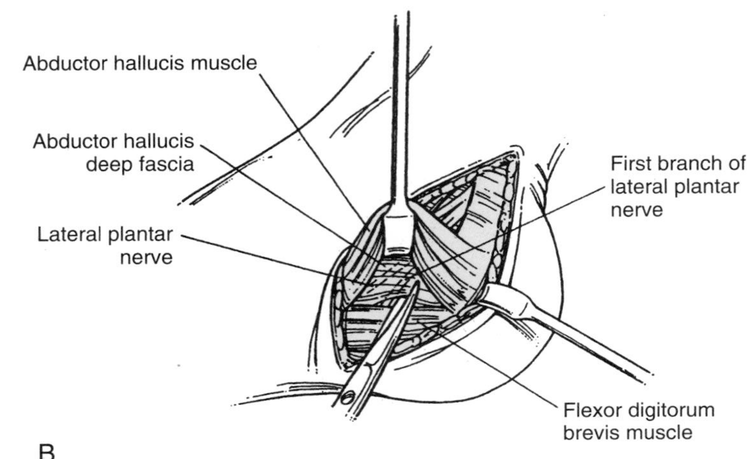

FIGURE 6–33 Incising the superficial fascia of the abductor hallucis muscle (**A**) and the deep fascia (**B**) is necessary to adequately release the lateral plantar nerve and its first branch. (From DiGiovanni BF, Gould JS: Tarsal tunnel syndrome and related entities. Foot Ankle Clin 3:405-426, 1998.)

difficulties, and dissatisfaction with physical appearance. The most common deformity of the foot and ankle is equinovarus. The equinus component is caused by overactivity of the gastrocnemius-soleus complex. The varus is due to relative overactivity of the tibialis anterior, with lesser contributions from the FHL, FDL, and tibialis posterior.

2. Treatment
   a. Nonoperative care—The key to nonoperative management is early intervention with physical therapy, stretching and strengthening, and maintenance of joint range of motion. Other modalities include splinting, serial casting, oral muscle relaxants, phenol and lidocaine nerve blocks, and botulinum toxin injections. Phenol blocks have a proven history, will often have longer-lasting effects, and are less expensive than botulinum toxin. The advantage of botulinum is the ease of delivery; it needs only an injection into the muscle belly, rather than a precise injection around the motor nerve.
   b. Surgical treatment—**Equinus deformity** is surgically addressed with lengthening of the Achilles tendon. The most common techniques are Z-lengthening, fractional lengthening, and percutaneous triple hemisectioning (Fig. 6–36). Varus deformity is addressed with a **split anterior tibialis tendon transfer** (SPLATT) to the lateral cuneiform or cuboid. Release of the toe flexors is sometimes required because toe flexion deformity occurs by a tenodesis effect as the ankle is brought into a more plantigrade position (Fig. 6–37). If a fixed bony component to the deformity exists, lateral closing wedge osteotomy, subtalar fusion, or calcaneal osteotomy may be necessary. Surgery for acquired spasticity should be delayed at least 6 months after onset to allow for maximum recovery.

F. Charcot-Marie-Tooth disease—**Charcot-Marie-Tooth** (CMT) disease is the most common inherited neuropathy, affecting approximately 1 in every 2500 people. There are many genetic variants of CMT disease, and more are described as diagnostic tools become more sophisticated.

1. Forms—In the autosomal dominant form of CMT disease, there is a duplication of chromosome 17. An abnormal myelin protein is the basis of CMT degenerative neuropathy. Males are more

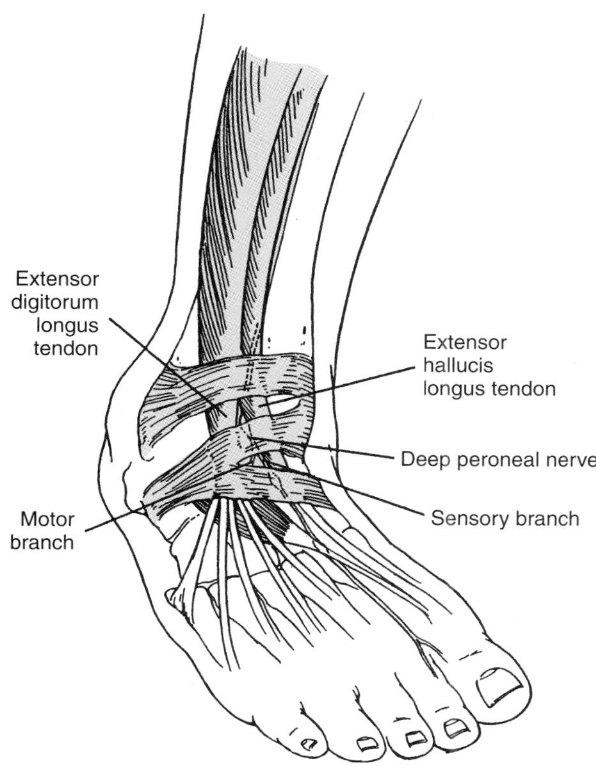

FIGURE 6–34 Anatomy of the deep peroneal nerve and the extensor retinaculum. (From Myerson MS: Foot and Ankle Disorders. Philadelphia, WB Saunders, 2000.)

commonly affected, but the disease is usually more severe in females. The earlier the onset, the more severe the neurologic findings. The autosomal recessive patients present the earliest, usually at less than 10 years of age. Sex-linked recessive inheritance usually presents in the second decade, and the autosomal dominant in the third decade. Sensory deficit is variable and may be manifested as proprioceptive loss more than pure sensory deficit. However, when sensory loss is severe, recurrent ulceration, deep infection, and even neuropathic arthropathy can mimic diabetic neurologic loss.

2. Diagnosis—Patients complain of deformity and awkward gait more often than pain. These complaints are manifestations of the common findings on physical examination. The physical examination reveals a symmetrical elevation of the arches, a plantar-flexed first ray, hindfoot varus, claw toes, decreased ankle jerks, and a flatfoot or toe-heel gait (marionette gait). In addition, the EDB and extensor hallucis brevis (EHB) are atrophied. The patient's thighs appear of normal size, but the lower legs appear smaller than normal. Prominent and tender calluses may be present beneath the metatarsal heads because of the cavus deformity associated with claw toes and distal migration of the forefoot pad. The toe extensors are recruited in the swing phase of gait as ankle dorsiflexors because of a weak tibialis anterior. Ankle eversion is weak owing to peroneus brevis atrophy, but the peroneus longus function remains strong. It is this imbalance from a weakened tibialis anterior compared with the peroneus longus that contributes to the plantar-flexed first metatarsal. With the first metatarsal plantar flexed and the forefoot pronated (valgus), the hindfoot supinates, compensatory hindfoot varus develops, and the distal tibia and fibula externally rotate. Once the spectrum of linked deformities develops, it is only a matter of time until they become fixed. It is this difference between fixed (cannot be passively corrected) and flexible (passively correctable) deformities that has such a profound effect on the treatment plan. The Coleman block test (Fig. 6–38) can be used to determine if a hindfoot varus deformity is fixed or flexible.
3. Treatment
   a. Flexible deformity—In an adolescent with closed physes and a supple deformity, surgical rather than brace management is currently recommended because of the progressive pattern of this disease. Surgical treatment involves (1) release of the plantar fascia,

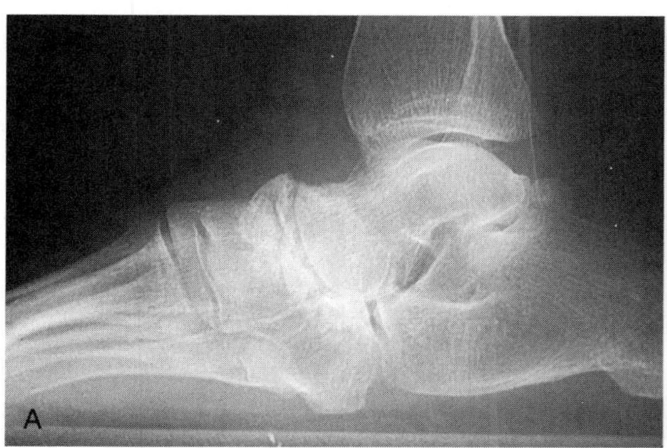

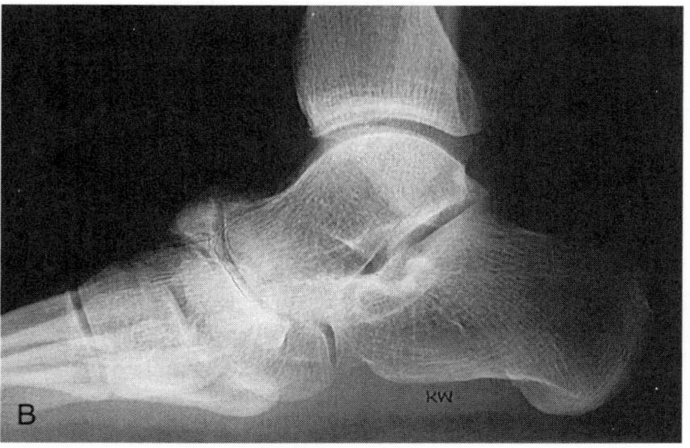

FIGURE 6–35 Arthritis of the talonavicular joint (**A**) or nonunion of a navicular fracture (**B**) can compress the deep peroneal nerve. (From Myerson MS: Foot and Ankle Disorders. Philadelphia, WB Saunders, 2000.)

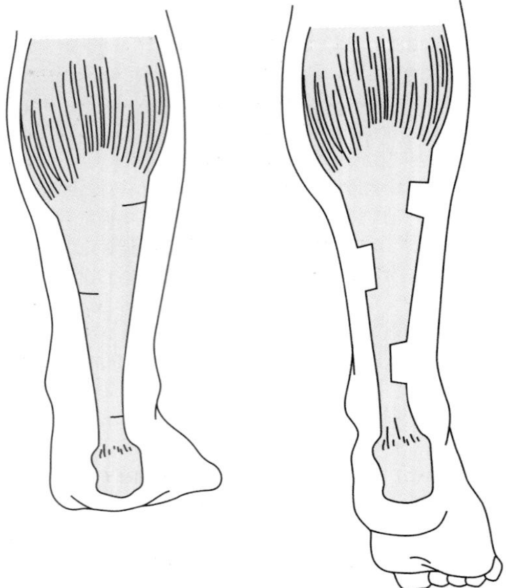

FIGURE 6–36 Triple hemisectioning of the Achilles tendon. (From Mann RA: Surgery of the Foot, 5th ed. St. Louis, CV Mosby, 1986.)

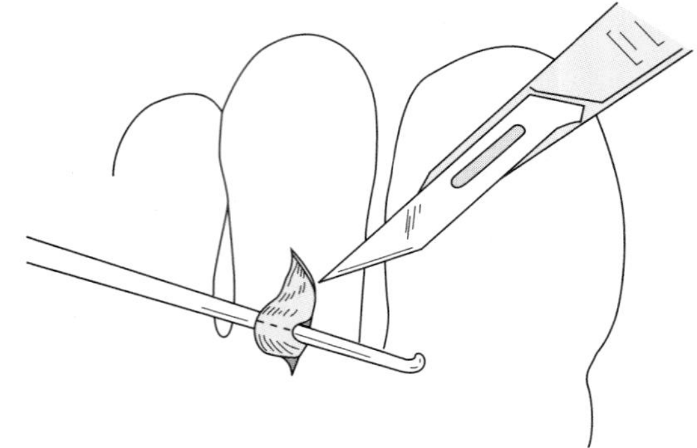

FIGURE 6–37 Toe flexor release. (From Keenan MAE, Botte MJ: Traumatic brain injury. In Nickel VL, Botte MJ, eds: Orthopaedic Rehabilitation, 2nd ed. New York, Churchill Livingstone, 1992.)

(2) closing-wedge dorsiflexion osteotomy of the first metatarsal (occasionally including the second metatarsal in older patients), (3) calcaneal sliding and closing-wedge osteotomies, (4) transfer of the peroneus longus into the peroneus brevis at the level of the distal fibula, and (5) frequently Achilles tendon lengthening (TAL). Clawing of the toes is improved by flexor-to-extensor transfers and extensor tendon lengthening or tenotomy.

b. Fixed deformity—If brace management is chosen, a locked-ankle, short-leg cast (ankle-foot orthosis) with an outside (varus-correcting or lateral) T-strap is recommended. A rocker sole also aids the gait and decreases the energy expended. Fixed deformities usually require a triple arthrodesis for hindfoot correction, with transfer of the posterior tibial tendon through the interosseous membrane and a TAL. A plantar fascia release, dorsiflexion osteotomy of the first or second metatarsal or both, and correction of the claw toe deformities might also be required. If many procedures are required to correct multiple fixed deformities, they should be staged. The clawed hallux can be surgically treated with a Jones procedure (arthrodesis of the interphalangeal joint and transfer of the EHL to the first metatarsal). Clawing of the lesser toes is improved by capsulotomies of the MTP joints, extensor tendon lengthening, and resection of the head and neck of the proximal phalanges. The younger the patient, the more

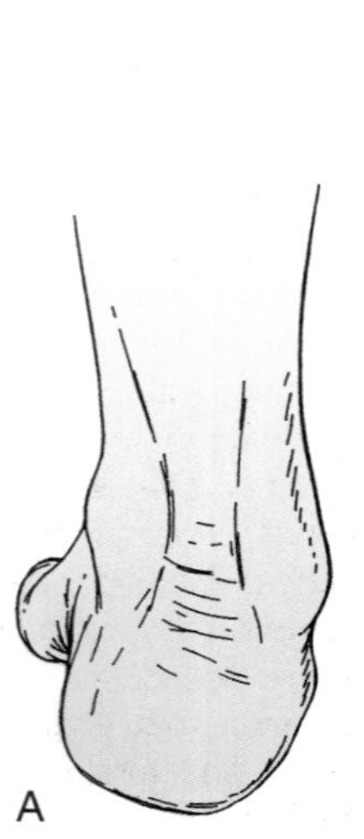

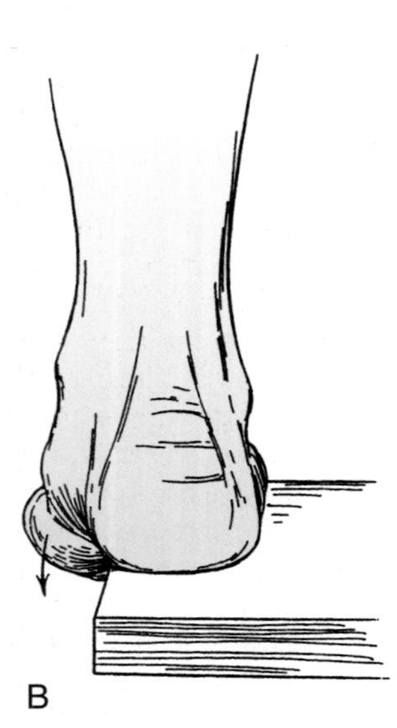

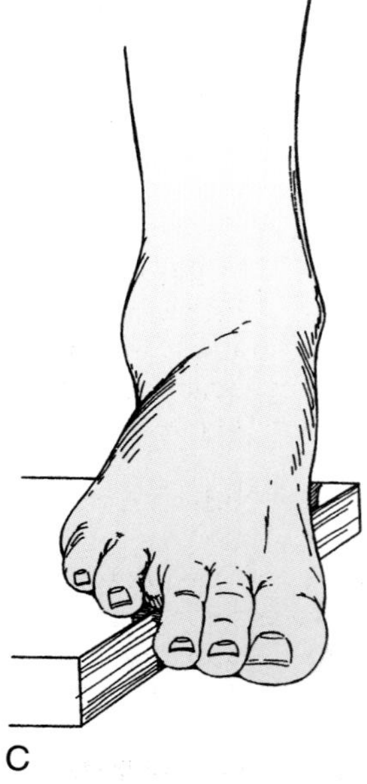

FIGURE 6–38 Coleman block test for determining flexibility of the hindfoot component of cavus deformity. **A**, Hindfoot varus. Posterior (**B**) and anterior (**C**) views of flexible hindfoot varus. (From Myerson MS: Foot and Ankle Disorders. Philadelphia, WB Saunders, 2000.)

important it is to try soft tissue releases, tendon transfers, and osteotomies to avoid degenerative arthritic changes in joints adjacent to those that have been fused. Even in mild fixed deformities, every effort should be made to preserve cartilage unless the deformities cannot be corrected without arthrodesis.

XII. Arthritic Disease

A. Crystalline disease

1. Gout

a. Pathology—**Gout** is a disease of abnormal purine metabolism that results in precipitation and deposition of monosodium urate crystals into synovium-lined joints. The deposition of these needle-shaped crystals into the joint fluid induces a severe inflammatory response. Gout may be induced by certain medications that increase serum uric acid, localized trauma, alcohol, or purine-rich foods as well as by the postsurgical state. Men are more commonly affected than women.

b. Diagnosis—The attack is sudden and very painful, with intense signs of inflammation (redness, swelling, warmth, tenderness). The great toe MTP joint is most often involved (50-75% of initial attacks), and over a chronic course, 90% of patients with gouty attacks will have one or more episodes involving the hallux MTP joint (podagra). Characteristic radiographic signs are inordinate soft tissue enlargement about the MTP joint and bony erosions at a distance from the joint articular surface as well as erosions on both sides of the joint. However, in the chronic condition, after a number of attacks and large deposits of gouty residue (tophi), extensive articular and periarticular destruction can occur. The diagnosis of gouty arthropathy is usually a clinical one, with a characteristic history (''Not even a sheet could touch it'') and physical findings. However, pathognomonic signs are needle-shaped monosodium urate crystals, which under polarized light are strongly negatively birefringent. The serum uric acid may or may not be elevated.

c. Treatment—An acute attack is usually treated with indomethacin or colchicine. If chronic gouty attacks have destroyed the joint or deposited large quantities of tophi, an arthrodesis, removal of quantities of tophaceous debris, or both may be required.

2. Pseudogout

a. Pathology—**Pseudogout (chondrocalcinosis)** commonly affects the knee but may present in an articulation of the foot or ankle. It may have a severe initial inflammatory response due to deposition of **calcium pyrophosphate dihydrate** (CPPD) crystals in or about a joint. Pseudogout is usually articular, with less periarticular soft tissue involvement than gout, although inflammatory signs may be striking.

b. Diagnosis—The diagnosis is confirmed by joint aspiration, which reveals weakly positive birefringent crystals under polarized light microscopy. These crystals may have varied shapes. The lesser MTP joints can be affected as well as the talonavicular and subtalar joints, whereas in gout, these joints usually are not involved. On radiographs, intra-articular calcifications are often seen, which are not characteristic of gout. Joint destruction can occur with recurrent attacks over a long period, but this is rare.

c. Treatment—Treatment is with rest, oral NSAIDs for acute chemical synovitis, and protected weight bearing.

B. **Seronegative spondyloarthropathy** (SNSA)

1. Diagnosis—These inflammatory arthritides are negative for rheumatoid factor and distinguished from RA clinically by a higher incidence of involvement of entheses (i.e., the interface between collagen and bone where ligament, tendon, and capsular tissue insert into bone). A predilection for involvement of this transitional tissue is found in psoriatic arthritis, ankylosing spondylitis, Reiter syndrome, and inflammatory bowel disease. These arthritides may also destroy articular cartilage but characteristically are more destructive toward collagen and fibrocartilage. Osteopenia is rare in these entities, and in contrast to RA, it often presents in the foot as plantar fasciitis or Achilles tendinitis. Psoriatic arthritis can present with swollen and inflamed distal joints or, more classically, as dactylitis, or ''sausage digit.'' Additional findings may include nail pitting, onycholysis, and keratosis. The posterior tibial tendon can become inflamed and attenuated as well. When periarticular, bony erosion does occur, the classic ''pencil-in-cup'' sign is typical of psoriatic arthritis (Fig. 6–39).

2. Treatment—NSAIDs are the mainstay of treatment. On occasion, methotrexate or sulfasalazine will be prescribed under the direction and observation of a rheumatologist. Recalcitrant Achilles tendinitis/tendinopathy and plantar fasciitis occasionally benefit from surgical intervention.

C. **Rheumatoid arthritis**—This condition is a chronic, symmetrical polyarthropathy that most commonly presents in the third and fourth decades and is more prevalent in women. Synovitis is the mechanism by which this systemic disease causes ligament and capsular laxity and cartilage and bony erosion. The vasculitis and soft tissue fragility that is common in patients with RA must be respected. Diligent care of the soft tissues during nonoperative and operative management is essential. Immune-mediating pharmacologic therapies (e.g., methotrexate) are routinely discontinued in the perioperative period.

1. Diagnosis—The majority of rheumatoid patients have difficulties with their feet. The forefoot is more commonly involved than the midfoot or hindfoot. The pathophysiology and symptomatology

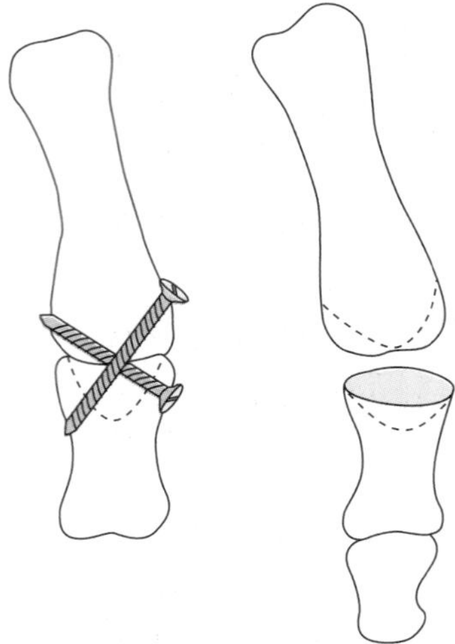

FIGURE 6–39 "Pencil-in-cup" technique for joint arthrodesis of the first MTP.

are initiated by synovitis (usually at the MTP joints). Chronic synovitis can lead to incompetence of the joint capsules and collateral ligaments. The toes tend to sublux and even dislocate dorsally, deviate laterally into valgus, and develop hammering (Fig. 6–40). The intrinsic muscles worsen the claw-toe deformity, and the plantar fat pad migrates distally and atrophies, allowing the metatarsal heads to apply more plantar pressure and form keratoses. As the lesser toes deviate laterally, the hallux moves into valgus alignment and transfer metatarsalgia worsens. The midfoot and hindfoot are less commonly and less severely involved in RA. When these joints are affected, the subtalar joint deviates into valgus, the talar head drops into plantar flexion, and the navicular is displaced laterally, resulting in a pes planovalgus foot.

2. Treatment—Synovitis can be treated conservatively with rest, NSAIDs, immune-modulating drugs under the direction of rheumatologists, toe taping, orthoses, and careful use of corticosteroid injections. Synovectomy of the MTP joints can provide symptomatic relief early in the course of the disease and may delay soft tissue and joint destruction. Once deformity has occurred, "rheumatoid forefoot reconstruction" is indicated (Fig. 6–41). This involves first MTP arthrodesis (resection and silicone arthroplasty have met with poor results due to cock-up deformity, silicone synovitis, and osteolysis), resection arthroplasty, and pinning of the lesser MTP joints and closed osteoclasis of the interphalangeal joints. This can be accomplished through two well-placed longitudinal dorsal incisions (Fig. 6–42). Extensor brevis

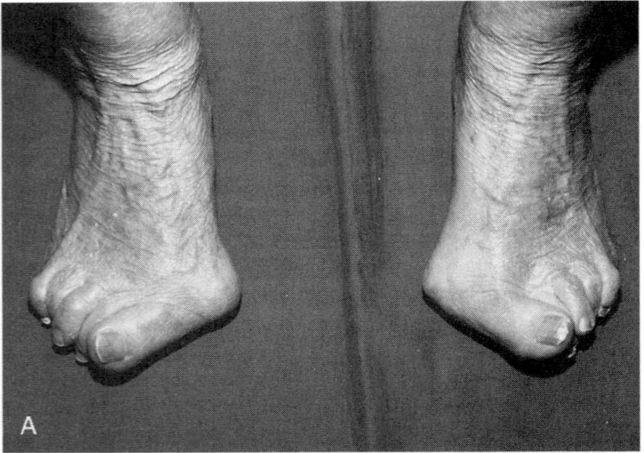

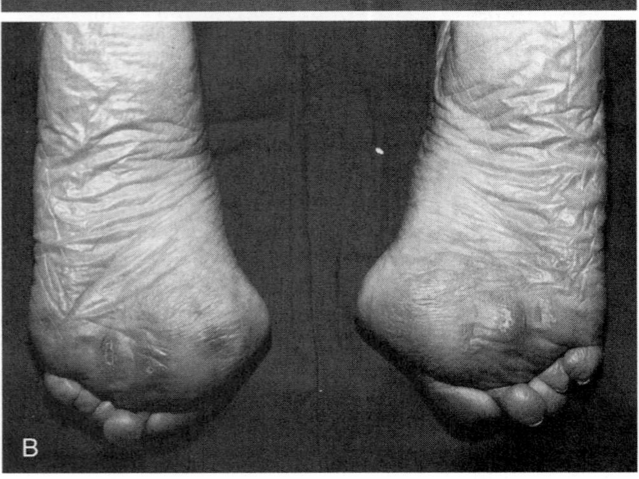

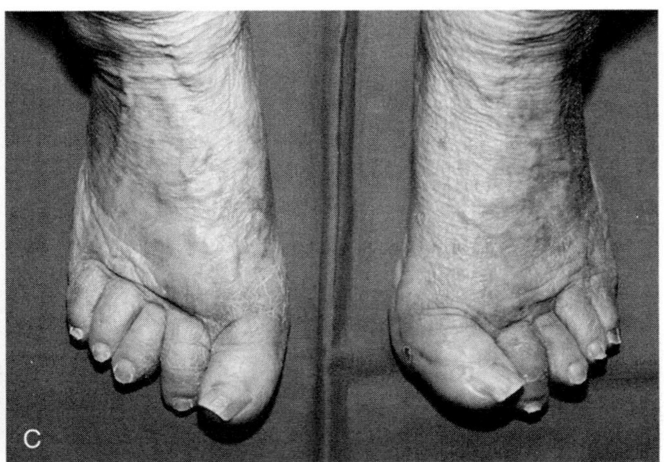

FIGURE 6–40 Clinical appearance of rheumatoid arthritis of the forefoot. (From Myerson MS: Foot and Ankle Disorders. Philadelphia, WB Saunders, 2000.)

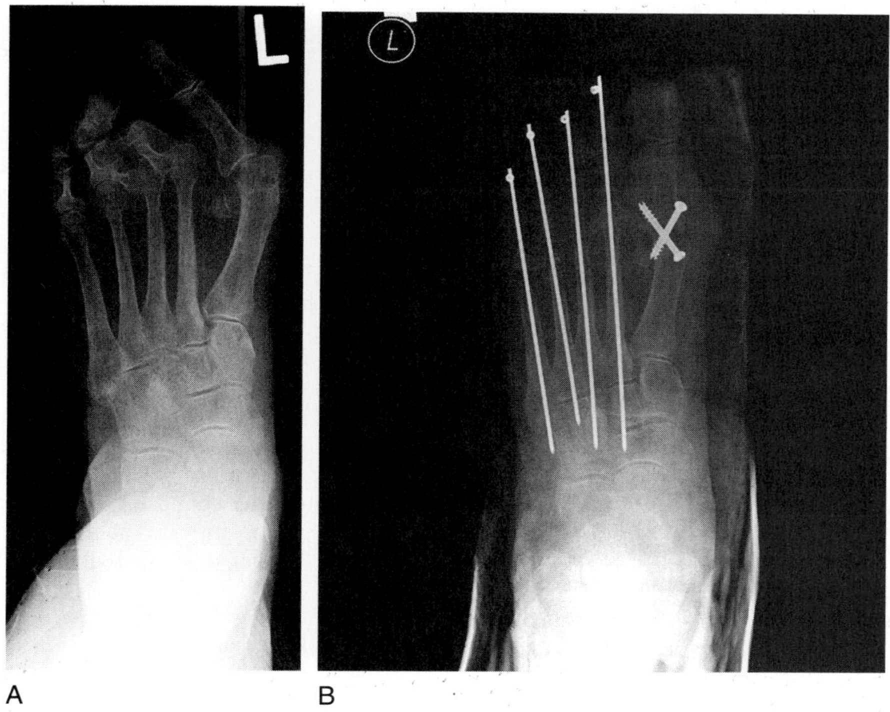

FIGURE 6–41 Preoperative (**A**) and postoperative (**B**) radiographs for rheumatoid forefoot reconstruction.

tenotomy, Z-lengthening of the extensor longus tendons, and resection of the base of the proximal phalanges may be necessary. A cup-in-cone technique for the first MTP fusion is helpful. The lesser MTPs should be pinned in position before the final hallux MTP position is chosen (approximately 15 degrees of valgus and 20-25 degrees of dorsiflexion relative to the metatarsal). If the patient has supple midfoot or hindfoot deformity, orthoses can provide adequate relief and maintenance of alignment. When the deformity is fixed, triple arthrodesis is recommended.

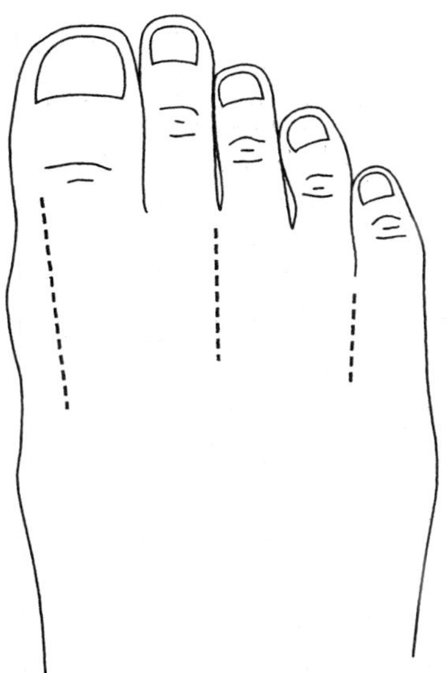

FIGURE 6–42 Incisions for first MTP joint arthrodesis and lesser MTP joint resection arthroplasty for rheumatoid arthritis.

D. Osteoarthritis—**Osteoarthritis** and **post-traumatic arthritis** share similarities in the mechanical nature of the problem, clinical presentation, and treatment algorithm. Whereas trauma is the most common cause of arthritis in the hindfoot and tibiotalar articulations, osteoarthritis commonly affects the first MTP joint and the midfoot joints (tarsometatarsal, intercuneiform, navicular-cuneiform, and talonavicular joints). In addition, other disorders, such as lateral ankle instability, posterior tibial tendon insufficiency, and neuromuscular deformities, can cause or contribute to degenerative arthritis.

1. Diagnosis—Patients have tenderness over the dorsum of the first MTP joint and limited dorsiflexion. The earliest radiographic sign may be a small depression in the dome of the metatarsal head. When the hallux is extended, abutment of the proximal phalanx against this lesion in the articular cartilage produces pain and instinctive flexion of the joint, thereby limiting extension. As the disease worsens, an osteophyte at the dorsal articular margin of the metatarsal head presents a mechanical block to extension. The severity of hallux rigidus is determined by radiographic appearance:
   - Grade I—Mild to moderate osteophyte formation with joint space preservation
   - Grade II—Moderate osteophyte formation with joint space narrowing and subchondral sclerosis
   - Grade III—Marked osteophyte formation and diminished joint space, including the inferior portion

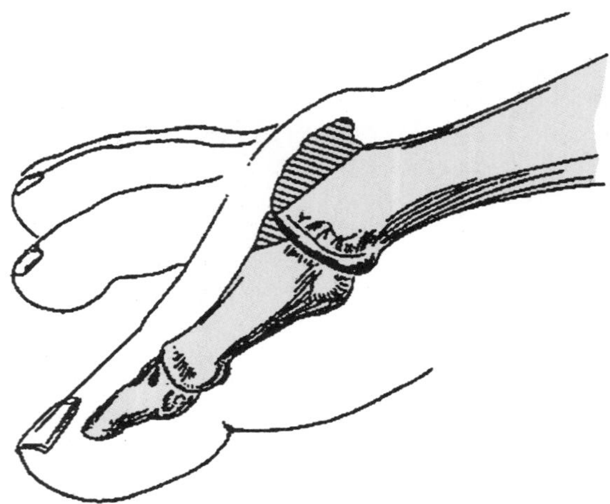

FIGURE 6–43 Standard cheilectomy for first MTP joint arthritis.

Most patients with grades I and II changes can be treated with cheilectomy (removal of the proliferative bone from around the metatarsal head), which removes the buttress preventing dorsiflexion of the proximal phalanx on the metatarsal head (Fig. 6–43). Some authors have reported that adding an extension osteotomy of the proximal phalanx improves patient satisfaction. Patients with grade III changes usually require arthrodesis or Keller resection arthroplasty (Table 6–6).

2. Treatment—Initial treatment should include anti-inflammatory medications, activity modification, and orthotic support or bracing. Hallux rigidus can be conservatively managed with a stiff foot plate with an extension under the great toe. Midfoot arthritis can also benefit from a stiff sole and possibly a rocker bottom. Hindfoot pain secondary to degenerative arthritis can be addressed with a University of California–Berkeley Biomechanics Laboratory (UCBL) orthosis. For ankle degeneration, an ankle-foot orthosis with a rocker bottom will often provide relief. Surgical management of foot and ankle osteoarthritis usually involves arthrodesis. Degenerative arthritis of the first MTP joint often results in hallux rigidus, in which motion of the joint is limited to varying degrees. A number of causative factors have been suggested, including trauma, repeated microtrauma, osteochondral fractures (particularly in adolescent and young-adult athletes), hyperextension of the first metatarsal, an abnormally long first metatarsal, and severe foot pronation.

XIII. Postural Disorders

A. Pes planus deformity—Pes planus (flatfoot) can be either a congenital or an acquired deformity. The acquired deformities are addressed in this section, and congenital deformities are reviewed in Chapter 3, Pediatric Orthopaedics. Flatfoot is further characterized as flexible or fixed.

1. Pathology—The most common cause of adult **acquired flatfoot** is posterior tibial tendinitis, a degenerative problem involving the primary dynamic support for the arch. The multifactorial etiology may include inflammatory disorders such as RA, a zone of hypovascularity 2-6 cm from the

TABLE 6-6 NONOPERATIVE AND ARTHRODESIS RECOMMENDATIONS FOR FOOT AND ANKLE ARTHRITIS

Joint/Condition	Brace/Orthosis	Position of Arthrodesis
Ankle arthritis	Fixed ankle-foot orthosis; double-upright brace applied to the shoe	Ankle arthrodesis 5° DF 5-10° ER Neutral varus/valgus Total ankle replacement: very limited role
Hindfoot arthritis (triple arthrodesis, all joints) Subtalar Talonavicular Calcaneocuboid	UCBL (University of California–Berkeley Biomechanics Laboratory	Subtalar arthrodesis 10° valgus 0° rotation Talonavicular 0° varus/valgus forefoot 0° talonavicular-1st MT angle Calcaneocuboid 0° varus/valgus forefoot
Tarsometatarsal joints (Lisfranc)	Rigid-soled shoe or carbon footplate	1st, 2nd, 3rd TMT arthrodesis 4th, 5th TMT resection arthroplasty with or without interposition graft
1st MTP arthritis	Rigid-soled shoe or carbon foot plate	1st MTP arthrodesis 10° DF in relation to floor or 25° DF in relationship to 1st MT 5-10° valgus (< 10° valgus puts more stress on IP joint with risk of IP arthritis) Neutral rotation Keller resection arthroplasty (see Adult Hallux Valgus) 1st MTP implant Not recommended

DF, dorsiflexion; ER, external rotation; IP, interphalangeal; MT, metatarsal; MTP, metatarsophalangeal; TMT, tarsometatarsophalangeal.

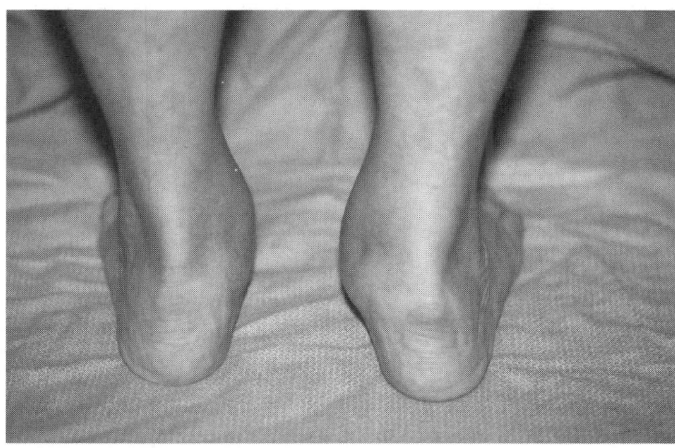

FIGURE 6–44 "Too many toes" sign with acquired flatfoot deformity.

attachment of the tendon on the navicular, and overload of the arch from activity or obesity. The posterior tibial tendon fires after the foot is flat to generate heel rise and locking of the transverse tarsal joint for a rigid, stable foot during push-off.

2. Diagnosis—The foot position during standing demonstates that the hindfoot is in valgus, the arch is depressed, and the forefoot is abducted, exposing "too many toes" when the foot is viewed posteriorly (Fig. 6–44). Flexible deformities are passively correctable to a plantigrade foot, and bracewear may improve the alignment and reduce pain. Fixed deformities are rigid malalignments of the hindfoot that are considered unbraceable and may require surgical correction. The rigid nature is often secondary to arthritis of the hindfoot joints. The four stages of tendinitis are listed along with the physical examination findings, symptoms, and treatment options in Tables 6–7 and 6–8.
3. Treatment—The most challenging decisions for surgery are with stages II and IV deformities. Stage II occurs when the tendon is tearing and functionally incompetent but passively correctable. The current recommendations include a medial tendon transfer (usually FDL to a tunnel in the navicular) and either a medial calcaneal displacement osteotomy or lateral column lengthening at the calcaneocuboid joint or through the distal calcaneus. A short gastrocnemius-soleus complex is considered a primary deforming force and is lengthened by the hemisection method or a gastrocnemius slide. Stage IV is characterized by deltoid ligament involvement and is best seen on a standing anteroposterior radiograph of the ankle demonstrating talar tilt in the ankle mortise. A reliable reconstruction of the deltoid ligament has not been clearly defined at this time, making complete correction of this deformity difficult.

B. Pes cavus deformity—**Pes cavus deformity** is a highly arched foot that most frequently occurs with neurological disorders producing soft tissue imbalance.
   1. Etiology—The etiology of the unilateral cavus foot needs to be investigated to rule out tethering of the spinal cord or spinal cord tumors. When the deformity is bilateral it is most often associated with a hereditary pattern of presentation, the most common being CMT disease (peroneal muscle atrophy), which affects 1 in 2500 people. The tibialis anterior, EDL, and peroneus brevis musculature are initially affected, leading to the cavus malalignment. The genetic workup can provide a diagnosis and inform the patient of the genetic influence of the disease and transmission pathway. The mixed motor sensory neuropathies such as CMT have variable penetrance; therefore, the severity of each cavus foot may differ.
   2. Diagnosis and treatment—There are multiple components to the cavus foot and therefore varying presenting symptoms, and the surgical approach is tailored to each case. The most common complaints are painful calluses under the first metatarsal, fifth metatarsal, and medial heel due to the plantar-flexed first ray and varus hindfoot. The Coleman block test (see Fig. 6–38) is used to assess the flexibility of the hindfoot (out of varus) when the first metatarsal plantar flexion (forefoot valgus) is eliminated. A wooden block is

TABLE 6-7 PHYSICAL EXAMINATION FOR POSTERIOR TIBIAL TENDON DYSFUNCTION

				Deformity			
Stage	**Symptoms**	**Pathology**	**Arch**	*Abducted Forefoot*	*Valgus Hindfoot*	*Single-Limb Heel-Rise*	*"Too Many Toes"*
I	Medial ankle pain, swelling	Synovitis	Normal	Negative	Negative	Normal	Negative
IIA	Medial ankle pain, swelling, ± sinus tarsi pain	Tenosynovitis and degeneration	Loss	Negative	Positive	Abnormal	Negative
IIB	Medial ankle pain, swelling, ± sinus tarsi pain	Tenosynovitis and degeneration	Loss	Positive	Positive	Abnormal	Positive
III	Sinus tarsi pain, fibular abutment pain	Degenerative arthritis of the hindfoot	Loss	Positive	Positive	Abnormal	Positive
IV	Sinus tarsi pain, fibular abutment pain, ankle pain	Degenerative arthritis of the hindfoot and deltoid insufficiency and talar tilt	Loss	Positive	Positive	Abnormal	Positive

TABLE 6-8 TREATMENT OF PES PLANUS DEFORMITY

Stage	Treatment	
	Nonoperative Treatment	*Operative Treatment*
I	Immobilize (cast, boot, brace); NSAIDs; medial heel and sole wedge orthosis	Synovectomy
IIA	Ankle brace (over-the-counter or custom); UCBL orthosis; short articulated AFO; medial heel and sole wedge orthosis	TAL or gastroc slide; FDL to navicular transfer Bone options Medial displacement calcaneal osteotomy Subtalar arthrodesis
IIB	Ankle brace (over-the-counter or custom); UCBL orthosis; short articulated AFO; medial heel and sole wedge orthosis	TAL or gastroc slide; FDL to navicular transfer Bone options Lateral column lengthening with or without medial displacement calcaneal osteotomy Subtalar arthrodesis
III	Articulated AFO; custom ankle brace	Triple arthrodesis; TAL or gastroc slide
IV	Nonarticulated AFO; custom ankle brace	Triple arthrodesis; TAL or gastroc slide; and deltoid ligament reconstruction

AFO, ankle-foot orthosis; FDL, flexor digitorum longus; gastroc, gastrocnemius; NSAIDs, nonsteroidal anti-inflammatory drugs; TAL, Achilles tendon lengthening; UCBL, University of California–Berkeley Biomechanics Laboratory.

placed just lateral to the first ray so that the first metatarsal head can lie off the block and the remainder of the block can be on the weight-bearing foot. If the hindfoot is passively correctable, the hindfoot will go into valgus. This would suggest that correction of the forefoot valgus with a first metatarsal dorsiflexion osteotomy would correct the foot position. If the hindfoot is not corrected with the block test, a calcaneal lateral closing wedge osteotomy or a subtalar fusion may be needed if arthritic symptoms are present. Other nonoperative and operative recommendations are presented in Table 6–9.

XIV. Tendon Disorders

A. Achilles tendon—The Achilles tendon is addressed in the section on heel pain.

B. Peroneal tendons
1. Diagnosis—The history reveals localized swelling and tenderness over peroneal tendons that may be chronic. The location of pain can be behind the fibula secondary to recurrent peroneal subluxation or dislocation or just distal to the fibula, a common location for peroneus brevis degenerative tears. Very rarely, an acute injury can occur to the peroneal tendons, resulting in an acute rupture of the peroneus longus tendon at or through a fracture of the os peroneum. Classically, radiographs show a retraction or fracture of the os peroneum, requiring acute repair.
2. Treatment
   a. Nonoperative treatment—Chronic peroneal tendinosis or tenosynovitis is initially treated nonoperatively with activity modification, NSAIDs, an ankle brace to decrease

TABLE 6-9 TREATMENT OF CAVUS FOOT

Component	Treatment	
	Nonoperative Treatment	*Operative Treatment*
Claw toe	Toe-tip Silipos sleeves	
Flexible claw toe		FDL tenotomies on toes 2-5
Fixed claw-toe deformity		PIP and DIP resections
Ankle instability	Ankle brace	
Painful plantar calluses of 1st and 5th rays	Total contact inserts	
Equinus deformity due to dorsiflexion weakness		Achilles tendon lengthening or gastrocnemius slide
Plantar-flexed ray		Dorsiflexion osteotomy of 1st (2nd and 3rd as needed) MT
Peroneus longus–deforming force on 1st ray		Peroneus longus–to–brevis transfer to aid in eversion
Uncorrectable hindfoot varus (unresponsive to Coleman block test) or subtalar arthrodesis for arthritis		Dwyer closing lateral wedge calcaneal osteotomy
Fixed hindfoot varus and fixed forefoot valgus with arthritis of the hindfoot joints		Triple arthrodesis

DIP, distal interphalangeal; FDL, flexor digitorum longus; MT, metatarsal; PIP, proximal interphalangeal.

subtalar motion and rest the tendons, and physical therapy. If 6-8 weeks of rest and physical therapy do not improve the symptoms, an MRI may reveal a tear, although false-negative results have been reported in the literature with MRI for longitudinal tears of the peroneal tendons.

b. Surgical treatment—Surgical treatment is indicated for resistant cases of peroneal tendinitis. The surgical procedure is based on the pathology: tenosynovectomy, débridement and repair of degenerative tears (usually the peroneus brevis), and/or tenodesis if there is a complete rupture or severely degenerative tendon, prohibiting repair. Hindfoot varus deformity is an etiologic factor in the occurrence of peroneal tendinitis and degenerative tears and should be corrected with a Dwyer osteotomy (lateral closing wedge osteotomy of the calcaneus) when they are present on physical examination. Peroneal subluxation or dislocation is also an etiologic factor and should be addressed if it is present on examination.

C. Posterior tibial tendon—The posterior tibial tendon is addressed in the section on pes planus deformity.

D. Anterior tibial tendon—Tenosynovitis of the anterior tibial tendon is uncommon but can be observed in patients with inflammatory arthritis. Immobilization in a walking cast or ankle-foot orthosis along with use of NSAIDs is recommended. Corticosteroid injections can provide relief but increase the risk of tendon rupture. Complete ruptures are rare and mainly occur in older patients.

E. FHL—Stenosing FHL tenosynovitis is usually seen in dancers on pointe. Patients have posterior ankle pain and triggering of the interphalangeal joint of the great toe. The location of the stenosis is most often between the posterolateral and posteromedial tubercles of the talus, where the FHL travels. Release of the fascia between these two structures can relieve the pain. There are limited nonoperative options, with the exception of activity modification.

XV. Heel Pain

A. Plantar heel pain

1. Neurologic causes—The neurologic causes include spinal nerve root and peripheral nerve entrapment.

a. **Plantar fasciitis**—Proximal plantar fasciitis is a painful heel condition that can affect both sedentary and active individuals and is most often seen in the adult population.

(1) Presentation—Typical presentation includes exquisite pain and tenderness over the plantar medial tuberosity of the calcaneus at the proximal insertion of the plantar fascia, which is often at its worst with the first step in the morning or after prolonged sitting. The pathology most likely involves microtears at the origin of the plantar fascia, which initiates inflammation and an injury-repair process that leads to a traction osteophyte. A significant number of patients will have bilateral symptoms. A small subset of patients may experience pain and tenderness at the origin of the abductor hallucis, which may indicate entrapment or inflammation of the first branch of the lateral plantar nerve. Approximately 10% of patients will develop persistent, disabling symptoms.

(2) Treatment—Nonoperative treatments include Achilles tendon stretching, cushioned heel inserts, night splints, walking casts, cortisone injections, and anti-inflammatory medications. Plantar fascia–specific stretching protocols have been found to be very effective, ameliorating the patient's pain, allowing greater activity, and improving overall satisfaction (Fig. 6–45). Refractory cases can be treated operatively with a limited (medial one third) release of the plantar fascia. Complete release can place the longitudinal arch of the foot at risk, overload the lateral column, and lead to dorsolateral foot pain. If entrapment of the lateral plantar nerve is suspected, concomitant release of the deep fascia of the abductor hallucis may be warranted.

2. Bony causes

a. Stress injury—**Calcaneal stress fractures** can be a cause of heel pain, especially in the active individual or military recruit. Although bone scintigraphy can be used to diagnose this condition, MRI is the more sensitive and specific test. Approximately half of these stress injuries are in the posterior aspect of the calcaneus and the other half in the anterior and middle portions of the bone.

b. **Periostitis**—Sometimes referred to as a "stone bruise," pain and tenderness in the

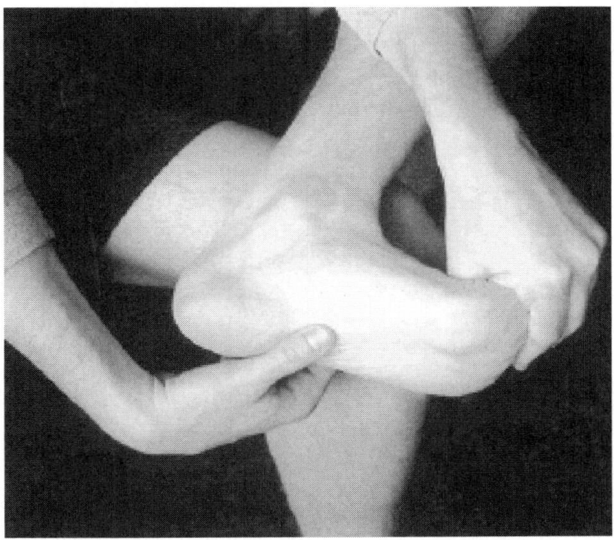

FIGURE 6–45 Plantar fascia-specific stretch. (Courtesy of Dr. Benedict F. DiGiovanni.)

central portion of the heel pad can represent traumatic periosteal or bursal inflammation secondary to a known injury or atrophic heel pad. Cushioned shoe inserts and a short course of treatment in a well-padded cast are appropriate interventions. The examiner should be vigilant for other signs or symptoms suggesting inflammatory arthritis.

B. Posterior heel pain

1. Anatomy—The anatomic structures at issue with posterior heel pain include the Achilles tendon (comprising the gastrocnemius and soleus tendons), the posterior calcaneus, the retrocalcaneal bursa, and the pretendon bursa. The Achilles tendon rotates distally and inserts on the posterior aspect of the calcaneal tuberosity, not the posterosuperior prominence (Fig. 6–46). The Achilles accepts 2000 to 7000 N of stress, depending on the applied load, and transfers forces of six to 10 times body weight during a running stride. When evaluating the tendon for contracture, the Silverscold test should be employed, assessing the degree of dorsiflexion with the knee extended and flexed as the gastrocnemius crosses two joints and is relaxed with knee flexion, thereby distinguishing Achilles contracture from gastrocnemius tightness.

2. **Retrocalcaneal bursitis/Haglund's deformity**

   a. Diagnosis—Inflammation of the bursa that lies between the anterior surface of the Achilles tendon and the posterosuperior aspect of the calcaneus often occurs along with insertional tendinitis and Haglund's deformity (prominence of the posterosuperior calcaneal tuberosity) (Fig. 6–47). Patients present with deep posterior heel pain, fullness and tenderness with palpation medial and lateral to the tendon, and increased pain with ankle dorsiflexion. Plain radiographs will demonstrate Haglund's deformity. MRI is rarely necessary to make the diagnosis.

   b. Treatment—Nonoperative management of this condition is similar to that for tendonitis. Steroid injection of the bursa can be helpful occasionally, but intratendon injection should be avoided because it is believed to increase the risk of rupture. Operative treatment includes débridement of the inflamed retrocalcaneal bursa along with excision of the Haglund deformity when present. If extensive débridement of the Achilles insertion is necessary, consideration can be made for reinforcing the repair with an FHL transfer, plantaris tendon graft, or fascial turndown.

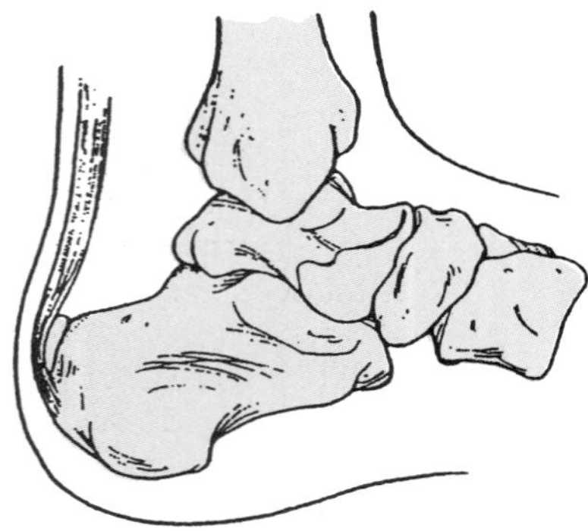

FIGURE 6–46 Insertion of the Achilles tendon on the middle third of the posterior calcaneus. (From DiGiovanni BF, Gould JS: Achilles tendonitis and posterior heel disorders. Foot Ankle Clin 2:411-428. 1997.)

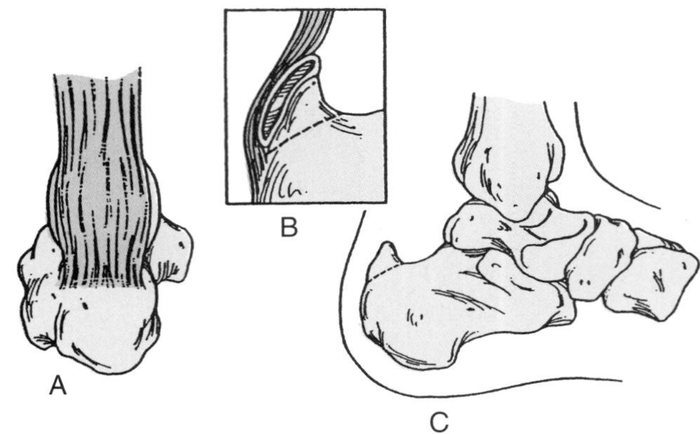

FIGURE 6–47 Retrocalcaneal bursitis and Haglund's deformity. **A**, Posterior hindfoot view. **B**, Inflammation of the retrocalcaneal bursa and line of bone resection. **C,** Prominent posterior superior calcaneal tuberosity. (From DiGiovanni BF, Gould JS: Achilles tendonitis and posterior heel disorders. Foot Ankle Clin 2:411-428. 1997.)

3. Insertional Achilles tendinitis

   a. Diagnosis—This tendinitis is an enthesopathy that presents with symptoms similar to those of noninsertional Achilles tendinitis but localized to the insertion of the tendon on the posterior calcaneus. Patients describe a progressive enlargement of the bony prominence of the heel along with pain caused by direct pressure from shoe wear. Imaging and histopathologic examination will often demonstrate attritional changes, tendinosis, cystic changes in the posterior tuberosity, bone spur formation, and/or intratendinous ossification (Fig. 6–48).

   b. Treatment—Nonoperative therapies are the mainstays of treatment and include ice, anti-inflammatory medications, modification of activity and shoe wear, heel lifts, stretching, and silicone heel sleeves/pads to decrease the pain from direct pressure. When operative intervention is indicated, a medial longitudinal incision with a transverse J component distally can provide excellent exposure while protecting the sural nerve and lateral blood supply to the tendon (Fig. 6–49). Through this approach the degenerative portions of the tendon can be excised, heterotopic bone can be removed, and any re-anchoring or repair of the Achilles can be performed. The duration of

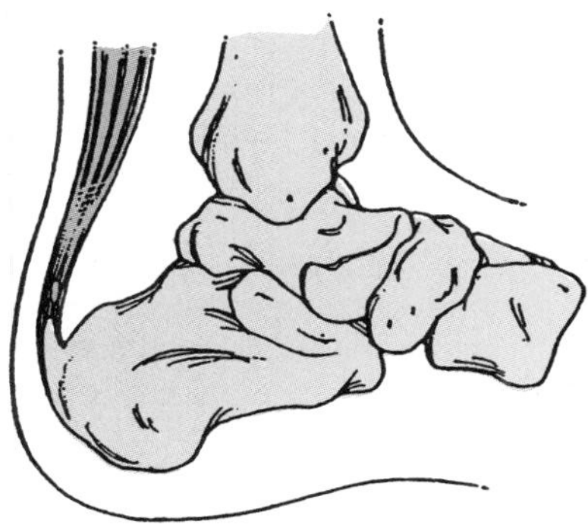

FIGURE 6–48 Insertional Achilles tendinitis with calcific tendinoplasty. (From DiGiovanni BF, Gould JS: Achilles tendonitis and posterior heel disorders. Foot Ankle Clin 2:411-428. 1997.)

postoperative immobilization with a heel lift may depend on whether a simple débridement or repair was performed.

4. Noninsertional Achilles tendinitis/tendinosis
   a. Diagnosis—Patients often present with pain, swelling, and warmth during and after running exercises. The etiology is thought to be multifactorial and may include training errors and poor lower extremity alignment. The pathology can include inflammation of the paratenon alone, peritendinitis with a component of tendinosis, or tendinosis alone. It is often localized approximately 2-6 cm proximal to the insertion of the tendon. Vascular studies have shown that the contributions to the blood supply to the tendon arise from the bony insertion, the musculotendinous junction, and the ventral mesotenal vessels. They are relatively sparse in the 2-6–cm region.
   b. Treatment—Nonoperative treatments include ice, anti-inflammatory medicines, stretching the Achilles, eccentric strengthening exercises, heel lifts that can be gradually shortened, and iontophoresis. When this disorder is recalcitrant to conservative care, operative interventions may include excision of the thickened and inflamed paratenon through a longitudinal incision just medial to the tendon. On the molecular level, the excessive repetitive loading of the Achilles tendon affects the collagen cross-linking and structural stability of the tendon that are thought to lead to the pathology of tendinosis. Débridement of the pathologic areas of the tendon through longitudinal incisions in the substance of the tendon, followed by repair, can also be performed when appropriate. For more than 50% degenerative involvement of the Achilles, a tendon transfer with FHL is recommended.

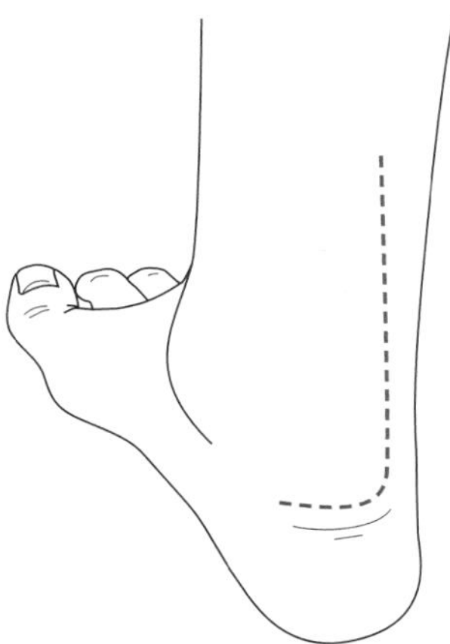

FIGURE 6–49 J-incision for treatment of posterior heel disorders and Achilles tendon débridement.

XVI. The Diabetic Foot

A. Pathophysiology

1. Diabetic neuropathy—Although diabetics have multisystem disease involving the cardiovascular system, kidneys, eyes, and intestines, it is the diagnosis of foot ulcerations that results in the greatest rate of hospital admissions and lower extremity amputations. The combination of neuropathy and excess pressure on the plantar foot leads to ulceration.
   a. Sensation and autonomic and motor components
      (1) Sensation—The polyneuropathic loss of sensation begins in a stocking distribution of the feet and progresses proximally. It is diagnosed by the inability to perceive the 5.07 Semmes-Weinstein monofilament. Ninety percent of patients who cannot feel the 5.07 monofilament have lost protective sensation to their feet and are at risk for ulceration. With the Therapeutic Shoe Bill, money is allocated for neuropathic patients to purchase extra-depth shoes and total contact inserts (three per year) for ulcer prevention.
      (2) Autonomic neuropathy leads to an abnormal sweating mechanism. The foot becomes dry and vulnerable to fissuring cracks, which then become portals for infection.
      (3) The most common peripheral nerve motor neuropathy involves the common peroneal nerve. This is expressed clinically by loss of tibialis anterior motor function and a foot drop. The small intrinsic musculature of the foot is also commonly affected and results in claw toes. These toe deformities can lead to toe-tip ulcerations due to excessive pressure.
   b. Hypomobility syndrome—This syndrome is the result of excessive glycosylation of the soft tissues of the extremities and leads to decreased joint range of motion.
   c. Peripheral vascular disease—This disease occurs in 60-70% of patients who have

had diabetes for over 10 years. The large and small vessels are diseased. With the absence of palpable pulses of the feet on physical examination, noninvasive vascular examination should be performed, which consists of waveforms (normal is triphasic), ankle-brachial indices (minimum for healing, 0.45; normal, 1.0), and absolute toe pressures (minimum for healing, 40 mm Hg; normal, 100 mm Hg). Transcutaneous oxygen measurements (pO_2) of the toes greater than 40 mm Hg have been found to be predictive of healing. Calcifications in the artery can falsely elevate the ankle-brachial index.

d. Immune system impairment—The diabetic patient is not more vulnerable to infection but is poor at fighting off infection once it has developed. This is due to poor cellular defenses such as abnormal phagocytosis, altered chemotaxis of the white blood cells, and a poor cytotoxic environment (due to hyperglycemia) to fight off bacteria.

e. Metabolic deficiency—Reduced total protein less than 6.0, WBC count less than 1500, and albumin levels less than 2.5 result in poor healing potential and can be found in diabetics who are depleted of protein in the urine.

B. Clinical problems

1. Ulcers

a. Classification—Additional factors important in healing rates include ulcer location (forefoot, midfoot, and heel) and the presence or absence of arterial disease (Table 6–10).

b. Treatment—Treatment is based on the depth of the ulcer, the presence or absence of infection, and structural deformity (e.g., midfoot collapse, equinus contractures, toe deformities). Options include ostectomies of bone prominence; arthrodeses; tendon lengthening; and joint resections or amputations to obtain a functional, plantigrade foot.

2. Charcot arthropathy—**Charcot arthropathy** is a chronic, progressive, destructive process affecting bone architecture and joint alignment in people lacking protective sensation. The etiologic factors leading to the progressive bone resorption have not been elucidated. The process is staged 0-3 and is related to the degree of warmth, swelling, and erythema as the process advances from bone resorption and fragmentation to bone formation and consolidation (Table 6–11). Treatment is based on the stage and the ability to maintain a plantigrade foot with or without brace wear. Surgery is reserved for the unbraceable limb. Surgical options include arthrodesis, osteotomy, soft tissue release, and tendon lengthening or amputation.

3. Infection

a. The diabetic foot—Diabetic foot infections occur contiguous to an open skin wound (ulceration, skin fissure, or cut). The hematogenous spread of infection and seeding of bacteria in the foot or ankle are extremely rare. If the foot is warm, erythematous, and swollen and there is not an open skin lesion, it most likely represents an initial presentation of Charcot arthropathy. Infections in the diabetic foot or ankle are either isolated soft tissue infections (cellulitis or abscess) or osteomyelitis.

(1) MRI is the appropriate study to assess the patient for an abscess if an isolated needle aspirate is not feasible. It has a high false-positive rate in the diagnosis

TABLE 6-10 WAGNER CLASSIFICATION OF DIABETIC ULCERS

Grade	Description	Treatment
Grade 0	Skin intact, but bony deformities produce a "foot at risk"	Extra-depth shoes, custom-molded pressure relief insoles, serial examinations
Grade 1	Localized, superficial ulcer	Débridement of the ulcer in the office. A total contact cast is recommended if palpable or strongly positive Doppler pulses and wound margins that bleed well with local débridement are present. The risk of loss of a vascularly compromised foot in an occlusive cast must be weighed against the risk of leaving the ulcer. The patient and physician make this decision together. The potential for healing even large, full-thickness ulcers is so high using total-contact casting that some degree of ischemia is acceptable. Also, the extent of possible tracking of the ulcer is important to document (Fig. 6–39). Initially, the cast is changed weekly, then biweekly until healing occurs. This usually can be done in the office.
Grade 2	Deep ulcer to tendon, bone, ligament, or joint	This usually requires formal débridement in the operating room, followed by a total-contact cast.
Grade 3	Deep abscess, osteomyelitis	If area of osteomyelitis can be locally débrided (with profound neuropathy this may be done in the office) and adequate bleeding is present, a total-contact cast is indicated. The cast is changed weekly or more often if drainage is initially extensive.
Grade 4	Gangrene of toes or forefoot	Because ischemia is present, vascular surgery consultation is required to decide if arteriovascular reconstruction is possible. If increased arterial flow can be established, the ulcer or a more limited partial foot amputation may heal.
Grade 5	Gangrene of entire foot	Major amputation; arterial bypass surgery may allow a below-knee amputation to heal.

TABLE 6-11 STAGES OF CHARCOT ARTHROPATHY (EICHENHOLTZ)*

Stage	Signs and Symptoms	Radiographs
0: Clinical (prefragmentation)	Acute inflammation; confused with infection	Regional bone demineralization
1: Dissolution (fragmentation)	Acute inflammation, swelling, erythema, warmth; confused with infection	Regional bone demineralization, periarticular fragmentation, joint dislocation
2: Coalescence	Less inflammation, less swelling, less erythema	Absorption of bone debris; early bone healing and periosteal new bone formation
3: Resolution	Resolved erythema, swelling, and warmth; consolidation of healing	Smoothed bone edges, bony/fibrous ankylosis

**Based on the signs, symptoms, and radiographic changes that occur with the neuropathic joint/fracture over time.*

of osteomyelitis, particularly with concurrent Charcot arthropathy.

(2) Sixty-seven percent of the foot ulcerations that probe to bone have contiguous osteomyelitis.

(3) An isolated technetium scan is not predictive of osteomyelitis. A WBC-labeled scan or dual-image Tc/In scan is more sensitive and specific for osteomyelitis in diabetics.

(4) Diabetic foot infections are polymicrobial, and a culture of the superficial wound does not identify the organism responsible for the infection and should not be performed. Initial broad-spectrum antibiotic coverage is initiated after surgical cultures are obtained. The antibiotics are adjusted when the sensitivity returns. Isolated cellulitis may be treated with antibiotics alone. In addition to treatment with antibiotics, abscesses are surgically irrigated and drained. Osteomyelitis is treated with débridement and antibiotics. The débridement may consist of an exostosectomy of bone or require a more extensive removal, resulting in an amputation.

XVII. Trauma

A. Phalangeal fractures

1. Diagnosis—**Phalangeal fractures** are the most common injuries to the forefoot; the proximal phalanx of the fifth toe is the one most often involved. Phalangeal fractures are usually caused by a stubbing mechanism (axial loading with varus or valgus force) or by a heavy load dropped on the foot. Presenting symptoms are pain, ecchymosis, and swelling.
2. Treatment—All nondisplaced phalangeal fractures, with or without articular involvement, can be treated with stiff-soled shoes and protected weight bearing. "Buddy taping" of the injured toe to an adjacent toe may improve pain relief and help stabilize potentially unstable fractures. Fractures with clinical deformity require reduction. Closed reduction with gravity traction and axial realignment is usually possible, and the reduction is usually stable. Fractures of the phalanges of the hallux carry greater functional significance than those of the lesser toes. Injuries to the distal phalanx are often the result of a crush mechanism, whereas those of the proximal phalanx are from axial loads (stubbing). Operative treatment is indicated for gross instability or intra-articular discontinuity. Fixation can be achieved with crossed K-wires or mini–fragment screws. The most common complication of these injuries is stiffness.

B. **Metatarsal fractures**—The five metatarsals are interconnected and stabilized by the bony architecture of the midfoot and the ligamentous attachments at the metatarsal bases and necks (intermetatarsal ligaments). For this reason, severe displacement of shaft fractures is uncommon unless multiple metatarsals are fractured. The mechanisms for metatarsal fracture include crush-type injury (which can result in severe soft tissue trauma), twisting forces, and chronic stresses. Anteroposterior, lateral, and oblique radiographs are usually suitable to detect fractures. Bone scans will aid in the detection of stress fractures. Stress fracture of the second metatarsal is the most common and is classically described in amenorrheal dancers. The first and fifth metatarsals have unique functions and are more mobile and susceptible to injury

1. Fracture of the first, second, third, and fourth metatarsals—The first metatarsal bears approximately one third of the body weight; therefore, maintenance of alignment is very important. Significant displacement or angulation of a first metatarsal shaft fracture should be treated with a mode of operative stabilization (percutaneous pinning, lag screw fixation, plate fixation, external fixation) dictated by the fracture pattern and comminution. The central three metatarsals (second, third, and fourth) have similar characteristics and can be treated similarly. The majority of central metatarsal shaft fractures are minimally displaced and can therefore be successfully treated with a short-leg cast, low-tide walking boot, or hard-soled shoe with arch support. Those with displacement greater than 3-4 mm, significant angulation less than 10 degrees, or intra-articular involvement are likely to benefit from operative stabilization. Care should be taken to maintain proper metatarsal length in order to minimize the risk of transfer metatarsalgia or plantar keratosis. Options include crossed K-wires, intramedullary pins, and mini–fragment plates and screws (Fig. 6–50). Fractures of the metatarsal bases (1-4) occur

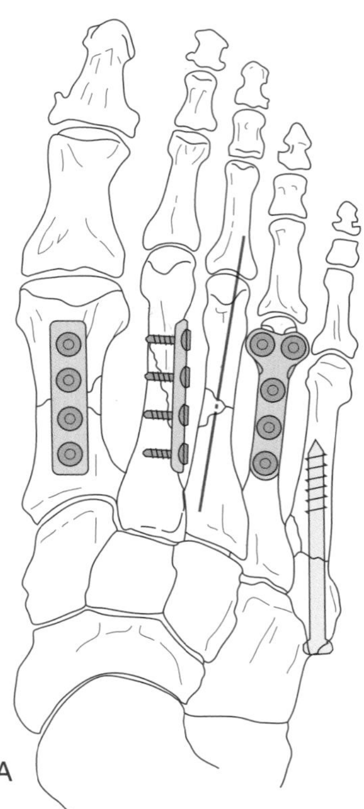

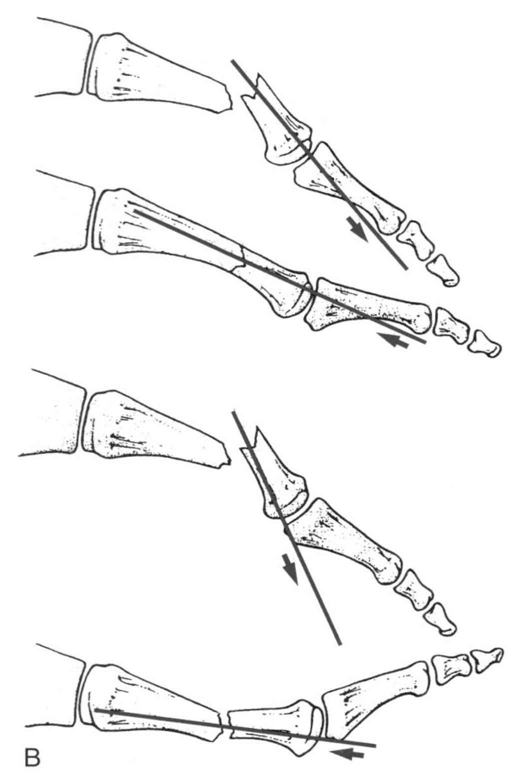

FIGURE 6–50 Various methods of internal fixation of metatarsal fractures. **A**, Plate and screw fixation, Kirschner wire fixation, and compression screw fixation. **B**, Antegrade-retrograde Kirschner wire technique. (From Browner BD, Jupiter JB, Levine AM, Trafton PG: Skeletal Trauma, 3rd ed. Philadelphia, WB Saunders, 2003.)

primarily through metaphyseal bone and heal rapidly. Oblique fractures heal more rapidly than transverse or comminuted fractures. When multiple metatarsals are fractured, a Lisfranc injury must be ruled out.

2. Fracture of the fifth metatarsal—Fifth metatarsal fractures represent a unique subset of forefoot injuries. They are often referred to as ''**Jones fractures**,'' but more accurate and anatomic descriptions of fifth metatarsal fractures have been created (Fig. 6–51). Zone 1 injuries are tuberous avulsion fractures that occur at the insertion of the peroneus brevis tendon, often from an inversion mechanism. Zone 2 injuries are the truly acute Jones fractures at the metaphyseal–diaphyseal junction. Stress fractures of the proximal diaphysis (zone 3) occur mostly in athletes, result from repetitive microtrauma, and occur in the vascular watershed region of the proximal fifth metatarsal, making these injuries slow to heal and producing a greater risk of nonunion.

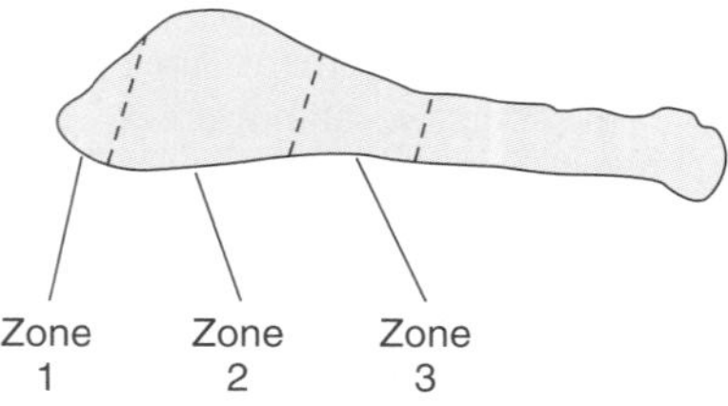

FIGURE 6–51 Three zones of fifth metatarsal fractures.

3. Avulsion fracture—Avulsion fractures can be treated in a weight-bearing cast, boot, or hard-soled shoe and activity advanced as tolerated. Acute Jones fractures and stress fractures can be treated for 6-8 weeks in a non–weight-bearing, short-leg cast. Due to the higher incidence of delayed unions and nonunions in this region of the metatarsal, some advocate early operative intervention with intramedullary screw fixation with or without bone grafting. This may offer an earlier return to activities in the active patient or athlete.

C. First MTP joint injuries—The hallux MTP dislocation is uncommon but more common than traumatic dislocation of the lesser MTPs. The hallux will typically dislocate dorsally due to hyperextension, and the volar plate will rupture at its insertion on the metatarsal neck. The sesamoids, conjoined tendons, and intersesamoidal ligament will either stay intact and inhibit reduction or fail and therefore make closed reduction successful (Fig. 6–52). The stability of the first MTP joint should be assessed after ''turf toe''–type injuries (Fig. 6–53).

D. Midfoot injuries—The midfoot is defined as the five bones distal to the Chopart joint and proximal to the Lisfranc joint (navicular, cuneiforms, and cuboid). It is a relatively immobile segment of the foot owing to the articulations and strong plantar ligaments, and it acts as a stout connection between the forefoot and hindfoot. There are no ground-contact, weight-bearing surfaces, but the

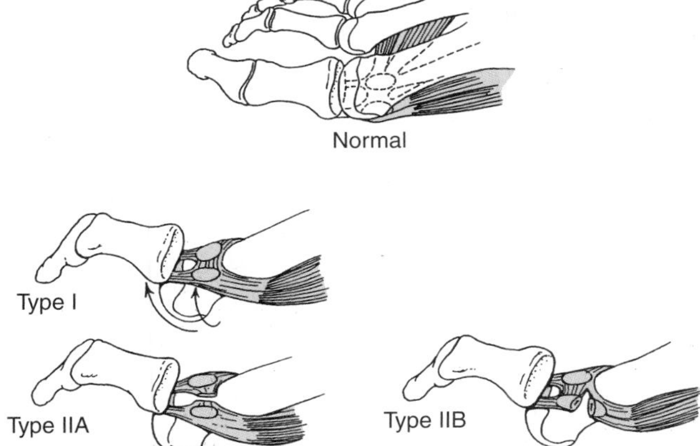

FIGURE 6–52 Jahss classification of first MTP joint dislocations. (Redrawn from Jahss MH: Disorders of the Foot and Ankle: Medical and Surgical Management. Philadelphia, WB Saunders, 1991.)

midfoot serves an important shock absorbing function. Chopart's and Lisfranc's joints are therefore of greater functional importance than the articulations among the midfoot bones (Fig. 6–54).

1. Cuboid injuries—These injuries can be isolated but more often are associated with other midfoot or Lisfranc fractures/dislocations. Radiographic evaluation should include anteroposterior, lateral, and oblique (30-degree medial oblique is ideal) views. Weight-bearing/stress views can help ascertain midfoot stability if there is clinical concern. CT allows for more precise evaluation of the fracture fragments and articular congruity. The majority of cuboid fractures are avulsions near the calcaneocuboid articulation due to an inversion force (lateral ankle sprain). They can be treated conservatively, with weight bearing as tolerated. The more significant cuboid fractures result from forced plantar flexion and abduction of the forefoot, which apply an axial load to the bone. The resulting comminuted, impacted fracture has been termed a "nutcracker" fracture (Fig. 6–55). The cuboid is critical to the integrity of the lateral column of the foot. This fracture requires operative fixation if the magnitude of comminution or displacement compromises the length and alignment of the lateral column. Cuboid syndrome is a painful subluxation seen in athletes, especially ballet dancers. The patient may have pain or a palpable "click" as the foot is brought from plantar flexion and inversion to dorsiflexion and eversion. Complete dislocation of the cuboid is extremely rare, is often due to higher-energy mechanisms, and is displaced in a plantar and medial direction.
2. Cuneiform injuries—Fractures and dislocations involving the cuneiform bones are relatively uncommon; isolated fractures or dislocations have been reported, but most occur in association with other midfoot injuries. Of the three cuneiform bones, the medial one is the most commonly injured. Displaced or unstable medial cuneiform injuries require anatomic reduction and stable fixation.
3. Navicular fractures
   a. Anatomy—The navicular articulates with the talar head on its concave proximal surface and with the three cuneiforms distally. It is rigidly fixed in the midfoot by dense ligamentous attachments. Because the majority of the hindfoot motion occurs through the talonavicular joint, anatomic reduction of fractures that disrupt this articulation is paramount. Vascular studies have demonstrated that the navicular receives its blood supply from the dorsalis pedis and plantar medial arteries and through a plexus near the tuberosity. The

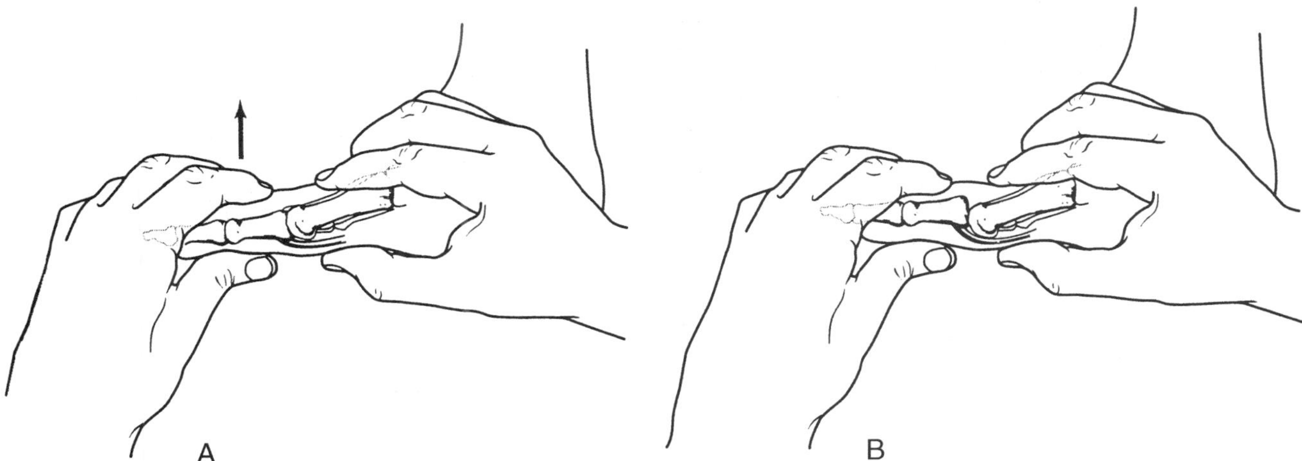

FIGURE 6–53 Test of stability of the MTP joint. **A**, Position of the hands to test dorsoplantar stability of the plantar complex. **B**, Direction of motion. (From Early JA: Fractures and dislocations of the midfoot and forefront. In Bucholz RW, Heckman JD, eds: Rockwood and Green's Fractures in Adults, 5th ed. Philadelphia, Lippincott Williams & Wilkins, 2001, p 2230.)

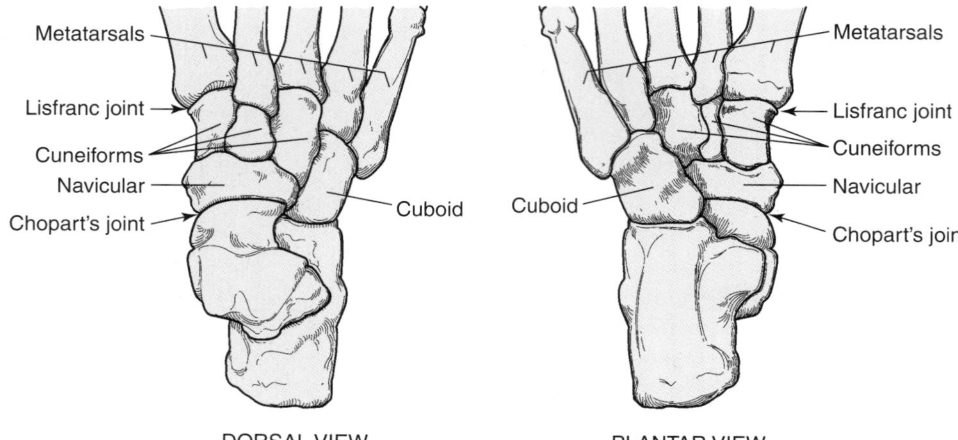

FIGURE 6–54 Bony anatomy of the midfoot. (From Early JS: Fractures and dislocations of the midfoot and forefoot. In Bucholz RW, Heckman JD, eds: Rockwood and Green's Fractures in Adults, 5th ed. Philadelphia, Lippincott Williams and Wilkins, 2001, p 2183.)

central portion of the bone is relatively less vascular and therefore at risk for stress injuries and nonunions. The two most common complications of navicular fractures are post-traumatic: degenerative arthritis and avascular necrosis.

b. Classification—Fractures of the navicular can be classified as avulsion, tuberosity, body, and stress injuries.
   (1) Avulsion fractures are the most common and the least significant. The ligamentous attachments avulse a fragment of bone during inversion, twisting, and hyper–plantar flexion injuries.
   (2) Acute eversion of the foot with simultaneous contraction of the tibialis posterior can avulse a portion of the tuberosity. The broad attachment of this tendon usually keeps the fragment from being significantly displaced. One should always look for a lateral injury because it is a common finding (anterior process of the calcaneus, cuboid fracture). Significantly displaced fractures can be treated with excision or surgical fixation, depending on the fragment size.
   (3) The body of the navicular can be fractured by a crushing mechanism or an axial load (a fall on a plantar-flexed foot). Type I injuries are in the coronal plane. Type II fractures are oriented from a dorsal-lateral to plantar-medial position and result in medialization (adduction) of the fragment and forefoot. Type III injuries involve notable comminution (Fig. 6–56). Open reduction and internal fixation (ORIF) of even minimally displaced fractures is recommended because of the importance of these joints to hindfoot motion.
   (4) Stress fractures of the navicular typically occur in the central portion of the bone secondary to repetitive trauma such as distance running. CT and bone scanning can aid in the diagnosis. Non–weight

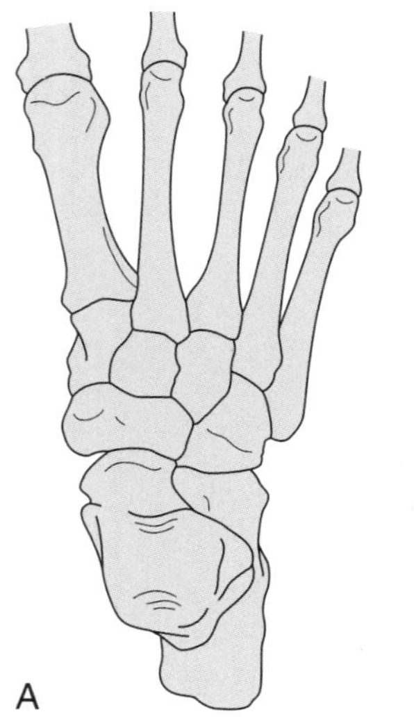

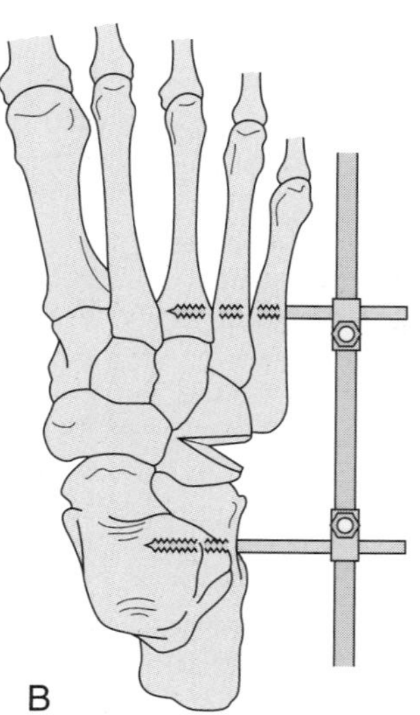

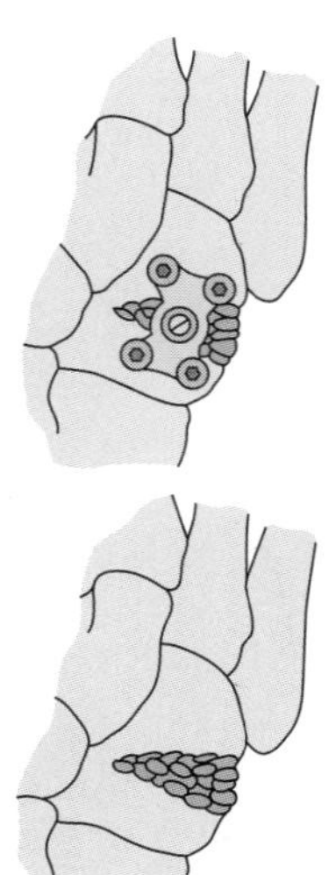

FIGURE 6–55 **A**, "Nutcracker" fracture of the cuboid. **B**, External fixation with bone grafting, often augmented by a small buttress plate. (From Browner BD, Jupiter JB, Levine AM, Trafton PG: Skeletal Trauma, 3rd ed. Philadelphia, WB Saunders, 2003.)

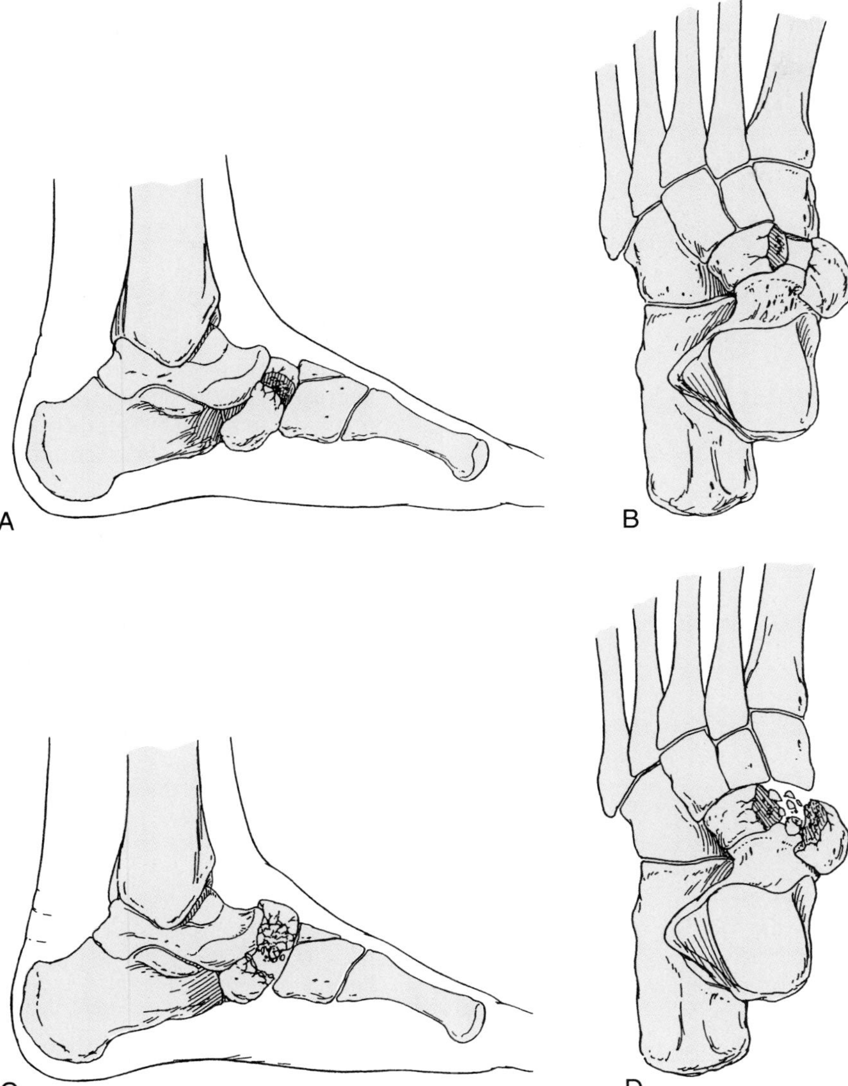

FIGURE 6–56 Navicular fracture classification. **A**, Type I. **B**, Type II. **C** and **D**, Type III. (From Myerson MS: Foot and Ankle Disorders. Maryland, Saunders, 2000.)

bearing is critical, and if healing does not occur, surgical fixation with bone grafting may be necessary.

E. Talus fractures

1. Anatomy—More than half of the surface area of the talus is covered by articular cartilage. The neck is angled in a medial and plantar direction relative to the axis of the body. There are no muscular or ligamentous attachments. The blood supply can be tenuous and is provided by three main vessels: the posterior tibial artery, the dorsalis pedis artery, and the perforating peroneal artery. The arteries of the tarsal sinus, the tarsal canal, and the deltoid are important branches of the main vessels. The artery of the tarsal canal carries the main supply to the talus, especially the body. The head and neck are vascularized by the artery of the tarsal sinus and the dorsalis pedis. A thorough understanding of the relationship between fracture displacement and those vessels that are disrupted is extremely important when operative approaches and fixation are planned.
2. Classification—Talar body fractures affect both the subtalar and tibiotalar articulations; consequently, restoration of articular congruity is essential. Fracture lines that enter the subtalar joint anterior to the lateral process are identified as neck fractures, and those that enter posterior to the lateral process are classified as body fractures. Figure 6–57 depicts a simple classification system.
3. Mechanism of injury—These injuries constitute less than 1% of all fractures but rank second (behind calcaneus fractures) among all tarsal bone injuries. Forceful dorsiflexion such as that which occurs during a fall from a significant height or a motor vehicle collision is a common mechanism. It is common to have coincidental malleolar fractures, which suggest that a

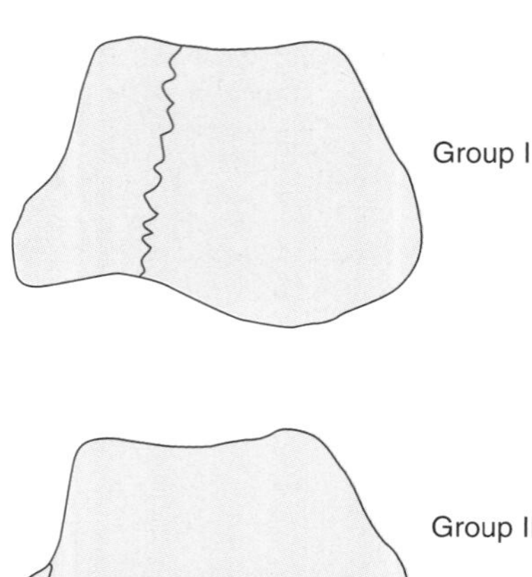

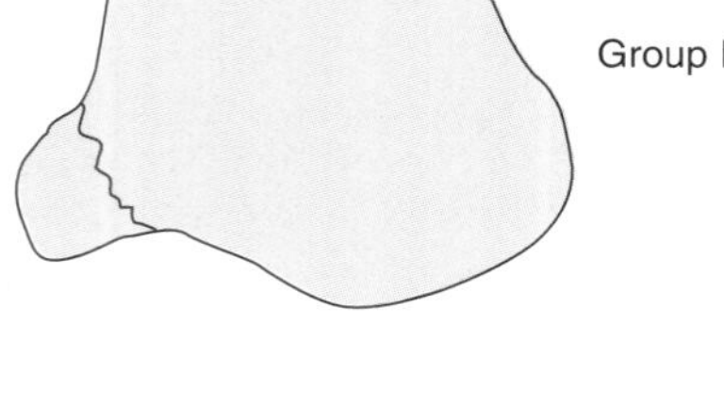

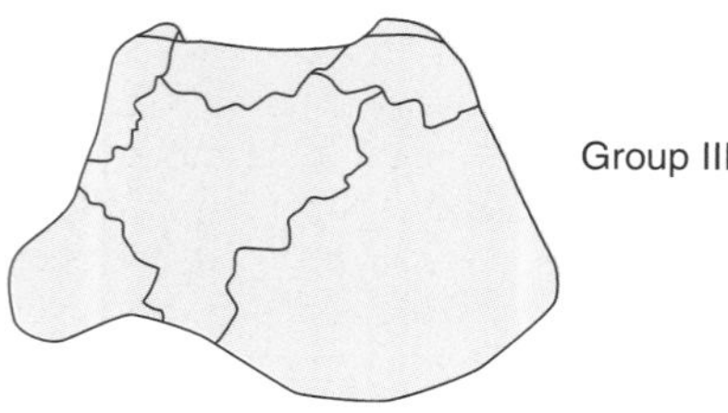

FIGURE 6–57 Classification of talar body fractures.

rotational force is often present and may be a significant contributor to displacement.

a. Talar neck fractures—These represent the most common talus injury. As the foot is forcefully dorsiflexed, the anterior tibia becomes impacted and fractures the relatively narrower, more trabecular bone of the neck. The energy propagates through the ligaments that stabilize the subtalar joint, leading to subluxation or dislocation of the body. If the hindfoot deviates into supination, the talar neck can fracture the medial malleolus, become impacted and comminuted, and result in talar head rotation and displacement.
   (1) Classification— Table 6–12 shows the Hawkins classification of talar neck fractures. Type I fracture lines exit between the middle and posterior facets. In theory, only one of the three sources of perfusion is disturbed. Any fracture that is more than 1 mm displaced should be treated as a type II injury. With these two types of injury, two sources of blood supply are disrupted. In Type III injuries, the body is usually extruded posteriorly and medially. In theory, the blood supply has been completely compromised. More then 50% of these injuries are open, and many result in infection. Type IV injuries include subluxation or dislocation of the talonavicular joint.

4. Diagnosis—Physical examination will demonstrate marked swelling and often gross deformity and soft tissue compromise with the higher-grade injuries. Attention should be paid to the spine because coincidental fractures are not uncommon. Anteroposterior, lateral, and Canale oblique (Fig. 6–58) radiographs should be routine. Talar head fractures can be easily overlooked if they are small or minimally displaced. CT scanning is very useful for evaluating the fracture pattern, comminution, and angulation during preoperative planning. The incidence of osteonecrosis is very low.
5. Treatment—The treatment goals for all types of talus fractures are anatomic reduction (length, rotation, angulation) and stabilization because even slight displacement can significantly alter the contact characteristics of the subtalar joint. If the fragment results in talonavicular incongruity or instability, operative fixation is warranted in order to minimize post-traumatic arthrosis. The talonavicular joint is critical to overall hindfoot

TABLE 6-12 HAWKINS CLASSIFICATION OF TALAR NECK FRACTURES

Type	Description	Treatment	Complications
I	Nondisplaced talar neck fracture	Non–weight-bearing cast until union (usually 6-8 wk)	AVN, 13% (fractures that develop AVN may have reduced spontaneously)
II	Displaced talar neck fracture with subluxation or dislocation of subtalar joint but intact ankle mortise	Occasionally closed reduction and internal fixation in sagittal plane with fluoroscopy (usually ORIF)	AVN, 30-45% Post-traumatic arthritis of the subtalar joint, 40-90%
III	Displaced talar neck fracture with dislocation of talar body from ankle mortise	ORIF	AVN, 90-100% Post-traumatic arthritis of the subtalar and tibiotalar joints, 40-90% Nonunion, 13% Malunion, 27%
IV	Displaced talar neck fracture with dislocation of talar body from ankle mortise and subluxation or dislocation of talonavicular joint	ORIF	AVN, 90-100% Post-traumatic arthritis of the subtalar and tibiotalar joints, 40-90% Nonunion, 13% Malunion, 27%

AVN, avascular necrosis; ORIF, open reduction with internal fixation.

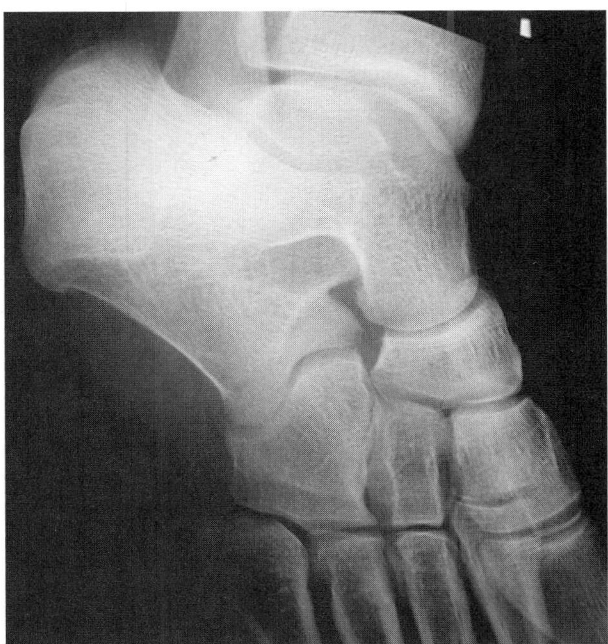

A

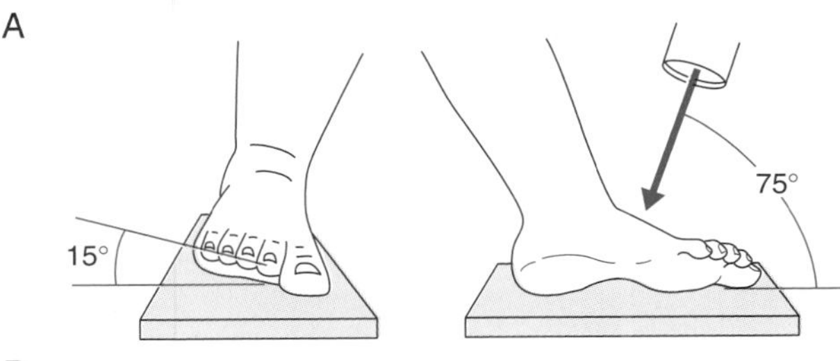

B

FIGURE 6–58 **A**, The Canale view of the talar neck. **B**, The angle at which the x-ray beam should be directed. (From Browner BD, Jupiter JB, Levine AM, Trafton PG: Skeletal Trauma, 3rd ed. Philadelphia, WB Saunders, 2003.)

motion; therefore, fusion for talar head fractures should be a salvage procedure.

a. Talar neck fractures
   (1) Type I—Type I fractures can be immobilized in a non–weight-bearing cast for 6-8 weeks, with frequent radiographs to monitor the injury for displacement.
   (2) Type II—Varus deformity of the talar neck is the most common malunion. It is commonly seen in type II fractures that are treated without reduction and stabilization and in fractures with medial neck comminution. If they heal in this position, the foot will be in relative cavus and supination and the lateral border of the foot will experience abnormal forces during ambulation. Corrective procedures include medial column lengthening, lateral column shortening, and/or talar neck osteotomy. Arthrodesis of degenerative joints is sometimes necessary, but it is crucial to rule out a large area of osteonecrosis because it may result in failure of fusion. Type II injuries require immediate reduction, which can be achieved by plantar flexing the foot and manipulating the heel. Because splinting/casting in plantar flexion is often needed to maintain reduction, it is another reason these fractures should be treated operatively. The medial approach is commonly used, but care should be taken to avoid stripping the medial blood supply. Other concerns include underestimating the degree of varus angulation and medial impaction (shortening). Medial compression screw fixation can worsen such malalignment. A lateral approach may allow easier evaluation of talar length and angulation. The approaches and screw placements include medial, lateral, and posterolateral directions/locations (Fig. 6–59). Type II fractures often involve the medial malleolus. If not, an osteotomy is sometimes necessary for adequate exposure. Again, care should be taken to preserve the remaining medial vascular supply. When the talar body has been completed extruded and is grossly contaminated, it may be appropriate to disregard the body and perform a delayed reconstruction because the rates of deep infection and overall failure are very high.
   (3) Type III—Displaced talar neck fractures with dislocation of the talar body from the ankle mortise also require immediate reduction. These are at significant risk for avascular necrosis (AVN), subtalar ankle post-traumatic arthritis, malunion, and nonunion.
   (4) Type IV—Type IV injuries may require stabilization of the talonavicular joint. Both the head and the body are at risk of avascular necrosis. Type IV injuries offer the worst prognosis.

b. Talar process and tubercle fractures—The treatment of talar process and tubercle fractures depends on the degree of articular involvement, displacement, and comminution. Nondisplaced fractures can be immobilized in a non–weight-bearing cast. Displaced fractures can be internally fixed, but highly comminuted fractures may need to be treated with excision. Cleavage fractures should be anatomically reduced and stabilized. Impacted fractures may require bone grafting for structural support. Medial malleolar osteotomy can help to provide adequate exposure.

6. Complications—The three main complications of talus fractures are osteonecrosis, post-traumatic arthrosis, and malunion. Table 6–12 correlates the type of talar neck fractures with the incidence of each of these complications. The "Hawkins sign" is the

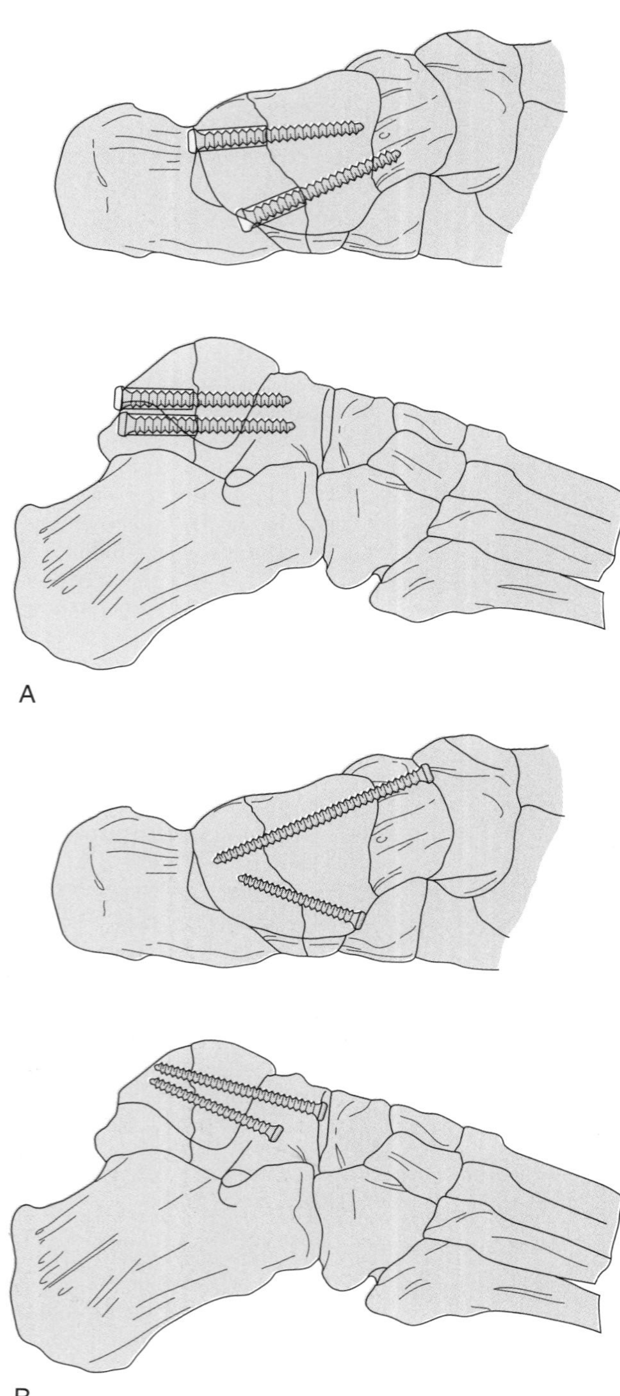

FIGURE 6–59 Internal fixation of talar neck fractures. Screws can be directed from anterior to posterior or from posterior to anterior. **A**, Posteroanterior screw fixation for talar neck and body fractures through a posterolateral or posteromedial approach. **B**, Anteroposterior compression screw fixation. (From Browner BD, Jupiter JB, Levine AM, Trafton PG: Skeletal Trauma, 3rd ed. Philadelphia, WB Saunders, 2003.)

radiolucency of the subchondral bone that can be visualized on the anteroposterior and mortise views. This is evidence of preserved vascularity of the talar body and is a good prognostic sign. The absence of this finding does not mean that osteonecrosis is inevitable. MRI is useful for evaluating osteonecrosis, but not during the first few weeks. These fractures can still heal in the setting of avascular necrosis.

F. Calcaneus fractures—Fractures are generally divided into articular and extra-articular fractures. Either kind can be displaced or nondisplaced and open or closed, which markedly affect clinical outcome.
   1. Extra-articular calcaneal fractures—Avulsion fractures of the tuberosity are caused by forceful Achilles tendon contraction. Anterior process fractures (beak fractures) are avulsions at the bifurcate ligament. These fractures can be treated nonoperatively with cast immobilization unless they are displaced. If a fracture of the tuberosity or an anterior process fracture is displaced more than 1 cm and the fragment is large enough to support internal fixation, the fragment should be replaced and fixed. If the fragment is displaced more than 1 cm but is too small for internal fixation, it should be excised. Isolated sustentaculum fractures without posterior facet involvement are rare. However, persistent medial hindfoot pain after an injury that should have a clinical resolution should be evaluated by CT scanning. Rarely will ORIF be required.
   2. Articular fractures
      a. Diagnosis—Approximately 75% of all fractures of the calcaneus are posterior facet fractures, and most of them have some degree of displacement. The classification system of Sanders (Fig. 6–60), based on CT scanning, is the most widely used, although the Essex-Lopresti (Fig. 6–61), based on radiographic appearance, is also helpful. Axial loading and shear forces account for the mechanism of injury, and one or more fragments of the posterior facet are impacted into the body of the calcaneus. This reduces or reverses the Böhler angle (Fig. 6–62), which is normally 25-40 degrees, and "bursts" the lateral wall of the calcaneus laterally beneath the fibula. This multiplanar disruption

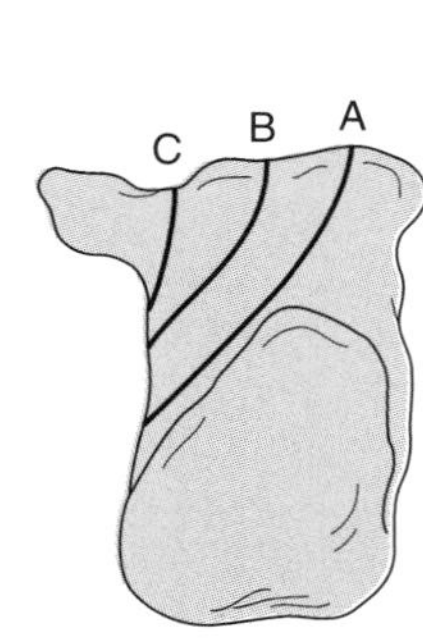

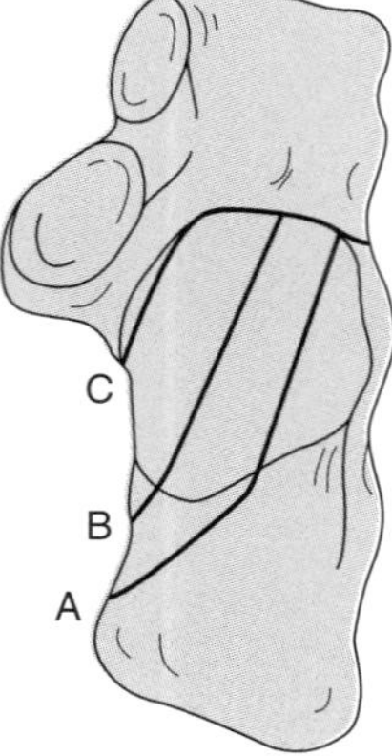

FIGURE 6–60 The Sanders classification of calcaneus fractures is based on the coronal images of the fracture line through the posterior facet. (From Browner BD, Jupiter JB, Levine AM, Trafton PG: Skeletal Trauma, 3rd ed. Philadelphia, WB Saunders, 2003.)

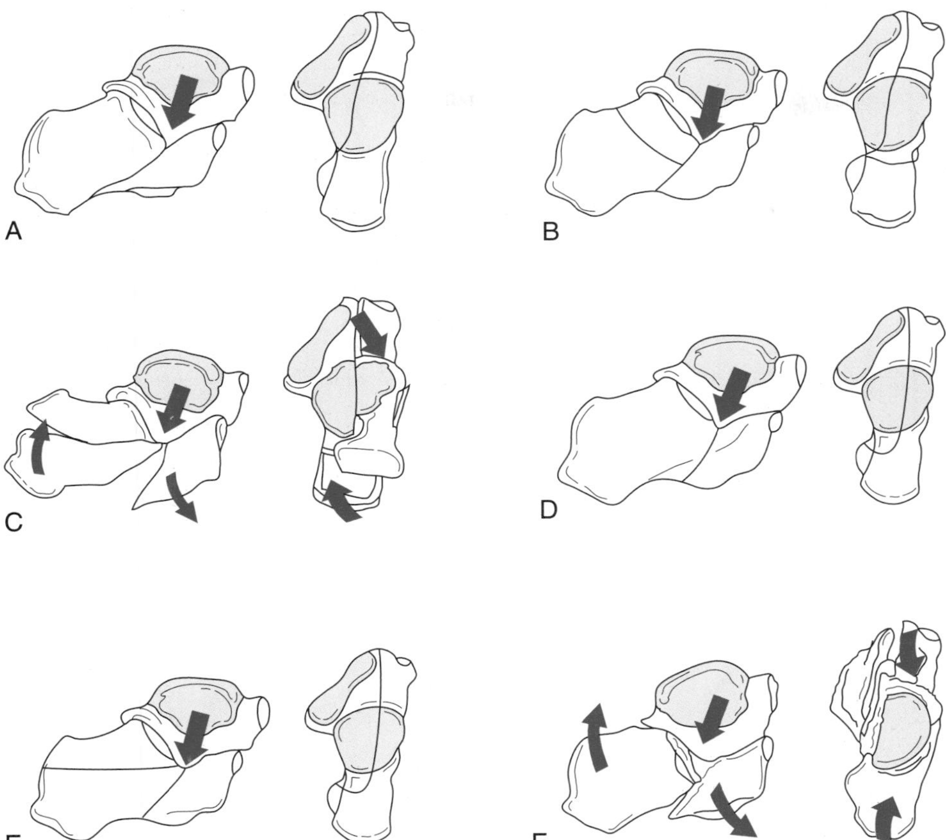

FIGURE 6–61 Essex-Lopresti classification. The tongue type: primary fracture line (**A**), posterior-exiting fracture line (**B**), further displacement (**C**). The joint-depression type: primary fracture line (**D**), superior-exiting fracture line (**E**), further depression of the posterior facet and separation from the tuberosity (**F**).

of the posterior facet can result in calcaneofibular abutment; peroneal tendon encroachment; articular pain; heel pad crush symptoms; and shoe-wear difficulty from a shortened, widened, and flattened calcaneus. Routine plain films (anteroposterior, lateral, oblique, and axial os calcis views) are helpful to evaluate the Böhler angle and the degree of calcaneal shortening. CT scanning in the coronal (posterior and middle facets) and axial (calcaneocuboid joint involvement and tuberosity displacement) planes is helpful in evaluating this multiplanar injury as well as in preoperative planning. If CT scanning is not available, a Broden oblique view

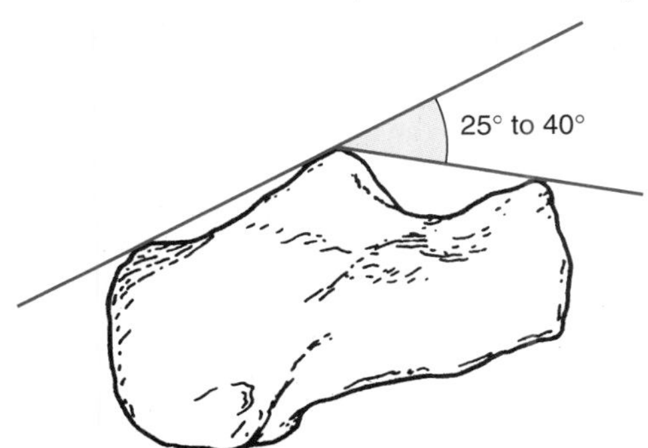

FIGURE 6–62 Böhler angle. (From Murphy GA: Fractures and dislocations of foot. In Canale ST, ed: Campbell's Operative Orthopaedics, 10th ed. St. Louis, CV Mosby, 2003, p 4233.)

(Fig. 6–63) of the ankle is helpful to evaluate posterior face displacement.

b. Prognosis and treatment—The prognosis for articular fractures of the calcaneus treated by either nonoperative or operative methods is guarded, and operative management is controversial in patients who smoke or are more than 50-60 years old. However, Sanders does not believe age should be a factor and reported approximately 75-80% good to excellent results in types II and III articular fractures treated with ORIF. Displacement of a posterior facet fracture of more than 2-3 mm is an indication for ORIF. The recommended treatment of type I fractures is non–weight bearing for 4-6 weeks and early motion after a short period of immobilization (2-3 weeks) for soft tissue stabilization. Type IV fractures are very comminuted and severely displaced and have a poor prognosis regardless of treatment. Restoration of calcaneal anatomy and primary arthrodesis of the posterior facet with bone grafting, if needed, are gaining popularity but are technically demanding procedures.

G. Peritalar (subtalar) dislocations

1. Medial dislocation—Medial peritalar dislocations are more common than lateral ones. They result from forceful inversion of the hindfoot, resulting in medial displacement of the

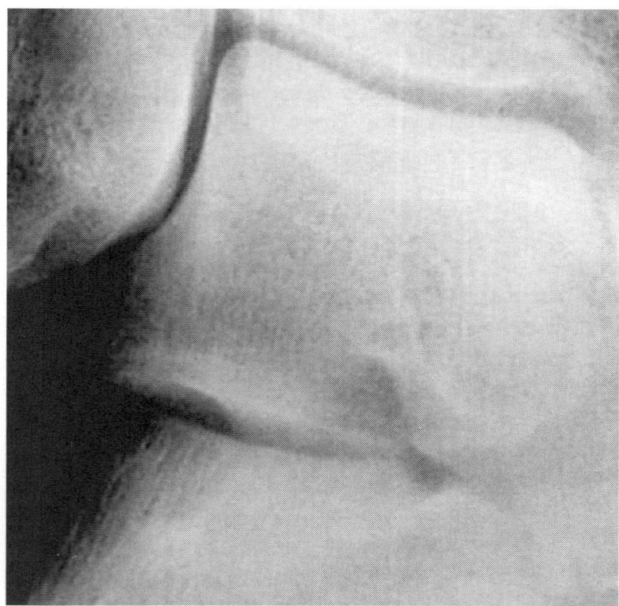

A

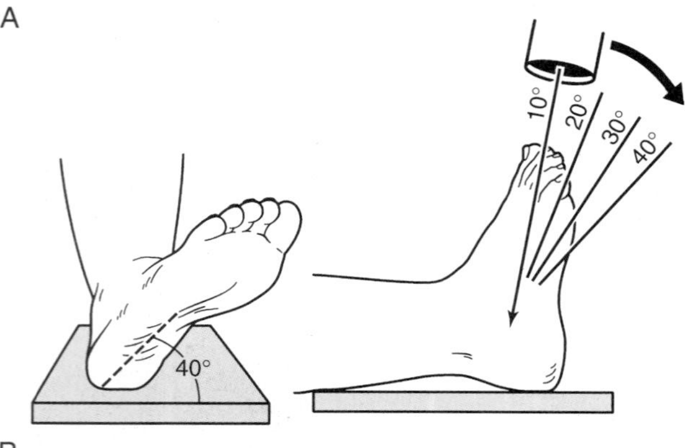

B

FIGURE 6–63 **A**, The Broden view of the subtalar joint. **B**, The angle at which the x-ray beam should be directed. (From Browner BD, Jupiter JB, Levine AM, Trafton PG: Skeletal Trauma, 3rd ed. Philadelphia, WB Saunders, 2003.)

calcaneus. Given the mechanism and resulting appearance of the foot, this injury has been referred to as a "basketball foot" or an "acquired clubfoot." Reduction can usually be accomplished under sedation or general anesthesia. The most common obstacles to reduction are the EDB, the extensor retinaculum, the peroneal tendons, and the talonavicular capsule.

2. Lateral dislocation—Lateral peritalar dislocation occurs with forceful eversion of the hindfoot. The calcaneus is displaced laterally, and the deformity has been termed an "acquired flatfoot." The most common obstacles to reduction are an interposed posterior tibial tendon and FHL tendon. All subtalar dislocations warrant a CT scan to rule out small intra-articular fragments.

H. Lisfranc injury

1. Anatomy—The Lisfranc articulation is a stable construct because of its bony architecture and strong plantar ligaments. The base of the second metatarsal fits into a mortise formed by the proximally recessed middle cuneiform. In addition, in the coronal plane, the second metatarsal base serves as the cornerstone in a "Roman arch" configuration (Fig. 6–64). The Lisfranc ligament is a stout band extending from the plantar-lateral aspect of the medial cuneiform to the base of the second metatarsal.

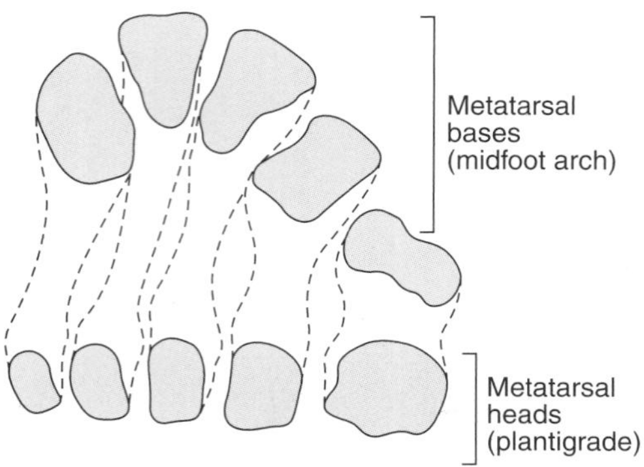

FIGURE 6–64 The "Roman arch" configuration of the metatarsal bases. (From Browner BD, Jupiter JB, Levine AM, Trafton PG: Skeletal Trauma, 3rd ed. Philadelphia, WB Saunders, 2003.)

2. Diagnosis—The patterns of TMT joint injuries can be highly variable, ranging from nondisplaced, purely ligamentous disruptions to severe fracture-dislocations. If the diagnosis is missed or improper treatment delivered, the patient may be left with a planovalgus deformity and post-traumatic arthritis. TMT injuries are more common in men. The trauma can be direct or indirect. Motor vehicle accidents, falls from a height, crush injuries, and athletics (axial loading of a plantar-flexed foot) (Fig. 6–65) are the most common mechanisms. Patients typically present with severe pain, an inability to bear weight, marked swelling, and tenderness. Plantar ecchymosis should raise suspicion for a TMT injury. All patients should be evaluated for compartment syndrome, and pressure measurement should be performed when appropriate. Anteroposterior, lateral, and oblique radiographs should be obtained. When the diagnosis is suspected but not confirmed by these initial views, weight-bearing or stress views (forefoot abduction) can be helpful. Figure 6–66 demonstrates the normal relationships among the metatarsal and tarsal bones that should be assessed. The "fleck sign" is a small, bony avulsion from the base of the second metatarsal seen in the first intermetatarsal space that is diagnostic of a Lisfranc injury. CT is very useful in both the diagnostic phases and during preoperative planning.
3. Classification—Multiple classification schemes have been described but are not useful for determining treatment and prognosis. All are based on the congruency of the articulations and the direction of metatarsal displacement. Descriptive terms have included isolated, homolateral, divergent, partially incongruent, totally incongruent, and purely ligamentous.

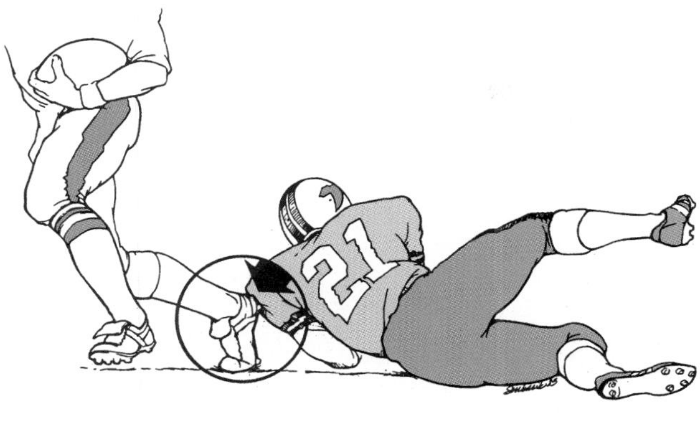

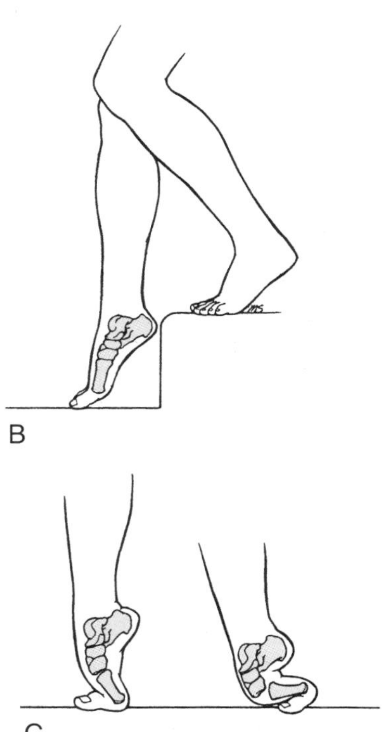

FIGURE 6–65 Mechanism of injury of tarsometatarsal joint can include axial load to the foot in fixed equinus (**A**), axial loading as in descending stairs (**B**), and axial loading resulting from a fall from a height (**C**). (From Early JS: Fractures and dislocations of the midfoot and forefoot. In Bucholz RW, Heckman JD, eds: Rockwood and Green's Fractures in Adults, 5th ed. Philadelphia, Lippincott Williams & Wilkins, 2001, p 2204.)

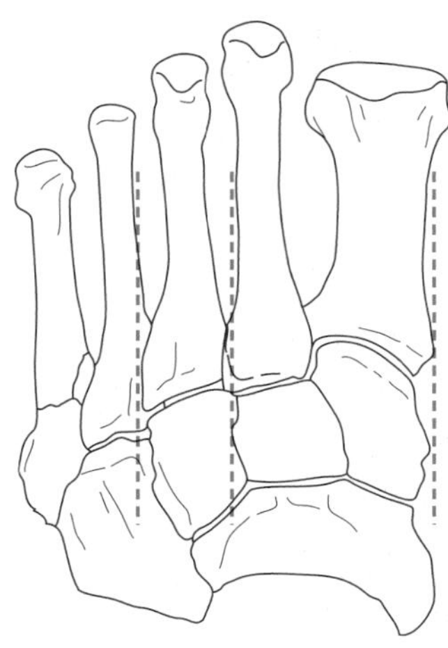

FIGURE 6–66 The normal radiographic lines seen on the oblique view of the foot.

4. Treatment—Regardless of classification, the goal of treatment is always the same: anatomic reduction and stable fixation. Therefore, nonsurgical management of TMT injuries should be limited to those cases with no displacement and good stability under stress (weight-bearing or forced-abduction radiographs). Operative intervention should be delayed until the soft tissue swelling has resolved and there is a return of skin wrinkles. The choice of hardware and method of fixation will depend greatly on the injury pattern. Figure 6–67 shows commonly used incisions and successful hardware configurations. In general, the medial column should be addressed first,

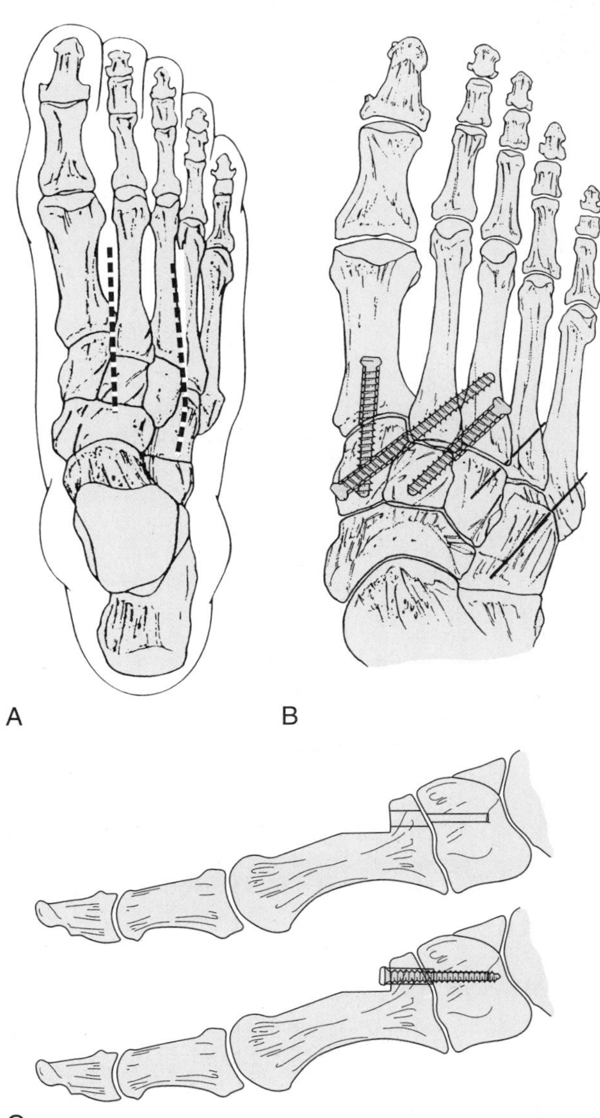

FIGURE 6–67 **A** through **C**, Incision and screw placement for open reduction and internal fixation of tarsometatarsal injuries. (From Browner BD, Jupiter JB, Levine AM, Trafton PG: Skeletal Trauma, 3rd ed. Philadelphia, WB Saunders, 2003.)

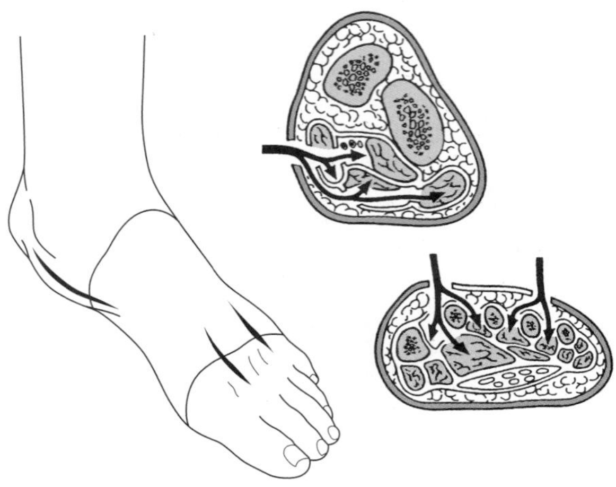

FIGURE 6–68 Releasing compartment syndrome of the foot through three incisions. (From Browner BD, Jupiter JB, Levine AM, Trafton PG: Skeletal Trauma, 3rd ed. Philadelphia, WB Saunders, 2003.)

with reduction and absolute stabilization (screw fixation). Then the lateral articulations (fourth and fifth) can be temporarily stabilized with percutaneous pins. Purely ligamentous injuries may have a slower healing potential. There may be a role for primary partial arthrodesis in these patients (Ly and Coetzee).

I. Compartment syndrome
   1. Anatomy—The medial compartment contains the abductor hallucis and FHB. The central compartment includes the FDB, the lumbricals, quadratus plantae, and adductor hallucis. The lateral compartment has the flexors, abductors, and opponens to the fifth toe. The interosseous compartment includes the seven interossei. The dorsalis pedis artery forms an anastomosis with the plantar arch by passing between the first and second metatarsal bases.
   2. Mechanism of injury—When the intracompartmental fluid pressure meets or exceeds the capillary filling pressure (perfusion pressure), irreversible muscle and nerve damage can occur. Most of the injuries that result in compartment syndrome are crush injuries. Calcaneus fractures carry a 10% incidence of compartment syndrome.
   3. Diagnosis—The clinician must maintain a high index of suspicion. Clinical findings include massive swelling, pain out of proportion to the injury that is not relieved by immobilization or appropriate analgesics, severe pain with passive motion of the toes (stretching the intrinsic muscles), and paresthesias and/or loss of light-touch and two-point discrimination. There are many cases of compartment syndrome with normal capillary refill and palpable and/or Doppler positive pulses. Intracompartmental pressure measurement is the gold standard for diagnosis. Values greater than 40 mm Hg, those within 30 mm Hg of the diastolic pressure, or those greater than 30 mm Hg for a prolonged period signify a compartment syndrome. The result of unrecognized and untreated compartment syndrome is claw toes.
   4. Treatment—Fasciotomies can be performed through three incisions: one over the second metatarsal, one over the fourth metatarsal, and a medial approach along the inferior border of the first metatarsal (Fig. 6–68). The wounds should be left open for approximately 5 days and may require skin grafting.

Selected Bibliography

ANATOMY AND BIOMECHANICS

Aktan Ikiz ZA, Ucerler H, Bilge O: The anatomic features of the sural nerve with an emphasis on its clinical importance. Foot Ankle Int 26:560–567, 2005.

Hunt AE, Smith RM, Torode M: Extrinsic muscle activity, foot motion, and ankle joint moments during the stance phase of walking. Foot Ankle Int 22:31–41, 2001.

Joseph B, Rebello G, Mayya S: The use of a working model for teaching functional and applied surgical anatomy of the subtalar joint. Foot Ankle Int 27:286–292, 2006.

Salathe EP, Arangio GA: A biomechanical model of the foot: the role of muscles, tendons, and ligaments. J Biomech Engl 124:281–287, 2002.

Ucerler H, Ikiz AA: The variations of the sensory branches of the superficial peroneal nerve course and its clinical importance. Foot Ankle Int 26: 942–946, 2005.

GAIT

Blackwood CB, Yuen TJ, Sangeorzan BJ, Ledoux WR: The midtarsal joint locking mechanism. Foot Ankle Int 26:1074–1080, 2005.

Brodsky JW: Preliminary gait analysis results after posterior tibial tendon reconstruction: A prospective study. Foot Ankle Int 25:96–100, 2004.

Chambers HG, Sutherland DH: A practical guide to gait analysis. J Am Acad Orthop Surg 10:222–231, 2002.

Cornwall MW, McPoil TG, Fishco WD, et al: The influence of first ray mobility on forefoot plantar pressure and hindfoot kinematics during walking. Foot Ankle Int 27:539–547, 2006.

Inman VT: Human locomotion. 1966. Clin Orthop Relat Res 288:3–9, 1993.

Kitaoka HB, Crevoisier XM, Hansen D, et al: Foot and ankle kinematics and ground reaction forces during ambulation. Foot Ankle Int 27:808–813, 2006.

Saunders JB, Inman VT, Eberhart HD: The major determinants in normal and pathological gait. J Bone Joint Surg [Am] 35:543–558, 1953.

HALLUX VALGUS AND VARUS

Aminian A, Kelikian A, Moen T: Scarf osteotomy for hallux valgus deformity: An intermediate follow-up of clinical and radiographic outcomes. Foot Ankle Int 27:883–886, 2006.

Aronson J, Nguyen LL, Aronson EA: Early results of the modified Peterson bunion procedure for adolescent hallux valgus. J Pediatr Orthop 21:65–69, 2001.

Coughlin MJ, Saltzman CL, Nunley JA II: Angular measurements in the evaluation of hallux valgus deformities: A report of the ad hoc committee of the American Orthopaedic Foot and Ankle Society on angular measurements. Foot Ankle Int 23:68–74, 2002.

Grimes JS, Coughlin MJ: First metatarsophalangeal joint arthrodesis as a treatment for failed hallux valgus surgery. Foot Ankle Int 27:887–893, 2006.

Lau JT, Myerson MS: Modified split extensor hallucis longus tendon transfer for correction of hallux varus. Foot Ankle Int 23:1138–1140, 2002.

Lorei TJ, Kinast C, Klarner H, Rosenbaum D: Pedographic, clinical, and functional outcome after scarf osteotomy. Clin Orthop Relat Res 451:161–166, 2006.

Kopp FJ, Patel MM, Levine DS, Deland JT: The modified Lapidus procedure for hallux valgus: A clinical and radiographic analysis. Foot Ankle Int 26:913–917, 2005.

Malal JJ, Varghese B: Blood flow to the metatarsal head after chevron bunionectomy. Foot Ankle Int 27:1011–1012, 2006.

Pinney S, Song K, Chou L: Surgical treatment of mild hallux valgus deformity: The state of practice among academic foot and ankle surgeons. Foot Ankle Int 27:970–973, 2006.

Pinney SJ, Song KR, Chou LB: Surgical treatment of severe hallux valgus: The state of practice among academic foot and ankle surgeons. Foot Ankle Int 12:1024–1029, 2006.

Richardson EG: Complications after hallux valgus surgery. Instr Course Lect 48:331–342, 1999.

Richardson EG, Donley BG: Disorders of hallux. In Canale ST, ed: Campbell's Operative Orthopaedics, 10th ed. St. Louis, CV Mosby, 2003.

Skalley TC, Myerson MS: The operative treatment of acquired hallux varus. Clin Orthop Relat Res 306:183–191, 1994.

Thordarson DB, Rudicel SA, Ebramzadeh E, Gill LH: Outcome study of hallux valgus surgery—an AOFAS multi-center study. Foot Ankle Int 22:956–959, 2001.

Veri JP, Pirani SP, Claridge R: Crescentic proximal metatarsal osteotomy for moderate to severe hallux valgus: A mean 12.2 year follow-up study. Foot Ankle Int 22:817–822, 2001.

LESSER-TOE DEFORMITIES

Cooper PS: Disorders and deformities of the lesser toes. In Myerson MS, ed: Foot and Ankle Disorders. Philadelphia, WB Saunders, 2000.

Coughlin MJ: Lesser toe abnormalities. Instr Course Lect 52:421–444, 2003.

Coughlin MJ, Dorris J, Polk E: Operative repair of the fixed hammertoe deformity. Foot Ankle 21:94–104, 2000.

Femino JE, Mueller K: Complications of lesser toe surgery. Clin Orthop 391:72–88, 2001.

Mizel MS, Yodlowski ML: Disorders of the lesser metatarsophalangeal joints. J Am Acad Orthop Surg 3:166–173, 1995.

Murphy GA: Lesser toe abnormalities. In Canale ST, ed: Campbell's Operative Orthopaedics, 10th ed. St. Louis, CV Mosby, 2003.

Murphy GA: Mallet toe deformity. Foot Ankle Clin 3:279, 1998.

Richardson EG: Lesser toe deformities: An overview. Foot Ankle Clin 3:195–198, 1998.

Richardson, EG: Orthopaedic Knowledge Update—Foot and Ankle 3. Rosemont, IL, American Academy of Orthopaedic Surgeons, 2004.

SESAMOIDS

Biedert R, Hintermann B: Stress fractures of the medial great toe sesamoids in athletes. Foot Ankle Int 24:137–141, 2003.

Richardson EG: Hallucal sesamoid pain: Causes and surgical treatment. J Am Acad Orthop Surg 7:270–278, 1999.

NEUROLOGIC DISORDERS

Coughlin MJ, Pinsonneault T: Operative treatment of interdigital neuroma: A long-term follow-up study. J Bone Joint Surg 83:1321–1328, 2001.

DiGiovanni BF, Gould JS: Tarsal tunnel syndrome and related entities. Foot Ankle Clin 3:405–426, 1998.

Myerson MS: Neuromuscular conditions in the adult. In Myerson MS, ed: Foot and Ankle Disorders. Philadelphia, WB Saunders, 2000.

Richardson EG: Neurogenic disorders. In Canale ST, ed: Campbell's Operative Orthopaedics, 10th ed. St. Louis, CV Mosby, 2003.

ARTHRITIC DISEASES

Brage M: Degenerative joint disease of the midfoot. Foot Ankle Clin 4:355–368, 1999.

Coughlin MJ: Rheumatoid forefoot reconstruction: A long-term follow-up study. J Bone Joint Surg 82:322–341, 2000.

Easley ME, Trnka HJ, Schon LC, Myerson MS: Isolated subtalar arthrodesis. J Bone Joint Surg 82:613–624, 2000.

Goucher NR, Coughlin MJ: Hallux metatarsophalangeal joint arthrodesis using dome-shaped reamers and dorsal plate fixation: A prospective study. Foot Ankle Int 27:869–876, 2006.

Ishikawa SN, Abidi A: Degenerative disease of the hindfoot. Foot Ankle Clin 4:369–394, 1999.

Kitaoka HB, Crevoisier XM, Harbst K, et al: The effect of custom-made braces for the ankle and hindfoot on ankle and foot kinematics and ground reaction forces. Arch Phys Med Rehab 87:130–135, 2006.

Knecht SI, Estin M, Callaghan JJ, et al: The Agility total ankle arthroplasty: Seven to sixteen-year follow-up. J Bone Joint Surg [Am] 86:1161–1171, 2004.

Richardson EG: Rheumatoid foot. In Canale ST, ed: Campbell's Operative Orthopaedics, 10th ed. St. Louis, CV Mosby, 2003.

Saltzman CL, Salamon ML, Blanchard GM, et al: Epidemiology of ankle arthritis: Report of a consecutive series of 639 patients from a tertiary orthopaedic center. Iowa Orthop J 25:44–46, 2005.

Sammarco VJ, Magur EG, Sammarco GJ, Bagwe MR: Arthrodesis of the subtalar and talonavicular joints for correction of symptomatic hindfoot malalignment. Foot Ankle Int 27:661–666, 2006.

Shereff MJ, Baumhauer JF: Hallux rigidus and osteoarthrosis of the first metatarsophalangeal joint. J Bone Joint Surg 80:898–908, 1998.

Smith RW, Shen W, Dewitt S, Reischl SF: Triple arthrodesis in adults with non-paralytic disease: A minimum ten-year follow-up study. J Bone Joint Surg [Am] 86:2707–2713, 2004.

PES PLANUS AND PES CAVUS

Alvarez RG, Marini A, Schmitt C, Saltzman CL: Stage I and II posterior tibial tendon dysfunction treated by a structured nonoperative management protocol: An orthosis and exercise program. Foot Ankle Int 27:2–8, 2006.

Dolan CM, Herring JA, Anderson JG, et al: Randomized prospective study comparing tri-cortical iliac crest autograft to allograft in the lateral column lengthening component for operative correction of adult acquired flatfoot deformity. Foot Ankle Int 28:8–12, 2007.

Giannini S, Ceccarelli F, Benedetti MG, et al: Surgical treatment of adult idiopathic cavus foot with plantar fasciotomy, naviculocuneiform arthrodesis, and cuboid osteotomy: A review of thirty-nine cases. J Bone Joint Surg [Am] 84(Suppl. 2):62–69, 2002.

Havenhill TG, Toolan BC, Draganich LF: Effects of a UCBL orthosis and a calcaneal osteotomy on tibiotalar contact characteristics in a cadaver flatfoot model. Foot Ankle Int 26:607–613, 2005.

Malicky ES, Crary JL, Houghton MJ, et al: Talocalcaneal and subfibular impingement in symptomatic flatfoot in adults. J Bone Joint Surg 84:2005–2009, 2002.

McCormack AP, Ching RP, Sangeorzan BJ: Biomechanics of procedures used in adult flatfoot deformity. Foot Ankle Clin 6:15–23, 2001.

Prado MP, de Carvalho AE Jr., Rodrigues CJ, et al: Vascular density of the posterior tibial tendon: A cadaver study. Foot Ankle Int 27:628–631, 2006.

Toolan BC, Sangeorzan BJ, Hansen ST Jr.: Complex reconstruction for the treatment of dorsolateral peritalar subluxation of the foot: Early results after distraction arthrodesis of the calcaneocuboid joint in conjunction with stabilization of and transfer of the flexor digitorum longus tendon to the midfoot to treat acquired pes planovalgus in adults. J Bone Joint Surg 81:1545–1560, 1999.

Wapner KL: Pes cavus. In Myerson MS, ed: Foot and Ankle Disorders. Philadelphia, WB Saunders, 2000.

Younger AS, Hansen ST Jr: Adult cavovarus foot. J Am Acad Orthop Surg 13:302–315, 2005.

TENDON DISORDERS

Coetzee JC, Hansen ST: Surgical management of severe deformity resulting from posterior tibial tendon dysfunction. Foot Ankle Int 22:944–949, 2001.

Cohen BE, Johnson JE: Subtalar arthrodesis for treatment of posterior tibial tendon insufficiency. Foot Ankle Clin 6:121–128, 2001.

Crates J, Richardson EG: Treatment of stage I posterior tibial tendon dysfunction with medial soft-tissue procedures. Clin Orthop 365:46–49, 1999.

Hockenbury RT, Sammarco GJ: Medial sliding calcaneal osteotomy with flexor hallucis longus transfer for the treatment of posterior tibial tendon insufficiency. Foot Ankle Clin 6:569–581, 2001.

Johnson JE, Cohen BE, DiGiovanni BF, Lamdan R: Subtalar arthrodesis with flexor digitorum longus transfer and spring ligament repair for treatment of posterior tibial tendon insufficiency. Foot Ankle Int 21:722–729, 2000.

Porter D, McCarroll J, Knapp E, Torma J: Peroneal tendon subluxation in athletes: Fibular groove deepening and retinacular reconstruction. Foot Ankle Int 26:436–441, 2005.

Redfern D, Myerson M: The management of concomitant tears of the peroneus longus and brevis tendons. Foot Ankle Int 25:695–707, 2004.

Selmani E, Gjata V, Gjika E: Current concepts review: Peroneal tendon disorders. Foot Ankle Int 27:221–228, 2006.

HEEL PAIN

Angerman P, Hovgaard D: Chronic Achilles tendinopathy in athletic individuals: Results of conservative and surgical treatments. Foot Ankle Int 20:304–306, 1999.

DiGiovanni BF, Gould JS: Achilles tendonitis and posterior heel disorders. Foot Ankle Clin 2:411–427, 1997.

Holmes GB, Lin J: Etiologic factors associated with symptomatic Achilles tendinopathy. Foot Ankle Int 27:952–959, 2006.

Myerson MS, Mandelbaum B: Disorders of the Achilles tendon and retrocalcaneal region. In Myerson MS, ed: Foot and Ankle Disorders. Philadelphia, WB Saunders, 2000.

Pfeffer GB: Plantar heel pain. Instr Course Lect 50:521–531, 2001.

Schepsis AA, Jones H, Haas LA: Achilles tendon disorders in athletes. Am J Sports Med 30:287–305, 2002.

Schneider W, Niehus W, Knahr K: Haglund's syndrome: Disappointing results following surgery—a clinical and radiographic analysis. Foot Ankle Int 21:26–30, 2000.

Tashjian RZ, Hur J, Sullivan RJ, et al: Flexor hallucis longus transfer for repair of chronic Achilles tendinopathy. Foot Ankle Int 24:673–676, 2003.

Watson TS, Anderson RB, Davis WH, Kiebzak GM: Distal tarsal tunnel release with partial plantar fasciotomy for chronic heel pain: An outcome analysis. Foot Ankle Int 23:530–537, 2002.

DIABETIC FOOT AND INFECTIONS

Baumhauer JF, Fraga CJ, Gould JS, Johnson JE: Total calcanectomy for the treatment of chronic calcaneal osteomyelitis. Foot Ankle Int 19:849–855, 1998.

Bollinger M, Thordarson DB: Partial calcanectomy: An alternative to below knee amputation. Foot Ankle Int 23:927–932, 2002.

Cavanagh PR, Owings TM: Nonsurgical strategies for healing and preventing recurrence of diabetic foot ulcers. Foot Ankle Clin 11:735–743, 2006.

Clare MP, Fitzgibbons TC, McMullen ST, et al: Experience with the vacuum assisted closure negative pressure technique in the treatment of non-healing diabetic and dysvascular wounds. Foot Ankle Int 23:896–901, 2002.

Guyton GP, Saltzman CL: The diabetic foot: Basic mechanisms of disease. Instr Course Lect 51:169–181, 2002.

Hastings MK, Sinacore DR, Fielder FA, Johnson JE: Bone mineral density during total contact cast immobilization for a patient with neuropathic (Charcot) arthropathy. Phys Ther 85:249–256, 2005.

Matricali GA, Dereymaeker G, Muls E, et al: Economic aspects of diabetic foot care in a multidisciplinary setting: A review. Diabetes Metab Res Rev 2006.

Mueller MJ, Sinacore DR, Hastings MK, et al: Effect of Achilles tendon lengthening on neuropathic plantar ulcers: A randomized clinical trial. J Bone Joint Surg [Am] 85:1436–1445, 2003.

Myerson MS, Alvarez RG, Lam PW: Tibiocalcaneal arthrodesis for the management of severe ankle and hindfoot deformities. Foot Ankle Int 21:643–650, 2000.

Simon SR, Tejwani SG, Wilson DL, et al: Arthrodesis as an early alternative to nonoperative management of Charcot arthropathy of the diabetic foot. J Bone Joint Surg 82:939–950, 2000.

FRACTURES AND DISLOCATIONS

Aktuglu K, Aydogan U: The functional outcome of displaced intra-articular calcaneal fractures: A comparison between isolated cases and polytrauma patients. Foot Ankle Int 23:314–318, 2002.

Armagan OE, Shereff MJ: Injuries to the toes and metatarsals. Orthop Clin North Am 32:1–10, 2001.

Berkowitz MJ, Kim DH: Process and tubercle fractures of the hindfoot. J Am Acad Orthop Surg 13:492–502, 2005.

Buckley R, Tough S, McCormack R, et al: Operative compared with non-operative treatment of displaced intra-articular calcaneal fractures: A prospective, randomized, controlled multicenter trial. J Bone Joint Surg 84:1733–1744, 2002.

Chiodo CP, Myerson MS: Developments and advances in the diagnosis and treatment of injuries to the tarsometatarsal joint. Orthop Clin North Am 32:11–20, 2001.

Coris EE, Lombardo JA: Tarsal navicular stress fractures. Am Fam Physician 67:85–90, 2003.

DiGiovanni CW, Benirschke SK, Hansen ST: Foot injuries. In Browner BD, et al, eds: Skeletal Trauma: Basic Science, Management, and Reconstruction, 3rd ed. Philadelphia, WB Saunders, 2003.

Fotin PT, Balazsy JE: Talus fractures: Evaluation and treatment. J Am Acad Orthop Surg 9:114–127, 2001.

Keener BJ, Sizensky JA: The anatomy of the calcaneus and surrounding structures. Foot Ankle Clin 10:413–424, 2005.

Larson CM, Almekinders LC, Taft TN, Garrett WE: Intramedullary screw fixation of Jones fractures: Analysis of failure. Am J Sports Med 30:55–60, 2002.

Ly TV, Coetzee JC: Treatment of primarily ligamentous Lisfranc joint injuries: Primary arthrodesis compared with open reduction and internal fixation. J Bone Joint Surg 88:514–520, 2006.

Murphy GA: Fractures and dislocations of the foot. In Canale ST, ed: Campbell's Operative Orthopaedics, 10th ed. St. Louis, CV Mosby, 2003.

Pinney SJ, Sangeorzan BJ: Fractures of the tarsal bones. Orthop Clin North Am 32:21–33, 2001.

Richter M, Wippermann B, Krettek C, et al: Fractures and fracture dislocations of the midfoot: Occurrence, causes, and long-term results. Foot Ankle Int 22:392–398, 2001.

Rosenberg GA, Sferra JJ: Treatment strategies for acute fractures and nonunions of the proximal fifth metatarsal. J Am Acad Orthop Surg 8:332–338, 2000.

Thompson MC, Mormino MA: Injury to the tarsometatarsal joint complex. J Am Acad Orthop Surg 11:260–267, 2003.

Thordarson DB: Talar body fractures. Orthop Clin North Am 32:65–77, 2001.

Torg JS, Balduini FC, Zelko RR, et al: Fractures of the base of the fifth metatarsal distal to the tuberosity: Classification and guidelines for non-surgical and surgical management. J Bone Joint Surg [Am] 661:209–214, 1984.

Weinfeld SB: Surgical approaches to the talus. Foot Ankle Clin 9:703–708, 2004.

CHAPTER 7

Hand, Upper Extremity, and Microvascular Surgery

Lance M. Brunton AND A. Bobby Chhabra

CONTENTS

I. Anatomy*

A. Extensor anatomy
1. Extensor (dorsal) compartments of the wrist are depicted in Figure 7–1 and Table 7–1.
2. The extensor retinaculum prevents tendon bowstringing.
3. The **juncturae tendinum** are tendon interconnections in the dorsum of the hand that may mask proximal tendon lacerations.
4. The **sagittal bands** center the **extensor digitorum communis** (EDC) at the **metacarpophalangeal** (MCP) joint and attach to the volar plate (Fig. 7–2).
5. The **central slip** of the EDC inserts on the base of the middle phalanx and extends the **proximal interphalangeal** (PIP) joint (Fig. 7–3).
6. The extensor mechanism of the digit receives contributions from the **interossei** and **lumbricals** (see Figs. 7–3 and 7–4).
7. The radial and ulnar **lateral bands** receive contributions from the central slip of the EDC and the intrinsic muscles and then converge to form the **terminal extensor tendon**, which inserts on the base of the distal phalanx (see Figs. 7–3 and 7–4).
8. The **transverse retinacular ligament** prevents dorsal subluxation of the lateral bands (see Fig. 7–4).
9. The **triangular ligament** prevents volar subluxation of the lateral bands (see Fig. 7–3).
10. The **oblique retinacular ligament** (ligament of Landsmeer) is the most distal structure of the extensor mechanism and helps link PIP and **distal interphalangeal** (DIP) joint extension. This ligament becomes contracted in chronic boutonniere deformities (see Fig. 7–4).
11. **Grayson's and Cleland's ligaments** attach the radial and ulnar aspects of the distal phalanx to the overlying skin and lie volar and dorsal to the digital neurovascular bundles, respectively (Grayson's, ground; Cleland's, ceiling).

*See also Chapter 2, Anatomy.

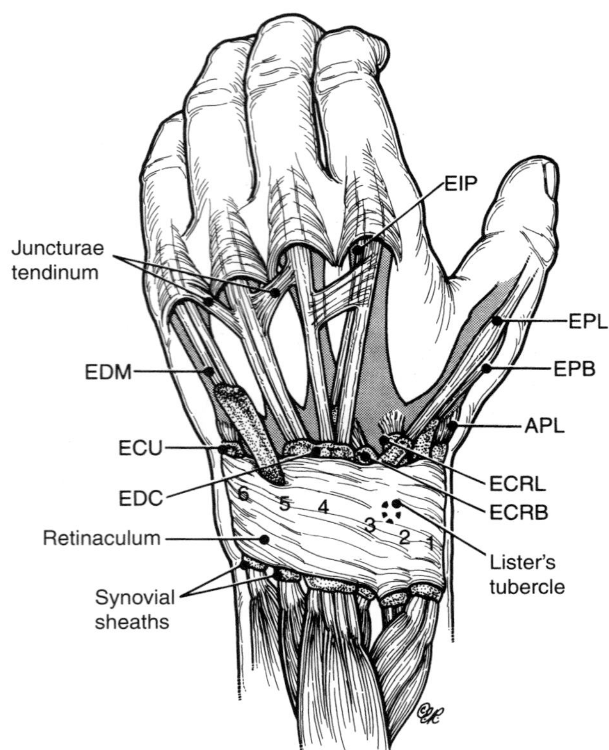

FIGURE 7–1 Dorsal compartments of the wrist and extensor tendons. The first compartment contains the abductor pollicis longus (APL) and extensor pollicis brevis (EPB); the second contains the radial wrist extensors, extensor carpi radialis longus (ECRL), and extensor carpi radialis brevis (ECRB); the third contains the extensor pollicis longus (EPL); the fourth contains the extensor digitorum communis (EDC) and extensor indicis proprius (EIP); the fifth contains the extensor digiti minimi (EDM); and the sixth contains the extensor carpi ulnaris (ECU). (From Doyle JR: Extensor tendons—Acute injuries. In Green DP, Hotchkiss RM, Pederson WC, eds: Green's Operative Hand Surgery, 4th ed, p 1951. New York, Churchill Livingstone, 1998.)

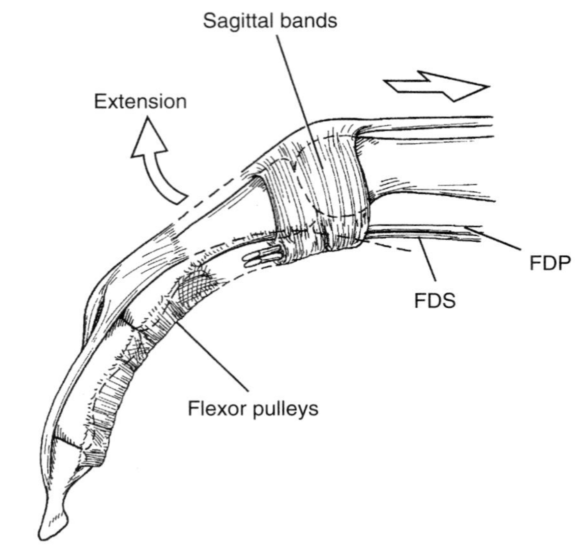

FIGURE 7–2 Sagittal bands of the extensor mechanism provide for extension of the metacarpophalangeal joint. FDP, flexor digitorum profundus; FDS, flexor digitorum superficialis. (From Trumble TE, ed: Principles of Hand Surgery and Therapy. Philadelphia, WB Saunders, 2000.)

B. Flexor anatomy
1. The **flexor digitorum profundus** (FDP) flexes the DIP joint, and the **flexor digitorum superficialis** (FDS) flexes the PIP joint. The small-finger FDS is absent in approximately 20% of people. The FDP tendon splits the FDS at **Camper's chiasma**, which is located at the level of the proximal phalanx (Fig. 7–5).
2. The digital flexor tendons are contained within sheaths distal to the MCP joints. Each of the four digits has five annular pulleys (A1-A5) and three cruciate pulleys (C1-C3). The A2 and A4 pulleys prevent flexor tendon bowstringing (Fig. 7–6). The thumb has two annular pulleys and an oblique pulley in between that prevents bowstringing.
3. The **carpal tunnel** contains the median nerve and nine flexor tendons (one **flexor pollicis longus** (FPL), four FDS, and four FDP tendons). The FPL tendon is the most radial structure. The FDS tendons of the long and ring digits are volar to the FDS tendons of the index and small digits. All four of the FDS tendons are volar to the FDP tendons (Fig. 7–7). The **Guyon canal** (ulnar tunnel) contains the ulnar nerve and artery.
4. The **palmaris longus** tendon, a common source of autograft for various reconstructive procedures in the upper extremity, is present in approximately 85% of people. The tendon becomes prominent with wrist flexion and thumb-to-small finger opposition.
5. The **flexor carpi radialis** (FCR) and the **flexor carpi ulnaris** (FCU) are the primary wrist flexors. The FCR inserts on the second metacarpal, and the

TABLE 7-1 EXTENSOR (DORSAL) COMPARTMENTS OF THE WRIST

Compartment	Tendons	Associated Pathology	Other Points
1	APL/EPB	de Quervain tenosynovitis	APL may have multiple slips or a separate compartment
2	ECRL/ECRB	Intersection syndrome	Radial to Lister's tubercle
3	EPL	Late rupture after closed treatment of distal radius fracture	Ulnar to Lister's tubercle; test by placing palm flat on table and lifting thumb
4	EDC/EIP	Extensor tenosynovitis	EIP ulnar to index EDC EDC to small finger in only 25%
5	EDM	Vaughn-Jackson syndrome	EDM ulnar to small EDC
6	ECU	ECU subluxation	ECU subsheath part of TFCC

APL, abductor pollicis longus; ECRB, extensor carpi radialis brevis; ECRL, extensor carpi radialis longus; ECU, extensor carpi ulnaris; EDC, extensor digitorum communis; EDM, extensor digiti minimi; EIP, extensor indicis proprius; EPB, extensor pollicis brevis; EPL, extensor pollicis longus; TFCC, triangular fibrocartilage complex.

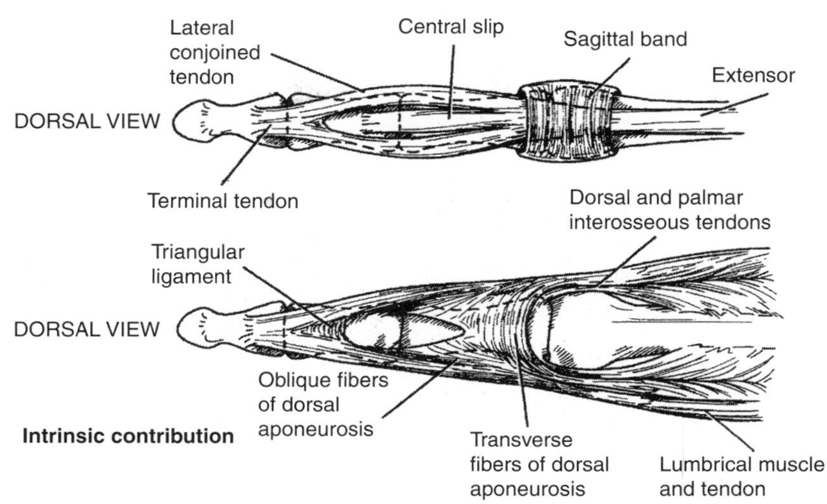

FIGURE 7–3 Dorsal view of the digital extensor tendon and intrinsics. (From Trumble TE, ed: Principles of Hand Surgery and Therapy. Philadelphia, WB Saunders, 2000.)

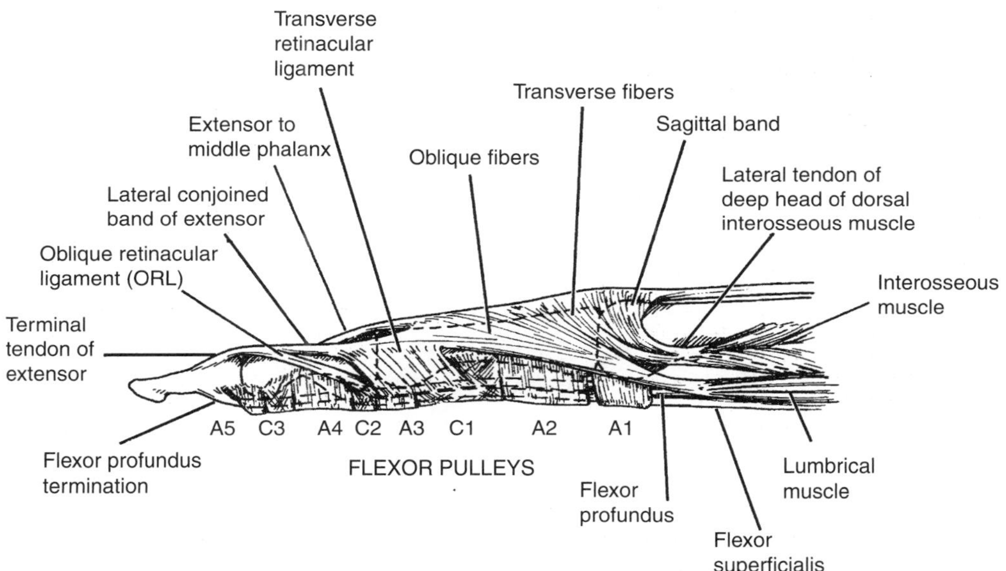

FIGURE 7–4 Lateral view of digital extensor tendons and intrinsics. (From Trumble TE, ed: Principles of Hand Surgery and Therapy. Philadelphia, WB Saunders, 2000.)

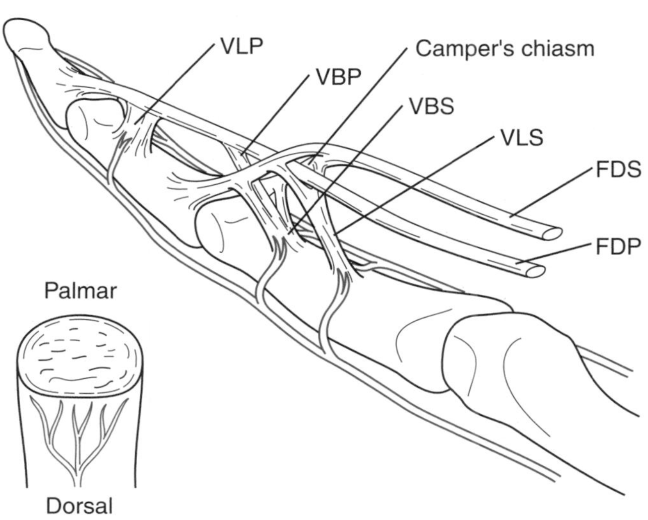

FIGURE 7–5 Decussation of the flexor digitorum superficialis produces Camper's chiasm. Both the flexor digitorum superficialis (FDS) and flexor digitorum profundus (FDP) receive their blood supply via the vinculum longus and brevis. VBP, vinculum brevis profundus; VBS, vinculum brevis superficialis; VLP, vinculum longus profundus; VLS, vinculum longus superficialis. (From Trumble TE, Budoff JE, Cornwall R, eds: Core Knowledge in Orthopaedics: Hand, Elbow, and Shoulder, p 190. Philadelphia, CV Mosby, 2006.)

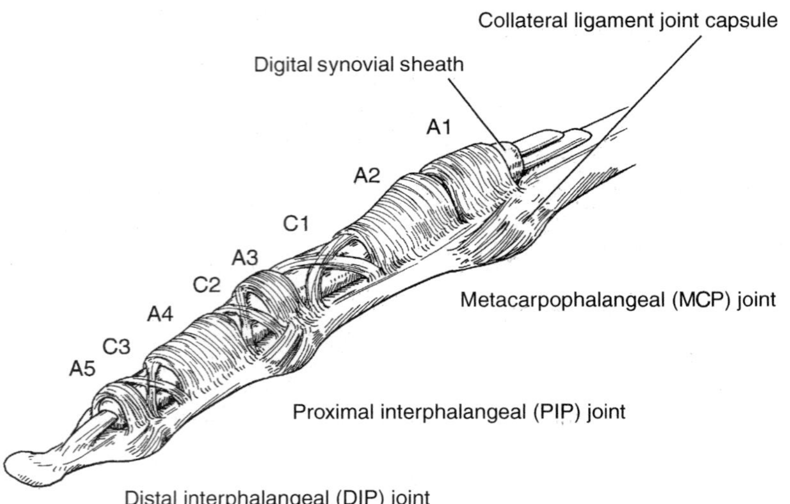

FIGURE 7–6 The flexor tendon sheath is composed of annular and cruciate pulleys. (From Trumble TE, ed: Principles of Hand Surgery and Therapy. Philadelphia, WB Saunders, 2000.)

Flexor retinaculum
Flexor carpi radialis
Transverse carpal ligament
Radial artery
Palmaris longus
Median nerve
Flexor pollicis longus
Flexor digitorum profundus
Flexor carpi ulnaris
Trapezium
Flexor digitorum superficialis
Trapezoid
Ulnar artery
Capitate
Ulnar nerve
Hamate
FDS
Palmaris longus
Median nerve
Ulnar artery
FCR
FCU
Radial artery
Pisiform
Triquetrum
FPL
FDP
Ulnar nerve

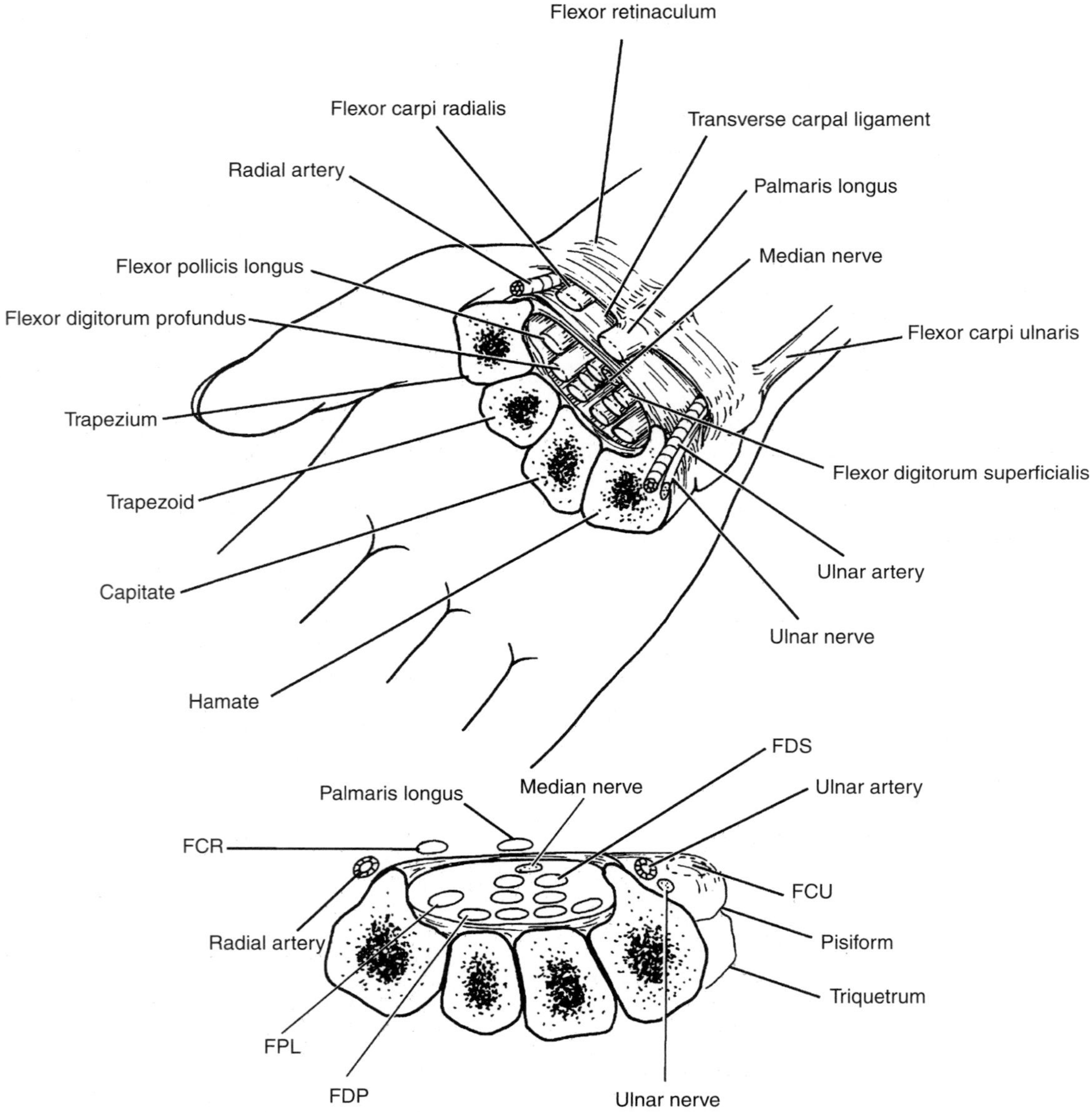

FIGURE 7–7 The median nerve, all of the digital flexor tendons, and the flexor pollicis longus (FPL) pass through the carpal tunnel. FCR, flexor carpi radialis; FCU, flexor carpi ulnaris; FDP, flexor digitorum profundus; FDS, flexor digitorum superficialis. (From Trumble TE, ed: Principles of Hand Surgery and Therapy. Philadelphia, WB Saunders, 2000.)

FCU inserts on the pisiform. The FCU is a more powerful wrist flexor, allowing for use of the FCR in tendon transfers and suspension arthroplasty of the thumb **carpometacarpal** (CMC) joint.

C. Intrinsic anatomy
   1. There are four dorsal and three palmar interosseous muscles. The dorsal interossei are finger abductors, and the palmar interossei are finger adductors. The interossei contribute to MCP joint flexion and interphalangeal (IP) joint extension. They are innervated by the ulnar nerve (Fig. 7–8).
   2. The four lumbrical muscles originate on the radial aspect of the FDP tendons and pass volar to the transverse metacarpal ligaments. The lumbricals help coordinate digital flexion and extension. They contribute to IP joint extension through their insertions on the radial lateral bands of the extensor mechanism. They simultaneously relax the extrinsic flexor system. The two radial lumbricals are innervated by the median nerve, and the two ulnar lumbricals by the ulnar nerve (Fig. 7–9).
   3. Intrinsic tightness is tested by comparing the amount of passive PIP flexion with the MCP joints in both flexion and extension. Because the intrinsic muscles are relaxed when the MCP joints are held in flexion, the test is positive if the amount of passive PIP flexion is less when the MCP joints are held in extension.

D. Neurovascular anatomy
   1. The hand is completely innervated by branches of the **median**, **ulnar**, and **radial nerves**. Figure 7–10 shows the sensory innervation to the hand.
   2. The **anterior interosseous** branch of the median nerve (AIN) innervates the FPL, index and long FDP, and pronator quadratus and is tested by asking the patient to make an "OK" sign. The **palmar cutaneous** branch of the median nerve usually lies between the palmaris longus and flexor carpi radialis at the level of the wrist flexion crease. The **recurrent motor branch** of the median nerve innervates the abductor pollicis brevis (APB), opponens pollicis, and superficial head of the flexor pollicis brevis (FPB).
   3. The ulnar nerve innervates all of the hypothenar and interossei muscles, the ring and small FDP and lumbricals, the FCU, the adductor pollicis, and the deep head of the FPB.
   4. Approximately 15% of the population has crossover variations between the median and ulnar nerves called Martin-Gruber anastomoses, which may create confusion during motor and sensory examination of the hand.
   5. The radial nerve innervates a portion of the brachialis muscle (the remainder is innervated by the musculocutaneous nerve). It also innervates the triceps, anconeus, brachioradialis, and extensor carpi radialis longus (ECRL) before dividing into the **superficial sensory branch** and the **posterior interosseous nerve**, which innervates the remaining extensor muscles of the forearm and hand.
   6. The digital nerves lie volar to the digital arteries. Major bleeding after a volar digital laceration typically indicates concurrent digital nerve injury.
   7. Vascular anatomy is further covered in Section IX, Vascular Disorders.

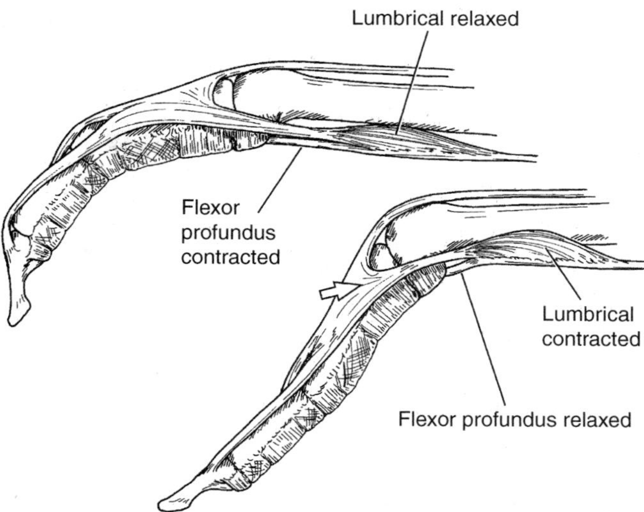

FIGURE 7–9 The lumbrical muscles flex the metacarpophalangeal joint and extend the proximal interphalangeal joint. (From Trumble TE, ed: Principles of Hand Surgery and Therapy. Philadelphia, WB Saunders, 2000.)

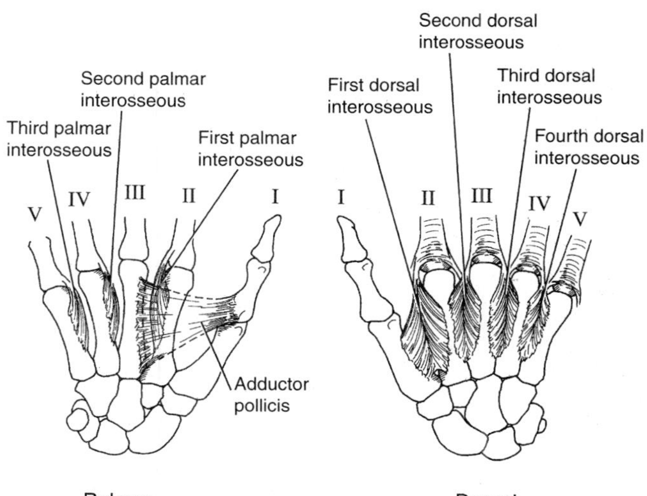

FIGURE 7–8 Four dorsal interossei provide abduction and three volar interossei provide adduction of the fingers. (From Trumble TE, ed: Principles of Hand Surgery and Therapy. Philadelphia, WB Saunders, 2000.)

II. Distal Radius Fractures

A. Introduction—The most common fracture of the upper extremity, with over 300,000 per year in the United States. These fractures typically result from high-energy trauma in young individuals and low-energy falls in older individuals with osteoporosis. The most prevalent group is Caucasian women over age 50. Successful treatment greatly depends on the patient profile, but restoration of normal anatomic relationships and articular surface congruity generally correlate with good outcomes.

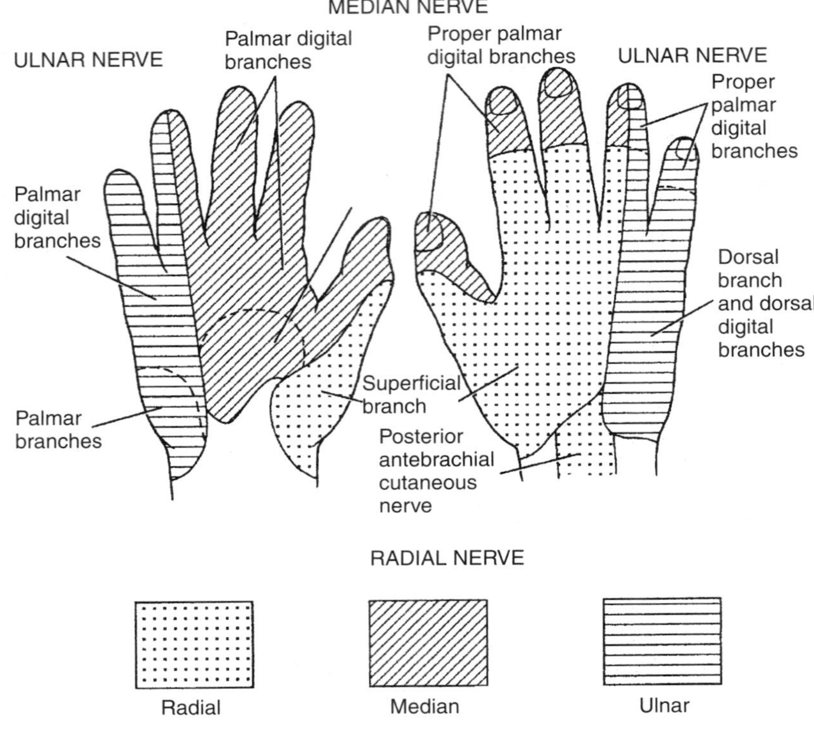

FIGURE 7–10 Sensory patterns of the median, ulnar, and radial nerves for the palm *(left)* and dorsum *(right)* of the hand. (From Trumble TE, ed: Principles of Hand Surgery and Therapy. Philadelphia, WB Saunders, 2000.)

B. Anatomy—The distal radius articular surface is biconcave, with separate facets for the scaphoid and lunate. It articulates with the distal ulna at the sigmoid notch. A small dorsal prominence called **Lister's tubercle** is a common landmark for dorsal surgical approaches. The metaphyseal portion of the distal radius has a thin cortex and is vulnerable to bending forces. The major deforming force in distal radius fractures is the insertion of the brachioradialis. In a normal wrist, 80% of the axial load is transmitted through the radius and 20% through the ulna and **triangular fibrocartilage complex** (TFCC). Altered anatomy leads to altered biomechanics and disproportionate axial load distribution.

C. Diagnosis
   1. Clinical—Pain, swelling, and deformity at the wrist are commonly seen. Open injuries are more common in young patients involved in motor vehicle accidents or falls from a height. Always examine the patient for concurrent snuffbox and ulnar-sided wrist tenderness. Evaluate the elbow and shoulder girdle as well. Median nerve function should be assessed before and after closed reduction. Acute carpal tunnel syndrome may develop in a small percentage of cases and requires emergent median nerve decompression.
   2. Radiographic—Anteroposterior, lateral, and oblique wrist radiographs should be obtained. Evaluate the following radiographic parameters in every distal radius injury:
      a. Intra-articular displacement and step-off—Check all views for extension of the fracture into the articular surface. Greater than 1 mm of articular step-off may lead to early posttraumatic radiocarpal arthrosis.
      b. Distal fragment displacement and angulation—Note the direction of displacement and degree of angulation (apex dorsal, Smith; apex volar, Colles) of the distal fragment on the lateral view. Greater than 20 degrees of initial apex volar angulation may correlate with instability and failure of closed treatment.
      c. Radial height—The distance between two parallel horizontal lines, one drawn tangential to the tip of the radial styloid and the other drawn tangential to the distal surface of the ulna on the anteroposterior view. The average distance is 11-13 mm. An attempt should be made to correct greater than 5 mm of radial shortening.
      d. Radial inclination—The angle between a horizontal line drawn tangential to the distal radius articular surface and another line drawn from the most ulnar aspect of the distal radius articular surface to the tip of the radial styloid on the anteroposterior view (Fig. 7–11). The average radial inclination is approximately 22 degrees; greater than 15 degrees is acceptable.
      e. Volar tilt (lunate fossa inclination)—On the lateral view, a vertical line is drawn parallel to the center of the radial shaft. A horizontal line is then drawn perpendicular to this line and tangential to the volar aspect of the lunate fossa. The angle between this horizontal line

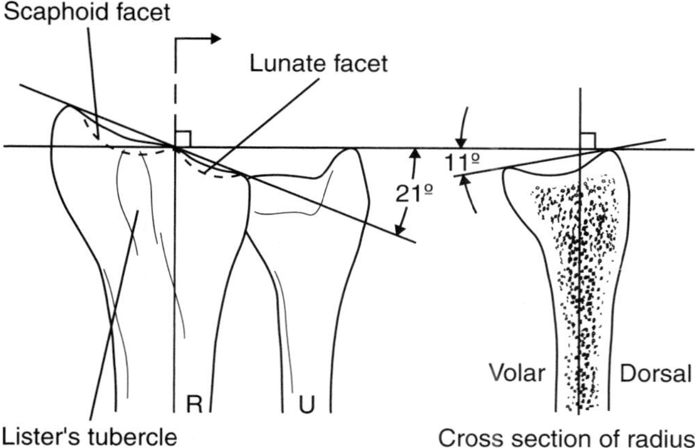

FIGURE 7–11 Schematic drawings of the average inclination and palmar tilt of the distal radius. R, radius; U, ulna. (From Trumble TE, Budoff JE, Cornwall R, eds: Core Knowledge in Orthopaedics: Hand, Elbow, and Shoulder, p 89. Philadelphia, CV Mosby, 2006.)

and a line connecting the volar and dorsal aspects of the lunate fossa measures the tilt of the articular surface, which averages 11 degrees volar (see Fig. 7–11). Up to 5 degrees of dorsal tilt or within 20 degrees of normal (compared with the contralateral uninjured side) is generally acceptable.

f. Ulnar variance—The relative length of the ulna compared with the length of the radius, as measured at the distal articular surface. Ulnar variance may be neutral (normal), positive, or negative (Fig. 7–12).
g. **Distal radioulnar joint** (DRUJ) involvement—Subluxation of the ulna in a dorsal or volar direction may be viewed on the lateral radiograph.
h. Other injuries—Coexisting fractures of the distal ulna or carpal bones may be present. Greater than 3 mm of widening between the scaphoid and lunate on the anteroposterior (AP) view may indicate scapholunate ligament disruption, which is commonly associated with the Hutchinson (''chauffeur's'') fracture.

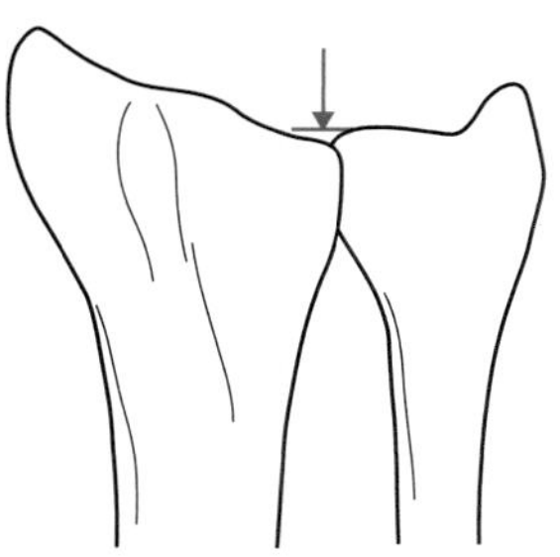

FIGURE 7–12 Ulnar variance of the distal radius. (From Trumble TE, Budoff JE, Cornwall R, eds: Core Knowledge in Orthopaedics: Hand, Elbow, and Shoulder, p 89. Philadelphia, CV Mosby, 2006.)

3. Other imaging studies—A **computed tomographic** (CT) scan provides superior bony detail and may aid in preoperative planning when complex fracture patterns are present. **Magnetic resonance imaging** (MRI) may be used to rule out an occult fracture or evaluate the surrounding soft tissues in patients with negative radiographs and persistent wrist pain after trauma. TFCC, scapholunate, or lunotriquetral ligament tears may be detected.

D. Classification—The common eponymic descriptions for distal radius fractures (e.g., Colles, Smith, Barton, Hutchinson) predate radiography. The most widely used classification of distal radius fractures remains purely descriptive. More than 10 other classification schemes exist (e.g., AO, Frykman, Fernandez, Melone, Mayo), but they largely fail to address prognosis or treatment considerations.

E. Treatment—The goals include maintaining reduction until union, restoring hand and wrist function, and preventing early radiocarpal arthritis. Factors such as age, general medical condition, activity demands, bone stock, fracture stability, and other associated injuries must be considered.

1. Closed reduction
   a. Indications—Definitive, closed treatment with cast immobilization is sufficient in low-energy injuries that are nondisplaced or minimally displaced after closed reduction, especially in functionally low-demand patients. Closed reduction is indicated in displaced fractures with unacceptable radiographic parameters. At the very least, an attempt should be made to restore radial height and volar tilt.
   b. Procedure—A hematoma block using local anesthetic can be administered dorsally to aid in patient comfort during the procedure. A combination of finger traps and an upper arm counterweight is commonly employed to achieve ligamentotaxis prior to manipulation. The reduction maneuver requires initial recreation and exaggeration of the deformity. The distal fragment is then manipulated on top of the radial shaft. A sugar tong plaster splint is applied with a three-point mold. The splint should not compromise MCP motion.
   c. Postreduction considerations—Radiographs should be obtained weekly for the first 3 weeks to make sure that reduction is maintained. Recent literature shows that loss of reduction correlates with increasing age. Immobilization continues for approximately 6-8 weeks. There is currently not enough evidence to determine the best method and duration of immobilization. Stiffness, muscle atrophy, and disuse osteopenia may result from closed treatment. Once immobilization is discontinued, an aggressive therapy regimen is critical to regain range of motion and grip strength. It is important to check active thumb extension at each visit

because extensor pollicis longus (EPL) tendon ruptures may occur from attrition and/or vascular insufficiency. The treatment is extensor indicis proprius (EIP)-to-EPL tendon transfer.

2. Surgical options—There are many options for surgical intervention. Systematic review of nearly 50 trials of various surgical methods for the treatment of distal radius fractures by the Cochrane Database group concluded that insufficient evidence exists to determine when or what type of surgery should be performed for the best overall clinical outcome. Treatment of these injuries should continue to be individually based and will certainly be guided by surgeon experience and preference.
   a. **Closed reduction and percutaneous pinning** (CRPP) with 0.062-inch K-wires—May be sufficient for extra-articular fractures. Kapandji intrafocal pinning employs K-wires as reduction tools to manipulate the distal fragment into anatomic alignment but is contraindicated in intra-articular fracture patterns and osteoporotic bone. These techniques may be supplemented by **external fixation**. The use of both the bridging (distal pins in the second metacarpal) and nonbridging (distal pins in the distal fragment) methods of external fixation have been advocated either alone or in combination with other treatment methods. Restoration of volar tilt and avoidance of joint distraction are technical challenges in bridging external fixation.
   b. **Open reduction with internal fixation** (ORIF)—Used for complex, unstable intra-articular fractures. It is also recommended for the Smith and Barton fracture patterns. A well-performed ORIF most reliably restores articular congruity. Dorsal-, volar-, and fragment-specific fixation methods have been employed, each with specific advantages and disadvantages. The main advantage of performing ORIF is to allow early wrist motion.
   c. **Dorsal plating**—Performed through a relatively simple approach between the third and fourth extensor compartments. The articular reduction is directly visualized. Although newer, lower-profile plates are now available, the historical disadvantages of this approach are extensor tendon irritation, potential tendon rupture, and the frequent need for hardware removal. These problems are avoided through a volar Henry approach between the FCR and radial artery. The classic indications for volar plating are the Smith and volar Barton fracture patterns. Newer fixed-angle locking plates allow for reduction and stabilization of dorsally displaced fractures. The volar approach may be complemented by wrist arthroscopy to aid in articular reduction. The fragment-specific fixation method, popularized by Medoff, uses low-profile constructs to restore anatomy but requires multiple incisions and is technically challenging. Intramedullary nails have been developed to allow for simple percutaneous fixation of minimally comminuted, extra-articular fracture patterns, but no long-term data exist to determine their efficacy. There is increased interest in percutaneously injected bone graft substitutes, such as calcium phosphate and coralline hydroxyapatite, but the supporting literature is limited to several observational case series.

F. Complications—Include nonunion, malunion, post-traumatic arthritis, carpal instability, EPL rupture, hardware failure, stiffness, and complex regional pain syndrome. Nonunion is uncommon. Asymptomatic malunion in a functionally low-demand patient does not require treatment. Low-demand patients with pain from ulnocarpal impaction may benefit from a distal ulna resection (Darrach procedure). A corrective radius osteotomy with ORIF and bone grafting may be indicated for higher-demand patients. Radiocarpal arthrosis is present in over 90% of patients with residual articular step-off of 1 mm and in 100% of patients with step-off of over 2 mm. Jupiter has determined that approximately two thirds of these patients will be symptomatic. EPL ruptures occur in approximately 3% of distal radius fractures during the course of treatment. When primary repair is not possible, a palmaris longus graft or EIP-to-EPL transfer is used.

III. Carpal Fractures and Instability

A. Anatomy—There are eight carpal bones aligned in two rows. The proximal row consists of the scaphoid, lunate, and triquetrum. The distal row contains the trapezium, trapezoid, capitate, and hamate. The scaphoid links the proximal and distal rows. The pisiform is a sesamoid bone within the FCU tendon. The carpus has a rich vascular supply with multiple anastomoses; however, the scaphoid, lunate, and capitate may each have a large area supplied by a single interosseous vessel. Ligamentous anatomy will be discussed later in this section.

B. Scaphoid fractures—The scaphoid is the most commonly fractured carpal bone (Table 7–2), accounting for up to 15% of all acute wrist injuries.

1. Anatomy—Approximately 75% of the scaphoid is covered by articular cartilage. The main blood supply to the scaphoid comes from a dorsal branch of the radial artery, enters at the dorsal ridge just distal to the waist, and flows in retrograde fashion toward the proximal pole. Additional branches off the superficial palmar branch of the radial artery enter at the distal tubercle and perfuse the distal third of the scaphoid. Because of this tenuous vascular anatomy, fractures of the waist and proximal pole are at risk for nonunion and post-traumatic osteonecrosis (Fig. 7–13).

TABLE 7-2 INCIDENCE OF CARPAL FRACTURES

Bone	Number of Fractures*	% of Total
Scaphoid	5036	78.8
Triquetrum	880	13.8
Trapezium	144	2.3
Hamate	95	1.5
Lunate	92	1.4
Pisiform	67	1.0
Capitate	61	1.0
Trapezoid	15	0.2
Total	**6390**	

**The number of fractures represents a total of 6390 fractures compiled from three referenced studies to accumulate incidence of carpal bone fractures.*

From Green DP, Hotchkiss RN, Pederson WC, et al: Green's Operative Hand Surgery, 5th ed, p 711. Philadelphia, Churchill Livingstone, 2005.

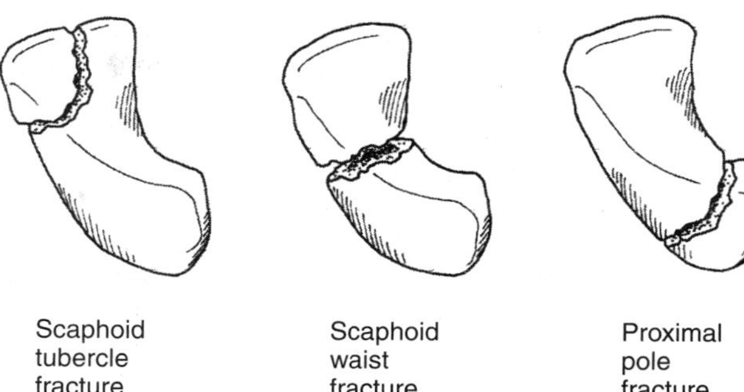

FIGURE 7–14 Scaphoid fractures can be simply described as involving the distal pole or tubercle, waist, or proximal pole. (From Trumble TE, ed: Principles of Hand Surgery and Therapy. Philadelphia, WB Saunders, 2000.)

2. Diagnosis—Scaphoid fractures must be suspected in anyone with radial wrist pain and swelling after injury. The most common mechanism is forced hyperextension and radial deviation of the wrist. Patients often have limited wrist range of motion secondary to pain. Tenderness may be elicited in the anatomic snuffbox dorsally but is more reliably elicited over the scaphoid tubercle volarly. A standard radiographic wrist trauma series, including posteroanterior, lateral, oblique, and scaphoid (30-degree wrist extension, 20-degree ulnar deviation) views, will be nondiagnostic in over 30% of cases on initial presentation. When standard radiographs are negative and a high clinical suspicion exists, there is controversy over the best adjunctive imaging modality to obtain for early diagnosis of a scaphoid fracture. Patients are typically placed in a thumb spica cast, and repeat radiographs are obtained between 2 and 3 weeks after injury. A bone scan, CT, and MRI have all been used for early diagnosis, with MRI appearing to provide the most accurate and cost-effective method. Waiting over 4 weeks to initiate treatment increases the overall nonunion rate from 5% to 45%.

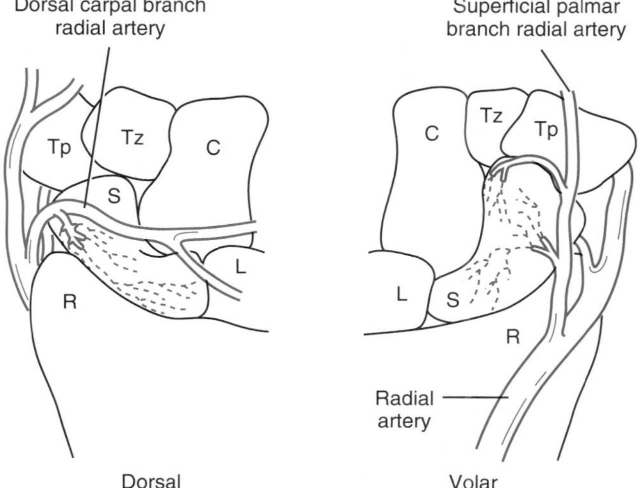

FIGURE 7–13 Dorsal and volar blood supply to the scaphoid from branches of the radial artery. C, capitate; L, lunate; R, radius; S, scaphoid; Tp, trapezium; Tz, trapezoid. (From Trumble TE, Budoff JE, Cornwall R, eds: Core Knowledge in Orthopaedics: Hand, Elbow, and Shoulder, p 117. Philadelphia, CV Mosby, 2006.)

3. Classification—Scaphoid fractures may be classified by their location: the tubercle, waist, and proximal pole (Fig. 7–14). Approximately two thirds of these injuries occur at the waist. Alternatively, scaphoid fractures may be classified by stability. Stable fractures are characterized by a transverse pattern, minimal comminution, and impaction. Unstable fractures often demonstrate more vertical or oblique patterns, significant comminution, and wide displacement.
4. Treatment
   a. Nonoperative treatment—This is best for nondisplaced fractures and consists of cast immobilization. The type of cast used (e.g., long-arm versus short-arm, standard versus thumb spica) is the clinician's preference. With nonoperative treatment, the expected time to union increases and the overall union rate decreases as the fracture becomes more proximal. Consequently, the length of cast immobilization should be greater for more proximal fractures.
   b. Surgical treatment—Union rates of over 90-95% have been consistently reported with operative treatment. Aggressive physical therapy is typically delayed until radiographic union is achieved. CT may be necessary to confirm the union.
      (1) Indications—The indications for surgery include fractures with greater than 1 mm of displacement, angulation greater than 15 degrees (**humpback deformity**), and trans-scaphoid perilunate dislocations. Proximal pole fractures represent another relative indication for acute surgical intervention.

(2) Techniques—Acute fractures with minimal displacement may be treated with percutaneous fixation techniques. Formal ORIF with compression screw fixation is favored for displaced fractures. The approach is dictated by the location of the fracture and surgeon preference.

5. Complications—Include nonunion, malunion, osteonecrosis, and post-traumatic arthritis. Symptomatic, early-stage scaphoid nonunion may be treated with ORIF and bone grafting. The inlay (Russe) technique is best used in cases with minimal deformity and a vascularized proximal pole, and the bone graft may be obtained from the distal radius or iliac crest. Scaphoid nonunion with an accompanying humpback deformity requires an opening-wedge interposition (Fisk) graft to restore scaphoid length and angulation. Although an interference fit is possible, most surgeons typically use a supplemental compression screw. The presence of intraoperative punctate bleeding is the most reliable sign of a vascular proximal pole. Vascularized bone grafting has become more popular in the treatment of scaphoid nonunion with an avascular proximal pole. The graft may be harvested from the distal radius and is based on the **1,2 intercompartmental supraretinacular artery** (1,2 ICSRA). Untreated, chronic nonunions develop a characteristic progression of arthritis called a **scaphoid nonunion advanced collapse (SNAC)** wrist. Options for treatment of a SNAC wrist include radial styloidectomy, proximal row carpectomy, scaphoid excision, four-corner fusion, and total wrist fusion, depending on the stage of presentation and surgeon preference.

C. Other carpal bone fractures—These fractures represent a small percentage of wrist injuries (see Table 7–2).

1. Lunate fractures—Rarely encountered in isolation, although they may be seen in the setting of a perilunate dislocation. Displaced fractures are treated with ORIF, and patients must be counseled on the high rate of post-traumatic osteonecrosis.
2. Capitate neck fractures—May occur in combination with scaphoid fractures or perilunate dislocations and are treated with ORIF or intercarpal fusion.
3. Triquetrum—The majority of injuries are dorsal capsular avulsion fractures and require only a brief period of immobilization.
4. Hook of the hamate—Patients often present with a history of blunt trauma to the palm, frequently associated with certain sports (e.g., golf, baseball, hockey, racquet sports). Accompanying paresthesias of the ring and small fingers are common. A carpal tunnel view may reveal the fracture, but a CT scan is the best confirmatory test (Fig. 7–15). Symptomatic patients who fail a trial of cast immobilization are treated with excision of the fracture fragment. ORIF has been described for larger fracture fragments but has a high complication rate and little clinical benefit. Be aware of the bipartite hamate, which may be differentiated from a fracture by smooth cortical surfaces.

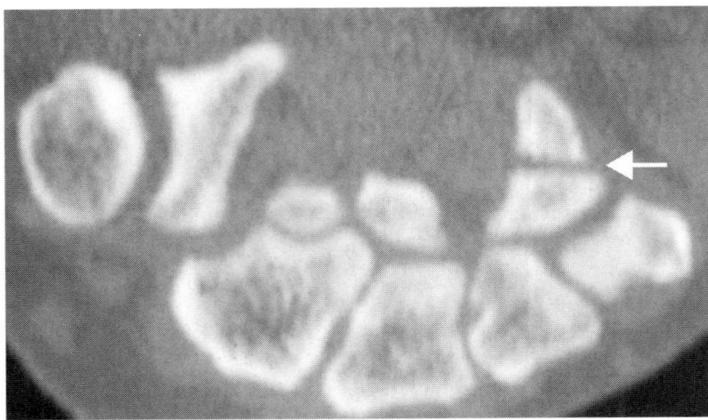

FIGURE 7–15 Sagittal computed tomographic scan of a hook-of-hamate fracture *(arrow)*. (From Trumble TE, ed: Principles of Hand Surgery and Therapy. Philadelphia, WB Saunders, 2000.)

5. Fractures of the trapezoid and pisiform—Very rare.

D. Carpal instability

1. Introduction—Carpal instability results from disruption of the normal kinematics of the wrist. It is characterized by wrist pain, loss of motion, weakness, degenerative arthritis, and disability. Abnormal carpal alignment may result in static or dynamic instability. Static instability can be detected on standard radiographs, whereas dynamic instability requires either stress radiographs or cineradiographic studies to become evident. **Carpal instability dissociative** (CID) describes instability between individual carpal bones of a single carpal row. Examples include the classic patterns of **dorsal intercalated segmental instability** (DISI) and **volar intercalated segmental instability** (VISI) (Fig. 7–16). **Carpal instability nondissociative** (CIND) describes instability between carpal rows, such as midcarpal or radiocarpal instability. Finally, perilunate dislocations are classified as carpal instability complex (CIC).
2. DISI—The most common form of carpal instability. It most often results from disruption of the scapholunate interosseous ligament. The extrinsic volar radiocarpal ligaments may also be involved. Loss of the normal ligamentous constraints leads to scaphoid hyperflexion and lunate hyperextension. Although the majority of cases result from traumatic injuries, attenuation of the ligament may also occur in some forms of inflammatory or crystalline arthropathy.
   a. Diagnosis—Physical examination findings are variable, although Watson's test is often positive. A palpable clunk may be felt while

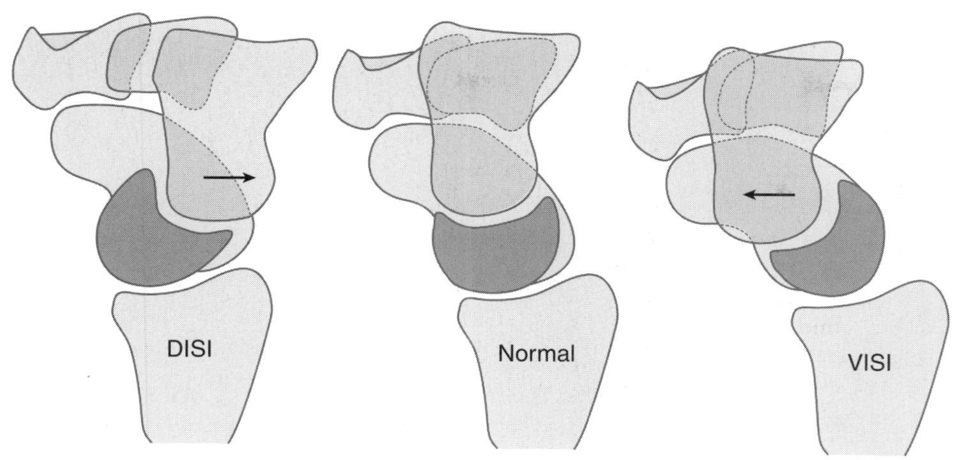

FIGURE 7–16 The two major patterns of sagittal malalignment as described by Dobyns and associates and Linscheid and coworkers. In dorsal intercalated segment instability (DISI) and volar intercalated segment instability (VISI, also known as PISI, for palmar), a midcarpal subluxation is possible *(arrow)*. (From Green DP, Hotchkiss RN, Pederson WC, Wolfe SW, eds: Green's Operative Hand Surgery, 5th ed, p 541. Philadelphia, Churchill Livingstone, 2005.)

applying dorsal pressure to the volar scaphoid tubercle as the wrist is moved from ulnar to radial deviation (Fig. 7–17). Standard radiographs may reveal an increased scapholunate angle (>70 degrees) or a widened scapholunate interval (> 3 mm). Bilateral clenched-fist views should be obtained and compared to confirm a scapholunate diastasis. Pathologic scaphoid hyperflexion may also be manifested as a "cortical ring sign" on the posteroanterior view (Fig. 7–18). MRI has become more sensitive for the detection of scapholunate ligament disruption. Wrist arthroscopy remains the gold standard for diagnosis.

b. Treatment—Treatment depends on the stage and type of instability. In cases of partial scapholunate ligament injury and occult instability, arthroscopic débridement and a

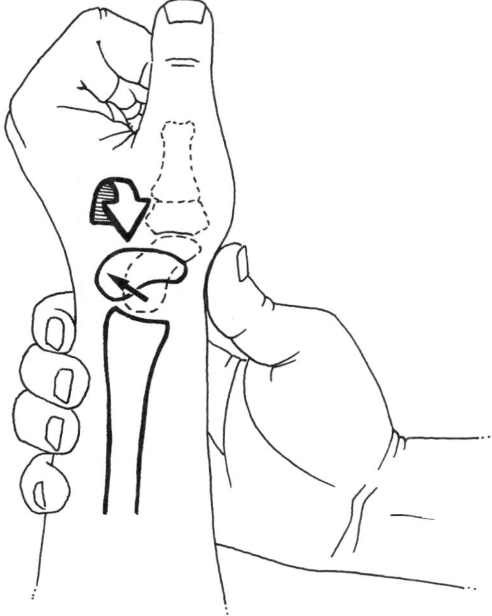

FIGURE 7–17 Watson's scaphoid shift test. Firm pressure is applied to the palmar tuberosity of the scaphoid while the wrist is moved from ulnar to radial deviation *(white arrow)*. In normal wrists, the scaphoid cannot flex because of the external pressure by the examiner's thumb. This may produce pain on the dorsal aspect of the scapholunate interval due to synovial irritation. A "positive" test is seen in a patient with a scapholunate tear or in lax patients; the scaphoid is no longer constrained proximally and will subluxate out of the scaphoid fossa *(black arrow)*. When pressure on the scaphoid is removed, the scaphoid goes back into position, and a typical snapping occurs. (From Green DP, Hotchkiss RN, Pederson WC, Wolfe SW, eds: Green's Operative Hand Surgery, 5th ed, p 557. Philadelphia, Churchill Livingstone, 2005.)

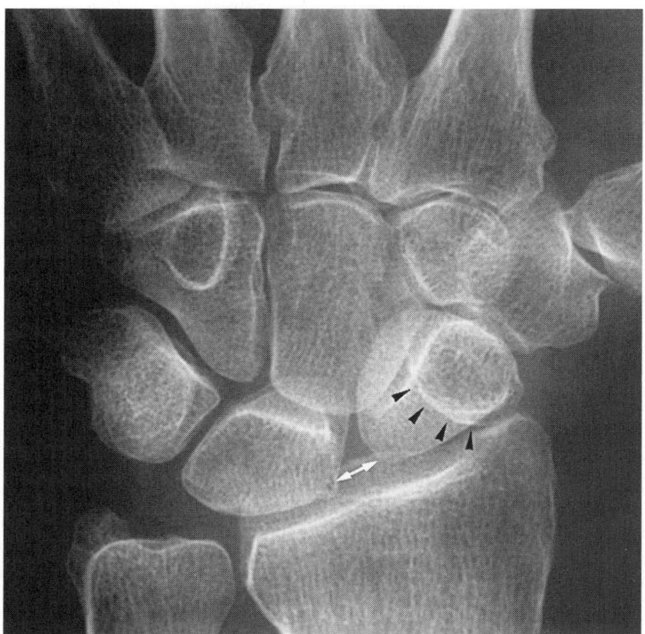

FIGURE 7–18 Posteroanterior view of the wrist of a 35-year-old man who sustained a hyperextension injury 4 months before seeking medical attention. Note the foreshortened scaphoid with the ring sign *(arrowheads)*, representing the frontal projection of the palmar tuberosity, and the increased scapholunate joint space *(white arrow)*, indicating the presence of scapholunate dissociation with rotatory subluxation of the scaphoid. (From Green DP, Hotchkiss RN, Pederson WC, Wolfe SW, eds: Green's Operative Hand Surgery, 5th ed, p 557. Philadelphia, Churchill Livingstone, 2005.)

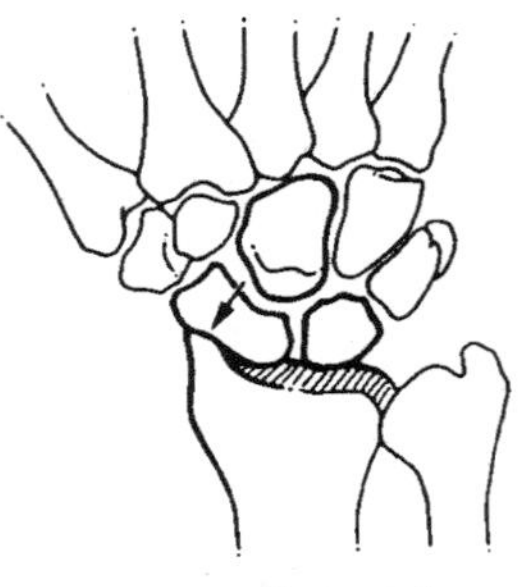
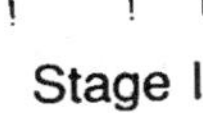

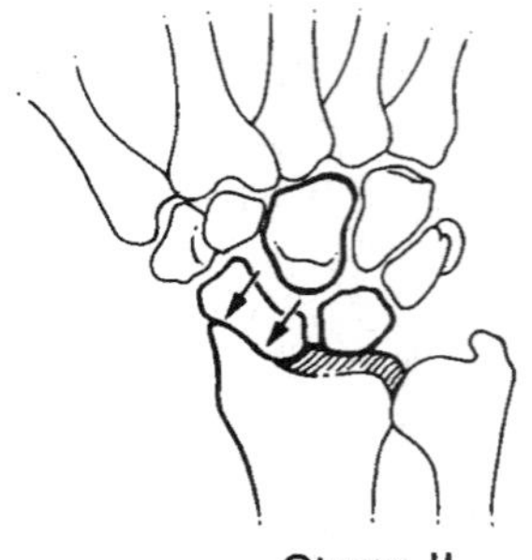

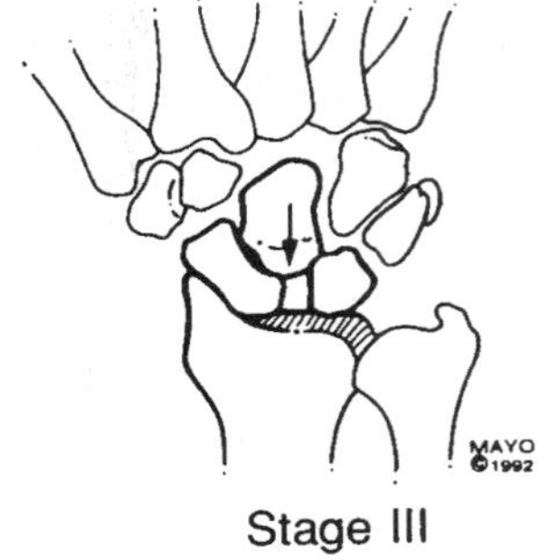

FIGURE 7–19 Stages of scapholunate advanced collapse. With advancing carpal collapse, the capitate may migrate proximally, resulting in midcarpal arthritis and disruption of the Gilula lines. (© Mayo Clinic. Reproduced with permission of the Mayo Foundation.)

period of postoperative immobilization may be sufficient. Acute scapholunate ligament ruptures may be amenable to primary repair. In cases of dynamic instability, multiple procedures have been described. Scapholunate ligament reconstruction and/or dorsal capsulodesis are commonly performed. Cases of chronic, static instability may result in **scapholunate advanced collapse (SLAC wrist)**. Three stages are described (Fig. 7–19). The radioscaphoid and capitolunate joints are affected, but the radiolunate joint is spared. Treatment depends on the condition of the capitate articular surface and the radioscaphocapitate ligament. Options include radial styloidectomy, proximal row carpectomy, scaphoid excision, four-corner fusion, and total wrist fusion.

3. VISI—The second most common form of carpal instability, although the overall incidence is still very low. It results from disruption of the lunotriquetral interosseous ligament. Accompanying injury of the dorsal radiocarpal ligaments may result in static instability. Both the scaphoid and lunate tilt in a volar direction.
   a. Diagnosis—Patients typically have ulnar-sided wrist pain. Possible radiographic findings include a break in Gilula's arc on the posteroanterior view and a scapholunate angle of less than 30 degrees on the lateral view. Arthroscopy is the gold standard for diagnosis.
   b. Treatment—Options for treatment include direct lunotriquetral ligament repair, FCU tendon augmentation, and lunatotriquetral arthrodesis. For patients with concurrent ulnocarpal impaction, an ulnar-shortening osteotomy may be performed, with reliably good relief of ulnar-sided wrist pain.
4. Midcarpal and radiocarpal instability
   a. CIND midcarpal instability—Patients present with a clunking wrist that may or may not be painful. Many of these patients have generalized ligamentous laxity. A history of trauma may not be present. Cineradiographic studies may show a sudden shift of the proximal carpal row, with active radial or ulnar deviation. Nonoperative management is maximized for these patients, and the majority will respond to periods of immobilization and therapy. If surgical intervention is necessary, a midcarpal fusion is the procedure of choice. Ligament reconstruction does not yield long-term success.
   b. CIND radiocarpal instability—This is more common than midcarpal CIND and results from malunion of the distal radius. Treatment is directed at correcting the malunion. Ulnar carpal translation is a radiocarpal CIND that occurs after global rupture of the extrinsic carpal ligaments. Radiographic diagnosis of ulnar translation is made when greater than 50% of the lunate width is translated in an ulnar direction relative to the lunate fossa of the radius. Immediate open repair, reduction, and pinning are indicated because late repairs yield poor results.
5. Perilunate dislocations—Potentially devastating injuries that result from forced dorsiflexion, ulnar deviation, and supination of the wrist. Approximately 25% of these injuries are missed in the emergency department. Mayfield described four stages of perilunar disruption of ligamentous constraints, proceeding in a counter-clockwise direction (from the radius to the ulna). In stages I through III, progressive disruption of the scapholunate, scaphocapitate, and lunotriquetral joints occurs. A volar lunate dislocation represents a stage IV injury and indicates complete circumferential ligamentous disruption (Fig. 7–20). Lesser-arc injuries involve purely ligamentous disruptions, while greater-arc injuries involve accompanying carpal bone fractures (e.g., trans-scaphoid or transcapitate perilunate dislocation). Emergent reduction and stabilization of these injuries are recommended. There is no role for closed treatment. ORIF of bony injuries and open ligamentous repair with percutaneous pinning of the involved joints are performed. Acute carpal tunnel syndrome is treated with emergent carpal tunnel release. Postoperative thumb spica cast immobilization is continued for approximately 8 weeks. Late diagnosis of these injuries results in consistently worse outcomes.

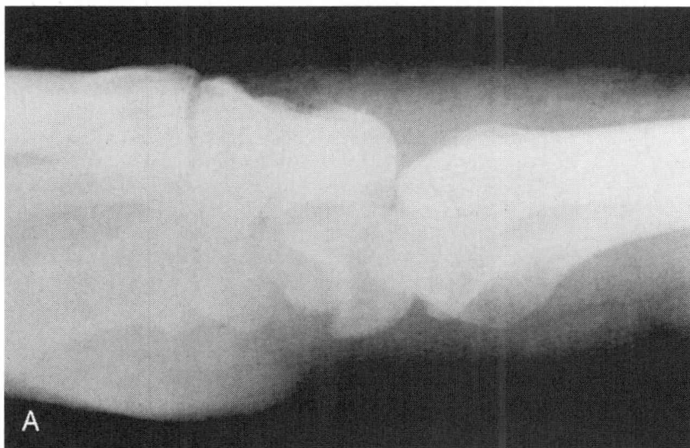

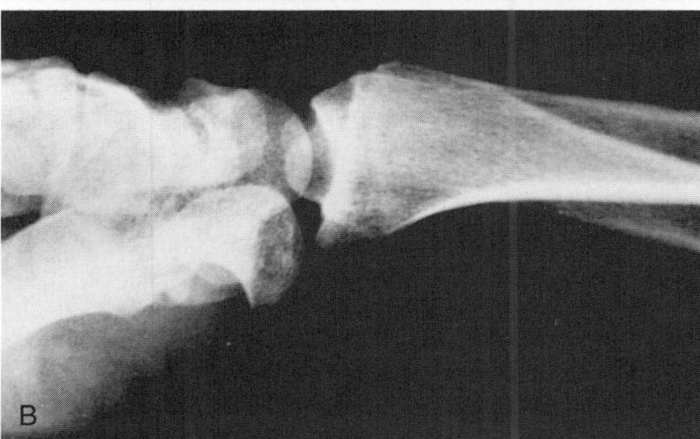

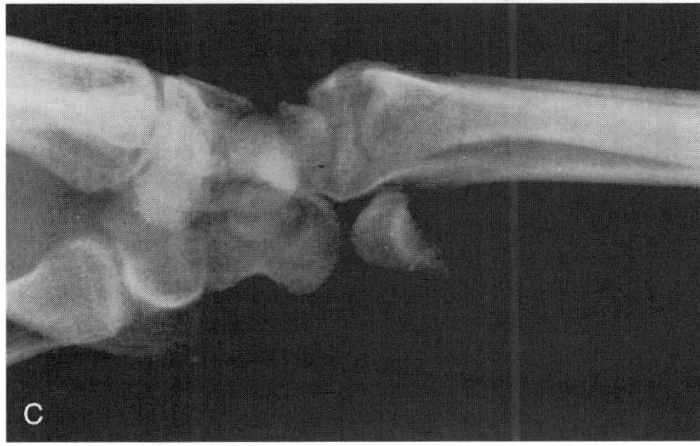

FIGURE 7–20 Carpal dislocations constitute a spectrum of injury, and the initial lateral radiograph in a patient with a carpal dislocation may depict a configuration at any point on that spectrum. **A**, A "pure" dorsal perilunate dislocation. **B**, An intermediate stage. **C**, A "pure" volar lunate dislocation. (From Green DP, Hotchkiss RN, Pederson WC, Wolfe SW, eds: Green's Operative Hand Surgery, 5th ed, p 592. Philadelphia, Churchill Livingstone, 2005.)

IV. Metacarpal and Phalangeal Injuries

A. Introduction—Fractures of the metacarpals and phalanges are the most frequently encountered injuries of the skeletal system. The vast majority of these injuries may be treated nonoperatively. The hand is splinted with the IP joints in full extension, the MCP joints in 70-90 degrees of flexion, and the wrist in 30 degrees of extension (intrinsic-plus position). The MCP joint collateral ligaments are relaxed in extension and taut in flexion. In general, immobilization should not last longer than 3 weeks. Surgical intervention may be necessary in open injuries, intra-articular fractures, irreducible fractures, and digit malrotation and when multiple fractures are present. The goals of treatment are stable reduction, edema control, and early range of motion.

B. Fractures, dislocations, and ligamentous injuries
   1. Metacarpal head—Rare intra-articular injury that most commonly occurs in the index finger. Be aware of associated "fight bites," which require surgical débridement. Greater than 1 mm of articular step-off may warrant ORIF with K-wires or mini–fragment screws. A highly comminuted or open fracture may be best treated with spanning external fixation.
   2. Metacarpal neck—The weakest portion of the metacarpal; most frequently involves the ring and small finger. **Boxer's fracture** technically describes a metacarpal neck fracture of the small finger. The intrinsic muscles are the major deforming force leading to apex dorsal angulation. Many of these injuries may be treated with closed reduction (Jahss maneuver) and 2-3 weeks of immobilization (Fig. 7–21). Acceptable angulation of each metacarpal neck is as follows: index and long fingers, less than 20 degrees; ring finger, less than 40 degrees; and small finger, less than 70 degrees. Percutaneous pinning is rarely necessary. Although malunion may be common, the functional deficits are minimal.
   3. Metacarpal shaft—These fractures may be described as transverse, oblique, or spiral. The latter two fracture patterns are associated with a higher incidence of rotational deformity. Acceptable angulation of each metacarpal shaft is as follows: index and long fingers, less than 10 degrees; and ring and small fingers, less than 30 degrees. No degree of malrotation can be accepted. All digits should point toward the scaphoid tubercle as a clenched fist is made. Comparison with the uninjured contralateral hand is recommended. Just 5 degrees of malrotation will result in 1.5 cm of digital overlap.

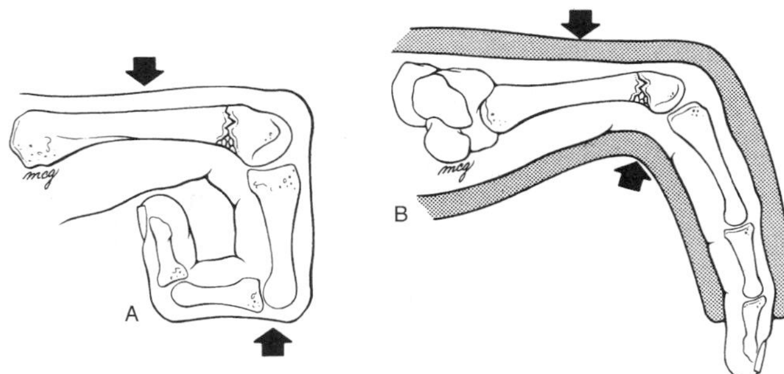

FIGURE 7–21 **A**, The Jahss maneuver for reduction of a metacarpal neck fracture. *Arrows* indicate the direction of pressure application for fracture reduction. **B**, After reduction, the fingers are held in an intrinsic-plus (safe) position in an ulnar gutter splint with molding as indicated by *arrows*. (From Green DP, Hotchkiss RN, Pederson WC, Wolfe SW, eds: Green's Operative Hand Surgery, 5th ed, p 283. Philadelphia, Churchill Livingstone, 2005.)

Every 2 mm of metacarpal shortening leads to 7 degrees of extensor lag, and up to 5 mm is acceptable without significant functional deficit. Irreducible fractures are treated with ORIF. Options include plate-screw constructs and intramedullary fixation. Prominent dorsal plates may interfere with extensor tendon function and necessitate later removal after union is obtained. Multiple metacarpal shaft fractures should be treated operatively regardless of whether displacement or rotational deformity is present.

4. Metacarpal base fracture and CMC joint dislocation—Stable, minimally displaced fractures of the metacarpal base are typically treated nonoperatively. Ring and small CMC joint fractures-dislocations are less common injuries that usually result from high energy and behave similar to a Lisfranc injury of the foot. A pronated 30-degree oblique radiograph provides the best view for diagnosis. A small-finger CMC joint fracture-dislocation is termed a "reverse" or "baby" Bennett fracture. The extensor carpi ulnaris (ECU) tendon is a major deforming force. Accompanying distal row carpal fractures may be seen. CMC dislocations must be percutaneously pinned for 6 weeks and then undergo aggressive range of motion.
5. Thumb metacarpal—The most common fracture pattern is the extra-articular epibasal fracture. Up to 30 degrees of angulation is acceptable secondary to compensatory CMC joint motion. However, excessive angulation may lead to MCP joint hyperextension and requires CRPP. A **Bennett** fracture is described as a fracture-dislocation of the base of the thumb metacarpal. The abductor pollicis longus (APL) causes proximal, dorsal, and radial displacement of the metacarpal base fragment. The adductor pollicis causes supination and adduction of the metacarpal shaft. The anterior oblique ligament keeps the volar ulnar base fragment reduced. CRPP or ORIF is chosen based on the size of the fracture fragments. A **Rolando** fracture is a comminuted intra-articular fracture that may be in the shape of a Y or a T (Fig. 7–22). The degree of comminution guides treatment because CRPP, ORIF, and external fixation all are viable options.
6. Skier's or gamekeeper's thumb—Acute (skier's) or chronic (gamekeeper's) injury to the thumb MCP joint **ulnar collateral ligament** (UCL). A competent UCL is critical for an effective pinch. The mechanism of injury is usually forced hyperextension of the thumb. Differentiation between complete and partial tears is difficult to determine by physical examination alone. Stress radiographs and/or MRI may aid in the diagnosis. A stress examination should not be performed until a bony injury is ruled out. If no fracture is present, the proximal phalanx is stressed radially with the MCP joint fully flexed and fully extended. Instability in full extension can be present only if the UCL and volar plate are completely ruptured. Otherwise, the degree of opening in flexion helps differentiate partial (< 30 degrees) from complete (> 30 degrees) injuries of the UCL. Partial injuries may be treated with thumb spica cast immobilization for 4-6 weeks. In 80% of cases, a complete injury is accompanied by a **Stener lesion**, in which the adductor pollicis aponeurosis is interposed between the avulsed UCL and its insertion site on the base of the proximal phalanx (Fig. 7–23). The presence of a Stener lesion will prevent proper healing of the UCL tear and requires surgical intervention to repair the ligament. A displaced avulsion fracture of the base of the proximal phalanx may occasionally require ORIF with a single screw if the fragment is large enough. Chronic UCL injuries require ligament reconstruction with the use of adjacent joint capsule or a tendon graft.
7. MCP joint dislocation— Classified as simple or complex. Dorsal dislocations are the most common, and the index finger is the most frequently involved. In a simple dislocation, skin dimpling is typically absent and closed reduction is possible. In a complex dislocation, skin dimpling is usually present, and interposition of the volar plate and/or sesamoids occurs. They are usually irreducible by closed means. Longitudinal traction and hyperextension of the MCP joint are avoided during closed reduction

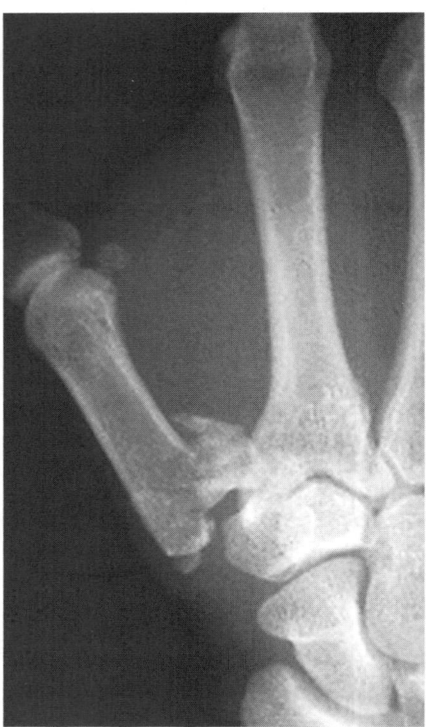

FIGURE 7–22 Comminuted metacarpal base fracture. (From Trumble TE, Budoff JE, Cornwall R, eds: Core Knowledge in Orthopaedics: Hand, Elbow, and Shoulder, p 66. Philadelphia, CV Mosby, 2006.)

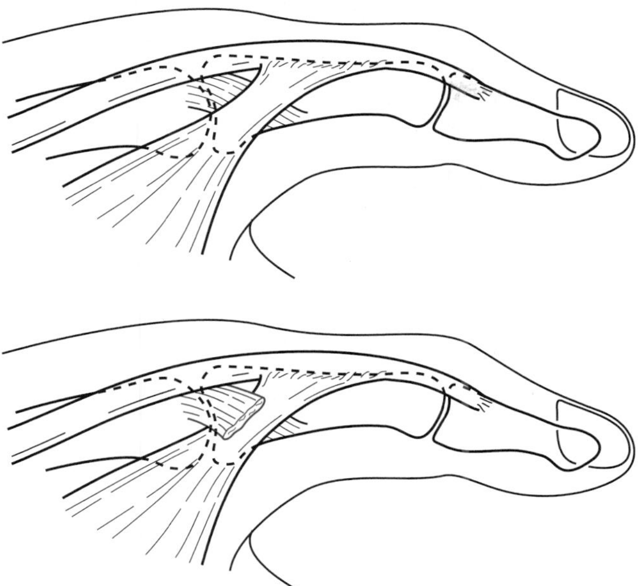

FIGURE 7–23 Stener lesion occurs when the proximal portion of the torn proper collateral ligament on the ulnar side of the thumb metacarpophalangeal joint comes to lie dorsal to the leading edge of the adductor aponeurosis. (From Trumble TE, Budoff JE, Cornwall R, eds: Core Knowledge in Orthopaedics: Hand, Elbow, and Shoulder, p 61. Philadelphia, CV Mosby, 2006.)

maneuvers. Direct pressure is placed over the proximal phalanx with the wrist held in flexion to relax the extrinsic flexors. Irreducible dislocations require open reduction through a dorsal or volar approach; however, the volar approach risks iatrogenic digital neurovascular injury.

8. Proximal (P1) and middle (P2) phalanges—Fractures of P1 will lead to apex volar angulation from proximal fragment flexion (interossei) and distal fragment extension (central slip). Fractures of P2 will lead to either apex dorsal (proximal to the FDS insertion) or apex volar (distal to the FDS insertion) angulation. The majority of these fractures are treated nonoperatively if less than 10 degrees of angulation is present and there is no rotational deformity. Three weeks of immobilization in the intrinsic-plus position is followed by aggressive therapy to restore range of motion. Radiographic union lags behind clinical union by several weeks. Unstable fracture patterns may require CRPP. Long oblique and spiral fracture patterns may be amenable to ORIF with interfragmentary lag screws or a mini–fragment plate-screw construct. External fixation is reserved for highly comminuted intra-articular fractures or those associated with gross contamination and segmental bone loss.
9. PIP joint dislocation—Simple dorsal dislocations are the most commonly encountered and are easily reduced with longitudinal traction. Short-term buddy taping is usually sufficient aftercare. Persistent instability after initial reduction may require 4 weeks of a dorsally based extension block splint. Volar dislocations result in central slip disruption and are much less common, but they often require temporary pinning when unstable after closed reduction. These injuries should be treated with PIP extension splinting for 6 weeks to allow the central slip to heal and prevent a boutonniere deformity. The dislocation is occasionally rotatory, with one of the condyles buttonholed between the central slip and the lateral band. Open reduction is generally required for these injuries.
10. PIP joint fracture-dislocation—Inappropriate recognition and treatment of these injuries may result in significant functional deficits. Dorsal dislocation is accompanied by fracture of the base of the middle phalanx (Fig. 7–24). These injuries have been classified by Hastings into three types based on the amount of P2 articular surface involved (Table 7–3). Treatment options include dorsal block splinting, ORIF, and volar plate arthroplasty. Highly comminuted "pilon" fractures of the base of the middle phalanx may be treated with the Suzuki dynamic traction method to allow early range of motion. Chronic PIP fracture-dislocations are best treated with a volar plate arthroplasty.
11. DIP dislocation and distal phalanx fractures—May accompany extensive soft tissue and/or nail bed disruption in severe fingertip injuries. Open injuries are initially treated with antibiotics, tetanus prophylaxis, thorough wound irrigation and débridement, DIP joint reduction, nail bed repair, and splinting. Unstable, displaced fractures of the distal phalanx may require percutaneous pinning to support the nail bed repair. A stable tuft fracture is more common with these injuries and requires no specific treatment apart from splinting. Soft tissue loss is treated accordingly. For further details see Section VII, Nail and Fingertip Injuries.

V. Tendon Injuries and Overuse Syndromes

A. Extensor tendon injury—Description and treatment are based on zones of injury (Fig. 7–25). The most commonly injured digit is the long finger. In general, partial lacerations constituting less than 50% of the tendon width do not require direct repair if the patient can extend the finger against resistance. These injuries may be treated with early protected motion to prevent adhesions. After direct suture repair of complete lacerations or those constituting greater than 50% of the tendon width, rehabilitation is based on the zone of injury.

1. Zone I injury (mallet finger)
   a. Diagnosis—Represents a disruption of the terminal extensor tendon at or distal to the DIP joint. These injuries often result from sudden forced flexion of the extended fingertip.
   b. Treatment—Treatment of a soft tissue mallet finger detected within 12 weeks of the injury involves extension splinting of the DIP joint for 6-8 weeks. There is no consensus on the best

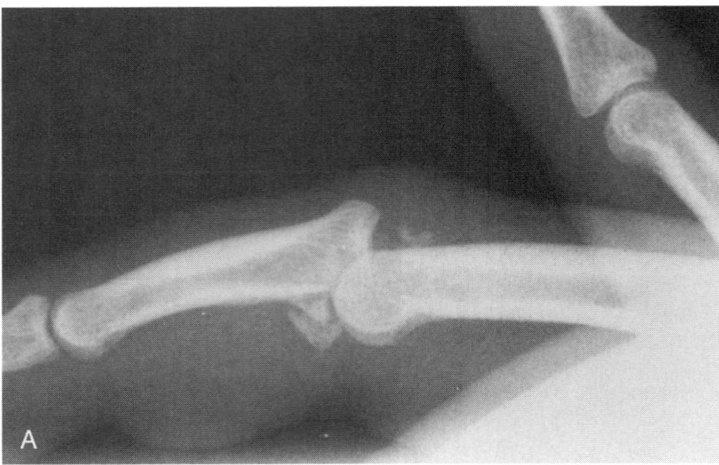

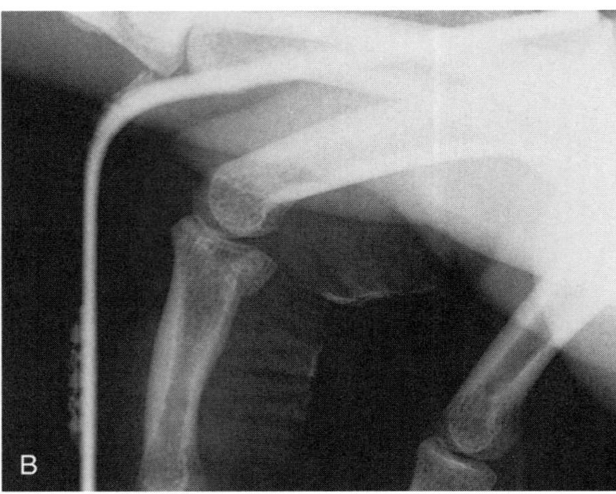

FIGURE 7–24 **A**, Type II fracture-dislocation of the proximal interphalangeal (PIP) joint in which approximately 40% of the volar articular surface is displaced by the fracture fragment. **B**, Fracture-dislocations with 40% or less of the articular surface involved may be successfully treated with dorsal extension block splinting. The patient is allowed to actively flex the PIP joint, which is progressively extended over the course of approximately 4 weeks. The key to this mode of treatment is concentric reduction of the PIP joint. (From Green DP, Hotchkiss RN, Pederson WC, Wolfe SW, eds: Green's Operative Hand Surgery, 5th ed, p 349. Philadelphia, Churchill Livingstone, 2005.)

type of splint to use, but hyperextension should be avoided. Noncompliance is common. A nondisplaced, bony mallet finger may also be treated with extension splinting. If there is volar subluxation of the distal phalanx, percutaneous pinning is required. ORIF should be performed for fragments constituting greater than 50% of the articular surface, and a number of techniques have been described. A chronic mallet finger detected more than 12 weeks after injury typically requires surgical intervention. If the DIP joint is supple and congruent and without arthritic changes, direct repair may be possible. Alternative options include tenodermodesis and **spiral oblique retinacular ligament** (SORL) reconstruction. Prolonged DIP flexion may result in a **swan-neck deformity** (Fig. 7–26), caused by attenuation of the volar plate and transverse retinacular ligament at the PIP joint and consequent dorsal subluxation of the lateral bands, resulting in PIP hyperextension. Contracture of the triangular ligament maintains the deformity. Options for correction of a swan-neck deformity include lateral band tenodesis, FDS tenodesis, and a Fowler central slip tenotomy. The best option for a painful, stiff, arthritic DIP joint is arthrodesis.

2. Zone II injury—Occurs over the middle phalanx of a digit or over the proximal phalanx of the thumb. The mechanism of injury usually involves a dorsal laceration or crush component. Partial disruptions (< 50%) are treated nonoperatively

TABLE 7-3 CLASSIFICATION OF PIP JOINT FRACTURE-DISLOCATIONS (HASTINGS)

Type	Amount of P2 Articular Surface Involved	Treatment
I—Stable	< 30%	Dorsally based extension block splint
II—Tenuous	30-50%	If reducible in flexion, dorsally based extension block splint
III—Unstable	> 50%	ORIF, hamate graft, or volar plate arthroplasty

ORIF, open reduction with internal fixation; PIP, proximal interphalangeal; P2, middle phalanx.

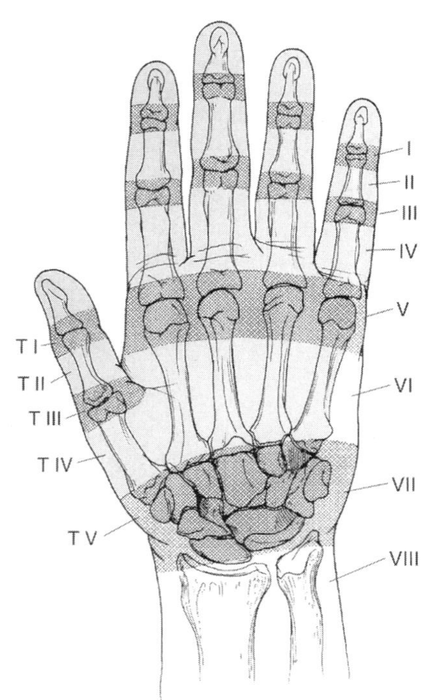

FIGURE 7–25 Zones of the extensor tendon system. (From Trumble TE, Budoff JE, Cornwall R, eds: Core Knowledge in Orthopaedics: Hand, Elbow, and Shoulder, p 203. Philadelphia, CV Mosby, 2006.)

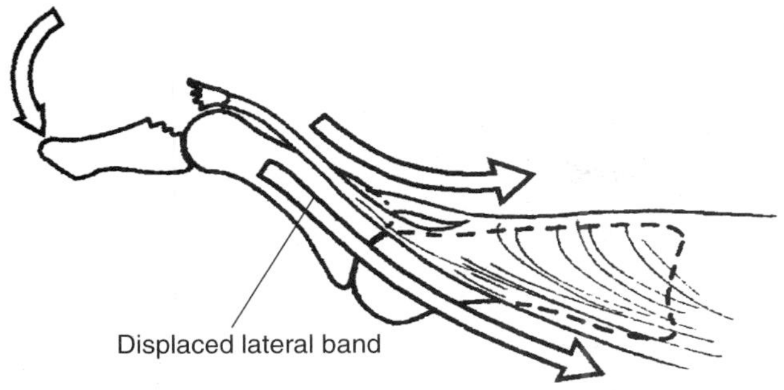

FIGURE 7–26 Swan-neck deformity from proximal migration of the lateral band complex after disruption of the distal extensor mechanism. The lateral bands move proximally into a more dorsal position and contract, which pulls the proximal interphalangeal joint into extension. (From Trumble TE, ed: Principles of Hand Surgery and Therapy. Philadelphia, WB Saunders, 2000.)

with local wound care and early mobilization. Otherwise, direct repair is performed in a manner similar to zone I injuries.

3. Zone III injury
   a. Diagnosis—A central slip rupture over the PIP joint of a digit or the MCP joint of the thumb. The Elson test is performed by flexing the patient's PIP joint 90 degrees over the edge of a table and asking him or her to extend the PIP joint against resistance (Fig. 7–27). The absence of PIP joint extension and fixed DIP joint extension are signs of central slip rupture. An acute **boutonniere deformity** results from attenuation of the triangular ligament and consequent volar subluxation of the lateral bands, resulting in PIP flexion and DIP hyperextension (Fig. 7–28). The deformity is maintained by contracture of the collateral ligaments, volar plate, and oblique retinacular ligament.
   b. Treatment—Treatment of closed injuries involves splinting the PIP joint in full extension for 6 weeks while maintaining active DIP joint flexion. Indications for operative intervention include an open injury and an accompanying displaced avulsion fracture. Loss of tendon substance may require a free-tendon graft or extensor mechanism turndown flap. Treatment of a chronic boutonniere deformity is best performed after attaining full passive PIP joint motion. The central slip is reconstructed, the contracted structures are released, and the lateral bands are repositioned. DIP hyperextension may be treated by releasing the terminal extensor tendon over the middle phalanx. The best option for a painful, stiff, arthritic PIP joint is arthrodesis.

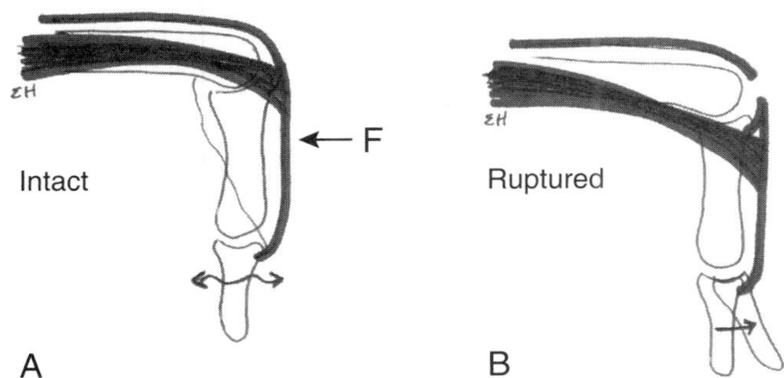

FIGURE 7–27 Elson test for acute rupture of the central slip. F, static force. (From Trumble TE, Budoff JE, Cornwall R, eds: Core Knowledge in Orthopaedics: Hand, Elbow, and Shoulder, p 206. Philadelphia, CV Mosby, 2006.)

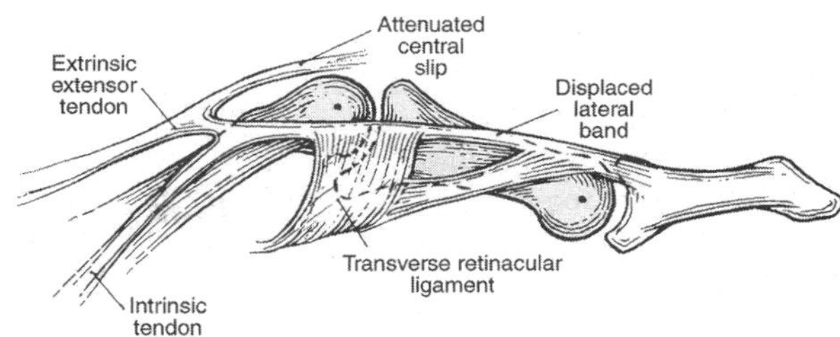

FIGURE 7–28 Boutonniere deformity showing volar migration of lateral bands after disruption of the central slip. As the lateral bands migrate volarly and contract, they produce a flexed posture of the proximal interphalangeal joint but an extended posture of the distal interphalangeal joint. (From Trumble TE, Budoff JE, Cornwall R, eds: Core Knowledge in Orthopaedics: Hand, Elbow, and Shoulder, p 206. Philadelphia, CV Mosby, 2006.)

4. Zone IV injury—Occurs over the proximal phalanx of a digit or over the metacarpal of the thumb. Treatment is similar to that for injuries in zone II. A common complication in this zone is adhesion formation, with resulting loss of digital flexion. Tenolysis may be required. Adhesion formation may be reduced with early protected range of motion and dynamic splinting. The preferred treatment for an unrecognized or chronic EPL rupture is EIP-to-EPL tendon transfer.
5. Zone V injury—Occurs over the MCP joint. Lacerations involving greater than 50% of the tendon substance should be repaired. Early mobilization and dynamic splinting is advocated. A fight bite requires surgical débridement of the MCP joint with delayed wound closure. Metacarpal head/neck fractures or MCP joint dislocations may be associated with these injuries and must be treated appropriately. **Sagittal band rupture** with dislocation of the extensor tendon usually occurs in the long digit. The radial fibers are frequently torn, causing ulnar dislocation of the tendon and an extensor lag. While acute injuries may be treated with 4-6 weeks of extension splinting of the MCP joint (one of the only exceptions to splinting the MCP joints in flexion), repair or reconstruction of the sagittal band is indicated for failed nonoperative treatment or chronic injury.
6. Zone VI injury—Occurs over the metacarpal and represents the most frequently injured zone. Associated lacerations of superficial sensory branches of the radial or ulnar nerves may occur. Direct repair is indicated when the disruption constitutes greater than 50% of the tendon

substance. Early protected motion and dynamic splinting are advocated postoperatively. The prognosis is good in the absence of concurrent skeletal injury.

7. Zones VII and VIII injury—Zone VII injury occurs at the level of the wrist joint, and zone VIII injury occurs in the distal forearm at the musculotendinous junction. Lacerations at the wrist level are usually associated with extensor retinaculum disruption, and postoperative adhesions are common. The retinaculum should be repaired to prevent tendon bowstringing. Static immobilization with the wrist held in extension and the MCP joints partially flexed is advised for the first 3 weeks, followed by protected motion. The results of surgical repair in these zones are not as good as those in zones IV, V, and VI.
8. Zone IX injury—Occurs in the extensor muscle bellies of the proximal forearm. These disruptions are often secondary to penetrating trauma and may be associated with neurovascular injury, which adversely affects the prognosis. Repair is performed with absorbable sutures or tendon grafts placed through the epimysium. The elbow and wrist are immobilized for at least 4 weeks postoperatively.

B. Flexor tendon injury—This injury usually results from volar lacerations, and concomitant neurovascular injury is common.

1. Physical examination—Thoroughly test DIP and PIP flexion of each digit in isolation when multiple digits are injured. Noting the resting position of the involved digit and checking the tenodesis effect of the hand may provide better information than probing the wounds.
2. Treatment overview—In general, partial lacerations constituting less than 25% of the tendon width may be trimmed. Epitenon repair is performed for lacerations involving between 25% and 50% of the tendon width. The standard of care for lacerations greater than 50% of the tendon width is simultaneous core and epitenon repair within 7-10 days of injury. The strength of repair is proportional to the number of suture strands that cross the repair site. In addition, dorsally placed core sutures are stronger. Epitenon repair decreases the gap size and increases the overall strength by 10-50%. An atraumatic minimal-touch technique minimizes adhesions. The A2 and A4 pulleys should be preserved in the digits, and the oblique pulley should be preserved in the thumb to prevent tendon bowstringing. The risk of tendon rupture is the greatest 3 weeks after repair, and failure typically occurs at the suture knots. In general, early protected range of motion is advocated to increase tendon excursion, decrease adhesion formation, and increase repair strength. However, children younger than age 6 require cast immobilization for 4 weeks.
3. Tendon healing factors—Abundant research continues to be focused on flexor tendon injuries. It is important to understand that no repair tissue matches the strength and stiffness of a normal uninjured tendon. Intrinsic healing is directed by tendon fibroblasts. Extrinsic healing potential is limited; there is only a small contribution from repair cells within the tendon sheath or from vascular invasion. Tendon healing is strongly influenced by biomechanical stimuli, and early mobilization has been shown to decrease adhesion formation and increase the strength of repair tissue. Many recent studies have investigated the use of growth factor augmentation of flexor tendon repair, but no definitive conclusions can be made at this point.
4. Treatment according to Verdan's zones (Fig. 7–29)
   a. Zone I injury (''rugger jersey'' finger)—FDP avulsion occurring distal to the FDS insertion. The mechanism of injury is forced extension of the DIP joint during grasping. The ring finger is involved in 75% of cases. These injuries have been classified by Leddy (Fig. 7–30). Type I injuries, in which the FDP is retracted to the palm, require direct repair within 7-10 days. Type II injuries may be directly repaired up to 6 weeks later, as the intact vincula prevent FDP retraction proximal to the PIP joint. Type III injuries require ORIF in addition to

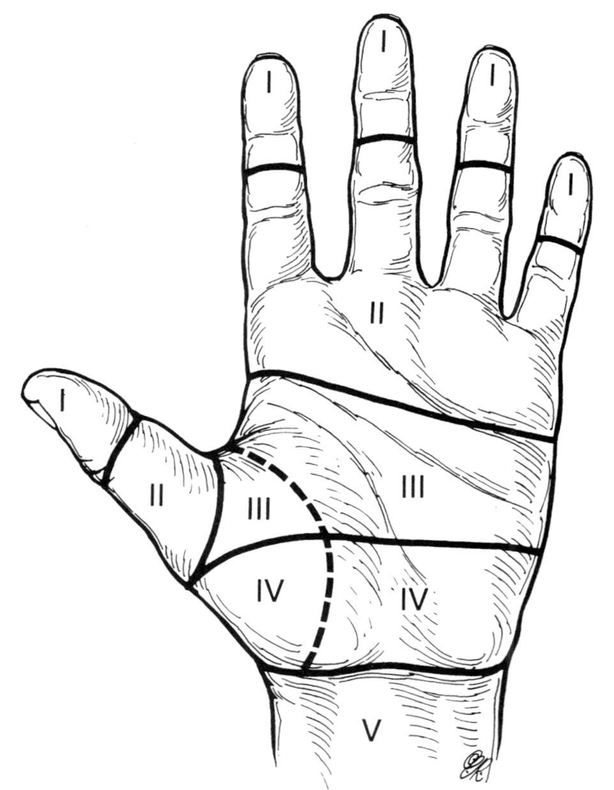

FIGURE 7–29 The flexor system has been divided into five zones or levels for the purposes of discussion and treatment. Zone II, which lies within the fibro-osseous sheath, has been called ''no man's land'' because it was once believed that primary repair should not be done in this zone. (From Green DP, Hotchkiss RN, Pederson WC, Wolfe SW, eds: Green's Operative Hand Surgery, 5th ed, p 221. Philadelphia, Churchill Livingstone, 2005.)

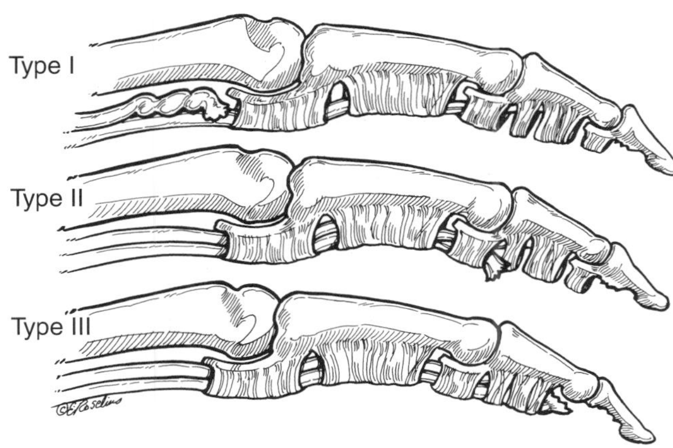

FIGURE 7–30 Profundus avulsion classification of Leddy and Packer. In type I, the flexor digitorum profundus is avulsed from its insertion and retracts into the palm. In type II, the profundus tendon is avulsed from its insertion, but the stump remains within the digital sheath, implying that the vinculum longus profundus is still intact. In type III, a bony fragment is attached to the tendon stump, which remains within the flexor sheath. Further proximal retraction is prevented at the distal end of the A4 pulley. (From Green DP, Hotchkiss RN, Pederson WC, Wolfe SW, eds: Green's Operative Hand Surgery, 5th ed, p 226. Philadelphia, Churchill Livingstone, 2005.)

tendon repair when applicable. Profundus advancement of 1 cm or more carries a risk of DIP joint flexion contracture or **quadrigia**. The latter phenomenon occurs because the FDP tendons share a common muscle belly, and distal advancement of one tendon will compromise flexion of the adjacent digits, resulting in forearm pain. If full PIP flexion is present, chronic type I injuries should be treated with observation. Otherwise, DIP arthrodesis in a functional position is preferred.

b. Zone II injury ("no man's land")—Occurs within the flexor tendon sheath between the FDS insertion and the distal palmar crease. Both the FDS and FDP are injured in this zone. The tendon lacerations may be at a different level than the skin laceration, depending on the position of the finger when the laceration occurred. Direct repair of both tendons with a core and epitendinous suture technique followed by an early mobilization protocol is advocated. The results of treatment in this zone have been historically poor and attributed to the high rate of adhesion formation at the pulleys and associated digital neurovascular injuries. Advances in postoperative rehabilitation have improved the clinical outcomes, although up to 50% of patients require subsequent tenolysis to enhance motion at least 3 months after repair.

c. Zone III injury—Occurs between the distal palmar crease and the distal end of the carpal tunnel. Compared with zone II injuries, the results of direct repair are much better. The lumbrical muscles originate from the radial aspect of the FDP tendons in zone III.

d. Zone IV injury—Occurs within the carpal tunnel. The transverse carpal ligament should be repaired in a lengthened fashion to prevent bowstringing and allow for immobilization of the wrist in flexion.

e. Zone V injury—Occurs between the proximal end of the carpal tunnel and the musculotendinous junction. Direct repair in this zone has a favorable prognosis. The results may be compromised by coexisting neurovascular injury.

5. Treatment specific to the FPL injury in the thumb—Direct repair of the FPL is advocated, although the rate of re-rupture is higher than it is in the digits.
   a. Zone I injuries—Occur distal to the IP joint crease
   b. Zone II injuries—Occur between the IP and MCP joint creases
   c. Zone III injuries—Occur beneath the thenar muscles
6. Flexor tendon reconstruction—Indicated for failed primary repair or chronic, untreated injuries. Requirements include supple skin, a sensate digit, adequate vascularity, and full passive range of motion of the adjacent joints. The majority of cases require a two-stage reconstruction. During stage I a temporary silicone rod is implanted, secured distally, and allowed to glide proximally. The A2 and A4 pulleys are either preserved or reconstructed. Stage II is performed at least 3 months later, after full passive range of motion has been attained and a sheath has formed around the silicone rod. The rod is removed, and a tendon autograft is passed through the sheath and underneath the pulley system. Extrasynovial graft choices include palmaris longus or plantaris or a toe extensor. Postoperative rehabilitation is intensive, and subsequent tenolysis is needed at least 50% of the time.
7. Kleinert and Duran protocols—The two most common postoperative rehabilitation protocols are those of Kleinert and Duran. The Kleinert protocol employs dynamic splinting, which allows for active digit extension and passive digit flexion. Synergistic splints also allow for active wrist motion to improve tendon excursion. The Duran protocol requires strict patient compliance because the other hand is used to perform passive digital flexion exercises. Both programs control motion for approximately 6 weeks. Newer protocols add components of early active digital flexion with the hope of further reducing adhesion formation and increasing tendon excursion. These protocols require stronger repair methods.

C. Stenosing tenosynovitis (trigger finger)
   1. Diagnosis—Caused by inflammation of the flexor tendon sheath, which inhibits the smooth gliding motion of flexor tendons in the digits or thumb. This common condition is initially characterized by pain and tenderness at the distal palm near the

TABLE 7-4 CLASSIFICATION OF TRIGGER DIGIT (GREEN)

Grade	Description
I	Pain and tenderness at the A1 pulley
II	Catching of digit
III	Locking of digit; passively correctable
IV	Fixed, locked digit

A1 pulley. If left untreated, stenosing tenosynovitis may lead to catching and locking of the digit as the space available for the flexor tendon narrows. The most widely used classification scheme was developed by Green (Table 7–4). The ring finger is the most commonly affected digit in adults (the thumb in children). Trigger finger occurs more frequently in middle-aged females, diabetics, and patients with rheumatoid arthritis. It may result from repetitive grasping activities.

2. Treatment—A great majority of patients, excluding the diabetic population, will respond favorably to corticosteroid injection into the flexor tendon sheath. For those who fail nonoperative management, open release of the A1 pulley yields a less than 10% recurrence rate. The adjacent digital neurovascular bundles must be well-protected during open release. A percutaneous technique with an 18-gauge needle is becoming more popular. Regardless of the technique, postoperative therapy is of paramount importance.

D. de Quervain tenosynovitis

1. Diagnosis—Affects the APL and extensor pollicis brevis (EPB) tendons in the first extensor compartment of the wrist. It commonly affects middle-aged women. New mothers, golfers, and racquet sport athletes are also affected. In addition to dorsoradial wrist tenderness and swelling, crepitus may be elicited over the tendons during thumb motion. Finkelstein's test places the first extensor compartment under maximum tension and exacerbates the symptoms. The examiner deviates the wrist in an ulnar direction while the patient holds his or her thumb within the palm.
2. Treatment—Nonoperative management includes rest, activity modification, thumb spica cast immobilization, **nonsteroidal anti-inflammatory drugs** (NSAIDs), and corticosteroid injections. When these measures fail, surgical release of the first extensor compartment may be performed. The dorsal aspect is released and the retinaculum preserved to prevent volar tendon subluxation. Anatomic variation within the first extensor compartment is frequently encountered in recalcitrant cases. The APL may have multiple slips, and the EPB may have its own separate compartment. Complications of operative treatment include superficial sensory radial nerve injury with neuroma formation, tendon subluxation, complex regional pain syndrome, and recurrence from incomplete release.

E. Intersection syndrome—Defined as tenosynovitis and/or bursitis occurring at the junction between the first and second extensor compartments, where the APL and EPB muscles cross the extensor carpi radialis longus and brevis (ECRL and ECRB, respectively) tendons. This overuse syndrome is seen in rowers, weightlifters, and golfers with some frequency. Tenderness, swelling, and crepitus are localized to an area approximately 4-5 cm proximal to the radiocarpal joint. When nonoperative measures fail, surgical release of the second extensor compartment and débridement of inflamed bursae may be effective.

F. FCR tendinitis—Overuse syndrome from repetitive resisted wrist flexion. Localized tenderness at the volar radial aspect of the wrist may be elicited and exacerbated by resisted wrist flexion. Nonoperative management with splint immobilization and corticosteroid injections is largely successful, but release of the FCR tendon sheath is required in a small percentage of resistant cases.

G. FCU calcific tendinitis—Characterized by the acute onset of volar ulnar wrist pain and swelling that may mimic pseudogout or septic arthritis in its severity. Fluffy calcium deposits may be seen on plain radiographs. The inflammation usually responds to ice, immobilization, and high doses of NSAIDs.

H. ECU tendinitis and subluxation—The ECU tendon is held tightly within a groove in the distal ulna, which is tethered by its fibro-osseous sheath. Overuse commonly leads to tendinitis. MRI may reveal splits or increased signal intensity within the tendon. Nonoperative management with rest, activity modification, splinting, NSAIDs, and corticosteroid injections is recommended. Traumatic subluxation of the ECU tendon may result from forceful hypersupination and ulnar deviation of the wrist. A painful snap or manual dislocation may be induced with the reproduction of this mechanism on physical examination. If diagnosed early, long-arm cast immobilization with the wrist held in pronation and slight radial deviation can be attempted. Chronic cases require either direct repair or reconstruction of the overlying extensor retinaculum, often accompanied by deepening of the ulnar groove. Wrist arthroscopy reveals concurrent TFCC tears in 50% of cases.

VI. Distal Radioulnar Joint, Triangular Fibrocartilage Complex, and Wrist Arthroscopy

A. Anatomy—The radius rotates about a fixed ulna at the DRUJ. Ulnar variance measures the distance in millimeters between the distal aspect of the ulnar head and the articular surface of the distal radius (Fig. 7–31). The amount is determined on a posteroanterior radiograph of the wrist with the forearm in a neutral position. There is relative positive ulnar variance with the forearm in pronation and negative ulnar variance with the forearm in supination. The TFCC stabilizes the DRUJ and transmits 20% of axial loads at the wrist (neutral ulnar variance). The components of the TFCC include the dorsal and volar radioulnar ligaments, the articular disk, a meniscus

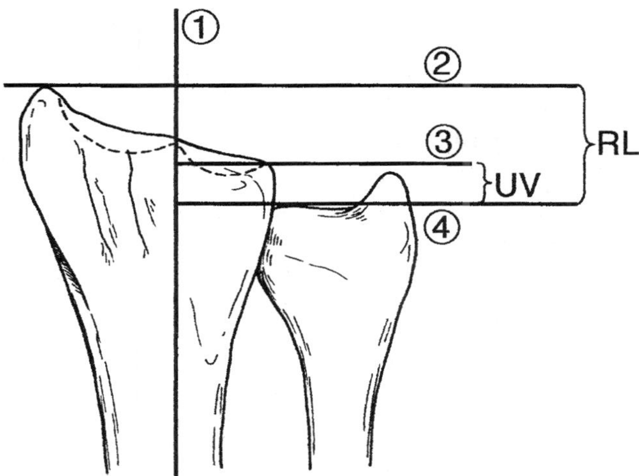

FIGURE 7–31 The relative length (RL) of the radius and ulna can be determined by measuring the distance from the tip of the radial styloid (line 2) drawn perpendicular to the long axis of the radius (line 1) and the distal end of the ulnar articular surface (line 4). The ulnar variance (UV) is measured as the distance between line 4 and line 3, the dense cortical line along the ulnar border of the distal radius articular surface. (From Trumble TE: Distal radioulnar joint and triangular fibrocartilage complex. In Principles of Hand Surgery and Therapy. Philadelphia, WB Saunders, 2000.)

homologue, the UCL, the ECU subsheath, and the origins of the ulnolunate and lunotriquetral ligaments. The periphery is well-vascularized, whereas the radial central portion is relatively avascular (Fig. 7–32).

B. DRUJ instability and post-traumatic osteoarthritis (OA)

1. Instability—Acute dislocation of the DRUJ can occur alone or in combination with ulnar styloid (base), radial shaft (Galeazzi), or Essex-Lopresti injuries. Isolated dislocations may be treated by closed reduction and immobilization (dorsal, forearm in supination; volar, forearm in pronation). Closed reduction may be impeded by interposition of the ECU tendon. Concurrent distal ulna fractures and TFCC tears may require open or arthroscopic treatment. In a **Galeazzi** injury, ORIF of the radial shaft is followed by assessment of DRUJ stability. An unstable DRUJ may require temporary radioulnar pinning proximal to the joint with the forearm immobilized in appropriate rotation. Chronic DRUJ instability may result from distal radius malunion, ulnar styloid nonunion, or large TFCC/ligamentous disruptions. Subtle chronic instability of the DRUJ may be evaluated on sequential CT scans with the forearm held in a neutral position, full supination, and full pronation and compared with the contralateral side. When chronic instability results from soft tissue incompetence, TFCC repair or ligament reconstruction with a palmaris tendon autograft may be indicated. A severely angulated distal radius malunion necessitates corrective osteotomy and appropriate treatment of resulting positive ulnar variance.
2. Post-traumatic DRUJ OA—A variety of treatment options exist for accompanying post-traumatic

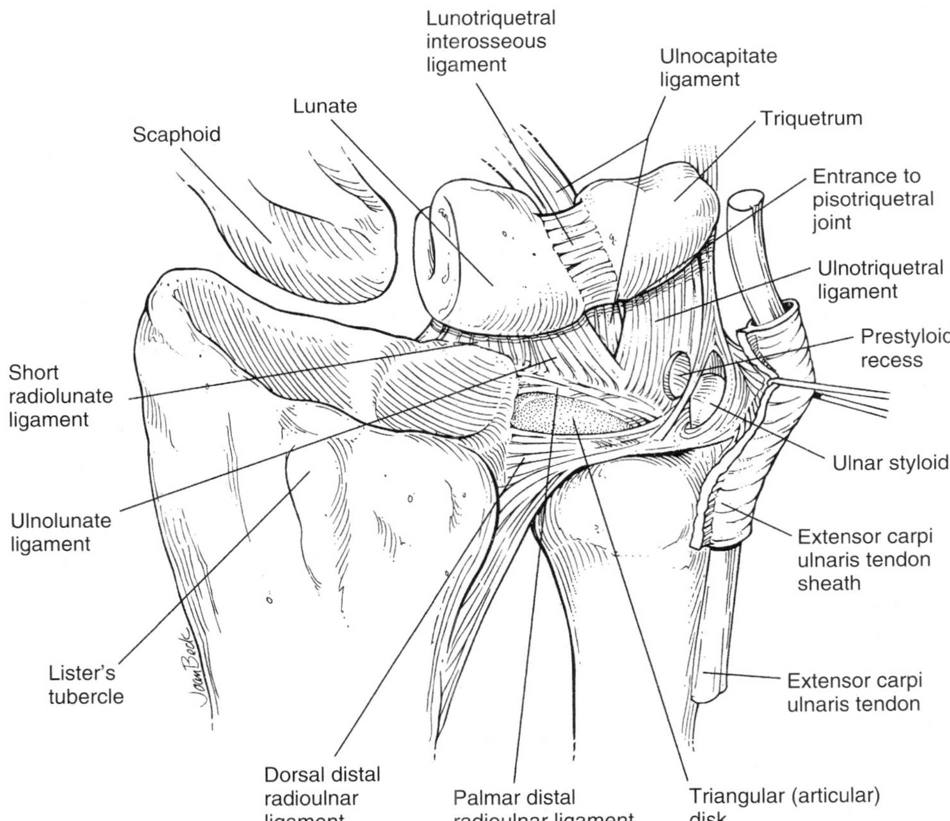

FIGURE 7–32 Anatomy of the triangular fibrocartilage complex. (From Cooney WP, Linscheid RL, Dobyns JH: The Wrist: Diagnosis and Operative Treatment. St. Louis, CV Mosby, 1998.)

DRUJ OA. Distal ulna resection (the Darrach procedure) is typically reserved for low-demand, elderly patients but may lead to painful proximal ulna stump instability. Hemiresection or interposition arthroplasty maintains the ulnar insertion of the TFCC and prevents radioulnar impingement by soft tissue (ECU tendon or capsular flap) interposition. In the Sauve-Kapandji procedure, the distal ulna is fused to the distal radius, and a pseudarthrosis is created at the ulnar neck. The early results of metallic ulnar head prosthetic replacement are promising, but no long-term studies have been performed to date. Creation of a one-bone forearm eliminates forearm rotation altogether and remains the ultimate salvage operation for persistent pain or other complications.

C. TFCC tears
 1. Classification and treatment—TFCC lesions are generally classified as traumatic (class I) or degenerative (class II) and have been further divided by Palmer into subtypes based on the specific location within the complex (Tables 7–5 and 7–6). The class and location of the tear have important implications for treatment. The value of MRI is increasing with regard to overall detection and localization of TFCC pathology. All acute traumatic lesions of the TFCC are initially managed with immobilization and NSAIDs. When nonoperative management fails to relieve persistent symptoms, wrist arthroscopy is indicated. The arthroscopic trampoline test is performed to assess the resiliency of the TFCC by balloting the central portion with a small probe.
  a. Class I—Central class IA tears are inherently stable and may simply be débrided when they are persistently symptomatic. A 2-mm peripheral rim must be maintained. Peripheral class IB tears are amenable to arthroscopic repair. Concurrent fractures of the ulnar styloid with persistent instability are either excised or internally fixed. The rare class IC tears are managed by either open or arthroscopic repair. Class ID tears are frequently associated with distal radius fractures and often respond to reduction of the radius. When operative intervention is necessary, both open and arthroscopic techniques have been described. Patients who undergo repair of a traumatic TFCC tear within 3 months of injury should expect to regain 80% of wrist range of motion and grip strength.
  b. Class II—Degenerative class II tears are associated with positive ulnar variance, increased ulnocarpal loading, and **ulnocarpal impaction syndrome** from abutment of the ulnar head into the proximal ulnar aspect of the lunate. Patients present with ulnar-sided wrist pain, which is increased with forearm pronation and grip, in the setting of positive ulnar variance on a posteroanterior wrist radiograph. In addition to detectable TFCC pathology, MRI may demonstrate focal increased signal in the lunate at the point of impaction. When conservative management fails, the goal of surgery is reduction of ulnocarpal loading. In the absence of DRUJ arthrosis, the most commonly performed procedure is an ulnar shortening osteotomy. DRUJ congruity should be preserved if overshortening is to be avoided. Alternatively, a simple wafer resection of the ulnar head dome has been described. Coexisting TFCC pathology is addressed by arthroscopic or open débridement. The treatment of class IIE lesions is somewhat controversial. Carpal instability from lunotriquetral disruption may require temporary percutaneous pinning after débridement of the TFCC and lunotriquetral ligament. In the setting of accompanying DRUJ arthrosis, the Darrach procedure, hemiresection arthroplasty, Sauve-Kapandji arthrodesis, and ulnar head replacement are all possible options.

D. Wrist arthroscopy—This procedure is indicated for the diagnosis of unexplained wrist pain and for the treatment of TFCC tears, osteochondral injuries, and intercarpal ligament tears (such as tears of the scapholunate ligament). It has also been used for excision of dorsal wrist ganglia, removal of intra-articular loose bodies, and septic wrist débridement. Wrist arthroscopy is useful to assess articular reduction

TABLE 7-5 CLASS I: TRAUMATIC TFCC INJURIES

Class	Characteristics	Treatment
IA	Central perforation or tear	Resection of an unstable flap back to a stable rim
IB	Ulnar avulsion with or without ulnar styloid fracture	Repair of the rim to its origin at the ulnar styloid
IC	Distal avulsion (origins of UL and UT ligaments)	Advancement of the distal volar rim to the triquetrum (bone anchor)
ID	Radial avulsion (involving the dorsal and/or volar radioulnar ligaments)	Direct repair to the radius to preserve the TFCC contribution to DRUJ stability

DRUJ, distal radioulnar joint; TFCC, triangular fibrocartilage complex; UL, ulnolunate; UT, ulnotriquetral.

TABLE 7-6 CLASS II: DEGENERATIVE TFCC TEARS (ULNOCARPAL IMPACTION SYNDROME)

Class	Characteristics
IIA	TFCC wear (thinning)
IIB	IIA + lunate and/or ulnar chondromalacia
IIC	TFCC perforation + lunate and/or ulnar chondromalacia
IID	IIC + LT ligament disruption
IIE	IID + ulnocarpal and DRUJ arthritis

DRUJ, distal radioulnar joint; LT, lunotriquetral; TFCC, triangular fibrocartilage complex.

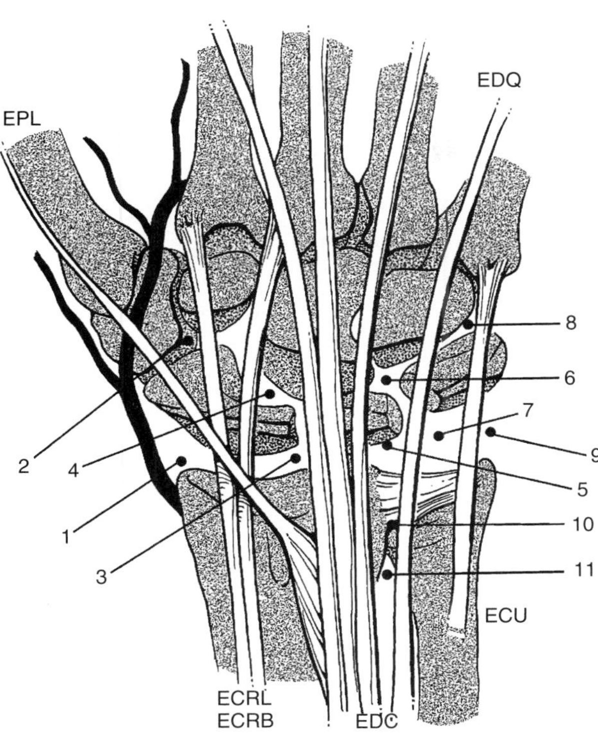

FIGURE 7–33 Diagram illustrating the six dorsal compartments of the wrist and their relationship to the underlying carpal bones and the extensor compartments. DRUJ, distal radioulnar joint; ECRB, extensor carpi radialis brevis; ECRL, extensor carpi radialis longus; ECU, extensor carpi ulnaris; EDC, extensor digitorum communis; EDQ, extensor digiti quinti; EPL, extensor pollicis longus; RMC, radial midcarpal; STT, scaphotrapeziotrapezoid; UMC, ulnar midcarpal. (From Green DP, Hotchkiss RN, Pederson WC, Wolfe SW, eds: Green's Operative Hand Surgery, 5th ed, p 770. Philadelphia, Churchill Livingstone, 2005.)

of distal radius and carpal bone fractures during or after ORIF. A traction tower is useful. The radiocarpal joint should be insufflated with saline or local anesthetic prior to trocar insertion. A 2.7-mm camera is used. Five radiocarpal portals are described with reference to the extensor tendon compartments, and each has anatomic structures at risk with their use (Fig. 7–33).

VII. Nail and Fingertip Injuries

A. Introduction—Fingertip injuries are the most common hand injuries seen in emergency departments. The long finger is the most commonly involved digit. These injuries may be broadly classified as those with and those without soft tissue loss. Crush injuries without extensive soft tissue loss may result in nail plate avulsions, nail matrix lacerations, and distal phalanx (tuft) fractures. Radiographs should always be obtained. Distal phalanx fractures are typically reduced when the nail bed is repaired, but large, displaced fragments may require percutaneous pinning. All smokers with distal finger injuries should be urged to stop smoking.

B. Nail structure—The nail plate is composed of keratin and originates from the ventral **germinal matrix** proximal to the nail fold. The **sterile matrix** lies directly beneath the nail plate and contributes keratin to increase the plate thickness. The crescent-shaped white lunula is seen through the proximal nail plate at the junction of the sterile and germinal matrices. The **hyponychium** lies between the distal nail bed and the skin of the fingertip, serving as a barrier to microorganisms. The **eponychium**, also called the cuticle, is at the distal margin of the proximal nail fold. The **paronychia** forms the lateral margins (Fig. 7–34).

C. Nail bed injury—A small subungual hematoma constituting less than 50% of the nail area may be treated without nail plate removal. The nail plate should be perforated with a sterile needle. Subungual hematomas that make up greater than 50% of the nail area require nail plate removal to

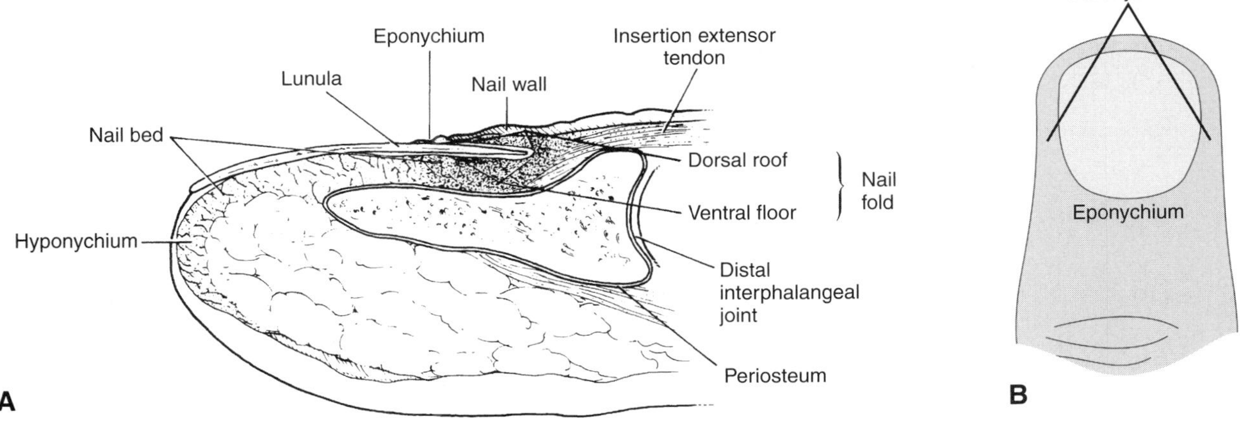

FIGURE 7–34 **A**, The anatomy of the nail bed is shown in sagittal section. **B**, The perionychium includes the paronychium, eponychium, hyponychium, and nail bed. (From Green DP, Hotchkiss RN, Pederson WC, Wolfe SW, eds: Green's Operative Hand Surgery, 5th ed. Philadelphia, Churchill Livingstone, 2005.)

repair significant underlying nail matrix lacerations. Acute repair offers the best results. Tetanus prophylaxis and antibiotics are given immediately. A digital block should be administered, and a Penrose drain may be used as a temporary finger tourniquet. If it is still available, the nail plate is removed and soaked in Betadine. The wounded area is débrided and thoroughly irrigated. The sterile and/or germinal matrix is repaired with 6-0 or smaller absorbable suture under loupe magnification. The eponychial fold is then splinted open with the Betadine-soaked nail plate or nonadherent gauze to allow a new nail to grow distal from the germinal matrix. If significant nail matrix has been lost, options include a split-thickness matrix graft from an adjacent injured finger or transfer of the nail matrix from the second toe. Nail plate deformities, especially nail ridging, are very common after nail bed repair. A hook nail may result from a tight nail bed repair, distal advancement of the matrix, or loss of underlying bony support. Patients should be counseled about a 50% incidence of fingertip hypersensitivity and/or cold intolerance. Complete growth of a new nail takes 3-6 months, depending on the age of the patient.

D. Fingertip injuries with tissue loss—Treatment of these injuries may be time intensive and challenging. The general principles of treatment include preservation of digit length, maintenance of sensate fingertip pulp, prevention of joint contracture, and eventual pain-free use of the digit. The correct characterization of the injury is critical and guides treatment.
   1. Fingertip injuries without exposed bone—These may be allowed to heal by second intention if less than 1 cm^2 of the tip or pulp is involved. Otherwise, skin or composite grafts may be required. Full-thickness skin grafts are best for the fingertip because they provide better durability, minimal contraction, and superior sensibility compared with the split-thickness variety.
   2. Fingertip injuries with exposed bone—It is best to characterize the injury by the orientation of tissue loss, such as volar oblique, dorsal oblique, or transverse.
      a. Volar oblique injury
         (1) Cross-finger flap—The treatment of choice for a volar oblique injury. Dorsal skin and subcutaneous tissue are elevated superficial to the paratenon from the adjacent digit to create a bed for the injured fingertip. The donor site is covered with a split-thickness skin graft. The flap is split during a separate procedure 2-3 weeks later (Fig. 7–35).
         (2) Thenar flap—Best reserved for volar index or long digit injuries. The flap is lifted parallel to the proximal thumb crease and split after 2-3 weeks (Fig. 7–36). Potential complications include donor site tenderness and PIP contracture (especially in older patients).

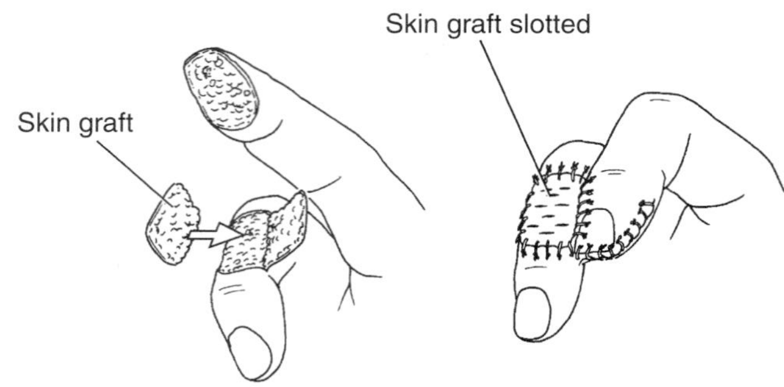

FIGURE 7–35 A cross-finger flap provides soft tissue coverage for the palmar aspect of the adjacent finger or thumb, but a full-thickness skin graft is required for the donor site. (From Trumble TE, ed: Principles of Hand Surgery and Therapy. Philadelphia, WB Saunders, 2000.)

         (3) Homodigital island flap—Raised on the digital artery of the involved finger and may maintain sensory innervation to the fingertip.
         (4) Heterodigital island flap—A neurovascular flap raised on the ulnar aspect of the long or ring finger and typically tunneled in the palm to provide coverage to the thumb.
         (5) Other possible donor sites—Include distant flaps in the chest, abdomen, and groin, although they may be cumbersome and too bulky for the fingertip.
      b. Transverse or dorsal oblique injury—A V-Y advancement may be performed to preserve length and cover transverse or dorsal oblique fingertip injuries. A wide volar flap is lifted off the distal phalanx, with a tapered base created at the level of the DIP crease. The flap is then advanced over the fingertip toward the dorsal side, and a tension-free closure is made (Fig. 7–37). Kutler popularized two separate smaller V-Y advancements from the lateral aspects of the digit to cover transverse fingertip injuries (Fig. 7–38).

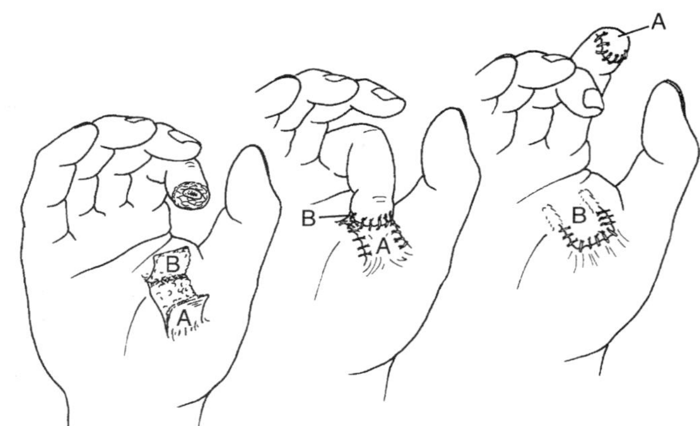

FIGURE 7–36 A thenar flap provides soft tissue coverage for the index and middle fingers without requiring a skin graft for the donor site. (From Trumble TE, ed: Principles of Hand Surgery and Therapy. Philadelphia, WB Saunders, 2000.)

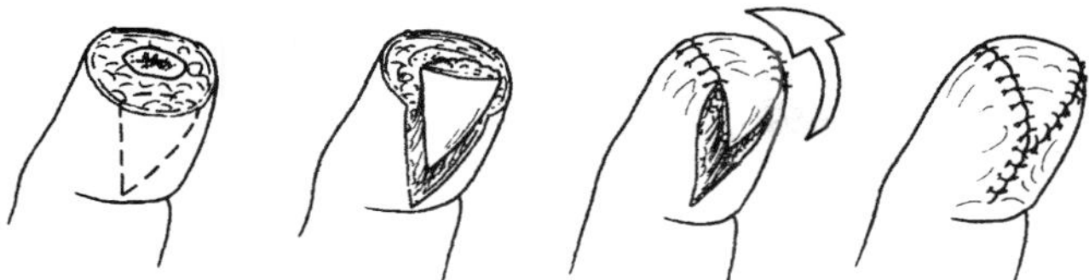

FIGURE 7–37 A V-Y flap provides sensate soft tissue coverage for the fingertip in small central deficits. (From Trumble TE, ed: Principles of Hand Surgery and Therapy. Philadelphia, WB Saunders, 2000.)

Alternatively, these injuries are treated by bone shortening and conversion to a volar coverage option. Shortening and closing an injury that acutely violates the FDP insertion may result in a **lumbrical-plus finger**. The FDP tendon retracts and creates tension on the extensor mechanism, causing paradoxical IP joint extension with active finger flexion. This is treated with release of the radial lateral bands.

c. Transverse or volar oblique thumb injury—The Moberg advancement flap is best used for transverse or volar oblique thumb injuries. The entire volar surface of the thumb with its neurovascular bundles is advanced (Fig. 7–39). Potential complications include flap necrosis and thumb flexion contracture.
d. Dorsal thumb injury—This injury may be covered with a first dorsal metacarpal artery kite flap.
e. Distal fingertip amputation—Composite flaps for distal fingertip amputations may be attempted in patients younger than 6 years old, but parents must be willing to see it fail.

VIII. Soft Tissue Coverage and Microsurgery

A. Upper extremity wounds

1. Introduction—The management of traumatic upper extremity wounds begins with a thorough assessment of the wound, including its size, location, involvement of deep structures, and the presence of contamination. The standard of care involves early débridement and administration of antibiotics. Complex wounds may require several surgical débridements to remove nonviable tissue. A clean wound bed is essential prior to any definitive coverage procedure. There are multiple

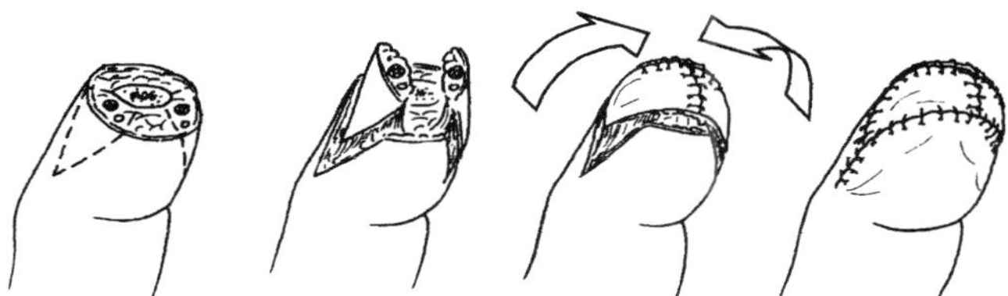

FIGURE 7–38 A Kutler flap provides sensate soft tissue coverage for the fingertip in small central defects. (From Trumble TE, ed: Principles of Hand Surgery and Therapy. Philadelphia, WB Saunders, 2000.)

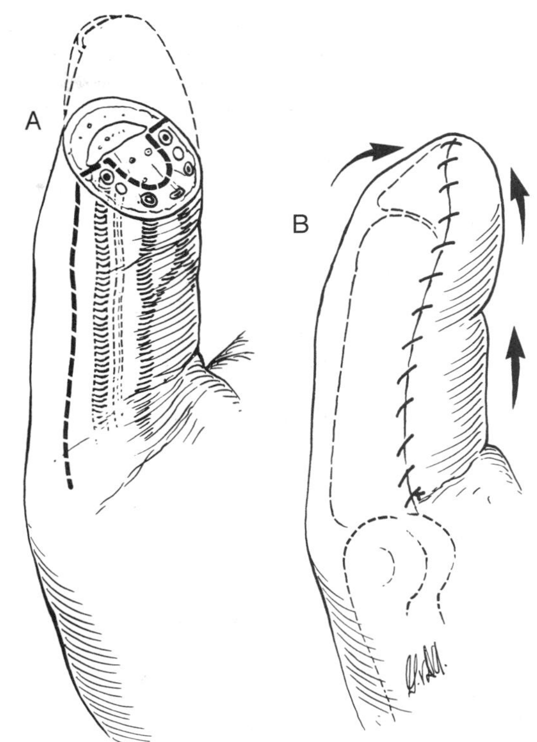

FIGURE 7–39 A Moberg advancement flap. **A**, Most useful for amputations distal to the thumb interphalangeal joint, the Moberg advancement flap is composed of the entire palmar skin of the thumb, including the neurovascular bundle. **B**, Flexion of the interphalangeal joint assists in coverage of the defect by the advancement flap. (Modified from Lister GD: The theory of the transposition flap and its practical application in the hand. Clin Plast Surg 8:115-128, 1981.)

advantages to early coverage of traumatic wounds. Infection rates increase dramatically if coverage is delayed longer than 1 week after injury. Infected wounds must be treated with culture-specific antibiotics.

2. The reconstructive ladder—The goals of soft tissue reconstruction in the upper extremity are to provide coverage of deep structures (e.g., bone, cartilage, tendons, nerves, blood vessels), create a barrier to microorganisms, restore dynamic function of the limb, and prevent joint contractures. Cosmetic appearance is a secondary priority. The options for soft tissue reconstruction, in order of increasing complexity, consist of primary closure, second intention, skin grafting, and flaps. The choice of definitive procedure is guided by wound characteristics and patient factors. Primary closure of a traumatic wound is generally not advised unless the wound is minimally contaminated and can be closed within 6 hours of the injury. Wounds may be allowed to heal by second intention, a process involving wound granulation, epithelialization, and contraction. Bone, nerve, tendon, or other deep structures must not be exposed. Regular dressing changes or vacuum-assisted closure devices are necessary to promote this type of healing.

3. Skin grafts—Autografts may be either **split-thickness skin grafts** (STSGs) or **full-thickness skin grafts** (FTSGs). Both types require a clean wound bed without exposed bone or tendon. Skin grafts are prone to early failure from shear stress and hematoma formation. STSGs are preferred for dorsal hand wounds. Meshed grafts provide a greater surface area and typically have better "take" because of a lower incidence of hematoma formation and infection. The anterolateral thigh is a common donor site for STSGs. FTSGs are preferred for volar wounds and the fingertip. They are more durable, contract less, and provide better sensibility. The proximal forearm and hypothenar aspect of the hand are common donor sites for FTSGs. Allografts may be used as a temporary measure to prepare a wound bed for later autografting. Xenografts are occasionally used as biologic dressings.
4. Flaps—A flap is a unit of tissue supported by blood vessels and moved from a donor site to a recipient site to cover a defect in tissue. This unit may be composed of one tissue type or a composite of several tissue types that may include the skin, fascia, muscle, tendon, nerve, or bone. The transfer of vascularized tissue to a defect promotes healing and lowers the secondary infection rate. Flap reconstruction is indicated when the wound has exposed bone (stripped of periosteum), tendon (stripped of paratenon), cartilage, or an orthopaedic implant. Flaps may be classified by their vascular supply, tissue type, donor site, and method of transfer.
   a. Flap classification by blood supply—**Axial-pattern flaps** have a single named arteriovenous pedicle. These flaps may be raised on their pedicle and transferred locally, or the pedicle can be divided and transferred to a distant site as a free flap. **Random-pattern flaps** do not have a single named arteriovenous pedicle but instead depend on the microcirculation for viability. Examples of random-pattern flaps are the cross-finger and thenar flaps. Axial-pattern flaps have a more predictable blood supply, greater mobility, and more effective resistance to infection than random-pattern flaps.
   b. Flap classification by tissue type—Flaps may be composed of a single tissue or a composite. Fascia flaps and muscle flaps are examples of single-tissue flaps. Composite flaps often allow for single-stage reconstructions. **Cutaneous flaps**, such as the thenar H flap, include skin and subcutaneous tissue. **Fasciocutaneous flaps**, such as the radial forearm flap, include the fascia with the overlying skin and subcutaneous tissue. **Musculocutaneous flaps** include muscle with the overlying skin, subcutaneous tissue, and fascia. An **osteocutaneous flap** is composed of a portion of bone (e.g., fibula) with overlying soft tissue. Innervated flaps preserve the nerve supply with the tissue unit. Either motor or sensory nerves may be preserved, depending on their anatomic location and the choice of flap to be transferred.
   c. Flap classification by donor site
      (1) Local flaps—Local flaps are provided by tissue that is adjacent to or near the defect. They may be further classified as transposition, rotation, advancement, axial flag, and fillet flaps. (a) **Transposition flaps** are geometric in their design and may be either axial or random pattern with regard to blood supply. A **Z-plasty** is a form of transposition flap. While the lengths of the **Z-plasty** limbs should always be equal, the angles may vary to change the amount of desired lengthening. The commonly used 60-degree angle theoretically yields 75% lengthening along the line of the central limb (Fig. 7–40). (b) **Rotation flaps** are not geometric and are universally random pattern with regard to blood supply. With this in mind, the length of the flap to be rotated should not exceed the width of its base, for doing so will exceed the capacity of the microcirculation to maintain tissue viability. (c) **Advancement flaps** such as the V-Y and Moberg types proceed in a straight line to fill the defect. (d) **Axial-flag flaps** are based on the dorsal digital artery (Fig. 7–41) and may be further characterized as **homodigital** (transferred to a defect on the same digit) or **heterodigital** (transferred to a different digit). (e) **A fillet flap**, taken from an amputated digit, is occasionally salvaged for initial coverage of a mangled hand.
      (2) Distant flaps—Distant flaps are used when local flaps are either inadequate

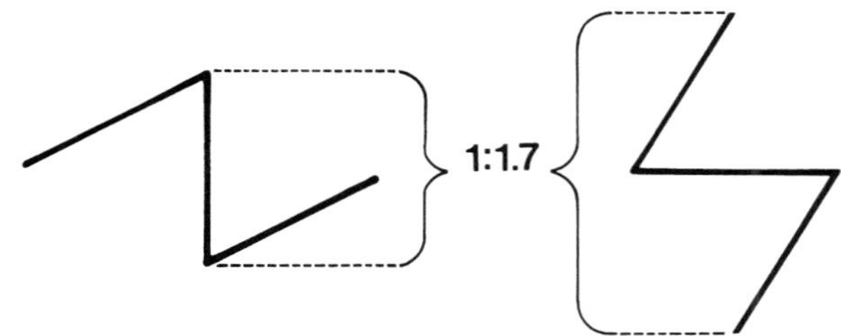

FIGURE 7–40 Standard 60-degree Z-plasty. Here all limbs of the Z-plasty are of equal length, and the angles between the limbs are 60 degrees. When the flaps are transposed, the lengthening that is achieved along the line of the central limb is 70-75% of its original length. (From Green DP, Hotchkiss RN, Pederson WC, Wolfe SW, eds: Green's Operative Hand Surgery, 5th ed, p 1655. Philadelphia, Churchill Livingstone, 2005.)

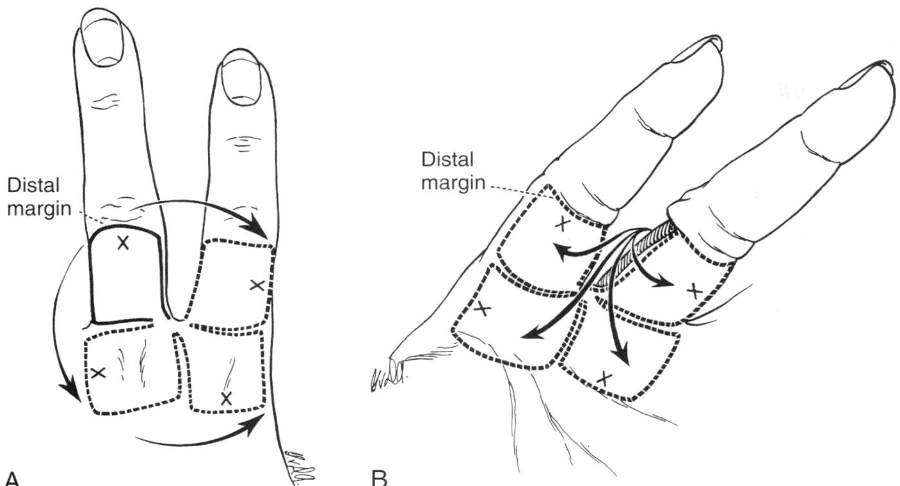

FIGURE 7–41 **A**, An axial flag flap raised on the dorsum of the middle finger can be rotated to cover defects on the proximal phalanx of the index finger or over the MCP joint of either of those two digits. **B**, By carrying the flap through the web space, it can reach defects on the palmar surface of the MCP joint of either the index or the middle finger. (Modified from Lister GD: The theory of the transposition flap and its practical application in the hand. Clin Plast Surg 8:115-128, 1981.)

or unavailable for soft tissue coverage. For example, a degloved or burned hand may be placed in a raised pocket of tissue in the abdomen or groin. Several weeks later, the flap is divided and the donor site either skin-grafted or allowed to heal by second intention. Alternatively, the defect site may be dissected away from the distant pocket of skin. In this case the donor site is primarily closed, and the defect may require a split-thickness skin graft over the vascularized granulation tissue.

d. Flap classification by method of transfer—Flap reconstruction may be performed in a single stage or in two stages, like the previously mentioned abdominal pocket flap. In most instances, the donor tissue remains attached to the native vasculature. Alternatively, **free flaps** (free tissue transfer) are distant axial-pattern flaps raised on a named arteriovenous pedicle; they are then divided and reanastomosed to donor vessels near the defect but away from the zone of injury. The most frequently used donors for use in the upper extremity include the gracilis (medial femoral circumflex artery), latissimus dorsi (thoracodorsal artery), and serratus anterior (the serratus branch of the subscapular artery) free flaps. Patients are typically monitored postoperatively for several days in some form of intensive care unit. The main cause of free flap failure is inadequate arterial blood flow. Persistent vasospasm may lead to thrombosis at the anastomosis. Hypotension must be avoided and the patient kept well hydrated. Vasoconstrictive agents such as nicotine and caffeine are restricted. Seroma or hematoma formation can also lead to flap demise.

B. Traumatic upper extremity amputation
1. Indications and contraindications—Primary indications to attempt replantation include multiple-digit amputations, thumb amputation, the level of amputation at or proximal to the wrist, and any amputation in a child. A relative indication is a level of amputation distal to the FDS insertion (zone I). Primary contraindications to replantation include a single-digit amputation (except for the thumb), crushed or mangled amputated parts, prolonged ischemia, segmental amputations, and a level of amputation that is proximal to the FDS insertion (zone II). Patients with multisystem traumatic injuries and those with multiple medical comorbidities or disabling psychiatric conditions may be poor candidates for attempted replantation.
2. Care of the amputated part—The amputated part should be wrapped in moist gauze (normal saline or lactated Ringer's solution) and placed within a sealed plastic bag, which is then placed in an ice-water bath. Although it is somewhat controversial, replantation is not recommended if warm ischemia time is more than 6 hours for an amputation level proximal to the carpus or more than 12 hours for an amputated digit. Cold ischemia times of less than 12 hours for an amputation level proximal to the carpus or less than 24 hours for an amputated digit may still permit successful replantation, highlighting the importance of appropriate cooling of the amputated part.
3. Operative sequence of replantation—(1) bone stabilization, (2) extensor tendon repair, (3) flexor tendon repair, (4) arterial reanastomosis, (5) venous reanastomosis, (6) nerve repair, and (7) skin approximation. For multiple-digit

amputations, the structure-by-structure technique is faster and has a higher viability rate. The priority for digit replantation is the thumb, followed by the long, ring, small, and index fingers. Arterial reanastomosis is performed first during limb replantation, and appropriate fasciotomies must be done to prevent reperfusion-induced compartment syndrome.

4. Postoperative care—Important considerations include maintaining a warm environment (~80° F) and adequate hydration. Medical therapies such as aspirin, dipyridamole, low-molecular-weight dextran and heparin may be given if necessary. There is a higher incidence of postoperative hemorrhage when using two anticoagulants with aspirin (53%) than when using one (2%). The hematocrit must be carefully monitored. Nicotine, caffeine, and vasopressors are prohibited.
5. Replantation monitoring—The most reliable methods are close observation of color, capillary refill, and tissue turgor. Measuring oxygen saturation by pulse oximetry and measuring skin surface temperature are safe, noninvasive, reproducible monitoring methods. Either a drop in temperature of greater than 2° C in 1 hour or a temperature lower than 30° C indicates decreased digital perfusion.
6. Complications—The most frequent cause of early (within 12 hours) replantation failure is **arterial thrombosis** from persistent vasospasm. Failure after 12 hours is typically secondary to **venous congestion or thrombosis**. Late complications include infection, hypersensitivity, and cold intolerance.
   a. Arterial insufficiency—Suggested by pale skin color, decreased or absent capillary refill, and loss of a Doppler-measurable pulse. If arterial insufficiency develops, consider measures such as releasing constricting bandages, placing the extremity in a dependent position, administering heparin, and performing a stellate ganglion block. If these maneuvers fail to promote arterial inflow, exploration and revision may be indicated.
   b. Inadequate venous outflow—Venous congestion is suggested by ruborous skin color, tissue engorgement, and increased capillary refill and may subsequently cause diminished arterial inflow and replantation failure. If first-line measures such as dressing removal and extremity elevation fail to resolve the problem, medicinal leeches (*Hirudo medicinalis*) may be employed. Leeches produce the anticoagulant hirudin, which yields 8-12 hours of sustained bleeding. *Aeromonas hydrophila* infection is a risk with leech use, so prophylactic antibiotics should be administered. If leeches are not available or tolerated by the patient or nursing staff, heparin-soaked pledgets can be used. Revision of the vascular anastomoses remains the last resort.
7. Results—The factor considered the most predictive of digital survival after replantation is the mechanism of injury. The outcome of replantation also depends on ischemia time. Clean, transverse amputations with cold ischemia of less than 8 hours survive replantation in 94% of cases. After 8 hours, the success rate drops to 74%. Replanted digits typically regain 50% of the total active motion and have static two-point discrimination of 10 mm.
8. Forearm and arm replantation—Arterial inflow is established before skeletal stabilization with the use of shunts, if necessary, to minimize ischemia time. Fasciotomies are always performed. Blood loss during the procedure must be closely monitored. Muscle necrosis may lead to myoglobinuria and life-threatening renal failure. An elevated postoperative serum potassium level may be prognostic of replantation failure. Late complications include infection, Volkmann's ischemic contracture, and insignificant functional recovery.
9. Hand allotransplantation—Controversial procedure that introduces potentially life-threatening complications from postoperative immunosuppression for a condition that is not itself life threatening.

C. Ring avulsion injuries—Ring finger injury occurs when skin, soft tissue, and neurovascular structures are forcibly avulsed from the underlying bone and deeper tissues. These injuries have been classified by Urbaniak. In class I injuries, circulation is adequate and the digit can usually be salvaged with standard treatment of the soft tissue injury. In class II injuries, circulation is compromised and inadequate. If there is no accompanying bone or tendon injury, revascularization is recommended. Finally, class III injuries are characterized by complete degloving and are treated with completion amputation.

IX. Vascular Disorders

A. Anatomy—The hand is supplied by the radial and ulnar arteries. Some individuals have a persistent median artery. The ulnar artery is dominant and is the main contributor to the superficial palmar arch. The radial artery is the main contributor to the deep palmar arch and the thumb via the princeps pollicis artery. A complete arch, present in 80% of hands, provides arterial branches to all five digits, and if either the radial or ulnar artery is injured proximally, sufficient digital perfusion remains through the uninjured artery and the complete arch. Individuals with an incomplete arch (20%) may have significant compromise of perfusion if the dominant artery is injured (Fig. 7–42).

B. Evaluation of vascular dysfunction
1. History and physical examination—Evaluation of vascular dysfunction begins with a thorough history and physical examination. **Allen's test** is a good screening tool. A positive test denotes absent arterial filling of the hand when either

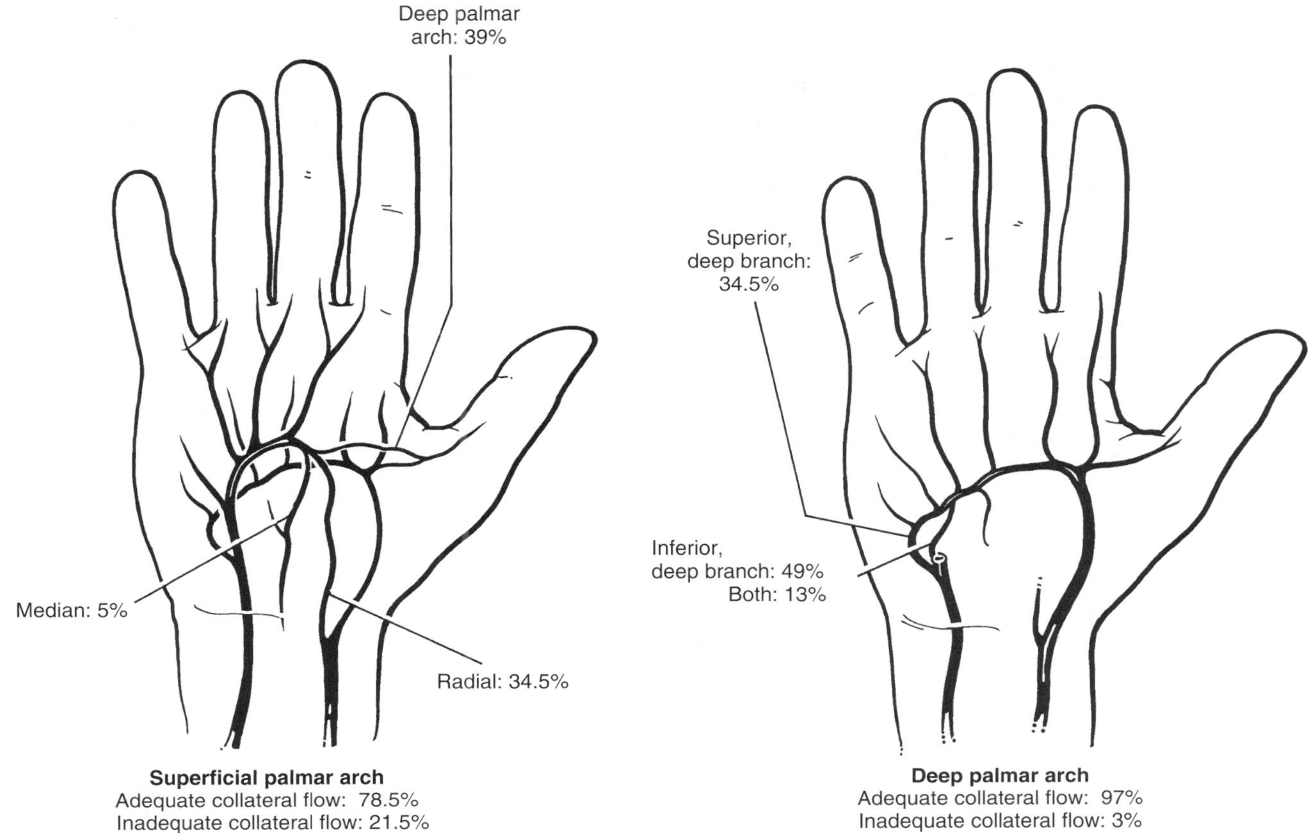

FIGURE 7–42 The superficial palmar arch is completed by branches from the deep palmar arch, radial artery, or median artery in 78.5% of patients; the remaining 21.5% are "incomplete." The deep palmar arch is completed by the superior branch of the ulnar artery, the inferior branch of the ulnar artery, or both in 98.5% of patients. (Modified from Koman LA, Urbaniak JR: Ulnar artery thrombosis. In Brunelli G [ed]: Textbook of Microsurgery. Milan, Masson, 1988, pp 75-83, with permission.)

the compressed radial or ulnar artery is released at the wrist. Cold stimulation testing may demonstrate autonomic vascular dysfunction. Patients with arterial disease require more than 20 minutes to return to pre-exposure temperatures when submersed in ice water for 20 seconds, compared with normal subjects, who require approximately 10 minutes.

2. Other testing—Findings can be further confirmed with a Doppler probe. Arteriography remains the gold standard for elucidating the nature and extent of thrombotic and embolic disease of the hand vasculature. It provides a roadmap for surgical intervention. Color duplex ultrasound has emerged as an excellent noninvasive study to help detect many forms of vessel pathology, with rates of sensitivity and specificity similar to those in arteriography (with experienced operators). Photoplethysmography (pulse volume recordings) demonstrates arterial insufficiency when there is loss of the dicrotic notch or a decreased rate of rise in the systolic peak. A three-phase bone scan may be a useful adjunctive test in certain clinical scenarios. Phase 1 images taken 2 minutes after radiotracer injection provide information similar to arteriography. Arterial occlusion, arteriovenous malformations (AVMs), and vascular tumors can be detected during this phase. After 5-10 minutes, phase II (soft tissue) images may show decreased perfusion when vasospastic disorders are present. Delayed phase III (skeletal) images are obtained 2-3 hours after injection but are not particularly helpful in vascular disorders.

C. Occlusive vascular disease—Etiologies include blunt or penetrating arterial trauma, atherosclerosis, aneurysm formation, emboli, and a variety of systemic diseases. The disease often presents with unilateral claudication, paresthesias, and/or cold intolerance. Ulcerations and gangrene are late findings of unrecognized vascular compromise.

1. Hypothenar hammer syndrome—The most common post-traumatic vascular occlusive condition of the upper extremity. Thrombosis or aneurysm formation of the distal ulnar artery occurs from blunt trauma to the hypothenar eminence. Clinical findings may include localized tenderness, cold intolerance, ischemic pain, and accompanying compression neuropathy of the ulnar nerve in the Guyon canal. Noninvasive vascular studies or arteriography may help confirm the diagnosis. Treatment

may involve resection and ligation of the thrombosed ulnar artery or reconstruction with a vein graft.

2. Embolic disease—The majority of arterial emboli to the upper extremity are of cardiac origin. Another subset of emboli originates from the subclavian system in cases of thoracic outlet syndrome. Emergent embolectomy is performed when feasible and followed by intravenous heparin therapy. Smaller vessels are treated with a thrombolytic agent such as tissue plasminogen activator, streptokinase, or urokinase if the diagnosis is made within 36 hours of occlusion. Warfarin is given for at least 3 months.
3. Small-vessel occlusive disease—May be seen in connective tissue diseases such as scleroderma, systemic lupus erythematosus, rheumatoid arthritis, Sjögren syndrome, and dermatomyositis. Another etiology is small-vessel arteritis from Buerger disease, which affects predominantly males who are heavy smokers. These conditions are often progressive despite treatment.

D. Vasospastic disease—Periodic digital ischemia may be induced by cold temperature or other sympathetic stimuli, such as pain or emotional stress. The digits initially turn white from vasospasm and cessation of flow, then blue from cyanosis and venous stasis, and finally red from rebound hyperemia. The last stage is often accompanied by dysesthesia. Vasospastic disease with a known underlying cause (Box 7–1) is termed the **Raynaud phenomenon** (Table 7–7). Some degree of vascular occlusive disease is always present, giving a combined clinical picture. Symptoms are usually asymmetrical, and peripheral pulses are often absent. Trophic changes may occur. Treatment is focused on the underlying disease. When no underlying cause is present, the clinical condition is known as **Raynaud disease** (see Table 7–7). The most commonly affected group is premenopausal women. The symptoms are usually bilateral, and peripheral pulses are often present. Calcium channel blockers may provide transient relief of symptoms. Biofeedback techniques may also be beneficial. Digital sympathectomy is considered in those severe cases in which conservative management fails. Smoking cessation and avoidance of cold exposure are imperative in both the Raynaud phenomenon and Raynaud disease.

Box 7–1 Causes of Secondary Vasospastic Disorder

- Connective tissue disease: scleroderma (incidence of Raynaud disease, 80-90%), SLE (incidence, 18-26%), dermatomyositis (incidence, 30%), RA (incidence, 11%)
- Occlusive arterial disease
- Neurovascular compression: thoracic outlet syndrome
- Hematologic abnormalities: cryoproteinemia, polycythemia, paraproteinemia
- Occupational trauma: percussion and vibratory tool workers
- Drugs and toxins: sympathomimetics, ergot compounds, beta-adrenergic blockers
- CNS disease: syringomyelia, poliomyelitis, tumors/infarcts
- Miscellaneous: RSD, malignant disease

CNS, central nervous system; RA, rheumatoid arthritis; RSD, reflex sympathetic dystrophy; SLE, systemic lupus erythematosus.

TABLE 7-7 RAYNAUD DISEASE VERSUS RAYNAUD PHENOMENON

Characteristic	Disease	Phenomenon
History		
Triphasic color change	Yes	Yes
Age > 40 years	No	Yes
Progression rapid	No	Yes
Underlying disease	No	Yes
Female predominance	Frequent	Occasional
Physical examination		
Tophic findings (ulcer, gangrene)	Infrequent	Frequent
Abnormal Allen test	No	Common
Asymmetrical findings	Infrequent	Frequent
Laboratory testing		
Blood chemistry	Normal	Frequently abnormal
Microangiology	Normal	Frequently abnormal
Angiography	Normal	Frequently abnormal

From Green DP, Hotchkiss RN, Pederson WC, et al: Green's Operative Hand Surgery, 5th ed, p 2304. Philadelphia, Churchill Livingstone, 2005.

E. Acute compartment syndrome—Surgical emergency resulting from increased pressure within a closed anatomic space, leading to reduced capillary blood flow below the threshold for local tissue perfusion. Prolonged ischemia secondary to a missed or delayed diagnosis may result in irreversible muscle or nerve damage within a compartment. Digital compartment syndromes are rare but certainly possible.

1. Compartments—The three forearm compartments include the mobile wad of three (brachioradialis, ECRL, and ECRB) and the dorsal and volar compartments. The deep muscles of the volar compartment incur the highest pressures. There are ten compartments in the hand: the adductor pollicis, thenar, hypothenar, four dorsal interosseous, and three volar interosseous compartments.
2. Diagnosis—Compartment syndrome is a clinical diagnosis, and a high index of suspicion is critical after crush injuries and limb reperfusion. The most common cause in children is a supracondylar humerus fracture. Compartment pressures should be measured in equivocal cases or in unresponsive patients. Compartment monitoring is also imperative after animal bites, high-energy trauma, and burn injuries. Increased pain with a passive stretch of the affected compartment is the most sensitive finding on physical examination. Paresthesias, pallor, pulselessness, and paralysis are late findings.
3. Treatment—Revascularization procedures in the upper extremity are often accompanied by the

appropriate fasciotomies. Forearm fasciotomies require three incisions over the three compartments; the ten compartments of the hand can be released with a total of five incisions. Two dorsal incisions are sufficient to release all seven interosseous compartments. Separate incisions are made over the thenar and hypothenar compartments (Fig. 7–43). Carpal tunnel release is also recommended after forearm fasciotomies. Digital fasciotomies are performed with radial incisions for the thumb and small finger and ulnar incisions for the other three digits. After fasciotomies of all the affected compartments, delayed wound closure is recommended. Skin grafting may be necessary. Early hand therapy is important, but the factor that affects prognosis the most is the time between tissue compromise and surgical intervention. Long-term sequelae of unrecognized and untreated acute compartment syndrome include muscle fibrosis and **Volkmann ischemic contracture**.

F. Volkmann ischemic contracture—Classic sequela of untreated acute compartment syndrome developing from advanced myonecrosis and muscle fibrosis in the forearm. The FDP and FPL are the most vulnerable and commonly affected muscles. Mild, moderate, and severe forms have been described. The mild form is manifested as mild flexion contractures of the ring and long DIP joints, but patients often have normal strength and sensibility. Progressively worsening contractures and sensorimotor deficits are seen in the moderate and severe forms. Chronic pain and significant hand dysfunction are common. Patients with the severe form often have an insensate hand with an intrinsic-minus ("claw hand") deformity. Contracture releases and tendon transfers are performed to help improve function, although the success of these procedures may be limited in severe cases. Nerve decompression may be necessary in patients with chronic neuropathic pain, especially when muscle fibrosis causes extrinsic compression on intrinsically compromised peripheral nerves.

G. Frostbite—Damage to tissue from prolonged exposure to subfreezing temperatures. Ice crystals

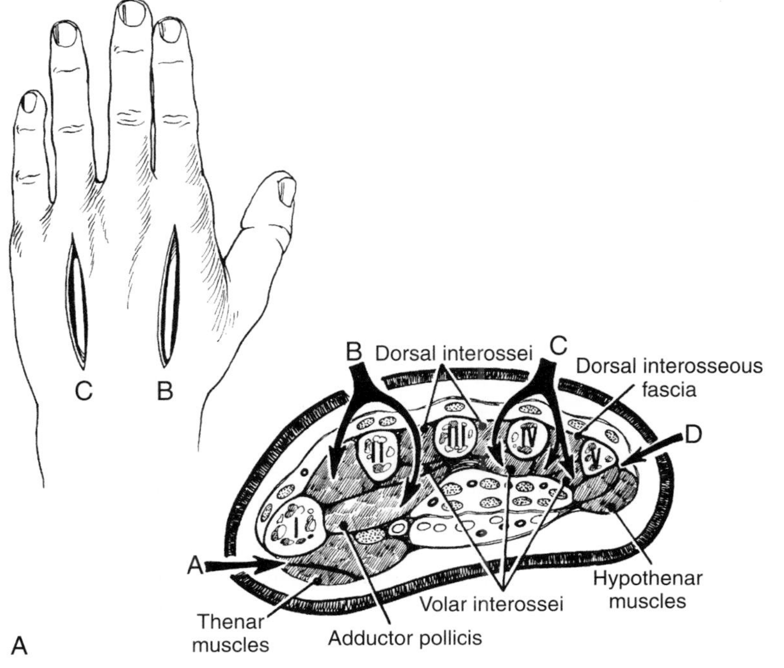

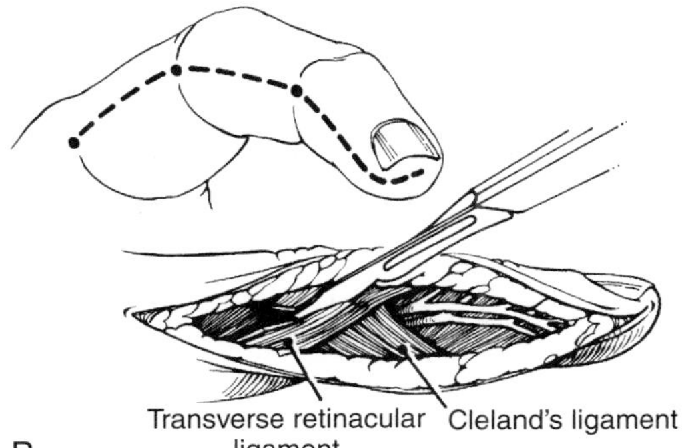

FIGURE 7–43 **A**, Both dorsal and volar interosseous compartments and the adductor compartment to the thumb can be released through two longitudinal incisions over the second and third metacarpals (B and C). The thenar and hypothenar compartments are opened through separate incisions (A and D). **B**, Correct placement of a midaxial incision in the finger. A flexion contracture of the finger may occur if the incision is placed too far volarward. (From Green DP, Hotchkiss RN, Pederson WC, Wolfe SW, eds: Green's Operative Hand Surgery, 5th ed, p 1993. Philadelphia, Churchill Livingstone, 2005.)

form within extracellular fluid, causing subsequent intracellular dehydration and cell death. Increased wind chill, skin contact with metal or ice, and alcohol intoxication exacerbate frostbite. After initial resuscitative management, rapid rewarming of the affected body part is performed in a water bath kept at 40-44°C. Intravenous analgesics or conscious sedation is usually necessary during this exquisitely painful process. Local wound management, limb elevation, splinting, and early therapy are routine aspects of care. Surgical débridement and amputation should be delayed until unequivocal tissue demarcation occurs, although escharotomy is required for constrictive, circumferential digital involvement. Chronic cold intolerance is common. Calcium channel blockers or surgical sympathectomy may be required for late, persistent vasospastic disease. Children may have premature growth plate closure.

Box 7–2 Nerve Compression Etiology

SYSTEMIC
Diabetes
Alcoholism
Renal failure
Raynaud

INFLAMMATORY
Rheumatoid arthritis
Infection
Gout
Tenosynovitis

FLUID IMBALANCE
Pregnancy
Obesity

ANATOMIC
Synovial fibrosis
Lumbrical encroachment
Anomalous tendon
Median artery
Fracture deformity

MASS
Ganglion
Lipoma
Hematoma

X. Compression Neuropathy

A. Introduction

1. Definition—Compression neuropathy is a chronic condition with sensory, motor, or mixed involvement. Sensory symptoms may include numbness and tingling, while motor symptoms range from weakness to paralysis. Pain results from direct trauma, vascular infarction, or systemic neuropathy and not from chronic compression. The first sensory perceptions to be lost are those of light touch, pressure, and vibration, and the last to be impaired are pain and temperature.
2. Pathology—Paresthesias result from early microvascular compression and neural ischemia. Intraneural edema increases over time and exacerbates microvascular compression. Pressure and vibratory thresholds are increased. Continued compression may lead to structural changes such as demyelination, fibrosis, and axonal loss. These changes may cause weakness or paralysis of the motor nerve. Abnormal two-point discrimination may also be evident after prolonged compression.
3. History—The patient's history may reveal night symptoms, dropping of objects, clumsiness, or weakness. If the onset of symptoms is preceded by viral illness and shoulder pain, consider **Parsonage-Turner syndrome**, a self-limiting inflammatory brachial plexopathy.
4. Physical examination—Observe the position and posture of the digits, hand, wrist, and elbow at rest. Changes in skin color, temperature, texture, and moisture may result from sympathetic nervous system dysfunction. Look for other clues that may indicate an associated systemic disease, such as diabetes, thyroid disease, inflammatory arthropathy, and vitamin deficiency (Box 7–2). Examine individual muscle strength (grades 0-5), pinch strength, and grip strength.
5. Neurosensory testing—This should be performed in the context of both dermatomal and peripheral nerve distributions. Semmes Weinstein monofilaments measure the cutaneous pressure threshold, a function of large nerve fibers (the first to be affected in compression neuropathy). Two-point discrimination should be measured on the fingertip pulp of each digit. The inability to perceive a difference of less than 5 mm is abnormal and constitutes a late finding in compression neuropathy. Pertinent provocative maneuvers are described for each nerve compression syndrome below.
6. Electrodiagnostic testing—Sensory and motor nerve function is tested by **electromyography** (EMG) and **nerve conduction studies** (NCSs). The results are often the only objective evidence of a neuropathic condition but to some extent are operator dependent. EMG is helpful in diagnosing cervical radiculopathy and myopathic conditions in which groups of muscles are affected. NCSs measure nerve conduction velocity, distal latency, and amplitude. Demyelination decreases conduction velocity (sensory fibers before motor fibers) and increases distal latency, and with axonal loss a decrease in sensory or motor potential amplitude may be evident. EMG and NCSs are useful adjunctive tests in certain conditions, but they may be associated with a high false-negative rate.
7. Compression neuropathy—Characterized by phases of the disease (Table 7–8). The appropriate treatment depends on the phase of the disease. Decisions are guided by history, physical examination, sensory threshold testing, and EMG and NCSs.
8. Double-crush phenomenon—Normal axonal function is dependent on factors synthesized in the nerve cell body. Blockage of axonal transport at one point makes the entire axon more susceptible to compression elsewhere. Cervical radiculopathy or proximal nerve entrapment may coexist with distal nerve compression

TABLE 7-8 COMPRESSION NEUROPATHY

Phase	Symptoms	NCV	EMG	Pathology	Treatment
Early	Intermittent	Normal or ↑ sensory latency	Normal	Edema	Nonoperative
Intermediate	Constant	+	±	Edema	Surgery
Late	Sensory and motor deficit	+	+	Fibrosis and axonal loss	Surgery—less predictable outcome

EMG, electromyography; NCV, nerve conduction velocity; ↑, increased.

in the double-crush syndrome. The outcome of surgical decompression may be disappointing unless all points of compression are addressed. It is logical to start with less complex distal releases first.

B. Median nerve
   1. Carpal tunnel syndrome (CTS)—The most common compressive neuropathy in the upper extremity.
      a. Anatomy—The volar boundary of the carpal tunnel is formed by the **transverse carpal ligament** (TCL), which attaches to the scaphoid tuberosity and trapezium radially and to the pisiform and hook of the hamate ulnarly. The floor of the carpal tunnel is formed by the proximal carpal row and deep volar carpal ligaments.
      b. History and physical examination—Risk factors include female sex, obesity, pregnancy, diabetes, hypothyroidism, chronic renal failure, inflammatory arthritis, storage diseases, smoking, alcoholism, advanced age, and repetitive wrist flexion during occupational activity. Acute CTS occurs in the setting of high-energy trauma, such as distal radius fractures and fracture-dislocation of the radiocarpal joint. Patients report paresthesias and pain (often at night) in the palmar aspect of the radial 3½ digits. Weakness and loss of fine motor control are late findings.
      c. Testing—The most sensitive provocative test is the carpal tunnel compression test (Durkin's test). Other provocative tests include Tinel and Phalen signs. Large sensory fibers (light touch, vibration) are affected before small fibers (pain and temperature). Semmes Weinstein monofilament testing is sensitive for diagnosing early CTS. Two-point discrimination of each digit should be checked on all patients. Look for thenar atrophy in severe denervation. EMG and NCSs are not necessary for the diagnosis of CTS, but they may help confirm the diagnosis in equivocal cases. Distal sensory latencies greater than 3.5 msec or motor latencies greater than 4.5 msec are abnormal. Increased conduction velocity and decreased peak amplitude are less specific. EMG may show fibrillation at rest, positive sharp waves, or complex repetitive discharges.
      d. Differential diagnosis—These include cervical radiculopathy, brachial plexopathy, thoracic outlet syndrome, pronator syndrome, ulnar neuropathy with Martin-Gruber anastomoses, and peripheral neuropathy of multiple etiologies.
      e. Nonoperative treatment—Nonsurgical alternatives include activity modification, night splints, and NSAIDs. Steroid injections yield transient relief in 80% of patients; only 22% are symptom free at 12 months, but 40% are symptom free for more than 12 months when they have symptoms for less than 1 year, normal two-point discrimination, no thenar atrophy, less than 1-2–msec prolongation of sensory/motor latencies, and no denervation potentials on EMG. Failure to improve after corticosteroid injection is a poor prognostic factor, and surgery is less successful in these cases.
      f. Surgical treatment—Surgical options are open or endoscopic release of the TCL. No additional benefit is gained from internal neurolysis or tenosynovectomy. Structures within the Guyon canal can be injured if the incision and approach are too ulnar. If the incision and approach are too radial, risk to the recurrent motor branch of the median nerve is increased (Fig. 7–44). There are three main variations of the recurrent motor branch course: extraligamentous (~50%), subligamentous (~30%), and transligamentous (~20%) (Fig. 7–45). The most common complication of endoscopic carpal tunnel release (ECTR) is incomplete division of the TCL. ECTR is associated with an earlier return to work and better early patient satisfaction scores; however, the complication rate appears higher. The long-term results of open carpal tunnel release (CTR) and ECTR are equivalent. Complication rates are most closely associated with the experience of the operating surgeon rather than the operative technique. After standard open release, pinch strength returns to the preoperative level in 6 weeks and grip strength in 3 months. Pillar pain in the palm adjacent to the incision is common for 3-4 months in open CTR. Persistent symptoms after CTR may be secondary to incomplete release of the

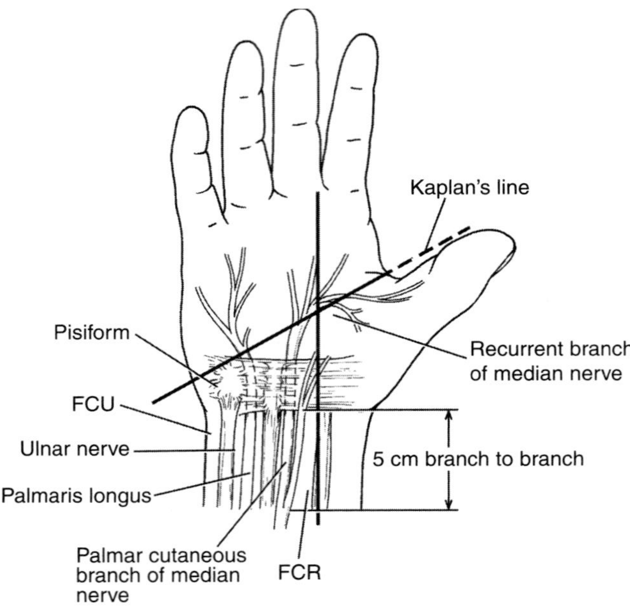

FIGURE 7–44 Kaplan's line is drawn along the ulnar border of the abducted thumb. The motor branch is identified as the intersection of Kaplan's line and a line drawn longitudinally in the web space of the index and middle fingers. FCR, flexor carpi radialis; FCU, flexor carpi ulnaris. (From Trumble TE, Budoff JE, Cornwall R, eds: Core Knowledge in Orthopaedics: Hand, Elbow, and Shoulder. Philadelphia, CV Mosby, 2006.)

TCL, iatrogenic median nerve injury, a missed double-crush phenomenon, concomitant peripheral neuropathy, or a space-occupying lesion. The success of revision CTR relies on identifying the underlying cause of the failure.

2. Pronator syndrome—Caused by compression of the median nerve more proximally, with anatomic sites including a supracondylar process (anterior distal humerus, which occurs in 1% of the population), the ligament of Struthers (courses between the supracondylar process and medial epicondyle), the bicipital aponeurosis (lacertus fibrosis), the space between the heads of the pronator teres, and the FDS aponeurotic arch (Fig. 7–46).
   a. Diagnosis—Pronator syndrome is differentiated from CTS by proximal volar forearm pain and sensory disturbances in the distribution of the palmar cutaneous branch of the median nerve. Test resisted elbow flexion with the forearm supinated (bicipital aponeurosis), resisted forearm pronation with the elbow extended (pronator teres) and resisted long-finger PIP joint flexion (FDS). Elbow radiographs are mandatory. Electrodiagnostic tests are usually normal.
   b. Treatment—The mainstays of treatment are activity modification, splints, and NSAIDs. Surgery is indicated for patients in whom nonoperative management has failed for 3-6 months and includes decompression of all potential sites of compression. The success rate is approximately 80% in most series. Pronator syndrome is also associated with medial epicondylitis and may improve by simply treating the latter condition.
3. Anterior interosseous nerve (AIN) syndrome—Involves motor loss of the FPL, the index and long FDP, and the pronator quadratus (PQ), without sensory disturbance. The FDP and FPL are tested by asking the patient to make an "OK" sign (precision tip-to-tip pinch). PQ involvement is tested by resisted pronation with the elbow maximally flexed. Bilateral AIN palsy may indicate Parsonage-Turner syndrome (viral brachial neuritis), especially if motor loss was preceded by intense pain in the shoulder region. Electrodiagnostic tests are helpful in confirming the diagnosis. It is important to rule out an isolated tendon disruption, such as FPL rupture in patients with rheumatoid arthritis (Mannerfelt syndrome). Apart from the aforementioned sites in pronator syndrome, additional sites of compression include an enlarged bicipital bursa and Gantzer's muscle (accessory head of the FPL). The vast majority of patients recover with observation. Nonoperative treatment involves activity modification and elbow splinting in 90 degrees of flexion. The results of surgical decompression are generally satisfactory if done within 3-6 months after the onset of symptoms.

C. Ulnar nerve
1. Cubital tunnel syndrome—The second most common compression neuropathy of the upper extremity. Sites of compression include the arcade of Struthers (fascial hiatus in the medial intermuscular septum as the ulnar nerve passes from the anterior to the posterior compartment 8 cm proximal to the medial epicondyle), medial intermuscular septum, medial head of the triceps, medial epicondyle, Osborne's ligament (cubital tunnel roof or retinaculum), anconeus epitrochlearis (anomalous muscle originating from the medial olecranon and inserting on the medial epicondyle), and FCU aponeurosis (Fig. 7–47). Other sources of compression include tumors, ganglions, osteophytes, heterotopic ossification, and medial epicondyle nonunion. Burns, cubitus varus or valgus deformities, medial epicondylitis, and repetitive elbow flexion/valgus stress during occupational or athletic activities are other associations.
   a. Diagnosis—Symptoms may include paresthesias of the ulnar 1½ digits and ulnar dorsal hand, intrinsic weakness with a positive Froment sign (compensatory thumb IP flexion during pinch owing to a weak adductor pollicis), and the Wartenberg sign (persistent abduction and extension of the small digit when asked to adduct the digits). Provocative tests include the ulnar nerve compression test or Tinel sign posterior to the

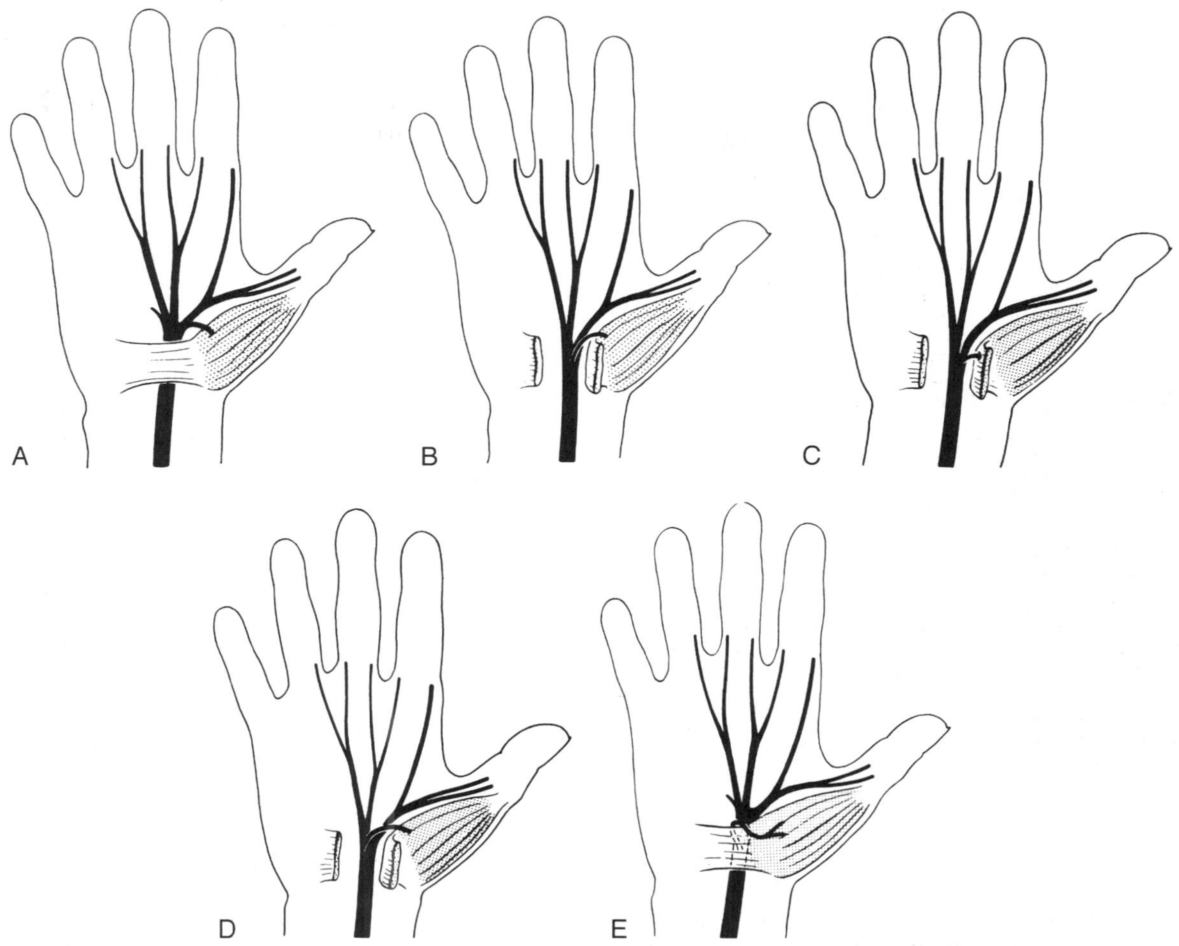

FIGURE 7–45 Variations in median nerve anatomy in the carpal tunnel. **A**, The most common pattern of the motor branch is extraligamentous and recurrent. **B**, Subligamentous branching of a recurrent median nerve. **C**, Transligamentous course of the recurrent branch of the median nerve. **D**, The motor branch can uncommonly originate from the ulnar border of the median nerve. **E**, The motor branch can lie on top of the transverse carpal ligament. (From Lanz U: Anatomical variations of the median nerve in the carpal tunnel. J Hand Surg [Am] 2:44-53, 1977.)

medial epicondyle and prolonged elbow flexion, each of which elicits worsening sensory disturbance or pain in an ulnar nerve distribution. Clawing of ulnar digits is a severe, late finding of ulnar neuropathy. Electrodiagnostic tests are helpful in confirming the clinical diagnosis.

b. Treatment—Nonoperative treatment includes activity modification, night splints (elbow held in 45 degrees of flexion), and NSAIDs. Numerous surgical techniques have been described, such as in situ cubital tunnel decompression, medial epicondylectomy, and anterior ulnar nerve transposition (subcutaneous, submuscular, or intramuscular). There is a high rate of recurrence of cubital tunnel syndrome (25-33%) with the different techniques, with anterior submuscular transposition and musculofascial lengthening producing the best results from meta-analyses. There are no prospective, randomized, controlled studies comparing the different techniques. In general, better results with fewer recurrences are obtained if surgery is performed prior to motor denervation. Persistent postoperative posterior elbow pain may indicate a neuroma of the medial antebrachial cutaneous nerve.

2. Ulnar tunnel syndrome—Compression neuropathy of the ulnar nerve in the Guyon canal. The most common cause of ulnar tunnel syndrome is a ganglion cyst (80% of nontraumatic cases). Other causative factors may include hook-of-hamate nonunion, ulnar artery thrombosis, palmaris brevis hypertrophy, or anomalous muscles.
   a. Anatomy—The borders of the Guyon canal are the volar carpal ligament (roof), the transverse carpal ligament (floor), the hook of the hamate (radial), and the pisiform and abductor digiti minimi muscle belly (ulnar) (Fig. 7–48). The ulnar tunnel is divided into three zones. Zone I is proximal to the bifurcation of the nerve and associated with mixed motor/sensory symptoms. Zone II surrounds the deep motor branch and is associated with pure motor symptoms. Ganglia and hook-of-hamate fractures are frequent causes in zones I and II. Zone III surrounds the superficial

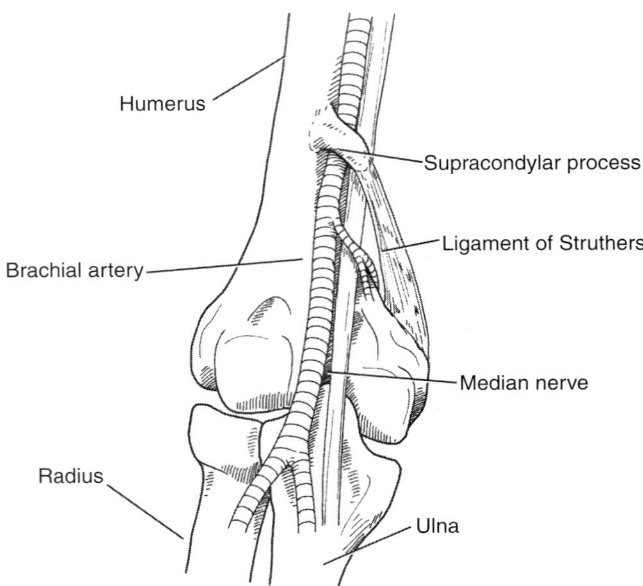

FIGURE 7–46 The ligament of Struthers bridges the supracondylar process of the humerus to the medial epicondyle or the origin of the humeral head of the pronator teres. (From Trumble TE, Budoff JE, Cornwall R, eds: Core Knowledge in Orthopaedics: Hand, Elbow, and Shoulder, p 243. Philadelphia, CV Mosby, 2006.)

sensory branch and is associated with pure sensory symptoms. Thrombosis of the ulnar artery is the most likely cause in zone III.

b. Diagnosis—Symptoms may be pure motor, pure sensory, or mixed, based on the location of compression. Useful adjunctive tests include CT for hook-of-hamate fracture, MRI for a ganglion cyst or other space-occupying lesion, and Doppler ultrasound for ulnar artery thrombosis.

c. Treatment—The success of treatment depends on identifying the cause. Nonoperative treatment includes activity modification, splints, and NSAIDs. Operative treatment involves decompressing the ulnar nerve by addressing the underlying cause. The Guyon canal is adequately decompressed by release of the transverse carpal ligament when concurrent CTS exists.

D. Radial nerve

1. Acute compression—Though rare, the radial nerve can be compressed by a fibrous arch from the lateral head of the triceps. Acute compression of the radial nerve is associated with the Holstein-Lewis fracture pattern at the junction of the middle and distal thirds of the humerus. Clinical findings include weakness in both radial nerve–innervated muscles (brachioradialis, ECRL) and muscles innervated by the **posterior interosseus nerve** (PIN). Sensory disturbances in the distribution of the radial nerve may be present. Electrodiagnostic tests are very helpful. Initial observation is warranted, but surgical decompression may be indicated if no recovery is seen by 3 months.

2. Posterior interosseous nerve compression syndrome—Symptoms include lateral elbow pain and distal muscle weakness. Look for radial deviation with active wrist extension because the radial wrist extensors are innervated by the radial nerve more proximally. The PIN innervates the ECRB, supinator, EIP, ECU, EDC, extensor digiti minimi (EDM), APL, EPB, and EPL. Patients may also have dorsal wrist pain, where the terminal nerve fibers provide sensory innervation to the dorsal wrist capsule. The terminal branch is located on the floor of the fourth extensor compartment. EMG and NCSs are usually diagnostic. The anatomic sites of compression include a fascial band at the radial head, the recurrent leash of Henry, the edge of the ECRB, the arcade of Frohse (the most common site, proximal edge of the supinator), and the distal edge of the supinator (Fig. 7–49). Unusual causes include chronic radial head dislocation, Monteggia

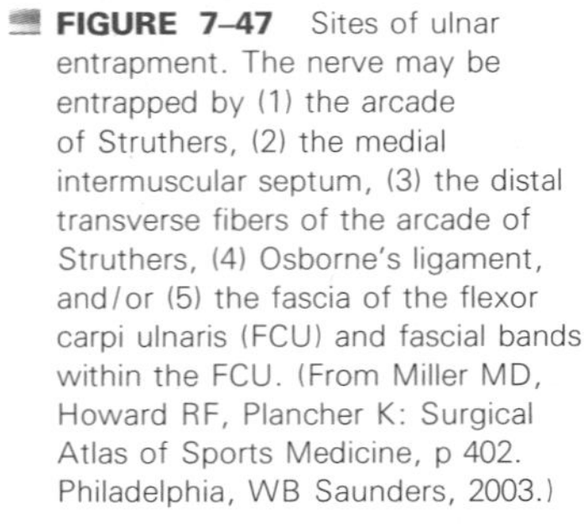

FIGURE 7–47 Sites of ulnar entrapment. The nerve may be entrapped by (1) the arcade of Struthers, (2) the medial intermuscular septum, (3) the distal transverse fibers of the arcade of Struthers, (4) Osborne's ligament, and/or (5) the fascia of the flexor carpi ulnaris (FCU) and fascial bands within the FCU. (From Miller MD, Howard RF, Plancher K: Surgical Atlas of Sports Medicine, p 402. Philadelphia, WB Saunders, 2003.)

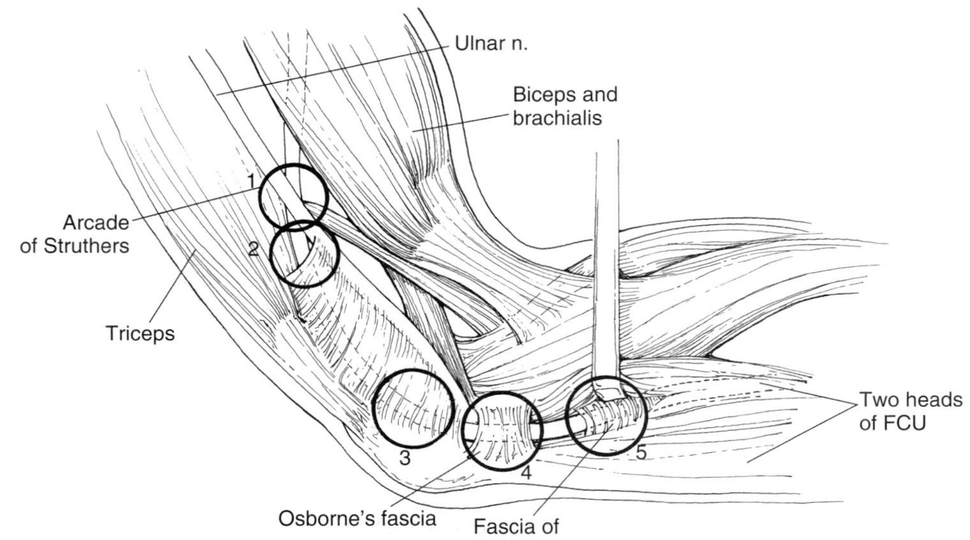

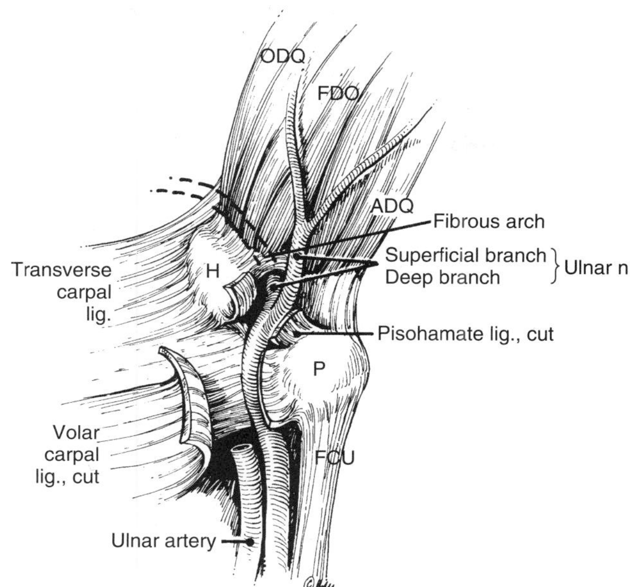

FIGURE 7–48 The ulnar nerve courses through the Guyon canal between the volar carpal ligament and the transverse carpal ligament. ADQ, abductor digiti quinti; FCU, flexor carpi ulnaris; FDQ, flexor digiti quinti; H, hamate; ODQ, opponens digiti quinti; P, pisiform. (From Green DP, Hotchkiss RM, Pederson WC, eds: Green's Operative Hand Surgery, 4th ed. New York, Churchill Livingstone, 1998.)

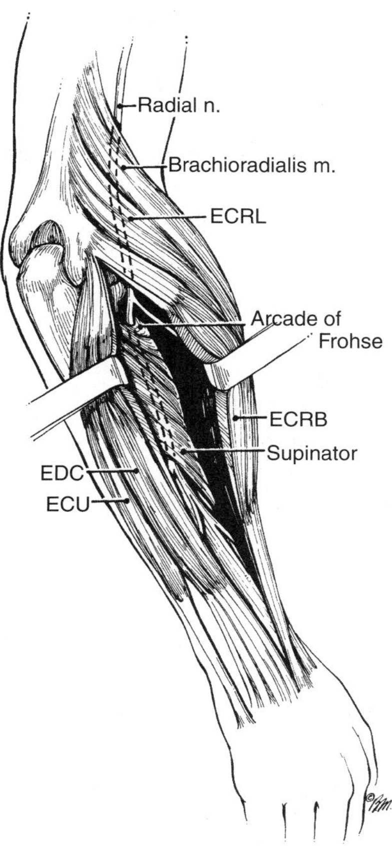

FIGURE 7–49 Extension of the posterior Thompson approach to the radial tunnel. ECRB, extensor carpi radialis brevis; ECRL, extensor carpi radialis longus; ECU, extensor carpi ulnaris; EDC, extensor digitorum communis. (From Green DP, Hotchkiss RN, Pederson WC, Wolfe SW, eds: Green's Operative Hand Surgery, 5th ed, p 1039. Philadelphia, Churchill Livingstone, 2005.)

fracture-dislocations, rheumatoid synovitis of the radiocapitellar joint, and a space-occupying elbow mass. PIN palsy is differentiated from extensor tendon rupture by a normal tenodesis test. Nonoperative treatment includes activity modification, splinting, and NSAIDs. If these modalities fail to provide recovery by 3 months, operative intervention is warranted. Surgical decompression of all anatomic sites of compression by either an anterior or a posterior approach provides good to excellent results for 85% of patients.

3. Radial tunnel syndrome—Characterized by lateral elbow and radial forearm pain without motor or sensory dysfunction. Provocative tests include resisted long-finger extension (positive if resistance reproduces pain at the radial tunnel) and resisted supination. Lateral epicondylitis coexists in a small percentage of patients. The point of maximum point tenderness is 1.5 cm anterior and distal to the lateral epicondyle in radial tunnel syndrome. Despite affecting the same nerve (PIN) and sites of compression, electrodiagnostic tests are typically normal. Prolonged nonoperative treatment for up to 1 year with activity modification, splints, NSAIDs, and local modalities is warranted. The success of surgical decompression is less predictable than for PIN syndrome, with good to excellent results of only 50-80% reported and maximum recovery not reached until 9-18 months postoperatively.
4. Cheiralgia paresthetica (Wartenberg syndrome)—Compressive neuropathy of the superficial sensory branch of the radial nerve. It is compressed between the brachioradialis and ECRL with forearm pronation (by a scissor-like action between the tendons). Symptoms include pain, numbness, and paresthesias over the radiodorsal hand. The provocative tests include forceful forearm pronation for 60 seconds and a Tinel sign over the nerve. This condition is initially treated by activity modification, splinting, and NSAIDs. Surgical decompression is warranted if a 6-month trial of nonoperative treatment fails.

E. Other compressive neuropathies

1. Suprascapular nerve entrapment syndrome—Presents with acute onset of deep, diffuse posterolateral shoulder pain. It occurs after trauma or aggressive athletic activity. The most consistent finding is pain with palpation over the suprascapular notch. Electrodiagnostic tests are helpful in establishing the diagnosis. Supraspinatus/infraspinatus muscle atrophy may occur secondary to a delay in diagnosis. Both muscles are affected when compression of the nerve occurs at the suprascapular notch. Isolated infraspinatus atrophy is most often secondary to a ganglion at the spinoglenoid notch, which may be visualized by MRI. Spinoglenoid notch ganglions are associated with

posterior labrum tears in almost 100% of cases. The current trend is toward early surgical decompression through a combined arthroscopic/open posterior approach.

2. Thoracic outlet syndrome—Two types exist: vascular and neurogenic. The vascular variety involves subclavian vessel compression or aneurysm and is diagnosed by physical examination and angiography. In the Adson test, the patient keeps the arm at the side, hyperextends the neck, and rotates the head to the affected side. A diminished radial artery pulse with inhalation is suggestive of subclavian artery compromise, but the test has questionable reliability. The neurogenic variety is an entrapment neuropathy of the lower trunk of the brachial plexus. It is infrequent and diagnosed by clinical examination alone (EMG and NCSs are rarely helpful). Sensory disturbances of the medial brachial and antebrachial cutaneous nerves may differentiate the condition from cubital tunnel syndrome. The Roos sign indicates heaviness or paresthesias in the hands after holding them above the head for at least 1 minute. Cervical and chest radiographs should be obtained to rule out a cervical rib or Pancoast tumor. Physical therapy focuses on shoulder girdle strengthening and proper posture and relaxation techniques. Transaxillary first rib resection by a thoracic surgeon yields good to excellent results in 90% of cases in which a cervical rib is the cause; however, the complications can be disastrous.

XI. Nerve Injuries and Tendon Transfers

A. Peripheral nerve injuries

1. Introduction—Peripheral nerve function may be compromised by a spectrum of mechanisms, such as compression, stretch, blast, crush, avulsion, transection, and tumor invasion. The evaluation and treatment of traumatic peripheral nerve dysfunction are guided by the mechanism of injury and the presence of other injuries. The most important factor determining the chance of nerve recovery is the age of the patient. There is a noticeable decline in prognosis after age 20. Additionally, the prognosis is better in stretch injuries; clean wounds; and early, direct surgical repair. Conversely, a poor outcome is expected in crush or blast injuries, infected or scarred wounds, and late surgical repair.

2. Classification—Peripheral nerve injuries were classified by Seddon in 1943 into neurapraxia, axonotmesis, and neurotmesis (Table 7–9).
   a. Neurapraxia is a mild nerve stretch or contusion that results in focal conduction block without wallerian degeneration. While there may be disruption of the myelin sheath, the epineurium, perineurium, and endoneurium are intact. The prognosis is excellent, with recovery expected within days to weeks.
   b. Axonotmesis is an incomplete nerve injury that produces wallerian degeneration distal to the site of injury and consequent conduction block. Even though axons are disrupted, recovery is expected because the endoneurium remains intact. This provides a conduit for nerve regeneration, which is followed by an advancing Tinel sign. However, fibroblast proliferation within the nerve sheath may impede nerve regrowth and lead to a neuroma-in-continuity.
   c. Neurotmesis is a complete nerve injury that results in disruption of all anatomic layers (epineurium, perineurium, and endoneurium), wallerian degeneration, and resulting conduction block. The proximal nerve end will form a neuroma and the distal end a glioma. Sutherland further classified neurotmesis into different degrees of injury based on sequential disruption of the anatomic layers (see Table 7–9). These injuries have the worst overall prognosis.

In axonotmesis and neurotmesis, the distal nerve segment undergoes wallerian degeneration. The degradation products are removed by phagocytosis. Myelin-producing Schwann cells proliferate and align themselves along the basement membrane, forming a tube that will receive regenerating axons. The nerve cell body enlarges as the rate of structural protein production increases. Each proximal axon forms multiple sprouts that connect to the distal stump and migrate at a rate of 1 mm/day.

3. Surgical repair—When surgical repair of a peripheral nerve injury is indicated, the best results are achieved when the repair is performed within 10-14 days of the injury. Repair should be performed

TABLE 7-9 CLASSIFICATION OF NERVE INJURY

Classification			
Seddon	*Sunderland*	**Injury**	**Prognosis**
Neurapraxia	First degree	Demyelination injury	Temporary conduction block; resolves in 1-2 days
Axonotmesis	Second degree	Axonal injury	Regeneration is usually complete but may take several weeks or months
Neurotmesis	Third degree	Endoneurium injured	Regeneration occurs but is not satisfactory
	Fourth degree	Perineurium injured	Spontaneous regeneration is unsatisfactory, resulting in neuroma in continuity
	Fifth degree	Severed nerve trunk	Spontaneous regeneration is not possible without surgery

From Trumble TE, Budoff JE, Cornwall R: Hand, Elbow, and Shoulder: Core Knowledge in Orthopaedics, p 227. Philadelphia, CV Mosby, 2006.

within a clean, well-vascularized wound bed and should be free of tension. Nerve length may be gained by neurolysis or transposition. Of the various repair techniques, such as epineural, individual fascicular, and group fascicular, no single technique has been shown to be superior. The use of nerve conduits has gained in popularity. Gaps of greater than 2.5 cm typically require nerve grafting. Options include autogenous grafts (e.g., sural nerve), vascularized nerve grafts, and bioactive conduits. Synthetic collagen tubes have demonstrated favorable outcomes for digital nerve repair of gaps of less than 4 mm. Growth factor augmentation (e.g., insulin-like, fibroblast) has been studied in animal models and shown to promote nerve regeneration. Chronic peripheral nerve injuries may be treated with neurotization and/or tendon transfers.

B. Traumatic brachial plexus injury—Knowledge of brachial plexus anatomy is critical for understanding the evaluation and diagnosis of brachial plexus lesions (Fig. 7–50). High-energy mechanisms are associated with more severe lesions, such as root avulsions and the rupture of entire segments of the plexus.

1. Diagnosis—The location and severity of injury should be well-characterized, with a comprehensive motor and sensory evaluation to assist in treatment planning and recovery assessment. Determine if the injury is supraclavicular or infraclavicular. Most supraclavicular injuries result from traction mechanisms. If the injury is supraclavicular, determine if it is pre- or postganglionic. Preganglionic lesions (nerve root avulsions) have the worst prognosis. Signs of severe injury include the presence of a Horner sign (ptosis, miosis, and anhidrosis), global motor dysfunction, complete sensory loss, and severe neuropathic pain. In cases of clinically complete brachial plexopathy, less than one-quarter of patients have avulsion of all five roots. A complete radiographic series should include the cervical spine, chest, and shoulder girdle. Inspiratory and expiratory chest radiographs may demonstrate a paralyzed hemidiaphragm, indicating a severe upper root injury. Root avulsions may be indicated by the presence of corresponding fractures of the transverse spinal processes. Scapulothoracic dissociation is often linked to multiple root avulsions and major vascular injury. MRI and CT myelography are often employed in the initial workup of traumatic brachial plexus injuries. EMG and NCSs may help localize the site of injury, and **somatosensory evoked potentials** (SSEPs) may help differentiate between pre- and postganglionic lesions. Sequential electrodiagnostic studies are performed to monitor recovery.
2. Timing of surgical treatment—Modern series reveal a reverse relationship between the time from injury to operative intervention and clinical outcome. Immediate surgical exploration may be indicated in cases of penetrating trauma or

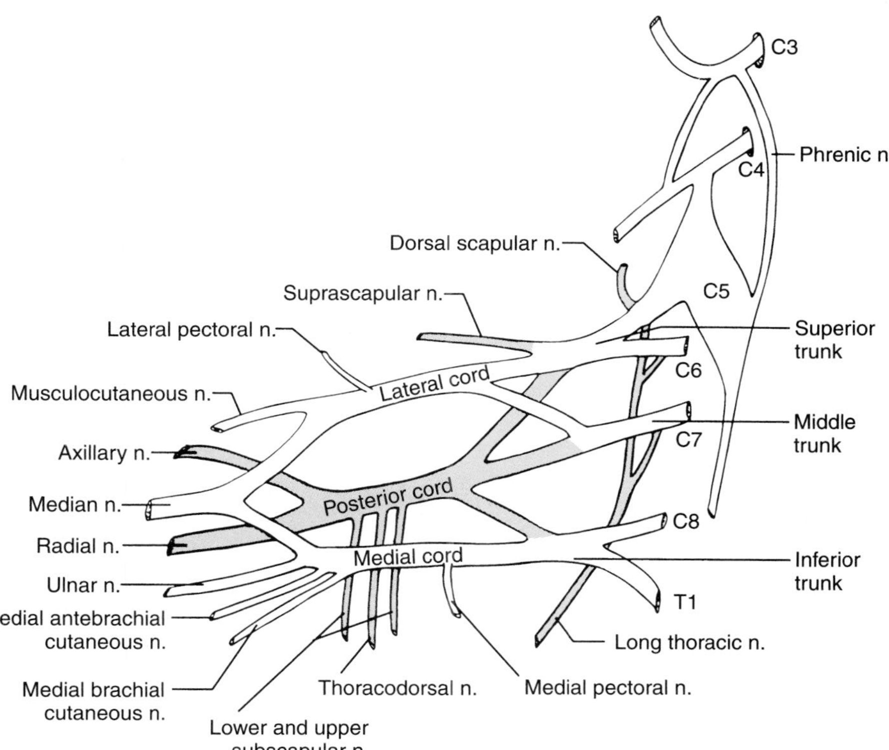

FIGURE 7–50 Brachial plexus anatomy. (From Brushart TM, Wilgus EF: Brachial plexus and shoulder girdle injuries. In Browner BD, Jupiter JB, eds: Skeletal Trauma, 2nd ed, p 1696. Philadelphia, WB Saunders, 1998.)

iatrogenic injuries. On the other hand, one study showed that many patients with gunshot wounds to the plexus improved over time without surgical exploration. It is reasonable to observe these patients for 3 months in the absence of a major vascular injury. Early surgical intervention (3 weeks to 3 months after injury) is indicated in patients with complete or near-complete injuries resulting from a high-energy mechanism. Patients with brachial plexus palsy resulting from low-energy mechanisms, especially in those with an incomplete upper plexus lesion, are best observed for at least 3-6 months for spontaneous recovery. Surgery may be warranted if recovery plateaus early. Nerve repair or reconstruction beyond 6 months from the time of injury has a less predictable clinical outcome. The most reliable clinical sign of nerve regeneration and recovery is an advancing Tinel sign. Muscle fibrosis occurs after 18-24 months.

3. Tendon/nerve transfers—An isolated C8-T1 injury is best treated with early tendon transfers. In these cases, full recovery is unlikely because of the distance between the lesion and the intrinsic muscles of the hand. For other lesions, nerve repair or reconstruction should be prioritized. The order of priority in brachial plexus surgery is (1) elbow flexion, (2) shoulder stabilization, and (3) hand function. Because direct repair is often compromised by excessive tension, neuroma excision and nerve cable grafting are the favored methods. Donor sites include the sural, medial brachial cutaneous, and medial antebrachial cutaneous nerves. The best outcomes are obtained in young patients and in those who undergo nerve grafting within 3 months after injury. Nerve transfers are indicated when an insufficient number of proximal axons are available, such as occurs in multiple root avulsions. The **Oberlin transfer** incorporates the ulnar nerve branch (fascicle) to the FCU into the musculocutaneous nerve to address biceps function. The descending branch of the spinal accessory nerve (cranial nerve [CN] XI) may be transferred to the suprascapular nerve to address shoulder function. Patients who do not show meaningful recovery of shoulder and elbow function after 6-12 months may be good candidates for shoulder arthrodesis and tendon transfers to increase the functional activities of daily living.

C. Neonatal brachial plexopathy—This condition is associated with high birth weight, shoulder dystocia, cephalopelvic disproportion, and forceps delivery. The muscle grading system used to evaluate these patients is as follows: M0, no contraction; M1, contraction without movement; M2, contraction with slight movement; and M3, complete movement. Complete recovery is possible if the biceps and deltoid are graded M1 by 2 months. Incomplete recovery can be expected if the biceps and deltoid do not contract within 3-6 months. Surgery is not recommended if biceps contraction is evident at 3 months. The results of nerve grafting are better in infants than adults, and reinnervation of the hand intrinsic muscles is possible.

D. Cerebral palsy

1. Introduction—The typical pattern of upper extremity deformity resulting from this nonprogressive central nervous system injury includes thumb-in-palm, clenched fist, wrist flexion, forearm pronation, elbow flexion, and shoulder internal rotation. Initial nonoperative management involves physical therapy and night-time static-extension splints.
2. Nonoperative treatment—Oral medications such as diazepam, baclofen, tizanidine, and dantrolene have been used to help decrease spasticity. Some patients may benefit from an intrathecal baclofen infusion pump. Botulinum toxin A is transiently effective (3-6 months) when severe spasticity is present.
3. Surgical treatment—Surgical correction of a deformity to improve function is best performed on children with higher IQs (over 50-70), voluntary muscle control, and good sensibility. A thumb-in-palm deformity is corrected by the release or lengthening of the adductor pollicis, first dorsal interosseous, FPB, and FPL muscles. This procedure is combined with a Z-plasty of the first web space and tendon transfers to augment thumb extension and abduction. Fractional or Z-plasty tendon lengthening may improve digital flexor tightness in patients with a clenched fist. This may be enhanced by neurectomy of the motor branch of the ulnar nerve to reduce intrinsic spasticity. Wrist extension is classically achieved with the Green transfer of the FCU to the ECRB around the ulnar border of the forearm.
4. Other surgical interventions—If the child is a poor candidate for correction of a deformity, other operative interventions may be performed for hygiene purposes. Shoulder contractures may be addressed with a derotational humeral osteotomy or lengthening of the subscapularis and/or pectoralis major muscles. Shoulder arthrodesis is also an option. Mild elbow contractures may be improved by musculocutaneous neurectomy. Severe contractures may be addressed by biceps and brachialis muscle lengthening combined with anterior joint capsulotomy. Wrist contractures are treated with arthrodesis. Digit flexion contractures are either lengthened or undergo FDS-to-FDP transfer.

E. Tendon transfers

1. Indications—These procedures are indicated to replace irreparably injured tendons/muscles, substitute for the function of a paralyzed muscle, and restore balance to a deformed hand. One of the most common indications for tendon transfers is to improve function after peripheral nerve injury of the upper extremity, when spontaneous recovery is unlikely. The timing of tendon transfers is controversial and depends on age, indication, and prognosis. Tendon transfers are generally deferred until tissue equilibrium is achieved, passive joint

mobility is restored, and donors with adequate power and excursion are available. This deferral may translate to over 12 months after brachial plexus injury or until spasticity resolves in a tetraplegic hand.

2. Key concepts—Important definitions to understand include force, amplitude (excursion), work capacity, and power. Force is proportional to the cross-sectional area of the muscle. The greatest force of contraction is exerted when the muscle is at its resting length. Amplitude or excursion is proportional to the length of the muscle. Smith's 3-5-7 rule estimates the excursion of the wrist flexors/extensors (3 cm), MCP extensors (5 cm), and the FDP (7 cm). Work capacity is force times length (F × L). Power is the amount of work performed in a unit of time.
3. The selection of a transfer is based on a careful assessment of the patient. The following questions are integral to the assessment. What function is missing? What tendons are available for transfer? What are the options for transfer? Classic transfers are outlined in Table 7–10. Some of the basic tenets of tendon transfers are expressed below.

   Select a donor muscle-tendon unit that is expendable but matches the qualities of the unit being replaced.

   A transfer should perform only one function.

   Wrist tenodesis should be preserved.

   After transfer, at least one wrist flexor/extensor and one digit flexor/extensor should remain.

   Synergistic actions are those that occur together in normal function (e.g., finger flexion and wrist extension). Synergistic transfers are easier to rehabilitate.

   One grade of motor strength is lost after tendon transfer.

   A straight line of pull is best.

   The most common cause of failure after tendon transfer is the development of motion-limiting adhesions, which require aggressive hand therapy and possible tenolysis if there is minimal improvement.

TABLE 7-10 CLASSIC TENDON TRANSFERS

Palsy	Loss	Transfer
Radial	Wrist extension	Pronator teres to ECRB
	Finger extension	FCU to EDC II-V, FCR to EDC II-V
		FDS III to EPL and EIP, FDS IV to EDC III-V
	Thumb extension	Palmaris longus to EPL
		FDS to radial lateral band
Low ulnar	Hand intrinsics (interosseous and ulnar lumbricals)	ECRL to lateral band
		EDQ EIP to lateral band FCR + graft to lateral band
		Metacarpal phalangeal capsulodesis
	Thumb adduction	ECRL + graft to adductor pollicis
		Brachioradialis + graft to adductor pollicis
	Index abduction	EIP to first dorsal interosseous
		Abductor pollicis longus to first dorsal interosseous
		ECRL to first dorsal interosseous
High ulnar	Low problems + FDP Ring and small fingers	Suture to functioning FDP index and long index and long finger.
Low median	Opposition	FDS ring to abductor pollicis brevis (FCU pulley)
		EIP to thumb proximal phalanx (routed around the ulna for line of pull)
		Abductor digiti quinti to abductor pollicis brevis
		Palmaris longus to abductor pollicis brevis
High median	Thumb IP flexion	Brachioradialis to flexor pollicis longus
	Index- and long-finger flexion	Suture to functioning FDP ring and small finger or ECRL to FDP index and long finger if additional power is needed.
Low median and ulnar	Thumb adduction	ECRB + graft to adductor tubercle of thumb
	Index abduction	Abductor pollicis longus to first dorsal interosseous
	Opposition	EIP to abductor pollicis brevis
	Clawed fingers	Brachioradialis + four-tailed free graft to the A2 pulley
	Volar sensibility	Neurovascular island flap from back of hand
High median and ulnar	Thumb adduction	ECRB + graft to adductor tubercle of thumb
	Thumb IP flexion	Brachioradialis to FPL
	Thumb abduction	EIP to abductor pollicis brevis
	Index abduction	Abductor pollicis longus to first dorsal interosseous
	Finger flexion	ECRL to FDP
	Clawed fingers	Tenodesis of all metaphalangeal joints, with free-tendon graft from dorsal carpal ligament routed deep to transverse metacarpal ligament to extensor apparatus
	Wrist flexion	ECU to FCU
	Volar sensibility	Neurovascular island flap from back of hand

ECRB, extensor carpi radialis brevis; ECRL, extensor carpi radialis longus; ECU, extensor carpi ulnaris; EDC, extensor digitorum communis; EDQ, extensor digiti quinti; EIP, extensor indicis proprius; EPL, extensor pollicis longus; FCR, flexor carpi radialis; FCU, flexor carpi ulnaris; FDP, flexor digitorum profundus; FDS, flexor digitorum superficialis; FPL, flexor pollicis longus.

XII. Arthritis

A. OA—Primary idiopathic degenerative joint disease that commonly affects the DIP joints and the **trapeziometacarpal** (TM) joint of the thumb. The erosive form more commonly affects the PIP joints. The MCP joints are not typically involved. OA of the wrist is usually post-traumatic. The hallmark symptoms of OA are pain, swelling, and decreased range of motion, and the classic radiographic findings are joint space narrowing, osteophytes, subchondral sclerosis, and subchondral cyst formation. Nonoperative management includes activity modification, NSAIDs, and intra-articular corticosteroid injections. Unique findings and specific operative treatments for the various involved joints follows.

1. DIP joint—Characterized by the presence of marginal osteophytes called **Heberden nodes**. Surgery may be warranted for uncontrollable pain, instability, or the presence of a symptomatic **mucous cyst**. The cyst may be excised, along with any accompanying osteophytes, for symptomatic relief. Occasionally, skin coverage with a local rotational flap is necessary after cyst excision. Severe arthritic changes or deformity may also require arthrodesis with Kirschner wires or a small cannulated screw in approximately 5-10 degrees of flexion.
2. PIP joint—Characterized by the presence of **Bouchard nodes**. Options for surgical intervention include arthrodesis and arthroplasty. Arthrodesis provides a more predictable outcome for the index PIP joint, where the lateral stresses associated with pinch may compromise the durability of arthroplasty. If arthrodesis is chosen, the joint should be fused in increasing degrees of flexion from radial to ulnar—index, 40 degrees; long, 45 degrees; ring, 50 degrees; and small, 55 degrees—to match the resting cascade of the hand. PIP arthroplasty is better reserved for the long, ring, and small digits, which are involved in power grasp. The operation may be performed through either a dorsal or a volar approach with the use of either silicone elastomer or pyrocarbon implants, and approximately 60 degrees of motion can be expected after a course of postoperative therapy.
3. MCP joint—Primary cases of OA involving this joint are rare; it may be involved in patients with hemochromatosis. It may be treated with silicone, pyrocarbon, or newer surface replacements to alleviate pain and preserve some functional range of motion. The use of surface replacement technology requires competent collateral ligaments. Arthrodesis of the MCP joints severely limits hand function but may be required secondary to septic arthritis or failed arthroplasty. Again, the digits are placed in increasing amounts of flexion—index, 25 degrees; long, 30 degrees; ring, 35 degrees; and small, 40 degrees.
4. Thumb MCP joint—Rarely involved in primary OA. Pain is reliably relieved by arthrodesis, with the joint placed in approximately 10-20 degrees of flexion.
5. Thumb TM joint—Also termed basal joint or CMC joint OA. Theorized by Pellegrini as resulting from attenuation of the anterior oblique ligament (beak ligament), leading to instability, dorsoradial subluxation, and articular cartilage degeneration. Pain and/or crepitus may be elicited with the grind test, using combined axial compression and circumduction. Metacarpal adduction, first web space contracture, and compensatory MCP hyperextension are late findings. Up to one half of all patients with thumb CMC OA also have CTS. Other conditions, such as adjacent joint arthritis, trigger thumb, and de Quervain's tenosynovitis, may coexist and must be addressed. Eaton and Littler described four stages of disease (Table 7–11). Heavy laborers may benefit from arthrodesis in the early stages of disease. The thumb TM joint is fused in 20 degrees of radial abduction and 40 degrees of palmar abduction. The most commonly performed surgical intervention for advanced-stage CMC OA is trapezium excision with **ligament reconstruction tendon interposition** (LRTI). The FCR is typically used to suspend the metacarpal, although a slip of the APL may be effectively used, as described by Thompson. If the thumb MCP joint hyperextends more than 30 degrees during pinch, concurrent fusion or volar capsulodesis is recommended to avoid excessive stress on the ligament reconstruction. The status of the scaphotrapezoidal joint must be assessed intraoperatively. Settling of the first metacarpal during pinch does not seem to correlate with clinical outcome. The past use of silicone arthroplasty has resulted in an unacceptably high failure rate from silicone synovitis or instability.

B. Rheumatoid arthritis—Systemic autoimmune inflammatory disease that primarily affects the synovium surrounding the small joints of the hand and wrist. The pathophysiology of rheumatoid arthritis is discussed in Chapter 1, Basic Sciences. Arthritis of the hand joints lasting for longer than 6 weeks is one of the seven diagnostic criteria used by the American

TABLE 7-11 EATON STAGES OF TRAPEZIOMETACARPAL OSTEOARTHRITIS

Stage	Description
I	Normal joint with the exception of possible widening from synovitis
II	Joint space narrowing, with debris and osteophytes < 2 mm
III	Joint space narrowing, with debris and osteophytes > 2 mm
IV	Involvement of scaphotrapezial joint space in addition to narrowing of the trapeziometacarpal joint

From Trumble TE, Budoff JE, Cornwall R: Core Knowledge in Orthopaedics: Hand, Elbow, and Shoulder, p 330. Philadelphia, CV Mosby, 2006.

College of Rheumatology. In contrast to OA, the DIP joints are usually spared.

1. Diagnosis—Patients typically present with symmetrical complaints of pain, morning stiffness, and significant swelling of the hands. Tenosynovitis, tendon rupture, and other soft tissue manifestations are also common. While serologic studies may be positive (rheumatoid factor in 70-90% of patients) within several months of disease onset, the classic radiographic features, including diffuse osteopenia, periarticular erosion, and joint subluxation, may not appear for several years (Fig. 7–51). MRI with intravenous contrast is more sensitive for detecting early disease, with findings of enhanced synovial proliferation, bone marrow edema, and periarticular erosion. Disability from joint destruction and deformity can be limited by early diagnosis and aggressive medical management with **disease modifying antirheumatic drugs** (DMARDs).
2. Treatment of common skeletal and soft tissue manifestations of rheumatoid arthritis in the upper extremity—Surgical intervention in patients with rheumatoid arthritis should be approached with caution.
   a. Rheumatoid nodules—Subcutaneous masses consisting of chronic inflammatory cells surrounded by a collagenous capsule. They are seen in 20-25% of patients with rheumatoid arthritis. These nodules constitute the most common extra-articular manifestation of the disease and are associated with aggressive disease. They occur over bony prominences on the extensor surfaces of the upper extremity. They may erode through the skin and cause a chronically draining sinus. Excision may be indicated for diagnostic biopsy, pain relief, or cosmetic improvement.
   b. Tenosynovitis—Hyperplasia and inflammatory cell infiltration of synovium-lined tendon sheaths that may precede joint manifestations in rheumatoid arthritis. It may involve the flexor and/or extensor tendons of the hand and wrist. Nonoperative management with rest, activity modification, splinting, and anti-inflammatory medication is attempted for at least 4-6 months. Tenosynovectomy is reserved for cases of failed conservative treatment or when impending tendon rupture is evident.
   c. Tendon rupture—May occur secondary to chronic tenosynovitis or mechanical abrasion over bony prominences. **Vaughn-Jackson syndrome** results from progressive rupture of extensor tendons, starting with the EDM and continuing radially, from attrition over a prominent distal ulnar head. The EPL may rupture from the same process occurring at Lister's tubercle. Finally, **Mannerfelt syndrome** results in FPL and/or index FDP rupture secondary to attrition over a volar scaphoid osteophyte. Direct repair is prone to failure in these cases, making tendon transfer the preferred method of treatment (Fig. 7–52). Tendon rupture must be clinically differentiated from sagittal band rupture with tendon subluxation, in which patients are unable to actively extend the affected digit at the MCP joint but can maintain extension when the tendon is relocated passively. It is also important to examine the tenodesis effect to help differentiate between rupture and neurologic deficit (PIN) in patients who are unable to extend their digits.
   d. Caput ulnae syndrome—End-stage finding of DRUJ instability in rheumatoid arthritis. DRUJ synovitis leads to surrounding capsular and ligamentous laxity. As the ECU subsheath stretches, the ECU tendon subluxes in an ulnar and volar direction. Subsequently, the carpus supinates on the radius and further stretches the dorsal restraints. As a result, the ulnar head subluxes dorsally and a "piano-key sign" may be elicited. The ulnar head may cause attritional rupture of extensor tendons (see above, Vaughn-Jackson syndrome), leading to supination of the carpus away from the ulnar head and further stretching the dorsal restraints. This developing instability allows

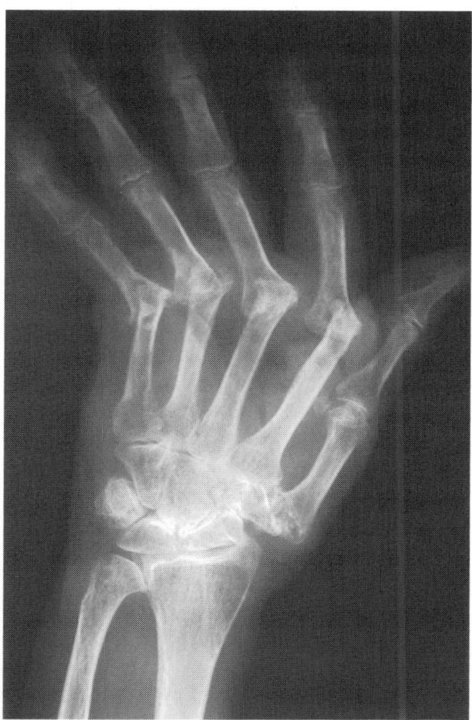

FIGURE 7–51 Radiograph showing distal radioulnar joint arthritis, ulnar translocation of the carpus, radial deviation of the metacarpals, and ulnar deviation and subluxation of the proximal phalanx. (From Trumble TE, Budoff JE, Cornwall R, eds: Core Knowledge in Orthopaedics: Hand, Elbow, and Shoulder, p 347. Philadelphia, CV Mosby, 2006.)

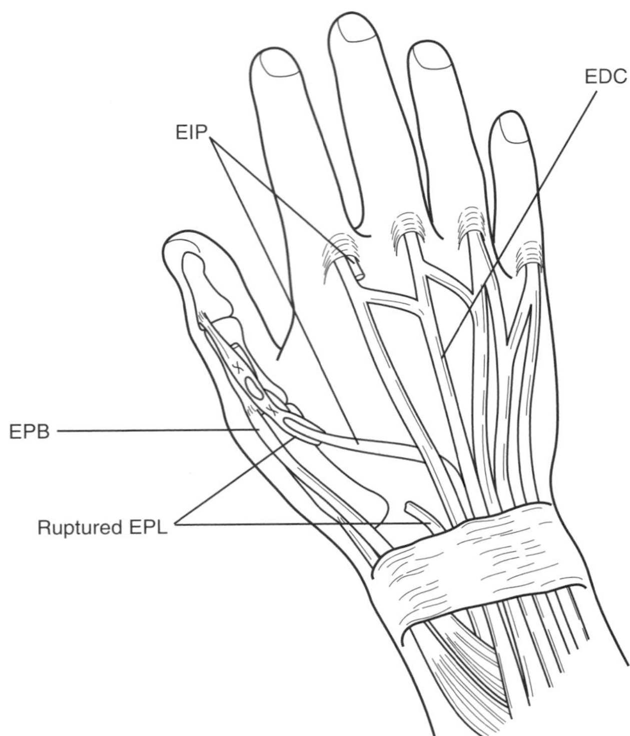

FIGURE 7–52 Transfer of the extensor indicis proprius (EIP) for an extensor pollicis longus (EPL) rupture. EDC, extensor digitorum communis; EPB, extensor pollicis brevis. (From Trumble TE, Budoff JE, Cornwall R, eds: Core Knowledge in Orthopaedics: Hand, Elbow, and Shoulder, p 365. Philadelphia, CV Mosby, 2006.)

the ulna to subluxate in a dorsal direction. When this occurs, it adds to increased pressure in the overlying extensor compartments, which are already elevated by synovitis. This increased pressure causes ischemic necrosis and rupture of the extensor tendons. Treatment options include a Darrach resection of the distal ulna, the Sauve-Kapandji procedure, resection hemiarthroplasty, and ulnar head replacement.

e. Rheumatoid wrist—Extensive synovitis and pannus formation weakens the capsular and ligamentous structures that stabilize the radiocarpal joints and DRUJs, and the carpus subluxes in a volar and ulnar direction. The carpus also supinates on the radius, as previously described. Chronic scapholunate ligament disruption can lead to rotatory subluxation of the scaphoid and progressive carpal collapse. Early synovectomy may delay severe joint destruction and deformity in some cases. Intermediate-stage disease may benefit from a radiolunate arthrodesis, which centralizes the lunate and diminishes further carpal subluxation. Wrist arthrodesis remains the gold standard for advanced radiocarpal destruction. Although motion is sacrificed, pain relief is reliable. Bilateral wrist fusions are not contraindicated. **Total wrist arthroplasty** is an option in low-demand patients with adequate bone stock, minimal deformity, and intact extensor tendon function. The advances of newer-generation metal/polyethylene combination implants are helping decrease the historically high rate of complications associated with total wrist arthroplasty.

f. MCP joint involvement—Leads to a deformity pattern of ulnar deviation and volar subluxation. Synovitis and pannus formation stretch the weaker radial sagittal bands, and the extensor tendons sublux in the ulnar aspect. There is concurrent loss of volar plate and collateral ligament integrity. The fingers are maintained in the deformed position by contracture of the intrinsic muscle tendons. Simultaneous wrist involvement leads to the characteristic Z deformity, with ulnar translation and supination of the carpus, radial deviation of the metacarpals, and ulnar deviation of the fingers. Early treatment with synovectomy and recentralization of the extensor tendons provides a temporary solution. **MCP arthroplasty** is the most common definitive treatment to relieve pain and improve cosmesis. Restoration of function is variable. Complications may include infection, implant failure, and recurrent deformity. Concomitant correction of wrist deformity is paramount to the success of MCP arthroplasty.

g. PIP joint involvement—Synovitis leads to attenuation of stabilizing structures, which may lead to either boutonniere or swan neck deformities.
   (1) **Boutonniere**—Attenuation of the central slip of the terminal extensor tendon leads to volar lateral band subluxation with PIP hyperflexion and consequent DIP hyperextension.
   (2) **Swan-neck**—Attenuation of the volar plate leads to dorsal lateral band subluxation with PIP hyperextension and consequent DIP hyperflexion.

h. Rheumatoid thumb—Classified into six types by Nalebuff (Table 7–12). The most common deformity is the type I boutonniere with hyperflexion of the MCP joint and hyperextension of the IP joint. The uncommon type II deformity is characterized by a boutonniere TM subluxation or dislocation. Type III is a swan-neck deformity with TM joint dislocation, MCP joint hyperextension, IP joint flexion, and metacarpal adduction. Type IV, also known as gamekeeper's thumb, consists of incompetence and instability in the MCP joint ulnar collateral ligament. The rare type V deformity is similar to the swan-neck without TM joint involvement or metacarpal adduction. Treatment is

TABLE 7-12 NALEBUFF CLASSIFICATION OF RHEUMATOID THUMB DEFORMITIES

Type	Description
I	Boutonniere
II	Boutonniere with carpometacarpal involvement
III	Swan-neck deformity
IV	Gamekeeper's deformity
V	Swan-neck deformity with no metacarpal adduction or carpometacarpal changes
VI	Skeletal collapse with loss of bone substance (arthritis mutilans)

From Trumble TE, Budoff JE, Cornwall R: Core Knowledge in Orthopaedics: Hand, Elbow, and Shoulder, p 368. Philadelphia, CV Mosby, 2006.

dictated by the deformity. Type VI, also known as arthritis mutilans, results in collapse of the thumb skeleton and requires a combination of arthrodeses.

C. Juvenile rheumatoid arthritis (JRA)—Age of onset is prior to 16 years. Other rheumatic diseases must be excluded. A classic difference between JRA and the adult form is radial deviation of the MCP joints and ulnar deviation of the wrist. Nonoperative treatment is favored in order to avoid damage to the growing physes. Three disease types are described: systemic (20%), polyarticular (40%), and pauciarticular (40%).
   1. Systemic form (Still disease)—It may be associated with transient arthritis in the setting of fever, anemia, hepatosplenomegaly, uveitis, and lymphadenitis. Rheumatoid factor is negative. Only one fourth of patients develop chronic, disabling arthritis.
   2. Polyarticular form—A symmetrical form of JRA affecting at least five joints. A small percentage of patients have a positive rheumatoid factor. It more closely resembles the adult form of the disease, and chronic progression is likely.
   3. Pauciarticular form—An asymmetrical form of JRA affecting less than five joints. This variant produces more large-joint and lower extremity involvement. Females typically have an earlier disease onset than males and may have a positive anti–nuclear antibody (ANA). An association with human leukocyte antigen (HLA)–B27 and sacroiliitis is more common in males.

D. Psoriatic arthritis—Seronegative spondyloarthropathy that affects approximately 20% of patients with psoriasis. Skin involvement precedes joint manifestations by several years. Classic clinical findings include nail pitting and sausage digits. Radiographs may show a DIP "pencil-in-cup" deformity in chronic cases, where the distal surface of the middle phalanx is eroded and the base of the distal phalanx is widened. When medical management with DMARDs is exhausted, operative treatment with osteotomy, arthroplasty, or fusion may be warranted.

E. Systemic lupus erythematosus (SLE)—Most often affects young women between the ages of 15 and 25 years. The majority of patients have a rheumatoid-like presentation of inflammatory small-joint hand arthritis. The MCP joints are characteristically deviated in the ulnar aspect and subluxed in a volar direction, although passive correction is often possible. Other potential findings in SLE include marked joint laxity, the Raynaud phenomenon, a facial butterfly rash, positive ANA, and anti-DNA antibodies. Radiographs may appear normal despite the clinical presentation. DMARDs are the mainstays of treatment. When operative intervention is necessary, arthrodesis is more reliable than arthroplasty.

F. Scleroderma (systemic sclerosis)—Hand manifestations include the Raynaud phenomenon, PIP flexion contractures, skin ulceration, fingertip pulp atrophy, and calcific deposits within the digits (calcinosis cutis). Absorption of the tufts of the distal phalanges may be seen radiographically. Periadventitial digital sympathectomy may be necessary for refractory cases of the Raynaud phenomenon. Arthrodesis is used for fixed PIP flexion contractures. Symptomatic calcific deposits may be excised. Fingertip ulcerations are best treated with limited amputation.

G. Gout—Caused by precipitation of monosodium urate crystals, which deposit in the joints and other tissues. 90% of cases occur in men. Elevated uric acid levels do not necessarily correlate with the prevalence of gouty attacks. Gout may be associated with any state of high metabolic turnover. Radiographs may show periarticular erosions and soft tissue tophi in chronic cases. The diagnosis is confirmed by joint aspiration, which shows negatively birefringent monosodium urate crystals. Acute attacks are treated with indomethacin or colchicine. Allopurinol is used for chronic prophylaxis against further attacks.

H. Calcium pyrophosphate deposition disease (CPPD, pseudogout)—Causes an acute monarticular arthritis that mimics septic arthritis. The wrist is the second most commonly affected joint. Aspiration yields positively birefringent calcium pyrophosphate dihydrate crystals. Radiographs may show chondrocalcinosis of the TFCC. Treat with high doses of NSAIDs.

XIII. Idiopathic Osteonecrosis of the Carpus

A. Kienböck disease (idiopathic osteonecrosis of the lunate)
   1. Etiology—It is more common in males between the ages of 20 and 40. This disease is rare in children, but the prognosis is better. It has a multifactorial etiology. Anatomic variability of lunate blood supply is a major factor. There are several known patterns of extraosseous and intraosseous blood supply that may increase susceptibility to repetitive microtrauma. The principal biomechanical factor is negative ulnar variance, which increases shear stress on the marginally perfused lunate. Lunate geometry and increased intraosseous pressure from venous stasis may also contribute.

TABLE 7–13 STAGES OF KIENBÖCK DISEASE

Stage	Description
I	Normal radiographs or linear fracture, abnormal but nonspecific bone scan, diagnostic appearance on magnetic resonance imaging (lunate shows low signal intensity on T1-weighted images; lunate may show high or low signal intensity on T2-weighted images, depending on extent of disease process)
II	Lunate sclerosis, one or more fracture lines with possible early collapse of lunate on radial border
III	Lunate collapse
A	Normal carpal alignment and height
B	Fixed scaphoid rotation (ring sign), carpal height decreased, capitate migrates proximally
IV	Severe lunate collapse with intra-articular degenerative changes at midcarpal joint, radiocarpal joint, or both

From Allan CH, Joshi A, Lichtman DM: Kienböck's disease: Diagnosis and treatment. J Am Acad Orthop Surg 9:128–136, 2001.

2. Diagnosis—Ulnar variance is determined with a posteroanterior view of the wrist in neutral rotation. Patients present with dorsal wrist pain, swelling, and limited range of motion. Grip strength may be markedly reduced in the later stages. Unexplained, persistent dorsal wrist pain in a young patient should prompt an MRI evaluation. The Lichtman classification is widely used (Table 7–13). Typical MRI findings in early Kienböck disease include diffuse low signal intensity throughout the lunate on T1- and T2-weighted images (Fig. 7–53). Increased signal intensity on T2-weighted images may indicate revascularization.
3. Treatment—Treatment is based on the Lichtman stage and ulnar variance. A 3-month trial of cast immobilization is appropriate for stage I disease, but the success of nonoperative treatment is limited. Operative treatment is indicated for patients who present with radiographic findings (stage II or higher) or those who fail a trial of immobilization. The first line of surgical treatment is a joint-leveling procedure. In patients with ulnar-negative variance, radial shortening with osteotomy is preferred over ulnar lengthening with a bone graft. Capitate shortening with capitohamate fusion is used for patients with ulnar-positive variance. Vascularized bone grafting has been used for stages I-IIIA. The preferred pedicle is from the 4,5 **intercompartmental supraretinacular artery** (4,5 ICSRA). The early results are encouraging, but long-term studies are still needed. Treatment of stage IIIB Kienböck disease must address the associated carpal instability. Options include scaphoid-trapezium-trapezoid (STT) fusion, scaphocapitate fusion, and a proximal row carpectomy (PRC). Stage IV disease with radiocarpal and/or midcarpal arthrosis typically requires either PRC or wrist fusion.

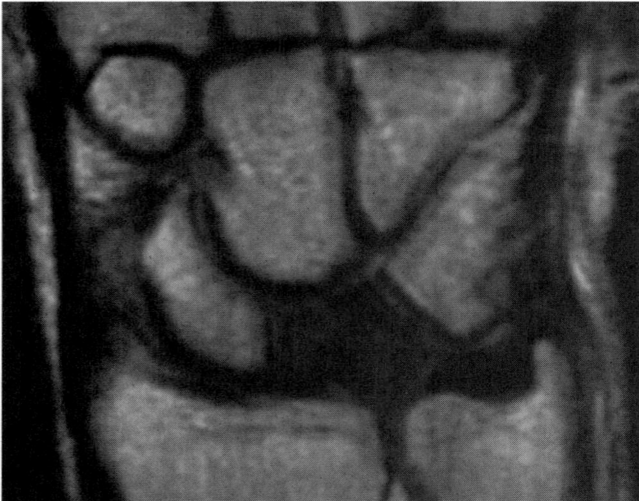

FIGURE 7–53 T1-weighted magnetic resonance image of the carpus revealing decreased signal within the lunate. (From Trumble TE, Budoff JE, Cornwall R, eds: Core Knowledge in Orthopaedics: Hand, Elbow, and Shoulder, p 179. Philadelphia, CV Mosby, 2006.)

B. Preiser disease (idiopathic osteonecrosis of the scaphoid)— This is a rare diagnosis based on radiographic evidence of sclerosis and fragmentation of the scaphoid without evidence of prior fracture. Predisposing vascular patterns have not been determined. The average age at onset is 45 years, and patients present with dorsoradial wrist pain. There is a four-stage radiographic classification similar to that developed for Kienböck disease. Preiser disease may also be classified into complete and partial involvement by MRI findings. It is first treated with cast immobilization, which is effective in only 20% of cases. Operative treatment may include drilling, curettage, allograft replacement, vascularized bone grafting, PRC, scaphoid excision, and four-corner fusion or total wrist fusion.

XIV. Dupuytren Disease

A. Introduction—Dupuytren disease is a benign fibroproliferative disorder of unclear etiology. It typically begins as a nodule in the palmar fascia and progresses insidiously to form diseased cords and finally digital flexion contractures, beginning at the MCP joint and progressing distally. The disease occurs predominantly in Caucasian males of northern European descent. Although an autosomal dominant inheritance pattern with variable penetrance is suspected, the offending gene has not been isolated, and sporadic cases are still more common. Dupuytren disease has been associated with tobacco and alcohol use, diabetes, epilepsy, chronic pulmonary disease, tuberculosis, and human immunodeficiency virus/acquired immunodeficiency syndrome (HIV/AIDS). No association with occupation has been determined.

B. Myofibroblast formation—A cytokine-mediated transformation of normal fibroblasts into myofibroblasts has been implicated in the disorder.

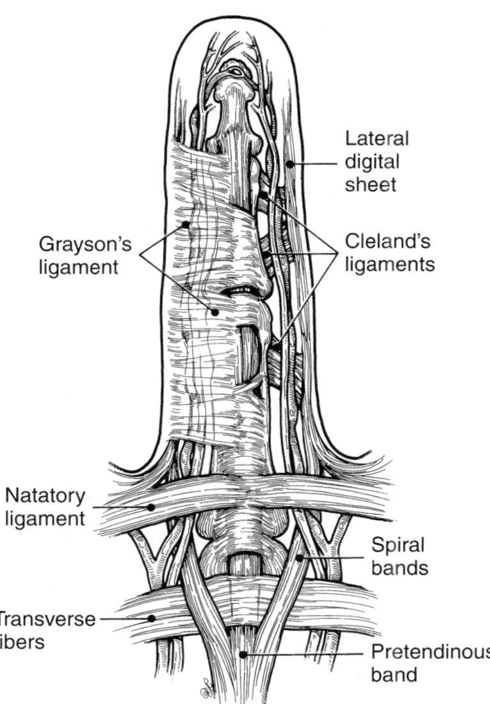

FIGURE 7–54 Parts of the normal digital fascia that become diseased. Grayson's ligament, shown on the left, is an almost continuous sheet of thin fascia in the same plane as the natatory ligament. Cleland's ligaments, shown on the right, do not become diseased. The lateral digital sheet receives fibers from the natatory ligament and the spiral bands. The spiral bands pass on either side of the metacarpophalangeal joint, deep to the neurovascular bundles, to reach the side of the finger. (From McFarlane RM: Patterns of the diseased fascia in the fingers in Dupuytren's contracture. Plast Reconstr Surg 54:31-44, 1974.)

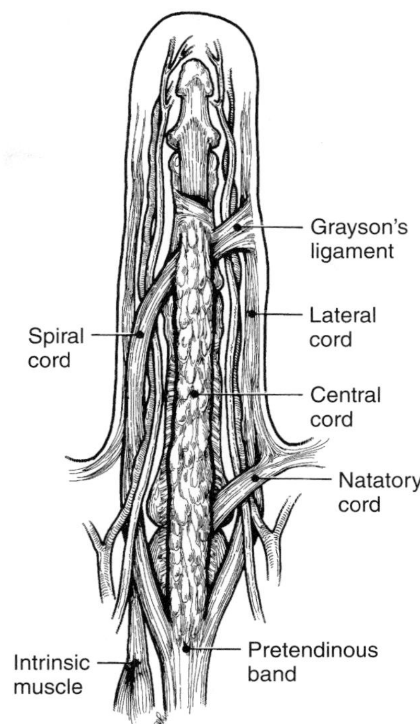

FIGURE 7–55 The change in the normal fascia bands to diseased cords. (From Green DH, Hotchkiss RM, Pederson WC, Lampert R, eds: Green's Operative Hand Surgery, 4th ed. New York, Churchill Livingstone, 1998. Courtesy of Dr. R. M. McFarlane.)

Myofibroblasts are the predominant cell type found histologically in the Dupuytren fascia, and their contractile properties are abnormal and exaggerated. There is an increase in the ratio of type III to type I collagen as well as an increase in free radical formation in the palm. Three stages of disease are recognized: proliferative, involutional, and residual.

C. Structural anomalies—Normal fascial structures that become involved in the disease process include the pretendinous band, natatory band, spiral band, Grayson ligament, retrovascular band, and lateral digital sheet (Fig. 7–54). The Cleland ligament is not involved in the disease process. Normal bands become diseased cords. The spiral cord, which leads to PIP contractures, consists of contributions from the pretendinous band, spiral band, lateral digital sheet, and Grayson ligament. Spiral cords put the neurovascular bundle at risk by displacing it more centrally and superficially as the PIP joint contracture increases. Other cords that may become diseased include the central cord, lateral cord, retrovascular cord, abductor digiti minimi cord, and intercommissural cord of the first web space (Fig. 7–55).

D. Diagnosis—Patients may present early with a tender palmar nodule or later with flexion contractures that impair simple activities of daily living. The distributions of digit involvement, in decreasing order of frequency, are the ring, small, long, thumb, and index digits. **Dupuytren diathesis** describes patients with early disease onset and rapid progression of joint contractures, often bilateral and including more radial digits. Additional extrapalmar locations may be involved, such as the dorsum of the PIP joint (Garrod knuckle pads), penis (Peyronie disease), and plantar surface of the foot (Ledderhose disease). Patients with Dupuytren diathesis should be counseled about higher recurrence rates after surgical intervention.

E. Treatment
   1. Nonsurgical options—Nonoperative treatment of Dupuytren disease is largely unsuccessful. Corticosteroid injections provide some relief of symptoms in early, localized disease or in areas of recurrence after operative treatment.
   2. Surgical treatment
      a. Indications—The indications for surgery include a positive tabletop test (the inability to place the hand flat on a tabletop), MCP flexion contracture of >30 degrees, and any PIP flexion contracture, all of which cause significant functional impairment.
      b. Procedures—Regional palmar fasciotomy of the involved digits is the procedure of

choice. Segmental aponeurectomy has been shown to be as effective as regional fasciotomy in two studies. Total palmar fasciotomy is no longer favored because it does not completely prevent recurrence and has a high complication rate. The open-palm technique of McCash may be the procedure of choice in older patients who are at high risk for stiffness. Leaving the wounds open reduces hematoma formation, decreases edema, and allows for early motion. The open-palm technique is associated with the lowest rate of complications. Dermofasciectomy is generally reserved for patients with Dupuytren diathesis or for recurrent cases. Skin deficits can be addressed with Z-plasty, V-Y advancement, full-thickness skin grafting, or healing by second intention.

c. Complications and postoperative care—The most common complication after operative treatment is recurrence, with long-term rates around 50% (higher in Dupuytren diathesis). Judicious postoperative therapy with active range of motion and splinting is critical for improved outcomes and the prevention or delay of recurrence. Early postoperative "flare reactions" are more common in women. Dorsal subluxation of the PIP joint can occur if the entire palmar plate is removed. Other potential complications include infection, digital neurovascular injury, complex regional pain syndrome, hematoma, skin loss, and amputation.

XV. Hand Tumors

A. Benign soft tissue tumors

1. Ganglion—The most common soft tissue mass of the hand and wrist. It contains either joint or tendon sheath fluid. The tissue encapsulating the fluid does not have a true epithelial lining. A traumatic etiology is suspected in many cases. Seventy percent of cases occur at the dorsal wrist, usually originating from the scapholunate articulation (Fig. 7–56). The majority of volar wrist ganglions originate from the radioscaphoid or scaphotrapezial joints (Fig. 7–57). Mucous cysts occur at the DIP joint in patients with OA, and retinacular cysts form from herniated tendon sheath fluid. The lesions are often firm and well-circumscribed and may transilluminate on physical examination. The overall recurrence rate after aspiration of ganglions is around 50%. Open excision is the surgical procedure of choice, although many dorsal ganglions can be effectively removed arthroscopically. It is critical to remove the stalk at the base of the cyst and a portion of the underlying joint capsule. Volar wrist ganglions have a higher recurrence rate, ranging from 15-20%.

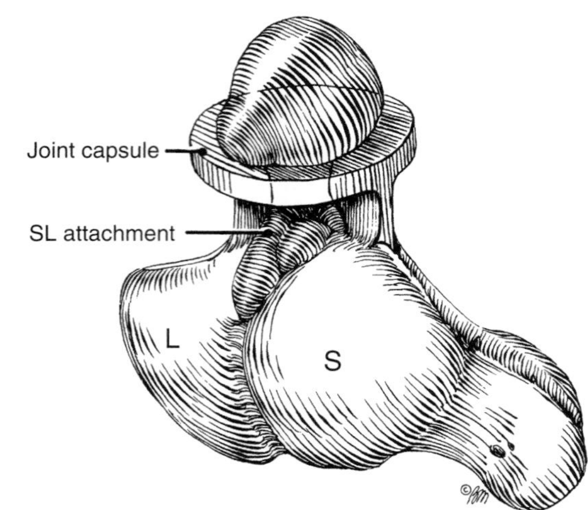

FIGURE 7–56 The ganglion and scapholunate (SL) attachments are isolated from the remaining, uninvolved joint capsule (not shown). L, lunate; S, scaphoid. (From Green DP, Hotchkiss RN, Pederson WC, Wolfe SW, eds: Green's Operative Hand Surgery, 5th ed, p 2229. Philadelphia, Churchill Livingstone, 2005.)

2. Giant cell tumor of tendon sheath—The second most common soft tissue mass of the hand. Other names include xanthoma and localized nodular synovitis. It presents as a slow-growing, nontender, multilobulated mass on the volar aspect of a digit. The mass contains multinucleated giant cells, xanthoma cells, and hemosiderin deposits. Treatment is through marginal excision. In contrast to a single tumor, lesions with multiple discrete tumors are associated with a higher recurrence rate, as high as 50% in some series.
3. Lipoma—Extremely common tumor of adipose cell origin. Though usually painless, they may reach substantial size over time. Lipomas in the palm may compress the carpal tunnel or the Guyon canal, leading to neurologic deficits. MRI may be helpful for preoperative planning in these cases. The lesions have the same bright signal characteristics as subcutaneous fat on T1-weighted images. Symptomatic lipomas are treated with marginal excision and have a low recurrence rate.
4. Epidermal inclusion cyst—A common, painless, slow-growing mass arising from a penetrating

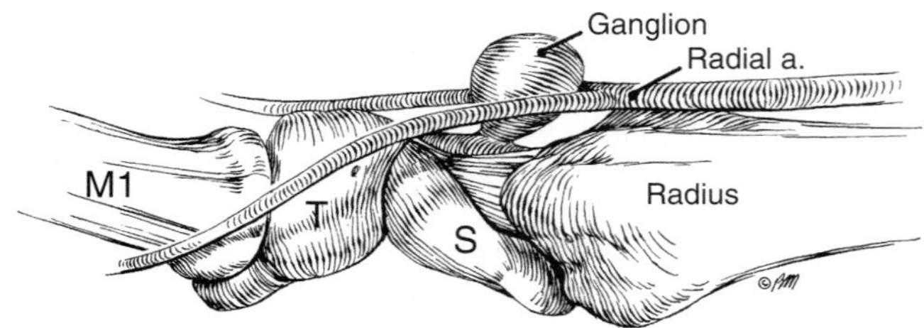

FIGURE 7–57 The usual relationship of the ganglion to the radial artery and volar joint capsule. S, scaphoid; T, trapezium; M1, first metacarpal. (From Green DP, Hotchkiss RN, Pederson WC, Wolfe SW, eds: Green's Operative Hand Surgery, 5th ed, p 2232. Philadelphia, Churchill Livingstone, 2005.)

injury that drives keratinizing epithelium into subcutaneous tissues. Curative treatment is with marginal excision.

5. Neurolemmoma (schwannoma)—The most common peripheral nerve tumor of the upper extremity. It presents with a painless mass, positive Tinel sign, and normal neurologic examination. The cell of origin is the myelin-forming Schwann cell. The tumor is composed of Antoni A (cellular) and Antoni B (matrix) regions. Treatment is with marginal excision. Because these tumors are eccentric and encapsulated, they can be shelled out of the nerve without disrupting the axons. Neurologic injury is seen in less than 5% of cases, and the recurrence rate is low.
6. Neurofibroma—Slow-growing, painless mass that arises from nerve fascicles. Although neurofibroma is known to occur more frequently in patients with neurofibromatosis, it may be solitary in the hand and wrist. A portion of the nerve is usually sacrificed during surgical excision, and grafting may be required.
7. Glomus tumor—Smooth muscle tumor of perivascular temperature–regulating bodies. It usually occurs in the subungual region of the hand and may cause nail ridging and erosions of the distal phalanx. The tumor is characterized by exquisite pain and cold intolerance. MRI with gadolinium is a helpful adjunctive diagnostic study. Treatment is with marginal excision, and the recurrence rate is low.
8. Hemangioma—Vascular proliferations that can be divided into capillary (superficial) and cavernous (deep) lesions. Many infantile hemangiomas become involuted by age 7, and those that arise during childhood are observed. Kasabach-Merritt syndrome is a rare complication resulting from entrapped platelets and a potentially fatal coagulopathy. In adults, MRI with gadolinium may help distinguish these benign vascular tumors from arteriovenous malformations and angiosarcomas. If the lesion is small and accessible, the treatment is with marginal excision. Embolization may be more feasible alternative for larger lesions.
9. Pyogenic granuloma—Rapidly growing, pedunculated lesion with friable tissue that bleeds easily. It is considered to be a disorder of angiogenesis and not of infectious or traumatic etiology. Treatment is with marginal excision.

B. Malignant soft tissue tumors

1. Squamous cell carcinoma (SCC)—The most common malignancy of the hand is squamous cell carcinoma. It is usually seen in elderly men with premalignant conditions such as actinokeratosis or chronic osteomyelitis. The primary risk factor is excessive exposure to ultraviolet radiation. SCC is also the most common subungual malignancy. It has a higher metastatic potential than basal cell carcinoma. Treatment is with wide excision or Mohs micrographic surgery. Lymph node biopsy may be necessary.
2. Sarcoma—The most common sarcomas are epithelioid and synovial. Other common sarcomas of the upper extremity include liposarcoma and malignant fibrous histiocytoma. Most soft tissue sarcomas metastasize to the lungs. Lymph nodes are the second most common area.
   a. Epithelioid sarcoma—Firm, slow-growing mass presenting in young to middle-aged adults. It may be located in the digits, palm, or forearm and may eventually ulcerate and drain. The mass commonly spreads to regional lymph nodes. MRI may help characterize the extent of the tumor. Histologically, the sarcoma is composed of malignant epithelial cells and central areas of necrosis. Treatment is with wide or radical excision accompanied by sentinel lymph node biopsy. Adjuvant chemotherapy or radiation therapy may be considered but remains somewhat controversial for this tumor.
   b. Synovial sarcoma—Firm, slow-growing mass that usually forms adjacent to the carpus. It also occurs in young to middle-aged adults. The mass is composed of epithelial and spindle cells with multiple histologic patterns. Treatment is with wide or radical excision, with 5-year survival rates of approximately 80%. More recently, adjuvant chemotherapy and external beam radiation have proven successful in reducing local recurrence rates.

C. Benign bone tumors

1. Enchondroma—The most common benign bone tumor of the upper extremity. It typically occurs in the second to fourth decades, and most cases are asymptomatic and discovered incidentally. The tumor arises from the metaphyseal medullary canal and spreads to the diaphysis. It is usually seen in the proximal phalanx and metacarpal (Fig. 7–58). Enchondroma causes symmetrical fusiform expansion of bone, with endosteal scalloping and intramedullary calcifications. It may present as a pathologic fracture. Histologically, enchondroma of the hand is characterized by benign cartilage of high cellularity. If mitotic figures are present, low-grade chondrosarcoma should be suspected. The recommended treatment is with curettage and bone grafting. Excision, intramedullary internal fixation, and bone cementing have also been successful in a small series.
2. Osteochondroma—Benign cartilage tumor characterized by a bony surface outgrowth capped by cartilage. It is rarely seen in the hand, except in multiple hereditary exostosis. The distal aspect of the proximal phalanx is the most common location of involvement in the hand. Malignant transformation of a hand osteochondroma has never been described. Asymptomatic lesions are observed.
3. Osteoid osteoma—May present with swelling without pain in the hand. It is usually found in

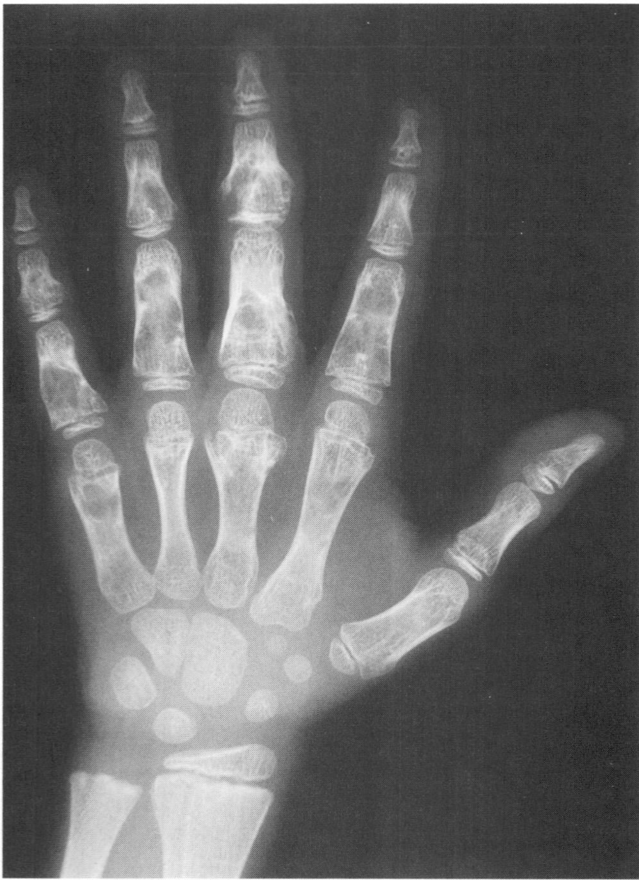

FIGURE 7–58 Multiple enchondromas (Ollier disease). (From Green DP, Hotchkiss RN, Pederson WC, Wolfe SW, eds: Green's Operative Hand Surgery, 5th ed, p 2250. Philadelphia, Churchill Livingstone, 2005.)

the carpus (scaphoid) and proximal phalanx. Diagnosis is made after identification of a radiolucent nidus within a sclerotic lesion. When nonoperative management fails, excision of the nidus is curative. Radiofrequency ablation may also be used effectively.

4. Unicameral bone cyst—Common tumor in children. It is occasionally seen in the metacarpals and phalanges or the metaphyseal distal radius. Most of these cysts resolve spontaneously. Treatment is with aspiration and injection of methylprednisolone acetate.
5. Giant cell tumor—Characterized as benign but may be locally aggressive. It is more common in young to middle-aged women and presents with pain, swelling, and occasionally pathologic fracture. The distal radius is the most common site of occurrence. An eccentric, lytic lesion is seen in the metaphysis and epiphysis. Cortical destruction and an associated soft tissue mass are not unusual. Osteoclast-like, multinucleated giant cells are abundant on histologic examination, and their nuclei match those of the surrounding stromal cells. Treatment with wide excision is preferred because curettage alone yields a high local recurrence rate. Packing the lesion with polymethylmethacrylate has been successful. Joint preservation is paramount. The distal radius must be occasionally reconstructed by using an allograft or a vascularized free fibula.

D. Malignant bone tumors—The most common hand malignancy is metastatic lung carcinoma, which is usually seen in the distal phalanx. The next most common primary sites of disease metastasizing to the hand are from the breast or kidney. Acral metastasis is a poor prognostic sign, with less than 6-month survival expected at the time of discovery. The three most common primary malignant bone tumors of the hand and wrist are chondrosarcoma, osteosarcoma, and Ewing sarcoma. When they occur, the most common sites are the phalanges and metacarpals. Treatment for each tumor is the same as their treatment elsewhere in the body.

XVI. Hand Infections

A. Introduction—Hand infections can involve any tissue type and a variety of pathogens (Table 7–14). *Staphylococcus aureus* is the most common pathogen, involved in 50-80% of all hand infections. *Streptococcus* organisms are the second most common. Gram-negative and anaerobic bacteria are seen in intravenous drug abusers, diabetics, and patients with farmyard injuries or bite wounds. Community-acquired, **methicillin-resistant *S. aureus*** (MRSA) is becoming more prevalent.

B. Paronychia/eponychia—The most common infections in the hand, infecting the nail fold and usually caused by *S. aureus*. They are treated by incision and drainage and partial or total nail plate removal, oral antibiotics, soaks, and dressing changes. It is important to preserve the eponychial fold by placing the old nail or nonadherent gauze between the skin and nail bed after débridement. Chronic cases in which oral antibiotic therapy fails are often secondary to *Candida albicans* and occur more commonly in diabetics. In rare cases marsupialization (excision of the dorsal eponychium) may be required to eradicate the infection.

C. Felon—Infection of the septated fingertip pulp. *S. aureus* is the most common pathogen. It is treated by incision and drainage through a midlateral incision and appropriate antibiotics. It is important to break up the septa to adequately decompress the fingertip; otherwise, local compartment syndrome can occur. Digital incisions are usually placed in the ulnar aspect, except for in the thumb and small digit, where they are placed in the radial aspect (Fig. 7–59). The incision should be left open and a change of dressing performed. Delayed diagnosis and treatment may lead to concurrent flexor tenosynovitis, osteomyelitis, or digital tip necrosis.

D. Human bite—Potentially serious infection treated promptly with incision and drainage, especially if a joint or tendon sheath is violated. It most commonly involves the third or fourth MCP joint (fight bite). Radiographs are mandatory to rule out fracture. The most frequently isolated

TABLE 7-14 HAND INFECTIONS

Type	Location	Pathogen	Antibiotic	Comment
Paronychia	Eponychium	*Staphylococcus aureus*	Dicloxacillin or clindamycin PO Nafcillin IV	Release eponychial fold May require nail removal
Felon	Pulp space	*S. aureus*	Dicloxacillin or clindamycin PO Nafcillin IV	Release all septa Volar incision preferred
Human bite	MCP and PIP	*Streptococcus* sp. *S. aureus* *Eikenella corrodens*	Ampicillin/sulbactam IV Penicillin for *E. corrodens*	Treatment failure with cephalosporins usually due to *E. corrodens*
Dog and cat bites	Varied	α-Hemolytic streptococci (46%) *Pasteurella multocida* (26%) *S. aureus* (13%) Anaerobes (41%)	Ampicillin/sulbactam IV or amoxicillin-clavulanic acid PO	Failure of oral treatment common
Necrotizing fasciitis	Varied	*Clostridia* Group A β-streptococci	Broad-spectrum triple antibiotic—penicillin, clindamycin, gentamicin	32% mortality Amputations frequent
Fungal	Cutaneous	*Candida albicans*	Topical antifungal	Common in diabetics with chronic paronychia
	Nail	*Trichophyton rubrum*	Ketoconazole or itraconazole PO	Pulse dosing 1 week per month
	Subcutaneous	*Sporothrix schenckii* *Mycoplasma* sp.	Based on culture	

IV, intravenously; MCP, metacarpophalangeal; PIP, proximal interphalangeal; PO, orally.

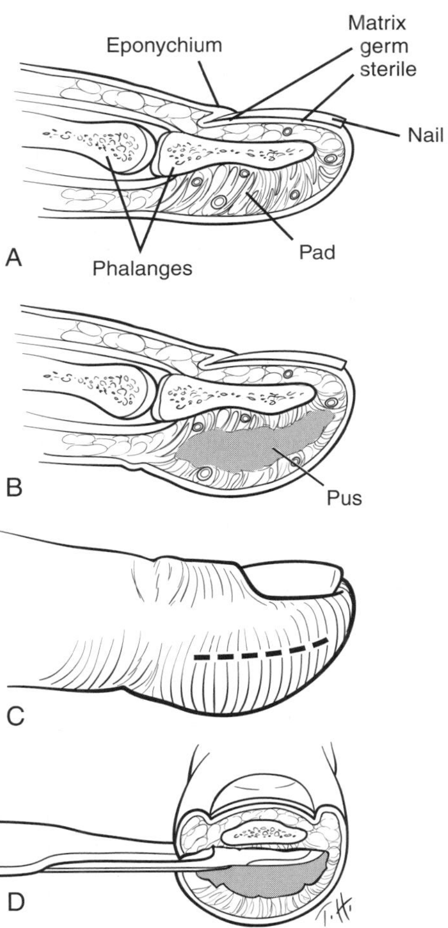

FIGURE 7–59 **A**, Cross section of the distal fingertip showing the septated anatomy of the pad. **B**, Collection of pus within the finger pulp space. **C**, Incision for drainage of felon. **D**, The incision should include all of the involved septal compartments. (From Green DP, Hotchkiss RN, Pederson WC, Wolfe SW, eds: Green's Operative Hand Surgery, 5th ed, p 61. Philadelphia, Churchill Livingstone, 2005.)

organisms are group A streptococcus and *S. aureus*. *Eikenella corrodens* and *Bacteroides* species must also be considered. The empirical antibiotics of choice are intravenous ampicillin/sulbactam and oral amoxicillin/clavulanate.

E. Dog and cat bites—Potentially serious injuries often requiring incision and drainage. Pure cellulitis is treated with splinting, elevation, soaks, and intravenous antibiotics. The frequency of various isolates is as follows: α-hemolytic streptococcus, 46%; anaerobes, 41%; *Pasteurella multocida*, 26%; and *S. aureus*, 13%. Ampicillin/sulbactam and amoxicillin/clavulanate are the empirical antibiotics of choice.

F. Pyogenic flexor tenosynovitis (FTS)—Infection of the flexor tendon sheath may occur in a delayed fashion after penetrating trauma. *S. aureus* is the most common pathogen. The four classic clinical signs have been described by **Kanavel**: (1) flexed, resting posture of the involved digit; (2) fusiform swelling of the digit; (3) tenderness of the flexor tendon sheath; and (4) pain with passive digit extension. If the infection is recognized early, the patient should be admitted and treated with splinting and intravenous antibiotics. If the signs improve within the first 24 hours, surgery may be avoided. Otherwise, the treatment of choice is incision and drainage and intravenous antibiotics. The flexor tendon sheath can be irrigated through small incisions placed distally (open A5 pulley) and proximally (open A1 pulley). Alternatively, a long midlateral incision can be used (Fig. 7–60). Continuous-drip irrigation with an indwelling catheter carries a risk for compartment syndrome. Index and thumb FTS can spread to the deep thenar space; long, ring, and small-finger FTS can spread to the midpalmar space; and small-finger FTS can also spread to the ulnar bursa. The classic "horseshoe abscess" is based on proximal

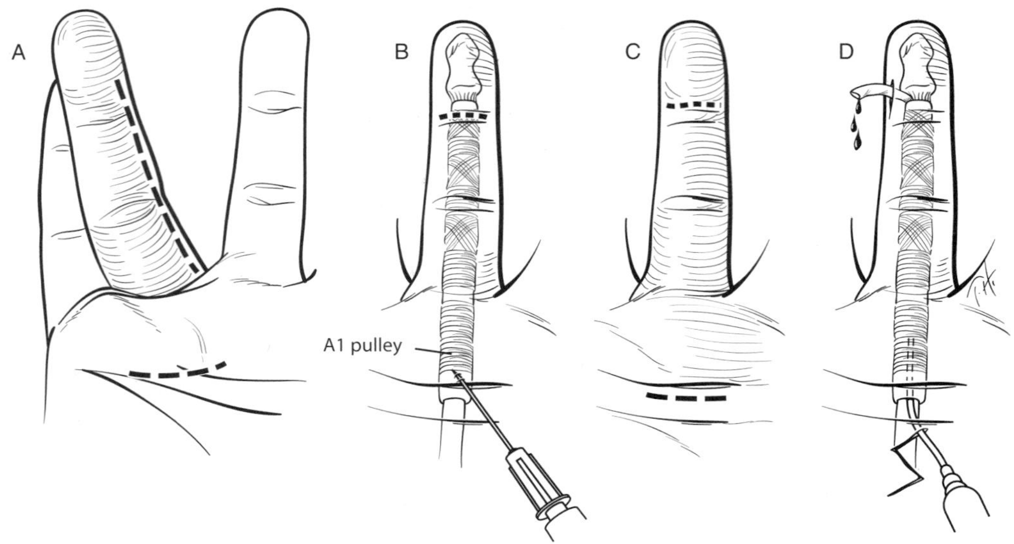

FIGURE 7–60 Incision for drainage of tendon sheath infections. **A**, Open drainage incisions through the midaxial approach. **B**, Sheath irrigation with distal opening of the sheath and proximal syringe irrigation. **C**, Incisions for intermittent through-and-through irrigation. **D**, Technique for closed tendon sheath irrigation. (From Green DP, Hotchkiss RN, Pederson WC, Wolfe SW, eds: Green's Operative Hand Surgery, 5th ed, p 67. Philadelphia, Churchill Livingstone, 2005.)

communication between the thumb and small-finger flexor tendon sheaths in the Parona space, a potential space between the PQ and FDP tendons. Aggressive postoperative hand therapy is paramount in order to prevent adhesions and digit stiffness.

G. Herpetic whitlow—Caused by herpes simplex virus (HSV) type. 1. It occurs with increasing frequency in dental hygienists and health care workers. This infection is also common in toddlers. It presents with digit pain and erythema and is followed by the formation of small vesicles that may coalesce into bullae. Herpetic whitlow may be accompanied by fever, malaise, and lymphadenitis. The diagnosis is confirmed by a Tzanck smear and antibody titers. The process is self-limiting, usually resolving in 7-10 days. Incision and drainage are not recommended because the rates of secondary bacterial infection are high. Treatment with acyclovir may shorten the duration of symptoms. Recurrence may be stimulated by fever, stress, and/or sun exposure.

H. Deep potential-space infections—A collar button abscess occurs in the web space between digits. It is treated by incision and drainage with volar and dorsal incisions (avoiding the skin in the web itself) and intravenous antibiotics. Midpalmar space infections are rare. Clinically, there is a loss of midline contour of the hand, and palmar pain elicited with flexion of the long, ring, and small fingers. Thenar and hypothenar space infections are also rare. They present with pain and swelling over their respective areas, which are exacerbated by flexion of the thumb or small finger. Incision and drainage and intravenous antibiotics are required for all of these deep potential-space infections (Fig. 7–61).

I. Necrotizing fasciitis—Severe infection with devastating outcomes when treatment is delayed. Group A β-hemolytic streptococcus is the most common organism. Suspicion should be raised in immunocompromised patients (those with diabetes, cancer, or AIDS) as well as alcoholics and intravenous drug abusers. This infection requires emergent, radical débridement and broad-spectrum intravenous antibiotic coverage that includes penicillin, clindamycin, metronidazole, and an aminoglycoside. Intraoperative findings may include liquefied subcutaneous fat, dishwater pus, muscle necrosis, and venous thrombosis. Hemodynamic monitoring is urgent. Amputation may be necessary. The mortality rate is high and correlates with the time to treatment.

J. Gas gangrene—Caused by *Clostridium perfringens* and other *Clostridium* species (gram-positive rods). This condition occurs in devitalized, contaminated wounds and leads to myonecrosis. Extensive surgical débridement is necessary to prevent systemic infection.

K. Fungal infection—Serious infection usually seen in immunocompromised patients. The areas of infection are divided into cutaneous, subcutaneous, and deep locations.
   1. Cutaneous infection—Chronic infection of the nail fold is usually caused by *C. albicans* and is treated with topical antifungal agents and nail marsupialization. **Onychomycosis** is a destructive, deforming infection of the nail plate that is usually caused by *Trichophyton rubrum*. This infection is also treated with topical antifungal agents; systemic therapy with griseofulvin or ketoconazole may be necessary in recalcitrant cases.
   2. Subcutaneous infection—Subcutaneous infections are usually caused by *Sporothrix schenckii*, which follows penetrating injury while handling plants or soil (the rose thorn is the classic

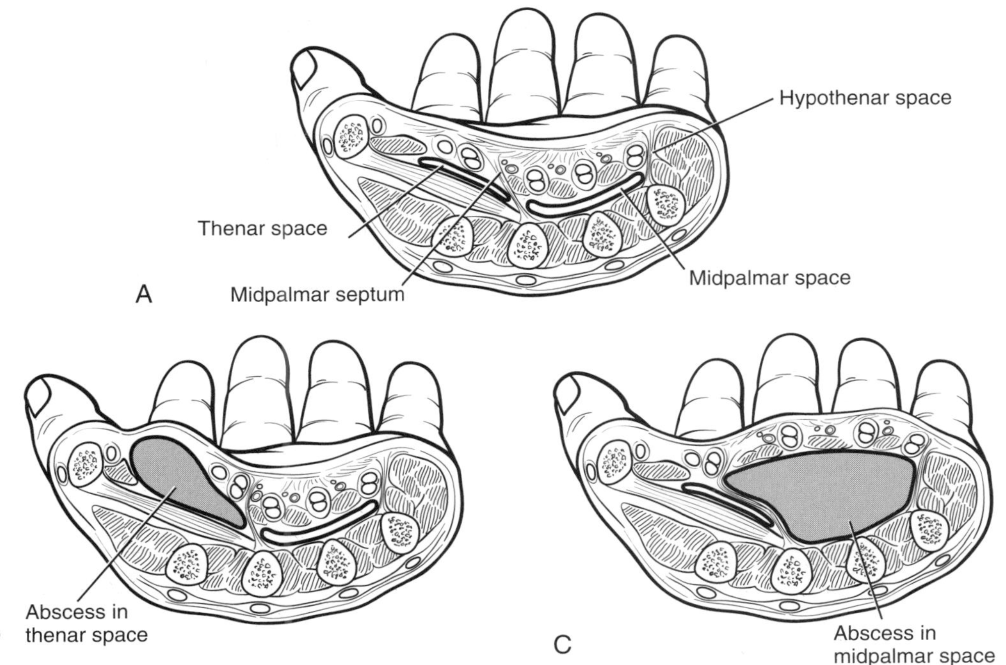

FIGURE 7–61 Deep palmar spaces. **A**, Potential spaces of the midpalm. **B**, Thenar space abscess. **C**, Midpalmar space abscess. (From Green DP, Hotchkiss RN, Pederson WC, Wolfe SW, eds: Green's Operative Hand Surgery, 5th ed, p 71. Philadelphia, Churchill Livingstone, 2005.)

vehicle of transmission). It starts with a papule at the site of inoculation, with subsequent lesions developing along the lymphatic vessels. Treatment is with potassium iodine solution.

3. Deep infection—Several forms of deep infection exist, including tenosynovitis, septic arthritis, and osteomyelitis. Treatment involves surgical débridement and culture-specific antifungal agents. Endemic pathogens include histoplasmosis, blastomycosis, and coccidioidomycosis. Opportunistic infections include aspergillosis, candidiasis, mucormycosis, and cryptococcosis.

L. Atypical mycobacterial infections—These organisms are widely distributed in the environment but are infrequent human pathogens. When they do infect humans, they are often indolent and fail to respond to usual treatments. The most common organisms include *Mycobacterium marinum, M. kansasii, M. terrae*, and *M. avium-intracellulare complex*. Musculoskeletal manifestations involve the wrist and hand in 50% of cases. *M. marinum* proliferates in freshwater and saltwater enclosures. *M. kansasii* and *M. terrae* are found in soil. *M. avium-intracellulare complex* is found in soil, water, and poultry and is the most frequently isolated organism in terminal AIDS patients. The diagnosis is based on biopsy for histopathology. Granulomas are common. Cultures and sensitivities are critical and require a special medium (Lowenstein-Jensen) at exact temperatures (32° C). A chest radiograph is mandatory to rule out hematogenous spread. Treatment generally requires surgical débridement and a culture-specific antibiotic such as rifampin, ethambutol, or tetracycline.

M. HIV and hand infections—The virulence of the offending organisms is enhanced by the immunocompromised state. The following organisms are frequent isolates: HSV, cytomegalovirus (CMV), *Candida, Cryptococcus, Histoplasma, Aspergillus*, and *Mycobacterium*. HSV is the most common hand infection in AIDS patients.

XVII. Congenital Hand Differences

A. Introduction—The limb bud appears during the fourth week of gestation. The hand begins as a paddle, with digital separation occurring between 47 and 54 days. Development of the lower limb lags behind by 48 hours. Congenital hand anomalies occur at a rate of 1 in 600 live births. The following broad classification scheme is widely used.

Failure of formation
Failure of differentiation
Duplication
Overgrowth
Undergrowth
Amnion disruption sequence
Generalized skeletal abnormalities

In general, surgical intervention to correct congenital hand differences should be performed before the child establishes compensatory mechanisms and before starting school. Cosmetic appearance should not be improved at the cost of further functional impairment. Early genetic counseling is a critical part of the care of a child with congenital hand differences in the setting of other extraskeletal anomalies.

B. Failure of formation
   1. Transverse absence—These deformities, also termed congenital amputations, usually occur at the proximal forearm level and are typically not part of a syndrome. The majority are unilateral and are thought to be the result of vascular insult to the **apical ectodermal ridge** (AER). Early prosthetic fitting is the treatment of choice.
   2. Longitudinal absence
      a. Radial dysplasia—Characterized by deficiency of the radius and radial carpal structures (Fig. 7–62). Thumb dysplasia is included in the spectrum of presentation (to be covered in the section on Undergrowth). Both extremities are affected in over 50% of cases. Associated systemic syndromes include Holt-Oram syndrome, thrombocytopenia with absent radius (TAR), Fanconi anemia, and VACTERL syndrome (**v**ertebral, **a**nal, **c**ardiac, **t**racheal, **e**sophageal, **r**enal, and **l**imb anomalies). Type I manifests a short radius with both physes present, type II has a hypoplastic radius, type III a partially absent radius, and type IV is characterized by total radial aplasia. Early therapy to preserve passive range of motion is critical. If adequate elbow range of motion is present, a centralization procedure to realign the carpus on the distal ulna may be attempted when the child is between 6 and 12 months of age.
      b. Ulnar dysplasia—Characterized by deficiency of the ulna or ulnar carpal structures. This type of dysplasia is tenfold less common than its radial counterpart and is not associated with systemic syndromes. Additional hand anomalies, such as digit absence and syndactyly, are prevalent. Elbow abnormalities are frequently evident. Other musculoskeletal anomalies, including proximal femoral focal deficiency, fibula deficiency, phocomelia, and scoliosis, are also common. Type I is characterized by a small ulna with both physes present. Types II and III relate to partial or complete absence of the ulna. Type IV includes radiohumeral synostosis. General clinical considerations include the position of the hand, function of the thumb, stability of the elbow, and presence of syndactyly. The condition of the thumb is the most important determinant of surgical intervention in ulnar dysplasia.
      c. Cleft hand—The true cleft hand is often bilateral and familial, involves the feet, and has associated absent metacarpals, differentiating it from symbrachydactyly. The severity of this anomaly varies widely from a cleft between the middle and ring fingers to absent radial digits and syndactyly of the ulnar digits. Cleft closure and thumb web construction are the top priorities. Syndactyly should be released early. Thumb reconstruction may require web space deepening, tendon transfer, rotational osteotomy, and/or toe-to-hand transfer. Web deepening should not precede cleft closure because it may compromise the flaps for cleft closure. Transverse bones should be removed because they widen the cleft as the child grows.

C. Failure of differentiation
   1. Radioulnar synostosis—The finding of bony bridging between the radius and ulna is bilateral in 60% of cases. Examination reveals a fixed pronation deformity. The radius is wide and bowed,

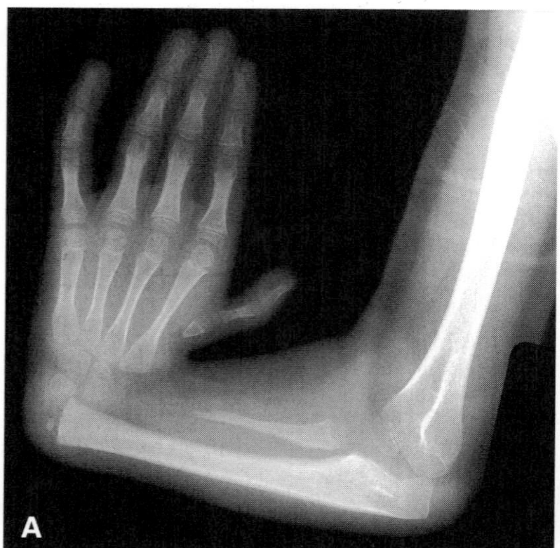

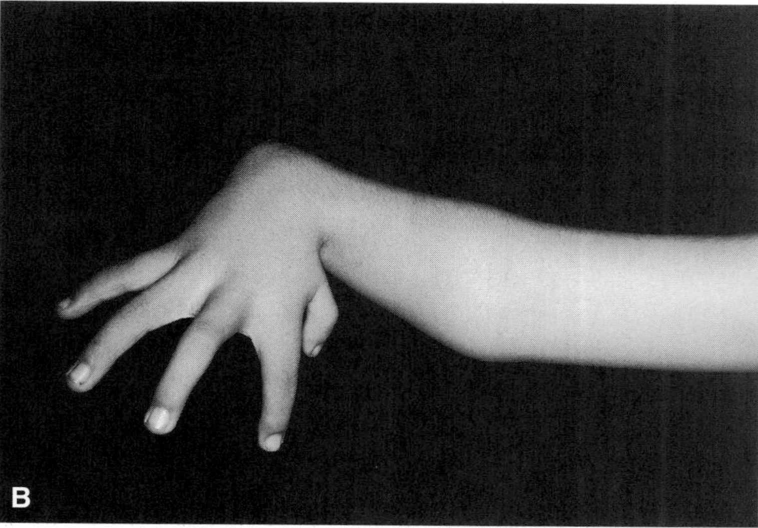

FIGURE 7–62 An 8-year-old child with Holt-Oram syndrome whose cardiac problems precluded earlier surgery. **A** and **B**, The deformity from his type 3 radius deficiency was too severe for single-stage centralization. (From Green DP, Hotchkiss RN, Pederson WC, Wolfe SW, eds: Green's Operative Hand Surgery, 5th ed, p 1473. Philadelphia, Churchill Livingstone, 2005.)

whereas the ulna is narrow and straight. If a significant pronation deformity exists, a rotational osteotomy may be done at about age 5.

2. Symphalangism (congenital digital stiffness)—Hereditary symphalangism is autosomal dominant and associated with correctable hearing loss. It is more common in the ulnar digits. Nonhereditary symphalangism is seen in conjunction with syndactyly, Apert syndrome, and Poland syndrome. The appearance and function of the digits may be improved by angular osteotomies toward the end of adolescent growth.
3. Camptodactyly (congenital digital flexion deformity)—Classically occurs at the small-finger PIP joint.
   - Type I is seen in infancy and affects the sexes equally; it responds to splinting and stretching.
   - Type II is seen in adolescent girls. The deformity results from either abnormal lumbrical insertion or an abnormal FDS origin and/or insertion. If full PIP extension can be achieved actively with the MCP held in flexion and there are no profound secondary radiographic changes, the digit can be explored and the abnormal tendon transferred to the radial lateral band.
   - Type III camptodactyly involves multiple digits with more severe flexion contractures and is usually associated with a syndrome.

   In general, nonoperative treatment is favored for all three types. If a functional deficit exists after skeletal maturity, corrective osteotomy may improve alignment and function.
4. Clinodactyly (congenital curvature of the digit in the radioulnar plane)
   - Type 1 clinodactyly is the most common, with minor angulation and normal digit length present.
   - Type II clinodactyly is present in 25% of the children with Down syndrome and is characterized by minor angulation and a short phalanx.
   - In type III clinodactyly there is marked angulation and a delta phalanx. The delta phalanx has a C-shaped epiphysis and a longitudinally bracketed diaphysis. Early excision is performed when the delta phalanx is a separate bone and the involved digit is excessively long. Otherwise, an opening wedge osteotomy may help correct the angulation.
5. Flexed thumb—The two main causes are congenital trigger thumb and congenital clasped thumb.
   a. Congenital trigger thumb—A congenital trigger thumb involves flexion at the IP joint. Most cases resolve spontaneously. Persistent trigger thumbs are treated with A1 pulley release when the child is between 6 and 12 months old.
   b. Congenital clasped thumb—A congenital clasped thumb results in deficient active thumb extension and slight limitation of passive extension. Supple clasped thumbs are usually caused by weak or absent EPL and EPB muscles and are treated with tendon transfers. The rigid variety is associated with hypoplastic extensors, MCP joint contractures, UCL deficiency, thenar muscle hypoplasia, and inadequate skin in the first web space. Complex cases may require any or all of the following: capsular release of the MCP or CMC joints; muscular release of the adductor pollicis, FPB, or first dorsal interosseous; Z-lengthening of the FPL; extensor or opposition tendon transfer; and/or deepening of the first web space.
6. Arthrogryposis (congenital curved joints)—Results from a defect in the motor unit and may be either neurogenic (90%) or myopathic (10%). Immobility in the womb results in symmetrical joint contractures. Arthrogryposis is classified into three types.
   - In type I arthrogryposis there is a single localized deformity such as forearm pronation or a complex clasped thumb. Surgical correction of an isolated deformity is often possible.
   - Type II arthrogryposis is characterized by full expression of the disorder, causing absence of shoulder musculature; thin, tubular limbs; elbow extension contractures; wrist flexion; and ulnar deviation contractures, finger flexion contractures, and thumb adduction contractures.
   - Type III arthrogryposis manifests the constellation of type II joint contractures along with polydactyly and involvement of other organ systems.

   Types II and III are treated with a combination of splinting, serial casts, and therapy to decrease the severity of joint contractures. Once passive joint mobility is restored, tendon transfers may be performed. An attempt is made to provide the child with functional elbows and wrists; however, arthrodesis may provide an improved ability to perform activities of daily living.
7. Syndactyly—The most common congenital hand anomaly (1 in 2500 live births) results from failure of apoptosis to separate the digits. It is classified based on the absence (simple) or presence (complex) of bony connections between the involved digits and whether the bony connections are complete or incomplete (Fig. 7–63). Acrosyndactyly refers to fusion between the more distal portions of the digit by proximal fenestration, often seen in constriction ring syndrome. Pure syndactyly is autosomal dominant, with reduced penetrance and variable expression that yield a positive family history in 10-40% of cases. The distribution of digit involvement is thumb-index (5%),

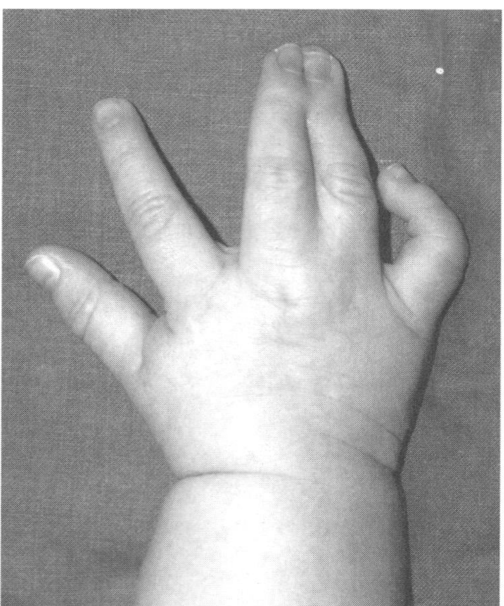

FIGURE 7–63 Simple and complete syndactyly between third and fourth rays. (From Green DP, Hotchkiss RN, Pederson WC, Wolfe SW, eds: Green's Operative Hand Surgery, 5th ed, p 1382. Philadelphia, Churchill Livingstone, 2005.)

index-long (15%), long-ring (50%), and ring-small (30%). In general, release of the digits is performed at around 1 year of age. Rays of unequal length should be released before 6 months. Cases of acrosyndactyly require distal release in the neonatal period. Syndactyly releases are performed in two stages, with only one side of the digit released during one operation, in order to preserve circulation of the digit. Full-thickness skin grafting is invariably required after full release is completed. Possible complications include web creep and nail deformities. Poland and Apert syndromes are commonly tested conditions that include syndactyly.

D. Duplication

1. Preaxial polydactyly (thumb duplication)—This congenital condition has been classified by Wassel (Table 7–15). Type IV is the most common (43%) and is characterized by a duplicated proximal phalanx (Fig. 7–64). Thumb duplication is usually unilateral, sporadic, and not associated with a syndrome

TABLE 7-15 PREAXIAL POLYDACTYLY THUMB CLASSIFICATION

Type	Description	Frequency
I	Bifid distal phalanx	2%
II	Duplicated distal phalanx	15%
III	Bifid proximal phalanx	6%
IV	Duplicated proximal phalanx	43% (most common)
V	Bifid metacarpal	10%
VI	Duplicated metacarpal	4%
VII	Triphalangia	20%

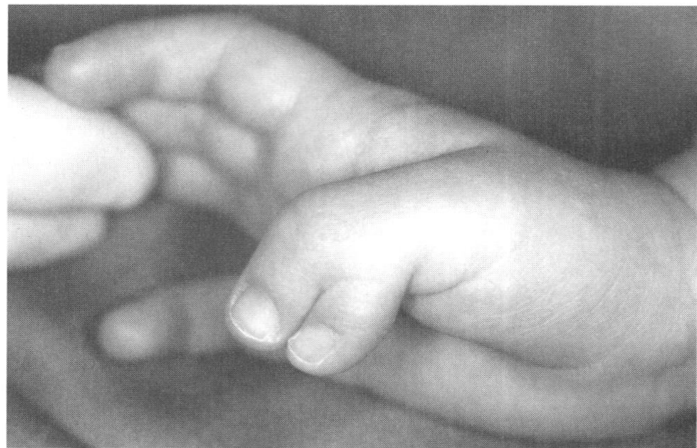

FIGURE 7–64 Type IV duplication with duplicated proximal and distal phalanges that articulate with a bifid metacarpal head. (Courtesy of Shriners Hospitals for Children, Philadelphia.)

except in type VII. Type VII associations include Holt-Oram syndrome, Fanconi anemia, Blackfan-Diamond anemia, hypoplastic anemia, imperforate anus, cleft palate, and tibial defects. The best possible thumb is reconstructed from the available anatomic structures. When duplicate thumbs of equal size are present, the radial thumb is removed. Reconstruction of all components is usually performed in one stage.

2. Postaxial polydactyly (small-finger duplication)—Type A is a well-formed duplicated digit, and type B is a rudimentary skin tag. This disorder is 10 times more common in African Americans than Caucasians. Associated anomalies are rare in African Americans because the condition is inherited as an autosomal dominant trait. However, in Caucasians a thorough genetic workup is mandatory because virtually every body system and 17 chromosomal abnormalities have been discovered. Vestigial digits are either tied off in the nursery or amputated before 1 year of age. The type A digit is managed by preservation of the radial digit and appropriate augmentation of soft tissue structures from the ulnar digit.

3. Central polydactyly—Usually associated with syndactyly. Early surgery is indicated to prevent angular deformity with growth. Impaired motion may result from interposed digits or symphalangism of adjacent digits. The tendons, nerves, and vessels may be shared to the point that only one finger from three skeletons may be obtainable. Angular deviation may require ligament reconstruction, osteotomy, or both.

E. Overgrowth

1. Macrodactyly—Characterized by nonhereditary congenital digital enlargement. Ninety percent of cases are unilateral, and 70% of cases involve multiple digits. The adult analogue is lipofibromatous hamartoma of the median nerve. Angular deviation, joint stiffness, and nerve compression syndromes also occur.

Static macrodactyly is present at birth, and growth is linear with the adjacent digits. Progressive macrodactyly is not always evident at birth, but exponential growth occurs thereafter. The most favorable outcome for a severely affected single digit is amputation. When the thumb or multiple digits are involved, the following procedures may offer improvement: epiphyseal ablation, angular and/or shortening osteotomies, longitudinal narrowing osteotomies, nerve stripping, and debulking. Stiffness and neurovascular compromise are common.

F. Undergrowth

1. Thumb hypoplasia—This congenital difference has been classified by Blauth (Table 7–16). The critical structure is the CMC joint. Type I manifests a smaller thumb with slender bones and normal thenar musculature and typically requires no treatment. Types II and IIIA are treated with stabilization of the MCP joint UCL, web deepening, and extrinsic extensor tendon reconstruction. Types IIIB-V are best treated with pollicization.

G. Amnion disruption sequence (constriction ring syndrome)—Sporadic occurrence with no evidence of hereditary predisposition. It is manifested in four ways: (1) simple constriction rings, (2) rings with distal deformity with or without lymphedema, (3) acrosyndactyly, and (4) amputation. Neonatal surgery is indicated when edema jeopardizes digital circulation. Release is accomplished by multiple circumferential Z-plasty. Acrosyndactyly is managed by early release, preferably in the neonatal period, as previously mentioned.

H. Generalized skeletal abnormalities

1. Congenital dislocation of the radial head—May be distinguished from a traumatic origin by bilateral involvement, other congenital anomalies (60%), and familial occurrence. It is typically irreducible by closed means. Some helpful radiographic clues include a hypoplastic capitellum, a short ulna with a long radius, and a convex radial head. Surgical indications include pain, limited motion, and cosmetic dissatisfaction. In these instances, radial head excision is performed once the child reaches skeletal maturity.
2. Madelung deformity—Results from disruption of the volar ulnar physis of the distal radius. As the child grows, the distal radius exhibits excessive radial inclination and a radiopalmar tilt. Symptoms arise from ulnocarpal impaction, restricted forearm rotation, and median nerve compression. If the deformity is not painful, no treatment is necessary. Otherwise, the procedure of choice is corrective osteotomy of the radius with or without distal ulna recession. Severe deformity may benefit from a distraction external fixator to avoid neurovascular compromise after correction.

TABLE 7-16 BLAUTH'S CLASSIFICATION OF THUMB HYPOPLASIA

Type	Characteristics
I	Minor hypoplasia, all structures present, small thumb
II	Adduction contracture, MCP joint ulnar collateral ligament instability, thenar hypoplasia, normal skeleton with respect to articulations
IIIA	Extensive intrinsic and extrinsic musculotendinous deficiencies, intact CMC joint
IIIB	Extensive intrinsic and extrinsic musculotendinous deficiencies, basal metacarpal aplasia, CMC joint not intact
IV	Total or subtotal aplasia of the metacarpal, rudimentary phalanges, thumb attached to hand by a skin bridge (pouce flottant)
V	Complete absence of thumb

CMC, carpometacarpal; MCP, metacarpophalangeal.

XVIII. Elbow

A. Articular and ligamentous anatomy

1. The three articulations at the elbow are the ulnohumeral, radiocapitellar, and proximal radioulnar joints. The articular surface of the distal humerus is angled 30 degrees anterior to the axis of the humeral shaft and is in approximately 6 degrees of valgus compared with the epicondylar axis. The normal range of elbow flexion/extension is 0-150 degrees, and the normal forearm rotation of both pronation and supination is 80 degrees. The functional range of motion is 30-130 degrees in flexion/extension and 50 degrees in both pronation and supination. The normal valgus carrying angle of the elbow is 5-10 degrees for males and 10-15 degrees for females. In full extension, 60% of the axial load is transmitted through the radiocapitellar joint.
2. The **medial (ulnar) collateral ligament** (MCL) consists of anterior, posterior, and transverse bundles (Fig. 7–65). The anterior bundle is the primary restraint to valgus stress within the functional range of the elbow. It originates on the medial epicondyle and inserts on the sublime tubercle on the medial side of the coronoid process. Secondary restraint to valgus stress is provided by the radial head. The posterior bundle of the MCL provides restraint to valgus stress with the elbow in full flexion. Stability in full extension is provided by the MCL, capsule, and congruity of the ulnohumeral joint.
3. The **lateral collateral ligament** (LCL) **complex** is composed of the **radial collateral ligament** (RCL), the **lateral ulnar collateral ligament** (LUCL), the **accessory collateral ligament**, and the **annular ligament** (Fig. 7–66). The LUCL originates on the lateral epicondyle and inserts on the crista supinatoris of the proximal ulna. The LUCL

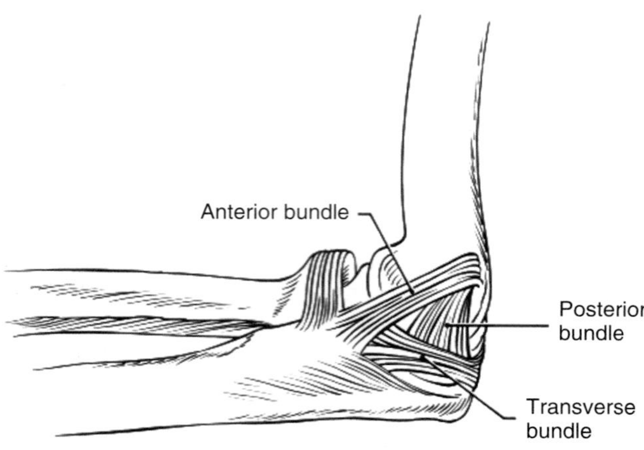

FIGURE 7–65 Medial collateral ligament complex. (From Trumble TE, Budoff JE, Cornwall R, eds: Core Knowledge in Orthopaedics: Hand, Elbow, and Shoulder, p 484. Philadelphia, CV Mosby, 2006.)

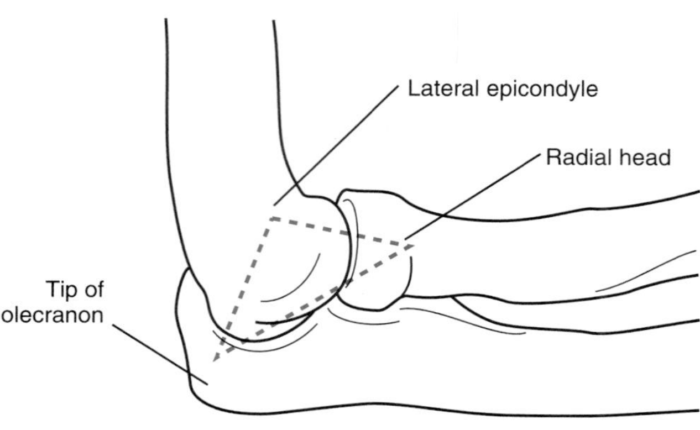

FIGURE 7–67 The anconeal soft spot (lateral infracondylar recess) is the most sensitive area in which to detect a joint effusion. This triangular area located on the lateral aspect of the elbow is outlined by the radial head, tip of the olecranon, and lateral epicondyle. (From Trumble TE, Budoff JE, Cornwall R, eds: Core Knowledge in Orthopaedics: Hand, Elbow, and Shoulder, p 489. Philadelphia, CV Mosby, 2006.)

provides the primary restraint to varus and external rotational stress.

B. Joint aspiration or injection—Best performed through the anconeal soft spot at the lateral aspect of the elbow between a triangle of bony landmarks: the radial head, lateral epicondyle, and tip of the olecranon (Fig. 7–67).

C. Elbow imaging
   1. Plain radiographs—Anteroposterior, lateral, and oblique views are usually sufficient to evaluate most elbow pathology.
   2. CT—Provides superior bony detail in complex fractures of the distal humerus, radial head, and coronoid process. It is also used for the detection of ossified loose bodies and to localize heterotopic ossification.
   3. MRI—Provides superior detail of soft tissue. It is considered the best imaging modality for the evaluation of ligamentous injuries, occult fractures, osteochondritis dissecans, nonossified loose bodies, tendon injury, and soft tissue masses.

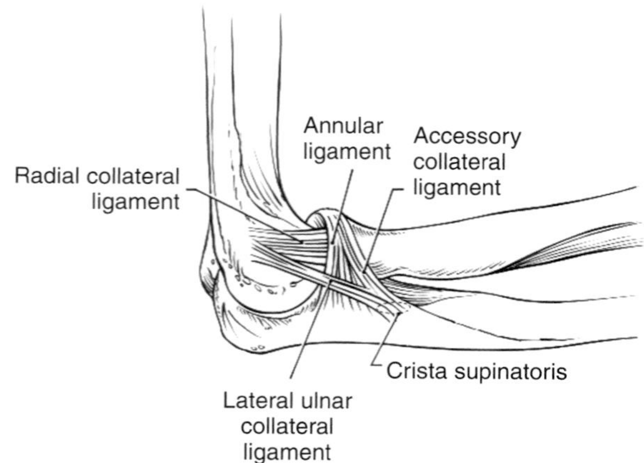

FIGURE 7–66 Lateral collateral ligament complex. (From Trumble TE, Budoff JE, Cornwall R, eds: Core Knowledge in Orthopaedics: Hand, Elbow, and Shoulder, p 484. Philadelphia, CV Mosby, 2006.)

D. Tendon disorders
   1. Lateral epicondylitis (tennis elbow)—Common tendinopathy of the ECRB caused by repetitive wrist extension and forearm rotation. This condition affects industrial workers with far greater prevalence than racket-sport athletes.
      a. Diagnosis—Patients present with lateral elbow pain. Tenderness is elicited at the lateral epicondyle and exacerbated by resisted wrist extension. Grip strength is greatly diminished with the elbow extended compared with the elbow flexed. Histologic examination reveals angiofibroblastic hyperplasia and not acute inflammation.
      b. Treatment—The mainstay of treatment is nonoperative intervention, with rest, counterforce bracing, NSAIDs, and local corticosteroid injections. The efficacy of corticosteroid injections has been recently debated. Rehabilitative exercises are initiated when symptoms permit. These measures should be exhausted for up to 12 months before surgical options are discussed. The concurrent causes of lateral elbow pain, such as radial tunnel syndrome, must be investigated and ruled out prior to surgery. The ECRB origin is identified through a lateral approach. An abnormal, friable tendon is safely removed by the Nirschl scratch test. Iatrogenic injury to normal tissue, such as the LCL complex, must be avoided. Minimal bony débridement is advocated. Incomplete removal of tendinosis is the most common reason for failed pain relief and revision surgery. Posterior tennis elbow is a similar condition affecting the insertion of the triceps tendon.

2. Medial epicondylitis—Similar but less common tendinopathy affecting the origin of the flexor-pronator mass at the medial epicondyle. Prolonged conservative management is recommended because the success of surgical débridement is less predictable than it is in lateral epicondylitis.
3. Distal biceps tendon rupture—Typically caused by eccentric loading of the flexed elbow during manual labor, weightlifting, or athletic activity. Patients may experience a painful "pop," and supination strength is diminished more than flexion strength. In complete ruptures, the biceps muscle belly may be retracted proximally. Risk factors include steroid and tobacco use. MRI may help distinguish complete from partial injuries in equivocal cases. Surgical repair is recommended in active individuals with a complete rupture. Single- and two-incision techniques have been employed for reattachment to the radial tuberosity, and each has had excellent functional results. The two-incision technique is associated with a higher rate of radioulnar synostosis. Chronic injuries may require free-tendon graft augmentation to provide length and appropriate biceps tension. The amount of strength before injury is rarely recovered in these cases.
4. Triceps tendon rupture—Rare injury caused by either a direct blow to the posterior elbow or sudden forceful flexion of an extended elbow. Rupture typically occurs at the musculotendinous junction. Patients cannot extend the elbow against gravity. Differentiation between partial and complete injuries is best assessed by MRI. Surgical repair should be performed in complete injuries and partial injuries constituting greater than 50% of the tendon, with concomitant loss of extension strength.

E. Elbow trauma

1. Distal humerus fractures
   a. Diagnosis—The anatomic morphology of the distal humerus may be thought of as two columns and a spool. Most fractures of the distal humerus in adults involve both columns and the articular surface. These fractures tend to occur in younger patients as the result of high-energy trauma and in elderly individuals with osteopenic bone from low-energy falls at ground level. CT scanning is tremendously helpful in characterizing the degree of comminution and articular step-off.
   b. Treatment—Nonoperative treatment may be appropriate for medically ill patients with low functional demands, but the vast majority of these injuries require ORIF. Surgical approaches include triceps sparing (Bryan-Morrey), triceps splitting, and olecranon osteotomy. Although the latter may provide the best visualization of the articular surface, nonunion and symptomatic hardware are potential complications. The standard fixation technique is 90-90 (orthogonal) double plating; however, parallel plating with interdigitation of screw threads may be biomechanically stronger in complex fracture patterns. Locking-plate technology should be considered for patients with poor bone quality. Elderly patients with severe comminution of the articular surface may be better served by a semiconstrained total elbow arthroplasty in order to allow early range of motion and reliable pain relief.
2. Radial head fractures—Typically result from a fall onto a flexed elbow.
   a. Classification—Classified by Mason and modified by Hotchkiss into types I-IV (Fig. 7–68).
      Type I injuries are nondisplaced or minimally displaced, with no mechanical block to forearm rotation.
      Type II fractures are displaced more than 2 mm and may have a mechanical block. A reliable evaluation of mechanical block may require aspiration of hemarthrosis and the intra-articular injection of local anesthetic.
      Type III fractures are comminuted.

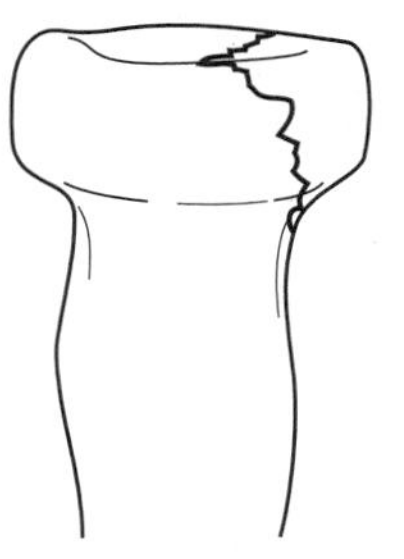
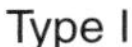

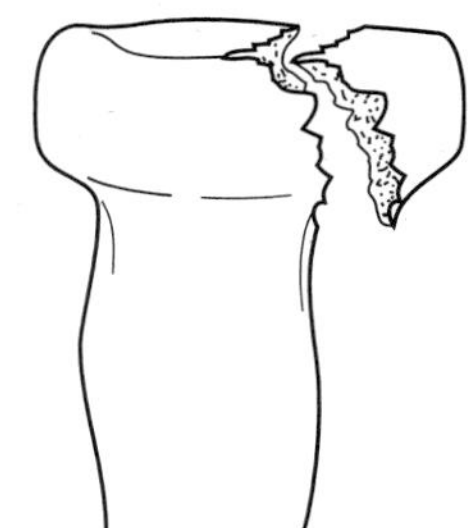

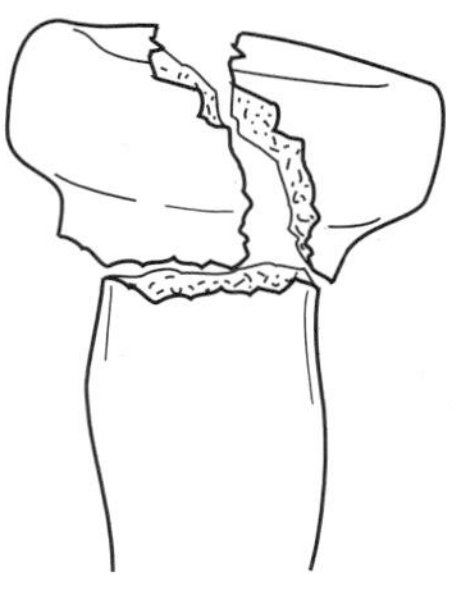

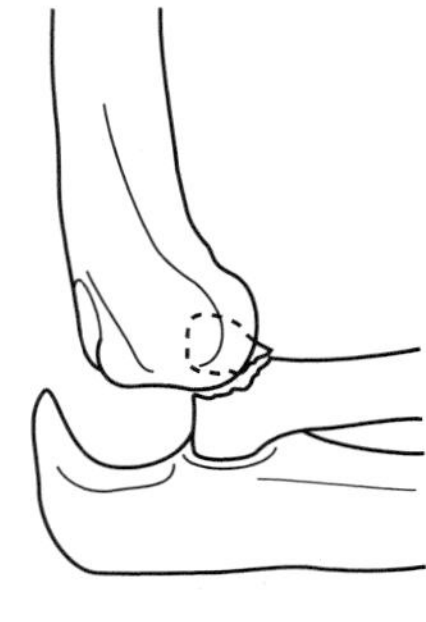

FIGURE 7–68 Radial head classification. (From Trumble TE, Budoff JE, Cornwall R, eds: Core Knowledge in Orthopaedics: Hand, Elbow, and Shoulder, p 526. Philadelphia, CV Mosby, 2006.)

Type IV fractures are associated with an elbow dislocation.

b. Diagnosis—Oblique radiographs or a CT scan may be necessary to evaluate alignment and displacement. Associated injuries are frequently encountered, including ligamentous or capsular disruption and other periarticular fractures. If wrist tenderness is elicited, radiographs should be obtained to rule out an **Essex-Lopresti** injury.

c. Treatment—Treatment of these injuries is focused on early range of motion to prevent stiffness. Type I fractures are typically managed nonoperatively. Most radial head nonunions are asymptomatic. Type II fractures with a mechanical block are treated with ORIF (insertion of headless screws or miniplates through a lateral Kocher approach). The safe zone for screw placement extends along a 110-degree arc, where the radial head is nonarticular. Treatment of type III fractures is accomplished with ORIF, excision, or metallic prosthetic head replacement. When more than three articular fragments are present, ORIF has a high rate of early failure and poor results. Excision is acceptable in the absence of MCL or interosseous ligamentous injury. A radial head prosthesis is always used in the setting of elbow fracture-dislocation. Avoid overstuffing the joint, which will lead to early capitellar wear and late instability.

3. Essex-Lopresti injury—Radioulnar instability caused by sequential injury to the DRUJ, interosseous membrane, and radial head. Disruption of the central third of the interosseous membrane can decrease radioulnar instability by 70%. All patients with radial head fractures should have a thorough clinical and radiographic evaluation in order to assess the DRUJ. The radial head must be either fixed or replaced to prevent proximal migration of the radius. Treat TFCC pathology concurrently. Failure to recognize this injury can lead to late longitudinal instability and ulnar impaction syndrome.

4. Coronoid fractures—Occur most often in the setting of elbow dislocation. These fractures are divided into types I-III based on the size of the proximal fragment. Treat with ORIF to help restore elbow stability. Small fragments may require braided suture fixation.

5. Olecranon fractures—Typically result from a direct blow to the proximal ulna. The proximal fragment is often displaced by the proximal pull of the triceps. The lateral radiograph is examined for fracture displacement, comminution, and articular congruity. Tension band constructs work well for simple transverse fracture patterns but are associated with a high rate of symptomatic hardware (> 50%) that requires later removal. Comminuted fractures with articular displacement are best treated with formal ORIF by using a plate-screw construct. Elderly patients who have severely comminuted fractures may benefit from excision of the proximal fragment and reattachment of the triceps tendon adjacent to the joint line.

6. Elbow dislocation—The site of injury is usually posterolateral. The dislocation is generally classified as simple or complex (with associated fractures). Closed reduction should be performed promptly after assessment of the neurovascular status. Test patient stability through range of motion. Simple dislocations should be splinted in 90 degrees of elbow flexion with the forearm pronated. Instability within 30 degrees of full extension may be an indication for acute ligamentous repair. The lateral ligamentous complex is always repaired, followed by the MCL if instability persists. A "**terrible triad**" injury consists of an elbow dislocation with fractures of the radial head and coronoid process. Treat this injury with ligamentous repair, ORIF of the coronoid, and either ORIF or prosthetic replacement of the radial head. Persistent instability may require placement of a hinged external fixator. The primary goal in all elbow dislocations is early motion.

7. Monteggia fracture-dislocations—The proximal third of the ulna shaft fracture is accompanied by radial head subluxation/dislocation. Monteggia fracture-dislocations are classified by Bado into types I-IV (Fig. 7–69). Anatomic plate fixation of the ulna usually reduces the radial head. Persistent instability may require annular ligament repair.

F. Elbow instability

1. Posterolateral rotatory instability—Caused by incompetence of the LUCL (Fig. 7–70). Patients relate a history of one or more elbow dislocations treated nonoperatively. This condition presents with pain and recurrent mechanical symptoms. The lateral pivot shift test reproduces the instability with a combination of supination, axial compression, and valgus loading as the elbow is brought from full extension to 40 degrees of flexion. The ulna rotates externally on the trochlea and produces posterior radial head subluxation. With increasing flexion, the triceps becomes taut and the radial head reduces with a palpable clunk. Patient apprehension is common, and either intra-articular local anesthetic or examination under general anesthesia may be necessary to confirm the diagnosis. Chronic instability may require reconstruction of the LUCL with a free-tendon graft.

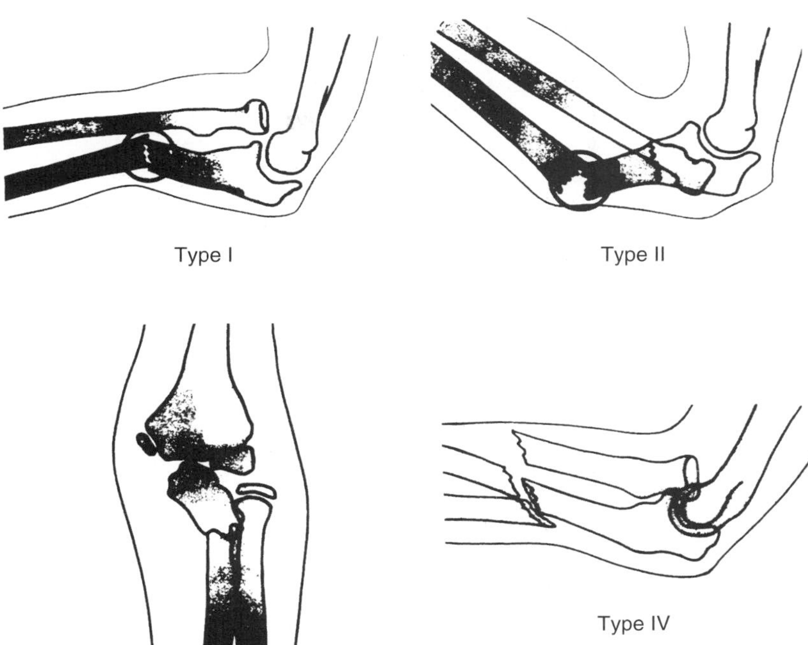

FIGURE 7–69 Classification of Monteggia fractures. (From Reckling FW, Cordell LD: Unstable fracture-dislocations of the forearm. Arch Surg 96:1004, 1968; reprinted by permission. Copyright 1968 American Medical Association.)

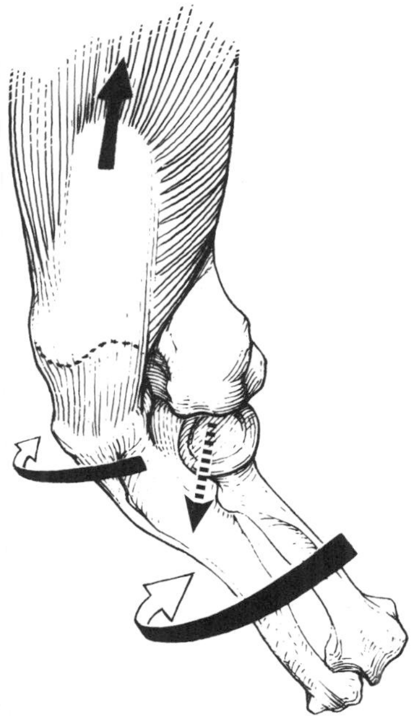

FIGURE 7–70 Mechanism of deforming torsional forces. With active triceps contraction *(solid straight arrow)* while extension is being resisted, the deforming forces and moments cause a medial pull and external rotation torsion on the ulna about its long axis *(small curved arrow)*. This not only moves the ulna into external rotation but also causes the radial head to rotate posterolaterally off the capitellum *(straight dashed arrow)*. These represent the initial kinematic displacements of posterolateral rotatory subluxation *(large curved arrow)*. Over time, these chronic forces cause attenuation of the lateral collateral ligament complex, including the ulnar part, leading to frank posterolateral rotatory subluxation. (From O'Driscoll SW, Spinner R, McKee M, et al: Tardy posterolateral rotatory instability of the elbow due to cubitus varus. J Bone Joint Surg [Am] 83: 1358-1369, 2001. Reproduced with permission from Mayo Foundation.)

2. Varus posteromedial rotatory instability—Results from a fracture of the anteromedial coronoid process and LUCL injury. Treatment requires ORIF of the coronoid and LUCL reconstruction.
3. Valgus instability—May be acute after elbow trauma or chronic from repetitive loading and attenuation of the MCL. Primary ligamentous repair or reattachment to the inferior aspect of the medial epicondyle with the use of suture anchors is performed in the acute setting. Chronic instability is common in overhead-throwing athletes such as baseball pitchers. Increased valgus stress is produced during the cocking phase of throwing. Unrecognized or untreated MCL insufficiency may lead to capitellar wear, posteromedial impingement, olecranon osteophyte formation, and loose-body formation. Arthroscopic débridement of osteophytes and loose-body removal may be effective. Concurrent cubital tunnel syndrome occurs in at least 25% of cases. MRI may be helpful to differentiate complete from partial tears of the MCL. If conservative management fails, MCL reconstruction with a free-tendon graft may be indicated, especially in competitive athletes.

G. Elbow contracture—Stiffness and loss of motion are frequent complications after elbow injury; for this reason, aggressive therapy is employed as early as possible. In the nonathletic population, a loss of 30 degrees of terminal extension is well tolerated. However, loss of flexion interferes with activities of daily living. Contributing intrinsic factors may include articular incongruity, loose bodies, synovitis, bony ankylosis, and capsular contracture, all of which may be initially addressed by arthroscopy. External factors such as heterotopic ossification, muscle fibrosis, and ligamentous contracture require open treatment. Heterotopic ossification occurs in over 75% of the cases of elbow injury with accompanying head trauma. If an aggressive course of therapy fails to restore functional range of motion, surgical treatment may be warranted. A more aggressive approach to the excision of heterotopic ossification is being advocated, typically between 3 and 6 months once the bone has matured. The ulnar nerve should be transposed during posterior approaches.

H. Elbow arthritis

1. Rheumatoid arthritis—The most prevalent type of elbow arthritis. The elbow is affected in up to 50% of patients with rheumatoid arthritis. Chronic inflammation and synovitis may lead to ligament attenuation, periarticular osteopenia, and joint contracture. In patients in whom medical management fails, initial surgical treatment may include synovectomy and radial head excision. Relief of pain and improved range of motion are reliable, but the effect is temporary. Semiconstrained total elbow arthroplasty provides more permanent relief of pain but a higher rate of complications. Progressive bone resorption limits the effectiveness of interposition arthroplasty in patients with rheumatoid arthritis.
2. Post-traumatic arthritis—The second most common type of elbow arthritis. Young, active patients are good candidates for interposition arthroplasty with the use of either autogenous tensor fasciae latae or an Achilles tendon allograft.
3. Primary OA—Uncommon form of elbow arthritis typically affecting middle-aged male laborers. Osteophyte formation may lead to a mechanical block of motion. Narrowing of the radiocapitellar joint space is a common radiographic finding. Open or arthroscopic ulnohumeral joint and osteophyte débridement may have some utility to delay arthroplasty.
4. Total elbow arthroplasty (TEA)—Indicated in refractory rheumatoid arthritis, OA (primary and post-traumatic), and chronic instability and more recently espoused as the primary treatment for complex distal humerus fractures in elderly patients with poor bone stock. TEA is contraindicated in cases of intractable septic arthritis, in which primary arthrodesis is favored. Patients must agree to a weightlifting restriction of less than 10 pounds. Two primary types of prosthesis are unconstrained (unlinked) and semiconstrained (linked). Unconstrained TEA is used in OA with competent collateral ligaments and good bone stock. Semiconstrained prostheses act as a "sloppy hinge," with limited rotational and coronal plane motion, and are best for rheumatoid arthritis, chronic instability, and distal humerus fractures in the elderly. Each prosthetic design has demonstrated the ability to provide significant pain relief. Surgical approaches from a posterior midline incision include the triceps-splitting and triceps-sparing (Bryan-Morrey) approaches. The radial head is often resected. Repair of the triceps mechanism is of paramount importance for good postoperative function. Complications include infection, nerve injury, instability, periprosthetic fracture, and implant loosening from polyethylene wear. Staged reimplantation after infection has a poor salvage rate.

Selected Bibliography

ANATOMY

Green DP, Hotchkiss RN, Pederson WG, eds: Green's Operative Hand Surgery, 5th ed. New York, Churchill Livingstone, 2005.

Trumble TE, ed: Principles of Hand Surgery and Therapy. Philadelphia, WB Saunders, 2001.

Trumble TE, Budoff JE, Cornwall R, eds: Core Knowledge in Orthopaedics: Hand, Elbow and Shoulder. Philadelphia, CV Mosby, 2006.

DISTAL RADIUS FRACTURES

Benson LS, Minihane KP, Stern LD, et al: The outcome of intra-articular distal radius fractures treated with fragment-specific fixation. J Hand Surg [Am] 31:1333–1339, 2006.

Boyer MI, Galatz LM, Borrelli J Jr, et al: Intra-articular fractures of the upper extremity: New concepts in surgical treatment. Instr Course Lect 52: 591–605, 2003.

Doi K, Hattori Y, Otsuka K, et al: Intra-articular fractures of the distal aspect of the radius: Arthroscopically-assisted reduction compared with open reduction and internal fixation. J Bone Joint Surg [Am] 81:1093–1110, 1999.

Fernandez DL: Malunion of the distal radius: Current approach to management. Instr Course Lect 42:99–113, 1993.

Goldfarb CA, Rudzki JR, Catalano LW, et al: Fifteen-year outcome of displaced intra-articular fractures of the distal radius. J Hand Surg [Am] 31:633–639, 2006.

Hanel DP, Jones MD, Trumble TE: Wrist fractures. Orthop Clin North Am 33:35–57, 2002.

Hartigan BJ, Cohen MS: Use of bone graft substitutes and bioactive materials in treatment of distal radius fractures. Hand Clin 21:449–454, 2005.

Nana AD, Joshi A, Lichtman DM: Plating of the distal radius. J Am Acad Orthop Surg 13:159–171, 2005.

Orbay JL, Touhami A: Current concepts in volar fixed-angle fixation of unstable distal radius fractures. Clin Orthop Relat Res 445:58–67, 2006.

Rozental TD, Blazar PE: Functional outcome and complications after volar plating for dorsally displaced, unstable fractures of the distal radius. J Hand Surg [Am] 31:359–365, 2006.

Ruch DS, Papadonikolakis A: Volar versus dorsal plating in the management of intra-articular distal radius fractures. J Hand Surg [Am] 31:9–16, 2006.

Skoff HD: Postfracture extensor pollicis longus tenosynovitis and tendon rupture: A scientific study and personal series. Am J Orthop 32: 245–247, 2003.

Smith DW, Henry MH: Volar fixed-angle plating of the distal radius. J Am Acad Orthop Surg 13:28–36, 2005.

Wolfe SW, Austin G, Lorenze M: A biomechanical comparison of different wrist external fixators with and without K-wire augmentation. J Hand Surg [Am] 24:516–524, 1999.

CARPAL FRACTURES AND INSTABILITY

Bednar JM, Osterman AL: Carpal instability. J Am Acad Orthop Surg 1: 10–17, 1993.

Cohen MS, Kozin SH: Degenerative arthritis of the wrist: Proximal row carpectomy versus scaphoid excision and four-corner fusion arthrodesis. J Hand Surg [Am] 26:94–104, 2001.

Gelberman RH, Wolock BS, Siegel DB: Current concepts review: Fractures and non-unions of the carpal scaphoid. J Bone Joint Surg [Am] 71:1560–1565, 1989.

Goldfarb CA, Stern PJ, Kiefhaber TR: Palmar midcarpal instability: The results of treatment with 4-corner arthrodesis. J Hand Surg [Am] 29:258–263, 2004.

Herbert TJ, Fischer WE: Management of the fractured scaphoid using a new bone screw. J Bone Joint Surg [Br] 66:114–123, 1984.

Lavernia CJ, Cohen MS, Taleisnik J: Treatment of scapholunate dissociation by ligamentous repair and capsulodesis. J Hand Surg [Am] 17:354–359, 1992.

Lichtman DM, Wroten ES: Understanding midcarpal instability. J Hand Surg [Am] 31:491–498, 2006.

Linschied RL, Dobyns JH, Beabout JW, et al: Traumatic instability of the wrist: Diagnosis, classification and pathomechanics. J Bone Joint Surg [Am] 54:1612–1632, 1972.

Mayfield JK, Johnson RP, Kilcoyne RK: Carpal dislocations: Pathomechanics and progressive perilunar instability. J Hand Surg 5:226–241, 1980.

Polsky MB, Kozin SH, Porter ST, Thoder JJ: Scaphoid fractures: Dorsal versus volar approach. Orthopaedics 25:817–819, 2002.

Ruby LK, Stinson J, Belsky MR: The natural history of scaphoid nonunion. J Bone Joint Surg [Am] 67:428–432, 1985.

Shin AY, Battaglia MJ, Bishop AT: Lunotriquetral instability: Diagnosis and treatment. J Am Acad Orthop Surg 8:170–179, 2000.

Steinmann SP, Bishop AT, Berger RA: Use of the 1,2 intercompartmental supraretinacular artery as a vascularized pedicle bone graft for difficult scaphoid nonunions. J Hand Surg [Am] 27:391–401, 2002.

Stern PJ, Agabegi SS, Kiefhaber TR, Didonna ML: Proximal row carpectomy. J Bone Joint Surg [Am] 87(Supp. 1[Part 2]):166–174, 2005.

Vigler M, Avileo A, Lee SK: Carpal fractures excluding the scaphoid. Hand Clin 22:501–516, 2006.

Walsh JJ, Berger RA, Cooney WP: Current status of scapholunate interosseous ligament injuries. J Am Acad Orthop Surg 10:32–42, 2002.

Watson HK, Ballet FL: The SLAC wrist: Scapholunate advanced collapse pattern of degenerative arthritis. J Hand Surg [Am] 9:358–365, 1984.

METACARPAL AND PHALANGEAL INJURIES

Freeland AE, Lindley SG: Malunions of the finger metacarpals and phalanges. Hand Clin 22:341–355, 2006.

Freeland AE, Orbay JL: Extra-articular hand fractures in adults: A review of new developments. Clin Orthop Relat Res 445:133–145, 2006.

Geissler WB: Cannulated percutaneous fixation of intra-articular hand fractures. Hand Clin 22:297–305, 2006.

Hamilton SC, Stern PJ, Fassler PR, Kiefhaber TR: Mini-screw fixation for the treatment of proximal interphalangeal joint dorsal fracture-dislocations. J Hand Surg [Am] 31:1349–1354, 2006.

Joseph RB, Linschied RL, Dobyns JH, et al: Chronic sprains of the carpometacarpal joints. J Hand Surg [Am] 6:172–180, 1981.

Peterson JJ, Bancroft LW: Injuries of the fingers and thumb in the athlete. Clin Sports Med 25:527–542, 2006.

Poolman RW, Goslings JC, Lee JB, et al: Conservative treatment for closed small finger metacarpal neck fractures. Cochrane Database Syst Rev 20: CD-003210, 2005.

Stern PJ: Management of fractures of the hand over the last 25 years. J Hand Surg [Am] 25:817–823, 2000.

Williams RM, Kiefhaber TR, Sommerkamp TG, Stern PJ: Treatment of unstable dorsal proximal interphalangeal fracture-dislocations using a hemi-hamate autograft. J Hand Surg [Am] 28:856–865, 2003.

TENDON INJURIES AND OVERUSE SYNDROMES

Bishop AT, Topper SM, Bettinger PC: Flexor mechanism reconstruction and rehabilitation. In Peimer CA, ed: Surgery of the Hand and Upper Extremity. New York, McGraw Hill, 1996.

Chester DL, Beale S, Beveridge L, et al: A prospective, controlled, randomized trial comparing early active extension with passive extension using a dynamic splint in the rehabilitation of repaired extensor tendons. J Hand Surg [Br] 27:283–288, 2002.

Garberman SF, Diao E, Peimer CA: Mallet finger: Results of early versus delayed closed treatment. J Hand Surg [Am] 19:850–852, 1994.

Gelberman RH, Vande Berg JS, Lundborg GN, et al: Flexor tendon healing and restoration of the gliding surface. J Bone Joint Surg [Am] 65:70–80, 1983.

LaSalle WE, Strickland JW: An evaluation of the two-stage flexor tendon reconstruction technique. J Hand Surg [Am] 8:263–267, 1983.

Leddy JP, Packer JW: Avulsion of the profundus tendon insertion in athletes. J Hand Surg 2:66–69, 1977.

Lilly SI, Messer TM: Complications after treatment of flexor tendon injuries. J Am Acad Orthop Surg 14:387–396, 2006.

Lister GD, Kleinert HE, Kutz JE, et al: Primary flexor tendon repair followed by immediate controlled mobilization. J Hand Surg [Am] 2:441–451, 1977.

Manske PR, Gelberman RH, Vande Berg JS, et al: Intrinsic flexor tendon repair. J Bone Joint Surg [Am] 66:385–396, 1984.

Newport ML: Extensor tendon injuries in the hand. J Am Acad Orthop Surg 5:59–66, 1997.

Parkes A: The lumbrical plus finger. J Bone Joint Surg [Br] 53:236–239, 1971.

Ryzewicz M, Wolf JM: Trigger digits: Principles, management and complications. J Hand Surg [Am] 31:135–146, 2006.

Soejima O, Diao E, Lotz JC, Hariharan JS: Comparative mechanical analysis of dorsal versus palmar placement of core suture for flexor tendon repairs. J Hand Surg [Am] 20:801–807, 1995.

Stern PJ, Kastrup JJ: Complications and prognosis of treatment of mallet finger. J Hand Surg [Am] 13:329–334, 1988.

Strickland JW, Glogovac SV: Digital function following flexor tendon repair in zone II: A comparison of immobilization and controlled passive motion techniques. J Hand Surg [Am] 5:537–543, 1980.

Strickland JW: Flexor tendon injuries: I. Foundations of treatment. J Am Acad Orthop Surg 3:44–54, 1995.

Strickland JW: Flexor tendon injuries. II. Flexor tendon injuries: Operative technique. J Am Acad Orthop Surg 3:55–62, 1995.

Strickland JW: Development of flexor tendon surgery: Twenty-five years of progress. J Hand Surg [Am] 25:214–235, 2000.

Tuttle HG, Olvey SP, Stern PJ: Tendon avulsion injuries of the distal phalanx. Clin Orthop Relat Res 445:157–168, 2006.

Verdan C: Syndrome of quadrigia. Surg Clin North Am 40:425–426, 1960.

Wehbe MA, Schneider LH: Mallet fractures. J Bone Joint Surg [Am] 66: 658–669, 1984.

DISTAL RADIOULNAR JOINT, TRIANGULAR FIBROCARTILAGE COMPLEX, AND WRIST ARTHROSCOPY

Adams BD, Berger RA: An anatomic reconstruction for the distal radioulnar ligaments for posttraumatic distal radioulnar joint instability. J Hand Surg [Am] 27:243–251, 2002.

Bernstein MA, Nagle DJ, Martinez A, et al: A comparison of combined arthroscopic triangular fibrocartilage complex débridement and arthroscopic wafer distal ulnar resection versus arthroscopic triangular fibrocartilage complex débridement and ulnar shortening osteotomy for ulnocarpal abutment syndrome. Arthroscopy 20:392–401, 2004.

Bowers WH: Distal radioulnar joint arthroplasty: The hemi-resection interposition technique. J Hand Surg [Am] 10:169–178, 1985.

Chidgey LK: The distal radioulnar joint: Problems and solutions. J Am Acad Orthop Surg 3:95–109, 1995.

Cober SR, Trumble TE: Arthroscopic repair of triangular fibrocartilage complex injuries. Orthop Clin North Am 32:279–294, 2001.

Cooney WP: Evaluation of chronic wrist pain by arthrography, arthroscopy and arthrotomy. J Hand Surg [Am] 18:815–822, 1993.

Cooney WP, Linscheid RL, Dobyns JH: Triangular fibrocartilage tears. J Hand Surg [Am] 19:143–154, 1994.

Palmer AK: Triangular fibrocartilage complex lesions: A classification. J Hand Surg [Am] 14:594–606, 1989.

Scheker LR, Babb BA, Killion PE: Distal ulnar prosthetic replacement. Orthop Clin North Am 32:365–376, 2001.

Tomaino MM, Elfar J: Ulnar impaction syndrome. Hand Clin 21:567–575, 2005.

NAIL AND FINGERTIP INJURIES

Ashbell TS, Kleinert HK, Putcha S, et al: The deformed fingernail, a frequent result of failure to repair nail bed injuries. J Trauma 7:177–190, 1967.

Fassler RR: Fingertip injuries: Evaluation and treatment. J Am Acad Orthop Surg 4:84–92, 1996.

Louis DS, Palmer AK, Burney RE: Open treatment of digital tip injuries. JAMA 244:697–698, 1980.

Schenck R, Cheema TA: Hypothenar skin grafts for fingertip reconstruction. J Hand Surg [Am] 9:750–753, 1984.

Shephard GH: Treatment of nail bed avulsions with split thickness nail bed grafts. J Hand Surg [Am] 8:49–54, 1983.

Shibata M, Seki T, Yoshizu T, et al: Microsurgical toenail transfer to the hand. J Plast Reconstr Surg 88:102–109, 1991.

Zook EG, Guy RJ, Russell RC: A study of nail bed injuries: Causes, treatment, and prognosis. J Hand Surg [Am] 9:247–252, 1984.

Zook EG, Van Beek AL, Russell RC, et al: Anatomy and physiology of the perionychium: A review of the literature and anatomic study. J Hand Surg 5:528–536, 1980.

SOFT TISSUE COVERAGE AND MICROSURGERY

Boulas HJ: Amputations of the fingers and hand: Indications for replantation. J Am Acad Orthop Surg 6:100–105, 1998.

Godina M: Early microsurgical reconstruction of complex trauma of the extremities. Plast Reconstr Surg 78:285–292, 1986.

Gupta A, Wolff TW: Management of the mangled hand and forearm. J Am Acad Orthop Surg 3:226–236, 1995.

Hans CS, Wood MB, Bishop AT, et al: Vascularized bone transfer. J Bone Joint Surg [Am] 74:1441–1449, 1992.

Lister G, Scheker L: Emergency free flaps to the upper extremity. J Hand Surg [Am] 13:22–28, 1988.

Lister GD, Kallisman M, Tsai T: Reconstruction of the hand with free microvascular toe to hand transfer: Experience with 54 toe transfers. Plast Reconstr Surg 71:372–384, 1983.

Manktelow RT, Zuker RM, McKee NH: Functioning free muscle transplantation. J Hand Surg [Am] 9:32–39, 1984.

Matev IB: Thumb reconstruction through metacarpal bone lengthening. J Hand Surg [Am] 5:482–487, 1980.

Morrison WA, O'Brien B, MacLeod AM: Thumb reconstruction with a free neurovascular wrap-around flap from the big toe. J Hand Surg 5: 575–583, 1980.

Scheker LR, Kleinert HE, Hanel DP: Lateral arm composite tissue transfer to ipsilateral hand defects. J Hand Surg [Am] 12:665–672, 1987.

Stern PJ, Lister GD: Pollicization after traumatic amputation of the thumb. Clin Orthop 155:85–94, 1981.

Urbaniak JR, Evans JP, Bright DS: Microvascular management of ring avulsion injuries. J Hand Surg [Am] 6:25–30, 1981.

Urbaniak JR, Roth JH, Nunley JA, et al: The results of replantation after amputation of a single finger. J Bone Joint Surg [Am] 67:611–619, 1985.

Wood MB, Irons GB: Upper extremity free skin flap transfer: Results and utility compared with conventional distant pedicle skin flaps. Ann Plast Surg 11:523–526, 1983.

VASCULAR DISORDERS

Flatt AE: Digital artery sympathectomy. J Hand Surg 5:550–556, 1980.

Jones NF: Acute and chronic ischemia of the hand: Pathophysiology, treatment, and prognosis. J Hand Surg [Am] 16:1074–1083, 1991.

Koman LA, Urbaniak JR: Ulnar artery insufficiency—a guide to treatment. J Hand Surg 6:16–24, 1981.

Lankford LL: Reflex sympathetic dystrophy. In Omer G, Spinner M, eds: Management of Peripheral Nerve Problems. Philadelphia, WB Saunders, 1986.

Phillips CS, Murphy MS: Vascular problems of the upper extremity: A primer for the orthopedic surgeon. J Am Acad Orthop Surg 6:401–408, 2002.

Tsuge K: Treatment of established Volkmann's contracture. J Bone Joint Surg [Am] 57:925–929, 1975.

COMPRESSION NEUROPATHY

Agee JM, McCarroll HR, Tortosa R, et al: Endoscopic release of the carpal tunnel: A randomized, prospective multicenter study. J Hand Surg [Am] 17:987–995, 1992.

Buch-Jaeger N, Foucher G: Correlation of clinical signs with nerve conduction tests in the diagnosis of carpal tunnel syndrome. J Hand Surg [Br] 19:720–724, 1994.

Dellon AL: Review of results for ulnar nerve entrapment at the elbow. J Hand Surg [Am] 14:670–688, 1989.

Gelberman RH, Pfeffer GB, Galbraith RT, et al: Results of treatment of severe carpal tunnel syndrome without internal neurolysis of the median nerve. J Bone Joint Surg [Am] 69:896–903, 1987.

Gundberg AB: Carpal tunnel decompression in spite of normal electromyography. J Hand Surg 8:348–349, 1983.

Hartz CR, Linschied RL, Gramse RR, et al: The pronator teres syndrome: Compressive neuropathy of the median nerve. J Bone Joint Surg [Am] 63:885–890, 1981.

Leffert RD: Anterior submuscular transposition of the ulnar nerve. J Hand Surg 7:147–155, 1982.

Lubahn JD, Cermak MB: Uncommon nerve compression syndromes of the upper extremity. J Am Acad Orthop Surg 6:378–386, 1998.

Posner MA: Compression ulnar neuropathies at the elbow: II. Treatment. J Am Acad Orthop Surg 6:289–297, 1998.

Posner MA: Compression ulnar neuropathy at the elbow: I. Etiology and diagnosis. J Am Acad Orthop Surg 6:282–288, 1998.

Ritts GD: Radial tunnel syndrome: A 10-year surgical experience. Clin Orthop 219:201–205, 1987.

Spinner M: The anterior interosseous nerve syndrome. J Bone Joint Surg [Am] 52:84–94, 1970.

Szabo, RM, Steinberg, DR: Nerve entrapment syndromes in the wrist. J Am Acad Orthop Surg 115–123, 1994.

Szabo RM, Slater RR Jr, Farver TB, et al: The value of diagnostic testing in carpal tunnel syndrome. J Hand Surg [Am] 24:704–714, 1999.

Trumble TE, Diao E, Abrams RA, Gilbert-Anderson MM: Single-portal endoscopic carpal tunnel release compared with open release: A prospective, randomized trial. J Bone Joint Surg [Am] 84:1107–1115, 2002.

Wood VE: Thoracic outlet syndrome. Orthop Clin North Am 19:131–146, 1988.

NERVE INJURIES AND TENDON TRANSFERS

Allen CH: Functional results of primary nerve repair. Hand Clin 16:67–72, 2000.

Aziz W, Singer RM, Wolff TW: Transfer of the trapezius for flail shoulder after brachial plexus injury. J Bone Joint Surg [Br] 72:701–704, 1990.

Brand P: Biomechanics of tendon transfers. Hand Clin 4:137–154, 1988.

Dellon AL, Curtis RM, Edgerton MT: Reeducation of sensation in the hand after nerve injury and repair. Plast Reconstr Surg 53:297–305, 1974.

Eversmann WW: Tendon transfers for combined nerve injuries. Hand Clin 4:187–199, 1988.

Freehafer AA: Tendon transfers in patients with cervical spinal cord injury. J Hand Surg [Am] 16:804–809, 1991.

Gellman H, Nichols D: Reflex sympathetic dystrophy in the upper extremity. J Am Acad Orthop Surg 5:313–322, 1997.

Hentz VR, Brown M, Keoshian LA: Upper limb reconstruction in quadriplegia: Functional assessment and proposed treatment modifications. J Hand Surg 8:119–131, 1983.

House JH, Shannon MA: Restoration of strong grasp and lateral pinch in tetraplegia: A comparison of two methods of thumb control in each patient. J Hand Surg [Am] 10:22–29, 1985.

Inglis AE, Cooper W: Release of the flexor-pronator origin for flexion deformities of the hand and wrist in spastic paralysis. J Bone Joint Surg [Am] 48:847–857, 1966.

Keenan ME, Korchek JI, Botte MJ, et al: Results of transfer of the flexor digitorum superficialis tendons to the flexor digitorum profundus in adults with acquired spasticity of the hand. J Bone Joint Surg [Am] 69:1127–1132, 1987.

Lee SK, Wolfe SW: Peripheral nerve injury and repair. J Am Acad Orthop Surg 8:243–252, 2000.

Leffert RD: Clinical diagnosis, testing and electromyographic study in brachial plexus traction injuries. Orthop Clin North Am 237:24–31, 1988.

Riordan DC: Tendon transfers in hand surgery. J Hand Surg 8:748–753, 1983.

Seddon H: Three types of nerve injury. Brain 66:237–288, 1943.

Sedel L: The results of surgical repair of brachial plexus injuries. J Bone Joint Surg [Br] 64:54–66, 1982.

Skoff H, Woodbury DF: Current concepts review: Management of the upper extremity in cerebral palsy. J Bone Joint Surg [Am] 67:500–503, 1985.

Smith RJ: Tendon Transfers of the Hand and Forearm. Boston, Little, Brown, 1987.

Stern PJ, Caudle RJ: Tendon transfers for elbow flexion. Hand Clin 4: 297–307, 1988.

Stewart JD: Electrodiagnostic techniques. Hand Clin 2:677–687, 1986.

Sunderland S: A classification of peripheral nerve injuries producing loss of function. Brain 74:491–516, 1951.

Szabo RM, Gelberman RH: Operative treatment of cerebral palsy. Hand Clin 1:525–543, 1985.

Terzis J, Faibisoff B, Williams HB: The nerve gap: Suture under tension versus graft. Plast Reconstr Surg 56:166–170, 1975.

ARTHRITIS

Bamberger HB, Stern PJ, Kiefhaber TR, et al: Trapeziometacarpal joint arthrodesis: A functional evaluation. J Hand Surg [Am] 17:605–611, 1992.

Brown FE, Brown ML: Long-term results after tenosynovectomy to treat the rheumatoid hand. J Hand Surg [Am] 13:704–708, 1988.

Burton RI, Pellegrini VD Jr: Surgical management of basal joint arthritis of the thumb. Part II: Ligament reconstruction with tendon interposition arthroplasty. J Hand Surg [Am] 11:324–332, 1986.

Carroll RE, Hill NA: Arthrodesis of the carpometacarpal joint of the thumb. J Bone Joint Surg [Br] 55:292–294, 1973.

Cobb TK, Beckenbaugh RD: Biaxial total wrist arthroplasty. J Hand Surg [Am] 21:1011–1021, 1996.

Day CS, Ramirez MA: Thumb metacarpophalangeal arthritis: Arthroplasty or fusion?. Hand Clin 22:211–220, 2006.

Eaton RG, Lane LB, Litter JW, et al: Ligament reconstruction for the painful thumb carpometacarpal joint: A long-term assessment. J Hand Surg [Am] 9:692–699, 1984.

Fulton DB, Stern PJ: Trapeziometacarpal joint arthrodesis in primary osteoarthritis: A minimum two-year follow-up. J Hand Surg [Am] 26:109–114, 2001.

Ghavami A, Oishi SN: Thumb trapeziometacarpal arthritis: Treatment with ligament reconstruction tendon interposition arthroplasty. Plast Reconstr Surg 117:116–128, 2006.

Goldfarb CA, Dovan TT: Rheumatoid arthritis: Silicone metacarpophalangeal joint arthroplasty indications, technique and outcomes. Hand Clin 22:177–182, 2006.

Goldfarb CA, Stern PJ: Metacarpophalangeal joint arthroplasty in rheumatoid arthritis: A long-term assessment. J Bone Joint Surg [Am] 85:1869–1878, 2003.

Imbriglia JE, Broudy AS, Hagberg WC, et al: Proximal row carpectomy: Clinical evaluation. J Hand Surg [Am] 15:426–430, 1990.

Kirschenbaum D, Schneider LH, Adams DC, et al: Arthroplasty of the metacarpophalangeal joints with use of silicone rubber implants in patients who have rheumatoid arthritis. J Bone Joint Surg [Am] 75: 3–12, 1993.

Mannerfelt L, Norman O: Attritional ruptures of the flexor tendons in RA caused by bony spurs in the carpal tunnel. J Bone Joint Surg [Br] 51: 270–277, 1969.

Millender LH, Nalebuff EA: Arthrodesis of the rheumatoid wrist. J Bone Joint Surg [Am] 55:1026–1034, 1973.

Papp SR, Athwal GS, Pichora DR: The rheumatoid wrist. J Am Acad Orthop Surg 14:65–77, 2006.

Wajon A, Ada L, Edmunds I: Surgery for thumb (trapeziometacarpal joint) osteoarthritis. Cochrane Database Syst Rev 19: CD-004631, 2005.

IDIOPATHIC OSTEONECROSIS OF THE CARPUS

Almquist EE: Capitate shortening in the treatment of Kienböck's disease. Hand Clin 9:505–512, 1993.

Gelberman RH, Bauman TD, Menon J, Akeson WH: The vascularity of the lunate bone and Kienböck's disease. J Hand Surg 5:272–278, 1980.

Shin AY, Bishop AT: Pedicled vascularized bone grafts for disorders of the carpus: Scaphoid nonunion and Kienböck's disease. J Am Acad Orthop Surg 10:210–216, 2002.

Trumble T, Glisson RR, Seaber AV, et al: A biomechanical comparison of methods for treating Kienböck's disease. J Hand Surg [Am] 11:88–93, 1986.

Weiss AP, Weiland AJ, Moore JR, et al: Radial shortening for Kienböck disease. J Bone Joint Surg [Am] 73:384–391, 1991.

DUPUYTREN DISEASE

Benson LS, Williams CS, Kahle M: Dupuytren's contracture. J Am Acad Orthop Surg 6:24–35, 1998.

Hueston J, Seyfer A: Some medicologic aspects of Dupuytren's contracture. Hand Clin 7:617–763, 1991.

Ketchum LD: The injection of nodules of Dupuytren's disease with triamcinolone acetonide. J Hand Surg [Am] 25:1157–1162, 2003.

Rayan GM: Dupuytren disease: Anatomy, pathology, presentation and treatment. J Bone Joint Surg [Am] 89:190–198, 2007.

Reilly RM, Stern PJ, Goldfarb CA: A retrospective review of the management of Dupuytren's nodules. J Hand Surg [Am] 30: 1014–1018, 2005.

Schneider LH, Hankin FM, Eisenberg T: Surgery of Dupuytren's disease: A review of the open palm method. J Hand Surg [Am] 11:23–27, 1986.

Strickland JW, Bassett RL: The isolated digital cord in Dupuytren's contracture: Anatomy and clinical significance. J Hand Surg [Am] 10:118–124, 1985.

HAND TUMORS

Amadio PC, Lombardi RM: Metastatic tumors of the hand. J Hand Surg [Am] 12:311–316, 1987.

Angelides AB, Wallace PF: The dorsal ganglion of the wrist: Its pathogenesis, gross and microscopic anatomy, and surgical treatment. J Hand Surg 1:228–235, 1976.

Athanasian EA: Aneurysmal bone cyst and giant cell tumor of bone of the hand and distal radius. Hand Clin 20:269–281, 2004.

Carroll RE, Berman AT: Glomus tumors of the hand. J Bone Joint Surg [Am] 54:691–703, 1972.

Creighton J, Peimer C, Mindell E, et al: Primary malignant tumors of the upper extremity: Retrospective analysis of one hundred twenty-six cases. J Hand Surg [Am] 10:808–814, 1985.

Doyle LK, Ruby LK, Nalebuff EA, et al: Osteoid osteoma of the hand. J Hand Surg [Am] 10:408–410, 1985.

Fleegler EJ, Zeinowicz RJ: Tumors of the perionychium. Hand Clin 6: 113–133, 1990.

Forthman CL, Blazar PE: Nerve tumors of the hand and upper extremity. Hand Clin 20:233–242, 2004.

Frassica FJ, Amadio PC, Wold LE, et al: Primary malignant bone tumors of the hand. J Hand Surg Am 14:1022–1028, 1989.

Hayden RJ, Sullivan LG, Jebson PJ: The hand in metastatic disease and acral manifestations of paraneoplastic syndromes. Hand Clin 20:335–343, 2004.

Kuur E, Hansen SL, Lindequist S: Treatment of solitary enchondromas in fingers. J Hand Surg [Br] 14:109–112, 1989.

McDermott EM, Weiss AP: Glomus tumors. J Hand Surg [Am] 31: 1397–1400, 2006.

Moore JR, Weiland AJ, Curtis RM: Localized nodular tenosynovitis: Experience with 115 cases. J Hand Surg [Am] 9:412–417, 1984.

Murray PM: Soft tissue sarcoma of the upper extremity. Hand Clin 20: 325–333, 2004.

Nahra ME, Bucchieri JS: Ganglion cysts and other tumor related conditions of the hand and wrist. Hand Clin 20:249–260, 2004.

O'Connor MI, Bancroft LW: Benign and malignant cartilage tumors of the hand. Hand Clin 20:317–323, 2004.

Rock M, Pritchard D, Unni K: Metastases from histologically benign giant cell tumor of bone. J Bone Joint Surg [Am] 64:269–274, 1984.

Sforzo CR, Scarborough MT, Wright TW: Bone-forming tumors of the upper extremity and Ewing's sarcoma. Hand Clin 20:303–315, 2004.

Steinberg B, Gelberman RH, Mankin H, et al: Epithelioid sarcoma in the upper extremity. J Bone Joint Surg [Am] 74:28–35, 1992.

Strickland JW, Steichen JB: Nerve tumors of the hand and forearm. J Hand Surg 2:285–291, 1977.

Walsh EF, Mechrefe A, Akelman E, Schiller AL: Giant cell tumor of tendon sheath. Am J Orthop 34:116–121, 2005.

HAND INFECTIONS

Abrams RA, Botte MJ: Hand infections: Treatment recommendations for specific types. J Am Acad Orthop Surg 4:219–230, 1996.
Chuinard RG, D'Ambrosia RD: Human bite infections of the hand. J Bone Joint Surg [Am] 59:416–418, 1977.
Glickel SZ: Hand infections in patients with acquired immunodeficiency syndrome. J Hand Surg [Am] 13:770–775, 1988.
Gunther SF, Elliott RC, Brand RL, et al: Experience with atypical mycobacterial infection in the deep structures of the hand. J Hand Surg 2:90–96, 1977.
Hitchcock TF, Amadio PC: Fungal infections. Hand Clin 5:599–611, 1989.
Louis DS, Silva J Jr: Herpetic whitlow: Herpetic infections of the digits. J Hand Surg 4:90–94, 1979.
Neviaser RJ: Closed tendon sheath irrigation for pyogenic flexor tenosynovitis. J Hand Surg 3:462–466, 1978.
Schecter W, Meyer A, Schecter G, et al: Necrotizing fasciitis of the upper extremity. J Hand Surg 7:15–19, 1982.

CONGENITAL HAND DIFFERENCES

Blauth W: The hypoplastic thumb. Arch Orthop Unfallchir 62:225–246, 1967.
Buck-Gramcko D: Congenital malformations (editorial). J Hand Surg [Am] 15:150–152, 1990.
Buck-Gramcko D: Pollicization of the index finger. J Bone Joint Surg [Am] 53:1605–1617, 1971.
Buck-Gramcko D: Radialization as a new treatment for radial club hand. J Hand Surg [Am] 10:964–968, 1985.
Cleary JE, Omer GE: Congenital proximal radioulnar synostosis. J Bone Joint Surg [Am] 67:539–545, 1985.
Eaton CJ, Lister GD: Syndactyly. Hand Clin 6:555–575, 1990.
Eaton CJ, Lister GD: Toe transfer for congenital hand defects. Microsurgery 12:186–195, 1991.
Gallant GG, Bora W: Congenital deformities of the upper extremity. J Am Acad Orthop Surg 4:162–171, 1996.
Gilbert A: Toe transfers for congenital hand defects. J Hand Surg 7:118–124, 1982.
Kleinman WB: Management of thumb hypoplasia. Hand Clin 6:617–641, 1990.
Lamb DW: Radial club hand. J Bone Joint Surg [Am] 59:1–13, 1977.
Light TR, Manske PR: Congenital malformations and deformities of the hand. AAOS Instr Course Lect 38:31–71, 1989.
Manske PR, McCarroll HR Jr: Reconstruction of the congenitally deficient thumb. Hand Clin 8:177–196.
Marks TW, Bayne LG: Polydactyly of the thumb: Abnormal anatomy and treatment. J Hand Surg 3:107–116, 1978.
Miller JK, Wenner SM, Kruger LM: Ulnar deficiency. J Hand Surg [Am] 11:822–829, 1986.
Siegert JJ, Cooney WP, Dobyns JH: Management of simple camptodactyly. J Hand Surg [Br] 15:181–189, 1990.
Swanson AB: A classification for congenital limb malformation. J Hand Surg 8:693–702, 1983.
Tada K, Yonenobu K: Duplication of the thumb: A retrospective review of 237 cases. J Bone Joint Surg [Am] 65:584–598, 1983.
Tsuge K: Treatment of macrodactyly. J Hand Surg [Am] 10:968–969, 1985.
Upton J, Tan C: Correction of constriction rings. J Hand Surg [Am] 16: 947–953, 1991.
Weckesser EC: Congenital clasped thumb. J Bone Joint Surg [Am] 37: 1417–1428, 1968.

ELBOW

Armstrong AD, Yamaguchi K: Total elbow arthroplasty and distal humerus elbow fractures. Hand Clin 20:475–483, 2004.
Brunton LM, Anderson MW, Pannunzio ME, et al: Magnetic resonance imaging of the elbow: Update on current techniques and indications. J Hand Surg [Am] 31:1001–1011, 2006.
Calfee R, Madom I, Weiss AP: Radial head arthroplasty. J Hand Surg [Am] 31:314–321, 2006.
Chafik D, Lee TQ, Gupta R: Total elbow arthroplasty: Current indications, factors affecting outcomes, and follow-up results. Am J Orthop 33: 496–503, 2004.
Cohen MS: Fractures of the coronoid process. Hand Clin 20:443–453, 2004.
Ferlic DC, Patchett CE, Clayton ML: Elbow synovectomy in rheumatoid arthritis: Long term results. Clin Orthop 220:119–125, 1987.
King GJ: Management of comminuted radial head fractures with replacement arthroplasty. Hand Clin 20:429–441, 2004.
Mansat P, Morrey BF: The column procedure: A limited lateral approach for extrinsic contracture of the elbow. J Bone Joint Surg [Am] 80: 1603–1615, 1998.
McCarty LP, Ring D, Jupiter JB: Management of distal humerus fractures. Am J Orthop 34:430–438, 2005.
Morrey BF, Askew LJ, An KN, et al: A biomechanical study of normal elbow motion. J Bone Joint Surg [Am] 63:872–877, 1981.
Nirschl RP, Pettrone FA: Tennis elbow. J Bone Joint Surg [Am] 61:832–839, 1979.
O'Driscoll SW: Supracondylar fractures of the elbow: Open reduction, internal fixation. Hand Clin 20:465–474, 2004.
O'Driscoll SW, Bell DF, Morrey BF: Posterolateral rotatory instability of the elbow. J Bone Joint Surg [Am] 73:440–446, 1991.
Steinmann SP, King GJ, Savoie FH III: Arthroscopic treatment of the arthritic elbow. Instr Course Lect 55:109–117, 2006.
Tan V, Daluiski A, Capo J, Hotchkiss R: Hinged elbow external fixators: Indications and uses. J Am Acad Orthop Surg 13:503–514, 2005.
Tashjian RZ, Katarincic JA: Complex elbow instability. J Am Acad Orthop Surg 14:278–286, 2006.

CHAPTER 8

Spine

William C. Lauerman AND Bradley P. Graw

CONTENTS

I. Introduction

A. Anatomy (see Chapter 2, Anatomy)

B. History and physical examination (Table 8–1)—A complete history and physical examination are critical to fully assess complaints and should include evaluation of localized pain (tumor, infection), mechanical pain (instability, discogenic disease), radicular pain (**herniated nucleus pulposus** [HNP], stenosis), night pain (tumor), and systemic symptoms such as fever or unexplained weight loss (infection, tumor). The physical examination must evaluate both the spine and the neurologic function of the extremities (Table 8–2). Localized hip and shoulder pathology may simulate spine disease and must also be evaluated.

C. Objective tests—Plain radiographs should be obtained 4–6 weeks after onset of symptoms; add flexion-extension views for suspected instability. **Magnetic resonance imaging** (MRI) is excellent for further imaging of HNP, stenosis, soft tissue, tumor, and infection. **Computed tomographic** (CT) scans with fine cuts with or without myelographic dye are particularly helpful to examine bony anatomy after previous surgery. A bone scan, which is helpful in evaluating metastatic disease, may be negative with multiple myeloma. Laboratory evaluation consists of C-reactive protein and erythrocyte sedimentation rate for infection; metabolic screening; serum/urine protein electrophoresis for myeloma; and a complete blood count (often a high-normal **white blood cell** [WBC] count with infection, anemia with myeloma).

D. Workup of back pain—Back pain is a ubiquitous complaint, second only to upper respiratory infection as a cause of office visits, with 60-80% lifetime prevalence. The standard workup begins with the history (most important) and progresses to physical examination (see Table 8–1). Radiographic and laboratory studies rarely help in acute case. The following considerations in the evaluation of back pain are important.

1. Age—Children may be affected by congenital or, more often, developmental disorders, infection, or primary tumors. Young adults are more likely to suffer from disc disease, spondylolisthesis, or acute fractures. In older adults, spinal stenosis, metastatic disease, and osteopenic compression fractures are more common.
2. Radicular signs and symptoms—Often associated with disc herniation or spinal stenosis. Intraspinal pathologic conditions or other entities associated with cord or root impingement may be responsible. Herpes zoster is a rare cause of lumbar radiculopathy, with pain preceding the skin eruption.
3. Systemic symptoms—Careful history-taking can lead to the diagnosis of metabolic disease, ankylosing spondylitis (young adults, men more than women), tumor, or infection (confirmed by laboratory studies). Associated signs and symptoms may be essential to the diagnosis (e.g., ophthalmologic symptoms with spondyloarthropathies; other joint involvement with **rheumatoid arthritis** [RA] or

TABLE 8-1 EXAMINATION OF PATIENTS WITH DISORDERS OF THE SPINE

Component	Features
Inspection	Overall alignment in sagittal and coronal planes (sciatic scoliosis)
Gait	Wide-based (myelopathy), forward-leaning (stenosis), antalgic
Palpation	Localized posterior swelling (trauma), acute gibbus deformity, tenderness
Range of motion	Flexion/extension, lateral bend, full versus limited
Neurologic function	Motor, sensory, reflexes, assessment of long-tract signs (see also Table 8–7)
Special tests	Straight-leg raise, Spurling test, Waddell signs of inorganic pathology

osteoarthritis). Metastatic tumor should be considered in patients with a history of cancer, pain at rest, and/or systemic symptoms and in those older than age 50. Many patients with fibromyalgia have chronic back pain often refractory to localized treatment. Fibromyalgia is more common in women and is associated with sleep disturbance, irritable bowel syndrome, and dysmenorrhea. Excessive generalized tenderness on both sides of the midline is the hallmark physical finding.

4. Referred pain—"Back pain" can often be viscerogenic, vascular, or related to other skeletal areas (especially with hip arthritis). Careful history-taking and physical examination are essential. Common sources of referred back pain include peptic ulcer disease, cholecystitis, nephrolithiasis, pancreatitis, pelvic inflammatory disease, and abdominal aortic aneurysm.
5. Psychogenic pain—Psychological disturbances play an important role in some patients with chronic low-back disorders. Evidence of secondary gain (especially workers' compensation or litigation) and inappropriate (Waddell) signs, symptoms, and maneuvers can help identify these patients. Nevertheless, one must be wary of real pathologic conditions, even in such patients.
6. History of back pain—Perhaps the most important risk factor for future pain, especially with frequent disabling episodes and short intervals between episodes. Availability of workers' compensation, history of smoking, and age over 30 are also associated with the development of persistent, disabling lower back pain. The incidence of disabling pain declines after age 60.

II. Cervical Spine

A. Cervical spondylosis—Chronic disc degeneration and associated facet arthropathy. The resulting syndromes include discogenic neck pain (axial pain), radiculopathy (root compromise), myelopathy (cord compression), and combinations of these conditions.

1. Epidemiology—Cervical spondylosis typically begins between the ages of 40 and 50, is seen in men more than women, and occurs at the C5-C6 level more frequently than at the C6-C7 level. Risk factors include frequent lifting, cigarette smoking, and a history of excessive driving.
2. Pathoanatomy—Cervical spondylosis involves the disc and four other articulations (Fig. 8–1): two facet joints and two uncovertebral joints (of Luschka). The facet joint capsules are known to have sensory receptors that may play a role in pain and proprioceptive sensation in the cervical spine. The cervical cord becomes compromised when the diameter of the canal (normally about 17 mm) is reduced to less than 13 mm (measurable on a plain lateral radiograph). With neck extension, the cord is pinched between the degenerative disc and spondylotic bar anteriorly and the hypertrophic facets and infolded ligamentum flavum posteriorly. With neck flexion, the canal dimension increases slightly to relieve pressure on the cord. Progressive collapse of the cervical discs results in loss of normal lordosis of the cervical spine and chronic anterior cord compression across the kyphotic spine/anterior chondro-osseous spurs. Spondylotic changes in the foramina, primarily from chondro-osseous spurs of the joints of Luschka, may restrict motion and lead to nerve root compression. Soft-disc herniation is usually posterolateral, between the posterior edge of the uncinate process and the lateral edge of the posterior longitudinal ligament, resulting in acute radiculopathy. Anterior herniation may cause dysphagia (rare). Myelopathy may be seen with large central herniation or spondylotic bars with a congenitally narrow canal. Ossification of the posterior longitudinal ligament, resulting in cervical stenosis and myelopathy, is common in Asians but may also be seen in non-Asians.

TABLE 8-2 FINDINGS IN NERVE ROOT COMPRESSION

Level	Root	Muscles Affected	Sensory Loss	Reflex
C3-C4	C4	Scapular	Lateral neck, shoulder	None
C4-C5	C5	Deltoid, biceps	Lateral arm	Biceps
C5-C6*	C6	Wrist extensors, biceps, triceps (supination)	Radial forearm	Brachioradialis
C6-C7	C7	Triceps, wrist flexors (pronation)	Middle finger	Triceps
C7-C8	C8	Finger flexors, interossei	Ulnar hand	None
C8-T1	T1	Interossei	Ulnar forearm	None

*Most common level.

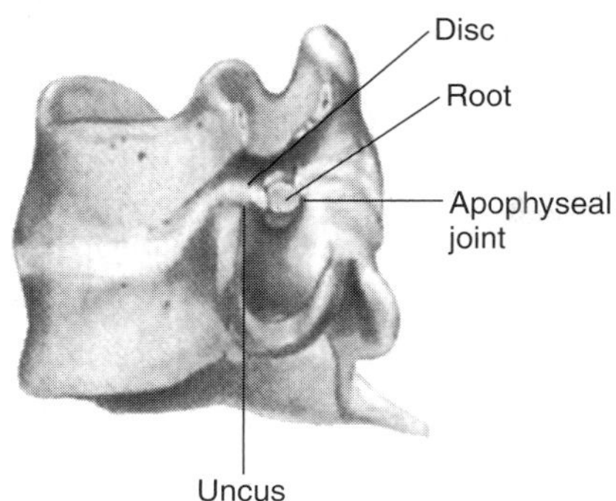

FIGURE 8–1 Cervical root impingement. (From Rothman RH, Simeone FA: The Spine, 2nd ed, p 452. Philadelphia, WB Saunders, 1982.)

3. Signs and symptoms—Degenerative discogenic neck pain may present with the insidious onset of neck pain without neurologic signs or symptoms, exacerbated by excess vertebral motion. Occipital headache is common. Radiculopathy can involve one or multiple roots, and symptoms include neck, shoulder, and arm pain; paresthesias; and numbness. Findings may overlap because of intraneural intersegmental connections of sensory nerve roots. Mechanical stress such as excessive vertebral motion, in particular rotation and lateral bend with a vertical compressive force (Spurling test), may exacerbate these symptoms. The lower nerve root at a given level is usually affected (see Table 8–2). Myelopathy may be characterized by weakness (upper more than lower extremity); decreased manual dexterity; an ataxic, broad-based, shuffling gait; sensory changes; spasticity; and (rarely) urinary retention. The most worrisome complaint is lower extremity weakness (corticospinal tracts). Patients may complain of urinary urgency or frequency. A "myelopathy hand" and the "finger escape sign" (small finger spontaneously abducts because of weak intrinsic muscles) suggest cervical myelopathy. Upper motor neuron findings such as hyperreflexia, the Hoffmann sign, inverted radial reflex (ipsilateral finger flexion when eliciting the brachioradialis reflex), clonus, or the Babinski sign may be present. Additionally, the upper extremities may have radicular (lower motor neuron) signs along with evidence of distal myelopathy. Funicular pain, characterized by central burning and stinging with or without the Lhermitte sign (radiating lightning-like sensations down the back with neck flexion), may also be present with myelopathy.
4. Diagnosis—Largely based on history and physical examination.
   a. Radiographs—Plain radiographs, including oblique views, should be assessed for changes in uncovertebral and facet joints, alignment, osteophytes (bars), and disc space narrowing and to measure the diameter of the sagittal canal. However, radiographic changes of the degenerated cervical spine may not correlate with symptoms: by the age of 70, 70% of patients will have degenerative changes on x-ray film.
   b. Other imaging studies—CT myelography or MRI effectively demonstrates neural compressive pathology, although false-positive MRI scans are common: 25% of asymptomatic patients over age 40 will have findings of either HNP or foraminal stenosis on cervical MRI. Therefore, correlation with history and physical examination is critical. MRI is also useful for detecting intrinsic changes in the spinal cord (myelomalacia—area of bright signal in the cord on T2) as well as disc degeneration. Discography is controversial and rarely used for cervical spine disorders.
   c. Electrodiagnostic studies—These have a high false-negative rate but may be helpful in select cases for differentiating peripheral nerve compression from radiculopathy and for detecting systemic neurologic disorders such as amyotrophic lateral sclerosis.
5. Nonsurgical treatment—**Nonsteroidal anti-inflammatory drugs** (NSAIDs), extraforaminal cervical nerve blocks, moist heat, cervical isometric exercises, the use of a collar, traction, and pain clinic modalities are helpful in most cases of discogenic neck pain and radiculopathy. Extraforaminal nerve blocks have been shown to be safe in large series of patients, with a less than 2% rate of minor complications.
6. Surgical treatment
   a. Indications—Indications for surgery include myelopathy with motor/gait impairment and radiculopathy with persistent, disabling pain and weakness. Surgery for discogenic neck pain is less rewarding.
   b. Procedures—Combined anterior (cervical) Smith-Robinson diskectomy and fusion (ACDF) is the preferred technique. Posterior foraminotomy is useful for single-level radiculopathy. For multilevel spondylosis and myelopathy, more extensive decompression is necessary. The anterior approach involves excision of osteophytes and corpectomy with a strut graft fusion with or without instrumentation. Anterior plating may increase the fusion rate in multilevel diskectomies with fusion and will protect a strut graft in multilevel corpectomies, although plating may actually contribute to nonunion after strut grafting. Adjunctive posterior plating may be employed in cases involving prior laminectomy or after multilevel corpectomy and strut grafting. Three-level ACDF with plating shows a 70% failure rate and should be supported with posterior instrumentation. Posterior approaches include canal-expansive laminoplasty (commonly used for ossification of the posterior longitudinal ligament), which can help decrease the incidence of instability associated with multilevel laminectomy.

Overall alignment should be lordotic for this approach to be successful.

c. Results and complications—Laminoplasty has been found to limit **range of motion** (ROM) postoperatively and has a significant rate of axial neck pain as well. Multilevel laminectomy may fail owing to failure to adequately relieve anterior compression or secondary to progressive kyphosis, which may require anterior decompression and fusion with a strut graft for salvage. Successful anterior decompression and fusion result in 70-90% improvement in pain and neurologic function. Complications of the anterior approach include neurologic injury (< 1%) and pseudarthrosis of 12% for single-level fusions, 30% for multilevel fusions (treated with posterior wiring or plating or repeat anterior fusion with plating if symptomatic), upper airway obstruction after multilevel corpectomy, and injury to other neck structures, including the recurrent laryngeal nerve (increased with right-sided approach). The complications of laminectomy include subluxation if the facets are sacrificed, leading to a swan-neck deformity, muscle ischemia, and direct spinal cord injury with quadriparesis. Radicular symptoms may be alleviated after decompression, but gait changes may not.

B. Cervical stenosis—May be congenital or acquired (traumatic, degenerative). Absolute stenosis (anteroposterior canal diameter < 10 mm) or relative stenosis (anteroposterior canal diameter 10- to 13-mm) predisposes the patient to the development of radiculopathy, myelopathy, or both from relatively minor soft- or hard-disc pathology or trauma. The Pavlov (Torg) ratio (canal/vertebral body width) should be 1.0. A ratio of less than 0.80 or a sagittal diameter of < 13 mm is considered a significant risk factor for later neurologic involvement. Minor trauma such as hyperextension may lead to a central cord syndrome, even without overt skeletal injury. In relative stenosis, radicular symptoms usually predominate. CT myelography and MRI are helpful. Evaluation may include somatosensory evoked potentials, which help identify cord compromise in absolute stenosis. Surgery may serve a prophylactic function but is usually reserved for patients who develop myelopathy or radiculopathy. The surgical approaches are similar to those previously described.

C. Rheumatoid spondylitis

1. Overview—Cervical spine involvement is common in RA (occurring in up to 90% of patients) and is more common with long-standing disease and multiple joint involvement. Neck pain, decreased ROM, crepitation, and occipital headaches are the most common complaints. Neurologic impairment (weakness, decreased sensation, hyperreflexia) in patients with RA usually occurs gradually and is often overlooked or attributed to other joint disease. Neurologic impairment with RA has been classified by Ranawat (Table 8–3). Surgery may not reverse significant neurologic deterioration, especially if a tight spinal canal is present, but it can stabilize it. Therefore, it is essential to look for subtle signs of early neurologic involvement and assess the **space available for the cord** (SAC), also known as the **posterior atlanto–dens interval** (PADI). Indications for surgical stabilization are instability, pain, neurologic deficit owing to neural compression, impending neurologic deficit (based on objective studies), and/or some combination of these conditions. Patients with RA should have flexion/extension films before elective surgery.

TABLE 8-3 RANAWAT'S CLASSIFICATION OF NEUROLOGIC IMPAIRMENT IN RA

Grade	Characteristics
I	Subjective paresthesias, pain
II	Subjective weakness; upper motor neuron findings
III	Objective weakness; upper motor neuron findings
IIIA	Ambulatory
IIIB	Nonambulatory

2. Atlantoaxial subluxation—Usually occurs in 50-80% of cases of RA. This condition is often the result of pannus formation at the synovial joints between the dens and the ring of C1, resulting in destruction of the transverse ligament, the dens, or both.

   a. Diagnosis—Anterior subluxation of C1 on C2 is the most common finding, but posterior and lateral subluxation can also occur. Findings on examination may include limitation of motion, upper motor neuron signs, and weakness. Plain radiographs that include patient-controlled flexion and extension views are evaluated to determine the **anterior atlanto–dens interval** (AADI) as well as the PADI. Instability is present with motion of more than 3.5 mm on flexion and extension views, although radiographic instability in RA is common and not necessarily an indication for surgery. C1-C2 motion of more than 9-10 mm or a PADI of less than 14 mm is associated with an increased risk of neurologic injury and usually requires surgical treatment. Myelopathy, progressive neurologic impairment, and progressive instability are also indications for surgical stabilization, usually a posterior C1-C2 fusion.

   b. Treatment—Transarticular screw fixation (Magerl) across C1-C2 eliminates the need for halo immobilization associated with wiring, but preoperative CT must be assessed to evaluate the position of the vertebral arteries. Atlantoaxial subluxation that is not reducible may require removal of the posterior arch of C1 for cord decompression followed by occiput–C2 fusion. Anterior cord compression because of pannus often resolves after **posterior spinal fusion** (PSF); odontoidectomy should be reserved as a secondary procedure and is only rarely necessary. Surgery is less successful in Ranawat grade IIIB patients but should be considered. Complications include pseudarthrosis (10-20%) and adjacent segment involvement on long-term follow-up. Extension of the fusion to the occiput lessens the nonunion rate. An SAC of less than 14 mm is a relative indication for prophylactic fusion, even in the absence of myelopathy.

3. Cranial settling (basilar invagination)—The second most common manifestation of RA (occurring in 40% of patients with RA). There is cranial migration of the dens from erosion and bone loss between the occiput and C1-C2. This condition is often seen in combination with fixed atlantoaxial subluxation. Measurements are shown in Figure 8–2. Landmarks may be difficult to identify, with the Ranawat line probably the most easily reproducible. Progressive cranial migration (> 5 mm) or neurologic compromise may require operative intervention (occiput–C2 fusion). Somatosensory evoked potentials may be helpful in evaluation. When brainstem compromise with functional impairment is significant, transoral or anterior retropharyngeal odontoid resection may be required. If there is any suggestion of cranial settling in cases of **atlantoaxial subluxation** (AAS), occipitocervical fusion is the conservative approach.
4. Subaxial subluxation—Occurs in 20% of cases of RA. It is commonly seen in combination with instability of the upper cervical spine. Because the joints of Luschka and facet joints are affected by RA, subluxation may occur at multiple levels. Involvement of the lower cervical spine is more common in males, with steroid use, with seropositive RA, in patients with rheumatoid nodules, and in those with severe RA. Subaxial subluxation of greater than 4 mm or more than 20% of the body is indicative of cord compression. A cervical height index (cervical body height/width) of less than 2.00 approaches 100% sensitivity and specificity in predicting neurologic compromise. Posterior fusion and wiring are sometimes required for subluxation greater than 4 mm with intractable pain and neurologic compromise.

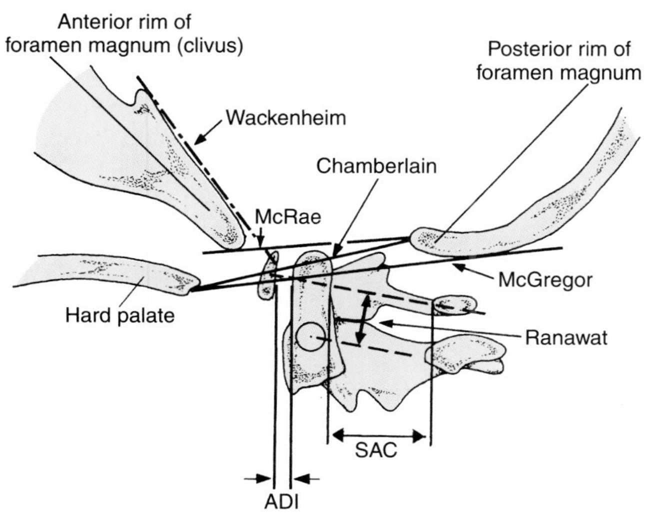

FIGURE 8–2 Common measurements in C1-C2 disorders. ADI, atlanto-dens interval; SAC, space available for the cord.

D. Cervical spine and cord injuries—See Chapter 11, Trauma, for classification and treatment of cervical spine injuries.

1. Epidemiology—Spinal cord injuries usually occur in young males involved in motor vehicle accidents, falls, and diving accidents. Gunshot wounds are an increasing cause. The findings may be subtle; the significant morbidity and mortality rates associated with missed injuries have led to the current emphasis on cervical spine protection after polytrauma. Missed cervical spine injuries are the most common in the presence of a decreased level of consciousness, alcohol/drug intoxication, and head injury and in patients with multiple injuries.
2. Progression of injury
   a. Spinal shock—Spinal shock usually involves a 24- to 72-hour period of paralysis, hypotonia, and areflexia. At its conclusion, spasticity, hyperreflexia, and clonus progress over days to weeks. The return of the bulbocavernosus reflex (anal sphincter contraction in response to squeezing the glans penis or tugging on the Foley catheter) signifies the end of spinal shock; for complete injuries, further neurologic improvement is minimal. Injuries below the thoracolumbar level (conus or cauda equina) may permanently interrupt the bulbocavernosus reflex.
   b. Neurogenic shock and hypovolemic shock—Neurogenic shock (secondary to loss of sympathetic tone) can be differentiated from hypovolemic shock based on the presence of relative bradycardia in neurogenic shock, in contrast to the presence of tachycardia and hypotension in hypovolemic shock. Swan-Ganz monitoring is helpful in this setting because neurogenic and hypovolemic shock often occur concurrently. Hypovolemic shock is treated with fluid resuscitation, whereas selective vasopressors are effective in neurogenic shock.
3. Physical and neurologic examination—Facial injuries, hypotension, and localized tenderness or spasm should be investigated. A careful neurologic examination to document the lowest remaining functional level and to assess the patient for the possibility of sacral sparing (sparing of posterior column function, indicating an incomplete spinal cord injury) is essential. The neurologic level, as defined by the standards of the American Spine Association, is the most caudal level with normal bilateral motor and sensory function.

4. Radiographic evaluation—Radiographic evaluation includes a complete cervical spine series (C1-T1), as multiple-level injuries occur in 10-20% of cases, and oblique views to investigate facet subluxation, dislocations, or fractures. Tomograms to evaluate dens fractures and facet joint injuries may be helpful. On the lateral view, 85% of cervical spine fractures are detected. CT scanning is useful for evaluating C1 fractures and assessing bone in the canal but may miss an axial plane fracture (type II odontoid). Fine-cut CT scanning is employed to assess areas of the cervical spine poorly visualized on plain film in the initial trauma workup. Myelography may be used in patients with an otherwise unexplained neurologic deficit. MRI has advantages for demonstrating posterior ligamentous disruption, disc herniation, canal compromise, and the status of the spinal cord.
5. Cord injuries—Cord injuries may be complete (no function below a given level) or incomplete (with some sparing of distal function). Most cord injury is due to contusion or compression, not transection. Sustained cord compression can lead to secondary injury and may result in more limited functional recovery. With complete injuries, an improvement of one nerve root level can be expected in 80% of the patients, and approximately 20% recover two functioning root levels. Several categories of incomplete lesions exist. These syndromes are classified based on the area of the spinal cord that has been the most severely damaged. A summary of the syndromes is presented in Table 8–4.
   a. Central cord syndrome—The most common, often seen in patients with preexisting cervical spondylosis who sustain a hyperextension injury. The cord is compressed anteriorly by osteophytes and posteriorly by the infolded ligamentum flavum. The cord is injured in the central gray matter, which results in proportionately greater loss of motor function to the upper extremities than to the lower extremities, with variable sensory sparing.
   b. Anterior cord syndrome—The second most common cord injury, in which the damage is primarily in the anterior two thirds of the cord, sparing the posterior columns (proprioception and vibratory sensation). These patients demonstrate greater motor loss in the legs than the arms. CT scan may demonstrate bony fragments compressing the anterior cord. The anterior cord syndrome has the worst prognosis.
   c. The Brown-Séquard syndrome—This damages half of the cord, causing ipsilateral motor loss, loss of position/proprioception, contralateral pain, and temperature loss (usually two levels below the insult). This injury, usually the result of penetrating trauma, has the best prognosis.
   d. Single-root lesions—These can occur at the level of the fracture, usually C5 or C6, leading to deltoid or biceps weakness; they are usually unilateral.
6. Treatment—See Chapter 11, Trauma.
   a. Medical treatment—For spinal cord injury presenting within 8 hours without contraindications, a bolus dose of methylprednisolone (30 mg/kg) should be given initially and then a drip (5.4 mg/kg) each hour for 23 hours if started within 3 hours or for 47 hours otherwise. Relative contraindications include pregnancy, age younger than 13 years, concomitant infection, penetrating spinal wounds, and uncontrolled diabetes. Gastrointestinal prophylaxis should be given.
   b. Other treatment—Immobilization is achieved with a collar for undisplaced, stable fractures, and with skeletal traction, a halo vest, or surgery for unstable fractures. Skeletal traction is applied immediately to realign the spine in the presence of a displaced fracture with or without neurologic injury. Skeletal traction requires the placement of Gardner-Wells tongs (pins parallel to the external auditory meatus) and the addition of 5-10 pounds initially, with 5-7 pounds per cervical level, with sequential radiographs between the additions of weight. Anterior decompression for incomplete injuries with persistent cord compression can lead to improvement of one to three levels, even with complete injuries. Also, stabilization may be indicated. Late decompression for up to 1 year may be effective in improving root return. Laminectomies are contraindicated except in the rare case of posterior compression from a fractured lamina.

TABLE 8-4 SPINAL CORD INJURY SYNDROMES

Syndrome	Pathology	Characteristics	Prognosis
Central	Age > 50, extension injuries	Affects upper > lower extremities; motor and sensory loss	Fair
Anterior	Flexion-compression	Incomplete motor and some sensory loss	Poor
Brown-Séquard	Penetrating trauma	Loss of ipsilateral motor function, contralateral pain, and temperature sensation	Best
Root	Foramina compression/herniated nucleus pulposus	Based on level (weakness)	Good
Complete	Burst/canal compression	No function below injury level	Poor

Gunshot injury to the spine is treated surgically if there is progression of neurologic injury or if the bullet rests in the spinal canal. Otherwise, these injuries should receive nonoperative treatment. Injuries accompanied by gastrointestinal perforation should be treated with antibiotics for 7-14 days.

7. Complications—Potentially negative outcomes are numerous and include neurologic injury, nonunion, and malunion. Autonomic dysreflexia can follow cervical and upper thoracic spinal cord injuries. It is commonly related to bladder overdistention or fecal impaction and is manifested by a pounding headache (from severe hypertension), anxiety, profuse head and neck sweating, nasal obstruction, and blurred vision. Urinary catheterization or amelioration of rectal impaction and supportive treatment usually relieve the symptoms. Instability in the cervical spine can occur late and is associated with greater than 3.5 mm of subluxation and greater than 11 degrees of difference in angulation between adjacent motion segments.
8. Prognosis—The Frankel classification is useful when assessing functional recovery from spinal cord injury (Table 8–5).

E. Sports-related cervical spine injuries
   1. Burner (stinger) syndrome—Common injury associated with stretching of the upper brachial plexus by bending the neck away from the depressed shoulder or neck extension toward the painful shoulder in the setting of foraminal stenosis (root irritation). The athlete will complain of burning dysesthesia with weakness in the involved extremity. Fracture or acute HNP should be ruled out. The athlete with a neck injury should be further evaluated for cervical pain, tenderness, or persisting neurologic symptoms.
   2. Transient quadriplegia—Usually seen after axial load injury (spearing) but may also be seen after forced hyperextension or hyperflexion. Transient quadriplegia presents with bilateral burning paresthesia and weakness or paralysis. There is an increased association with cervical stenosis (Torg ratio, < 0.8) as well as instability, HNP, and congenital fusions. The third and fourth cervical levels are the most commonly affected. It has no definitive association with future permanent neurologic injury. Patients with concurrent pathologic conditions, including instability, HNP, degenerative changes, and symptoms that last more than 36 hours, should be prohibited from contact sports.

TABLE 8-5 FRANKEL CLASSIFICATION OF CERVICAL SPINE INJURIES

Frankel Grade	Function
A	Complete paralysis
B	Sensory function only below injury level
C	Incomplete motor function (grades 1-2 of 5) below injury level
D	Fair to good (useful) motor function (grades 3-4 of 5) below injury level
E	Normal function (grade 5 of 5)

F. Other cervical spine problems—Ankylosing spondylitis and neuromyopathic conditions can cause severe flexion deformities of the cervical spine.
   1. Ankylosing spondylitis—Patients with ankylosing spondylitis must be carefully evaluated for occult fracture because of the problem of pseudarthrosis and progressive kyphotic deformity. A severe chin-on-chest deformity in ankylosing spondylitis, with the inability to look straight ahead, occasionally represents a major functional limitation and is often associated with severe hip flexion contractures as well as a flexion deformity of the lumbar spine. Treatment usually begins by addressing the hip and lumbar disorder but may ultimately require cervicothoracic laminectomy, osteotomy, and fusion for correction of the neck deformity. This procedure is performed under local anesthesia with brief general anesthesia, and postoperative immobilization is carried out in a halo cast.
   2. Neuromyopathic conditions—Traction, surgical release of contracted sternocleidomastoid muscles, and posterior fusion are sometimes required for severe neuromyopathic conditions. Internal fixation should be used in these cases to prevent subluxation, delayed union, nonunion, loss of correction, or neurologic injury. This treatment can reliably improve sagittal balance and horizontal gaze as well as help decrease neck pain, eating problems, and neurologic decline.

III. Thoracic/Lumbar Spine

A. Differential diagnosis—The physical examination, imaging studies, and laboratory tests assist with the differential diagnosis (Table 8–6).

B. Herniated nucleus pulposus
   1. Introduction—Disc degeneration with aging includes loss of water content, annular tearing, and myxomatous changes, resulting in herniation of nuclear material. Changes in proteoglycan metabolism, secondary immunologic factors, and structural factors also play a role. Discs can protrude (bulging nucleus, intact annulus), extrude (through the annulus but confined by the posterior longitudinal ligament), or be sequestrated (disc material free in canal). HNP is usually a disease of young and middle-aged adults; in older patients the disc nucleus desiccates and is less likely to herniate.
   2. Thoracic disc disease—Relatively uncommon (1% of all HNPs), it usually involves the middle to lower thoracic levels, with most herniations occurring at T11-T12 and 75% occurring at T8-T12. Thoracic HNP can be divided into central, posterolateral, and lateral herniations.

TABLE 8-6 DIFFERENTIAL DIAGNOSIS OF DISORDERS IN THE LUMBAR SPINE

	Disorder						
Parameter	*HNP*	*Spinal Stenosis*	*Spondylolisthesis/ Instability*	*Tumor*	*Spondyloarthropathy*	*Metabolic Abnormality*	*Infection*
Predominant pain (leg versus back)	Leg	Leg	Back	Back	Back	Back	Back
Constitutional symptoms				+	+		+
Tension sign	+						
Neurologic examination		+	+ after stress				
Plain x-ray studies		+	+	±	+	+	±
Lateral motion x-ray studies				+			
CT scan	+	+		+			+
Myelogram	+	+					
Bone scan				+	+	+	+
ESR				+	+		+
Ca/P/alk phos				+			

Ca/P/alk phos, calcium, phosphorus, alkaline phosphatase; CT, computed tomography; ESR, erythrocyte sedimentation rate; HNP, herniated nucleus pulposus; +, present; ±, present or absent.

Modified from Weinstein JN, Wiesel SW: The Lumbar Spine, p 360. Philadelphia, WB Saunders, 1990.

a. Diagnosis—It usually presents with the onset of back or chest pain that may progress to radicular symptoms (bandlike chest or abdominal discomfort, numbness, paresthesias, leg pain) and/or myelopathy (sensory changes, paraparesis, bowel/bladder/sexual dysfunction). Physical findings may be difficult to elicit but may include localized tenderness, sensory pinprick level, upper motor neuron signs with leg hyperreflexia, weakness, and an abnormal rectal examination (with normal upper extremity findings). Radiographs may show disc narrowing and calcification or osteophytic lipping. Underlying Scheuermann disease may predispose patients to develop HNP. CT myelography or MRI should demonstrate thoracic HNP. MRI is useful for ruling out cord disorder, but there is a high false-positive rate, requiring close clinical correlation.

b. Treatment—Immobilization, analgesics, and nerve blocks are sometimes helpful for radiculopathy. Surgery, usually performed through an anterior transthoracic approach or costotransversectomy (including anterior diskectomy and hemicorporectomy as needed), is recommended in the presence of myelopathy or persistent, unremitting pain with documented pathologic conditions. Thoracoscopic diskectomy can also be employed. The posterior approach to a thoracic HNP is contraindicated because of the high rate of neurologic injury.

3. Lumbar disc disease

a. Introduction—A major cause of morbidity with a major financial impact in the United States. This disc disease usually involves the L4-L5 disc (the "backache disc"), followed closely by L5-S1. Most herniations are posterolateral (where the posterior longitudinal ligament is the weakest) and may present with back pain and nerve root pain/sciatica involving the lower nerve root at that level (L5 at the L4-L5 level). Central prolapse is often associated with back pain only; however, acute insults may precipitate a cauda equina compression syndrome (Fig. 8–3). This syndrome is a surgical emergency that usually presents with bilateral buttock and lower extremity pain as well as bowel or bladder dysfunction (usually urinary retention), saddle anesthesia, and varying degrees of loss of lower extremity motor or sensory function. Digital rectal examination and evaluation of perianal sensation are important for the immediate diagnosis. Immediate myelography (or MRI) and surgery (if the test results are positive) are indicated in order to arrest progression of neurologic loss, although the prognosis for recovery is guarded in most cases.

b. Patient history—An acute injury or precipitating event should be sought, and the location of symptoms (especially pain radiating to the extremity), the character of pain, postural changes (neurogenic claudication), the effect of increased intrathecal pressure, and a complete review of symptoms (including psychiatric history) should be elicited. Occupational risks, such as those associated with jobs requiring prolonged sitting and repetitive lifting, are also important factors.

c. Physical examination—Intradiscal pressure is the lowest when one lies in the supine position and the highest when one sits and is flexed forward with weights in hands. Referred pain in mesodermal tissues of the same embryologic origin, often to the buttocks or posterior thighs, must be differentiated from true radicular pain due to nerve root impingement, with symptoms that

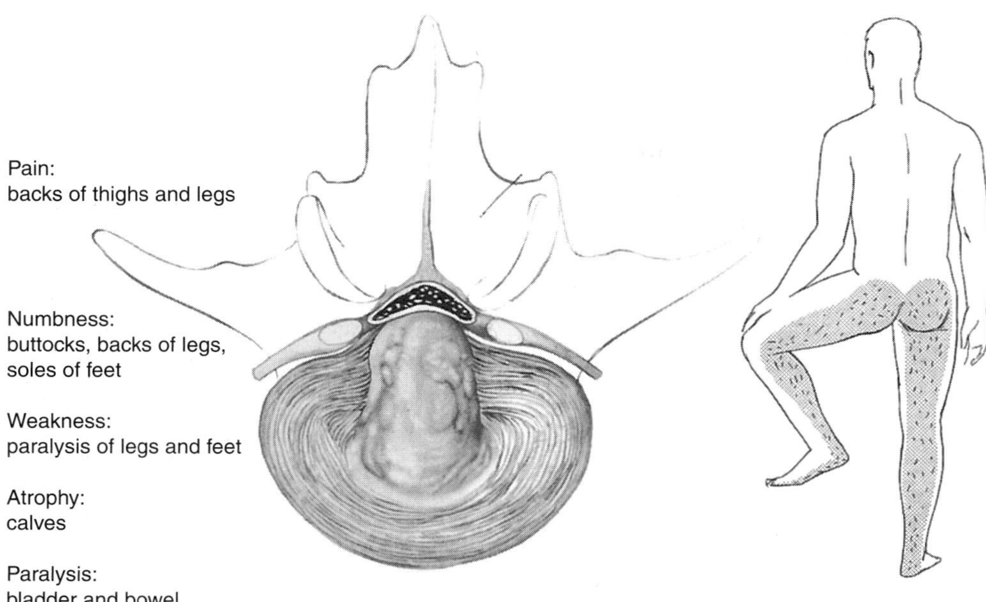

FIGURE 8–3 Cauda equina syndrome. (From DePalma AF, Rothman RH: The Intervertebral Disc, p 194. Philadelphia, WB Saunders, 1970.)

typically reach distal to the knee. Psychosocial evaluation, pain drawings, and psychological testing are helpful in some cases. The finding of an "inverted V" triad of hysteria, hypochondriasis, and depression on the Minnesota Multiphasic Personality Inventory has been identified as a significant adverse risk factor in lumbar disc surgery. Physical examination should include observation (change in posture, gait), palpation of the posterior spine (spasm, localized tenderness), measurement of ROM (decreased flexion), hip examination, vascular evaluation (distal pulses), abdominal and rectal examinations, and neurologic evaluation. Tension signs such as straight-leg raising or the bowstring sign (L4-L5 or L5-S1) and the femoral nerve stretch test (L2-L3 or L3-L4) are important findings that suggest HNP and are essential when a candidate for diskectomy is considered. A positive contralateral straight-leg raising test (pain in the affected buttock/leg when the opposite leg is raised) is the most specific test for HNP. Specific findings by level are presented in Table 8–7. A large central disc herniation at one level may impinge on more than one nerve root. Inappropriate signs and symptoms (Waddell) are also important to note. Inappropriate symptoms include pain at the tip of the "tailbone," pain plus numbness, and giving way of the whole leg. Nonorganic physical signs include tenderness with light touch in nonanatomic areas, simulation (light axial loading), distraction testing, pain with pelvic rotation, a negative sitting (and positive supine) straight-leg raising test, regional nonanatomic disturbances (such as a stocking-glove distribution), and overreaction.

d. Diagnostic tests
   (1) Plain radiography—Plain radiographs are indicated before proceeding with special tests to rule out other disorders, such as isthmic defects. However, most plain radiographic findings are nonspecific, and plain radiography can usually be deferred for 6 weeks.
   (2) CT and myelography—These are effective when used as confirmatory studies.

TABLE 8–7 FINDINGS IN LUMBAR DISC DISEASE

Level	Nerve Root	Sensory Loss	Motor Loss	Reflex Loss
L1-L3	L2,L3	Anterior thigh	Hip flexors	None
L3-L4	L4	Medial calf	Quadriceps, tibialis anterior	Knee jerk
L4-L5	L5	Lateral calf, dorsal foot	EDL, EHL	None
L5-S1	S1	Posterior calf, plantar foot	Gastrocnemius/soleus	Ankle jerk
S2-S4	S2,S3,S4	Perianal	Bowel/bladder	Cremasteric

EDL, extensor digitorum longus; EHL, extensor hallucis longus.

CT is noninvasive and helpful for demonstrating bony stenosis and identifying lateral pathologic conditions. Imaging of neural compression may be improved if combined with myelography.

(3) MRI—MRI is the neuroradiographic test of choice in most cases and is superior for identifying cord disorders, neural tumors, and disc disorders. It is noninvasive, involves no ionizing radiation, and gives a "myelogram" effect on the T2 images. Multiplanar views allow imaging of central, foraminal, and extraforaminal stenosis. In addition, MRI demonstrates the state of hydration of the discs and visualizes the marrow of the vertebral bodies, thus representing an excellent modality to screen for tumor or infection. False-positive MRI is common (occurring in 35% of those < 40 years old and in 93% of those > 60 years old) and therefore requires correlation with the history and physical examination. MRI is the imaging modality of choice for most back disorders.

(4) Other testing—**Electromyography** (EMG) and **nerve conduction velocity** (NCV) testing (which demonstrate fibrillations 3 weeks after nerve root pressure) are not usually helpful and rarely provide more information than a good physical examination. Thermography does not have proven efficacy in the evaluation of disc disease or any other disorder of the spine.

e. Nonoperative treatment—Activity modification, NSAIDs, moist heat, and progressive ambulation are successful in returning most patients to their normal function. Bed rest is shown to be no more effective than continued normal activity in terms of patient improvement. More than half of the patients who seek treatment for low-back pain recover in 1 week, and 90% recover within 1-3 months. Half of the patients with sciatica recover in 1 month. This treatment is followed by back rehabilitation and a fitness program. Aerobic conditioning and education are the most important factors in avoiding missed workdays due to disc disease and returning patients to work. Instruction should include avoiding rotation and flexion to avoid the increased disc pressure associated with these activities. If patients fail to improve within 6 weeks of conservative care, further evaluation is indicated. Those patients with predominantly low-back pain may require bone scan, MRI, and medical workup to rule out spinal tumors or infection. If these study results are normal, back rehabilitation will continue. In patients who have predominantly leg pain (sciatica) and in whom conservative therapy fails, a trial of lumbar epidural steroids may be helpful, although they are helpful in only 40-60% of patients. Additional studies (CT [with or without myelogram] or MRI) are undertaken in patients who after 6-12 weeks continue to be symptomatic with pain, neurologic deficits, and positive nerve tension signs. As a rule, these studies are preoperative tests and should be done to confirm clinical suspicions.

f. Surgical diskectomy—Patients with positive study results, neurologic findings, tension signs, and predominantly sciatic symptoms without mitigating psychosocial factors are the best candidates for surgical diskectomy. Standard partial laminotomy and diskectomy are the most commonly performed surgical procedures. Operative positioning requires the abdomen to be free to decrease pressure on the inferior vena cava and consequently on the epidural veins. With the proper indications, 95% of patients have initially good or excellent results, although as many as 15-20% of patients have significant backache on long-term follow-up. Patient prognosis depends on the anatomy of the disc at surgery, with recurrence rates being higher for patients with massive posterior annulus loss or without a contained defect (20-40%). Contained disc defects or disc fissuring correlates with better clinical outcomes and lower recurrence of symptoms (1-10%).

g. Minimally invasive surgical treatment—Percutaneous diskectomy currently has limited indications in the treatment of lumbar disc disease, with no long-term follow-up studies proving its efficacy. It is contraindicated in the presence of a sequestered fragment or spinal stenosis. Endoscopic diskectomy does allow direct visualization and can address sequestered fragments and lateral recess stenosis. Intradiscal enzyme therapy has fallen out of favor because of its questionable efficacy and serious complications (anaphylaxis and transverse myelitis). The indications for all of these minimally invasive treatments for disc herniations (leg pain, tension signs, neurologic deficits, positive study results) are similar to those for open surgery.

h. Complications—Fortunately rare, but can be devastating.

4. Vascular injury—May occur during attempts at disc removal if curettes are allowed to penetrate the anterior longitudinal ligament. Intraoperative pulsatile bleeding due to deep penetration is treated with rapid wound closure, intravenous fluids and blood, repositioning the patient, and a transabdominal approach to find and stop the source of bleeding. Mortality may exceed 50%.

Late sequelae of vascular injuries may include delayed hemorrhage, pseudoaneurysm, and arteriovenous fistula formation.

5. Nerve root injury—More common with anomalous nerve roots. Dural tears (1-4% incidence) should be repaired primarily when they occur to avoid the development of a pseudomeningocele or spinal fluid fistula. Adequate exposure as well as hemostasis, proper lighting, magnification, and a careful surgical technique is important for diminishing the incidence of the "battered root syndrome."
6. Failed back syndrome—Often the result of poor patient selection, but other causes include recurrent herniation (usually acute recurrence of signs/symptoms after a 6- to 12-month pain-free interval), herniation at another level, diskitis (3-6 weeks postoperatively, with rapid onset of severe back pain), unrecognized lateral stenosis (may be the most common), and vertebral instability. Epidural fibrosis occurs at about 3 months postoperatively and may be associated with back or leg pain; it responds poorly to re-exploration. Scarring can be differentiated from recurrent HNP with a gadolinium-enhanced MRI.
7. Dural tear—More common during revision surgery; it should be repaired immediately if it is recognized. Fibrin adhesive sealant may be a useful adjunct for effecting dural closure. Bed rest and subarachnoid drain placement are advocated if cerebrospinal fluid leak is suspected postoperatively.
8. Wound infection (approximately 1% in open diskectomy)—Similar to infection elsewhere. There is an increased risk in diabetics. Incision and drainage and removal of loose graft material may be required.
9. Cauda equina syndrome—Secondary to extruded disc, surgical trauma, and hematoma. It should be suspected with postoperative urinary retention. Digital rectal examination is used for the initial diagnosis. Further imaging may be necessary.

C. Discogenic back pain

1. Diagnosis—Patients complain that back pain is greater than leg pain and may have a paucity of physical findings, no radiculopathy, and negative tension signs. X-rays are negative for instability but may show disc space narrowing or other stigmata of spondylosis. MRI reveals decreased signal intensity in the disc space on T2 (dark disc). Discography is a useful preoperative study to correlate MRI findings with a clinically significant pain generator. The study should be performed at multiple levels to include all abnormal levels and one or more normal levels on MRI. To be considered reliably positive, the procedure should elicit pain after injection similar to that usually described by the patient (concordant pain) and should involve at least one minimally painful, nonconcordant level.
2. Treatment
   a. Conservative treatment—Treatment consists of conservative measures, with NSAIDs, physical therapy, and conditioning.
   b. Interbody fusion—If extended nonoperative treatment has failed and the patient has a positive MRI and discogram, interbody fusion can be performed from either an anterior or a retroperitoneal approach or through a posterior midline (posterior lumbar) or posterior transforaminal (TLIF) approach. Fusion is performed with structural constructs (femoral ring allografts or interbody fusion cages) in the disc space.
   c. **Intradiscal electrothermy** (IDET)—IDET involves percutaneously heating the fibers of the annulus fibrosus to reconfigure the collagen fibers, restoring the mechanical integrity of the disc. This may be effective in early conditions (< 50% loss of disc height) but not in more advanced disease; long-term follow-up suggests that symptomatic improvement often lasts less than 1 year, and this procedure has been largely abandoned.
   d. **Total disc replacement** (TDR)—The FDA has recently approved TDR as another surgical option for patients with degenerative disc disease at a single level (L4-S1) in the lumbar spine with the absence of spondylolisthesis and no relief from 6 months of nonoperative therapy. In direct comparison with anterior interbody fusion, the TDR showed equivalent clinical results and no catastrophic failures at 2-year follow-up. Significant concerns include long-term results, design issues, cost, and the safety of revision procedures.

D. Lumbar segmental instability—Present when normal loads produce abnormal spinal motion.

1. Diagnosis—The most common symptom is mechanical back pain, although "dynamic" stenosis can occur, leading to radicular symptoms. The most consistent clinical sign is the "instability catch" (sudden, painful catch with extension from a flexed position). Degenerative lumbar disc disease is indicated by disc space narrowing. A combination of annulus damage and disc space narrowing may reduce the disc's ability to resist rotatory forces. Continuing degeneration or facet subluxation may then lead to instability. Radiographically, traction spurs (horizontal and below disc margin), angular changes greater than 10 degrees (20 degrees at L5-S1) on flexion films, and translational motion greater than 3-4 mm (6 mm at L5-S1) with flexion-extension views are characteristic of lumbar instability but are difficult to quantify and may not correlate with clinical symptoms. Iatrogenic instability can occur after removal of one or more facet joints during surgery.

2. Treatment—Surgical treatment options do not have clearly defined indications, but posterolateral fusion is the standard treatment. The use of pedicle screw instrumentation is well established, with fusion rates approaching 90% in nonsmokers for one- or two-level fusions. The anatomic landmark for pedicle screw insertion in the lumbar spine is the intersection of the transverse process, pars intra-articularis, and lateral aspect of the superior articular facet. Pseudarthrosis and adjacent-level degeneration can occur in these patients. In achieving fusion, a posterior iliac crest bone graft is associated with a significantly lower risk of postoperative complications than an anterior iliac crest bone graft. The use of NSAIDs, including aspirin and Toradol, has been shown to decrease spinal fusion rates, but COX-2 inhibitors have not been shown to have the same inhibitory effect. In large studies, the rates of symptomatic degeneration at an adjacent spinal level are 15% at 5 years and about 40% at 10 years, with no correlation with the number of levels fused or preoperative degeneration.

E. Spinal stenosis

1. Introduction—Spinal stenosis is narrowing of the spinal canal or neural foramina, producing nerve root compression, root ischemia, and a variable syndrome of back and leg pain. Central stenosis produces compression of the thecal sac, whereas lateral stenosis involves compression of individual nerve roots either in the subarticular (lateral) recess (by the medial overgrowth of the superior articular facet at a given facet joint) or in the intervertebral foramen. Stenosis does not usually become symptomatic until patients reach late middle age; it affects men somewhat more often than women.

2. Central stenosis

   a. Introduction—Central stenosis can be congenital (idiopathic or developmental in achondroplastic dwarfs) or acquired. Acquired stenosis, the more common type, is usually degenerative owing to enlargement of osteoarthritic facets with medial encroachment, but it can be secondary to degenerative spondylolisthesis or can be post-traumatic, postsurgical, or the result of various disease processes (e.g., Paget disease, fluorosis). Preexisting "trefoil" canal shapes, a congenitally narrow canal, or medially placed facets may limit the canal's ability to tolerate minor acquired encroachment. Central stenosis represents compression of the thecal sac, with absolute stenosis defined as a cross-sectional area of < 100 mm^2 or < 10 mm of anteroposterior diameter as seen on CT cross section. Soft tissue structures, including the hypertrophied ligamentum flavum, facet capsule, and bulging disc, may contribute as much as 40% to thecal sac compression. Central stenosis is more common in men because their spinal canal is smaller at the L3-L5 levels than that of women, and it affects an older population more than lateral recess stenosis does.

   b. Patient history and physical examination—Symptoms include insidious pain and paresthesias with ambulation or prolonged standing and are relieved by sitting or with flexion of the spine. Patients commonly complain of lower extremity pain, usually in the buttock and thigh; numbness; or "giving way." Although it is typical in patients with HNP, a history of radiating leg pain in a true dermatomal distribution is relatively uncommon in those with spinal stenosis. Neurogenic claudication, which occurs in about 50% of patients with stenosis, can usually be differentiated from vascular claudication by history. Physical examination is also important. Stenosis patients will typically have pain with extension, normal extremity perfusion and pulses, and few neurologic findings. An abnormal neurologic examination is found in fewer than 50%. Tension signs are rarely positive. Standing treadmill tests can be a sensitive (greater than 90%) provocative evaluation of neurogenic claudication (Table 8–8).

   c. Imaging—Further workup may include plain radiographs on which disc degeneration, interspace narrowing, medially placed facets, and flattening of the lordotic curve are commonly seen; subluxation and degenerative changes of the facet joints may also be seen. Plain CT, postmyelographic CT, and MRI are standard imaging modalities. Careful inspection of these studies is necessary to assess lateral nerve root entrapment by medial hypertrophy of the superior facet or the tip of the superior facet, soft tissue thickening, osteophyte formation off the posterior vertebral body (uncinate spur), or a combination of these problems. Central stenosis is a diminution in the area of the thecal sac and is produced by thickening of the ligamentum flavum and/or posterior protrusion of the disc in combination with enlarged facet joints. Simply looking for the

TABLE 8-8 FINDINGS ON TREADMILL TESTS IN NEUROGENIC CLAUDICATION

	Finding	
Activity	*Vascular Claudication*	*Neurogenic Claudication*
Walking	Distal-proximal pain, calf pain	Proximal-distal thigh pain
Uphill walking	Symptoms develop sooner	Symptoms develop later
Rest	Relief with sitting or bending	
Bicycling	Symptoms develop	Symptoms do not develop
Lying flat	Relief	May exacerbate symptoms

"bony" measurements results in underestimating the degree of stenosis; a soft tissue contribution to thecal sac narrowing must be considered. A bone scan or MRI may help rule out malignancy. EMG/NCV testing may be used, but sensitivity is variable and depends on the examiner. NCV testing is sometimes helpful in differentiating radiculopathy from peripheral neuropathy.

d. Treatment—Rest, Williams flexion exercises, NSAIDs, and weight reduction are important in the management of patients with stenosis. Lumbar epidural steroids may be helpful for short-term relief but have shown variable results in controlled studies. A transforaminal nerve block can be effective when the involved roots can be identified and should be considered in most cases before moving to surgery. Surgery is indicated in patients with positive study results and a persistent, unacceptably impaired quality of life. Adequate decompression of the identified disorder typically includes laminectomy and partial medial facetectomy, which can usually be done without destabilizing the spine, thus avoiding fusion. Fusion is indicated in patients with surgical instability (removal of one facet or more), pars defects (including those that are postsurgical) with disc disease, symptomatic radiographic instability, degenerative or isthmic spondylolisthesis, and degenerative scoliosis.

3. Lateral stenosis—Lateral stenosis is impingement of nerve roots lateral to the thecal sac as they pass through the lateral recess and into the neural foramen; it is often associated with facet joint arthropathy (superior articular process enlargement) and disc disease (Fig. 8–4). The three-joint complex (disc and both facets) must be considered when evaluating lateral stenosis. Nerve root compression can occur at more than one level and must be completely decompressed to relieve the symptoms. Subarticular compression (lateral recess stenosis) consists of compression between the medial aspect of a hypertrophic superior articular facet and the posterior aspect of the vertebral body and disc. Hypertrophy of the ligamentum flavum and/or ventral facet joint capsule and vertebral body osteophyte/disc exacerbates the stenosis. Foraminal stenosis can be produced by intraforaminal disc protrusion, impingement of the tip of the superior facet, uncinate spurring, or a combination. Subarticular stenosis, which is more common, affects the traversing (lower) nerve root (L5 root at L4-L5), whereas foraminal stenosis affects the exiting (upper) root (L4 at L4-L5) at a motion segment. Lateral stenosis is most often seen in combination with central stenosis but can appear as an isolated entity usually involving middle-aged or even young adults with symptoms of radicular pain unrelieved by rest and without tension signs. Lower lumbar areas are usually involved because the foramina decrease in size as the size of the nerve root increases. Pain may be the result of intraneural edema and demyelination. Substance P may be released as a response to irritation of the spinal nerve root. After failure of nonoperative treatment, decompression of the hypertrophied lamina and ligamentum flavum and partial facetectomy are usually successful. Fusion may be necessary if instability is present or created.

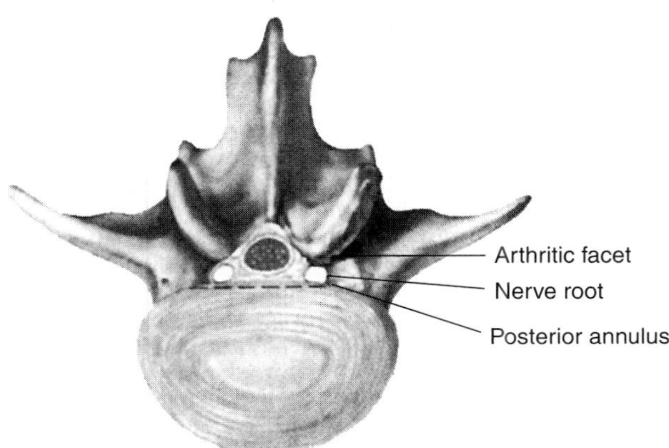

FIGURE 8–4 Lateral stenosis. Note nerve root entrapment laterally on the right by the arthritic facet and bulging posterior annulus. (From Rothman RH, Simeone FA: The Spine, 2nd ed, p 194. Philadelphia, WB Saunders, 1982.)

4. Extraforaminal lateral root compression ("far out syndrome" [Wiltse])—Involves L5 root impingement between the sacral ala and the L5 transverse process. It is usually seen in degenerative scoliosis, isthmic spondylolisthesis, and extraforaminal herniated discs. It must be specifically sought on special radiographs (25-degree caudocephalic [Ferguson] view), CT, or MRI.

F. Spondylolysis and spondylolisthesis

1. Spondylolysis—Spondylosis is a defect in the pars interarticularis. It is one of the most common causes of low-back pain in children and adolescents. The defect in the pars is thought to be a fatigue fracture from repetitive hyperextension stresses (the most common in gymnasts and football linemen), to which there may be a hereditary predisposition. Plain lateral radiographs demonstrate 80% of the lesions, with another 15% visible on oblique radiographs, which show a defect in the neck of the "Scottie dog," as described by Lachapelle (Fig. 8–5). CT, bone scanning, and (more recently) **single-photon emission computed tomography** (SPECT) may be helpful in identifying subtle defects; increased uptake is more compatible with acute lesions that have the potential to heal. Bracing or casting (a single-thigh pantaloon spica) has been advocated for acute lesions, but treatment is usually aimed at symptomatic relief rather than fracture healing and includes activity restriction, flexion exercises, and bracing. Nonunion is common and may not show on scans.

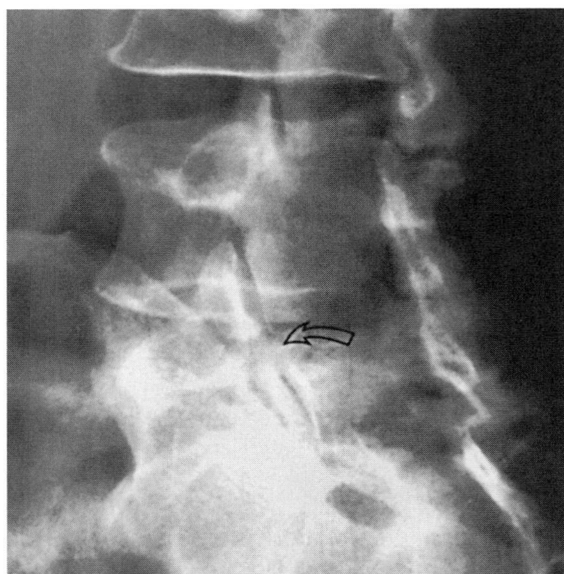

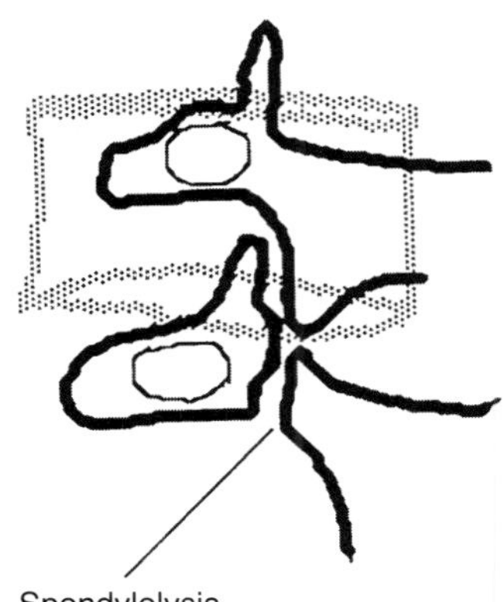

FIGURE 8–5 Spondylolysis. Note disruption of the neck of the "Scottie dog" *(arrow)*. (From Helms CA: Fundamentals of Skeletal Radiology, p 101. Philadelphia, WB Saunders, 1989.)

2. Spondylolisthesis—Spondylolisthesis, forward slippage of one vertebra on another, can be classified into six types etiologically (Newman, Wiltse, McNab) (Table 8–9; Figs. 8–6 and 8–7) and into five grades according to severity (Meyerding). The severity of the slip in spondylolisthesis is based on the amount or degree (compared with S1 width):
   Grade I—0-25%
   Grade II—25-50%
   Grade III—50-75%
   Grade IV—> 75%
   Grade V—> 100% (spondyloptosis)
   Other measurements, including the sacral inclination (normally > 30 degrees) and the slip angle (normally < 0 degrees, signifying lordosis at the L5-S1 disc), are also useful for quantifying lumbopelvic deformity, which affects cosmesis as well as prognosis (Fig. 8–8). The natural history of the disorder is that unilateral pars defects almost never slip and that the progression of spondylolisthesis slows over time. However, in adulthood, degeneration and narrowing of the disc (usually L5-S1) are common and lead to narrowing of the neural foramen and compression of the exiting (L5) root that causes the radicular symptoms.
3. Childhood spondylolisthesis—Usually at L5-S1 and typically type II; usually presents with back pain (instability), hamstring tightness, deformity, or alteration in gait ("pelvic waddle"). Although symptoms may begin at any time in life, screening studies identify the slippage as occurring most commonly at 4-6 years. Spondylolisthesis occurs most often in Caucasians, boys, and youngsters involved in hyperextension activities and is remarkably frequent in some Eskimo tribes (> 50%). It is thought to result from shear stress at the pars interarticularis and to be associated with repetitive hyperextension. Severe slips are rare and may be associated with radicular findings (L5), cauda equina dysfunction, kyphosis of the lumbosacral junction, and "heart-shaped" buttocks. Spina bifida occulta, thoracic hyperkyphosis, and Scheuermann disease are associated with spondylolisthesis.
   a. Low-grade disease (< 50% slip)—Spondylolysis or mild spondylolisthesis may require a bone or CT scan for diagnosis and usually responds to nonoperative treatment consisting of activity modification and exercise. Adolescents with a grade I slip may return to normal activities, including contact sports, once they are asymptomatic. Those with asymptomatic grade II spondylolisthesis are restricted from activities such as gymnastics or football. Progression is uncommon, but risk factors for progression include young

TABLE 8-9 TYPES OF SPONDYLOLISTHESIS

Type	Age	Pathology/Other
I—Dysplastic	Child	Congenital dysplasia of S1 superior facet
II—Isthmic*	5-50 yr	Predisposition leading to elongation/fracture of pars (L5-S1)
III—Degenerative	>40 yr	Facet arthrosis leading to subluxation (L4-L5)
IV—Traumatic	Any age	Acute fracture other than pars
V—Pathologic	Any age	Incompetence of bony elements
VI—Postsurgical	Adult	Excessive resection of neural arches/facets

**Most common type.*

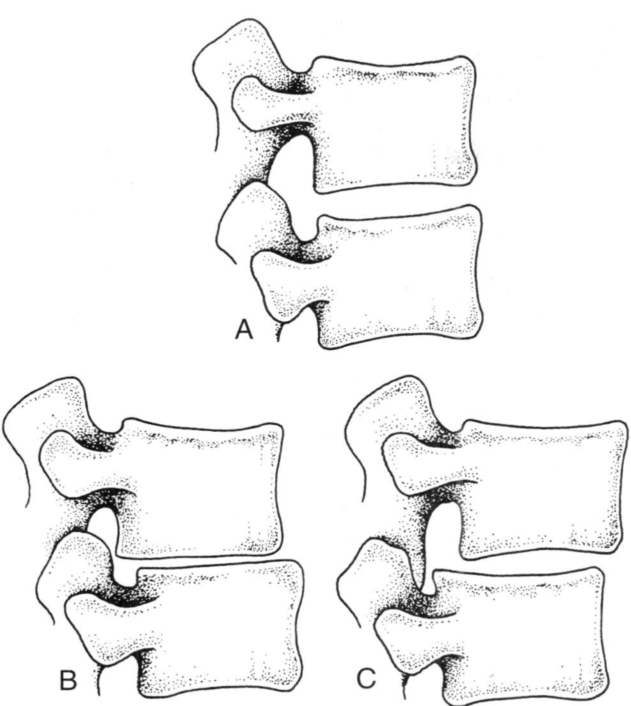

FIGURE 8–6 Degenerative spondylolisthesis. **A**, Normal. **B**, Retrolisthesis: disc narrowing is greater than posterior joint degeneration. **C**, Anterolisthesis: posterior joints are more degenerated than the disc. (From Weinstein JN, Wiesel SW: The Lumbar Spine, p 84. Philadelphia, WB Saunders, 1990.)

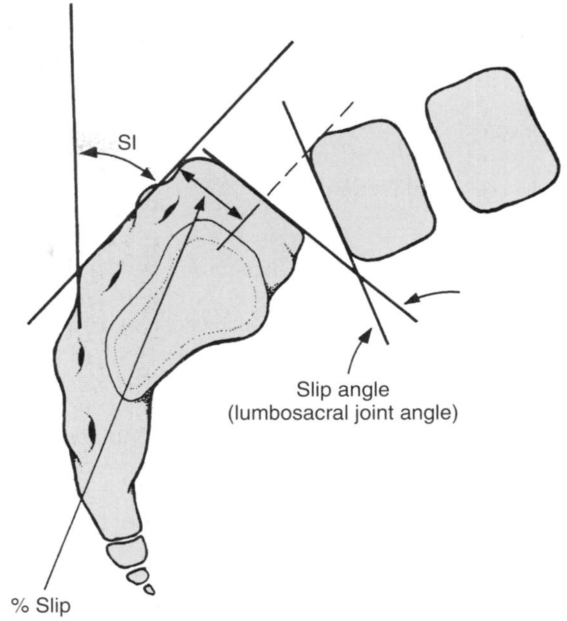

FIGURE 8–8 Measurements used for evaluation of spondylolisthesis. SI, sacroiliac. (Modified from Wiltse LL, Winter RB: Terminology and measurement of spondylolisthesis. J Bone Joint Surg [Am] 65:768-772, 1983.)

age at presentation, female gender, a slip angle of greater than 10 degrees (see Fig. 8–8), a high-grade slip, and a dome-shaped or significantly inclined sacrum (> 30 degrees beyond vertical position). Furthermore, patients with type I or dysplastic spondylolisthesis are at a higher risk for slip progression and the development of cauda equina dysfunction because the neural arch is intact. Patients with a greater than 25% slip, or with L4-L5 or L3-L4 spondylolisthesis, have a higher risk of low-back pain than the general population. Surgery for patients with a low-grade slip generally consists of L5-S1 posterolateral fusion in situ and is usually reserved for those with intractable pain in whom nonoperative treatment has failed or those demonstrating progressive slippage. Wiltse has popularized a paraspinal muscle–splitting approach to the lumbar transverse process and sacral alae that is frequently used in this setting. L5 radiculopathy is uncommon in children with low-grade slips and rarely if ever requires decompression. Repair of the pars defect with the use of a lag screw (Buck) or tension band wiring (Bradford) with bone grafting has been reported. It may be indicated in young patients with slippage less than 25% and a pars defect at L4 or above.

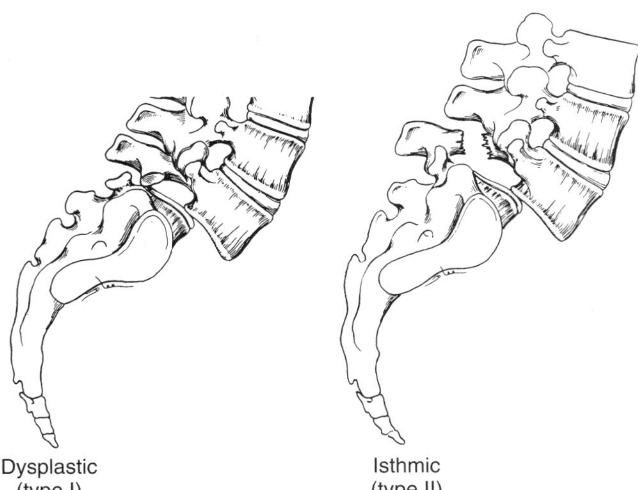

FIGURE 8–7 Spondylolisthesis. (From Rothman RH, Simeone FA: The Spine, 2nd ed, p 264. Philadelphia, WB Saunders, 1982.)

b. Grades III and IV spondylolisthesis and spondyloptosis (grade V)—These commonly cause neurologic abnormalities. L5-S1 isthmic spondylolisthesis causes an L5 radiculopathy (contrast with S1 radiculopathy in L5-S1 HNP). Prophylactic fusion is recommended in children with slippage of more than 50%. It often requires in situ bilateral posterolateral fusion, usually at L4-S1 (L5 is too far anterior to effect L5-S1 fusion) with or without instrumentation. Nerve root exploration is controversial but usually limited to children with clear-cut radicular pain or significant weakness. Reduction of spondylolisthesis has been associated with a 20-30% incidence of L5 root injuries (most are transient) and should be used cautiously. A cosmetically unacceptable deformity and L5-S1 kyphosis so severe that the posterior fusion mass from L4 to the sacrum would be under tension without reversal of the kyphosis are the most commonly cited indications. In situ fusion leaves a patient with a high-grade slip and lumbosacral kyphosis with such severe compensatory hyperlordosis above the fusion that long-term problems frequently ensue. Reduction in this setting is gaining widespread acceptance. Close neurologic monitoring is needed during the procedure and for several days afterward to identify postoperative neuropathy. Posterior decompression, fibular interbody fusion, and posterolateral fusion without reduction have been reported, with excellent long-term results (Bohlman). The Gill procedure, consisting of removal of the loose elements without fusion, is contraindicated.

4. Degenerative spondylolisthesis—More common in African Americans, diabetics, and women over age 40; it occurs most often at the L4-L5 level (see Fig. 8–6). It is reported to be more common in patients with transitional L5 vertebrae and sagittally oriented facet joints. Degenerative spondylolisthesis frequently results in central and lateral recess stenosis with L5 radiculopathy owing to root compression in the lateral recess between the hypertrophic and subluxated inferior facet of L4 and the posterosuperior body of L5. The operative treatment for degenerative spondylolisthesis involves decompression of the nerve roots and stabilization by posterolateral fusion.
5. Adult isthmic spondylolisthesis—While it is often asymptomatic, isthmic spondylolisthesis in an adult may cause back and radicular pain. Nonoperative treatment includes rest, a corset, NSAIDs, and flexion exercises. It is essential to assess the patient for other common sources of back pain before assuming that spondylolisthesis is the cause; MRI is useful in this setting. Isthmic L5-S1 spondylolisthesis frequently causes radicular symptoms in the adult that result from compression of the exiting L5 root in the L5-S1 foramen. Compression may involve hypertrophic fibrous repair tissue at the pars defect, uncinate spur formation off the posterior L5 body, and bulging of the L5-S1 disc. Operative treatment is favored in the presence of radicular symptoms and usually involves thorough foraminal decompression and fusion with or without pedicular screw fixation. Compromised results in workers' compensation patients have been reported.

G. Thoracolumbar injuries

1. Introduction—The thoracolumbar spine is the most common site for vertebral column injuries. Although the classification and treatment of these injuries is included in Chapter 11, Trauma, some points need to be emphasized here. The upper thoracic spine (T1-T10) is stabilized by the ribs and the facet orientation as well as the sternum and is less susceptible to trauma. However, at the thoracolumbar junction there is a fulcrum of increased motion, and this area is more commonly affected by spinal trauma. Two anatomic points also bear mention: (1) the middle thoracic spine is a vascular "watershed" area, and vascular insult can lead to cord ischemia; and (2) the spinal cord ends and the cauda equina begins at the level of L1-L2, so lesions below the L1 level have a better prognosis because the nerve roots (not the cord) are affected.
2. Stable versus unstable injuries—The three-column system (Denis) has been proposed for evaluating spinal injuries and determining which are stable and which unstable. The anterior column is composed of the anterior longitudinal ligament and the anterior two thirds of the annulus and vertebral body. The middle column consists of the posterior third of the body and annulus and the posterior longitudinal ligament. The posterior column comprises the pedicles, facets, spinous processes, and posterior ligaments, including the interspinous and supraspinous ligaments, ligamentum flavum, and facet capsules. There is only moderate reliability and repeatability of the Denis classification of spinal fractures. Disruption of the middle column (seen as widening of the interpedicular distances on anteroposterior radiographs or a change in height of the posterior cortex of the body on lateral views) suggests an unstable injury that may require operative fixation. In a lumbar burst fracture, the anterior and middle columns are compromised, potentially resulting in canal stenosis. The burst fracture is a dynamic event, with maximum canal occlusion and neural element compression during the moment of impact. In addition, disruption of the posterior ligamentous complex in the presence of anterior fracture or dislocation is a strong indication of instability and the potential need for surgical stabilization. Exceptions may include the upper thoracic spine, which is inherently more stable, and bony Chance fractures. Nonpathologic compression fractures of three sequential vertebrae lead to an increased risk of post-traumatic kyphosis.
3. Treatment
    a. Indications—Stable fractures with a well-aligned spine with less than 20-30 degrees of kyphosis and no neurologic compromise may be treated either operatively or nonoperatively (bracing or casting). However, stable burst fractures are best treated nonoperatively. The goals of surgery include stabilization of the fracture and preservation or improvement of neural function in all patients as well as more rapid entry into rehabilitation and a shorter hospital stay for patients with complete injuries. Rehabilitation after spinal cord injury is

discussed more fully in Chapter 10, Rehabilitation: Gait, Amputations, Prostheses, Orthoses, and Neurologic Injury.

b. Procedures—Operative intervention includes decompression for progressive neurologic deficit (emergency) or incomplete neurologic deficit, which may be accomplished anteriorly via vertebrectomy and stabilization or posteriorly via a transpedicular route. In midlumbar burst fractures there is no advantage to adding anterior stabilization to a posterior construct. Posterior instrumentation with restoration of height and sagittal alignment may decompress the canal by repositioning the posterolateral complex. Historically, posterior instrumentation and fusion have extended three levels above and two levels below the injury to stabilize the fracture. Constructs are created in either compression (fractures/dislocations, Chance fractures, or shear fractures) or distraction (burst fractures) in order to reduce and stabilize the injury. Newer, more rigid segmental systems with multiple hooks, wires, and screws or rod-sleeve constructs have supplanted the standard Harrington system and allow restoration of the normal sagittal contour of the spine. Pedicle screw systems purport to limit instrumentation levels to one above and one below the injury. High rates of screw breakage and progressive kyphosis have been reported.

4. Complications—In the short term, respiratory failure is a significant problem for the multiply injured patient with a thoracolumbar fracture. The risk is multifactorial, but the only independent risk factor under the surgeon's control is the interval before surgery, which should be less than 48 hours after admission. The most common long-term complication of a thoracolumbar fracture, treated with or without surgery, is pain. Unfortunately, the relationships among chronic pain, "stability," deformity, pseudarthrosis, and many other factors are unclear. Various types of post-traumatic deformity are noted, including scoliosis caudal to a complete injury (an age-related phenomenon with 100% occurrence in those < 10 years old) and progressive kyphosis (common in unrecognized posterior ligamentous injury). A symptomatic flat back of the lumbar spine results in a forward-flexed posture and easy fatigue (occurs with uncontoured distraction instrumentation). Other complications include late progressive neurologic loss and pain due to the development of post-traumatic syringomyelia. Late development of a neuropathic spine, with gross bony destruction and bony spicules in the soft tissue, has also been described.

H. Other thoracolumbar disorders

1. Destructive spondyloarthropathy—This disorder, seen in hemodialysis patients with chronic renal failure, typically involves three adjacent vertebrae and two intervening discs. Changes include subluxation, degeneration, and narrowing of the disc height. Although the process may resemble infection, it probably represents crystal or amyloid deposition.

2. Facet syndrome—Inflammation or degenerative osteoarthritis of the lumbar facet joints may cause pain that is characteristically in the lower back, with radiation down one or both buttocks and posterior thighs that is worse with extension. Selective injections of local anesthetics can be helpful in the diagnosis of this condition, but anesthetic/steroid injections into the facet joint as a treatment modality are less effective (< 20% with excellent pain relief). The significance of the facet syndrome is debated, and no widely accepted treatment regimen exists. There is no proof that surgery (facet rhizotomy or fusion) is beneficial.

3. **Diffuse idiopathic skeletal hyperostosis** (DISH)—Also known as Forestier disease, DISH is defined by the presence of nonmarginal syndesmophytes (differentiated from ankylosing spondylitis, which has marginal syndesmophytes [Fig. 8–9]) at three successive levels. DISH can occur anywhere in the spine but usually in the thoracic region and is more often seen on the right side. DISH is associated with chronic low-back pain and is more common in patients with diabetes and gout. The prevalence of DISH has been found to be as high as 28% in autopsy specimens. Although there appears to be no relationship between DISH and spinal pain, DISH is associated with extraspinal ossification at several joints, including an increased risk of heterotopic ossification after total hip surgery.

4. Ankylosing spondylitis—Patients positive for **human leukocyte antigen–B27** (HLA-B27) are usually young men who present with the insidious onset of back and hip pain during the third or fourth decade of life. Sacroiliac joint obliteration and marginal syndesmophytes allow radiographic differentiation from DISH. Ankylosing spondylitis may result in fixed cervical, thoracic, or lumbar hyperkyphosis. It occasionally causes marked functional limitation, primarily due to the inability of affected patients to face forward. Extension osteotomy and fusion of the lumbar spine with compression instrumentation can successfully balance

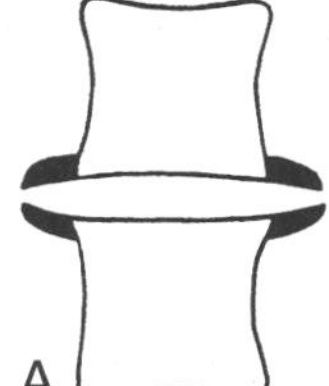

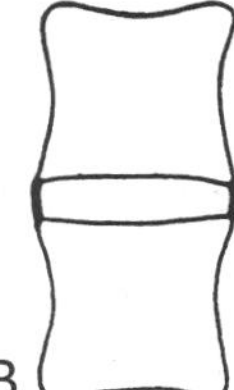

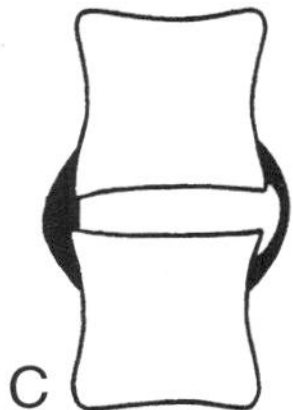

FIGURE 8–9 **A**, Osteophytes (present in degenerative joint disease). **B**, Marginal syndesmophytes (present in ankylosing spondylitis). **C**, Nonmarginal syndesmophytes (present in DISH). (From Rothman RH, Simeone FA: The Spine, 2nd ed, p 924. Philadelphia, WB Saunders, 1982.)

the head over the sacrum. Assessment of the patient for hip flexion contractures or cervicothoracic kyphosis is mandatory. The cervical spine may be corrected by a C7-T1 osteotomy and fusion under local anesthesia. The complications of osteotomy include nonunion, loss of correction, and neurologic and aortic injury. It has multiple medical associations, most notably pulmonary fibrosis and aortic regurgitation.

5. Adult scoliosis—Usually defined as scoliosis in patients over age 20, it is more symptomatic than its childhood counterpart (discussed in Chapter 3, Pediatric Orthopaedics). The cause is usually idiopathic but can also be neuromuscular, degenerative (secondary to degenerative disc disease or osteoporosis), post-traumatic, or postsurgical. The curves are usually thoracic (secondary to unrecognized adolescent scoliosis) or lumbar/thoracolumbar (most common in adults). The association between pain and scoliosis in the adult is controversial; adults with scoliosis have recently been shown to have an increased incidence of back pain, although it is rarely severe or precludes working.
   a. Diagnosis—Back pain is the most common presenting complaint and appears to be related to curve severity and location (lumbar curves more painful). Pain usually begins in the convexity of the curve and later moves to the concavity, reflecting a more refractory condition. Radicular pain and stenosis can occur and may require surgical decompression. Other complaints include cosmetic deformity, cardiopulmonary problems (thoracic curves > 60-65 degrees may alter pulmonary function tests; curves > 90 degrees may affect mortality), and neurologic symptoms (secondary to stenosis). There is no demonstrated association between curve progression and pregnancy. Progression is unlikely in curves of less than 30 degrees. Right thoracic curves of greater than 50 degrees are at the highest risk for progression (usually 1 degree/year), followed by right lumbar curves. Myelography with CT or MRI is useful for the evaluation of nerve root compression in stenosis. MRI, facet injections, and/or discography may be used to evaluate symptoms in the lumbar spine.
   b. Treatment
      (1) Nonoperative treatment—The uncertain correlation between adult scoliosis and back pain makes conservative management essential; this includes a thorough evaluation for other common causes of back pain. Nonoperative treatment includes NSAIDs, weight reduction, therapy, muscle strengthening, facet joint injections, and orthoses (used with activity).
      (2) Operative treatment—Surgery is usually reserved for young adults with symptomatic curves of greater than 50-60 degrees, for older patients with curves of 90 degrees and higher, and for those with progressive curves, cardiopulmonary compromise (worsening pulmonary function tests in severe curves), and refractory spinal stenosis. Nonsurgically treated adults with late-onset idiopathic scoliosis are highly productive at 50-year follow-up, with a slightly increased risk of shortness of breath with activity and chief complaints of back pain and poor cosmesis. Operative risk for these patients is high (up to a 25% complication rate in older patients); complications include pseudarthrosis (15% with posterior fusion only; the highest risk at the TL junction and at L5-S1), urinary tract infection, instrumentation problems, infection (up to 5%), and neurologic deficits. Additionally, long convalescence is usually required. Combined anterior release and fusion and posterior fusion and instrumentation may be beneficial for large (> 70-degree), more rigid curves (as determined on side-bending films) or curves in the lumbar spine. Preservation of normal sagittal alignment with fusion is critical. Fusion to the sacrum is associated with more complications (pseudarthrosis, instrumentation failure, loss of normal lordosis, and pain) and should be avoided when possible. Achieving a successful result, including fusion to the sacrum, is enhanced by combined anterior and posterior fusion. The ideal implant for instrumentation in these cases has not been found; commonly used instrumentation for sacral fixation includes the Galveston fixation and sacral pedicle or alar screw constructs. There is clinical and experimental evidence demonstrating the benefit of structural interbody grafting (femoral ring allograft or mesh cage) at L5-S1 and L4-L5 to decrease the stress on the sacropelvic fixation.

6. Postlaminectomy deformity—Progressive deformity (usually kyphosis) resulting from a prior wide laminectomy. In children this procedure is followed by a high risk (90%) of deformity. Fusion plus internal fixation may be considered prophylactic for young patients who require extensive decompression. Fusion using pedicular screw fixation is best for reconstruction in the adult lumbar spine.

I. Kyphosis
1. Introduction—Kyphosis in adults may be idiopathic (old Scheuermann's disease [since adolescence]), post-traumatic, secondary to trauma or ankylosing spondylitis, or the result of metabolic bone disease. Progressive kyphosis secondary to multiple osteoporotic compression fractures is usually treated with exercise, bracing, and medical management of the

underlying bone disease. Prevention of compression fractures has been successful with bisphosphonate treatment, with a decreased incidence of vertebral fractures of 65% at 1 year and 40% at 3 years. Surgical attempts at correction and stabilization are marked by a high complication rate. An underlying malignancy as a cause of the osteopenia should be considered; evaluation with MRI is sensitive for determining the presence of tumor. Vertebroplasty and kyphoplasty, percutaneous techniques designed to relieve pain, have been proposed for acute and subacute compression fractures; kyphoplasty has also been proposed to correct deformity. The precise indications for these techniques, such as the number of levels and timing, have not been defined, and long-term outcome data regarding their efficacy are lacking. In the short term, both techniques are able to improve pain and quality of life for at least 6 months. To respond to either technique, a fracture must still be in the active healing phase, which is best demonstrated on MRI. A patient with a painful but healed fracture is unlikely to improve.

2. Nontraumatic adult kyphosis—Severe idiopathic or congenital kyphosis may be a source of back pain in the adult, particularly when it is present in the thoracolumbar or lumbar spine. When the symptoms fail to respond to nonoperative management (see the preceding discussion on adult scoliosis), posterior instrumentation and fusion of the entire kyphotic segment with a compression implant may be indicated. Anterior fusion is performed in conjunction for curves not correcting to 55 degrees or less on hyperextension lateral radiographs.
3. Post-traumatic kyphosis—Post-traumatic kyphosis may be seen after fractures of the thoracolumbar spine treated without surgery, particularly when the posterior ligamentous complex has been disrupted; fractures treated by laminectomy without fusion; and fractures for which fusion has been performed unsuccessfully. Progressive kyphosis may produce pain at the fracture site, with radiating leg pain and/or neurologic dysfunction if there is associated neural compression. Operative options include posterior fusion with compression instrumentation for milder deformities; combined anterior and posterior osteotomies, instrumentation, and fusion for more severe deformities; and anterior spinal cord or cauda equina decompression combined with posterior instrumentation and fusion for cases involving neurologic dysfunction. Some all-posterior approaches, such as pedicle subtraction osteotomy, address anterior pathology and can achieve 30 degrees of correction per level. Patient comorbidities, pseudarthrosis in the thoracic spine, and adjacent-level disease are major concerns with the pedicle subtraction osteotomy.

IV. Sacrum and Coccyx

A. Sacroiliac joint pain—Elicited with the patient lying on the affected side without support (Gaenslen test); by direct compression; or with the flexion, abduction, and external rotation (FABER) test of the involved extremity. Local injections may have diagnostic and therapeutic roles. Orthotic management (trochanteric cinch) can be helpful. Fusion is not indicated unless an infection is present.

B. Idiopathic coccygodynia—Pain and point tenderness over the coccyx. The condition is more common in women and may occur after pregnancy or minor trauma or idiopathically. It is occasionally associated with a fracture; four types have been identified based on the morphology of the coccyx. The symptoms may last 1-2 years but are almost always self-limiting. Treatment should be conservative and may include a sitting donut, NSAIDs, stretching exercises, and local injection. Surgery is associated with a high failure rate and significant risk of complications.

C. Sacral insufficiency fracture—Occurs in older patients with osteopenia, often without a history of trauma. Complaints include low-back and groin pain. This fracture is diagnosed with a technetium bone scan (H-shaped uptake pattern is diagnostic) or CT scan. Treatment is nonoperative, with rest, analgesic medication, and ambulatory aids until the symptoms resolve.

V. Tumors and Infections of the Spine

A. Introduction—The spine is a frequent site of metastasis, and certain tumors with a predilection for the spine have unique manifestations in vertebrae. Tumors of the vertebral body include histiocytosis X, giant cell tumor, chordoma, osteosarcoma, hemangioma, metastatic disease, and marrow cell tumors. Tumors of the posterior elements include aneurysmal bone cysts, osteoblastoma, and osteoid osteoma. Radiographic changes include an absent pedicle, cortical erosion or expansion, and vertebral collapse. Bone scans can be helpful in cases of protracted back pain or night pain. MRI is the diagnostic test of choice. Malignant tumors have decreased T1 and increased T2 intensity, the sensitivity of which is increased with the use of gadolinium. Malignant tumors occur more frequently in the lower (lumbar > thoracic > cervical) spinal levels and in the vertebral body. Complete surgical excision is difficult and usually consists of tumor debulking and stabilization. Adjuvant therapy is essential. For more details on these tumors, refer to Chapter 9, Orthopaedic Pathology.

B. Metastasis—The most common tumors of the spine, spreading to the vertebral body first and later to the pedicles.

1. Diagnosis—Red flags for possible spinal metastasis include a history of cancer, recent unexplained weight loss, night pain, and age over 50 years. Most tumors are osteolytic and not demonstrated on plain films until over 30% destruction of the vertebral body has occurred.

Breast, lung, and prostate metastases are the most common, the latter of which are blastic. CT-guided needle biopsy is often possible, and surgery for diagnosis can be avoided. A poor prognosis is associated with neurologic dysfunction, proximal lesions, long duration of symptoms, and rapid growth of the metastasis.

2. Treatment
   a. Nonsurgical treatment—Radiation therapy and chemotherapy are the mainstays of treatment unless the tumor is destabilizing and progressive or causes spinal cord or cauda equina dysfunction. In the case of epidural spinal cord compression, radiation therapy should be combined with direct surgical decompression for the best clinical outcomes. Radiosensitivity varies among primary tumor types: prostate and lymphoid tumors are radiosensitive, breast cancer is 70% sensitive and 30% resistant; and gastrointestinal and renal cell tumors are radioresistant.
   b. Surgical treatment—Surgical indications include progressive neurologic dysfunction that is unresponsive to radiation therapy, persistent pain despite radiation therapy, the need for a diagnostic biopsy, and pathologic instability. Vertebroplasty is gaining favor in cases of metastatic disease of the spine (myeloma, breast) without instability or neurologic compromise and represents a minimally invasive alternative to open surgery. In cases of neurologic deficit and/or spinal instability, anterior decompression and stabilization (preserving intact posterior structures) may result in recovery of neurologic function. Posterior stabilization or a circumferential approach is indicated in cases of multiple levels of destruction, involvement of both the anterior and posterior columns, or translational instability. Life expectancy should play an important role with regard to whether surgical treatment is performed. Methylmethacrylate may be useful as an anterior strut but should be used only as an adjunct because of the high complication rate. Iliac crest grafting is preferred if life expectancy is more than 6 months. Anterior internal fixation may be indicated in order to maximize immediate stability and rehabilitation.

C. Primary tumors
   1. Osteoid osteoma and osteoblastoma—Common in the spine. These tumors may present with painful scoliosis in a child. Pain is typically relieved by aspirin. A bone scan can help localize the level, and thin-cut CT scans can direct surgical excision. Scoliosis (the lesion is typically at the apex of the convexity) resolves with early resection (within 18 months) in a child under 11 years of age. If there is no scoliosis, NSAIDs are the mainstay of treatment. If they do not alleviate the pain, resection may be required. Osteoblastomas typically occur in the posterior elements in older patients, with neurologic involvement in more than half. This presentation typically requires resection and posterior fusion.
   2. Aneurysmal bone cyst—May represent degeneration of more aggressive tumors. These cysts typically occur during the second decade of life, arising in the posterior elements but possibly also involving the anterior elements. Treatment is excision and/or radiation therapy.
   3. Hemangioma—Typically seen in asymptomatic patients. Symptomatic patients over age 40 may seek treatment after small spinal fractures. The classic patient with hemangioma has "jailhouse striations" on plain films and "spikes of bone" demonstrated on CT. Vertebrae are typically of normal size and not expanded (as in Paget disease). Treatment is observation or radiation therapy in cases of persistent pain after pathologic fracture. Anterior resection and fusion are reserved for refractory cases or pathologic collapse and neural compression, but massive bleeding may be encountered.
   4. Eosinophilic granuloma—Usually seen in children younger than 10 years. This tumor is seen more often in the thoracic spine and may present with progressive back pain. This tumor classically results in vertebral flattening (vertebra plana [Calvé disease]), which is seen on lateral radiographs. Biopsy may be required for diagnosis unless the radiographic picture is classic or histiocytosis has already been diagnosed. Chemotherapy is useful for the systemic form. Bracing may be indicated in children to prevent progressive kyphosis. Low-dose radiation therapy may be indicated in the presence of neurologic deficits; otherwise, symptoms are usually self-limiting. At least 50% reconstitution of vertebral height may be expected.
   5. Giant cell tumor—Usually seen in the fourth and fifth decades of life. It destroys the vertebral body in an expansile fashion. Surgical excision and bone grafting constitute the usual recommended treatment. A high recurrence rate is reported. Radiation therapy should be avoided because of the possibility of malignant degeneration of the tumor.
   6. Plasmacytoma/multiple myeloma—Also common in the spine, causing osteopenic, lytic lesions. Pain, pathologic fractures, and diffuse osteoporosis frequently occur. Increased calcium and decreased hematocrit levels as well as abnormal protein studies are common. Treatment is with radiation therapy (3000-4000 cGy) with or without chemotherapy. Surgery is reserved for patients with spinal instability and those with refractory neurologic symptoms.
   7. Chordoma—A classically slow-growing lytic lesion in the midline of the anterior sacrum or the base of the skull. It may occur in other

vertebrae (cervical spine most common). Patients with these tumors may present with intra-abdominal complaints and a presacral mass. Radiation therapy and surgery are preferred. Surgical excision can include up to half of the sacral roots (i.e., all roots on one side) and the patient still maintain bowel and bladder function. The recurrence rate is high, but aggressive attempts at surgical excision are indicated. Although a complete cure is rare, patients typically survive 10-15 years after diagnosis.

8. Osteochondroma—Arises in the posterior elements. It is frequently seen in the cervical spine. Treatment is by excision, which may be necessary to rule out sarcomatous changes.
9. Neurofibroma—Can present with enlarged intervertebral foramina seen on oblique radiographs.
10. Malignant primary skeletal lesions—Osteosarcoma, Ewing sarcoma, and chondrosarcoma are uncommon in the spine. When they occur they are associated with a poor prognosis. Chemotherapy and irradiation are the mainstays of treatment, but aggressive surgical excision may have a role. The lesions may actually be metastases, which are treated palliatively.
11. Lymphoma—Can present with "ivory" vertebrae. Usually associated with a systemic disease, lymphoma is treated after histologic diagnosis by irradiation and/or chemotherapy.
12. Fibrous dysplasia—At least 60% of patients with polyostotic fibrous dysplasia will have spinal involvement, mostly in the posterior elements. There is a strong correlation between the presence of a lesion and scoliosis, making scoliosis screening very important in the population with polyostotic disease.

D. Spinal infections

1. Disc space infection—Blood-borne infection can primarily invade the disc space in children. *Staphylococcus aureus* is the most common offender, but gram-negative organisms are common in older patients. Although all age groups are affected, children (mean age, 7 years) commonly present with an inability to walk, stand, or sit; back pain/tenderness; and restricted ROM. Laboratory studies may be normal except for an elevated erythrocyte sedimentation rate, C-reactive protein, and WBC count (often high normal or mildly elevated). Radiographic findings include disc space narrowing and end plate erosion, but these findings do not occur until 10 days to 3 weeks after onset and their absence is unreliable. MRI is the diagnostic test of choice, although a bone scan is also useful in the diagnosis. Treatment includes bed rest, immobilization, and antibiotics.
2. Pyogenic vertebral osteomyelitis—Seen with increasing frequency but still associated with a significant (6- to 12-week) delay in diagnosis.
   a. Patient history and physical examination—Older debilitated patients and intravenous drug users are at increased risk. The condition is more common in patients with a history of pneumonia, urinary tract infection, skin infection, or immunologic compromise (transplant, RA, **diabetes mellitus** [DM], human immunodeficiency virus [HIV: CD4+ > 200]). The organism is usually hematogenous in origin (*S. aureus*, 50-75% of cases). Fungal spondylitis can be seen in patients with immunologic compromise, and performing fungal cultures in this population may shorten the time to diagnosis. A history of unremitting spinal pain at any level is characteristic, and tenderness, spasm, and loss of motion are seen. Forty percent of neurologic deficits are seen in older patients, patients with infections at more cephalic levels of the spine, patients with debilitating systemic illnesses such as diabetes or RA, and those with delayed diagnoses.
   b. Diagnosis—Plain radiographic findings include osteopenia, paraspinous soft tissue swelling (loss of a psoas shadow), erosion of the vertebral end plates, and disc destruction. Disc destruction, seen on plain radiographs or MRI, is atypical of neoplasms. Bone scanning is sensitive for a destructive process. MRI is both sensitive for detecting infection and specific in differentiating infection from tumor. Gadolinium enhances the sensitivity. Tissue diagnosis via blood cultures or aspirate of the infection is mandatory.
   c. Treatment—Following tissue diagnosis, 6-12 weeks of intravenous antibiotics is the treatment of choice. Bracing may be used adjunctively. Open biopsy is indicated when a tissue diagnosis has not been made, and an anterior approach or costotransversectomy is used. Anterior débridement and strut grafting are reserved for refractory cases that are typically associated with abscess formation or cases involving neurologic deterioration, extensive bony destruction, or marked deformity. Posterior surgery is usually ineffective for débridement; posterior stabilization is only occasionally required after anterior débridement and strut grafting.
3. Spinal tuberculosis—The most common extrapulmonary location of tuberculosis is in the spine. It may be seen in the HIV positive population with a CD4+ count of 50 to 200. Originating in the metaphysis of the vertebral body and spreading under the anterior longitudinal ligament, spinal tuberculosis can cause destruction of several contiguous levels or result in skip lesions (15%) or abscess formation (50%) (Fig. 8–10). On early plain x-ray studies, anterior vertebral body destruction, with preservation of the disc, distinguishes tuberculosis from pyogenic infection. About two thirds of patients have abnormal chest radiographs, and

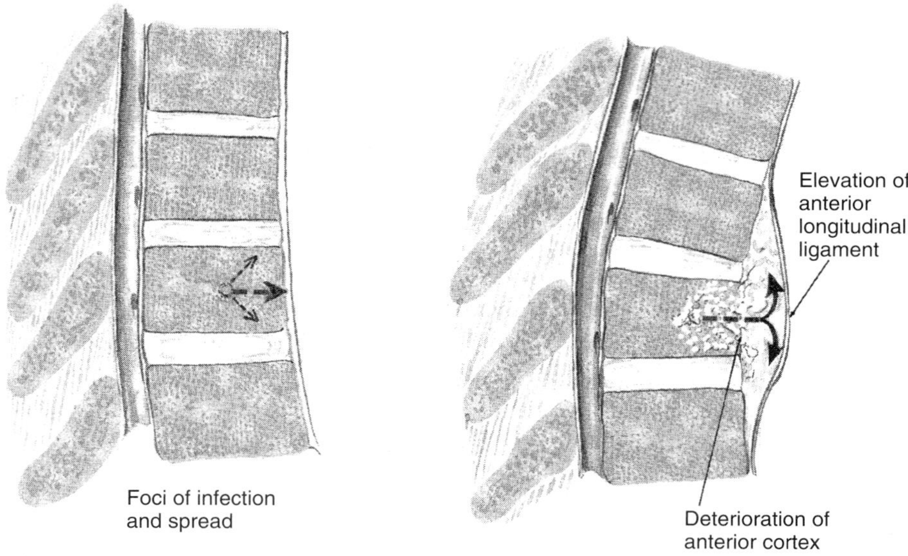

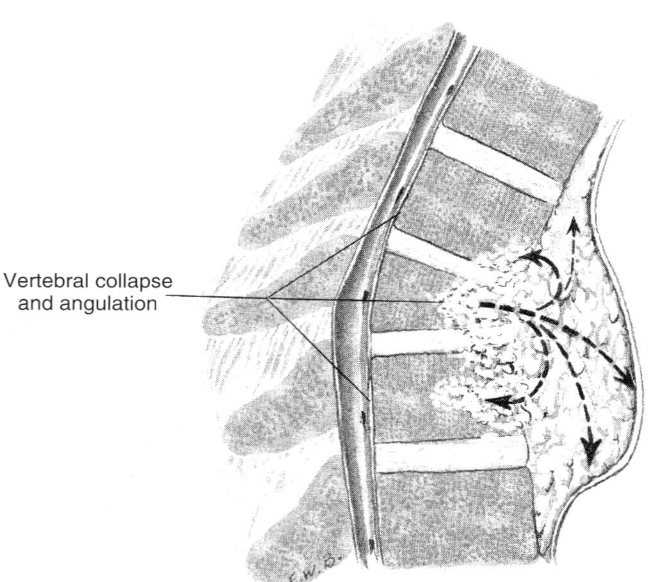

FIGURE 8–10 Pathogenesis of spinal tuberculosis. (From Herring JA: Tachdjian's Pediatric Orthopaedics, 3rd ed, p 1832. Philadelphia, WB Saunders, 2002.)

20% have a negative test for **purified protein derivative of tuberculin** (PPD) or are anergic. Severe kyphosis, sinus formation, and (Pott) paraplegia are late sequelae. Spinal cord injury may occur secondary to direct pressure from the abscess, bony sequestra (good prognosis), or (rarely) meningomyelitis (poor prognosis). Chemotherapy is the mainstay of treatment. Surgical indications are neurologic deficit; spinal instability; progressive kyphosis; and advanced disease with caseation, fibrosis, and avascularity that limits antibiotic penetration. Radical anterior débridement of the infection followed by uninstrumented autogenous strut grafting (Hong Kong procedure) is the accepted surgical treatment. Advantages include less progressive kyphosis, earlier healing, and a decrease in sinus formation. Adjuvant chemotherapy beginning 10 days before surgery is recommended.

Selected Bibliography

GENERAL INFORMATION

Recent Articles

Sidhu KS, Herkowitz HH: Spinal instrumentation in the management of degenerative disorders of the lumbar spine. Clin Orthop 335:39–53, 1997.

Classic Articles

Boden SD, Davis DO, Dina TS, et al: Abnormal magnetic resonance scans of the lumbar spine in asymptomatic subjects. J Bone Joint Surg [Am] 72:403–408, 1990.
Boden SD, McCown PR, Davis DO, et al: Abnormal MRI scans of cervical spine in asymptomatic subjects: A prospective investigation. J Bone Joint Surg [Am] 72:1178–1184, 1990.
Garfin SR, Bottle MJ, Walters RL, et al: Complications in the use of the halo fixation device. J Bone Joint Surg [Am] 68:320–325, 1986.
MacNab I, Dall D: The blood supply of the lumbar spine and its application to the technique of intertransverse lumbar fusion. J Bone Joint Surg [Br] 53:628–638, 1971.
White AA III, Johnson RM, Panjabi MM, et al: Biomechanical analysis of clinical stability in the cervical spine. Clin Orthop 109:85–96, 1975.

Review Articles

Boden SD: The use of radiographic imaging studies in the evaluation of patients who have degenerative disorders of the lumbar spine. J Bone Joint Surg [Am] 78:114–125, 1996.
Boden SD, Wiesel SW: Lumbar spine imaging: Role in clinical decision making. J Am Acad Orthop Surg 4:238–248, 1996.
Brodke DS, Ritter SM: Nonoperative management of low back pain and lumbar disc degeneration. J Bone Joint Surg [Am] 86:1810–1818, 2004.

DISC DISEASE

Recent Articles

Atlas SJ, Deyo RA, Keller RB, et al: The Maine lumbar spine study. Part II. Spine 21:1777–1786, 1996.
Brown CW, Deffer PA, Akmakjian J, et al: The natural history of thoracic disc herniations. Spine 17:S97–S102, 1992.
Butterman GR: Treatment of lumbar disc herniation: Epidural steroid injection compared with discectomy. J Bone Joint Surg [Am] 86:670–679, 2004.
Ghiselli G, Wang JC, Bhatia NN, et al: Adjacent segment degeneration after lumbar discectomy for sciatica: the effects of fragment type and annular competence. J Bone Joint Surg [Am] 85:102–108, 2003.
Kawaguchi Y, Kanamori M, Ishihara H, et al: Clinical and radiographic results of expansive lumbar laminoplasty in patients with spinal stenosis. J Bone Joint Surg [Am] 86:1698–1703, 2004.
Komori H, Shinomiya K: The natural history of HNP with radiculopathy. Spine 21:225–229, 1996.
Riew KD, Park J, Cho Y, et al: Nerve root blocks in the treatment of lumbar radicular pain. J Bone Joint Surg [Am] 88:1722–1725, 2006.
Stillerman CB, Chen TC, et al: Experience in the surgical management of 82 symptomatic thoracic disc herniations and review of the literature. J Neurosurg 88:623–633, 1998.
Toyone T, Tanaka T, Kato D, Kaneyama R: Low-back pain following surgery for lumbar disc herniation. J Bone Joint Surg [Am] 86:893–896, 2004.
Yukawa Y, Lenke LG, Tenhula J, et al: A comprehensive study of patients with surgically treated lumbar spinal stenosis with neurogenic claudication. J Bone Joint Surg [Am] 84:1954–1959, 2002.

Classic Articles

Albrand OW, Corkill G: Thoracic disc herniation: Treatment and prognosis. Spine 4:41–46, 1979.
Bell GR, Rothman RH: The conservative treatment of sciatica. Spine 9:54–56, 1984.
Bohlman HH, Zdeblick TA: Anterior excision of herniated thoracic discs. J Bone Joint Surg [Am] 70:1038–1047, 1988.
Hanley EN, Shapiro DE: The development of low back pain after excision of a lumbar disk. J Bone Joint Surg [Am] 71:719–721, 1989.
Kostuik JP, Harrington I, Alexander D, et al: Cauda equina syndrome and lumbar disc herniation. J Bone Joint Surg [Am] 68: 386–391, 1986.
Waddell G, Kummell EG, Lotto WM, et al: Failed lumbar disk surgery and repeat surgery following industrial injuries. J Bone Joint Surg [Am] 61:201–207, 1979.
Weber H: Lumbar disc herniation: A controlled, prospective study with ten years of observation. Spine 8:131–140, 1983.

Review Articles

Eismont FJ, Currier B: Current concepts review: Surgical management of lumbar intervertebral-disc disease. J Bone Joint Surg [Am] 71:1266–1271, 1989.
Rhee JM, Schaufele M, Abdu WA: Radiculopathy and the herniated lumbar disc. J Bone Joint Surg [Am] 88:2070–2080, 2006.
Vanichkachorn JS, Vaccaro A: Thoracic Disk Disease: Diagnosis and Treatment. J Am Acad Orthop Surg 8:159–169, 2000.

DEFORMITY

Recent Articles

Barr JD, Barr MS, et al: Percutaneous vertebroplasty for pain relief and spinal stabilization. Spine 25:923–928, 2000.
Belanger TA, Milam RA IV, Roh JS, Bohlman HH: Cervicothoracic extension osteotomy for chin-on-chest deformity in ankylosing spondylitis. J Bone Joint Surg [Am] 87:1732–1738, 2005.
Bridwell KH, Lewis SJ, Lenke LG, et al: Pedicle subtraction osteotomy for the treatment of fixed sagittal imbalance. J Bone Joint Surg [Am] 85:454–463, 2003.
Dickson JH, Mirkovic S: Results of operative treatment of idiopathic scoliosis in adults. J Bone Joint Surg [Am] 77:513–523, 1995.
Kim YJ, Bridwell KH, Lenke LG, et al: Pseudarthrosis in adult spinal deformity following multisegmental instrumentation and arthrodesis. J Bone Joint Surg [Am] 88:721–728, 2006.
Korosvessis P, Baikousis A, Zacharatos S, et al: Posterior short-segment instrumentation and fusion provides better results than combined anterior plus posterior stabilization for mid-lumbar (L2-L4) burst fractures. Spine 31:859–868, 2006.
Lieberman IH, Dudeney S, Reinhardt MK, Bell G: Initial outcome and efficacy of "kyphoplasty" in the treatment of painful osteoporotic compression fractures. Spine 26:1631–1638, 2001.
Potter BK, Lenke LG, Kuklo TR: Prevention and management of iatrogenic flat back deformity. J Bone Joint Surg [Am] 86:1793–1808, 2004.
Weinstein SL, Dolan LA, Spratt KF, et al: Health and function of patients with untreated idiopathic scoliosis: A 50-year natural history study. JAMA 289:559–567, 2003.

Classic Articles

Allen BL Jr., Ferguson RL: The Galveston technique of pelvic fixation with L-rod instrumentation of the spine. Spine 9:388–394, 1984.
Bradford DS, Moe JH, Montalvo FJ, et al: Scheuermann's kyphosis and roundback deformity: Results of Milwaukee brace treatment. J Bone Joint Surg [Am] 56:740, 1974.
Jackson RP, Simmons EH, Stripinis D: Incidence and severity of back pain in adult idiopathic scoliosis. Spine 8:749–756, 1983.
Lauerman WC, Bradford DS, Ogilvie JW, et al: Results of lumbar pseudarthrosis repair. J Spinal Disord 5:128–136, 1992.
Lauerman WC, Bradford DS, Transfeld EE, et al: Management of pseudarthrosis after arthrodesis of the spine for idiopathic scoliosis. J Bone Joint Surg [Am] 73:222–236, 1991.
Luque ER: Segmental spinal instrumentation of the lumbar spine. Clin Orthop 203:126–134, 1986.

Murray PM, Weinstein SL, Spratt KF: The natural history and long term follow-up of Scheuermann's kyphosis. J Bone Joint Surg [Am] 75:236–248, 1993.

Sponseller PD, Cohen MS, Nachemson AL, et al: Results of surgical treatment of adults with idiopathic scoliosis. J Bone Joint Surg [Am] 69:667–675, 1987.

Swank S, Lonstein JE, Moe JH, et al: Surgical treatment of adult scoliosis: A review of two hundred and twenty-two cases. J Bone Joint Surg [Am] 63:268–287, 1981.

Weinstein SL, Ponseti IV: Curve progression in idiopathic scoliosis. J Bone Joint Surg [Am] 65:447–455, 1983.

Winter RB, Lonstein JE, Denis F: Pain patterns in adult scoliosis. Orthop Clin North Am 19:339–345, 1988.

Review Articles

Bradford DS: Adult scoliosis: Current concepts of treatment. Clin Orthop Relat Res 229:70–87, 1988.

Bridwell KH: The pros and cons to saving the L5-S1 motion segment in a long scoliosis fusion construct. Spine 28:S234–S242, 2003.

Tribus CB: Degenerative lumbar scoliosis: Evaluation and management. J Am Acad Orthop Surg 11:174–183, 2003.

Tribus CB: Scheuermann's kyphosis in adolescents and adults: Diagnosis and management. J Am Acad Orthop Surg 6:36–43, 1998.

COMPLICATIONS

Recent Articles

Carreon LY, Puno RM, Dimar JR II, et al: Perioperative complications of posterior lumbar decompression and arthrodesis in older adults. J Bone Joint Surg [Am] 85:2089–2092, 2003.

Eck K, Bridwell KH, Ungacta FF, et al: Complications and results of long adult deformity fusions down to L4, L5 and the sacrum. Spine 26:E182–E191, 2001.

Edwards CC II, Karpitskaya Y, Cha C, et al: Accurate identification of adverse outcomes after cervical spine surgery. J Bone Joint Surg [Am] 86:251–256, 2004.

Klein JD, Hey LA: Perioperative nutrition and postoperative complications in patients undergoing spinal surgery. Spine 21:2676–2682, 1996.

McDonnell MF, Glassman SD: Perioperative complications of anterior procedures on the spine. J Bone Joint Surg [Am] 78:839–847, 1996.

Wang JC, Bohlman HH, Riew KD: Dural tears secondary to operations on the lumbar spine: Management and results after a two-year minimum follow-up of eighty-eight patients. J Bone Joint Surg 80:1728–1732, 1998.

Classic Articles

Detwiler KN, Loftus CM, Godersky JC, et al: Management of cervical spine injuries in patients with ankylosing spondylitis. J Neurosurg 72:210–215, 1990.

Deyo RA, Cherkin DC, Loeser JD, et al: Morbidity and mortality in association with operation on the lumbar spine. J Bone Joint Surg [Am] 74:536–543, 1992.

Eismont FJ, Wiesel SW, Rothman RH: The treatment of dural tears associated with spinal surgery. J Bone Joint Surg [Am] 63:1132–1136, 1981.

Farey ID, McAfee PC, Davis RF, Long DM: Pseudarthrosis of the cervical spine after anterior arthrodesis: Treatment by posterior nerve-root decompression, stabilization and arthrodesis. J Bone Joint Surg [Am] 72:1171–1177, 1990.

Flynn JC, Price CT: Sexual complications of anterior fusion of the lumbar spine. Spine 9:489–492, 1984.

Graham B, Can Peteghem PK: Fractures of the spine in ankylosing spondylitis: Diagnosis, treatment, and complications. Spine 14:803–807, 1989.

Kurz LT, Garfin SF, Both RE: Harvesting autologous iliac bone grafts: A review of complications and techniques. Spine 14:1324–1331, 1989.

Simpson JM, Silveri CP, Balderston MD, et al: The results of operation on the lumbar spine in patients who have diabetes mellitus. J Bone Joint Surg [Am] 75:1823–1829, 1993.

Simmons EH: Kyphotic deformity of the spine in ankylosing spondylitis. Clin Orthop 128:65–77, 1977.

CERVICAL SPONDYLOSIS, STENOSIS

Recent Articles

Bernhardt M, Hynes RA, Blume HW, White AA: Cervical spondylotic myelopathy. J Bone Joint Surg [Am] 75:119–128, 1993.

Bohlman HH, Emery SE, Goodfellow DB, et al: Robinson anterior cervical diskectomy and arthrodesis for cervical radiculopathy. J Bone Joint Surg [Am] 75:1298–1307, 1993.

Emery SE, Bohlman HH, Bolesta MJ, et al: Anterior cervical decompression and arthrodesis for the treatment of cervical spondylotic myelopathy: Two to seven year follow-up. J Bone Joint Surg [Am] 80:941–951, 1998.

Ghanayem AJ, Leventhal M, Bohlman HH: Osteoarthrosis of the atlanto-axial joints: Long-term follow-up after treatment with arthrodesis. J Bone Joint Surg [Am] 78:1300–1308, 1996.

Iwasaki M, Ebara S: Expansive laminoplasty for cervical radiculomyelopathy due to soft disc herniation. Spine 21:32–38, 1996.

Johnson MJ, Lucas GL: Value of cervical spine radiographs as a screening tool. Clin Orthop 340:102–108, 1997.

Ma DJ, Gilula LA, Riew KD: Complications of fluoroscopically guided extraforaminal cervical nerve blocks: An analysis of 1036 injections. J Bone Joint Surg [Am] 87:1025–1030, 2005.

McAfee PC, Bohlman HH, Ducker TB, et al: One-stage anterior cervical decompression and posterior stabilization: A study of one hundred patients with minimum two years of follow-up. J Bone Joint Surg [Am] 77:1791–1800, 1995.

Zdeblick TA, Hughes SS, Riew KD, et al: Failed anterior cervical discectomy and arthrodesis: Analysis and treatment of thirty-five patients. J Bone Joint Surg [Am] 79:523–532, 1997.

Classic Articles

Emery SE: Cervical spondylotic myelopathy: Diagnosis and treatment. J Am Acad Orthop Surg 9:376–388, 2001.

Fielding JW, Hensinger RN, Hawkins RJ: Os odontoideum. J Bone Joint Surg [Am] 62:376–383, 1980.

Gore DR, Sepic SB: Anterior cervical fusion for degenerated or protruded discs: A review of one hundred forty-six patients. Spine 9:667–671, 1984.

Gore DR, Sepic SB, Gardner GM, et al: Neck pain: A long-term follow-up of 205 patients. Spine 12:1–5, 1987.

Herkowitz HN, Kurz LT, Overholt DP: Surgical management of cervical soft disk herniation: A comparison between anterior and posterior approaches. Spine 15:1026–1030, 1990.

Hirabayashi K, Satomi K: Operative procedure and results of expansive open-door laminoplasty. Spine 13:870–876, 1988.

Smith GW, Robinson RA: The treatment of certain cervical spine disorders by anterior removal of the intervertebral disk and interbody fusion. J Bone Joint Surg [Am] 40:607–623, 1958.

Zdeblick TA, Bohlman HH: Cervical kyphosis and myelopathy: Treatment by anterior corpectomy and strut-grating. J Bone Joint Surg [Am] 71:170–182, 1989.

Review Articles

Bohlman HH: Cervical spondylosis and myelopathy. AAOS Instr Course Lect 44:81–98, 1995.

Law MD, Bernhardt M, White AA: Evaluation and management of cervical spondylotic myelopathy. AAOS Instr Course Lect 44:99–110, 1995.

Levine MJ, Albert TJ, Smith MD: Cervical radiculopathy: Diagnosis and nonoperative management. J Am Acad Orthop Surg 4:305–316, 1996.

Rao RD: Neck pain, cervical radiculopathy, and cervical myelopathy: Pathophysiology, natural history, and clinical evaluation. J Bone Joint Surg [Am] 84:1872–1881, 2002.

Rao RD, Gourab K, David KS: Operative treatment of cervical spondylotic myelopathy. J Bone Joint Surg [Am] 88:1619–1640, 2006.

RHEUMATOID SPONDYLITIS

Recent Articles

Boden SD, Dodge LD, Bohlman HH, et al: Rheumatoid arthritis of the cervical spine: A long-term analysis with predictors of paralysis and recovery. J Bone Joint Surg [Am] 75:1282–1297, 1993.

Classic Articles

Brooks AL, Jenkins EB: Atlanto-axial arthrodesis by the wedge compression method. J Bone Joint Surg [Am] 60:279–284, 1978.

Clark CR, Goetz DD, Menezes AH: Arthrodesis of the cervical spine in rheumatoid arthritis. J Bone Joint Surg [Am] 71:381–392, 1989.

Pellicci PM, Ranawat CS, Tsairis P, et al: A prospective study of the progression of rheumatoid arthritis of the cervical spine. J Bone Joint Surg [Am] 63:342–350, 1981.

Rana NA: Natural history of atlanto-axial subluxation in rheumatoid arthritis. Spine 14:1054–1056, 1989.

Ranawat CS, O'Leary P, Pellicci P, et al: Cervical spine fusion in rheumatoid arthritis. J Bone Joint Surg [Am] 61:1003–1010, 1979.

Review Articles

Monsey RD: Rheumatoid arthritis of the cervical spine. J Am Acad Orthop Surg 5:240–248, 1997.

CERVICAL SPINE INJURY

Recent Articles

Anderson PA, Bohlman HH: Anterior decompression and arthrodesis of the cervical spine: Long-term motor improvement. Part II: Improvement in complete traumatic quadriplegia. J Bone Joint Surg [Am] 74:683–692, 1992.

Bohlman HH, Anderson PA: Anterior decompression and arthrodesis of the cervical spine: Long term motor improvement. Part I: Improvement in incomplete traumatic quadriparesis. J Bone Joint Surg [Am] 74:671–682, 1992.

Hoffman JR, Mower WR, Wolfson AB, et al: Validity of a set of clinical criteria to rule out injury to the cervical spine in patients with blunt trauma. N Engl J Med 343:94–99, 2000.

McAfee PC, Bohlman HH, Ducker TB, et al: One-stage anterior cervical decompression and posterior stabilization. J Bone Joint Surg [Am] 77:1791–1800, 1995.

Torg JS, Naranja RJ, Pavlov H, et al: The relationship of developmental narrowing of the cervical spinal canal to reversible and irreversible injury of the cervical spinal cord in football players: An epidemiological study. J Bone Joint Surg [Am] 78:1308–1314, 1996.

Classic Articles

Allen BL Jr., Ferguson RL, Lehmann TR, et al: A mechanistic classification of closed, indirect fractures and dislocation of the lower cervical spine. Spine 7:1–27, 1982.

Anderson LD, D'Alonzo RT: Fractures of the odontoid process of the axis. J Bone Joint Surg [Am] 56:1663–1674, 1974.

Bohlman HH: Acute fractures and dislocations of the cervical spine: An analysis of 300 hospitalized patients and review of the literature. J Bone Joint Surg [Am] 61:1119–1142, 1979.

Clark CR, White AA III: Fractures of the dens: A multicenter study. J Bone Joint Surg [Am] 67:1340–1348, 1985.

Fielding JW, Hawkins RJ: Atlanto-axial rotatory fixation: Fixed rotatory subluxation of the atlanto-axial joint. J Bone Joint Surg [Am] 59:37–44, 1977.

Gallie WE: Fractures and dislocations of the cervical spine. Am J Surg 46:495, 1939.

Johnson RM, Hart DL, Simmons EF, et al: Cervical orthoses: A study comparing their effectiveness in restricting cervical motion in normal subjects. J Bone Joint Surg [Am] 59:332–339, 1977.

Kang JE, Figgie MP, Bohlman HH: Sagittal measurements of the cervical spine in subaxial fractures and dislocations: An analysis of two hundred eighty-eight patients with and without neurologic deficits. J Bone Joint Surg [Am] 76:1617–1628, 1994.

Levine AM, Edwards CC: The management of traumatic spondylolisthesis of the axis. J Bone Joint Surg [Am] 67:217–226, 1985.

Torg S, Pavlov H, Genuario SE, et al: Neurapraxia on the cervical spinal cord with transient quadriplegia. J Bone Joint Surg [Am] 68: 1354–1370, 1986.

LUMBAR STENOSIS

Recent Articles

Grob D, Humke T, Dvorak J: Degenerative lumbar spinal stenosis: Decompression with and without arthrodesis. J Bone Joint Surg [Am] 77:1036–1041, 1995.

Katz JN, Lipson SJ: Seven to ten year outcome of decompressive surgery for degenerative lumbar spinal stenosis. Spine 21:92–98, 1996.

Riew KD, Yin Y, Gilula L, et al: The effect of nerve-root injection on the need for operative treatment of lumbar radicular pain: A prospective, randomized, controlled, double-blind study. J Bone Joint Surg [Am] 82:1589–1593, 2000.

Stewart G, Sachs BL: Patient outcomes after reoperation on the lumbar spine. J Bone Joint Surg [Am] 78:706–711, 1996.

Classic Articles

Kirkaldy-Willis WH: The relationship of structural pathology to the nerve root. Spine 9:49–52, 1984.

Kirkaldy-Willis WH, Wedge JH, Yong-Hing K, et al: Pathology and pathogenesis of lumbar spondylosis and stenosis. Spine 3:319–328, 1978.

Spengler DM: Current concepts review: Degenerative stenosis of the lumbar spine. J Bone Joint Surg [Am] 69:305–308, 1987.

Recent Articles

Yuan PS, Albert TJ: Nonsurgical and surgical management of lumbar spinal stenosis. J Bone Joint Surg [Am] 86:2319–2330, 2004.

Spivak JM: Degenerative lumbar spinal stenosis. J Bone Joint Surg [Am] 80:1053–1067, 1998.

BACK PAIN

Recent Articles

Bono CM: Low-back pain in athletes. J Bone Joint Surg [Am] 86:382–396, 2004.

Jensen ME, Brant-Zawadzki MN, Obuchowski N, et al: Magnetic resonance imaging of the lumbar spine in people without back pain. N Engl J Med 331:69–73, 1994.

Rozenberg S, Delval C, Rezvani Y: Bed rest or normal activity for patients with acute low back pain: A randomized controlled trial. Spine 27:1487–1493, 2002.

Classic Articles

Deyo RH, Diehl AK, Rosenthal M: How many days of bed rest for acute low back pain? A randomized clinical trial. N Engl J Med 315:1064–1070, 1986.

Frymoyer JW: Back pain and sciatica. N Engl J Med 318:291–300, 1988.

Frymoyer JW, Pope MH, Clements JH, et al: Risk factors in low back pain: An epidemiological survey. J Bone Joint Surg [Am] 65:213–218, 1983.

Nachemson A: Work for all: For those with low back pain as well. Clin Orthop 179:77–85, 1983.

Review Articles

Botte MJ, Byrne TP, Abrams RA, et al: Halo skeletal fixation: Techniques of application and prevention of complications. J Am Acad Orthop Surg 4:44–53, 1996.

Slucky AV, Eismont FJ: Treatment of acute injury of the cervical spine. AAOS Instr Course Lect 44:67–80, 1995.

Torg JS, Guille JT, Jaffe S: Injuries to the cervical spine in American football players. J Bone Joint Surg 84:112–122, 2002.

SPONDYLOLISTHESIS

Classic Articles

Boxall D, Bradford DS, Winter RB, Moe JH: Management of severe spondylolisthesis in children and adolescents. J Bone Joint Surg [Am] 61:479–495, 1979.

Bradford DS: Closed reduction of spondylolisthesis and experience in 22 patients. Spine 13:580–587, 1988.

Bradford DS, Boachie-Adjei O: Treatment of severe spondylolisthesis by anterior and posterior reduction and stabilization: A long-term follow-up study. J Bone Joint Surg [Am] 72:1060–1066, 1990.

Frederickson BW, Baker D, McHolick WJ, et al: The natural history of spondylolysis and spondylolisthesis. J Bone Joint Surg [Am] 66:699–707, 1984.

Gill GG, Manning JG, White HL: Surgical treatment of spondylolisthesis without spine fusion. J Bone Joint Surg [Am] 37:493–520, 1955.

Harris IE, Weinstein SD: Long-term follow-up of patients with grade III and IV spondylolisthesis: Treatment with and without posterior fusion. J Bone Joint Surg [Am] 69:960–969, 1987.

Osterman K, Lindholm TS, Laurent LE: Late results of removal of the loose posterior element (Gill's operation) in the treatment of lytic lumbar spondylolisthesis. Clin Orthop Relat Res 117:121–128, 1976.

Peek RD, Wiltse LL, Reynolds JB, et al: In situ arthrodesis without decompression for grade III or IV isthmic spondylolisthesis in adults who have severe sciatica. J Bone Joint Surg [Am] 71:62–68, 1989.

Saraste H: The etiology of spondylolysis: A retrospective radiographic study. Acta Orthop Scand 56:253–255, 1985.

Wiltse LL, Winter RB: Terminology and measurement of spondylolisthesis. J Bone Joint Surg [Am] 65:768–772, 1983.

Wiltse LL, Guyer RD, Spencer CW, et al: Alar transverse process impingement of the L5 spinal nerve: The far-out syndrome. Spine 9:31–41, 1984.

Recent Articles

Bjarke CF, Stender HE, Laursen M, et al: Long term functional outcomes of pedicle screw instrumentation as a support for posterolateral spinal fusion: Randomized clinical study with a 5-year follow-up. Spine 27:1269–1277, 2002.

Carpenter CT, Dietz JW: Repair of a pseudarthrosis of the lumbar spine: A functional outcome study. J Bone Joint Surg [Am] 78:712–720, 1996.

Carragee EJ: Single-level posterolateral arthrodesis, with or without posterior decompression, for the treatment of isthmic spondylolisthesis in adults: A prospective, randomized study. J Bone Joint Surg [Am] 79:1175–1180, 1997.

Fischgrund JS, Mackay M, Herkowitz HN, et al: Degenerative lumbar spondylolisthesis with spinal stenosis: A prospective, randomized study comparing decompressive laminectomy and arthrodesis with and without spinal instrumentation. Spine 22:2807–2812, 1997.

Goel VK, Gilbertson LG: Basic science of spinal instrumentation. Clin Orthop 335:10–31, 1997.

Herkowitz HN, Kurz LT: Degenerative lumbar spondylolisthesis with spinal stenosis: A prospective study comparing decompression with decompression and intertransverse process arthrodesis. J Bone Joint Surg [Am] 73:802–808, 1991.

Jinkins JR, Rauch A: Magnetic resonance imaging of entrapment of lumbar nerve roots in spondylolytic spondylolisthesis. J Bone Joint Surg 76:1643–1648, 1994.

Thomsen K, Christensen FB: The effect of pedicle screw instrumentation on functional outcome and fusion rates in posterolateral lumbar spinal fusion: A prospective, randomized clinical study. Spine 22:2813–2822, 1997.

Zdeblick T: A prospective randomized study of lumbar fusion. Spine 18:983–991, 1993.

Review Articles

Hensinger RN: Current concepts review: Spondylolysis and spondylolisthesis in children and adolescents. J Bone Joint Surg [Am] 71:1098–1107, 1989.

Larsen JM, Capen DA: Pseudarthrosis of the lumbar spine. J Am Acad Orthop Surg 5:153–162, 1997.

Lauerman WC, Cain JE: Isthmic spondylolisthesis in the adult. J Am Acad Orthop Surg 4:201–208, 1996.

THORACOLUMBAR INJURY

Recent Articles

Carlson GD, Gorden CD, Oliff HS, et al: Sustained spinal cord compression. Parts I and II: Time-dependent effect on long-term pathophysiology. J Bone Joint Surg [Am] 85:86–101, 2003.

Delamarter RB, Sherman J, Carr JB: Pathophysiology of spinal cord injury: Recovery after immediate and delayed decompression. J Bone Joint Surg [Am] 77:1042–1049, 1995.

Henry TP, Mirza SK, Wang J, et al: Risk factors for respiratory failure following operative stabilization of thoracic and lumbar spine fractures. J Bone Joint Surg [Am] 88:997–1005, 2006.

Kaneda K, Taneichi H: Anterior decompression and stabilization with the Kaneda device for thoracolumbar burst fractures associated with neurological deficits. J Bone Joint Surg [Am] 79:69–83, 1997.

Wilcox RK, Boerger TO, Allen DJ, et al: A dynamic study of thoracolumbar burst fractures. J Bone Joint Surg [Am] 85:2184–2189, 2003.

Wood KB, Khanna G, Vaccaro AR, et al: Assessment of two thoracolumbar fracture classification systems as used by multiple surgeons. J Bone Joint Surg [Am] 87:1423–1429, 2005.

Wood K, Buttermann G, Mehbod A, et al: Operative compared with nonoperative treatment of a thoracolumbar burst fracture without neurological deficit: A prospective, randomized study. J Bone Joint Surg [Am] 85:773–781, 2003.

Classic Articles

Bohlman HH, Eismont FJ: Surgical techniques of anterior decompression and fusion for spinal cord injuries. Clin Orthop Relat Res 154:57–67, 1981.

Bracken MB, Shepard MJ, Collins WF, et al: A randomized, controlled trial of methylprednisolone or naloxone in the treatment of acute spinal cord injury. N Engl J Med 322:1405–1411, 1990.

Cain JE, DeJung JT, Divenberg AS, et al: Pathomechanical analysis of thoracolumbar burst fracture reduction: A calf spine model. Spine 18:1640–1647, 1993.

Cammissa FP Jr., Eismont FJ, Green BA: Dural laceration occurring with burst fractures and associated laminar fractures. J Bone Joint Surg [Am] 71:1044–1052, 1989.

Denis F: The three-column spine and its significance in the classification of acute thoracolumbar spinal injuries. Spine 8:817–831, 1983.

Ferguson RL, Allen BL Jr.: A mechanistic classification of thoracolumbar spine fractures. Clin Orthop Relat Med 189:77–88, 1984.

Holdsworth FW: Fractures, dislocations, and fracture-dislocations of the spine. J Bone Joint Surg [Am] 52:1534–1551, 1970.

Kaneda K, Abumi K, Fujiya M: Burst fractures with neurologic deficits of the thoracolumbar-lumbar spine: Results of anterior decompression and stabilization with anterior instrumentation. Spine 9:788–795, 1984.

McAfee PC, Bohlman HH, Yuan HA: Anterior decompression of traumatic thoracolumbar fractures with incomplete neurologic deficit using a retroperitoneal approach. J Bone Joint Surg [Am] 67:89–104, 1985.

Mumfred J, Weinstein JN, Spratt KF, et al: Thoracolumbar burst fractures: The clinical efficacy and outcome of nonoperative management. Spine 18:955–970, 1993.

Review Articles

Bohlman HH: Current concepts review: Treatment of fractures and dislocations of the thoracic and lumbar spine. J Bone Joint Surg [Am] 67:165–169, 1985.

Slucky AV, Potter HG: Use of magnetic resonance imaging in spinal trauma: Indications, techniques, and utility. J Am Acad Orthop Surg 6:134–145, 1998.

Vaccaro AR, Kim DH, Brodke DS, et al: Diagnosis and management of thoracolumbar spine fractures. J Bone Joint Surg [Am] 85:2456–2470, 2003.

SACRUM

Classic Articles

Denis F, Davis S, Comfort T: Sacral fractures: An important problem—retrospective analysis of 236 cases. Clin Orthop 227:67–81, 1988.

Newhouse KE, El-Khoury GY, Buckwalter JA: Occult sacral fractures in osteopenic patients. J Bone Joint Surg [Am] 75:1472–1477, 1992.

Postacchini F, Massobrio M: Idiopathic coccygodynia: Analysis of fifty-one operative cases and a radiographic study of the normal coccyx. J Bone Joint Surg [Am] 65:1116–1124, 1983.

INFECTIONS, TUMORS

Recent Articles

Bauer HC: Posterior decompression and stabilization for spinal metastases: Analysis of sixty-seven consecutive patients. J Bone Joint Surg [Am] 79:514–522, 1997.

Carragee EJ: Pyogenic vertebral osteomyelitis. J Bone Joint Surg [Am] 79:874–880, 1997.

Frazier DD: Fungal infections of the spine. J Bone Joint Surg [Am] 83:560, 2001.

Hulen CA, Temple HT, Fox WP, et al: Oncologic and functional outcome following sacrectomy for sacral chordoma. J Bone Joint Surg [Am] 88:1532–1539, 2006.

Leet AI, Magur E, Lee JS, et al: Fibrous dysplasia in the spine: Prevalence of lesions and association with scoliosis. J Bone Joint Surg [Am] 86:531–537, 2004.

Patchell RA, Tibbs PA, Regine WF, et al: Direct decompressive surgery and radiation therapy improved walking ability in metastatic epidural spinal cord compression. Lancet 266:643–648, 2005.

Weinstein MA, Eismont FJ: Infections of the spine in patients with human immunodeficiency virus. J Bone Joint Surg [Am] 87:604–609, 2005.

Classic Articles

Allen AR, Stevenson AW: A ten-year follow-up of combined drug therapy and early fusion in bone tuberculosis. J Bone Joint Surg [Am] 49:1001, 1967.

Batson OB: The function of the vertebral veins and their role in the spread of metastases. Ann Surg 112:138–149, 1940.

Bohlman HH, Sachs BL, Carter JR, et al: Primary neoplasms of the cervical spine: Diagnosis and treatment of twenty-three patients. J Bone Joint Surg [Am] 68:483–494, 1986.

Eismont FJ, Bohlman HH, Soni PL, et al: Pyogenic and fungal vertebral osteomyelitis with paralysis. J Bone Joint Surg [Am] 65:19–29, 1983.

Emery SE, Chan DPK, Woodward HR: Treatment of hematogenous pyogenic vertebral osteomyelitis with anterior débridement and primary bone grafting. Spine 14:284–291, 1989.

Hodgson AR, Stock FE, Fang HSY, et al: Anterior spinal fusion: The operative approach and pathological findings in 412 patients with Pott's disease of the spine. Br J Surg 48:172–178, 1960.

Kostulk JP, Errica TJ, Gleason TF, et al: Spinal stabilization of vertebral column tumors. Spine 13:250–256, 1988.

McAfee PC, Bohlman HH: One-stage anterior cervical decompression and posterior stabilization with circumferential arthrodesis: A study of twenty-four patients who had a traumatic or neoplastic lesion. J Bone Joint Surg [Am] 71:78–88, 1989.

Siegal T, Tiqva P, Siegal T: Vertebral body resection for epidural compression by malignant tumors: Results of forty-seven consecutive operative procedures. J Bone Joint Surg [Am] 67:375–382, 1985.

Weinstein JN, MacLain RF: Primary tumors of the spine. Spine 12:843–851, 1987.

OTHER

Recent Articles

Ahlmann E, Patzakis M, Roidis N, et al: Comparison of anterior and posterior iliac crest bone grafts in terms of harvest-site morbidity and functional outcomes. J Bone Joint Surg [Am] 84:716–720, 2002.

Blumenthal S, McFee PC, Guyer RD, et al: A prospective, randomized, multicenter food and drug administration investigational device exemptions study of lumbar total disc replacement with the CHARITE artificial disc versus lumbar fusion. Parts I and II. Spine 30:1565–1583, 2005.

Chen C, Lu Y, Kallakuri S, et al: Distribution of A-delta and C-fiber receptors in the cervical facet joint capsule and their response to stretch. J Bone Joint Surg [Am] 88:1807–1816, 2006.

McKiernan F, Faciszewski T, Jensen R: Quality of life following vertebroplasty. J Bone Joint Surg [Am] 86:2600–2606, 2004.

Reuben SS, Ekman EF: The effect of cyclooxygenase-2 inhibition on analgesia and spinal fusion. J Bone Joint Surg [Am] 87:536–542, 2005.

Riew KD, Long J, Rhee J, et al: Time-dependent inhibitory effects of indomethacin on spinal fusion. J Bone Joint Surg [Am] 85:632–634, 2003.

Tropiano P, Huang RC, Girardi FP, et al: Lumbar total disc replacement: Seven to eleven-year follow-up. J Bone Joint Surg [Am] 87:490–496, 2005.

Review Articles

Belanger TA, Rowe DE: Diffuse idiopathic skeletal hyperostosis: Musculoskeletal manifestations. J Am Acad Orthop Surg 9:258–267, 2001.

Edwards CC, Karpitskaya Y, Cha C, et al: Accurate identification of adverse outcomes after cervical spine surgery. J Bone Joint Surg [Am] 86:251–256, 2004.

Kambin P, McCullen G, Parke W, et al: Minimally invasive arthroscopic spinal surgery. AAOS Instr Course Lect 46:143–161, 1997.

Mason NA, Phillips FM: Minimally invasive techniques for the treatment of osteoporotic vertebral fractures. J Bone Joint Surg [Am] 88:1862–1872, 2006.

Regan JJ, Yuan H, McCullen G: Minimally invasive approaches to the spine. AAOS Instr Course Lect 46:127–141, 1997.

Rao RD, Singrakhia MD: Painful osteoporotic vertebral fracture: Pathogenesis, evaluation, and roles of vertebroplasty and kyphoplasty in its management. J Bone Joint Surg [Am] 85:2010–2022, 2003.

Tay BKB: Spinal infections. J Am Acad Orthop Surg 10:188–197, 2002.

CHAPTER 9

Orthopaedic Pathology

Frank J. Frassica, Deborah A. Frassica, AND Edward F. McCarthy

CONTENTS

I. Introduction

A. Staging—Staging systems may be useful for developing evaluation strategies, planning treatment, and predicting prognosis. For musculoskeletal lesions, the staging systems of the Musculoskeletal Tumor Society (also called the Enneking system) and the **American Joint Commission on Cancer** (AJCC system) are the most popular. In the Enneking system there are two separate systems for benign and malignant lesions. For malignant lesions, the system is based on knowing the histologic grade of the lesion (low or high), the anatomic features (intracompartmental or extracompartmental), and the absence (M_0) or presence (M_1) of metastases.

1. Enneking system—The Enneking staging system can be synthesized into six distinct stages (Table 9–1).
2. Variables of AJCC system—The most recent edition of the AJCC system has become more popular among medical oncologists and many orthopaedic oncologists. A working knowledge of both systems is necessary for examinations. To use this system, one must know the grade, the size, the presence or absence of discontinuous tumor (skip metastases), and the absence or presence of systemic metastases. The various stages are shown in Table 9–2. One should remember the order of importance for the variables of the AJCC staging system: stage (takes into account all factors), presence of metastases, discontinuous tumor, grade, and size.

B. Grading—Grading can be difficult and is based on nuclear anaplasia (degree of loss of structural differentiation), pleomorphism (variations in size and shape), and nuclear hyperchromasia (increased nuclear staining). Grading of tumors requires a morphologic range. Most grading systems are based on three grades: grade I, well differentiated; grade II, moderately differentiated; and grade III, poorly differentiated. The grade of the tumor most strongly correlates with the potential for metastasis: grade I (low grade), less than 10%; grade 2 (intermediate grade), 10-30%; and grade III (high grade), greater than 50%. Most malignant lesions are high grade (G_2); low-grade malignant (G_1) lesions are less common. Commonly graded lesions are shown in Table 9–3.

C. Tumor site—The plain radiographs and special studies, such as computed tomography (CT) and magnetic resonance imaging (MRI), are used to determine whether the tumor is situated within the bone compartment (intracompartmental, or T1) or has left the confines of the bone (extracompartmental, or T2). Preoperative MRI scans are used to determine the anatomic features of the tumor and plan surgical margins. A T1-weighted coronal MRI is obtained to determine the intramedullary extent of the tumor and detect skip metastases (discontinuous tumor).

D. Metastases—For most lesions, a chest radiograph and CT scan of the chest are performed to search for pulmonary lesions. A technetium bone scan is used to exclude the presence of other bone lesions.

TABLE 9–1 STAGING SYSTEM OF THE MUSCULOSKELETAL TUMOR SOCIETY (ENNEKING SYSTEM)

Stage	GTM	Description
IA	$G_1T_1M_0$	Low grade Intracompartmental No metastases
IB	$G_1T_2M_0$	Low grade Extracompartmental No metastases
IIA	$G_2T_1M_0$	High grade Intracompartmental No metastases
IIB	$G_2T_2M_0$	High grade Extracompartmental No metastases
IIIA	$G_{1/2}T_1M_1$	Any grade Intracompartmental With metastases
IIIB	$G_{1/2}T_2M_1$	Any grade Extracompartmental With metastases

Grade system (G): Low grade (G_1) and high grade (G_2). High-grade lesions are intermediate between low-grade, well-differentiated tumors and high-grade, undifferentiated tumors.

Tumor size (T): The size of the tumor is determined by using specialized procedures, including radiography, tomography, nuclear studies, computed tomography (CT), and magnetic resonance imaging (MRI). Compartments are used to describe the tumor site. These compartments are usually easily defined based on fascial borders in the extremities. Of note, the skin and subcutaneous tissues are classified as a compartment, and the potential periosseous space between cortical bone and muscle is often considered a compartment as well. T_0 lesions are confined within the capsule and within its compartment of origin. T_1 tumors have extracapsular extension into the reactive zone around it, but both the tumor and the reactive zone are confined within the compartment of origin. T_2 lesions extend beyond the anatomic compartment of origin by direct extension or some other means (e.g., trauma, surgical seeding). Tumors that involve major neurovascular bundles are almost always classified as T_2 lesions.

Metastases (M): Both regional and distal metastases have ominous prognoses; therefore, the distinction is simply between no metastases (M_0) and the presence of metastases (M_1).

TABLE 9–3 TYPICAL LOW- AND HIGH-GRADE BONE AND SOFT TISSUE TUMORS

Low-Grade Tumors	High-Grade Tumors
Bone	
Parosteal osteosarcoma	Intramedullary (classic) osteosarcoma
Primary chondrosarcoma	
Secondary chondrosarcoma	Postradiation sarcoma
Hemangioendothelioma	Paget sarcoma
Chordoma	Fibrosarcoma
Adamantinoma	Malignant fibrous histiocytoma
Soft Tissue	
Myxoid liposarcoma	Malignant fibrous histiocytoma
Lipoma-like liposarcoma	Pleomorphic liposarcoma
Angiomatoid malignant fibrous histiocytoma	Synovial sarcoma
	Rhabdomyosarcoma
	Alveolar cell sarcoma

E. Evaluation

1. Clinical presentation—Most patients with bone tumors present with musculoskeletal pain. The pain is similar whether the bone destruction is secondary to a primary mesenchymal tumor (e.g., osteosarcoma, chondrosarcoma) or results from metastatic bone disease, myeloma, or lymphoma. The pain is typically deep-seated and dull and may resemble a toothache. Initially, the pain may be intermittent and related to activity, a work injury, or a sporting injury. The pain usually progresses in intensity and becomes constant. Many patients experience pain at night. As the pain progresses, it is not relieved by **nonsteroidal anti-inflammatory drugs** (NSAIDs) or weaker narcotics (such as acetaminophen [Tylenol] with codeine). Most patients with a high-grade sarcoma will present with a 1- to 3-month history of pain. In contrast, with low-grade tumors, such as chondrosarcoma, adamantinoma, and chordoma, there may be a long history of mild to moderate pain (6-24 months).
2. Physical examination—Patients with suspected bone tumors should be examined carefully. The affected site is inspected for soft tissue masses, overlying skin changes, adenopathy, and general

TABLE 9–2 AMERICAN JOINT COMMITTEE ON CANCER STAGING SYSTEM FOR PRIMARY MALIGNANT TUMORS OF BONE FOR THOSE TUMORS DIAGNOSED ON OR AFTER JANUARY 1, 2003

Stage	Tumor	Lymph Node	Metastases	Grade
IA	T1	N0	M0	G1 or G2
IB	T2	N0	M0	G1 or G2
IIA	T1	N0	M0	G3 or G4
IIB	T2	N0	M0	G3 or G4
III	T3	N0	M0	Any G
IVA	Any T	N0	M1a	Any G
IVB	Any T	N1	Any M	Any G
	Any T	Any N	M1b	Any G

Tx = primary tumor cannot be assessed; T0 = no evidence of primary tumor; T1 = tumor 8 cm or less in greatest dimension; T2 = tumor more than 8 cm in greatest dimension; T3 = discontinuous tumors in the primary bone; Nx = regional lymph nodes not assessed; N0 = no regional lymph node metastases; N1 = regional lymph node metastasis; Mx = distant metastasis cannot be assessed; M0 = no distant metastasis; M1 = distant metastasis; M1a = lung; M1b = other distant sites; Gx = grade cannot be assessed; G1 = well differentiated (low grade); G2 = moderately differentiated (low grade); G3 = poorly differentiated (high grade); G4 = undifferentiated (high grade).

From American Joint Committee on Cancer. Bone. In Greene FL, Page DL, Fleming ID, et al, eds: AJCC cancer staging manual, pp 213–219. New York, Springer-Verlag, 2002.

musculoskeletal condition. When metastatic disease is suspected, the thyroid gland, abdomen, prostate, and breasts should be examined, as appropriate.

3. Imaging studies—Radiographs in two planes are the first imaging studies to be performed. When the clinician suspects malignancy and the radiographs are normal, selected studies may follow. A technetium bone scan is an excellent modality to search for occult bone involvement. In patients with myeloma for whom scan results may be negative, a skeletal survey is more sensitive. MRI is an excellent modality for screening the spine for occult metastases, myeloma, or lymphoma. A chest radiograph should be obtained in all age groups when the clinician suspects a malignant lesion. The radiographs must be carefully inspected to formulate a working diagnosis. The working diagnosis then guides the clinician during further evaluation and treatment. Formulation of the differential diagnosis is based on several clinical and radiographic parameters.
   a. Age of the patient—Knowledge of common diseases in defined age groups is the first step. Certain diseases are uncommon in particular age groups (Table 9–4).
   b. Number of bone lesions—Is the process monostotic or polyostotic? If there are multiple destructive lesions in middle-aged and older patients (ages 40-80 years), the most likely diagnosis is metastatic bone disease, multiple myeloma, or lymphoma. In young patients (ages 15-40 years), multiple lytic and oval lesions are most likely a vascular tumor (hemangioendothelioma). In children below age 5, multiple destructive lesions may represent metastatic disease such as neuroblastoma or a Wilms' tumor. Histiocytosis X (**Langerhans cell histiocytosis** [LCH]) may also lead to multiple lesions in the young patient. Fibrous dysplasia and Paget disease may present with multiple lesions in all age groups.
   c. Anatomic location within bone—Certain lesions have a predilection for occurring within a certain bone or a particular part of the bone. Adamantinoma is a malignant tumor that usually occurs in the tibia in young patients. Chondroblastoma most often occurs within the epiphysis of long bones. A giant cell tumor typically begins in the metaphysis and extends through the epiphysis to lie just below the cartilage. A Ewing tumor frequently involves the diaphysis. Osteogenic sarcoma usually occurs in the metaphysis of the distal femur and proximal tibia but occurs within the diaphysis in about 7% of patients with long-bone lesions.
   d. Effect of the lesion on bone—High-grade malignant lesions generally spread rapidly through the medullary cavity. Cortical bone destruction occurs early, and the process spreads into the adjacent soft tissues. Low-grade malignant lesions tend to spread slowly, but they also can destroy the cortical bone and produce a soft tissue mass.
   e. Response of the bone to the lesion—With high-grade lesions there is often little ability of the host bone to contain the process. The result is rapid destruction of cortical bone and the presence of a soft tissue mass. In contrast, with low-grade lesions, the host bone can often contain the lesion with a thickened cortex or rim of periosteal bone. With benign or low-grade lesions, there is often a thick periosteal response about the lesion.
   f. Matrix characteristics—If the lesion produces a matrix, it is helpful to determine whether the matrix is cartilage calcification or mineralization of osteoid. Cartilage calcification often appears stippled or may show arcs or rings; osteoid mineralization is often cloudlike.

TABLE 9-4 AGE DISTRIBUTION OF VARIOUS BONE LESIONS

	Type of Lesion	
Age	*Malignant*	*Benign*
Birth to 5 yr	Leukemia Metastatic neuroblastoma Metastatic rhabdomyosarcoma	Osteomyelitis Osteofibrous dysplasia
10-25 yr	Osteosarcoma Ewing tumor Leukemia	Eosinophilic granuloma Osteomyelitis Enchondroma Fibrous dysplasia
40-80 yr	Metastatic bone disease Myeloma Lymphoma Chondrosarcoma Malignant fibrous histiocytoma Paget sarcoma Postradiation sarcoma	Hyperparathyroidism Paget disease Mastocytosis Enchondroma Bone infarct

4. Laboratory studies—Blood tests are often nonspecific. A set of routine studies should be obtained when there is not an obvious diagnosis. The studies can be grouped into those for younger patients (up to age 40) and those for older patients (40-80 years) (Box 9–1).
5. Biopsy—Biopsy is generally performed after complete evaluation of the patient. It is of great benefit to both the pathologist and surgeon to have a narrow working diagnosis because it allows accurate interpretation of the frozen-section analysis and allows definitive treatment of some lesions based on the frozen section. There are several surgical principles that the clinician must follow.
   a. The orientation and location of the biopsy tract are critical. If the lesion proves to be malignant, the entire biopsy tract must be removed with the underlying lesion. Transverse incisions should be avoided (Fig. 9–1).
   b. The surgeon must maintain meticulous hemostasis to prevent hematoma formation and subcutaneous hemorrhage. When possible, biopsies are done through muscles so that

the muscle layer can be closed tightly. Tourniquets are used to obtain tissue in a bloodless field and then are released so that bleeding points can be controlled. Avitene, Gelfoam, and Thrombostat sprays are used as necessary. If hemostasis cannot be achieved, a small drain should be brought out of the corner of the wound to prevent hematoma formation. A compression dressing is routinely used on the extremities.

c. A frozen-section analysis is done on all biopsy samples to ensure that adequate diagnostic tissue is obtained. Before biopsy, the surgeon should review the radiographs with the pathologist to plan the biopsy site. When possible, the soft tissue component rather than the bony component should be sampled.

d. All biopsy samples should be submitted for bacteriologic analysis if the frozen section does not reveal a neoplasm. Antibiotics should not be delivered until the cultures are obtained.

e. Needle biopsy is an excellent method for achieving a tissue diagnosis and providing minimum tissue disruption. Careful correlation of the small tissue sample with the radiographs will often yield the correct diagnosis. When the nature of the lesion is obvious based on the radiographic features and when adequate tissue can be obtained with needle biopsy, the needle biopsy technique is safe to use. The pathologist must be experienced and comfortable with the small sample of tissue. When the diagnoses of needle biopsy and imaging studies are not concordant, an open biopsy should be done to establish the diagnosis. Open biopsy is often necessary in low-grade tumors and when the needle biopsy does not provide a definitive diagnosis.

F. Treatment

1. Surgical procedures—The goal of the treatment of malignant bone tumors is to remove the lesion with minimal risk of local recurrence. Limb salvage is performed when two essential criteria are met: (1) local control of the lesion must be at least equal to that of amputation surgery; and (2) the limb that has been saved must be functional. A wide surgical margin (a cuff of normal tissue around the tumor) is the surgical goal. Surgical margins are graded according to the system of the Musculoskeletal Tumor Society (Fig. 9–2).

a. Intralesional margin—The plane of dissection goes directly through the tumor. When the surgery involves malignant mesenchymal tumors, an intralesional margin results in 100% local recurrence.

b. Marginal margin—A marginal line of resection goes through the reactive zone of the tumor; the reactive zone contains inflammatory cells, edema, fibrous tissue, and satellites of tumor cells. When malignant mesenchymal tumors are resected, a plane of dissection through the reactive zone will probably result in a local recurrence rate of 25-50%. A marginal margin may be safe and effective if there has been an excellent response to preoperative chemotherapy (95-100% tumor necrosis).

c. Wide margin—A wide surgical resection is accomplished when the entire tumor is removed with a cuff of normal tissue. The local recurrence rate drops below 10% when such a surgical margin is achieved.

d. Radical margin—A radical margin is achieved when the entire tumor and its compartment

Box 9–1 Laboratory Evaluations for Young and Middle-Aged Patients

AGES 5-40 YEARS

Complete blood count with differential
Peripheral blood smear
Erythrocyte sedimentation rate

AGES 40-80 YEARS

Complete blood count with differential
Erythrocyte sedimentation rate
Chemistry group: calcium and phosphate
Serum or urine protein electrophoresis
Urinalysis

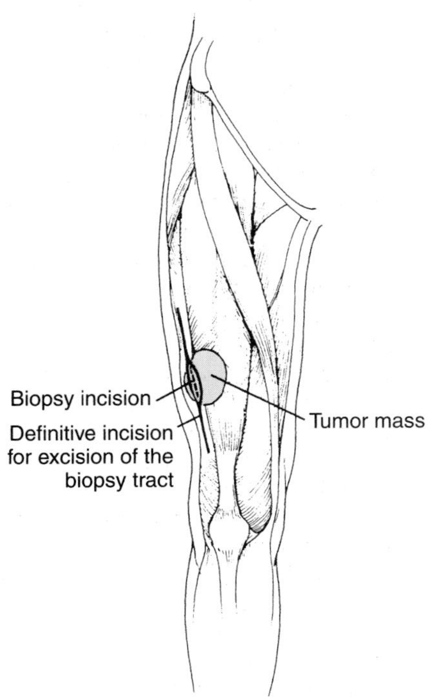

FIGURE 9–1 Lesion in the lateral aspect of the quadriceps mechanism. A short longitudinal incision is made over the lesion. Before the skin incision, a second incision line should be drawn to demonstrate how the biopsy tract can be removed at the time of the definitive surgery. (From Sim FH, Frassica FJ, Frassica DA: Soft tissue tumors: Diagnosis, evaluation and management. AAOS 2:209, 1994. ©1994 American Academy of Orthopaedic Surgeons. Reprinted with permission.)

(all surrounding muscles, ligaments, and connective tissues) are removed.

2. Adjuvant therapy
   a. Chemotherapy—Multiagent chemotherapy has a significant impact on both the efficacy of limb salvage and disease-free survival for osteogenic sarcoma and a Ewing tumor. The common mechanism of action for chemotherapy drugs is the induction of programmed cell death (apoptosis). Most protocols use preoperative regimens (called neoadjuvant chemotherapy) for 8-24 weeks. The tumor is then restaged and, if appropriate, limb salvage is performed. Next, patients undergo maintenance chemotherapy for 6-12 months. Patients with localized osteosarcoma or a Ewing tumor have up to a 60-70% chance for long-term disease-free survival with the combination of multiagent chemotherapy and surgery. The role of chemotherapy for soft tissue sarcoma remains more controversial.
   b. Radiation therapy—External beam irradiation is used for local control of a Ewing tumor, lymphoma, myeloma, and metastatic bone disease. It is also used as an adjunct for the treatment of soft tissue sarcomas, in which it is used in combination with surgery. The mechanism of action of external beam irradiation is the production of free radicals and direct genetic damage. There are several complications of radiation therapy.
      (1) Postirradiation sarcoma—This is a devastating complication in which a spindle sarcoma occurs within the field of irradiation for a previous malignancy (e.g., a Ewing tumor, breast cancer, Hodgkin disease). The histology is usually that of an osteosarcoma, fibrosarcoma, or malignant fibrous histiocytoma. Postirradiation sarcomas are probably more frequent in patients who undergo intensive chemotherapy (especially with alkylating agents) and irradiation.
      (2) Late stress fractures—These also may occur in weight-bearing bones to which high-dose irradiation has been applied. The subtrochanteric region and the diaphysis of the femur are common sites.

G. Molecular biology—Several bone and soft tissue neoplasms have been associated with tumor suppressor genes or specific genetic defects. A low level of the **retinoblastoma** (RB) gene has been associated with osteosarcoma. The *TB53* gene has also been found to have low levels in both rhabdomyosarcoma and osteosarcoma. Gene translocations have been found in Ewing sarcoma of bone (11:22) and several soft tissue sarcomas: myxoid liposarcoma (12:16), synovial sarcoma (X:18), and rhabdomyosarcoma (2:13).

II. Soft Tissue Tumors

A. Introduction—Soft tissue tumors are common. Patients may have small lumps or large masses.

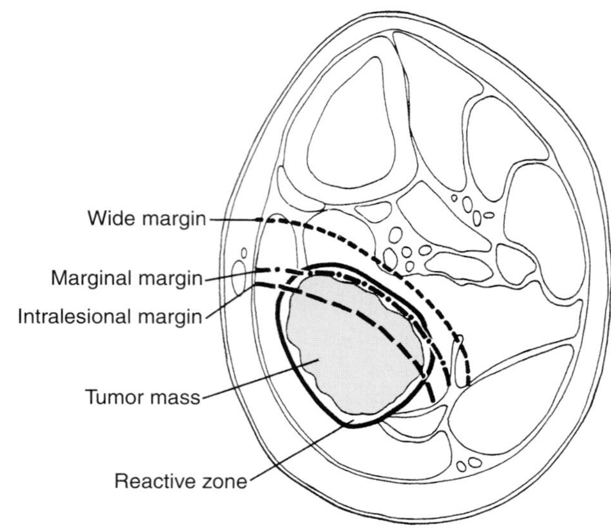

FIGURE 9–2 Types of surgical margins. An intralesional line of resection enters the substance of the tumor. A marginal line of resection travels through the reactive zone of the tumor. A wide surgical margin removes the tumor with a cuff of normal tissue. (From Sim FH, Frassica FJ, Frassica DA: Soft tissue tumors: Diagnosis, evaluation and management. AAOS 2:209, 1994. ©1994 American Academy of Orthopaedic Surgeons. Reprinted with permission.)

1. Classification—Soft tissue tumors can be broadly classified as benign or malignant (sarcoma) or characterized by reactive tumor–like conditions (Box 9–2). Lesions are classified according to the direction of differentiation of the lesion—the tumor tends to produce collagen (fibrous lesion), fat, or cartilage.
   a. Benign soft tissue tumors—These tumors may occur in all age groups. The lesions vary in their biologic behavior, from those that are asymptomatic and self-limiting (Enneking stage I—inactive) to those that are growing and symptomatic (Enneking stage II—active). Occasionally, benign lesions grow rapidly and invade adjacent tissues (Enneking stage III—aggressive).
   b. Malignant soft tissue tumors (sarcomas)—Sarcomas are rare tumors of mesenchymal origin. In the United States, there are approximately 9000 new cases of soft tissue sarcoma each year.
      (1) Diagnosis—Patients often experience an enlarging painless or painful soft tissue mass. Most sarcomas are large (> 5 cm), deep, and firm. In some instances they are small and may be present for a long time before recognition. Lesions that may be initially small include synovial sarcoma, rhabdomyosarcoma, epithelioid sarcoma, and clear cell sarcoma. Initial radiographic evaluation begins with plain radiographs in two planes. An MRI is the best imaging modality to define the anatomy and help characterize the lesion. When a

mass is judged to be indeterminate, an open incisional or needle biopsy is performed. A definitive histologic diagnosis must be established before planning treatment.

(2) Treatment—Radiation therapy is an important adjunct to surgery in the treatment of soft tissue sarcomas. The ionizing irradiation can be delivered preoperatively, perioperatively with brachytherapy after loading tubes, or postoperatively. Treatment regimens are often designed to use combinations of the three types of preoperative, postoperative, and external beam irradiation. Poor prognostic factors include the presence of metastases, high grade, size greater than 5 cm, and location below the deep fascia.

2. Diagnosis—The evaluation of patients with soft tissue tumors must be systematic to avoid errors. Unplanned removal of a soft tissue sarcoma is the most common error made by surgeons. A delay in diagnosis may also occur if the clinician does not recognize that the lesion is malignant. Patients who have a new soft tissue mass or one that is growing or causing pain should undergo MRI. The MRI should be carefully reviewed with a radiologist to characterize the nature of the mass. If it can be determined that the lesion is a benign process such as a lipoma, ganglionic cyst, or muscle tear, then it is classified as a *determinate lesion* and treatment can be planned without doing a biopsy. In contrast, if the exact nature of a lesion cannot be determined, the lesion is classified as *indeterminate*, and either a needle or open biopsy is necessary to determine the exact diagnosis. Then treatment can be planned. Excisional biopsy should not be performed when the clinician does not know the etiology of a soft tissue tumor.

B. Tumors of fibrous tissue—Fibrous tumors are common, and there is a wide range, from small, self-limiting, benign conditions to aggressive, invasive, benign tumors. The malignant fibrous tumors are fibrosarcoma and malignant fibrous histiocytoma.

1. Calcifying aponeurotic fibroma—This entity presents as a slowly growing, painless mass in the hands and feet in children and young adults ages 3-30 years. Radiographs may reveal a faint mass with stippling. Histologic examination shows a fibrous tumor with centrally located areas of calcification and cartilage formation. Local excision often results in recurrence in up to 50% of cases; however, the condition appears to resolve with maturity.
2. Fibromatosis
   a. Palmar (Dupuytren) and plantar (Lederhosen) fibromatosis—These disorders consist of firm nodules of fibroblasts and collagen that develop in the palmar and plantar fascia. The nodules and fascia become hypertrophic, producing contractures.
   b. Extra-abdominal desmoid tumor—This tumor is the most locally invasive of all benign soft tissue tumors. It commonly occurs in adolescents and young adults. On palpation the tumor has a distinctive "rock-hard" character. Multiple lesions may be present in the same extremity (10-25%). Histologically, the tumor consists of well-differentiated fibroblasts and abundant collagen. The lesion infiltrates adjacent tissues. Surgical treatment is aimed at resecting the tumor with a wide margin. Local recurrence is common. Radiotherapy has been used as an adjunct to prevent recurrence and progression. The behavior of the tumor is capricious in that recurrent nodules may remain dormant for years or grow rapidly for some time and then stop growing.
3. Nodular fasciitis—Nodular fasciitis is a common reactive lesion that presents as a painful, rapidly enlarging mass in a young person (ages 15-35 years). Half of these lesions occur in the upper extremity. Short, irregular bundles and fascicles; a dense reticulum network; and only small amounts of mature collagen characterize the lesion histologically. Mitotic figures are common, but atypical mitoses are never seen. Treatment consists of excision with a marginal line of resection.
4. Malignant fibrous soft tissue tumors—Malignant fibrous histiocytoma and fibrosarcoma are the two malignant fibrous lesions.
   a. Diagnosis—They have a similar clinical and radiographic presentation and are treated in a similar manner. Patients are generally between the ages of 30 and 80 years. The most common presentation is an enlarging, generally painless mass. When the mass reaches a substantial size (> 10 cm), the patient often experiences symptoms. Plain radiographs are usually normal except in advanced cases, in which there may be bone erosion or destruction. MRI often shows a deep-seated, inhomogeneous mass that is low on T1-weighted images and high on T2-weighted images. The two lesions may be similar histologically, but there are distinctive features. In *malignant fibrous histiocytoma*, the spindle and histiocytic cells are arranged in a storiform (cartwheel) pattern. Short fascicles of cells and fibrous tissue appear to radiate about a common center around slitlike vessels. Chronic inflammatory cells may also be present. In *fibrosarcoma* there is a fasciculated growth pattern, with fusiform or spindle-shaped cells, scanty cytoplasm, and indistinct borders, and the cells are separated by interwoven collagen fibers. In some cases the tissue is organized into a herringbone pattern, which consists of intersecting fascicles in which the nuclei in one fascicle are viewed transversely but in an adjacent fascicle are viewed longitudinally.

Box 9–2 Classification of Soft Tissue Tumors

TUMORS AND TUMOR-LIKE LESIONS OF FIBROUS TISSUE

Benign

Fibroma
Nodular fasciitis
Proliferative fasciitis

Fibromatoses

Superficial fibromatoses
- Palmar and plantar fibromatoses
- Knuckle pads

Deep fibromatoses (extra-abdominal fibromatoses)

Malignant

Adult fibrosarcoma
Postradiation fibrosarcoma

FIBROHISTIOCYTIC TUMORS

Benign

Fibrous histiocytoma
Atypical fibroxanthoma

Intermediate

Dermatofibrosarcoma protuberans

Malignant (Malignant Histiocytoma)

Storiform-pleomorphic
Myxoid (myxofibrosarcoma)
Giant cell (malignant giant cell tumor of soft parts)
Inflammatory (malignant xanthogranuloma, xanthosarcoma)

TUMORS AND TUMOR-LIKE CONDITIONS OF ADIPOSE TISSUE

Benign

Lipoma (cutaneous, deep, and multiple)
Angiolipoma
Spindle cell and pleomorphic lipoma
Lipoblastoma and lipoblastomatosis
Intra- and intermuscular lipoma
Hibernoma

Malignant

Liposarcoma
- Well-differentiated (lipoma-like, sclerosing, inflammatory)
- Myxoid
- Round cell (poorly differentiated myxoid)
- Pleomorphic
- Dedifferentiated

TUMORS OF MUSCLE TISSUE

Smooth Muscle

Benign

Leiomyoma (cutaneous and deep)
Angiomyoma (vascular leiomyoma)

Malignant

Leiomyosarcoma

Striated Muscle

Benign

Adult rhabdomyoma

Malignant

Rhabdomyosarcoma–predominantly embryonal (including botryoid), alveolar, pleomorphic, and mixed

TUMORS OF LYMPH VESSELS

Benign (lymphangioma)

Cavernous
Cystic (cystic hygroma)

Malignant

Lymphangiosarcoma
Postmastectomy lymphangiosarcoma

TUMORS AND TUMOR-LIKE LESIONS OF SYNOVIAL TISSUE

Benign

Giant cell tumor of tendon sheath
- Localized (nodular tenosynovitis)
- Diffuse (florid synovitis)

Malignant

Synovial sarcoma (malignant synovioma), predominantly biphasic or monophasic (either fibrous or epithelial)
Malignant giant cell tumor of tendon sheath

TUMORS AND TUMOR-LIKE LESIONS OF PERIPHERAL NERVES

Benign

Traumatic neuroma
Morton neuroma
Neurilemoma (benign schwannoma)
Neurofibroma, solitary
Neurofibromatosis (von Recklinghausen disease)
- Localized
- Plexiform
- Diffuse

Malignant

Malignant schwannoma
Peripheral tumors of primitive neuroectodermal tissues

TUMORS AND TUMOR-LIKE LESIONS OF CARTILAGE AND BONE-FORMING TISSUES

Benign

Panniculitis ossificans
Myositis ossificans
Fibrodysplasia (myositis) ossificans progressiva
Extraskeletal chondroma
Extraskeletal osteoma

Malignant

Extraskeletal chondrosarcoma
- Well-differentiated
- Myxoid (choroid sarcoma)
- Mesenchymal

Extraskeletal osteosarcoma

TUMORS AND TUMOR-LIKE LESIONS OF PLURIPOTENTIAL MESENCHYME

Benign mesenchymoma
Malignant mesenchymoma

Box 9-2 Classification of Soft Tissue Tumors—cont'd

TUMORS AND TUMOR-LIKE CONDITIONS OF BLOOD VESSELS

Benign

Hemangioma
Deep hemangioma (intramuscular, synovial, perineural)
Glomus tumor

Intermediate

Hemangioendothelioma

Malignant

Hemangiosarcoma
Malignant hemangiopericytoma

TUMORS AND TUMOR-LIKE CONDITIONS OF DISPUTED OR UNCERTAIN HISTOGENESIS

Benign

Tumoral calcinosis
Myxoma (cutaneous and intramuscular)

Malignant

Alveolar soft-part sarcoma
Epithelioid sarcoma
Clear cell sarcoma of tendons and aponeuroses
Extraskeletal Ewing sarcoma

UNCLASSIFIED SOFT TISSUE TUMORS AND TUMOR-LIKE LESIONS

b. Treatment—Treatment is by wide local excision. Radiation therapy is employed in many cases when the size of the tumor exceeds 5 cm. A common scenario is to deliver radiation preoperatively (5000 cGy), followed by resection of the lesion. A final radiation boost (1400-2000 cGy) is then given postoperatively or with brachytherapy afterloading tubes if the margins are very close or positive. Postoperative external beam irradiation (6300-6600 cGy) yields equal local control rates, with a lower postoperative wound complication rate but a higher incidence of postoperative fibrosis.

5. Dermatofibrosarcoma protuberans—This lesion is a rare, nodular, cutaneous tumor that occurs in early to middle adult life. The lesion is low grade. It has a tendency to recur locally, but it only rarely metastasizes, often after repeated local recurrence. In 40% of the cases it occurs on the upper or lower extremities. The tumor grows slowly but progressively. The central portion of the nodules shows uniform fibroblasts arranged in a storiform pattern around an inconspicuous vasculature. Wide resection is the best form of treatment.

C. Tumors of fatty tissue—There is a wide spectrum of benign and malignant tumors of fat origin. Each has a particular biologic behavior that guides evaluation and treatment.

1. Lipomas—Lipomas are common benign tumors of mature fat. They may occur in a subcutaneous, intramuscular, or intermuscular location. Patients often describe a long history of a mass and sometimes one that was only recently discovered. Most are not painful. Plain radiographs may show a radiolucent lesion in the soft tissues if the lipoma is deep within the muscle or between the muscle and bone. CT or MRI shows a well-demarcated lesion with the same signal characteristics as those of mature fat on all sequences. With fat suppression sequences, the lipoma has a uniformly low signal. If the patient experiences no symptoms and the radiographic features are diagnostic of lipoma, no treatment is necessary. If the mass is growing or causing symptoms, excision with a marginal line of resection or an intralesional margin is all that is necessary. Local recurrence is uncommon. There are several variants of which the surgeon must be aware.

a. Spindle cell lipoma—This lesion commonly occurs in male patients (ages 45-65 years). The tumor presents as a solitary, painless, growing, firm nodule. Histologically, there is a mixture of mature fat cells and spindle cells. There is a mucoid matrix with a varying number of birefringent collagen fibers. Treatment is excision with a marginal margin.

b. Pleomorphic lipoma—This lesion is common in middle-aged patients and presents as a slowly growing mass. There are lipocytes; spindle cells; and scattered, bizarre, giant cells histologically. The lesion may be confused with different types of liposarcoma. Treatment is by excision with a marginal margin.

c. Angiolipoma—This lesion is the only lipoma that is very painful when palpated. Patients usually present with small nodules in the upper extremity that are intensely painful. MRI may show a small, fatty nodule or completely normal results. Histologically, the lesion consists of mature fat cells (as in a typical lipoma) and nests of small arborizing vessels.

2. Liposarcomas—Liposarcomas are a type of sarcoma in which the direction of differentiation is toward fatty tissue. These lesions form a heterogeneous group of tumors, having in common the presence of lipoblasts (signet ring–type cells) in the tissue. Liposarcomas virtually never occur in the subcutaneous tissues. They are classified into the following types.

- Well-differentiated liposarcoma (low grade)
  - Lipoma-like
  - Sclerosing
  - Inflammatory
- Myxoid liposarcoma (intermediate grade)
- Dedifferentiated (high grade)
- Round-cell liposarcoma (high grade)
- Pleomorphic liposarcoma (high grade)

Liposarcomas metastasize according to the grade of the lesion: well-differentiated liposarcomas have a very low rate of metastasis (< 10%), the metastasis rate of intermediate-liposarcomas is 10-30%, and that of high-grade liposarcomas is > 50%.

D. Tumors of neural tissue—The two benign neural tumors are neurilemoma and neurofibroma. Their malignant counterpart is neurofibrosarcoma.

1. Neurilemoma (benign schwannoma)—This lesion is a benign nerve sheath tumor. It occurs in young to middle-aged adults (20-50 years) and is usually asymptomatic except for the presence of the mass. The tumor grows slowly and may wax and wane in size (cystic changes). MRI studies may demonstrate an eccentric mass arising from a peripheral nerve or show only an indeterminate soft tissue mass (low on T1- and high on T2-weighted images). Histologically, the lesion is composed of Antoni's A and B areas.
   a. Antoni A—Compact spindle cells usually having twisted nuclei; indistinct cytoplasm; and occasionally clear, intranuclear vacuoles. When the lesion is highly differentiated, there may be nuclear palisading, whorling of cells, and Verocay bodies. When the lesion is predominantly cellular (Antoni A), the tumor may be confused with a sarcoma. Treatment consists of removing the eccentric mass while leaving the nerve intact.
   b. Antoni B—Less orderly and cellular, these cells are arranged haphazardly in the loosely textured matrix (with microcystic changes, inflammatory cells, and delicate collagen fibers); the vessels are large and irregularly spaced.
2. Neurofibroma—This lesion may be solitary or multiple (neurofibromatosis). Most are superficial, grow slowly, and are painless. When they involve a major nerve, they may expand it in a fusiform fashion. Histologically, there are interlacing bundles of elongated cells with wavy, dark-staining nuclei. The cells are associated with wirelike strands of collagen. Small to moderate amounts of mucoid material separate the cells and collagen. Treatment consists of excision with a marginal margin. Neurofibromatosis (von Recklinghausen disease) is an autosomal dominant trait, with both peripheral and central forms of the disease. In addition to neurofibromas, patients have café au lait spots and variable skeletal abnormalities (nonossifying fibromas, scoliosis, and long-bone bowing). Malignant changes occur in 5-30% of patients. The presence of pain and an enlarging soft tissue mass may herald conversion to a sarcoma.
3. Neurofibrosarcoma—This sarcoma is a rare tumor that arises de novo or in the setting of neurofibromatosis. Neurofibrosarcomas are high-grade sarcomas and are treated in a fashion similar to that for other high-grade sarcomas.

E. Tumors of muscle tissue—These tumors are uncommon and range from benign leiomyoma and rhabdomyoma to the malignant entities of leiomyosarcoma and rhabdomyosarcoma. The benign entities seldom occur on the extremities.

1. Leiomyosarcoma—This tumor may present as a small nodule or a large extremity mass. The lesions may or may not be associated with blood vessels. They may be either low or high grade and are treated as other low and highgrade sarcomas.
2. Rhabdomyosarcoma—This highly malignant tumor is the most frequently occurring one in young patients (< 20 years of age). It is the most common sarcoma in young patients and may grow rapidly. Histologically, the lesion is composed of spindle cells in parallel bundles, multinucleated giant cells, and racquet-shaped cells. The histologic hallmark is the appearance of cross-striations within the tumor cells (rhabdomyoblasts). Rhabdomyoblasts may be difficult to find. Rhabdomyosarcomas are sensitive to multiagent chemotherapy. Wide surgical resection is performed after induction of chemotherapy. External beam irradiation plays a prominent role in the treatment of this tumor.

F. Vascular tumors—Hemangiomas and glomus tumors are the two principal benign entities, and hemangiopericytoma and angiosarcoma are the less common malignant entities.

1. Hemangioma—This soft tissue tumor is commonly seen in children and adults. The lesion may occur in a cutaneous, subcutaneous, or intramuscular location. Patients with large tumors have symptoms of vascular engorgement (aching, heaviness, swelling). MRI scans demonstrate a heterogeneous lesion with numerous small blood vessels and fatty infiltration. The clinician should examine the patient in both the supine and standing positions. Hemangiomas in the lower extremity will often fill with blood after several minutes. Plain radiographs may reveal small phleboliths. Nonoperative treatment consisting of NSAIDs, vascular stockings, and activity modification is chosen if local measures adequately control discomfort. Many patients can be treated by sclerosing the hemangioma with a sclerosing agent such as alcohol. This therapy is performed by interventional radiologists. Wide surgical resection is used for resistant cases, but the local recurrence rate is high.
2. Hemangiopericytoma—This rare tumor of the pericytes of blood vessels appears in benign and malignant forms. Within the malignant group, there is a morphologic range from intermediate- to high-grade malignancy. Patients present with a slowly enlarging, painless mass. Hemangiopericytoma is malignant and is treated similar to other sarcomas, with wide resection and radiation therapy in selected cases.
3. Angiosarcoma—In this rare tumor, the tumor cells resemble the endothelium of blood vessels. Angiosarcomas are highly malignant lesions that

are very infiltrative, with a high local failure rate. Amputation surgery is frequently necessary to achieve local control. Pulmonary metastases are common.

G. Synovial disorders—These entities include benign conditions, such as that affecting the ganglia, and synovial proliferative disorders, such as pigmented villonodular synovitis and synovial chondromatosis.

1. Ganglia—This disorder presents as an out-pouching of the synovial lining of an adjacent joint. The most common locations include the wrist, foot, and knee. The cyst is filled with gelatinous, mucoid material. Histologically, the cyst wall is made up of paucicellular connective tissue without a true epithelial lining. With MRI scanning, a homogeneously low signal on T1-weighted images and a very bright signal on T2-weighted images are found. A contrast agent such as gadolinium is useful in differentiating a cyst from a solid neoplasm because the cyst will not enhance (except for a small rim at the periphery) but active neoplasms usually will.
2. Pigmented villonodular synovitis—This reactive condition (not a true neoplasm) is characterized by an exuberant proliferation of synovial villi and nodules. The process may occur locally within a joint or diffusely. The knee is affected most often, followed in frequency by the hip and shoulder. Patients present with pain and swelling in the affected joint. Recurrent, atraumatic hemarthrosis is the hallmark of this disorder. Arthrocentesis demonstrates a bloody effusion. Cystic erosions may occur on both sides of the joint. Histologically, there are highly vascular villi lined with plump, hyperplastic synovial cells; hemosiderin-stained, multinucleated giant cells; and chronic inflammatory cells. Treatment is aimed at complete synovectomy. Knee synovectomy can be accomplished by arthroscopy for resection of all the intra-articular disease, followed by open posterior synovectomy to remove the posterior extra-articular extension. Local recurrence is common (30-50%) despite complete synovectomy. External beam irradiation (3500-4000 cGy) can reduce the rate of local recurrence to 10-20%.
3. Giant cell tumor of tendon sheath—This benign nodular tumor occurs along the tendon sheaths of the hands and feet. Histologically, the lesion is moderately cellular (sheets of rounded or polygonal cells). There are hypocellular, collagenized zones. Multinucleated giant cells are common, as are xanthoma cells. Treatment consists of resection with a marginal margin. Local recurrence is common and usually treated with repeat excision.
4. Synovial chondromatosis—This synovial proliferative disorder occurs within joints or bursae, ranging in appearance from metaplasia of the synovial tissue to firm nodules of cartilage. The lesion typically affects young adults, who present with pain, stiffness, and swelling. The knee is the most common location. Radiographs may demonstrate fine, stippled calcification. Treatment consists of removing the loose bodies and synovectomy.
5. Synovial sarcoma—This highly malignant, high-grade tumor occurs near joints but rarely arises from an intra-articular location. The tumor may be present for years or present as a rapidly enlarging mass. Regional lymph nodes may be involved. Synovial sarcoma is the most common sarcoma in the foot. Radiographs may show mineralization within the lesion in up to 25% of cases. The spotty mineralization may even resemble the peripheral mineralization seen in heterotopic ossification. Histologically, the tumor is biphasic, with both epithelial and spindle cell components. The epithelial component may show epithelial cells that form glands or nests, or they may line cystlike spaces. The tumor may also be composed of a single type of cell (monophasic), with the monophasic fibrous type being much more common than the monophasic epithelial type. A translocation between chromosome 18 and the X chromosome is always present, and the tumor cells stain positive for keratin and epithelial membrane antigen. Wide surgical resection with adjuvant radiotherapy is the most common method of treatment. Metastases develop in 30-60% of the cases. Larger tumors (> 5-10 cm) are more prone to distant spread.

H. Other rare sarcomas

1. Epithelioid sarcoma—This rare nodular tumor commonly occurs in the upper extremities of young adults. It may also occur about the buttock/thigh, knee, and foot. Epithelioid sarcoma is the most common sarcoma of the hand. The lesion may ulcerate and mimic a granuloma or rheumatoid nodule. Lymph node metastases are common. Histologically, the cells range from ovoid to polygonal, with deeply eosinophilic cytoplasm. Cellular pleomorphism is minimal. The lesions are often misdiagnosed as benign processes. Wide-margin surgical resection is necessary to prevent local recurrence.
2. Clear cell sarcoma—This tumor presents as a slowly growing mass associated with tendons or aponeuroses. The lesion usually occurs about the foot and ankle but may also involve the knee, thigh, and hand. Microscopically, it is characterized by compact nests or fascicles of rounded or fusiform cells with clear cytoplasm. Multinucleated giant cells are common. Wide surgical resection with adjuvant irradiation is the treatment of choice.
3. Alveolar cell sarcoma—This type of sarcoma presents as a slowly growing, painless mass in young adults (ages 15-35 years). It usually occurs in the anterior thigh. Microscopically, it appears as dense, fibrous trabeculae dividing the tumor into an organoid or nestlike arrangement. Cells are large and rounded and contain one or more vesicular nuclei with small nucleoli. Vascular invasion is prominent. Treatment consists of wide-margin surgical resection with adjuvant irradiation in selected cases.

I. Post-traumatic conditions
1. Hematoma—Hematoma may occur after trauma to the extremity. The lesion organizes and resolves with time. Sarcomas may spontaneously hemorrhage into the body of the tumor or after minor trauma and masquerade as a benign process. Clinicians should follow patients with hematomas at 6-week intervals until the mass resolves. MRI scanning is often not able to distinguish a simple hematoma from a sarcoma with spontaneous hemorrhage.
2. Myositis ossificans (heterotopic ossification)—This condition develops after single or repetitive episodes of trauma. Occasionally, patients cannot recall the traumatic episode. The most common locations are over the diaphyseal segment of long bones (in the middle aspect of the muscle bellies). As maturation progresses, radiographs show peripheral mineralization with a central lucent area. In most cases the lesion is not attached to the underlying bone, but in some cases it may become fixed to the periosteal surface. Histologically, there is a zonal pattern, with mature, trabecular bone at the periphery and immature tissue in the center. When the diagnosis is apparent, nonoperative treatment is all that is necessary.

III. Bone Tumors

A. Nomenclature—Primary bone lesions can be classified into three types: malignant bone tumors (sarcomas), benign bone tumors, and lesions that simulate bone tumors (reactive and miscellaneous conditions). Common lesions that are not of mesenchymal origin include metastatic bone disease, myeloma, and lymphoma. A common classification system for bone tumors is shown in Table 9-5.
1. Sarcomas—These are malignant neoplasms of connective tissue (mesenchymal) origin. Sarcomas generally exhibit rapid growth in a centripetal fashion and invade adjacent normal tissues. Each year in the United States there are about 2800 new bone sarcomas. High-grade, malignant bone tumors tend to destroy the overlying cortex and spread into the soft tissues. Low-grade tumors are generally contained within the cortex or the surrounding periosteal rim. Bone sarcomas metastasize primarily via the hematogenous route, with the lungs being the most common site. Osteosarcoma and Ewing sarcoma may also metastasize to other bone sites either at the initial presentation or later in the disease.
2. Benign bone tumors—These may be small and have a limited growth potential or may be large and destructive.
3. Tumor simulators and reactive conditions—These processes occur in bone but are not true neoplasms (e.g., osteomyelitis, aneurysmal bone cyst, bone island).

B. Bone-producing lesions—There are three lesions in which the tumor cells produce osteoid: osteoid osteoma, osteoblastoma, and osteosarcoma.

TABLE 9-5 CLASSIFICATION OF PRIMARY TUMORS OF BONE*

Histologic Type	Benign	Malignant
Hematopoietic		Myeloma Lymphoma
Chondrogenic	Osteochondroma Chondroma Chondroblastoma Chondromyxoid fibroma	Primary chondrosarcoma Secondary chondrosarcoma Dedifferentiated chondrosarcoma Mesenchymal chondrosarcoma Clear cell chondrosarcoma
Osteogenic	Osteoid osteoma Osteoblastoma	Osteosarcoma Parosteal osteosarcoma Periosteal osteosarcoma
Unknown origin	Giant cell tumor (Fibrous) histiocytoma	Ewing tumor Malignant giant cell tumor Adamantinoma
Fibrogenic	Fibroma Desmoplastic fibroma	Fibrosarcoma Malignant fibrous histiocytoma
Notochordal		Chordoma
Vascular	Hemangioma	Hemangioendothelioma Hemangiopericytoma
Lipogenic	Lipoma	
Neurogenic	Neurilemoma	

Classification is based on that advocated by Lichtenstein L: Classification of primary tumors of bone. Cancer 4:335–341, 1951.

1. Osteoid osteoma—This self-limiting benign bone lesion produces pain in young patients (ages 5-30 years), although all age groups may be affected.
a. Diagnosis—Patients present with pain that increases with time. Most patients have pain at night, which may be relieved by salicylates and other NSAIDs. The pain may be referred to an adjacent joint, and when the lesion is intracapsular, it may simulate arthritis. The tumor may produce painful scoliosis, growth disturbances, and flexion contractures. Common locations include the proximal femur, tibial diaphysis, and spine (Fig. 9–3). The radiographs usually show intensely reactive bone and a radiolucent nidus (Fig. 9–4). It may be possible to detect the lesion only with tomograms, CT scans, or MRI scans, because of the intense sclerosis. The nidus is by definition always less than 1.5 cm, although the area of reactive bone sclerosis may be long. The results of a technetium bone scan are always positive and show intense focal uptake. CT scans are superior to MRI scans in detecting and characterizing osteoid osteomas because the CT scans provide better contrast between the lucent nidus and the reactive bone than the MRI scan does. Microscopically, there is a distinct demarcation between the nidus and the reactive bone. The nidus consists of an interlacing network of osteoid trabeculae with variable mineralization. The trabecular organization is

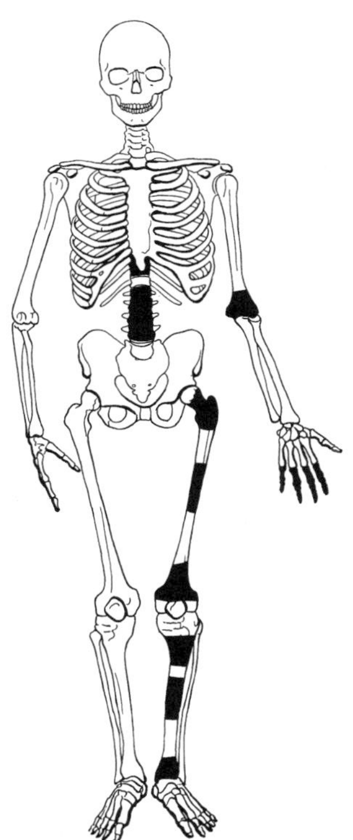

FIGURE 9–3 Skeletal distribution of the most common sites of osteoid osteoma. (From McCarthy EF, Frassica FJ: Pathology of Bone and Joint Disorders. Philadelphia, WB Saunders, 1998.)

haphazard, and the greatest degree of mineralization is in the center of the lesion.

b. Treatment—Patients can be treated with three different methods: NSAIDs, CT-guided radiofrequency ablation, and open surgical removal. About 50% of patients treated with NSAIDs will have their lesions burn out, with no further medical or surgical treatment necessary. CT-guided radiofrequency ablation has become the dominant method of treatment. Under CT guidance, a radiofrequency probe is placed into the lesion, and the nidus is heated to 80°C. About 90% of selected patients can be successfully treated with one or two radiofrequency ablations. The radiofrequency probe must be insulated to prevent thermal necrosis of normal structures such as the skin, subcutaneous tissues, neural elements, and blood vessels. Open surgical treatment consists of complete removal of the nidus by curettage with hand and power instruments. This procedure should be performed when radiofrequency ablation is not feasible or available or has failed.

2. Osteoblastoma—This rare bone-producing tumor can attain a large size and is not self-limiting. Patients present with pain, and when the lesion involves the spine, neurologic symptoms may be present. Common locations include the spine, proximal humerus, and hip (Fig. 9–5). Radiographically, there is bone destruction with or without the characteristic reactive bone formation in osteoid osteoma. The bone destruction occasionally has a moth-eaten or permeative character simulating a malignancy. Histologically, the lesions show regularly shaped nuclei containing little chromatin but abundant cytoplasm. The tissue is loosely arranged, with numerous blood vessels. The lesion does not permeate the normal trabecular bone but instead merges with them. Treatment consists of curettage or marginal excision.

3. Osteosarcoma—Spindle cell neoplasms that produce osteoid are arbitrarily classified as osteosarcoma. There are many types of osteosarcoma (Box 9–3 and Fig. 9–6). Lesions that must be recognized include high-grade intramedullary osteosarcoma (ordinary or classic osteosarcoma), parosteal osteosarcoma, periosteal osteosarcoma, telangiectatic osteosarcoma, osteosarcoma occurring with Paget disease, and osteosarcoma after irradiation. Historically, osteosarcoma was treated by amputation; long-term studies show a survival rate of only 10-20%, with the pulmonary system being the most common site of failure. Multiagent chemotherapy has dramatically improved long-term survival and the potential for limb salvage. It effectively destroys the malignant cells, and in many patients there is total necrosis of the tumor. The chemotherapy both kills the micrometastases that are present in 80-90% of the patients at presentation and sterilizes the reactive zone around the tumor. Preoperative chemotherapy is delivered for 8-12 weeks, followed by resection of the tumor. Staging studies are performed at the end of chemotherapy to ensure that the lesion is resectable. Maintenance chemotherapy is then given for 6-12 months. Long-term survival is approximately 60-70% with these regimens. Prognostic factors that adversely affect survival include (1) expression of P-glycoprotein, high serum alkaline phosphatase, high lactic dehydrogenase, vascular invasion, and no alteration of DNA ploidy after chemotherapy and (2) the absence of anti–shock protein 90 antibodies after chemotherapy.

a. High-grade intramedullary osteosarcoma—Also called "ordinary" or "classic" osteosarcoma, this neoplasm is the most common type of osteosarcoma and usually occurs about the knee in children and young adults (Fig. 9–7). Other common sites include the proximal humerus, proximal femur, and pelvis. Patients present primarily with pain. More than 90% of intramedullary osteosarcomas are high-grade and penetrate the cortex early to form a soft tissue mass (stage IIB lesion). About 10-20% of patients have pulmonary metastases at presentation. Plain radiographs demonstrate a lesion in

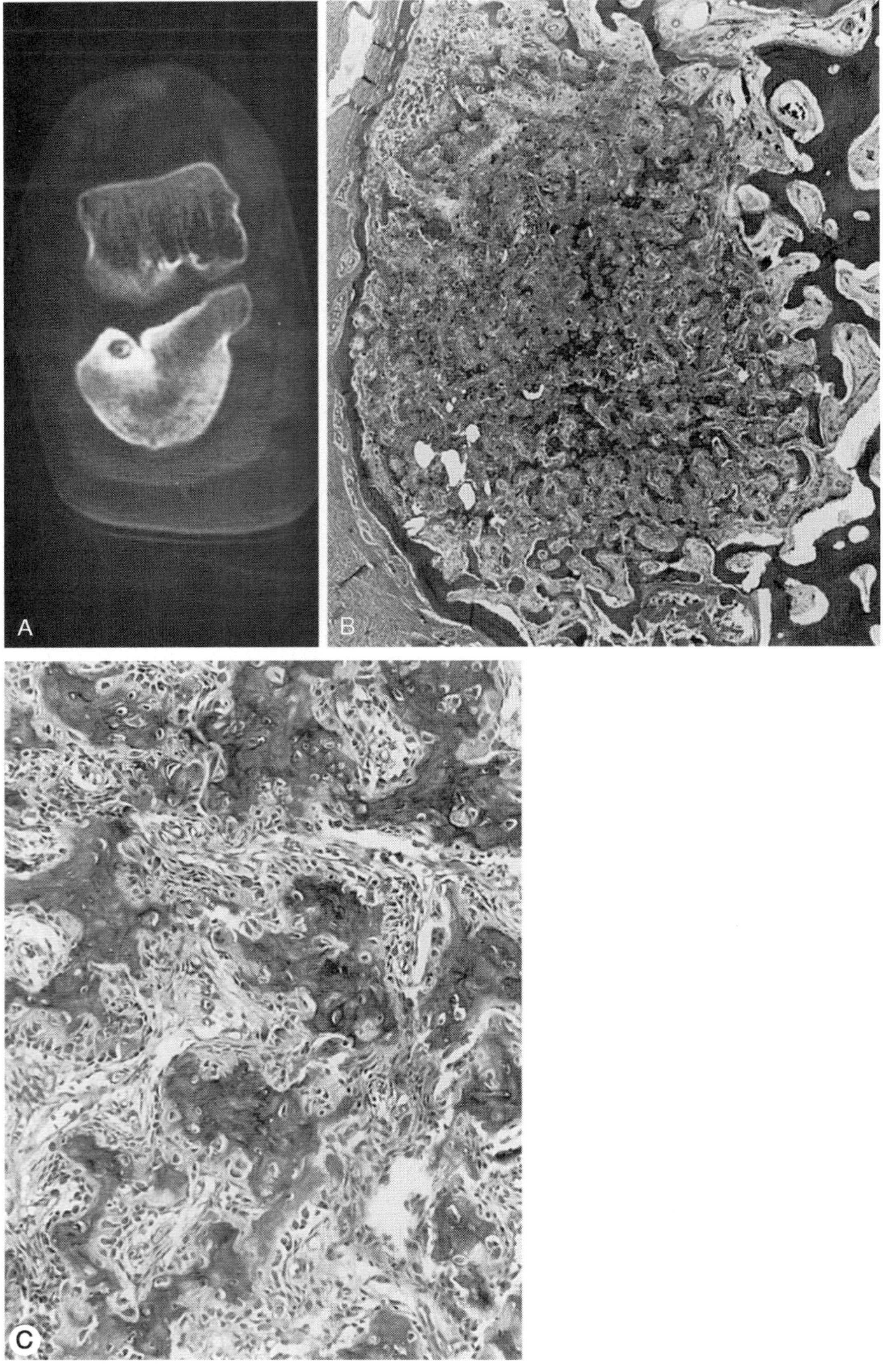

FIGURE 9–4 Osteoid osteoma of the calcaneus. **A**, Radiograph shows a well-circumscribed lytic lesion with dense surrounding bone and a central nidus. **B**, Low-power photomicrograph (× 25) shows the nidus. **C**, Higher-power photomicrograph (× 160) shows mineralizing new bone with a loose fibrovascular stroma.

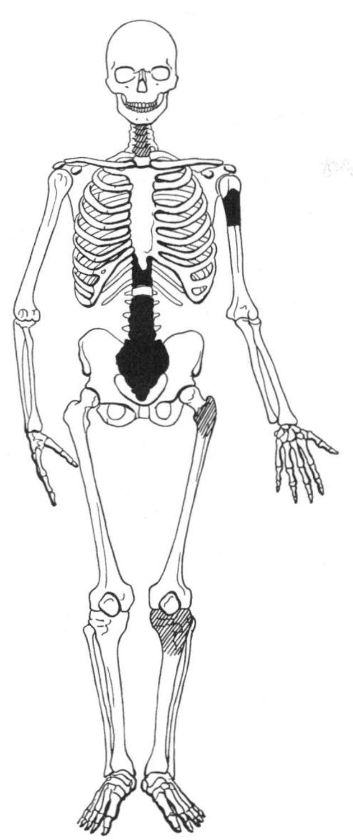

FIGURE 9–5 Skeletal distribution of the most common sites of osteoblastoma. (From McCarthy EF, Frassica FJ: Pathology of Bone and Joint Disorders. Philadelphia, WB Saunders, 1998.)

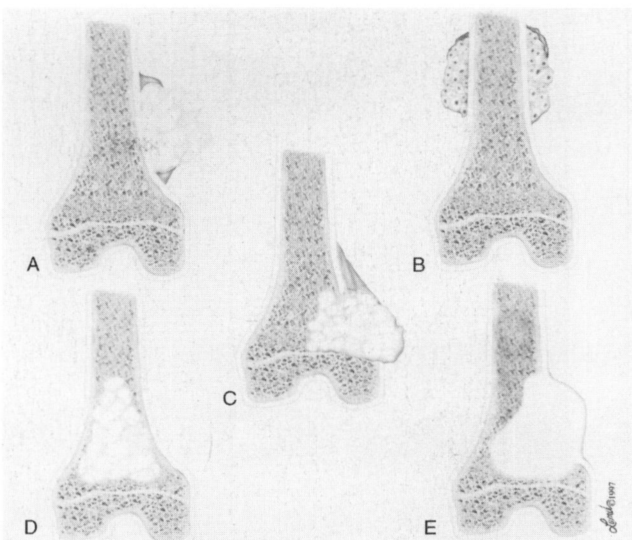

FIGURE 9–6 **A,** Parosteal osteosarcoma arises from the surface of the bone with broad cortical attachment. The tumor grows in a lobulated fashion. **B,** Periosteal osteosarcoma. Poorly mineralized lesion on the surface of the bone. **C,** High-grade intramedullary osteosarcoma. The cortical bone destruction and extension into the soft tissues is typical. **D,** Well-differentiated intramedullary osteosarcoma stays within the medullary cavity and usually does not break through the cortex. **E,** Telangiectatic osteosarcoma, a destructive lytic lesion with no bone production. The overlying cortex has been destroyed, with extension into the soft tissue. (From McCarthy EF, Frassica FJ: Pathology of Bone and Joint Disorders. Philadelphia, WB Saunders, 1998.)

which there is bone destruction and bone formation (Fig. 9–8). Occasionally, the lesion is purely sclerotic or lytic. MRI or CT scans are useful for defining the anatomy of the lesion with regard to intramedullary extension, involvement of neurovascular structures, and muscle invasion. Two criteria are used histologically: (1) the tumor cells produce osteoid, and (2) the stromal cells are frankly malignant. The lesions may be highly heterogeneous in appearance, with some lesions being predominantly chondroblastic, osteoblastic, or fibroblastic. Other lesions may contain large numbers of giant

Box 9–3 Classification of Osteosarcoma

High-grade central osteosarcoma
Low-grade central osteosarcoma
Telangiectatic osteosarcoma
Surface osteosarcoma
Parosteal osteosarcoma
Periosteal osteosarcoma
High-grade surface osteosarcoma
Osteosarcoma of the jaw
Multicentric osteosarcoma
Secondary osteosarcoma
- Osteosarcoma in Paget disease
- Postradiation osteosarcoma

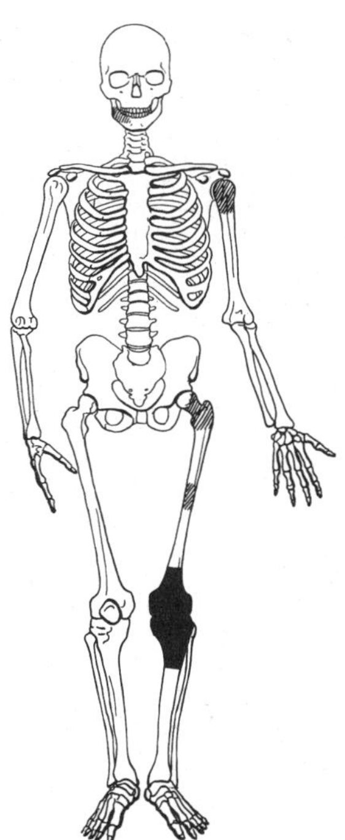

FIGURE 9–7 Skeletal distribution of the locations of conventional osteosarcoma. (From McCarthy EF, Frassica FJ: Pathology of Bone and Joint Disorders. Philadelphia, WB Saunders, 1998.)

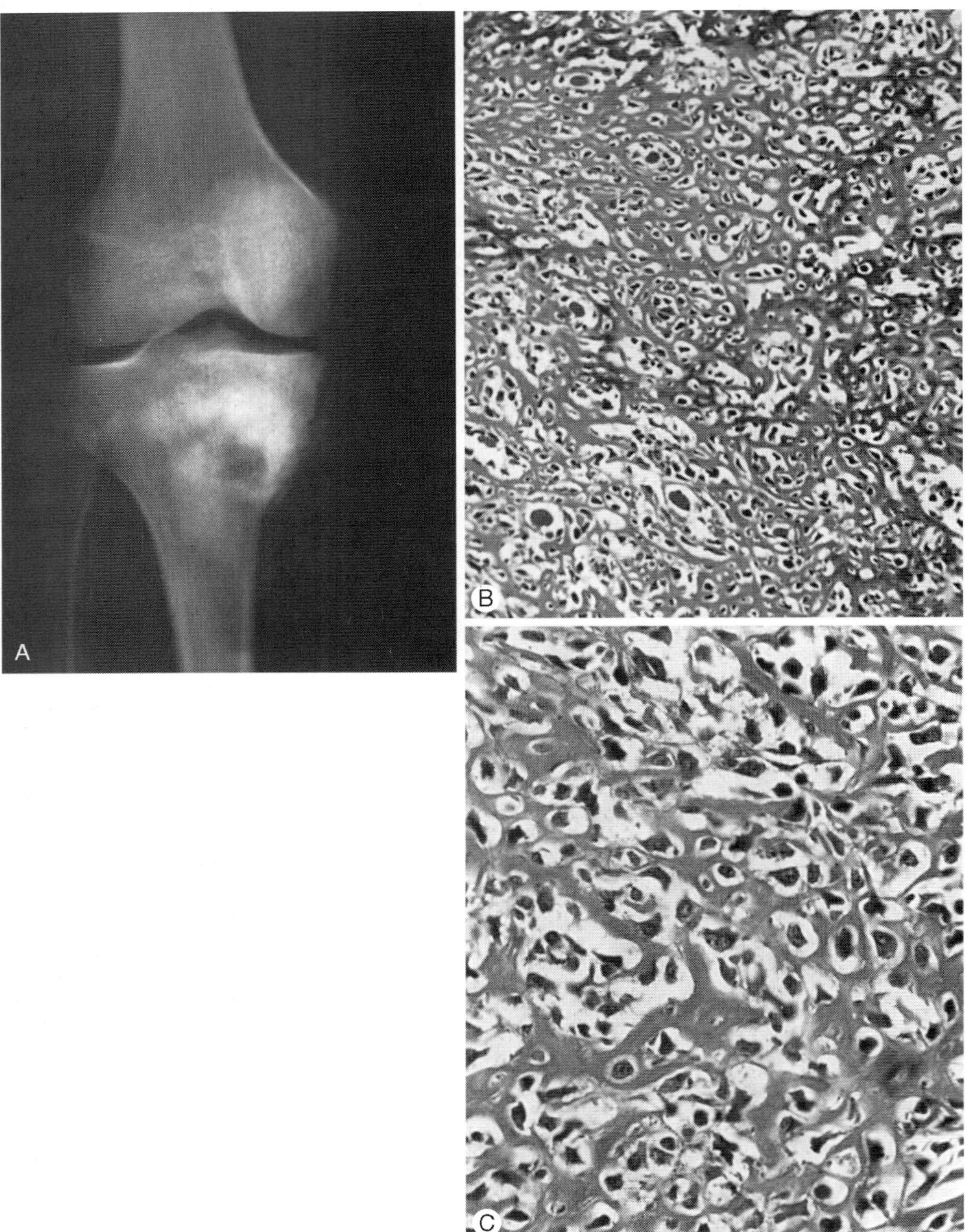

FIGURE 9–8 Conventional osteoblastic osteosarcoma of the proximal tibia. **A**, Radiograph shows a poorly defined osteoblastic lesion in the proximal tibial metaphysis. **B**, Low-power photomicrograph (× 160) shows lacelike mineralizing osteoid surrounding atypical osteoblasts. **C**, Higher-power photomicrograph (× 400).

cells or predominantly small cells rather than spindle cells.

b. Parosteal osteosarcoma—This low-grade osteosarcoma occurs on the surface of the metaphysis of long bones. Patients often complain of a painless mass. The most common sites are the posterior aspect of the distal femur, proximal tibia, and proximal humerus (Fig. 9–9); the lesion is more common in females than males. The radiographic appearance is characteristic in that it demonstrates a heavily ossified, often lobulated mass arising from the cortex (Fig. 9–10). Histologically, the most prominent feature is regularly arranged osseous trabeculae. Between the nearly normal trabeculae are slightly atypical spindle cells, which typically invade skeletal muscle found at the periphery of the tumor. Interestingly, cartilage is frequently present and may be arranged as a cap over the lesion. Treatment of parosteal osteosarcoma is by resection with a wide margin, which is usually curative. In approximately one sixth of the lesions that appear radiographically to be parosteal osteosarcoma, there is a high-grade malignancy. In this setting the lesion is called a dedifferentiated parosteal osteosarcoma. For typical low-grade parosteal osteosarcomas, chemotherapy or irradiation is not needed. However, the prognosis is much worse for dedifferentiated parosteal osteosarcomas, and multiagent chemotherapy is an important component of therapy. When local control has been achieved in parosteal osteosarcoma, the prognosis is excellent, with a long-term survival rate of over 95%. Invasion into the medullary cavity does not adversely affect long-term survival.

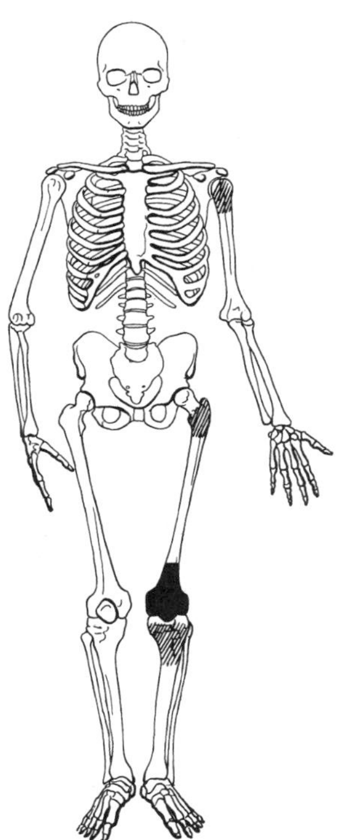

FIGURE 9–9 Skeletal distribution of the most common sites of parosteal osteosarcoma. (From McCarthy EF, Frassica FJ: Pathology of Bone and Joint Disorders. Philadelphia, WB Saunders, 1998.)

c. Periosteal osteosarcoma—This rare surface form of osteosarcoma occurs most often in the diaphysis of long bones (typically the femur or tibia) (Fig. 9–11). The radiographic appearance is fairly constant: a sunburst-type lesion rests on a saucerized cortical depression (Fig. 9–12). Histologically, the lesion is predominantly chondroblastic, and the grade of the lesion is intermediate (grade II). Highly anaplastic regions are not found. The prognosis for periosteal osteosarcoma is intermediate between very-low-grade parosteal osteosarcoma and high-grade intramedullary osteosarcoma. Preoperative chemotherapy, resection, and maintenance chemotherapy constitute the preferred treatment. The risk of pulmonary metastasis is 15-25%.

d. Telangiectatic osteosarcoma—The tissue of the lesion can be described as a bag of blood with few cellular elements. If present, these elements are highly malignant in appearance. The radiographic features of telangiectatic osteosarcoma are those of a destructive, lytic, expansile lesion. Telangiectatic osteosarcomas occur in the same locations as aneurysmal bone cysts (Fig. 9–13), and their radiographic appearances can be confused with each other.

C. Chondrogenic lesions—The principal benign cartilage lesions are chondroma, osteochondroma, chondroblastoma, and chondromyxoid fibroma (Fig. 9–14). The common malignant cartilage tumors are intramedullary chondrosarcoma and dedifferentiated chondrosarcoma. Clear cell chondrosarcoma and mesenchymal chondrosarcoma are rare forms.

1. Chondroma

a. Histologic and radiographic features—When these benign cartilage tumors occur on the surface of the bone they are called *periosteal chondroma*. They most often occur on the surfaces of the distal femur, proximal humerus, and proximal femur (Fig. 9–15). When chondromas are localized in the medullary cavity in the metaphysis of long bones, especially the proximal femur and humerus and the distal femur, they are called *enchondromas* (Fig. 9–16). Enchondromas are common in the hand, where they usually occur in the diaphysis and metaphysis. Involvement of the epiphysis is rare. Lesions in the hand may be hypercellular

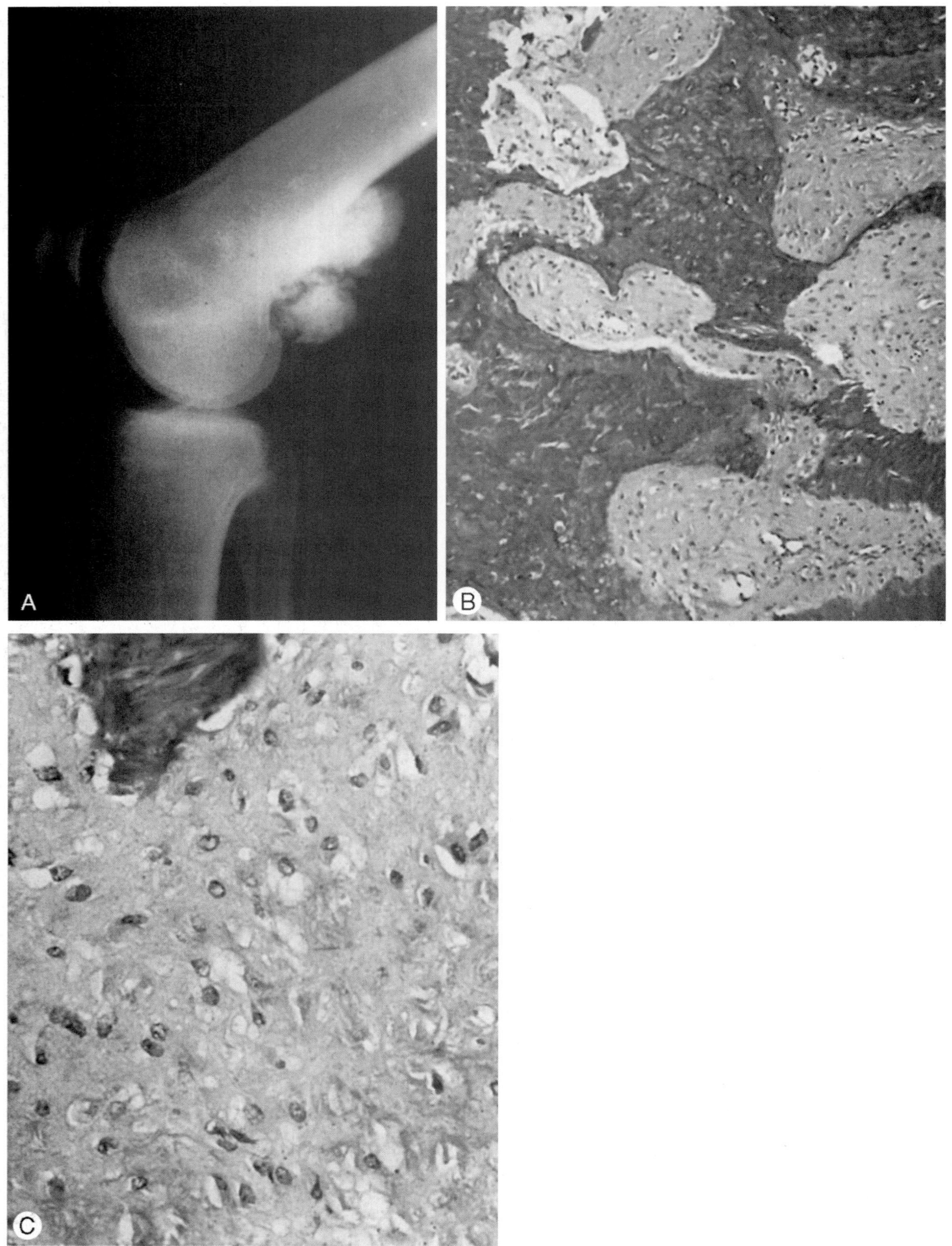

FIGURE 9–10 Parosteal osteosarcoma of the distal femur. **A**, Radiograph shows an exophytic, bony mass in the posterior distal femur. **B**, Low-power photomicrograph (× 160) shows plates of new bone in a fibrous matrix. **C**, Higher-power photomicrograph (× 400) shows a fibrous stroma with atypical cells.

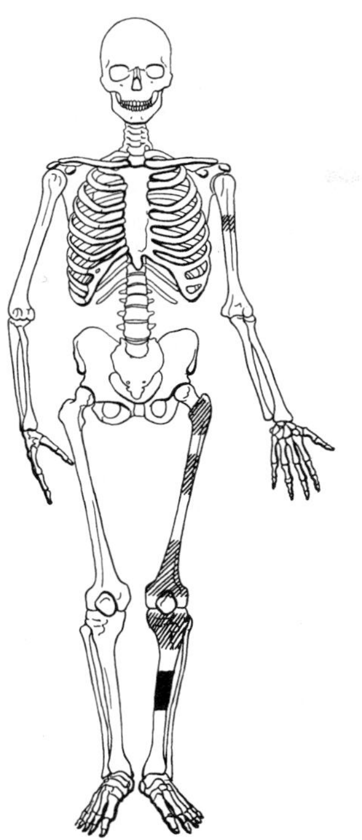

FIGURE 9–11 Skeletal distribution of the most common sites of periosteal osteosarcoma. (From McCarthy EF, Frassica FJ: Pathology of Bone and Joint Disorders. Philadelphia, WB Saunders, 1998.)

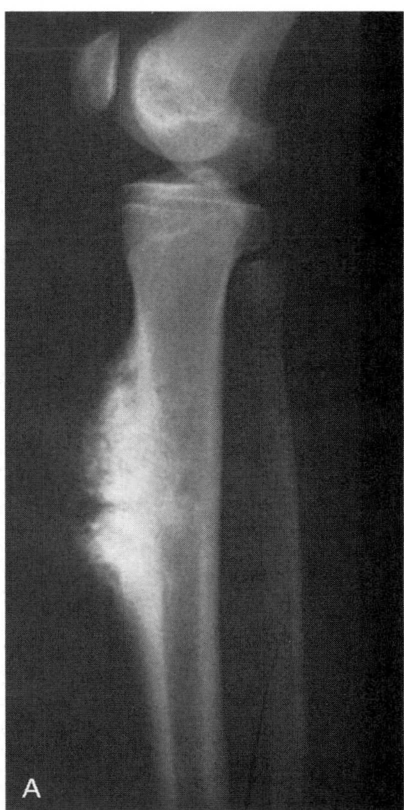

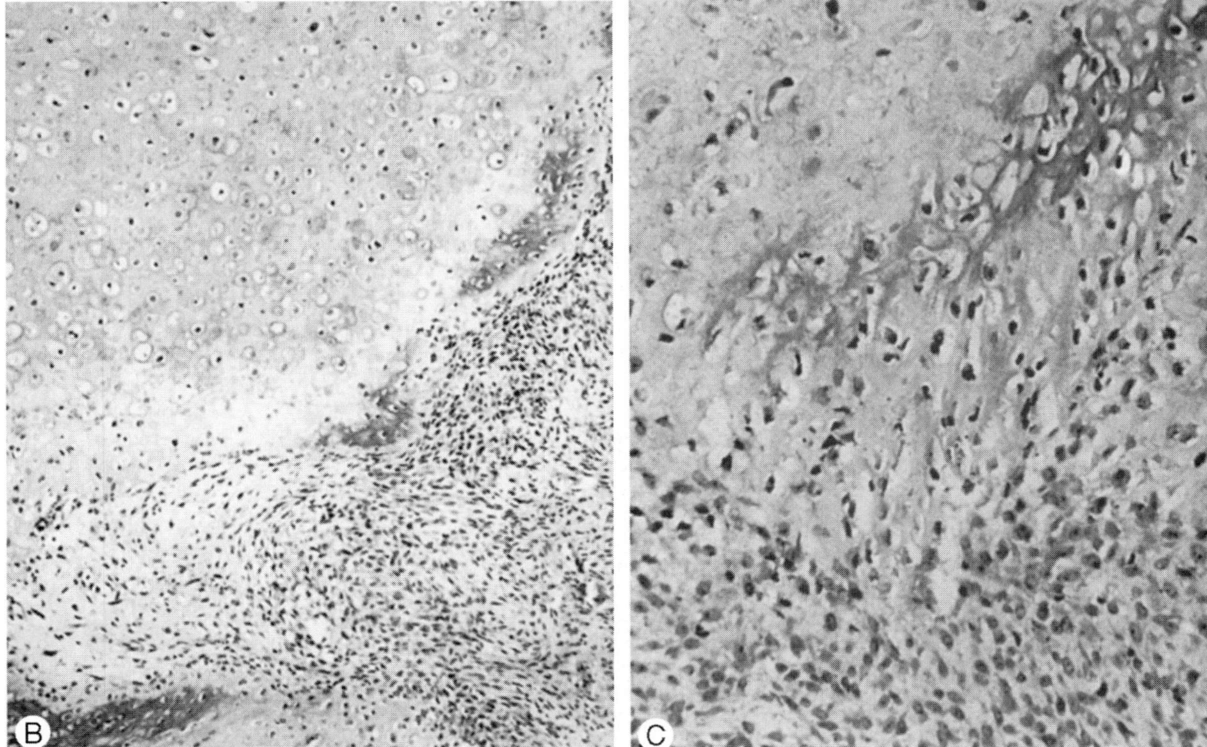

FIGURE 9–12 Periosteal osteosarcoma of the diaphysis of the tibia. **A**, Lateral radiograph showing a surface lesion with bone formation. **B**, Low-power photomicrograph (× 160) showing cartilage and bone formation. **C**, Higher-power photomicrograph showing pleomorphism and direct production of osteoid by the tumor cells.

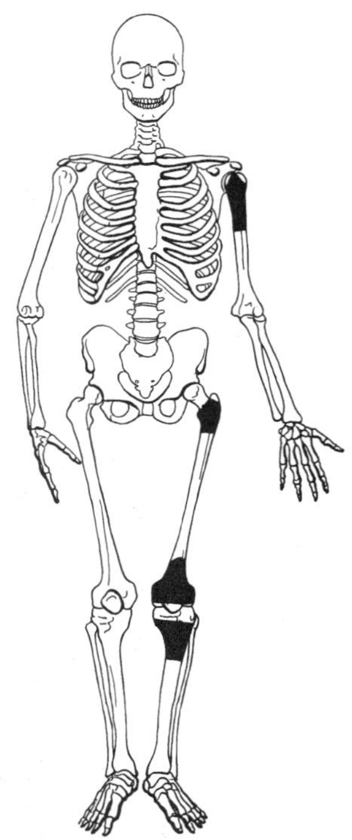

FIGURE 9–13 Skeletal distribution of the locations of telangiectatic osteosarcoma. (From McCarthy EF, Frassica FJ: Pathology of Bone and Joint Disorders. Philadelphia, WB Saunders, 1998.)

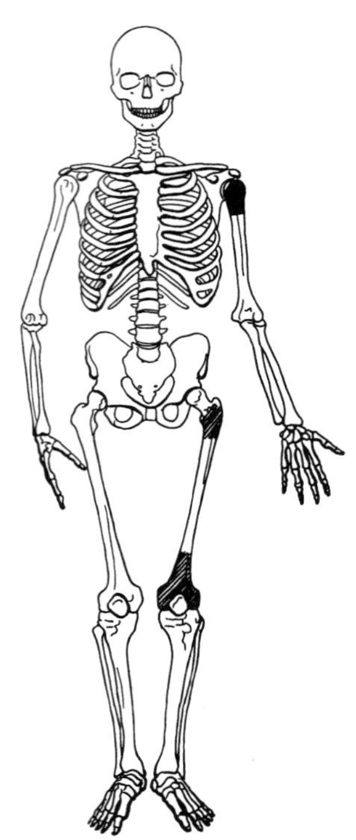

FIGURE 9–15 Skeletal distribution of the most common sites of periosteal chondroma. (From McCarthy EF, Frassica FJ: Pathology of Bone and Joint Disorders. Philadelphia, WB Saunders, 1998.)

and display worrisome histologic features, and pathologic fractures in the hand are common. Most enchondromas in long bones are asymptomatic. In long bones, radiographically there may be a prominent stippled or mottled calcified appearance (Fig. 9–17). Occasionally, active lesions are purely lytic without evidence of mineralization. Histologically, they are composed of small cells that lie in lacunar spaces. The lesion is usually hypocellular, and the cells have a bland appearance (no pleomorphism, anaplasia, or hyperchromasia). In contrast, in periosteal chondroma there is usually a well-demarcated, shallow cortical defect and a slight buttress of cortical bone at

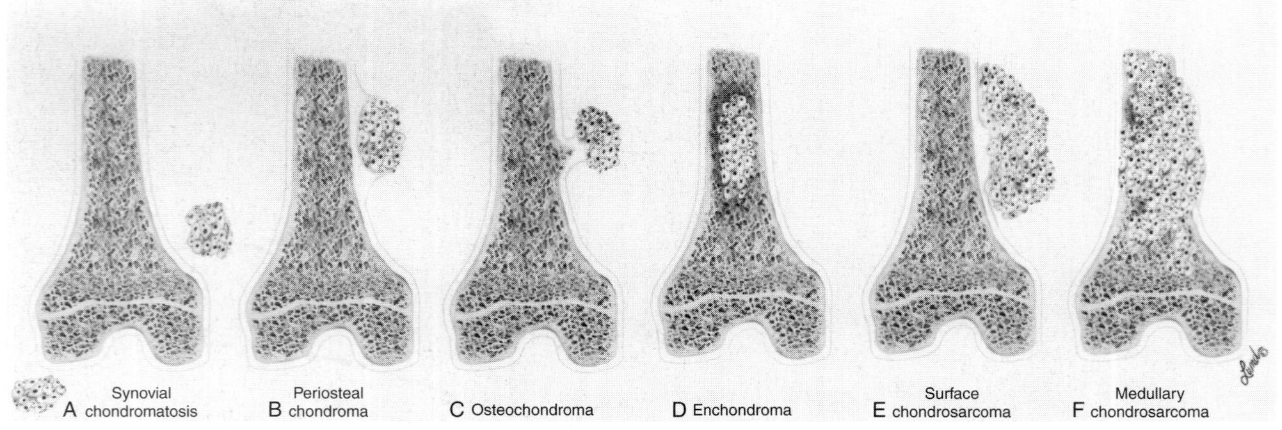

FIGURE 9–14 The common types of cartilage tumors. **A**, Lobular pattern of cartilage in synovial chondromatosis. **B**, Surface tumor of bone composed of mature cartilage that sits in a saucer-shaped depression on the bone's surface. These lesions are called periosteal chondromas. **C**, Surface tumor in which the cortices are continuous between the surface lesion and the host cortex. On top of the bone sits a thin rim of cartilage (1-3 mm). This lesion is called an osteochondroma and is one of the most common benign cartilage tumors. **D**, Enchondroma. Notice that this benign cartilage tumor sits in the medullary cavity in a quiescent manner. There are no cortical changes, such as erosions, cortical thickening, or cortical bone destruction. **E**, Surface chondrosarcoma is a rare malignant bone tumor in which there is a malignant cartilage mass on the surface of the bone. **F**, In medullary chondrosarcoma with active growth, there may be destruction of the cortex and extension into the soft tissues. In this instance the cartilage is growing and destroying the bone rather than being quiescent. (From McCarthy EF, Frassica FJ: Pathology of Bone and Joint Disorders. Philadelphia, WB Saunders, 1998.)

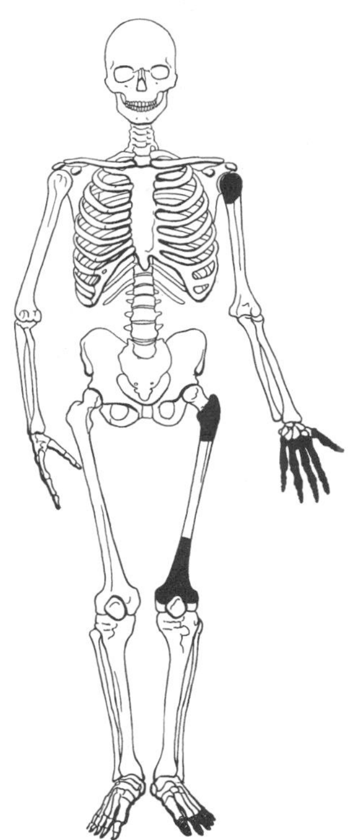

FIGURE 9–16 Skeletal distribution of the most common sites of enchondromas. Note the common location in the phalanges of the hand, the proximal humerus, and the distal femur. (From McCarthy EF, Frassica FJ: Pathology of Bone and Joint Disorders. Philadelphia, WB Saunders, 1998.)

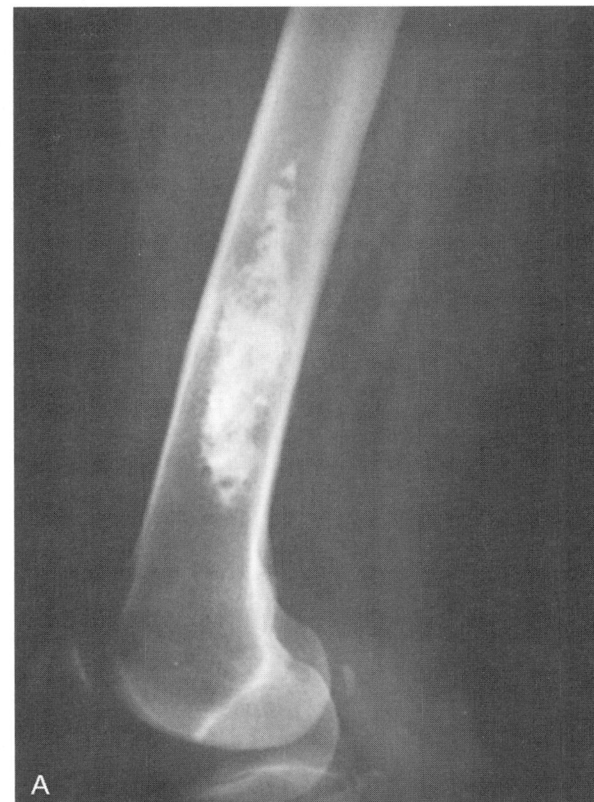

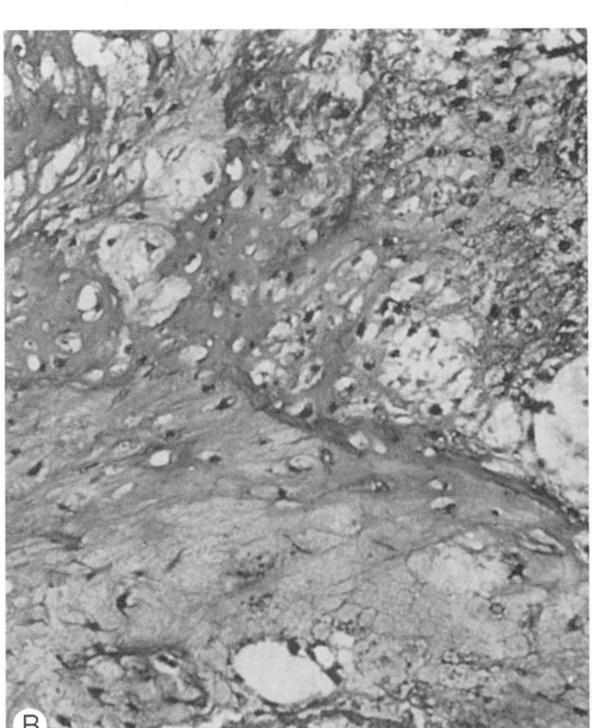

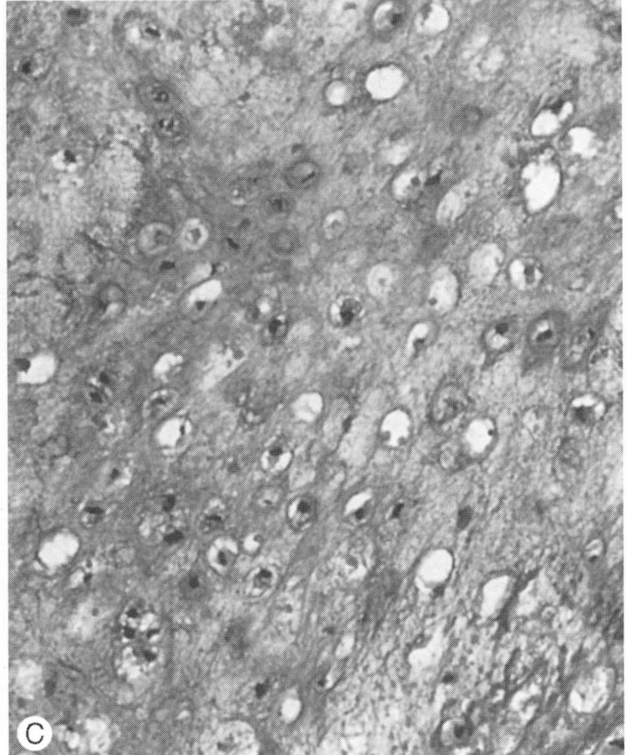

FIGURE 9–17 Enchondroma of the distal femur. **A**, Radiograph shows densely mineralized medullary lesion. **B**, Low-power (× 160) photomicrograph shows mineralized hyaline cartilage. **C**, Higher-power (× 250) photomicrograph shows bland chondrocytes in lacunae.

the edges of the lesion. About one third of the periosteal chondromas have a mineralized cartilaginous matrix on the radiograph (Fig. 9–18), whereas two thirds have no apparent radiographic mineralization. When lesions are not causing pain, serial radiographs are obtained to ensure that the lesions are inactive (not growing). Radiographs are obtained every 3-6 months for 1 to 2 years, then annually as necessary. The radiographic distinction between enchondroma and low-grade chondrosarcoma can be made on serial plain radiographs. With low-grade chondrosarcomas, one can see cortical bone changes (large erosions [> 50%] of the cortex, cortical thickening, and destruction) or lysis of the previously mineralized cartilage.

b. Diagnosis—Enchondromas may be multiple in the same extremity. When there are many lesions, the involved bones are dysplastic, and the lesions tend toward unilaterality, the diagnosis of multiple enchondromatosis, or Ollier disease, is made. The inheritance pattern is sporadic. If soft tissue angiomas are also present, the patient has the Maffucci syndrome. Chondrosarcomas virtually never occur in the setting of a previous enchondroma; however, patients with multiple enchondromatosis are at increased risk

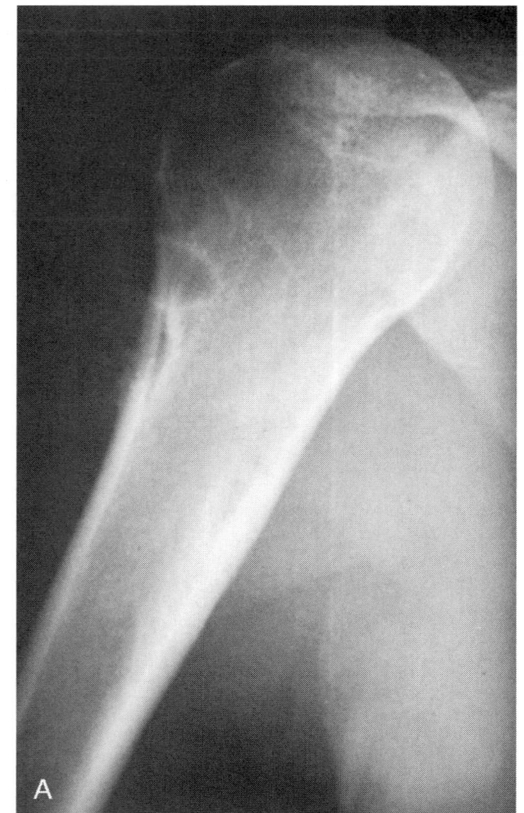

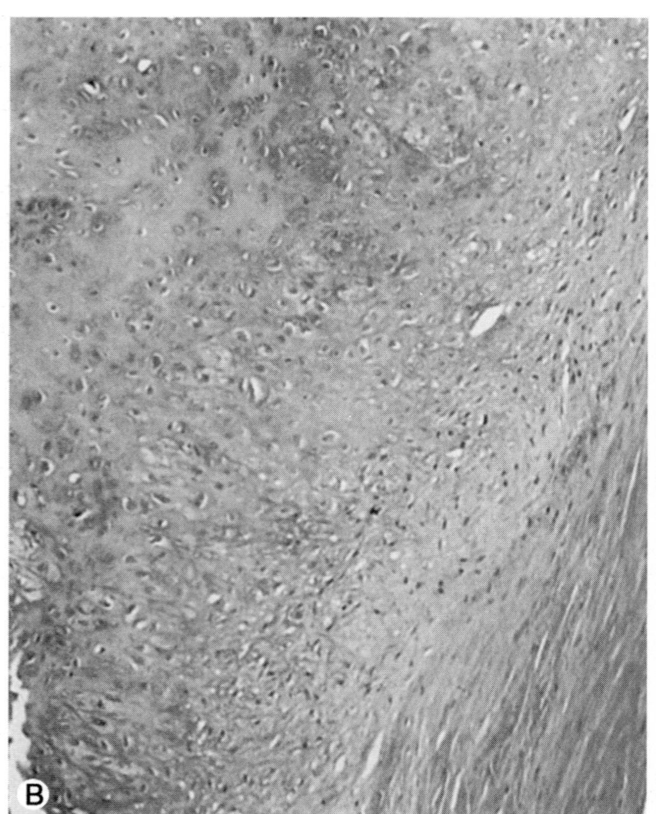

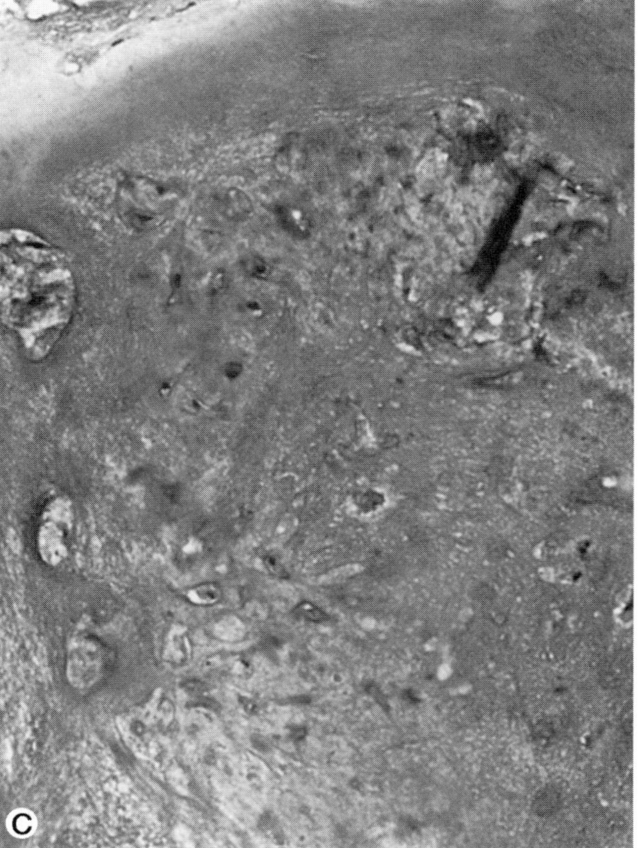

FIGURE 9–18 Periosteal chondroma of the proximal humerus. **A**, Radiograph shows surface lesion with stippled calcifications scalloping the cortex. **B**, Low-power photomicrograph (× 100) shows bland hyaline cartilage. **C**, Higher-power photomicrograph (× 250).

(Ollier disease, 30%; Maffucci syndrome, 100%). Patients with Maffucci syndrome also have a markedly increased risk of visceral malignancies, such as astrocytomas and gastrointestinal malignancies.

c. Treatment—Most enchondromas require no treatment other than observation. When surgical treatment is necessary, enchondromas are treated by curettage and bone grafting. Periosteal chondromas are usually excised with a marginal margin.

2. Osteochondroma
   a. Benign form—These benign surface lesions probably arise secondary to aberrant cartilage (from the perichondrial ring) on the surface of bone. Patients usually present with a painless mass after trauma, or the mass is discovered incidentally when a radiograph is obtained for another reason. Osteochondromas usually occur about the knee, proximal femur, and proximal humerus (Fig. 9–19). The characteristic appearance is a surface lesion in which the cortex of the lesion and the underlying cortex are continuous and the medullary cavity of the host bone also flows into (is continuous with) the osteochondroma (Fig. 9–20). The osteochondroma may have a narrow stalk (pedunculated) or a broad base (sessile). These lesions typically occur at the site of tendon insertions, and the affected bone is abnormally wide. Histologically, the underlying cortex is covered by a thin cap of cartilage. Grossly, the cartilage cap is usually only 2-3 mm thick. In a growing child the cap may exceed 1-2 cm. Histologically, the chondrocytes are arranged in linear clusters, with an appearance resembling that of the normal physis. When they are asymptomatic, these lesions are treated with observation only. Patients may experience pain secondary to muscle irritation, mechanical trauma (contusions), or an inflamed bursa over the lesion. In this scenario, excision is a logical alternative.

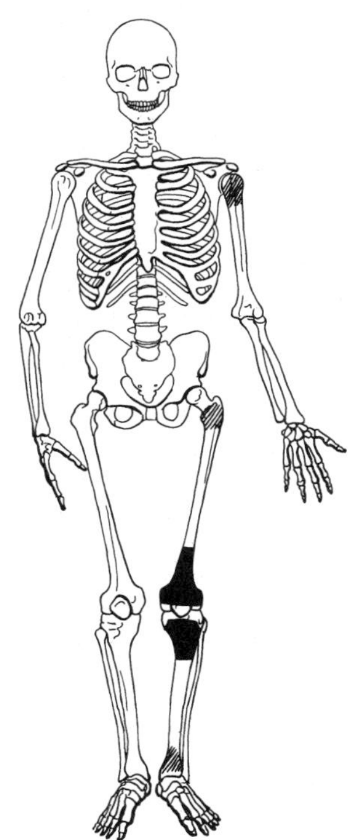

FIGURE 9–19 Skeletal distribution of the most common sites of osteochondromas. (From McCarthy EF, Frassica FJ: Pathology of Bone and Joint Disorders. Philadelphia, WB Saunders, 1998.)

   b. Malignant transformation—Pain in the absence of mechanical factors is a warning sign of malignant change. The development of a sarcoma in an osteochondroma is rare, far less than 1%. Destruction of the subchondral bone, mineralization of a soft tissue mass, and an inhomogeneous appearance are radiographic changes of malignant transformation. When malignant change occurs, a low-grade chondrosarcoma is usually present, although a dedifferentiated chondrosarcoma may rarely occur. When a chondrosarcoma develops in an osteochondroma, the lesion is termed a "secondary chondrosarcoma." The prognosis is usually excellent; these low-grade tumors seldom metastasize. Multiple exostoses represent a common disorder characterized by multiple osteochondromas. The inheritance pattern is autosomal dominant. The osteochondromas are often sessile and large. This is an autosomal dominant condition with mutations in the *EXT1* and *EXT2* gene loci. Approximately 10% of patients with multiple exostoses develop a secondary chondrosarcoma. The *EXT2* mutation is associated with a greater burden of disease and risk of malignancy.

3. Chondroblastoma—These benign cartilage tumors are centered in the epiphysis in young patients, usually with open physes. The most common locations are the distal femur, proximal tibia, and proximal humerus (Fig. 9–21). Although the lesion is usually in the epiphysis, it may also occur in an apophysis. Another common location is the triradiate cartilage of the pelvis. Patients usually present with pain referable to the involved joint. Radiographically, there is a central region of bone destruction that is usually sharply demarcated from the normal medullary cavity by a thin rim of sclerotic bone (Fig. 9–22). There may or may not be mineralization within the lesion. Histologically, the basic proliferating cells are thought to be chondroblasts. There are scattered multinucleated giant cells throughout the lesion and zones of chondroid substance. Mitotic figures may be found. Chondroblastomas are treated by curettage (intralesional margin) and bone grafting. About 2% of benign chondroblastomas metastasize to the lungs. There may be genetic abnormalities in chromosomes 5 and 8.

4. Chondromyxoid fibroma—These rare, benign cartilage tumors contain variable amounts of

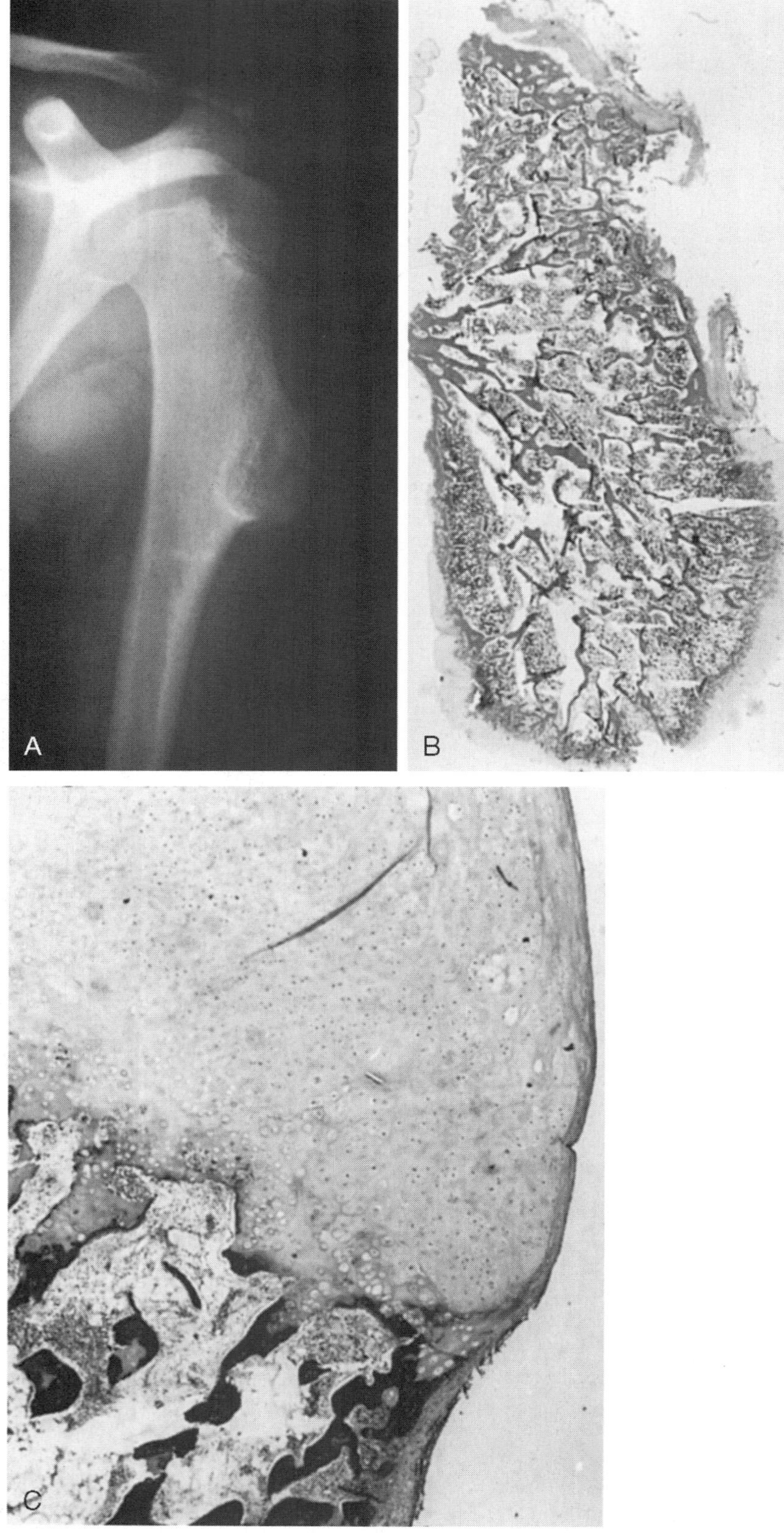

FIGURE 9–20 Osteochondroma of the proximal humerus. **A**, Radiograph shows sessile osteochondroma of the proximal humerus. **B**, Photomicrograph (× 6) shows the osteochondroma with a cartilaginous cap. **C**, Higher-power photomicrograph (× 25) shows the cartilage cap, which is undergoing endochondral ossification.

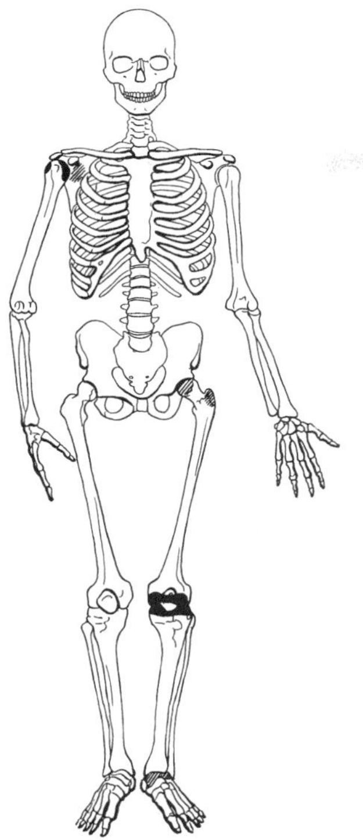

FIGURE 9–21 Skeletal distribution of the most common sites of chondroblastomas. Chondroblastomas begin in either the epiphysis or apophysis. They commonly occur in the distal femur; proximal tibia; femoral head; greater trochanteric apophysis; and proximal humeral epiphysis. Chondroblastomas in the proximal humeral epiphysis are called Codman's tumor. (From McCarthy EF, Frassica FJ: Pathology of Bone and Joint Disorders. Philadelphia, WB Saunders, 1998.)

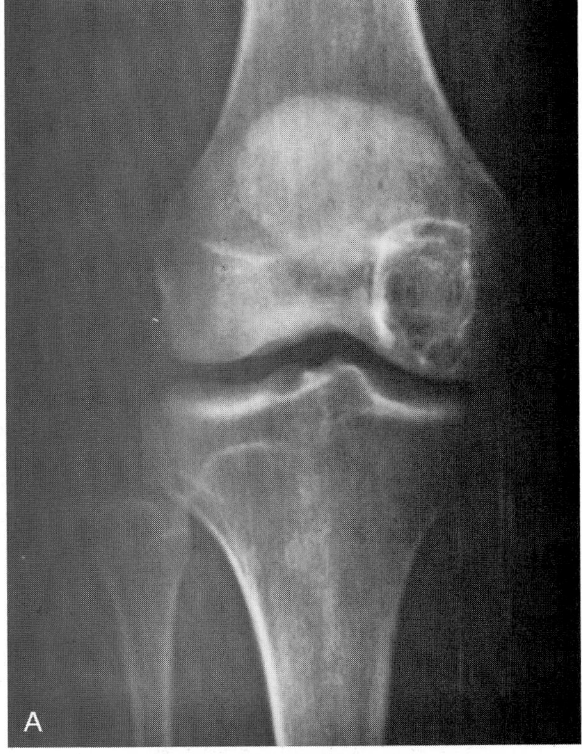

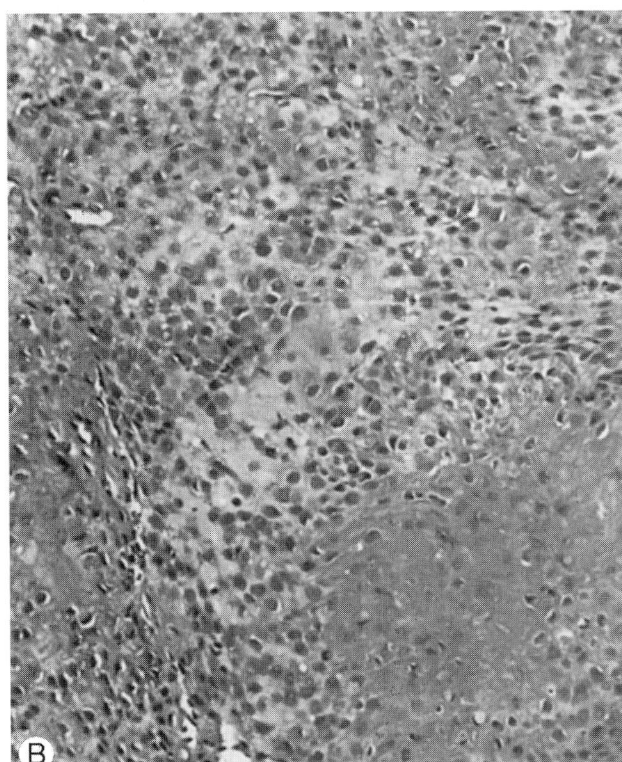

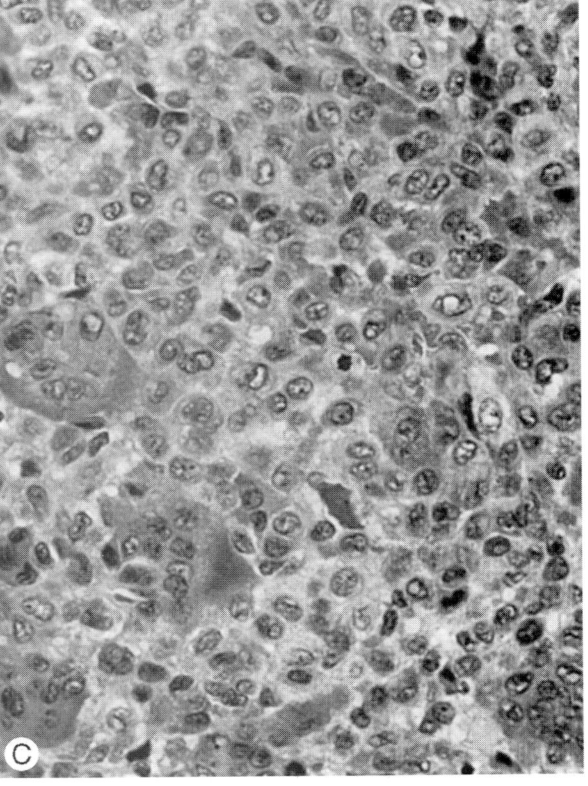

FIGURE 9–22 Chondroblastoma of the distal femur. **A**, Radiograph shows a well-circumscribed lytic lesion with a sclerotic rim in the distal femoral epiphysis. **B**, Low-power photomicrograph (× 160) shows cellular stroma in a chondroid matrix. **C**, Higher-power photomicrograph (× 400) shows rounded stromal cells with multinucleated giant cells.

chondroid, fibromatoid, and myxoid elements. The lesion is more common in males and tends to involve long bones (especially the tibia). The pelvis and distal femur are other common locations (Fig. 9–23). Patients present with pain of variable duration (months to years). Radiographically, there is a lytic, destructive lesion that is eccentric and sharply demarcated from the adjacent normal bone (Fig. 9–24). There is usually no matrix mineralization seen radiographically. The tumor grows in lobules, and there is often a condensation of cells at the periphery of the lobules. The chondroid element may vary from small to heavy concentrations. Treatment is by curettage and grafting. There may be a genetic rearrangement on chromosome 6 at position q13 (6q13).

5. Intramedullary chondrosarcoma—This malignant neoplasm of cartilage occurs in adults in the older age groups. The most common locations include the shoulder and pelvic girdles, knee, and spine. Patients may have pain or a mass. Plain radiographs are usually diagnostic, with bone destruction, thickening of the cortex, and mineralization consistent with cartilage within the lesion (Fig. 9–25). About 85% of patients will have prominent cortical changes. A soft tissue mass is often present in patients who have had symptoms for a long time. It may be extremely difficult to differentiate malignant cartilage based on histologic features alone. The clinical, radiographic, and histologic features of a particular lesion must be combined to avoid incorrect diagnosis. The criteria for the diagnosis of malignancy include (1) many cells with plump nuclei, (2) more than an occasional cell with two such nuclei, (3) especially large cartilage cells with large single or multiple nuclei containing clumps of chromatin, and (4) infiltration of the bone trabeculae. Chondromas of the hand (enchondromas)—the lesions in patients with Ollier disease and the Maffucci syndrome—and periosteal chondromas may have atypical histopathologic features (Fig. 9–26). However, their behavior is that of a benign cartilage lesion, and hence they are not malignant lesions. In intramedullary chondrocarcinoma there may be hypercellularity and worrisome nuclear features; however, the biologic behavior is innocent. More than 90% of chondrosarcomas are grade I or II lesions. Grade III lesions are uncommon and behave as other highly malignant bone tumors. Treatment consists of wide-margin surgical resection. For typical low-grade (grades I and II) chondrosarcoma, there is no role for chemotherapy or irradiation.

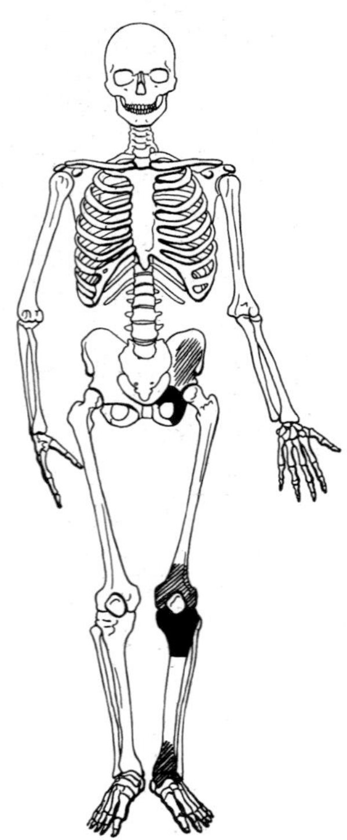

FIGURE 9–23 Skeletal distribution of the most common sites of chondromyxoid fibroma. The tibia and pelvis are common locations. (From McCarthy EF, Frassica FJ: Pathology of Bone and Joint Disorders. Philadelphia, WB Saunders, 1998.)

6. Dedifferentiated chondrosarcoma—These lesions are the most malignant cartilage tumors. The most common locations include the distal and proximal femur and the proximal humerus (Fig. 9–27). They have a bimorphic histologic and radiographic appearance. Histologically, there is a low-grade cartilage component that is intimately associated with a high-grade spindle cell sarcoma (osteosarcoma, fibrosarcoma, malignant fibrous histiocytoma). Radiographically, in more than 80% of the lesions there is a typical chondrosarcoma with a superimposed, highly destructive area (Fig. 9–28). Patients present with a picture similar to that of low-grade chondrosarcoma, including pain and decreased function. The prognosis is poor, and long-term survival is less than 10%. Wide-margin surgical resection and multiagent chemotherapy are the principal methods of treatment.

D. Fibrous lesions—There are three fibrous lesions of bone: metaphyseal fibrous defect (fibroma), desmoplastic fibroma, and fibrosarcoma.

1. Metaphyseal fibrous defect—This lesion commonly occurs in young patients. Most of these lesions resolve spontaneously and are probably not true neoplasms. Typical names for this lesion include nonossifying fibroma, nonosteogenic fibroma, cortical desmoid, fibromatosis, and xanthoma. The most common locations are the distal femur, distal tibia, and proximal tibia. Most patients are asymptomatic, and the lesion is discovered incidentally. The radiographic appearance is characteristic, with a lucent lesion that is metaphyseal, eccentric, and surrounded by a sclerotic rim (Fig. 9–29). The cortex may be slightly expanded and thinned. Histologically, there is a cellular, fibroblastic connective tissue background, with the cells arranged in whorled bundles. There are numerous giant cells, lipophages,

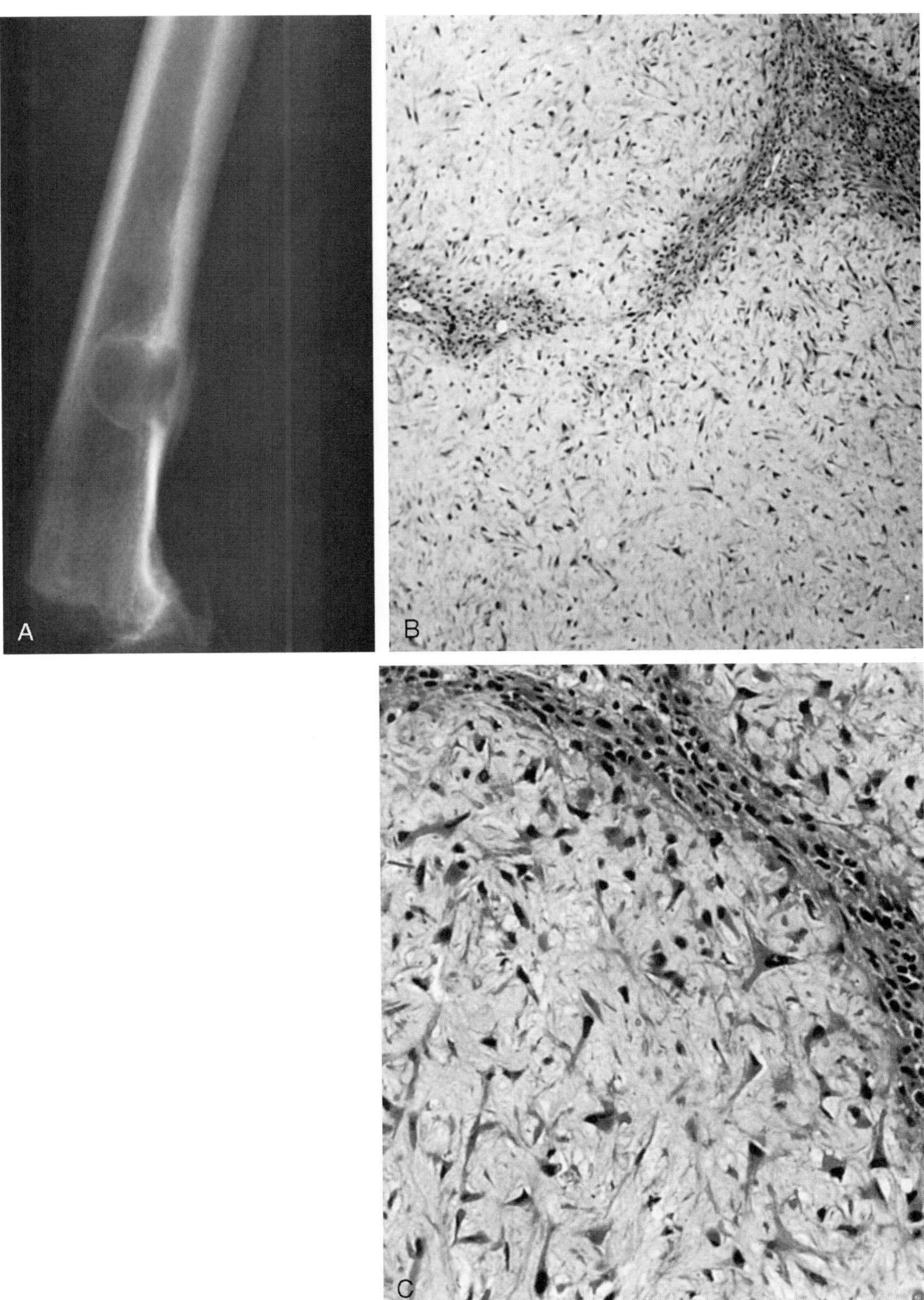

FIGURE 9–24 Chondromyxoid fibroma of the femur. **A**, Radiograph shows a well-circumscribed lytic lesion in the distal femur, with a rim of sclerotic bone. **B**, Low-power photomicrograph (× 100) shows lobules of fibromyxoid tissue. **C**, Higher-power photomicrograph (× 250) shows myxoid stroma with stellate cells.

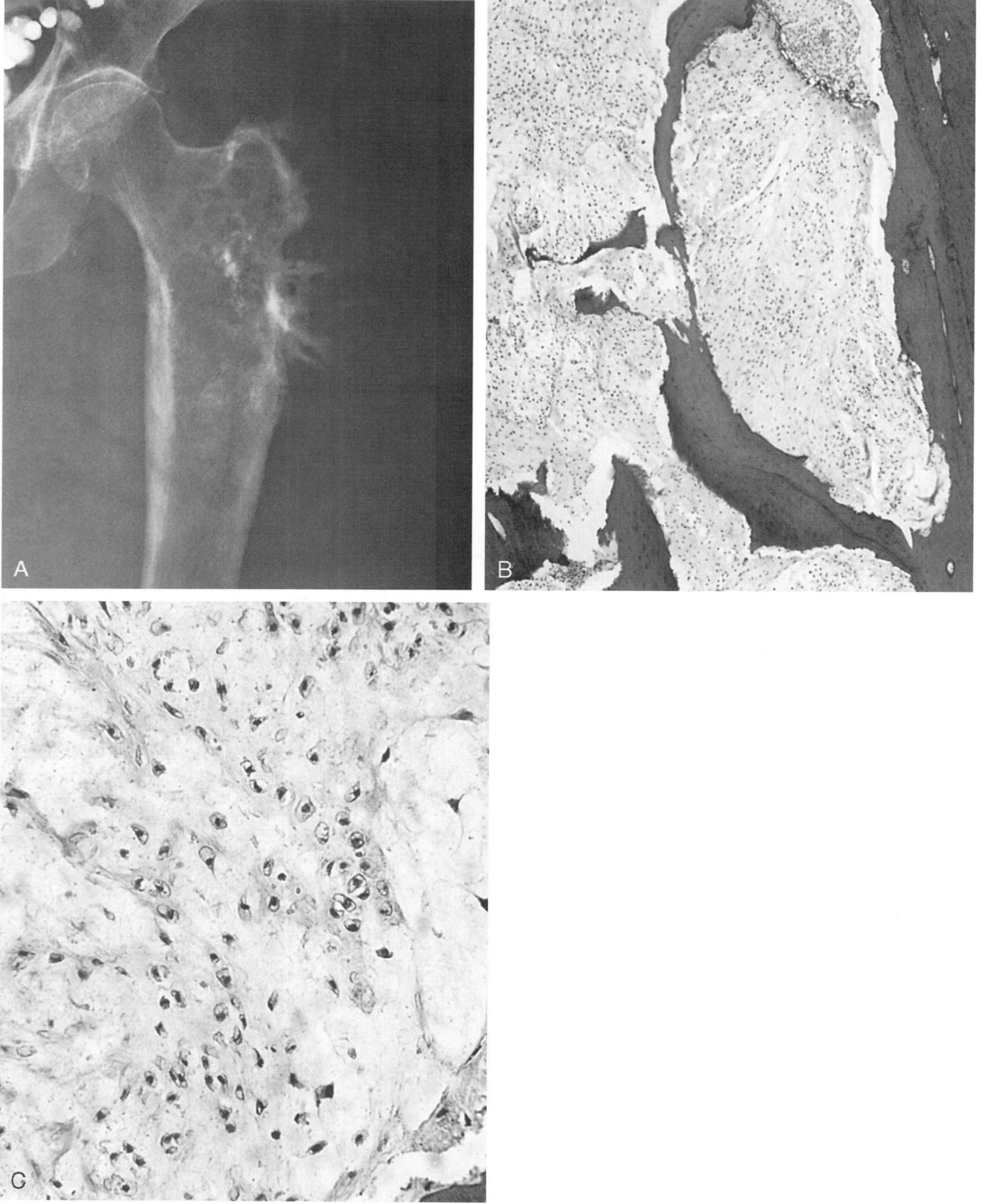

FIGURE 9–25 Central (intramedullary) chondrosarcoma of the proximal femur. **A**, Radiograph shows an expansile lytic lesion in the proximal femur with stippled calcifications. **B**, Low-power photomicrograph (× 40) shows cartilage with a permeative growth pattern. **C**, Higher-power photomicrograph (× 250) shows cellular cartilage.

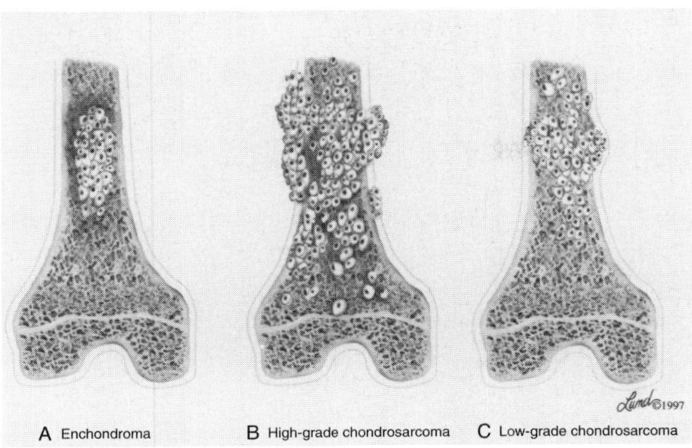

FIGURE 9–26 The three types of intramedullary cartilage tumors: enchondroma, high-grade chondrosarcoma, and low-grade chondrosarcoma. **A**, Enchondromas are inactive intramedullary tumors of the hyaline cartilage. Note that the cortices are not involved. There is no cortical erosion, thickening, expansion, or breakthrough. **B**, In contrast, high-grade chondrosarcoma shows destruction of the cortex and extension into the soft tissues. **C**, Low-grade chondrosarcoma. Note the cortical erosion, with expansion of the cortex but no breakthrough. (From McCarthy EF, Frassica FJ: Pathology of Bone and Joint Disorders. Philadelphia, WB Saunders, 1998.)

and various amounts of hemosiderin pigmentation. Treatment is with observation if the radiographic appearance is characteristic and there is not an excessive risk of pathologic fracture. If more than 50-75% of the cortex is involved and the patient is symptomatic, curettage and bone grafting are performed.

2. Desmoplastic fibroma—This lesion is a rare and low-grade but aggressive fibrous tumor of bone. Radiographically, the lesion is purely lytic. Because the process is low grade, there will often be residual or reactive trabeculated (or corrugated) bone. Histologically, this lesion is composed of abundant collagen and mature fibroblasts with no cellular atypia. Curettage and preservation of the joint may be performed, but there is a high risk of local recurrence. Wide resection results in the lowest risk of local recurrence but requires removal of the joint in young patients.
3. Fibrosarcoma—This malignant tumor of bone has a presentation and localization similar to that of osteosarcoma. The tumor affects primarily an older age group but does occur during all decades of life. Patients present with pain and swelling, as with any other malignant bone tumor. There is bone destruction radiographically, typically in a permeative pattern (Fig. 9–30). The histologic features are the same as those of soft tissue fibrosarcoma, with spindle cells, variable collagen production, and a herringbone pattern. Treatment consists of wide-margin surgical resection. Although the prognosis is poor, the role of chemotherapy has not been fully defined; effective regimens for the older patient have not been adequately explored.

E. Histiocytic lesions (malignant fibrous histiocytoma) —The most common locations include the distal femur, proximal tibia, proximal femur, ilium, and proximal humerus (Fig. 9–31). These malignant bone tumors have proliferating cells with a histiocytic quality. The nuclei are often indented, the cytoplasm is usually abundant and may be slightly foamy, the nucleoli are often large, and multinucleated giant cells are usually a prominent feature. There may be variable amounts of fibrous tissue found within the lesion, and the fibrogenic areas have a storiform appearance. Chronic inflammatory cells are frequently found. Patients present with pain and swelling. Radiographs usually demonstrate a destructive lesion, with either purely lytic bone destruction or a mixed pattern of bone destruction and formation (Fig. 9–32). Treatment is by wide surgical excision. Most patients are candidates for multiagent chemotherapy, although few studies have shown chemotherapy to be efficacious for this tumor.

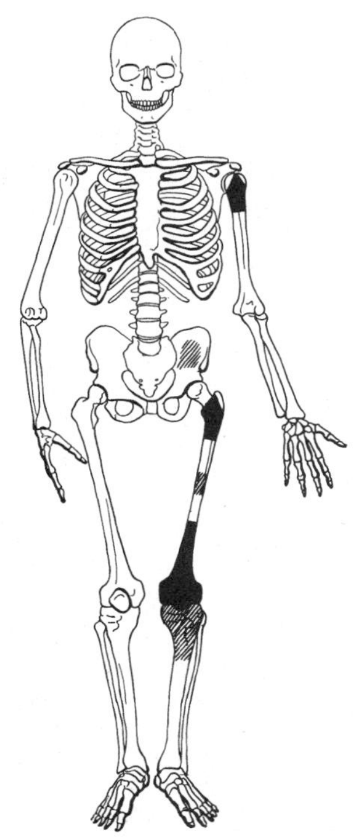

FIGURE 9–27 Skeletal distribution of the most common sites of dedifferentiated chondrosarcoma. The femur and humerus are the most common sites. (From McCarthy EF, Frassica FJ: Pathology of Bone and Joint Disorders. Philadelphia, WB Saunders, 1998.)

F. Notochordal tissue—Chordoma is a malignant neoplasm in which the cell of origin derives from primitive notochordal tissue. This lesion occurs predominantly at the ends of the vertebral column (spheno-occipital region and sacrum) (Fig. 9–33). About 10% of chordomas occur in the vertebral bodies (cervical, thoracic, and lumbar regions). Patients present with an insidious onset of pain. Lesions in the sacrum may present as pelvic pain, low-back pain, hip pain, or primarily gastrointestinal symptomatology (obstipation, constipation, loss of rectal tone). When vertebral bodies are involved, there may be a wide variation in neurologic symptoms because of nerve compression. Patients with a long-standing history of undiagnosed pelvic or

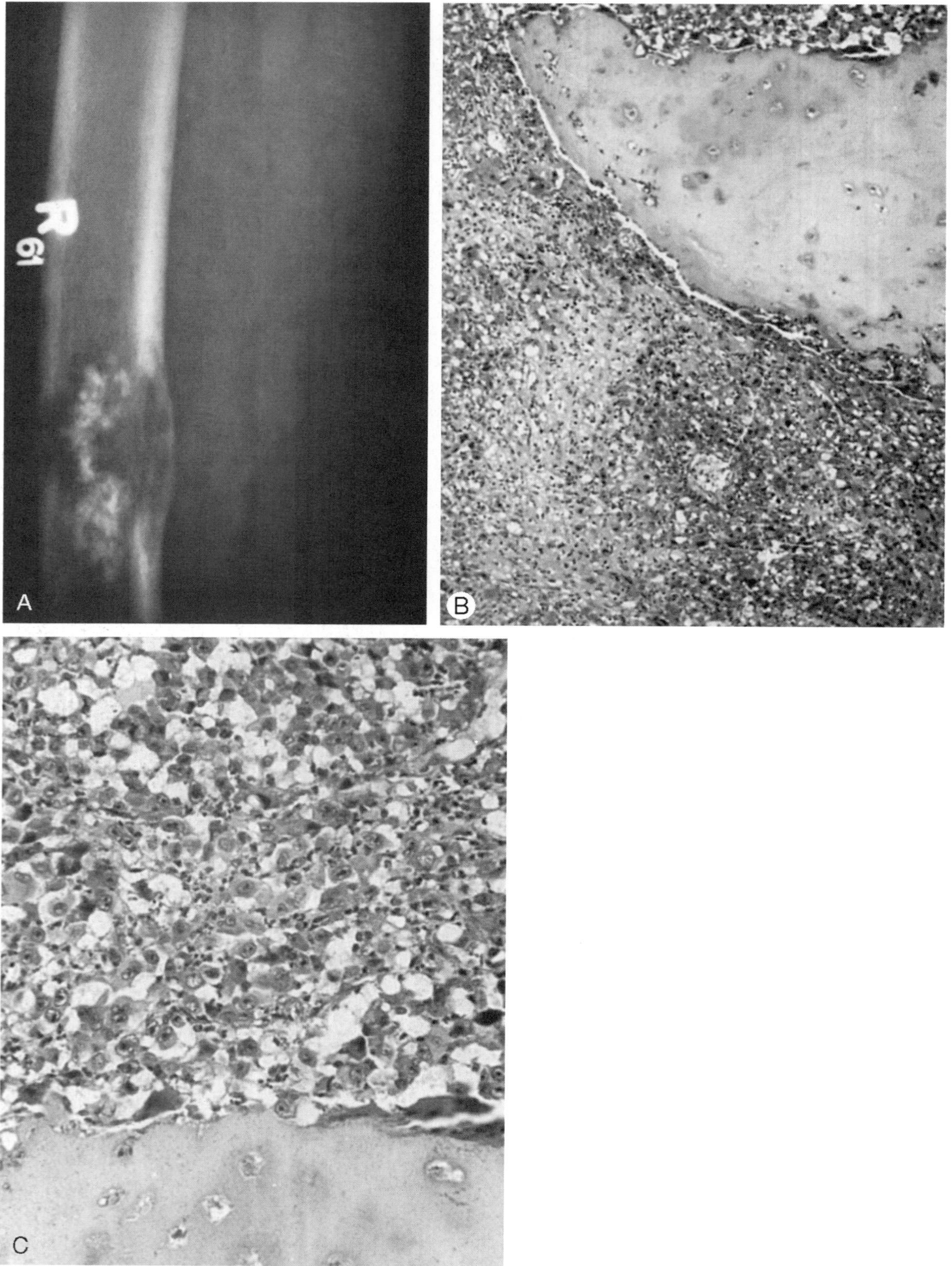

FIGURE 9–28 Dedifferentiated chondrosarcoma of the femur. **A**, Radiograph shows focal dense mineralization surrounded by a poorly defined lytic lesion. **B**, Low-power photomicrograph (× 100) shows an island of hyaline cartilage surrounded by a cellular neoplasm. **C**, Higher-power photomicrograph (× 250) shows hyaline cartilage adjacent to pleomorphic rounded cells.

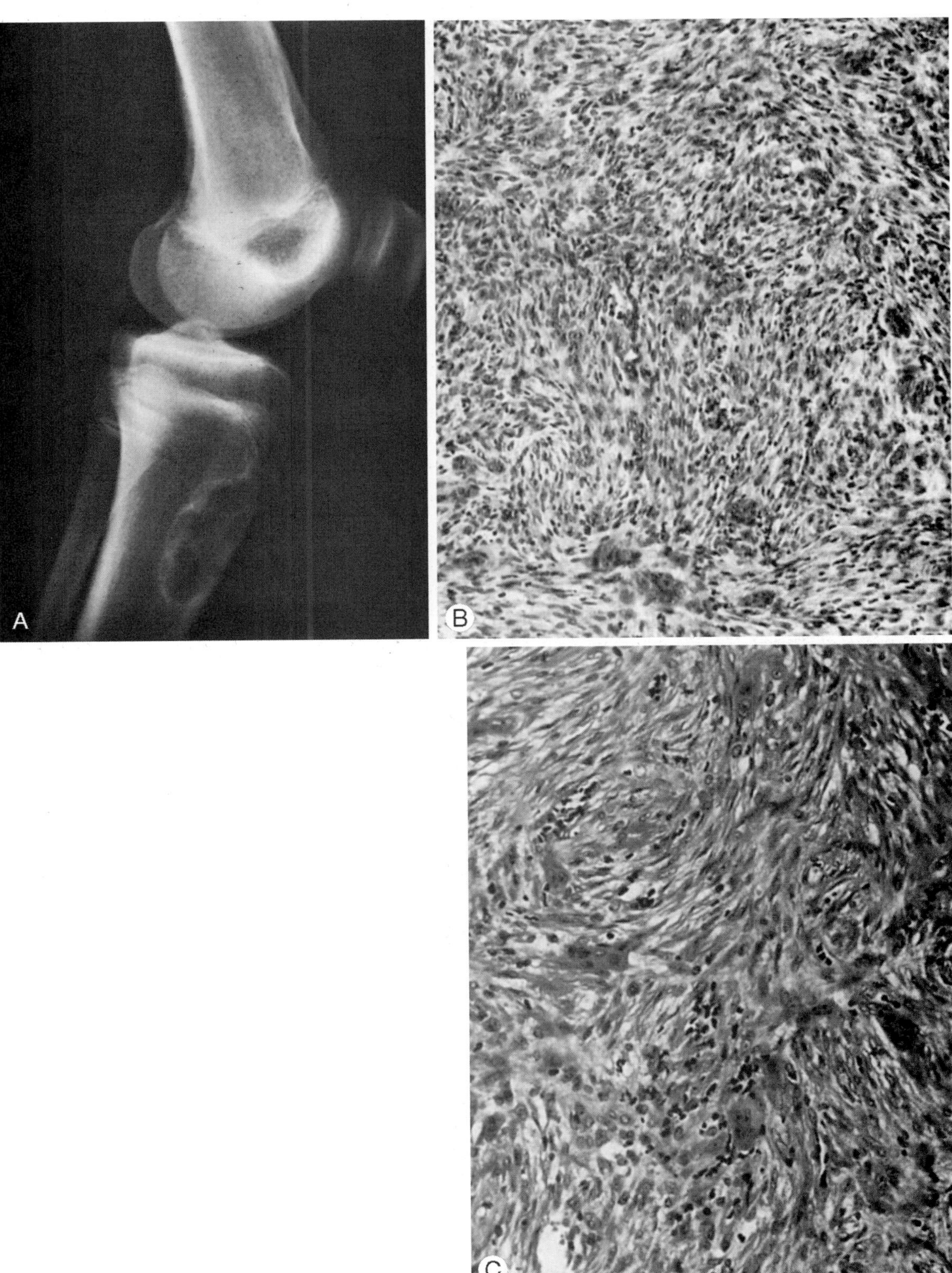

FIGURE 9–29 Nonossifying fibroma of the proximal tibia. **A**, Radiograph shows a scalloped, well-circumscribed lesion with a sclerotic rim in the proximal tibial metaphysis. **B**, Low-power photomicrograph (× 160) shows spindle cells in a storiform pattern and occasional multinucleated giant cells. **C**, Higher-power photomicrograph (× 250).

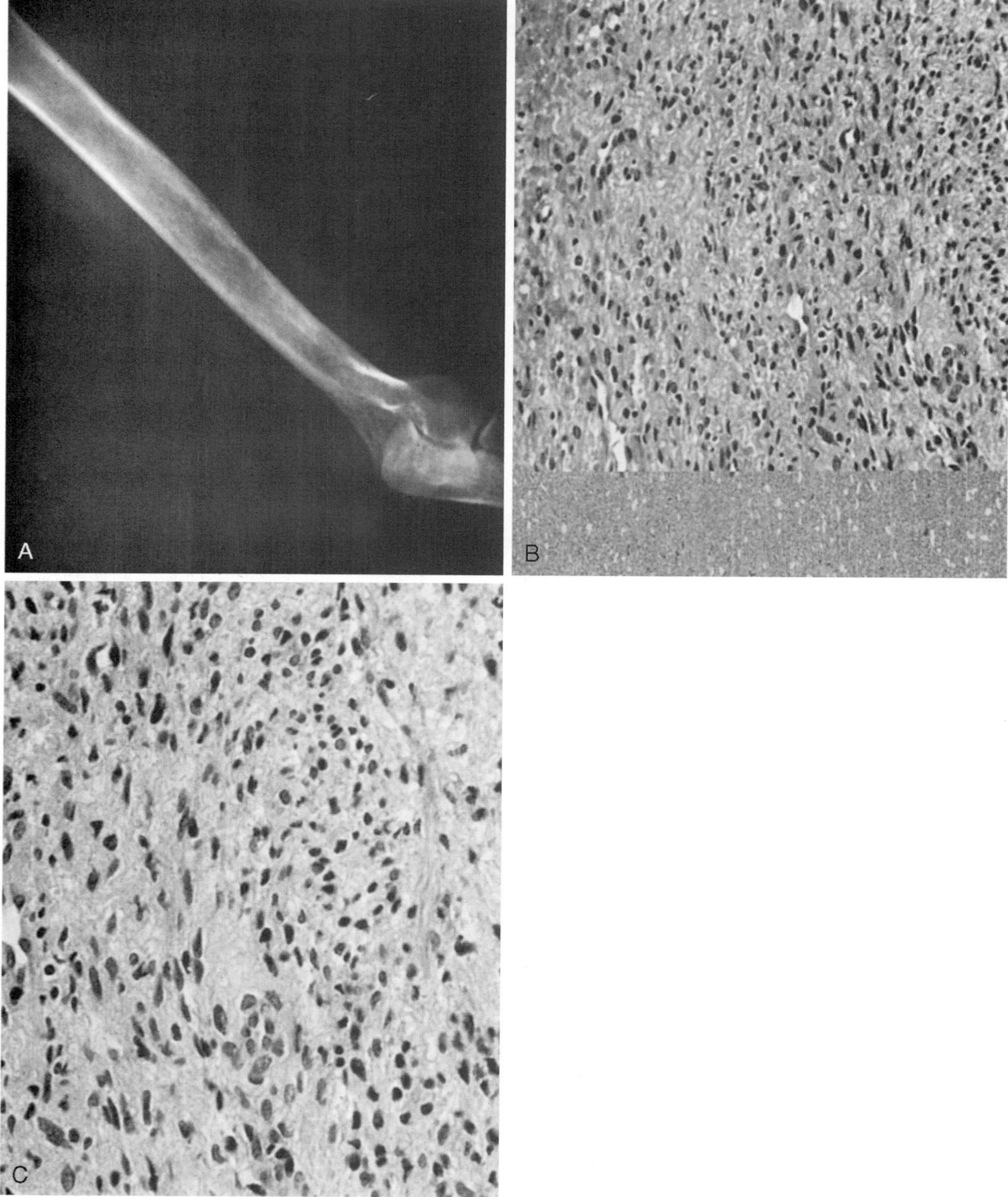

FIGURE 9–30 Fibrosarcoma of the humerus. **A**, Radiograph shows a permeative lesion in the midshaft of the humerus. **B**, Low-power photomicrograph (× 250) shows atypical spindle cells. **C**, Higher-power photomicrograph (× 400).

low-back pain should undergo a rectal examination because more than half of the sacral chordomas are palpable on digital examination. Plain radiographs often do not reveal the true extent of sacrococcygeal chordomas. The sacrum is difficult to evaluate on plain radiographs because of overlying bowel gas and fecal material and the angulation of the sacrum away from the x-ray beam on the anteroposterior view. In addition, the anteroposterior pelvic view reveals bone destruction only at the sacral cortical margins and neural foramina; these areas are not typically involved early. CT scans show midline bone

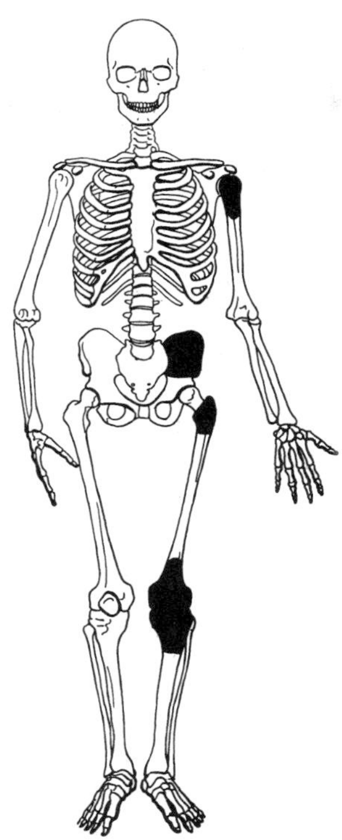

FIGURE 9–31 Skeletal distribution of the most common sites of malignant fibrous histiocytoma. (From McCarthy EF, Frassica FJ: Pathology of Bone and Joint Disorders. Philadelphia, WB Saunders, 1998.)

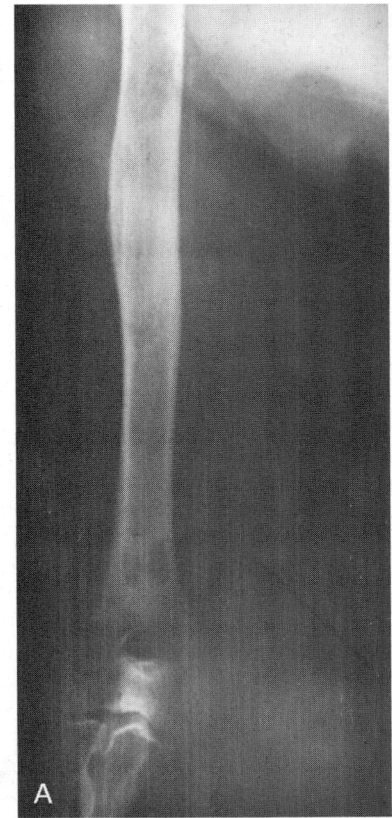

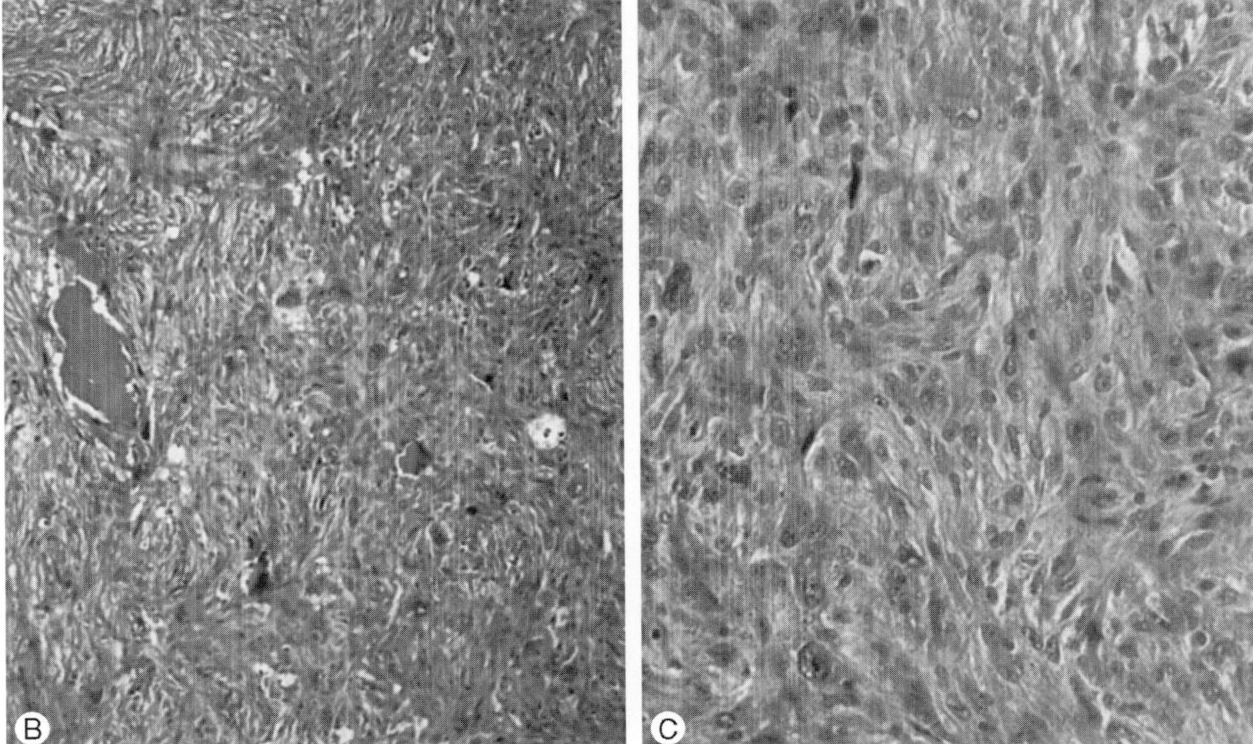

FIGURE 9–32 Malignant fibrous histiocytoma of the humerus. **A**, Radiograph shows poorly defined lytic lesions in the proximal and distal humerus. **B**, Low-power photomicrograph (× 200) shows spindle cells arranged in a storiform pattern. **C**, Higher-power photomicrograph (× 400) shows a uniform population of pleomorphic cells.

destruction and a soft tissue mass (Fig. 9–34). An MRI scan is an excellent modality to both detect a chordoma and define the anatomic features of the tumor. The signal characteristics show a low signal on T1-weighted images and a very bright signal on T2-weighted images. The sacrum is often expanded, and the soft tissue mass may show irregular mineralization. In the vertebral bodies, areas of lytic bone destruction or a mixed pattern of both bone formation and bone destruction are often seen. The tumor grows in distinct lobules. The chordoma cells sometimes have a vacuolated appearance and are called physaliferous cells. They are often arrayed in strands in a mass of mucous. Treatment is by resection with a wide surgical margin. Radiation therapy may be added if a wide margin is not achieved. Chordomas metastasize late in the course of the disease, and local extension can be fatal.

G. Vascular tumors—Vascular tumors of bone represent a heterogeneous group of disorders. Benign conditions include hemangioma, lymphangioma, and perhaps vanishing bone disease (Gorham disease or massive osteolysis). Malignant entities include hemangioendothelioma (hemangiosarcoma) and hemangiopericytoma.

1. Hemangioma (Fig. 9–35)—These tumors usually occur in vertebral bodies. Patients may present with pain or pathologic fracture. Vertebral hemangiomas have a characteristic appearance, with lytic destruction and vertical striations or a coarsened honeycomb appearance. Occasionally, more than one bone is involved. Histologically, there are numerous blood channels. Most lesions are cavernous, although some may be a mixture of capillary and cavernous blood spaces.
2. Hemangioendothelioma—Malignant vascular tumors of bone are rare. Patients may be in any age group and present with pain. Multifocal involvement of the bones of the same extremity is common. Radiographs show a predominantly oval lytic lesion with no reactive bone formation. The low-grade lesions often have residual trabecular bone. Histologically, the tumor cells form vascular spaces. The lesions range from very well differentiated tumors (easily recognizable vascular spaces) to very undifferentiated tumors (difficult to recognize their vasoformative quality). Low-grade multifocal lesions may be treated with radiation alone.

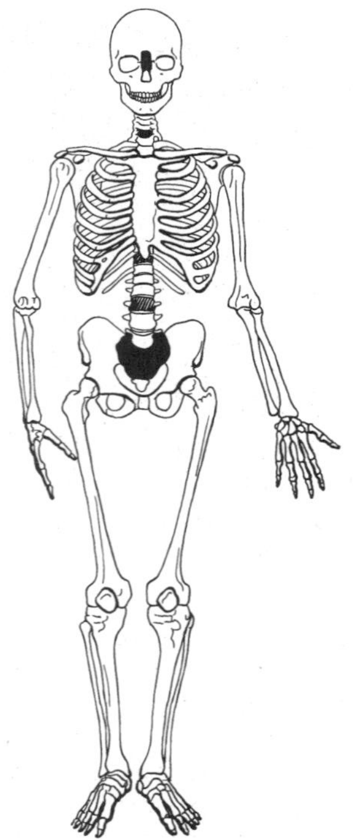

FIGURE 9–33 Skeletal distribution of the most common sites of chordoma. Chordomas occur exclusively in the spine, with 50% being sacrococcygeal, 40% in the spheno-occipital region, and 10% in the vertebra. (From McCarthy EF, Frassica FJ: Pathology of Bone and Joint Disorders. Philadelphia, WB Saunders, 1998.)

H. Hematopoietic tumors—Lymphoma and myeloma are two malignant hematopoietic tumors that may involve bone.

1. Lymphoma—Lymphoma of bone is uncommon and occurs in three scenarios: (1) as a solitary focus (primary lymphoma of bone), (2) in association with other osseous sites and nonosseous sites (nodal disease and soft tissue masses), and (3) as metastatic foci. The most common locations include the distal femur, proximal tibia, pelvis, proximal femur, vertebra, and shoulder girdle (Fig. 9–36). Malignant lymphoma of bone affects individuals during all decades of life. Patients generally present with pain. Large soft tissue masses may be present. The radiographs often show a lesion that involves a large portion of the bone (long lesion) (Fig. 9–37). Bone destruction is common and often has a mottled appearance. Reactive bone formation admixed with bone destruction is common. The cortex may be thickened. A mixed cellular infiltrate is usually present. Most lymphomas of bone are diffuse, large B-cell lymphomas. Treatment generally combines multiagent chemotherapy and consolidative irradiation. Surgery is generally used only to stabilize fractures.
2. Myeloma—Plasma cell dyscrasias represent a wide range of conditions, from **monoclonal gammopathy of undetermined significance** (MGUS [Kyle disease]) to multiple myeloma. There are three plasma cell dyscrasias with which the orthopaedist must be familiar: multiple myeloma, solitary plasmacytoma of bone, and osteosclerotic myeloma.
   a. Multiple myeloma—This malignant plasma cell disorder commonly occurs in patients between 50 and 80 years of age. Patients usually present with bone pain, usually in the spine and ribs, or a pathologic fracture. Fatigue is a common complaint secondary to the associated anemia. Symptoms may be related to complications such as renal insufficiency, hypercalcemia, and the deposition of amyloid. Serum creatinine levels are elevated in about 50% of patients. Hypercalcemia is present in about a third of

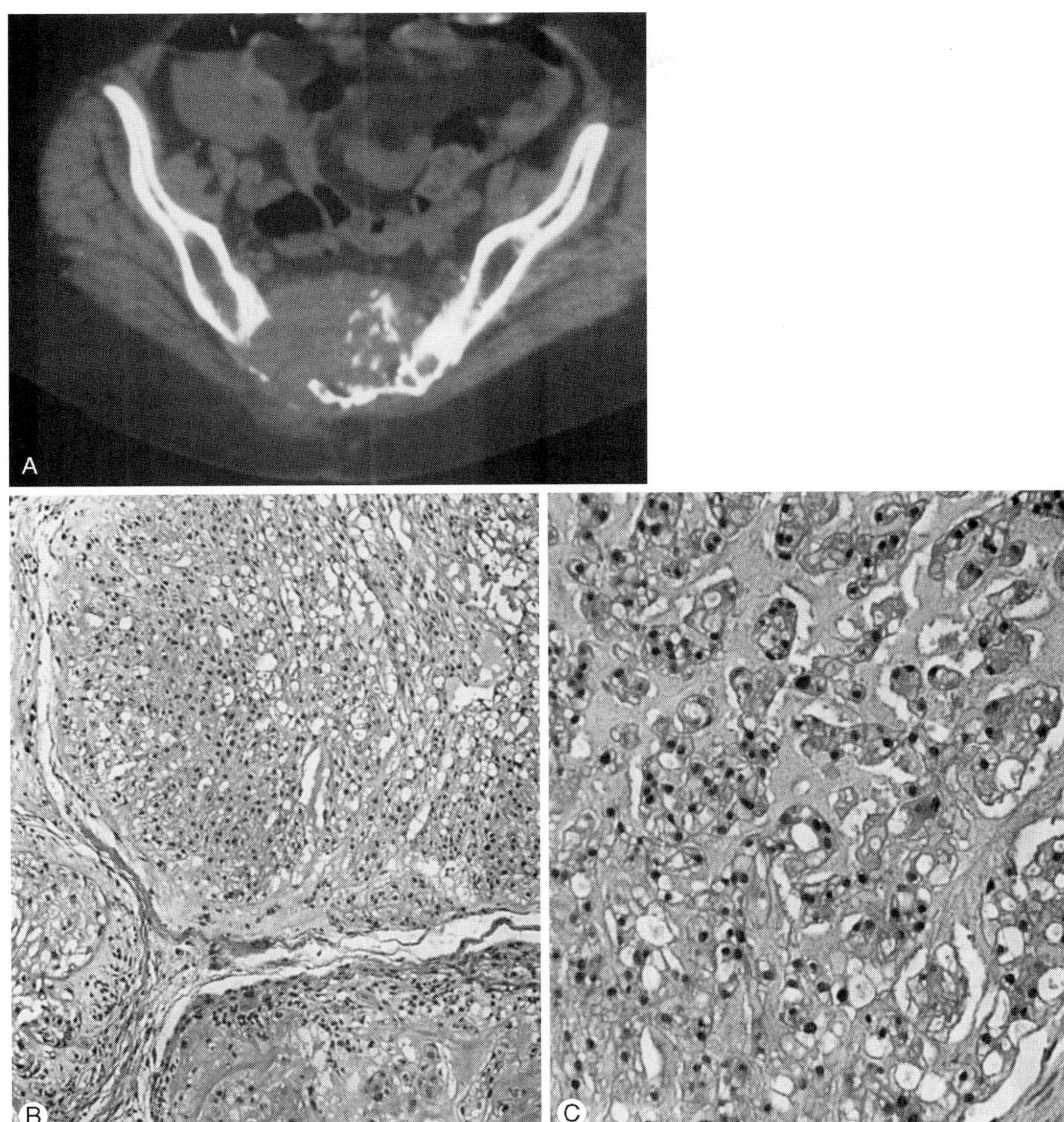

FIGURE 9–34 Chordoma of the sacrum. **A**, CT scan shows a destructive lesion in the sacrum. **B**, Low-power photomicrograph (× 100) shows a lobular arrangement of tissue. **C**, Higher-power photomicrograph (× 250) shows nests of physaliferous cells.

patients. The classic radiographic appearance is punched-out, lytic lesions (Fig. 9–38). The involved bone may show expansion and a "ballooned" appearance. Osteopenia may be the only finding. Histologically, the classic appearance is sheets of plasma cells that are monoclonal with immunostaining. Well-differentiated plasma cells have an eccentric nucleus and a peripherally clumped, chromatic "clock face" (Fig. 9–39). There is a perinuclear clear zone (halo) that represents the Golgi apparatus. In contrast, undifferentiated tumors lack some or all of these features, and the cells are anaplastic. The treatment of myeloma is with systemic therapy; surgical stabilization with irradiation is used for impending and complete fractures. Radiotherapy is also used for palliation of pain and treatment of neurologic symptoms. The prognosis is related to the stage of disease, with an overall median survival time of 18-24 months.

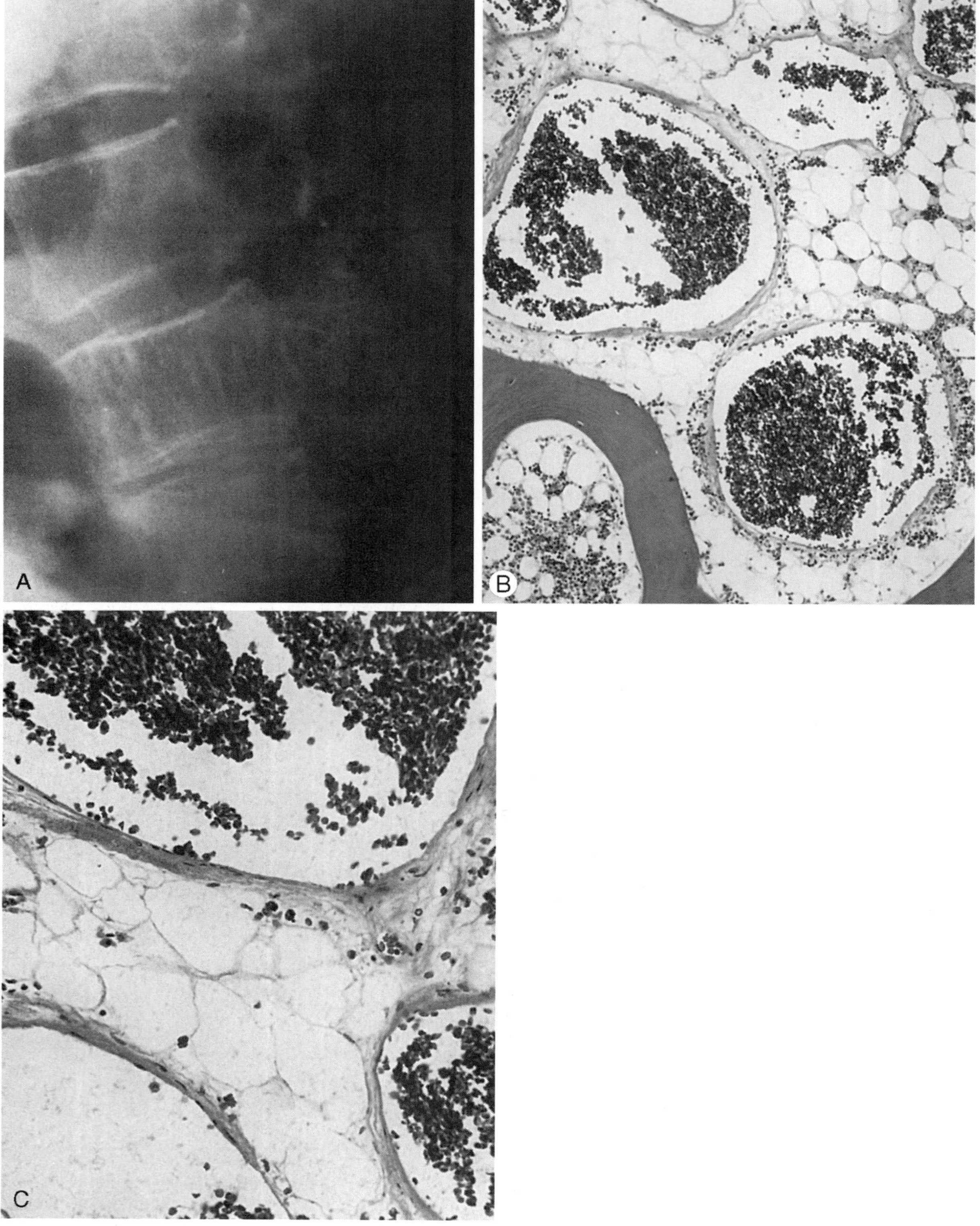

FIGURE 9–35 **A**, Hemangioma of the vertebra. **B**, Low-power photomicrograph shows dilated vascular spaces in the marrow (× 50). **C**, Higher-power photomicrograph (× 100) shows endothelium-lined spaces.

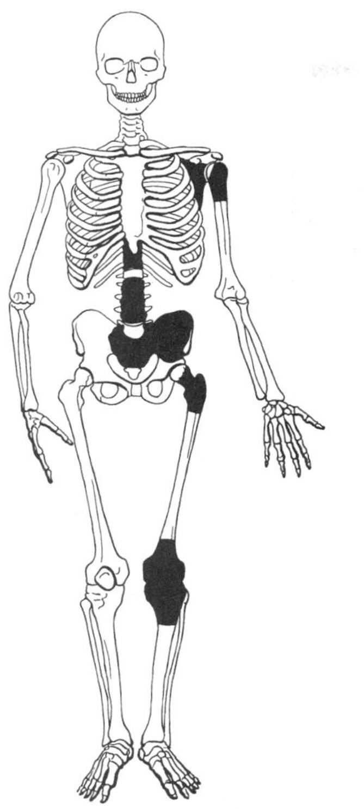

FIGURE 9–36 Skeletal distribution of the most common sites of lymphoma of the bone. The knee, pelvis, and vertebra are common sites. (From McCarthy EF, Frassica FJ: Pathology of Bone and Joint Disorders. Philadelphia, WB Saunders, 1998.)

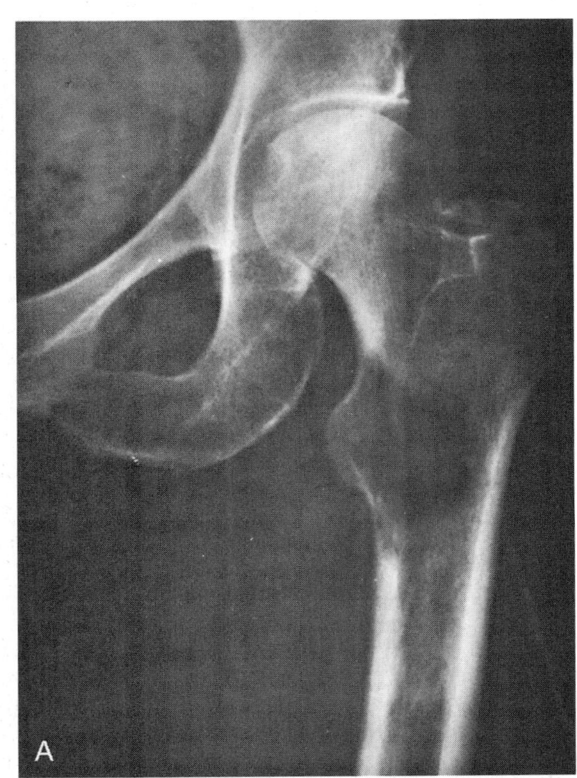

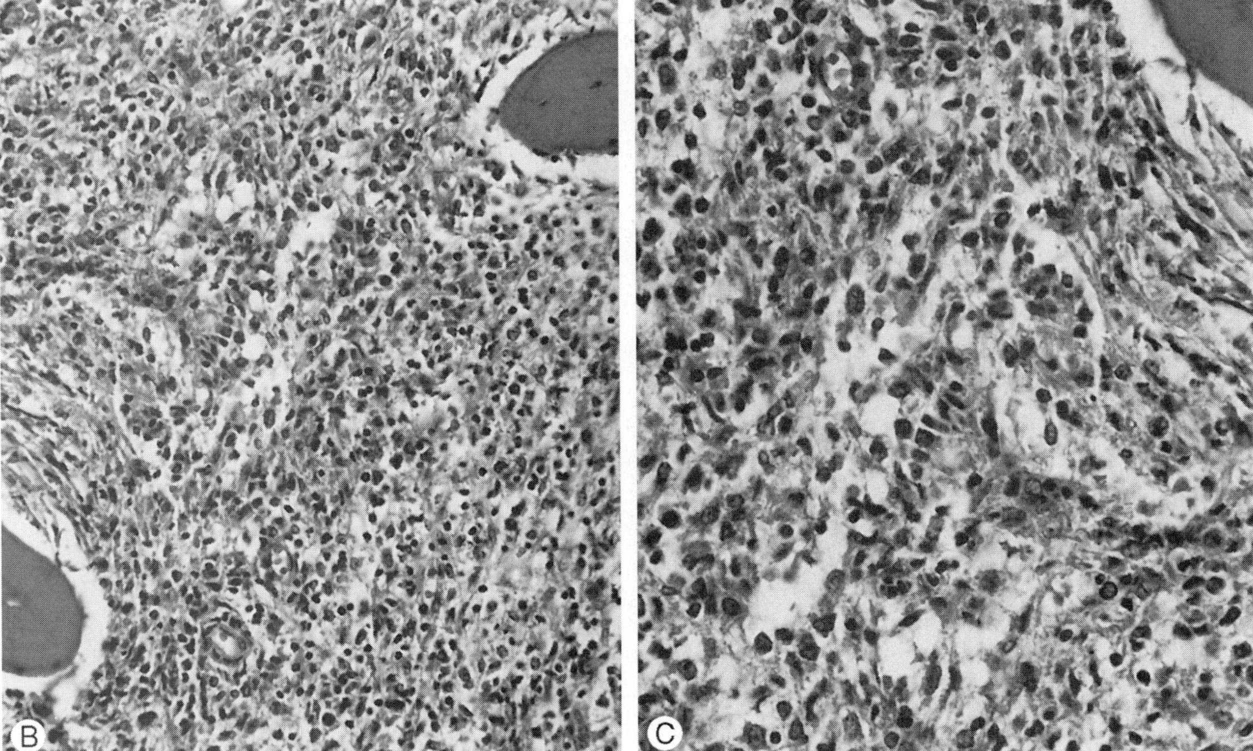

FIGURE 9–37 Lymphoma of bone. **A**, Radiograph shows a poorly circumscribed lytic lesion in the proximal femur and the ischium. **B**, Low-power photomicrograph (× 200) shows marrow replacement by a uniform population of lymphoid cells. **C**, Higher-power photomicrograph (× 400).

b. Solitary plasmacytoma of bone—It is important to differentiate solitary myeloma from multiple myeloma because of the more favorable prognosis in patients with the former. Diagnostic criteria include (1) a solitary lesion on skeletal survey, (2) histologic confirmation of plasmacytoma, and (3) bone marrow plasmacytosis of 10% or less. Patients with serum protein abnormalities and Bence Jones proteinuria of less than 1 g/24 hr at presentation are not excluded if they meet the aforementioned criteria. An MRI of the spine should be obtained because it is much more sensitive in detecting vertebral involvement. The radiographic and histologic features are the same as those for multiple myeloma. Treatment is with external beam irradiation to the lesion (4500-5000 cGy); when necessary, prophylactic internal fixation is performed. Approximately 50-75% of patients with solitary myeloma progress to multiple myeloma.

c. Osteosclerotic myeloma—This form of myeloma is a rare variant in which bone lesions are associated with a chronic inflammatory demyelinating polyneuropathy. The diagnosis of osteosclerotic myeloma is not generally made until the polyneuropathy is recognized and evaluated. Sensory symptoms (tingling, pins and needles, coldness) are noted first, followed by motor weakness. Both the sensory and motor changes begin distally, are symmetrical, and proceed

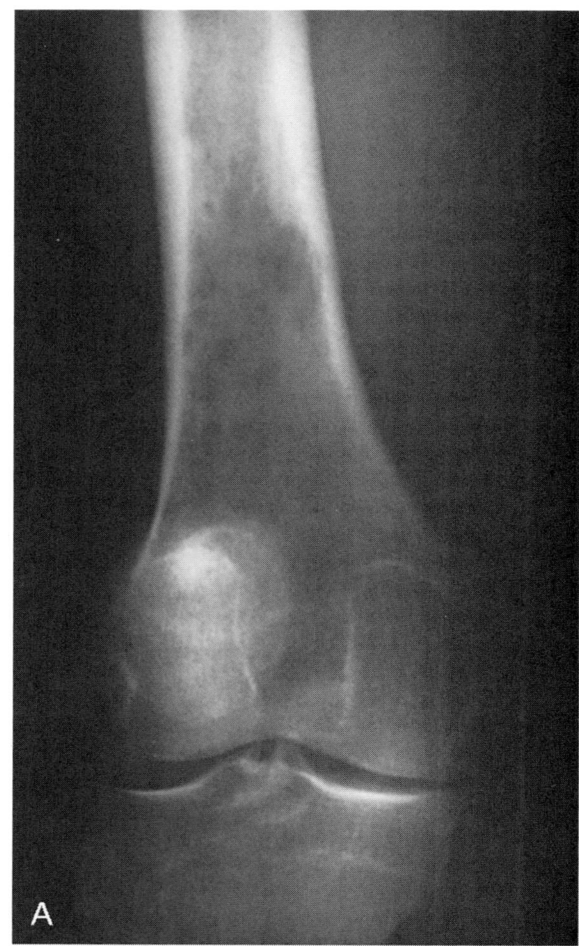

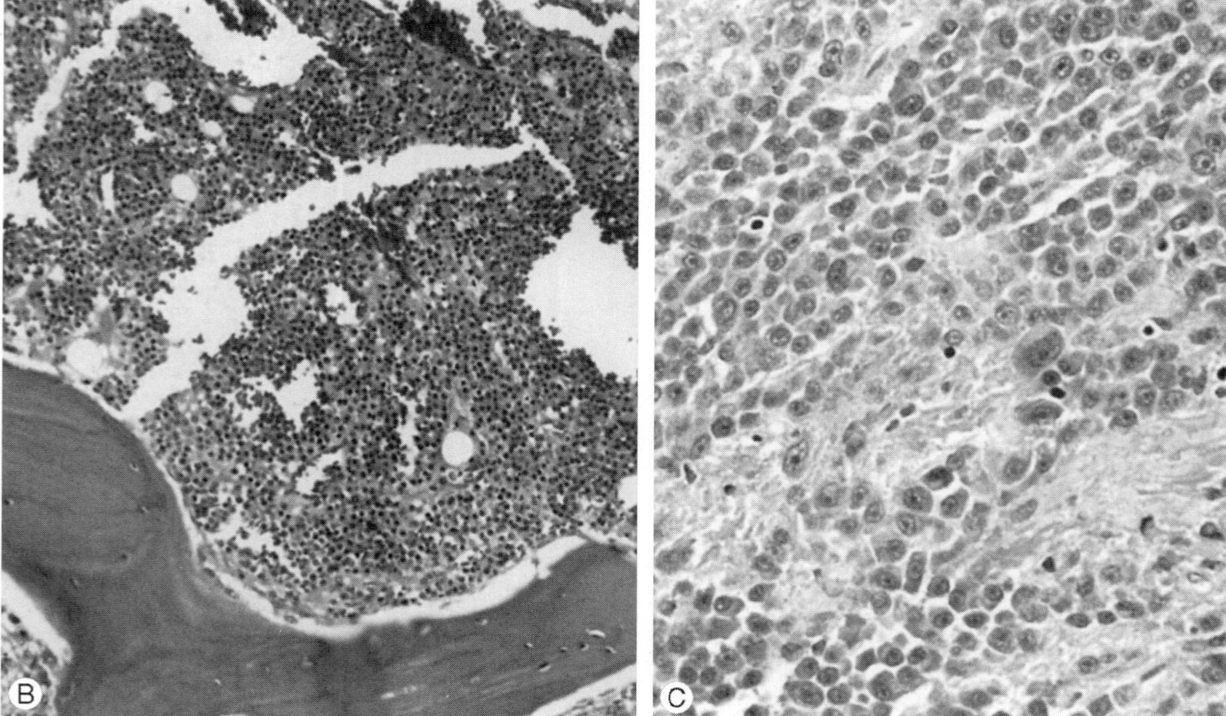

FIGURE 9–38 Multiple myeloma in the femur. **A**, Radiograph shows a poorly circumscribed lytic lesion in the distal femur. **B**, Low-power micrograph shows marrow replacement by a uniform population of cells. **C**, Higher-power photomicrograph (× 400) shows sheets of atypical plasma cells.

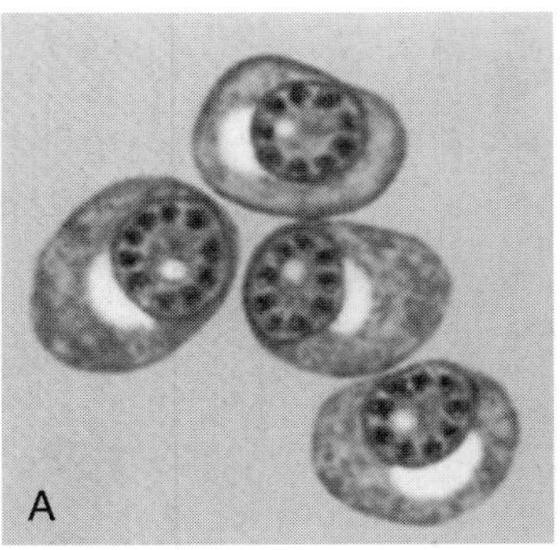

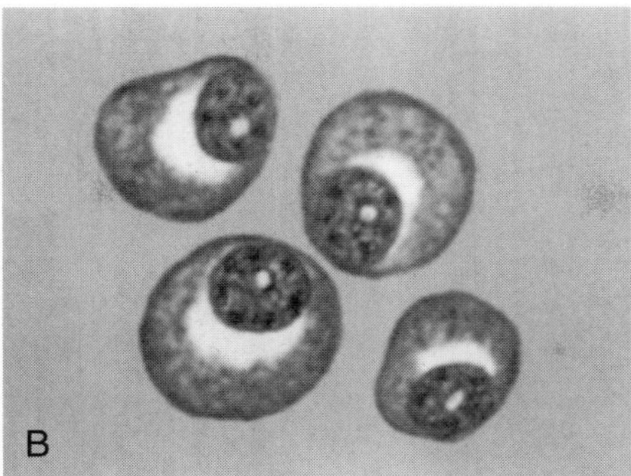

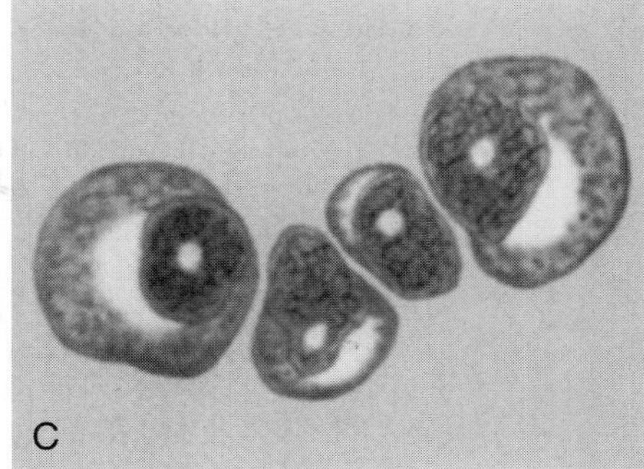

FIGURE 9–39 Myeloma cells. **A**, Plasma cells from a well-differentiated case of myeloma. They resemble the plasma cells seen in benign inflammatory cases. **B**, Plasma cells of intermediate maturity. **C**, Plasma cells that are immature and less well differentiated. (From Frassica FJ, Frassica DA, Sim FH: Myeloma of bone. In Stauffer, RN, ed: Advances in Operative Orthopaedics, vol 2, p 362. St. Louis, Mosby-Year Book, 1994.)

proximally. Severe weakness is common, but bone pain is not characteristic. Radiographic studies may show a spectrum from purely sclerotic to a mixed pattern of lysis and sclerosis. The lesions usually involve the spine, pelvic bones, and ribs; the extremities are generally spared. Patients may have abnormalities outside the nervous system and have a constellation of findings termed the POEMS syndrome (**p**olyneuropathy, **o**rganomegaly, **e**ndocrinopathy, **M**-protein, and **s**kin changes). Treatment is with a combination of chemotherapy, radiotherapy, and plasmapheresis. The neurologic changes may not improve with treatment.

I. Tumors of unknown origin—The three principal tumors of unknown origin are giant cell tumor, Ewing tumor, and adamantinoma.

1. Giant cell tumor
   a. Benign form—This distinctive neoplasm has poorly differentiated cells. The lesion is benign but aggressive. Further confusion results from the fact that this benign tumor may rarely (< 2% of the time) metastasize to the lungs (benign metastasizing giant cell tumor). The lesion is the most common in the epiphysis of long bones, and about 50% of lesions occur about the knee; the vertebra and sacrum are involved in about 10% of cases (Fig. 9–40). The sacrum is the most common axial location of giant cell tumors of bone. Unlike most bone tumors, which occur more often in males, giant cell tumors are more common in females. The lesion is uncommon in children with open physes. Multicentricity occurs in less than 1% of patients. Patients present with pain that is usually referable to the joint involved. Radiographs show a purely lytic destructive lesion in the metaphysis that extends into the epiphysis and often borders the subchondral bone (Fig. 9–41). Early in the symptomatic phase, the radiographs may appear normal; a small lytic focus is difficult to detect. The basic proliferating cell has a round to oval or even spindle-shaped nucleus. The giant cells appear to have the same nuclei as the proliferating mononuclear cells. Mitotic figures may be numerous. Giant cell tumors may undergo a number of secondary degenerative changes, such as aneurysmal bone cyst formation, necrosis, fibrous repair, foam cell formation, and reactive new bone (Fig. 9–42). Treatment is aimed at removing the lesion, with preservation of the involved joint. Extensive exteriorization (removal of a large cortical window over the lesion), curettage with hand and power instruments, and chemical cauterization with phenol are performed. The resulting large defect is usually reconstructed with subchondral bone grafts and methylmethacrylate. Local control with this treatment regimen has a success rate of 85-90%.
   b. Malignant form—Malignancy may occur in two forms in giant cell tumor: primary and secondary malignant giant cell tumors. In primary malignant giant cell tumor of bone, there is a coexisting, benign giant cell tumor and high-grade sarcoma (occurs in about 1% of giant cell tumors). Secondary malignant giant cell tumor occurs after radiation to treat a giant cell tumor or after multiple local recurrences. The most common scenario is that a patient has a large, aggressive, inoperable giant cell tumor. The patient then receives irradiation, and a sarcoma (osteosarcoma, fibrosarcoma, or malignant fibrous histiocytoma) develops in the irradiated field 3-50 years after the irradiation (called the latency period). A small number of patients may develop a high-grade sarcoma after multiple local recurrences in the absence of prior radiotherapy.
2. Ewing tumor
   a. Diagnosis—This distinctive small round cell sarcoma occurs most often in children and young adults; most children are older than 5 years. When a small blue cell tumor is found in a child younger than 5 years, metastatic neuroblastoma and leukemia should be excluded. In patients older than 30 years

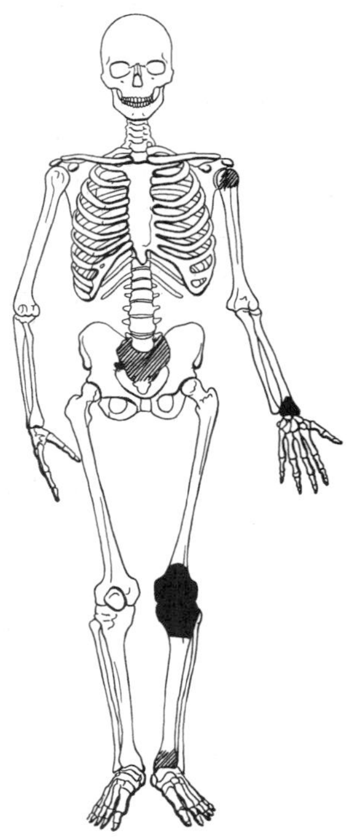

FIGURE 9–40 Skeletal distribution of the most common sites of giant cell tumor of the bone, which are the knee, distal radius, and proximal humerus. (From McCarthy EF, Frassica FJ: Pathology of Bone and Joint Disorders. Philadelphia, WB Saunders, 1998.)

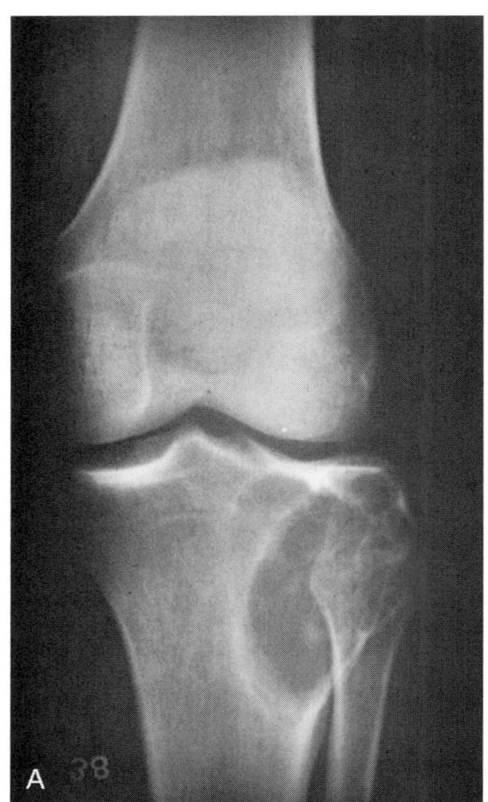

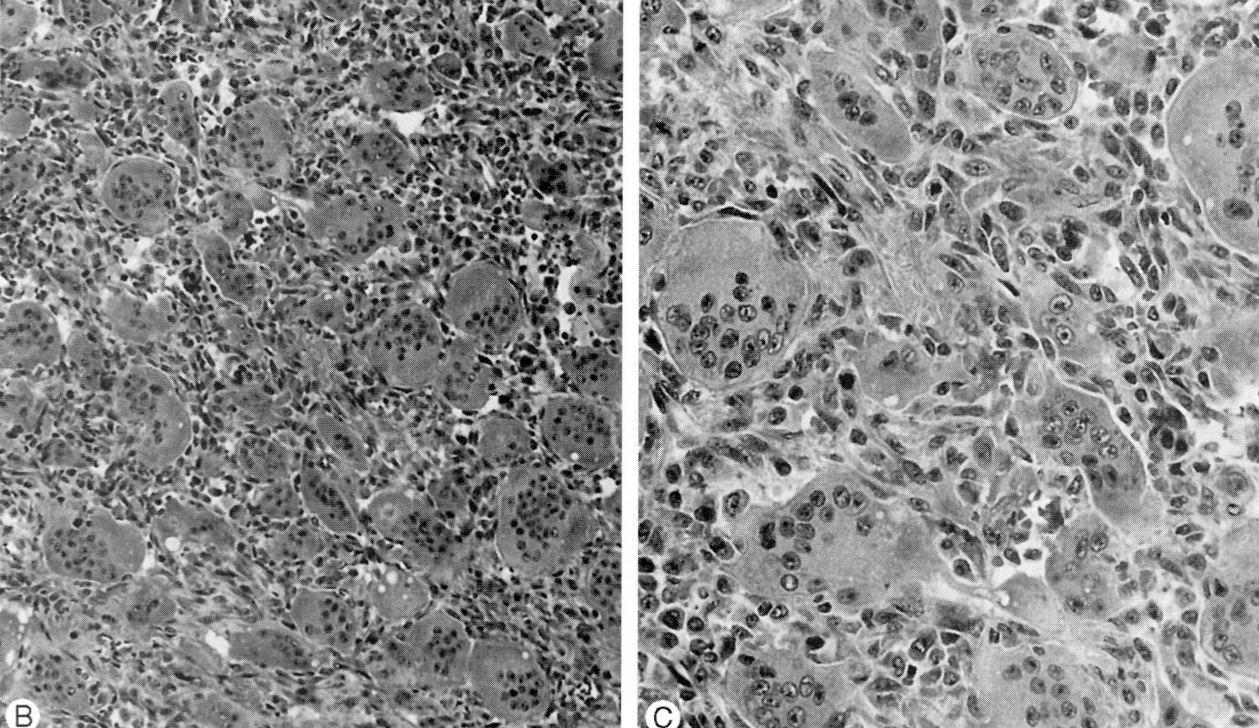

FIGURE 9–41 Giant cell tumor of the proximal tibia. **A**, Radiograph shows a well-circumscribed lytic lesion in the proximal tibia involving both the epiphysis and the metaphysis. **B**, Low-power photomicrograph (× 160) shows sheets of multinucleated giant cells. **C**, Higher-power photomicrograph (× 300).

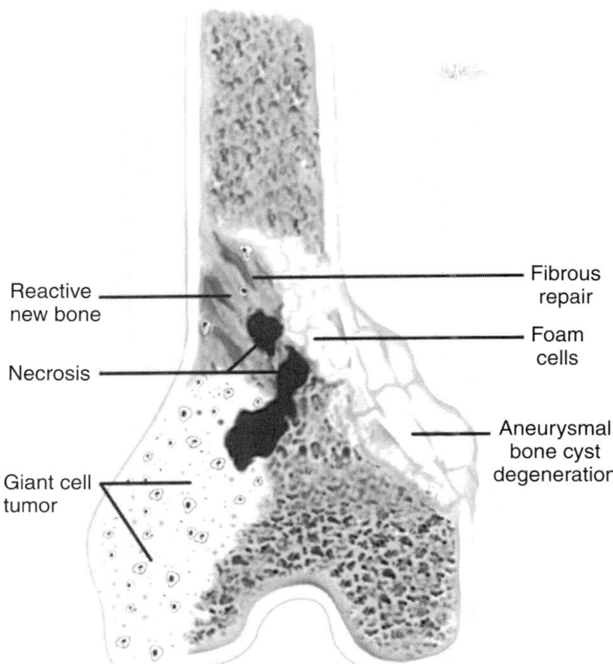

FIGURE 9–42 The secondary changes seen in giant cell tumor of the bone. This tumor may undergo many secondary changes, including aneurysmal bone cyst formation, in which the tumor causes marked expansion of the bone with resulting ballooning out of the cortex. Necrosis and cyst formation are also common. Fibrous repair, reactive new bone, and foam cells may often be found. (From McCarthy EF, Frassica FJ: Pathology of Bone and Joint Disorders. Philadelphia, WB Saunders, 1998.)

of age, metastatic carcinoma must be excluded. The most common locations include the pelvis, distal femur, proximal tibia, femoral diaphysis, and proximal humerus (Fig. 9–43). Patients generally present with pain, and fever may be present. Laboratory tests may show an elevated erythrocyte sedimentation rate, leukocytosis, anemia, and an elevated white blood cell count. Radiographs often show a large destructive lesion that involves the metaphysis and diaphysis; the lesion may be purely lytic or have variable amounts of reactive new bone formation (Fig. 9–44). The periosteum may be lifted off in multiple layers, giving a characteristic but uncommon onionskin appearance. There is often a large soft tissue component.

b. Treatment—Treatment involves a multimodality approach with multiagent chemotherapy, irradiation, and surgical resection. Most lesions have traditionally been treated with chemotherapy and irradiation, but the role of surgery is evolving. In some centers chemotherapy and surgery are the major forms of treatment, whereas in others traditional chemotherapy and external beam irradiation are preferred. The major benefits of wide surgical resection are a decrease in the risk of local recurrence and the avoidance of the potential for postirradiation sarcoma.

c. Survival—Long-term survival with multimodality treatment may be as high as 60-70%. There is a consistent chromosomal translocation (11:22) with the formation of a fusion protein (EWS-FLI 1). Poor prognostic factors include (1) spine and pelvic tumors, (2) tumors greater than 100 cm^3, (3) a poor response to chemotherapy (less than 90% necrosis), and (4) elevated lactic dehydrogenase levels (Temple). The *P53* mutation and gene fusion products other than EWS-FLI 1 are also poor prognostic factors.

3. Adamantinoma—This rare tumor of long bones contains epithelium-like islands of cells. The tibia is the most common site, although other long bones are infrequently involved (fibula, femur, ulna, radius) (Fig. 9–45). Most patients are young adults and present with pain over months to years. The typical radiographic appearance is that of multiple sharply circumscribed, lucent defects of different sizes, with sclerotic bone interspersed between the zones and extending above and below the lucent zones (Fig. 9–46). Typically, one of the lesions in the midshaft is the largest and is associated with cortical bone destruction. Histologically, the cells have an epithelial quality and are

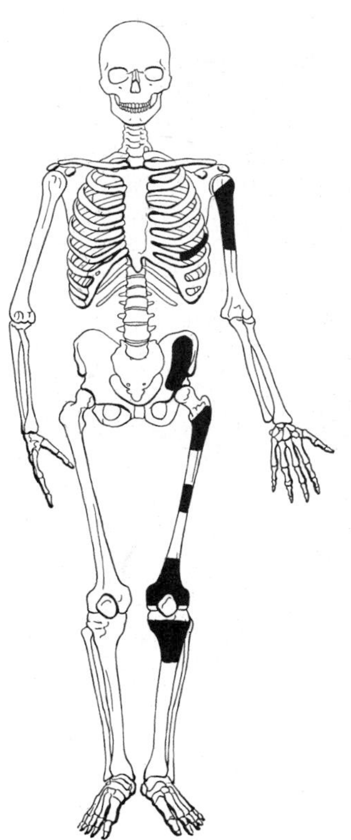

FIGURE 9–43 Skeletal distribution of the most common sites of Ewing tumor of the bone. The femur, pelvis, ribs, and humerus are common sites. (From McCarthy EF, Frassica FJ: Pathology of Bone and Joint Disorders. Philadelphia, WB Saunders, 1998.)

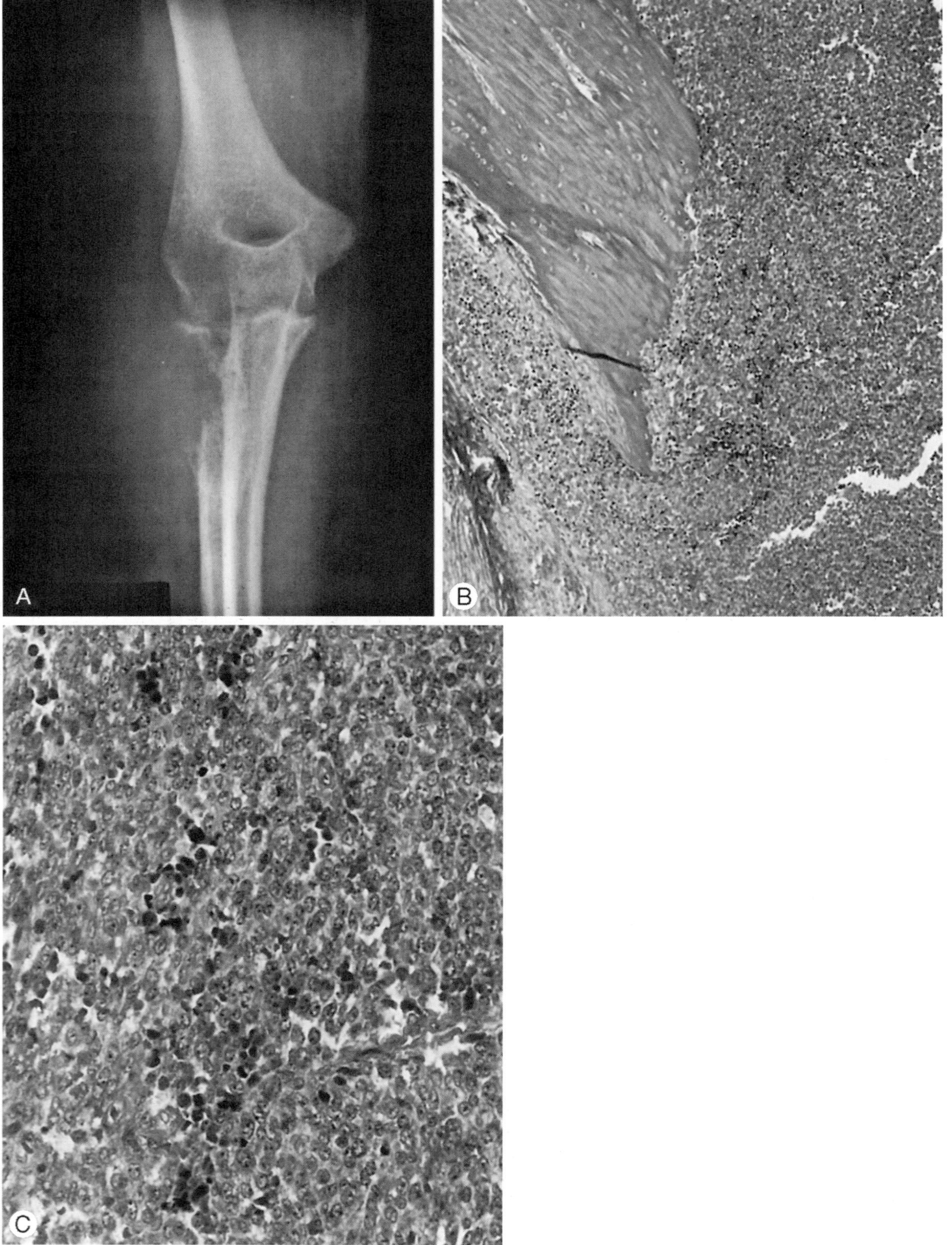

FIGURE 9–44 Ewing sarcoma of the proximal radius. **A**, Radiograph shows a destructive expansile lesion in the proximal radius. **B**, Low-power photomicrograph (× 100) shows bone surrounded by a highly cellular neoplasm. **C**, Higher-power photomicrograph (× 400) shows sheets of rounded cells.

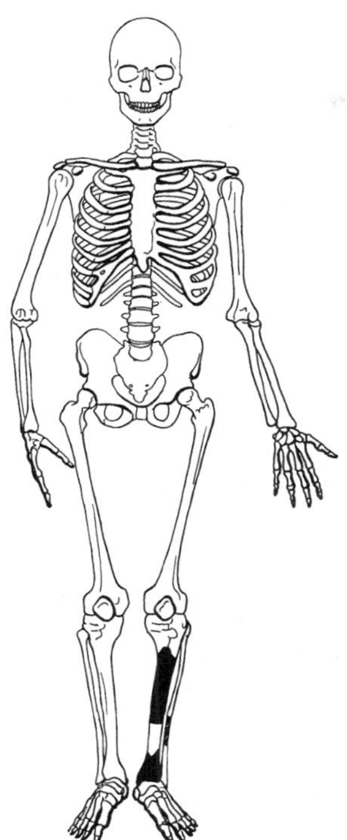

FIGURE 9–45 Skeletal distribution of the most common sites of adamantinoma. This peculiar tumor most often affects the tibia. (From McCarthy EF, Frassica FJ: Pathology of Bone and Joint Disorders, Philadelphia, WB Saunders, 1998.)

arranged in a palisading or glandular pattern; the epithelial cells occur in a fibrous stroma. The treatment of this low-grade, malignant lesion is by wide-margin surgical resection. The lesion may metastasize either early or after multiple failed attempts at local control.

J. Tumor-like conditions—There are many lesions that simulate primary bone tumors and must be considered in the differential diagnosis (Box 9–4). These lesions range from metastases to reactive conditions.

1. Aneurysmal bone cyst—This non-neoplastic reactive condition may be aggressive in its ability to destroy normal bone and extend into the soft tissues. The lesion may arise primarily in bone or be found in association with other tumors, such as giant cell tumor, chondroblastoma, chondromyxoid fibroma, and fibrous dysplasia. It may also occur within a malignant tumor. Three fourths of the patients with an aneurysmal bone cyst are less than 20 years of age. Patients experience pain and swelling, which may have been present for months or years. The characteristic radiographic finding is an eccentric, lytic, expansile area of bone destruction in the metaphysis; in classic cases there is a thin rim of periosteal new bone surrounding the lesion (Fig. 9–47). The plain radiograph may demonstrate the periosteal bone if it is mineralized, and the MRI scan usually shows the periosteal layer going all around the lesion. Fluid-fluid levels present on T2-weighted MRI scans are characteristic of aneurysmal bone cysts. The essential histologic features are cavernous blood-filled spaces without an endothelial lining. There are thin strands of bone present in the fibrous tissue of the septa. Benign giant cells may be numerous. Treatment is with careful curettage and bone grafting. Local recurrence is common in children with open physes.
2. Unicameral bone cyst—This lesion occurs most often in the proximal humerus and is characterized by symmetrical cystic expansion with thinning of the involved cortices; other common sites are the proximal femur and distal tibia. The cause is unknown, but it probably results from some disturbance of the physis. Patients generally present with pain, usually after a fracture due to minor trauma (e.g., sporting event, throwing a baseball, wrestling). The radiographic picture is characteristic, with a central lytic area and symmetrical thinning of the cortices (Fig. 9–48). The bone is often expanded; however, the bone is generally no wider than the physis. The lesion often appears trabeculated. When the cyst abuts the physeal plate, the process is called *active*; when there is normal bone intervening, the cyst is termed *latent*. Histologically, the cyst has a thin fibrous lining containing fibrous tissue, giant cells, hemosiderin pigment, and a few chronic inflammatory cells. The treatment of unicameral bone cysts begins with aspiration to confirm the diagnosis, followed by methylprednisolone acetate injection. Curettage and bone grafting are reserved for recalcitrant lesions in the proximal humerus. Unicameral bone cysts of the proximal femur are often treated with curettage, grafting, and internal fixation to avoid fracture. A fracture of the proximal femur may result in avascular necrosis of the femoral head and severe disability.
3. Histiocytosis X (LCH)—Lichtenstein originally divided this disorder into three entities: eosinophilic granuloma (monostotic bone disease), Hand-Schüller-Christian disease (multiple bone lesions and visceral disease), and Letterer-Siwe disease (a fulminating condition in young children). This condition is now usually referred to as LCH. The cellular abnormality is a proliferation of the Langerhans cells of the dendritic system. Eosinophilic granuloma of bone is analogous to monostotic LCH, while Hand-Schüller-Christian disease could be called polyostotic LCH with visceral involvement.
   a. Diagnosis—Eosinophilic granuloma of bone is the most common manifestation, in which only a single bone or occasionally multiple bones are involved. Patients present with pain and swelling. The radiographs often show a highly destructive lesion with well-defined margins (Fig. 9–49). The cortex may be destroyed by a periosteal

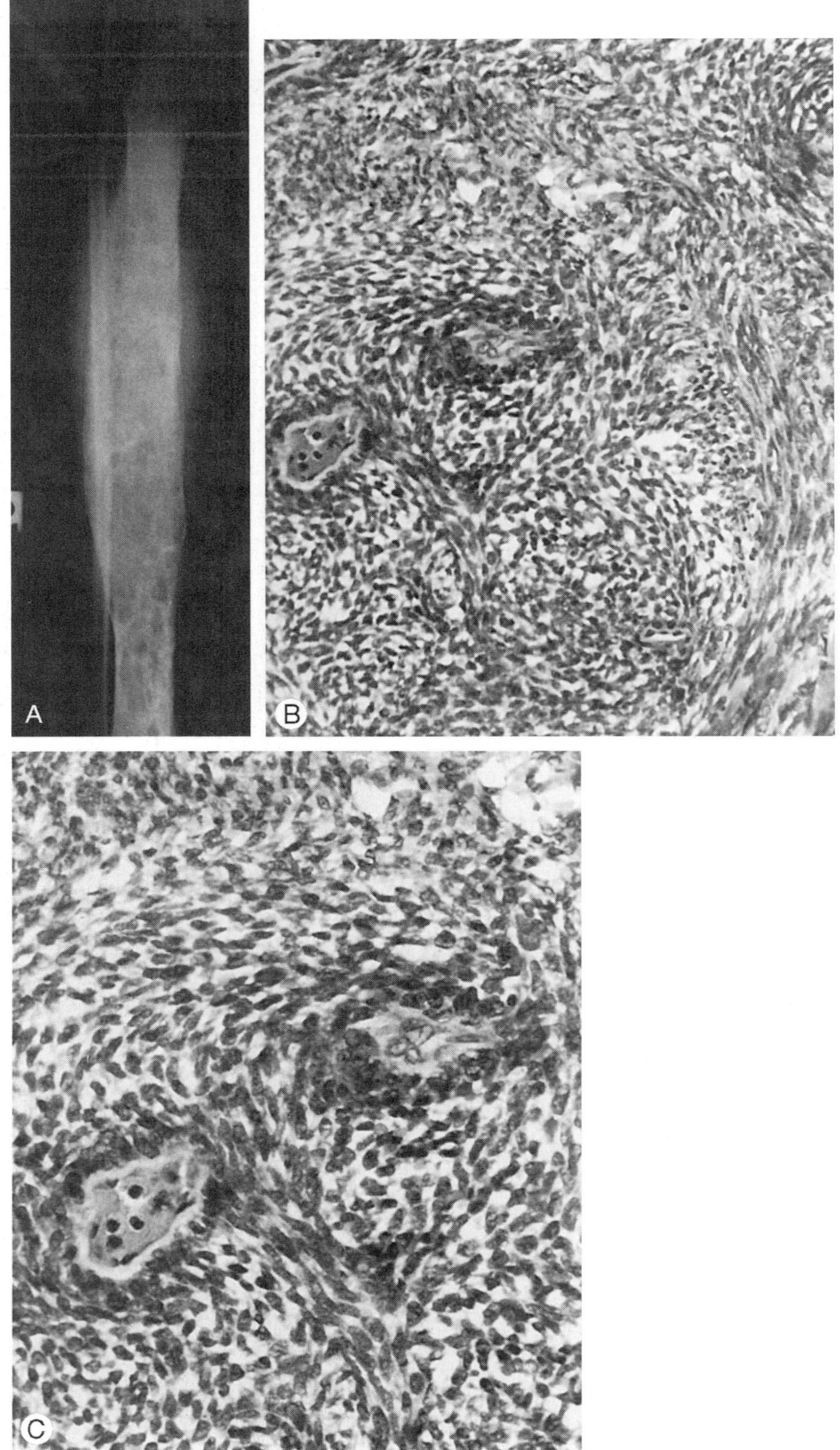

FIGURE 9–46 Adamantinoma of the tibia. **A**, Radiograph shows a bubbly, symmetrical lytic lesion in the tibial diaphysis. **B**, Low-power photomicrograph (× 250) shows biphasic differentiation, with spindle cells and epithelioid cells. **C**, Higher-power photomicrograph (× 400).

Box 9–4 Tumor-like Conditions (Tumor Simulators)

YOUNG PATIENT

Eosinophilic granuloma
Osteomyelitis
Avulsion fractures
Aneurysmal bone cyst
Fibrous dysplasia
Osteofibrous dysplasia
Heterotopic ossification
Unicameral bone cyst
Giant cell reparative granuloma
Exuberant callus

ADULT

Synovial chondromatosis
Pigmented villonodular synovitis
Stress fracture
Heterotopic ossification
Ganglionic cyst

OLDER ADULT

Mastocytosis
Hyperparathyroidism
Paget disease
Bone infarcts
Bone islands
Ganglionic cyst
Cyst secondary to joint disease
Epidermoid cyst

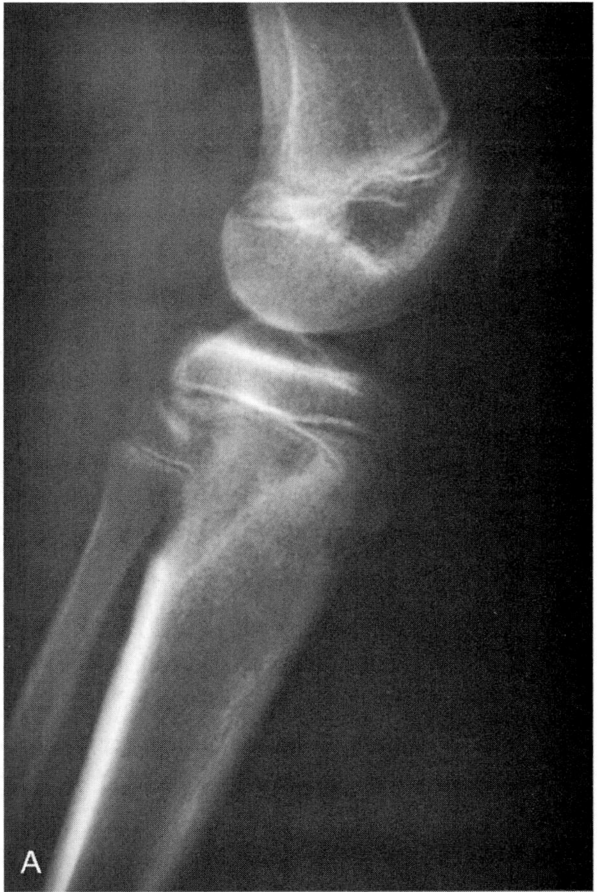

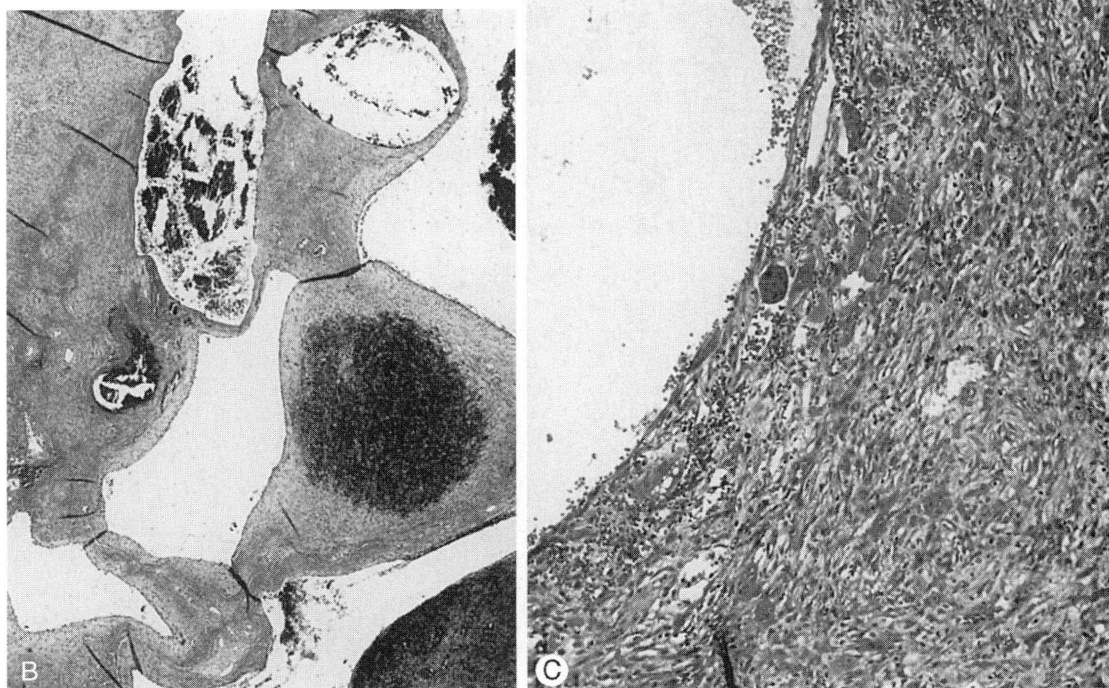

FIGURE 9–47 Aneurysmal bone cyst of the proximal tibia. **A**, Radiograph shows a well-defined lytic lesion in the posterior tibial metaphysis. **B**, Low-power photomicrograph (× 25) shows blood-filled lakes. **C**, Higher-power photomicrograph (× 50) shows the wall of the cyst, with fibroblasts and occasional multinucleated giant cells.

reaction, and there may be a soft tissue mass simulating a malignant bone tumor. There is a different amount of bone destruction of the involved cortices, resulting in the appearance of a bone within a bone. There may be expansion of the involved bone. Any bone may be involved. Histologically, the proliferating Langerhans cell, with an indented or grooved nucleus, is the characteristic cell. The cytoplasm is eosinophilic, and the nuclear membrane has a crisp border. Mitotic figures may be common. Bilobed eosinophils with bright, granular, eosinophilic cytoplasm are present in large numbers.

b. Treatment—Eosinophilic granuloma is a self-limiting process, and several forms of treatment have been successful, including corticosteroid injection, low-dose irradiation (600-800 cGy), curettage and bone grafting, and observation. When the articular surface is in jeopardy or an impending fracture is a possibility, concomitant curettage and bone grafting is a logical choice. Low-dose irradiation is effective for most lesions that cannot be injected and is associated with low morbidity. Hand-Schüller-Christian disease is characterized by both bone lesions and visceral involvement; the classic triad,

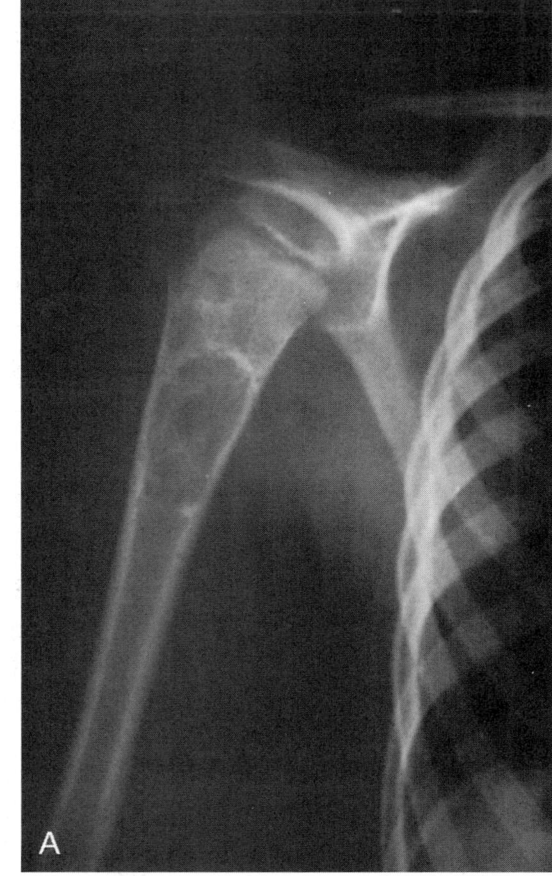

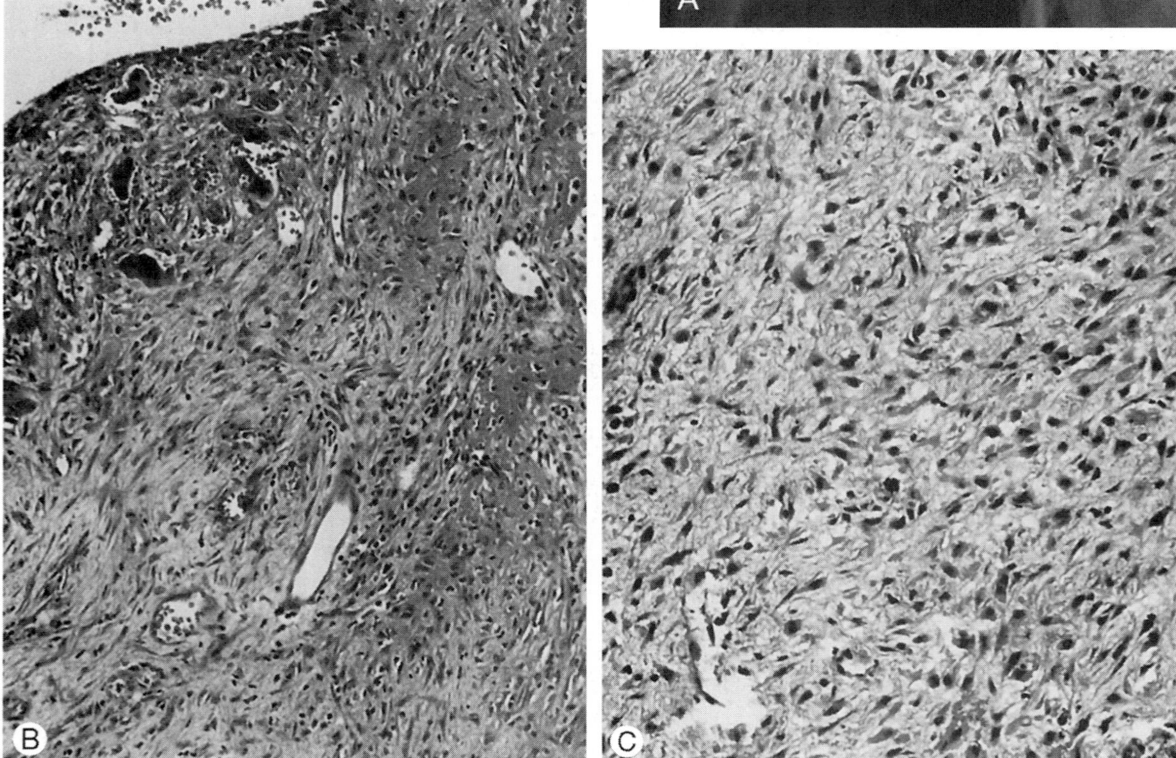

FIGURE 9–48 Unicameral bone cyst of the humerus. **A**, Radiograph shows a symmetrical, midline, well-circumscribed lytic lesion in the humeral metaphysis. **B**, Low-power photomicrograph (× 160) shows the fibrous tissue membrane, with reactive bone and occasional multinucleated giant cells. **C**, High-power field shows a uniform population of spindle cells without nuclear atypia.

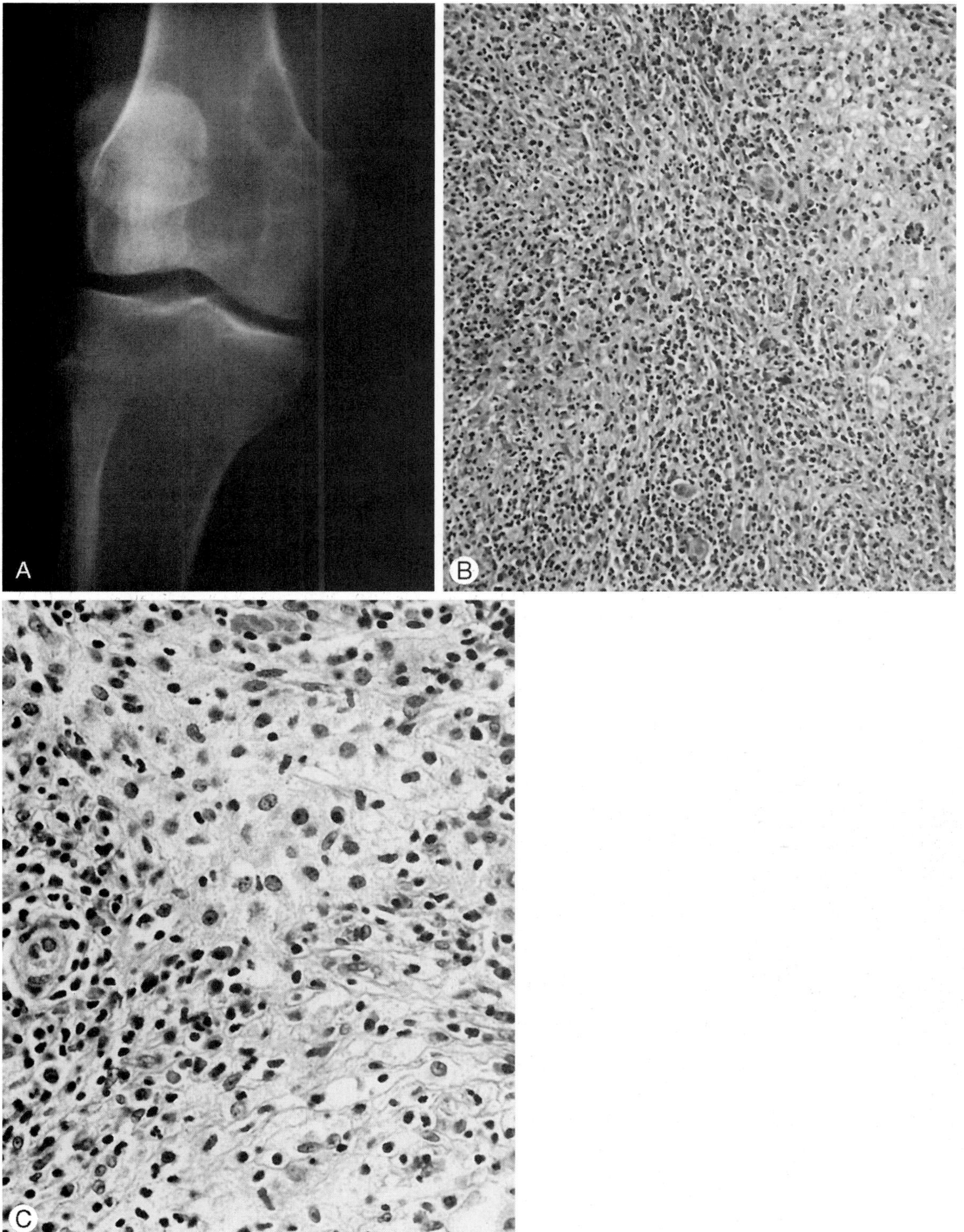

FIGURE 9–49 Eosinophilic granuloma of the distal femur. **A**, Radiograph shows a well-circumscribed lesion with a sclerotic rim in the femoral metaphysis. **B**, Low-power photomicrograph (× 160) shows a heterogeneous population of inflammatory cells, with an aggregation of histiocytes. **C**, Higher-power photomicrograph (× 400) shows nests of Langerhans histiocytes.

which occurs in fewer than one fourth of patients, includes exophthalmos, diabetes insipidus, and lytic skull lesions. Letterer-Siwe disease occurs in young children and is usually fatal.

4. Fibrous dysplasia—This developmental abnormality of bone is characterized by monostotic or polyostotic involvement. Yellow or brown patches of skin may accompany the bone lesions. There is a failure of the production of normal lamellar bone. The genetic mutation is an activating mutation of the GS alpha surface protein, resulting in increased production of **cyclic adenosine monophosphate** (cAMP). When endocrine abnormalities (especially precocious puberty) accompany multiple bone lesions and skin abnormalities, the condition is called McCune-Albright syndrome. Virtually any bone may be involved, with the proximal femur being the most common. Radiographs may show a variable appearance (looks highly lytic or like ground glass) (Fig. 9–50). There is often a well-defined rim of sclerotic bone around the lesion. The major histologic feature is proliferation of fibroblasts, which produces a dense collagenous matrix. There are often trabeculae of osteoid and bone within the fibrous stroma. Cartilage may be present in variable amounts. The bone fragments are present in a disorganized fashion and have been likened to "alphabet soup" and "Chinese letters." The treatment of fibrous dysplasia is predicated on the presence of symptoms and the risk of fracture. Internal fixation and bone grafting are used in areas of high stress where nonoperative treatment would not be effective; most patients do not need surgical treatment. Autogenous cancellous bone grafting is never used because the transplanted bone is quickly transformed into the woven bone of fibrous dysplasia. Cortical or cancellous allografts are usually used. Diphosphonate therapy has been shown to be effective in decreasing pain and reducing bone turnover in patients with polyostotic fibrous dysplasia.
5. Osteofibrous dysplasia—This uncommon entity primarily involves the tibia and is usually confined to the anterior tibial cortex. Bowing is very common, and children may develop pathologic fractures. The lesion typically presents in children younger than age 10. This diagnosis can be made radiographically. In general, biopsy is not necessary. When it is performed, the biopsy shows fibrous tissue stroma and a background of bone trabeculae with osteoblastic rimming. Nonoperative treatment is preferred until the child reaches maturity. These lesions usually regress and do not cause problems in adults.
6. Paget disease—This condition is characterized by abnormal bone remodeling. The disease is usually diagnosed during the fifth decade of life. The process may be monostotic or polyostotic. Radiographs demonstrate coarsened trabeculae and remodeled cortices. The coarsened trabeculae give the bone a blastic appearance. Histologically, the characteristic features are irregular, broad trabeculae; reversal or cement lines; osteoclastic activity; and fibrous vascular tissue between the trabeculae. Patients usually present with pain. Medical treatment of Paget disease is aimed at retarding the activity of the osteoclasts; the agents used include diphosphonates and calcitonin. The older diphosphonates (e.g., etidronate [Didronel]) stopped both osteoclastic activity and new bone formation; etidronate may cause osteomalacia and cannot be used for more than 6 months. Pamidronate, which can be used only intravenously, does not inhibit bone formation and has become one of the most useful agents in the diphosphonate class of medications. Oral agents may also be used. Patients may present with degenerative joint disease, fracture, or neurologic encroachment; joint degeneration is common in the hip and knee. Prior to replacement, arthroplasty patients should be treated with diphosphonates to decrease bleeding at the time of surgery. Less than 1% of patients with Paget disease develop malignant degeneration with the formation of a sarcoma within a focus of Paget disease. The symptoms of a Paget sarcoma are the abrupt onset of pain and swelling. The radiographs usually demonstrate cortical bone destruction and the presence of a soft tissue mass. Paget sarcomas are deadly tumors with a poor prognosis (long-term survival is < 20%).
7. Metastatic bone disease—This disease is the most common entity that destroys the skeleton in older patients. When a destructive bone lesion is found in a patient over age 40, metastases must be considered first. The five carcinomas that are most likely to metastasize to bone are those of the breast, lung, prostate, kidney, and thyroid. The most common locations are the pelvis, vertebral bodies, ribs, and proximal limb girdles. The pathogenesis of skeletal metastases is probably related to the Batson vertebral vein plexus. The venous flow from the breast, lung, prostate, kidney, and thyroid drains into the vertebral vein plexus (Fig. 9–51). The plexus has intimate connections to the vertebral bodies, pelvis, skull, and proximal limb girdles. Radiographs usually demonstrate a destructive lesion that may be purely lytic, a mixed pattern of bone destruction and formation, or a purely sclerotic lesion (Fig. 9–52). The histologic hallmark is the appearance of epithelial cells in a fibrous stroma; the epithelial cells are often arranged in a glandular pattern. Interestingly, the bone destruction is caused not by the tumor cells themselves but by activation of osteoclasts

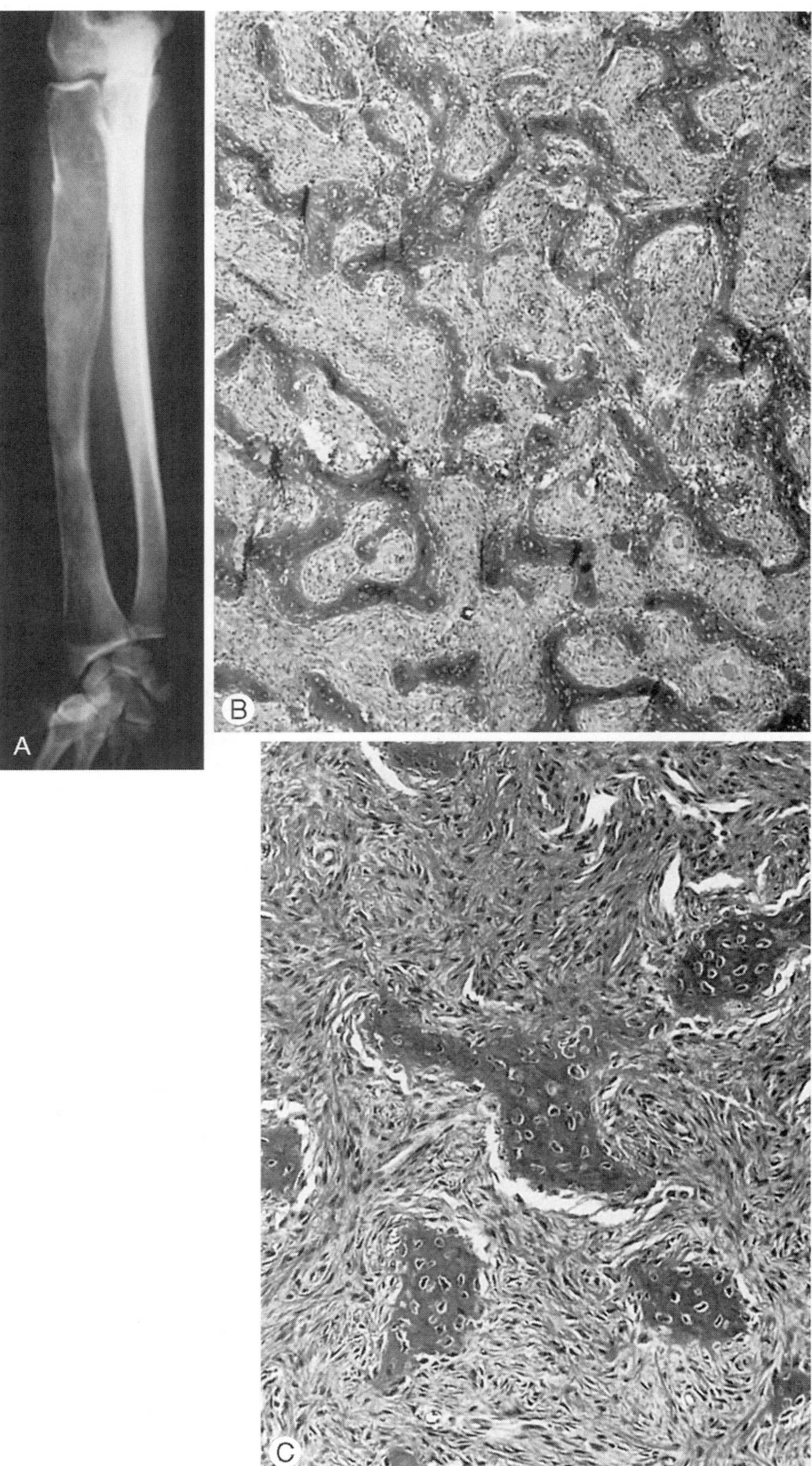

FIGURE 9–50 Fibrous dysplasia of the radius. **A**, Radiograph shows a long, symmetrical, ground-glass lytic lesion of the radius. **B**, Low-power photomicrograph (× 50) shows seams of osteoid in a fibrous background. **C**, Higher-power photomicrograph (× 160) shows osteoid surrounded by bland fibrous tissue.

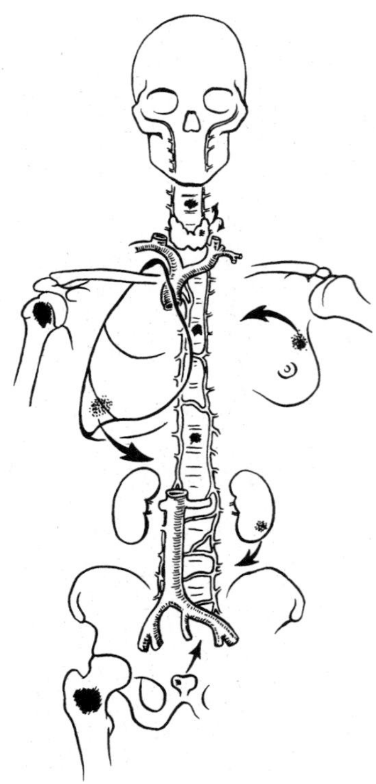

FIGURE 9–51 Batson venous plexus. This plexus is longitudinal and valveless and extends from the sacrum to the skull. The breast, lung, kidney, prostate, and thyroid glands connect to this system. Tumor cells can enter this system and spread to the vertebrae, ribs, pelvis, and proximal limb girdle. (From McCarthy EF, Frassica FJ: Pathology of Bone and Joint Disorders. Philadelphia, WB Saunders, 1998.)

(Fig. 9–53). In breast carcinoma, the tumor cells secrete parathyroid hormone–related peptide (PTHrP), which stimulates the release of the RANKL (receptor activator for nuclear factor κ B ligand) from the osteoblasts and marrow stromal cells. The RANKL attaches to the RANK receptor on the osteoclast precursor cells. In the presence of macrophage colony–stimulating factor, the osteoclast precursor cells differentiate into active osteoclasts that resorb the trabecular and cortical bone. With bone resorption, transforming growth factor–β, insulin-like growth factor–1, and calcium are released, and these factors stimulate the tumor cells to multiply and release more PTHrP. Guise has termed this process as the "vicious cycle" of metastatic bone disease. To combat the osteoclastic bone destruction, many patients are now treated with antiresorptive agents (diphosphonates) such as intravenous pamidronate and zoledronic acid. The treatment of metastatic bone disease is aimed at controlling pain and maintaining the independence of the patient. Prophylactic internal fixation is performed when impending fracture is deemed likely. There are many suggested criteria for fixation. The following conditions put the patient most at risk for fracture:

- More than 50% destruction of the diaphyseal cortices
- Permeative destruction of the subtrochanteric femoral region
- More than 50-75% destruction of the metaphysis
- Persistent pain after irradiation
- Weight-bearing pain (especially lower extremity pain with every footstep)

Patients older than age 40 with a single destructive bone lesion but without a known primary tumor must still be considered to have metastatic disease. Simon outlined a diagnostic strategy that identifies the primary lesion in up to 80-90% of patients (Box 9–5).

8. Osteomyelitis—Bone infections often simulate primary tumors. Occult infections may occur in all age groups. Patients may present with fever, chills, and/or bone pain. However, patients usually present with bone pain without systemic symptoms. The radiographs may be nonspecific. Bone destruction and formation are usually the characteristic findings of chronic infections; acute infections often produce cortical bone destruction and periosteal elevation. Serpiginous tracts and irregular areas of bone destruction suggest infection rather than neoplasm. Histologically, the lesion is usually apparent with (1) edema of the granulation tissue; (2) numerous new blood vessels; and (3) a mixed cell population of inflammatory cells, plasma cells, polymorphonuclear leukocytes, eosinophils, lymphocytes, and histiocytes. A chronic infection with long-standing wound drainage is occasionally complicated by a squamous cell carcinoma. One should always biopsy material that has been sent for culture and culture material that has been sent for biopsy. The treatment of osteomyelitis is removal of all dead tissue and appropriate antibiotic therapy.

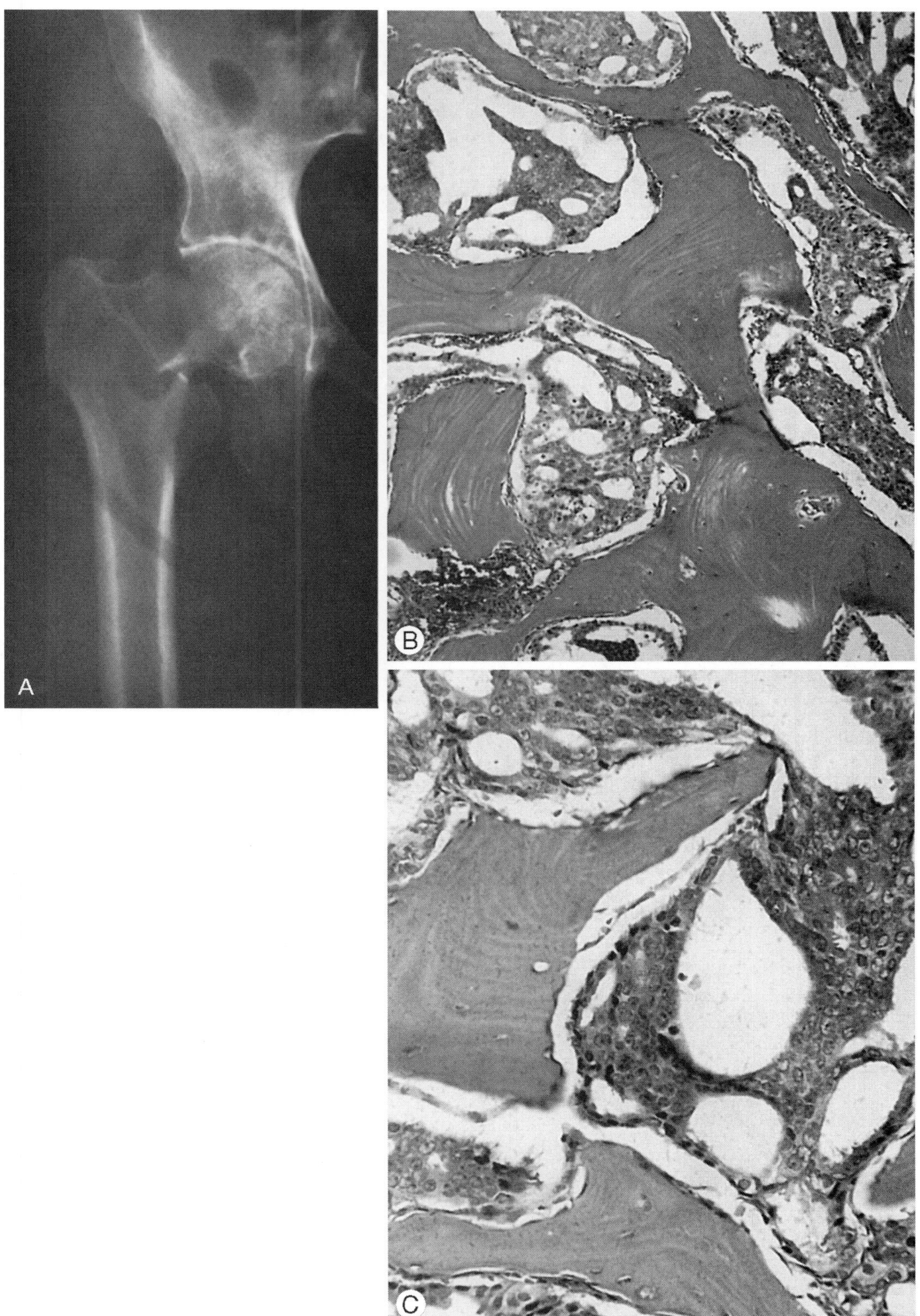

FIGURE 9–52 Metastatic carcinoma. **A**, Radiograph shows a lytic lesion in the femoral neck and the ilium. **B**, Low-power photomicrograph (× 100) shows the glandular arrangement of cells in the marrow space. **C**, Higher-power photomicrograph (× 400).

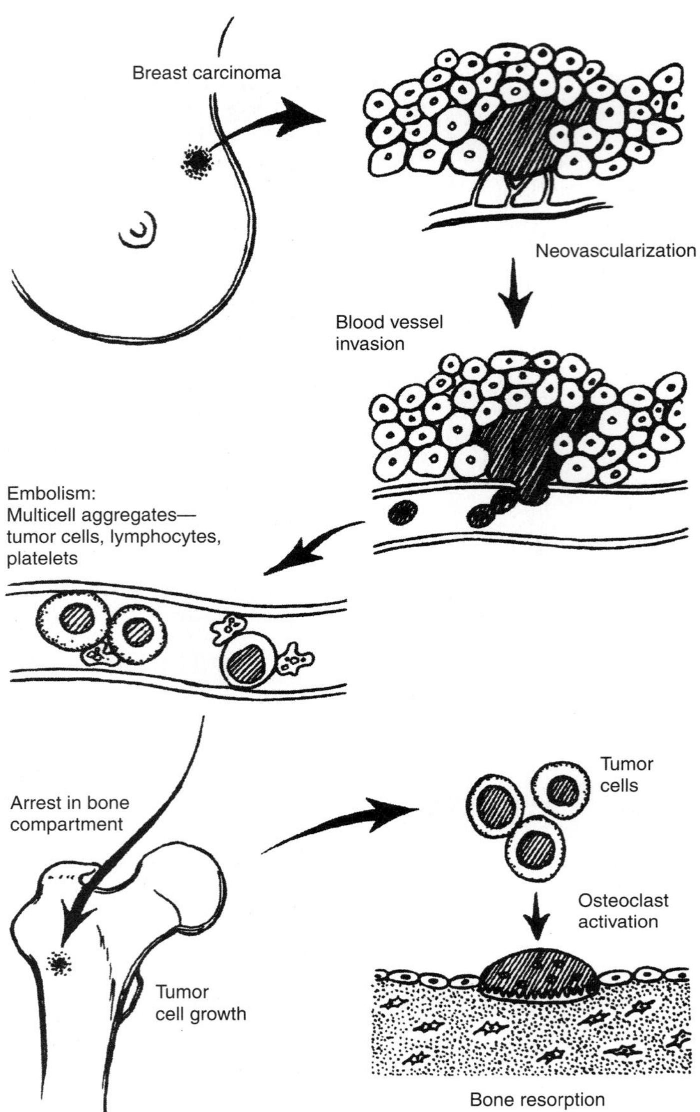

FIGURE 9–53 The mechanism of bone metastasis is complex. Metastatic cells spread into the venous system by vascular invasion and lodge in the medullary cavity. These tumor cells activate osteoclasts, which resorb the host bone. (From McCarthy EF, Frassica FJ: Pathology of Bone and Joint Disorders. Philadelphia, WB Saunders, 1998.)

Box 9–5 Evaluation of the Older Patient with a Single Bone Lesion and Suspected Metastases of Unknown Origin

Plain radiographs in two planes of the affected limb
Technetium bone scan to detect multiple lesions
Radiographic studies to search for occult neoplasms
Chest radiograph and CT of the chest to search for occult lung cancer
CT of the abdomen or ultrasonography of the abdomen to detect renal cell cancer or lymphoma
Skeletal survey if myeloma is suspected
Screening laboratory studies
Complete blood count with differential
Erythrocyte sedimentation rate
Chemistry group: liver function test, calcium, phosphorus, alkaline phosphatase
Serum or urine immunoelectrophoresis

CT, computed tomography.

IV. Tumor Tables*

TABLE 9-6 MOST COMMON MUSCULOSKELETAL TUMORS

Tumor Type	Tumor Name
Soft tissue tumor (children)	Hemangioma
Soft tissue tumor (adults)	Lipoma
Malignant soft tissue tumor (children)	Rhabdomyosarcoma
Malignant soft tissue tumor (adults)	Malignant fibrous histiocytoma
Primary benign bone tumor	Osteochondroma
Primary malignant bone tumor	Osteosarcoma
Secondary benign lesion	Aneurysmal bone cyst
Secondary malignancies	1. Malignant fibrous histiocytoma 2. Osteosarcoma 3. Fibrosarcoma
Phalangeal tumor	Enchondroma
Sarcoma of the hand and wrist	Epithelioid sarcoma
Sarcoma of the foot and ankle	Synovial sarcoma

Courtesy of Luke S. Choi, MD, Resident, Department of Orthopaedic Surgery, University of Virginia.

TABLE 9-7 COMMON TUMOR-ASSOCIATED GENETIC TRANSLOCATIONS

Tumor Type	Genetic Translocation
Myxoid liposarcoma	t(12;16)
Ewing's sarcoma	t(11;22)
Synovial sarcoma	t(X;18)
Myxoid chondrosarcoma	t(9;22)
Rhabdomyosarcoma	t(1;13) or t(2;13)

Courtesy of Luke S. Choi, MD, Resident, Department of Orthopaedic Surgery, University of Virginia.

TABLE 9-8 SPINAL TUMORS

Anterior Spine	Posterior Spine
Giant cell tumor	Aneurysmal bone cyst
Hemangioma	Osteoid osteoma
Eosinophilic granuloma	Osteoblastoma
Metastases	
Chordoma	
Multiple myeloma	

Courtesy of Luke S. Choi, MD, Resident, Department of Orthopaedic Surgery, University of Virginia.

TABLE 9-9 SMALL ROUND BLUE CELL TUMORS

Children	Adult
Ewing's sarcoma	Plasmacytoma/multiple myeloma
Neuroblastoma	Lymphoma
	Small round cell carcinoma

Courtesy of Luke S. Choi, MD, Resident, Department of Orthopaedic Surgery, University of Virginia.

TABLE 9-10 TUMOR IMMUNOSTAINS

Tumor	Immunostain
Langerhans cell histiocytosis	S100, +CD1A
Lymphoma	+CD20
Ewing's sarcoma	+CD99
Chordoma	Keratin, S100
Myeloma	+CD138
Adamantinoma	Keratin

Courtesy of Luke S. Choi, MD, Resident, Department of Orthopaedic Surgery, University of Virginia.

*Contributed by Luke S. Choi, MD

Selected Bibliography

Recent Articles

Bacci G, Longhi A, Ferrari S, et al: Prognostic factors in non-metastatic Ewing's sarcoma tumor of bone: An analysis of 579 patients treated at a single institution with adjuvant or neoadjuvant chemotherapy between 1972 and 1998. Acta Oncol 45:469–475, 2006.

Bell RS, O'Sullivan B, Liu FF, et al: The surgical margin in soft tissue sarcoma. J Bone Joint Surg [Am] 71:370–375, 1989.

Berrey BH Jr., Lord CF, Gebhardt MC, et al: Fractures of allografts: Frequency, treatment, and end results. J Bone Joint Surg [Am] 72:825–833, 1990.

Choong PFM, Pritchard DJ, Rock MG, et al: Survival after pulmonary metastectomy in soft tissue sarcoma: Prognostic factors in 214 patients. Acta Orthop Scand 66:561–568, 1995.

Frassica FJ, Frassica DA, Pritchard DJ, et al: Ewing sarcoma of the pelvis: Clinicopathological features and treatment. J Bone Joint Surg [Am] 75:1457–1465, 1993.

Frassica FJ, Waltrip RL, Sponseller PD, et al: Clinicopathologic features and treatment of osteoid osteoma and osteoblastoma in children and adolescents. Orthop Clin North Am 27:559–574, 1996.

Fuchs B, Dickey ID, Yaszemki MJ, et al: Operative management of sacral chordoma. J Bone Joint Surg [Am] 87:2211–2216, 2005.

Greene FL, Page DL, Fleming ID, et al. In AJCC Cancer Staging Manual, 6th ed, pp 221–228. New York, Springer Publishing Co, 2002.

Jemal A, Siegel R, Ward E, et al: Cancer statistics, 2006. CA Cancer J Clin 56:106–130, 2006.

O'Connor MI, Sim FH: Salvage of the limb in the treatment of malignant pelvic tumors. J Bone Joint Surg [Am] 71:481–494, 1989.

Peabody T, Monson D, Montag A, et al: A comparison of the prognoses for deep and subcutaneous sarcomas of the extremities. J Bone Joint Surg [Am] 76:1167–1173, 1994.

Quershi AA, Shott S, Mallin BA, Gitelis S: Current trends in the management of adamantinoma of long bones: An international study. J Bone Joint Surg [Am] 82:1122–1131, 2000.

Rock MG, Sim FH, Unni KK, et al: Secondary malignant giant cell tumor of bone: Clinicopathologic assessment of nineteen patients. J Bone Joint Surg [Am] 68:1073–1079, 1986.

Rougraff BT, Kneisl JS, Simon MA: Skeletal metastases of unknown origin: A prospective study of a diagnostic strategy. J Bone Joint Surg [Am] 75:1276–1281, 1993.

Rosenthal DI, Hornicek FJ, Wolfe MW, et al: Percutaneous radiofrequency coagulation of osteoid osteoma compared with operative treatment. J Bone Joint Surg [Am] 80:815–821, 1998.

Scully SP, Ghert MA, Zurakowski D, et al: Pathologic fracture in osteosarcoma: Prognostic importance and treatment implications. J Bone Joint Surg [Am] 84:49–57, 2002.

Simon MA, Bierman JS: Biopsy of bone and soft tissue lesions. J Bone Joint Surg [Am] 75:616–621, 1993.

Temple HT, Clohisy DR: Musculoskeletal oncology. In Menendez LR, ed, for the Musculoskeletal Tumor Society: Orthopaedic Knowledge Update (Chapter 17). Rosemont, IL, American Academy of Orthopaedic Surgeons, 2002.

Weber KL: What's new in musculoskeletal oncology. J Bone Joint Surg [Am] 87:1400–1410, 2005.

Yaw KM, Wurtz D: Resection and reconstruction for bone tumor in the proximal tibia. Orthop Clin North Am 22:133–148, 1991.

Yazawa Y, Frassica FJ, Chao EYS, et al: Metastatic bone disease: A study of the surgical treatment of 166 pathological humeral and femoral shaft fractures. Clin Orthop Relat Res 251:213–219, 1990.

Classic Articles

Bell RS, O'Sullivan B, Liu FF, et al: The surgical margin in soft tissue sarcoma. J Bone Joint Surg [Am] 71:370–375, 1989.

Berrey BH Jr., Lord CF, Gebhardt MC, et al: Fractures of allografts: Frequency, treatment, and end results. J Bone Joint Surg [Am] 72:825–833, 1990.

Eilber FR, Eckhardt J, Morton DL: Advances in the treatment of sarcomas of the extremity: Current status of limb salvage. Cancer 54:2695–2701, 1984.

Enneking WF, Spanier SS, Goodman MA: A system for the surgical staging of musculoskeletal sarcoma. Clin Orthop 153:106–120, 1980.

Enneking WF, Spanier SS, Malawer MM: The effect of the anatomic setting on the results of surgical procedures for soft parts sarcoma of the thigh. Cancer 47:1005–1022, 1981.

Heare TC, Enneking WF, Heare MJ: Staging techniques and biopsy of bone tumors. Orthop Clin North Am 20:273–285, 1989.

Madewell JE, Ragsdale BD, Sweet DE: Radiologic and pathologic analysis of solitary bone lesions. Part I: Internal margins. Radiol Clin North Am 19:715–748, 1981.

Mankin HJ, Doppelt SH, Sullivan TR, et al: Osteoarticular and intercalary allograft transplantation in the management of malignant tumors of bone. Cancer 50:613–630, 1982.

Mankin HJ, Lange TA, Spanier SS: The hazards of biopsy in patients with malignant primary bone and soft tissue tumors. J Bone Joint Surg [Am] 64:1121–1127, 1982.

Medsger TA Jr.: Twenty-fifth rheumatism review: Paget's disease. Arthritis Rheum 26:281–283, 1983.

Merkow RL, Lane JM: Current concepts of Paget's disease of bone. Orthop Clin North Am 15:747–764, 1984.

Miller MD, Yaw KM, Foley HT: Malpractice maladies in the management of musculoskeletal malignancies. Contemp Orthop 23:577–584, 1991.

Pritchard DJ, Lunke RJ, Taylor WF, et al: Chondrosarcoma: A clinicopathologic and statistical analysis. Cancer 45:149–157, 1980.

Ragsdale BD, Madewell JE, Sweet DE: Radiologic and pathologic analysis of solitary bone lesions. Part II: Periosteal reactions. Radiol Clin North Am 19:749–783, 1981.

Sim FH, Beauchamp CP, Chao EYS: Reconstruction of musculoskeletal defects about the knee for tumor. Clin Orthop 221:188–201, 1987.

Simon MA: Biopsy of musculoskeletal tumors. J Bone Joint Surg [Am] 64:1253–1257, 1982.

Simon MA: Current concepts review: Limb salvage for osteosarcoma. J Bone Joint Surg [Am] 70:307–310, 1988.

Simon MA, Nachman J: The clinical utility of pre-operative therapy for sarcomas. J Bone Joint Surg [Am] 68:1458–1463, 1986.

Springfield DS, Schmidt R, Graham-Pole J, et al: Surgical treatment for osteosarcoma. J Bone Joint Surg [Am] 70:1124–1130, 1988.

Sweet DE, Madewell JE, Ragsdale BD: Radiologic and pathologic analysis of solitary bone lesions. Part III: Matrix patterns. Radiol Clin North Am 19:785–814, 1981.

Wuisman P, Enneking WF: Prognosis for patients who have osteosarcoma with skip metastasis. J Bone Joint Surg [Am] 72:60–68, 1990.

Zimmer WD, Berquist TH, McLeod RA, et al: Bone tumors: Magnetic resonance imaging versus computed tomography. Radiology 155:709–718, 1985.

Review Articles

American Joint Committee on Cancer: Soft tissues. In Beahrs OH, Myers M, eds: Manual for Staging of Cancer, 3rd ed. Philadelphia, JB Lippincott, 1988.

Enneking WF: Clinical Musculoskeletal Pathology, 3rd ed. Gainesville, FL, University of Florida Press, 1990.

Frassica FJ, Chang BW, Ma LD, et al: Soft tissue sarcomas: General features, evaluation, imaging, biopsy, and treatment. Curr Orthop 11:105–113, 1997.

Frassica FJ, Gitelis SG, Sim FH: Metastatic Bone Disease: General Principles, Pathogenesis, Pathophysiology and Biopsy. Instr Course Lect 41:293–300, 1992.

Mindell ER: Chordoma. J Bone Joint Surg [Am] 63:501–505, 1981.

Orthopaedic Knowledge Update Home Study Syllabus I, II, III. Chicago, American Academy of Orthopaedic Surgeons, 1984, 1987, 1990.

Sim FH, Frassica FJ, Frassica DA: Soft tissue tumors: Evaluation, diagnosis, and management. J Am Acad Orthop Surg 2:202–211, 1994.

Simon MA: Current concepts review: Biopsy of musculoskeletal tumors. J Bone Joint Surg [Am] 64:1253–1257, 1982.

Textbooks

McCarthy EF, Frassica FJ: Pathology of Bone and Joint Disorders. Philadelphia, WB Saunders, 1998.

Mirra JM: Bone Tumors: Clinical, Radiologic, and Pathologic Correlations. Philadelphia, Lea and Febiger, 1989.

Sim FH: Diagnosis and Management of Metastatic Bone Disease: A Multidisciplinary Approach. New York, Raven Press, 1988.

Simon MA, Springfield D: Surgery for Bone and Soft Tissue Tumors. Philadelphia, Lippincott-Raven, 1998.

Unni KK: Dahlin's Bone Tumors: General Aspects and Data on 11,087 Cases. Philadelphia, Lippincott-Raven, 1996.

Wold LE, McLeod RA, Sim FH, et al: Atlas of Orthopaedic Pathology. Philadelphia, WB Saunders, 1990.

CHAPTER 10

Rehabilitation: Gait, Amputations, Prostheses, Orthoses, and Neurologic Injury

Frank A. Gottschalk

CONTENTS

I. Gait

A. Walking

1. Definitions—**Walking** is the repetitive process of sequential lower limb motion to move the body from one location to another while maintaining upright stability. Walking is a cyclic, energy-efficient activity. It requires that one foot be in contact with the ground at all times (single-limb support), with a period when both limbs are in contact with the ground (double-limb support) (Fig. 10–1). The **step** is the distance between initial swing and initial contact of the same limb. **Stride** is initial contact to initial contact of the same limb (Fig. 10–2). **Velocity** is a function of cadence (steps per unit time) and stride length. **Running** involves a period when neither limb is in contact with the ground.
2. Phases—Prerequisites for normal gait include **stance-phase stability, swing-phase ground clearance, the correct position of the foot before initial contact, and energy-efficient step length and speed**. The stance phase occupies 60% of the cycle, starting from initial contact and progressing through loading response, midstance, terminal stance, and preswing. The swing phase is 40% of the cycle and starts at initial swing (toe-off) and proceeds with limb acceleration to midswing, when the limb decelerates at terminal swing before the next cycle (Figs. 10–3 and 10–4). During initial swing, the hip and knee flex and the ankle begins to dorsiflex.

B. Gait dynamics—The combined phases of gait contribute to an energy-efficient process by **lessening excursion** of the center of body mass. The head, neck, trunk, and arms represent 70% of body weight. The trunk center of gravity of this mass is located just anterior to T10, which is 33 cm above the hip joints in an individual of average height (184 cm). The body's line of gravity is anterior to S2 and provides a reference for the moment arm to the center of the joint under consideration. The resulting gait pattern resembles a sinusoidal curve.

C. Determinants of gait (motion patterns)—In mechanical terms there are six independent degrees of freedom.

1. Pelvic rotation—The pelvis rotates horizontally about a vertical axis, alternately to the left and

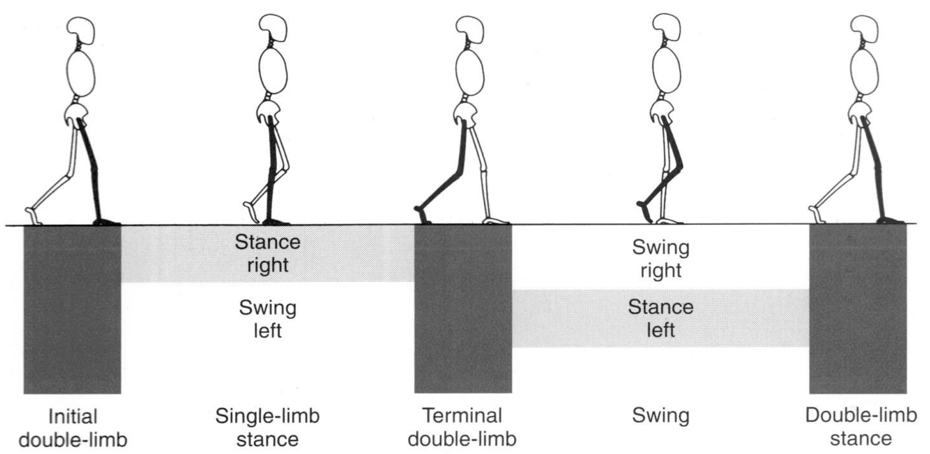

FIGURE 10–1 Subdivisions of stance and their relationships to the pattern of bilateral floor contact. (Adapted from Perry J: Gait Analysis: Normal and Pathological Function, 1992, with permission from SLACK, Inc.)

right of the line of progression, lessening the center-of-mass deviation in the horizontal plane and reducing the impact at initial floor contact.

2. Pelvic list—The non–weight-bearing, contralateral side drops 5 degrees, reducing superior deviation.
3. Knee flexion at loading—The stance-phase limb is flexed 15 degrees to dampen the impact of initial loading.
4. Foot and ankle motion—Through the subtalar joint, damping of the loading response occurs, leading to stability during midstance and efficiency of propulsion at push-off.
5. Knee motion—The knee works together with the foot and ankle to decrease necessary limb motion. The knee flexes at initial contact and extends at midstance.
6. Lateral pelvic displacement—This relates to the transfer of body weight onto the limb. The motion is 5 cm over the weight-bearing limb, narrowing the base of support and increasing stance-phase stability.

D. Muscle action—Agonist and antagonist muscle groups work in concert during the gait cycle to effectively advance the limb through space. The hip flexors advance the limb forward during the swing phase and are opposed during terminal swing, before initial contact by the decelerating action of the hip extensors. Most muscle activity is **eccentric**, which is muscle lengthening while contracting, and allows an antagonist muscle to dampen the activity of an agonist and act as a "shock absorber" (Fig. 10–5). **Isocentric** contraction is muscle length remaining constant during contraction (Table 10–1). Some muscle activity can be **concentric**, in which the muscle shortens to move a joint through space.

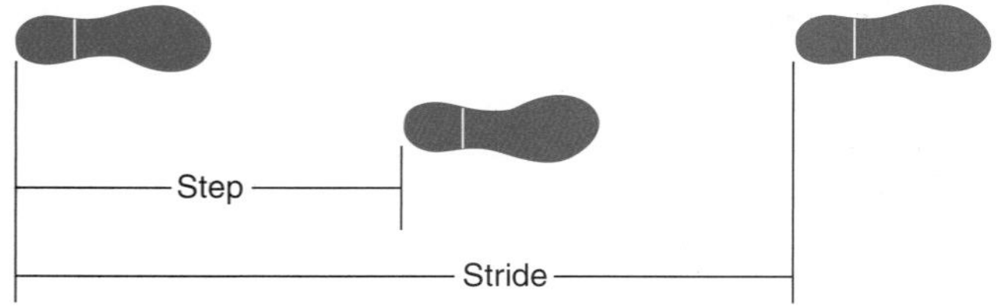

FIGURE 10–2 Step versus stride. (Adapted from Perry J: Gait Analysis: Normal and Pathological Function, 1992, with permission from SLACK, Inc.)

E. Pathologic gait—Abnormal gait patterns are caused by the following factors.

1. Muscle weakness or paralysis—Decreases the ability to normally move a joint through space. A walking pattern develops based on the specific muscle or muscle group involved and the ability of the individual to acquire a substitution pattern to replace that muscle's action (Table 10–2).
2. Neurologic conditions—May alter gait by producing muscle weakness, loss of balance, reduced coordination between agonist and antagonist muscle groups (i.e., spasticity), and joint contracture. **Hip scissoring** is associated with overactive adductors, and knee flexion contracture may be caused by hamstring spasticity. **Equinus deformity** of the foot and ankle may result in a steppage gait and back setting of the knee.
3. Pain in a limb—Creates an antalgic gait pattern, in which the individual shortens the stance phase to lessen the time that the painful limb is loaded. The contralateral swing phase is more rapid.
4. Joint abnormalities—Alter gait by changing the range of motion of that joint or producing pain. **Arthritis** of the hip and knee may have joint contractures and reduced range of motion. An **anterior cruciate–deficient knee** has quadriceps-avoidance gait, which is a net quadriceps moment during midstance that is lower than normal.
5. Hemiplegia—Characterized by prolongation of stance and double-limb support. Gait impairment may be excessive plantar flexion, weakness, and balance problems. Associated problems are ankle equinus, limitation of knee flexion, and increased hip flexion. Surgical correction of equinus is done 1 year after onset.
6. Crutches and canes—Devices that ameliorate instability and pain, respectively. Crutches increase stability by providing two additional loading points. A cane helps shift the center of gravity to the affected side when the cane is used in the

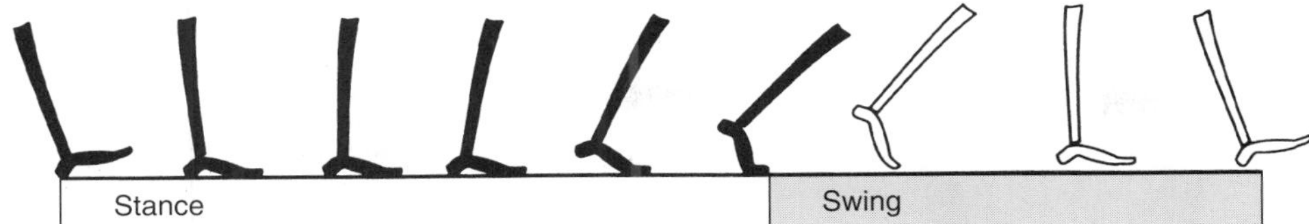

FIGURE 10–3 Divisions of the gait cycle. Clear and shaded bars represent the duration of each phase. (Adapted from Perry J: Gait Analysis: Normal and Pathological Function, 1992, with permission from SLACK, Inc.)

Right heel contact
Left heel contact
Right heel contact
Right step length
Left step length
Right step length
Cycle length (stride)
A

Right heel contact
Left toe-off
Left heel contact
Right toe-off
Right heel contact
Left toe-off
0%
50%
100%
Time, percent of cycle
Double support
Right single support
Double support
Left single support
Double support
Right stance phase
Right swing phase
Left swing phase
Left stance phase
B
Cycle (stride) duration

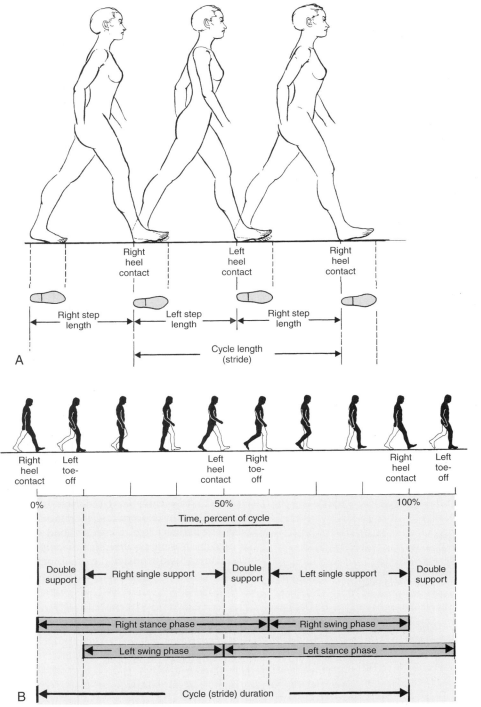

FIGURE 10–4 Distance (**A**) and time (duration) (**B**) dimensions of the walking cycle. (From Inman VT, Ralston H, Todd F: Human Walking, p 26. Baltimore, Williams & Wilkins, 1982.)

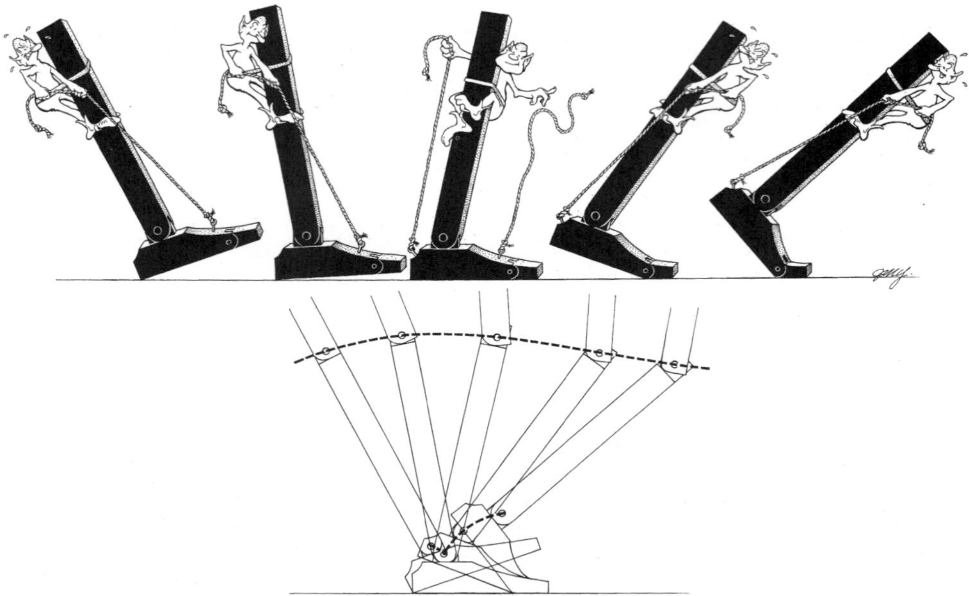

FIGURE 10–5 Effect of ankle motion, controlled by muscle action, on the pathway of the knee. The smooth and flattened pathway of the knee during the stance phase is achieved by forces acting from the leg on the foot. Foot slap is restrained during initial lowering of the foot; afterward, the plantar flexors raise the heel. (From Inman VT, Ralston H, Todd F: Human Walking, p 11. Baltimore, Williams & Wilkins, 1982.)

opposite hand. This decreases the joint reaction forces of the lower limb and reduces pain.

7. Arthritis—Forces across the knee may be 4-7 times those of body weight; 70% of the load across the knee occurs through the medial compartment.

II. Amputations

A. Introduction—All or part of a limb is amputated to treat peripheral vascular disease, trauma, tumor, infection, or a congenital anomaly. It is often an alternative to limb salvage and should be considered a reconstructive procedure. Because of the psychological implications and the alteration of body self-image, a multidisciplinary-team approach should be instituted to manage the patient.

B. Metabolic cost of amputee gait—The metabolic cost of walking is increased with proximal-level amputations and is inversely proportional to the length of the residual limb and the number of functional joints preserved. With a proximal amputation, patients have a decreased self-selected, maximum walking speed. Oxygen consumption increases the higher the amputation (or the shorter the stump); thus, the transfemoral amputee with peripheral vascular disease uses close to maximum energy expenditure during normal self-selected–velocity walking (Table 10–3).

C. Load transfer

1. Soft tissue envelope—The **soft tissue envelope** acts as an interface between the bone of the residual limb and the prosthetic socket. Ideally, it is composed of a mobile, securely attached muscle mass covering the bone end and full-thickness skin that tolerates the direct pressures and "pistoning" (mobility) within the prosthetic socket. It is rare for the prosthetic socket to achieve a perfect, intimate fit. A nonadherent soft tissue envelope allows some degree of mobility of the skin and muscle, thus eliminating the shear forces that produce tissue breakdown and ulceration.

2. Direct and indirect load transfer—**Load transfer** (i.e., weight bearing) occurs either directly or indirectly. **Direct load transfer** (i.e., terminal weight bearing) occurs in knee or ankle disarticulation (Syme amputation). For direct load transfer, intimacy of the prosthetic socket is necessary only for suspension. When the amputation is performed through a long bone (i.e., transfemoral or transtibial), the end of the stump does not take all the weight, and the load is transferred indirectly by the total contact method. This process requires an intimate fit of the prosthetic socket, 7-10 degrees of flexion of the knee for transtibial amputation,

TABLE 10-1 MUSCLE ACTION AND FUNCTION

Muscle	Action	Function
Gluteus medius	Eccentric	Controls pelvic tilt (midstance)
Gluteus maximus	Concentric	Powers hip extension
Iliopsoas	Concentric	Powers hip flexion
Hip adductors	Eccentric	Control lateral sway (late stance)
Hip abductors	Eccentric	Control pelvic tilt (midstance)
Quadriceps	Eccentric	Stabilizes knee at heel-strike
Hamstrings	Eccentric	Control rate of knee extension (stance)
Tibialis anterior	Concentric	Dorsiflexes ankle at swing
	Eccentric*	Slows plantar flexion rate (heel-strike)
Gastrocnemius/soleus	Eccentric	Slows dorsiflexion rate (stance)

*Predominant role.

TABLE 10-2 GAIT ABNORMALITIES CAUSED BY MUSCLE WEAKNESS

Weak Muscle	Phase	Direction	Type of Gait	Treatment
Gluteus medius	Stance	Lateral	Abductor lurch	Cane
Gluteus maximus	Stance	Backward	Lurch (hip hyperextension)	
Quadriceps	Stance	Forward	Lurch/back knee gait	AFO
	Swing	Forward	Abnormal hip rotation	
Gastrocnemius/soleus	Stance	Forward	Flatfoot (calcaneal) gait	± AFO
	Swing	Forward	Delayed heel rise	
Tibialis anterior	Stance	Forward	Foot drop/slap	AFO
	Swing	Forward	Steppage gait	

AFO, ankle-foot orthosis; ±, with or without.

and 5-10 degrees of adduction and flexion of the femur for transfemoral amputation (Fig. 10–6).

D. Amputation wound healing—The healing of amputation wounds depends on several factors, which include **vascular supply, nutrition**, and an **adequate immune status.**

1. Nutrition and immune status—Patients with malnutrition or immune deficiency have a high rate of wound failure or infection. A serum albumin level below 3.5 g/dL indicates a malnourished patient. An absolute lymphocyte count below 1500/mm^3 is a sign of immune deficiency. If possible, amputation surgery should be delayed in patients with stable gangrene until these values can be improved by nutritional support, usually in the form of oral hyperalimentation. In severely affected patients, nasogastric or percutaneous gastric feeding tubes are sometimes essential. When infection or severe ischemic pain requires urgent surgery, open amputation at the most distal, viable level, followed by open wound management, can be accomplished until wound healing can be optimized.
2. Vascular supply—Oxygenated blood is a prerequisite for wound healing, and a hemoglobin concentration of more than 10 g/dL is necessary. Amputation wounds generally heal by collateral flow, so arteriography is rarely useful for predicting wound healing.
   a. Doppler ultrasonography—Standard Doppler ultrasonography measures arterial pressure and has been used as the measure of vascular inflow to predict wound healing in the ischemic limb. An absolute Doppler pressure measurement of 70 mm Hg was originally described as the minimum inflow to support wound healing. The **ischemic index** is the ratio of the Doppler pressure at the level being tested to the brachial systolic pressure. It is generally accepted that patients require an ischemic index of 0.5 or greater at the surgical level to support wound healing. The ischemic index at the ankle (i.e., the ankle-brachial index) is the most accepted method for assessing adequate inflow to the ischemic limb. In the normal limb, the area under the Doppler waveform tracing is a measure of flow. These values are falsely elevated and not predictive in at least 15% of patients with diabetes and peripheral vascular disease because of the incompressibility and loss of compliance of calcified peripheral arteries. The ischemic index for toe pressure is more accurate in these patients and, if greater than 0.45, is usually predictive of adequate blood flow.
   b. **Transcutaneous partial pressure of oxygen**—$TcpO_2$ is the present gold standard for measurement of vascular inflow. It records the oxygen-delivering capacity of the vascular system to the level of contemplated surgery. Values greater than 40 mm Hg correlate with acceptable wound-healing rates without the false-positive values seen in noncompliant peripheral vascular diseased vessels. Pressures less than 20 mm Hg are predictive of poor healing potential.

TABLE 10-3 ENERGY EXPENDITURE FOR AMBULATION

Amputation Level	% Energy Above Baseline	Speed (m/min)	O_2 Cost (mL/kg/m)
Long transtibial	10	70	0.17
Average transtibial	25	60	0.20
Short transtibial	40	50	0.20
Bilateral transtibial	41	50	.20
Transfemoral	65	40	0.28
Wheelchair	0-8	70	0.16

E. Pediatric amputation—Pediatric amputations are usually the result of congenital limb deficiencies, trauma, or tumors. Congenital amputations are the result of failure of formation. The present classification system is based on the original work of the 1975 Conference of the **International Society for Prosthetics and Orthotics** (ISPO) and the subsequent standard developed by the **International Organization for Standardization** (ISO). Deficiencies are either longitudinal or transverse, with the potential for intercalary deficits. Amputation is rarely indicated in congenital upper limb deficiency; even rudimentary appendages can be functionally useful. In the lower limb, amputation of an unstable segment may allow direct load

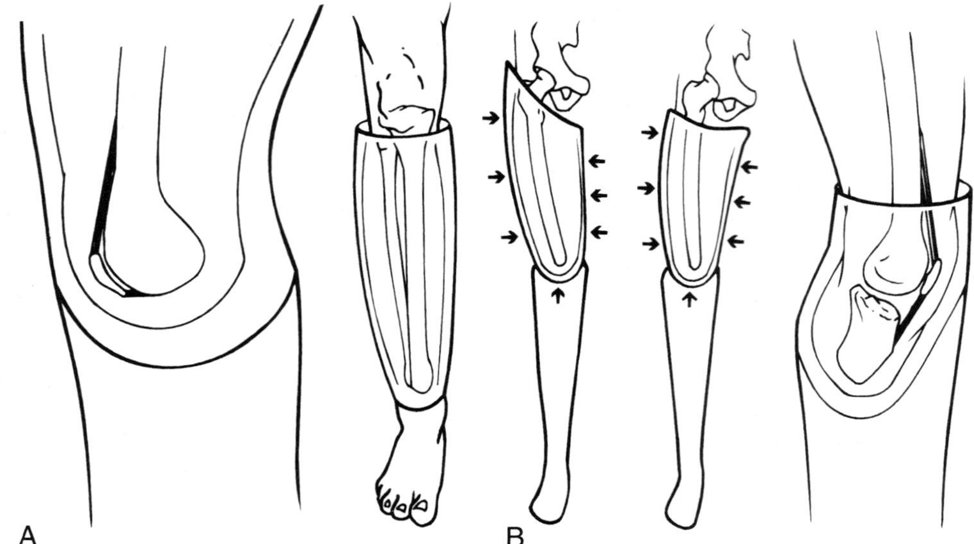

FIGURE 10–6 **A**, Direct load transfer is accomplished in the through-knee *(left)* and Syme ankle disarticulation *(right)* amputations. **B**, Indirect load transfer is accomplished in above-knee amputations with either a standard quadrilateral socket *(left)* or an adducted, narrow mediolateral socket *(center)*. The below-knee amputation *(right)* transfers weight indirectly with the knee flexed approximately 10 degrees. (From Pinzur M: New concepts in lower limb amputation and prosthetic management. Instr Course Lect 39:361, 1990.)

transfer and enhanced walking (e.g., Syme amputation for fibular hemimelia). In the growing child, disarticulations should be performed only when it is possible to maintain maximum residual limb length and prevent terminal bony overgrowth. Such overgrowth usually occurs in the humerus, fibula, tibia, and femur, in that order; it is typical in diaphyseal amputations. Numerous surgical procedures have been described to resolve this problem, but the best method is surgical revision of the residual limb with adequate resection of bone or autogenous osteochondral stump capping (Fig. 10–7).

F. Amputation after trauma—The grading scales for evaluating mangled extremities are not absolute predictors but provide reasonable guidelines for determining whether salvage is appropriate.

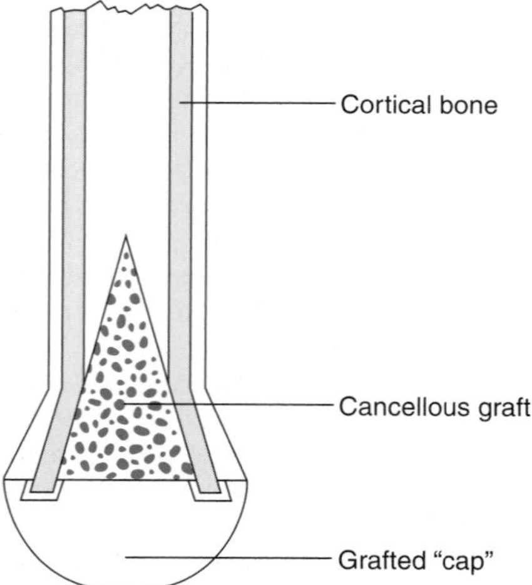

FIGURE 10–7 Diagram of the stump-capping procedure. The bone end has been split longitudinally. (Adapted from Bernd L, Blasius K, Lukoschek M, et al: The autologous stump plasty: treatment for bony overgrowth in juvenile amputees. J Bone Joint Surg [Br] 73:203-206, 1991.)

1. Indications—The absolute indication for amputation after trauma is **an ischemic limb with a vascular injury that cannot be repaired.** The guidelines for immediate or early amputation of mangled limbs differ between upper and lower limbs. Early amputation in the appropriate patient may prevent emotional, marital, financial, and addictive problems. Most grades IIIB and IIIC tibia fractures occur in young males who are laborers and may be more likely to return to gainful employment after amputation and prosthetic fitting. Sensation is not as crucial in the lower limb as in the upper limb, and current prostheses more closely approximate normal function.
   a. Disadvantages of limb salvage—Severe open tibia fractures that are managed by limb salvage rather than amputation are often associated with **high mortality and morbidity** owing to infection, increased energy expenditure for ambulation, and decreased potential to return to work. Gustillo-Anderson grades IIIB and IIIC open fractures of the tibia and fibula treated by limb salvage generally have poor functional outcomes and multiple complications and surgeries. The salvaged lower extremity with an insensate plantar weight-bearing surface (loss of posterior tibial nerve), with associated major functional muscle and bone loss, is unlikely to provide a durable limb for stable walking and is a potential source of early or late sepsis.
2. Contraindications
   a. Upper limb—When a salvaged upper limb remains sensate and has prehensile function, it will often function better than an

amputation with prosthetic replacement. Maintaining as much length as possible is the key to subsequent prosthetic use.

b. Lower limb—Lack of plantar sensation is not an indication to amputate because it may result from neurapraxia that can resolve. In the absence of other major factors, amputation should not be done.

G. Risk factors

1. Cognitive deficits—In order for patients to learn to walk with a prosthesis and care for their stumps and prostheses, they must possess certain cognitive capacities: memory, attention, concentration, and organization. Patients with cognitive deficits or psychiatric disorders have a low likelihood of becoming successful prosthesis users.
2. Diabetes—A majority of amputation patients are diabetic, with inherent immune deficiency. The most important risk factors for amputation in diabetic patients are the **presence of peripheral neuropathy** and development of deformity and infection.
3. Peripheral vascular disease—Most of the other amputation patients are malnourished patients with peripheral vascular disease of sufficient magnitude to require amputation, and they have disease in their coronary and cerebral arteries. Appropriate consultation with physical therapy, social work, and psychology departments is important to determine **rehabilitation potential.** Medical consultation will help determine cardiopulmonary reserve. The vascular surgeon should determine whether vascular reconstruction is feasible or appropriate. The **biologic amputation level** is the most distal functional amputation level with a high probability of supporting wound healing. This level is determined by the presence of adequate, viable local tissue to construct a residual limb capable of supporting weight bearing; an adequate vascular inflow; and serum albumin and a total lymphocyte count sufficient to aid surgical wound healing. The selection of an appropriate amputation level is determined by combining the biologic amputation level with the rehabilitation potential in order to choose the level that maximizes ultimate functional independence. Morbidity and mortality rates have remained unchanged for several decades. Thirty percent of patients with peripheral vascular disease die in the first 3 months and nearly 50% within the first year. Overall prosthetic use is 43%.

H. Musculoskeletal tumors

1. Goal of surgery—The primary goal of tumor surgery is to remove the tumor with adequate surgical margins.
2. Amputation versus limb salvage—Advances in chemotherapy and allograft or prosthetic reconstruction have made limb salvage a viable option in extremity sarcomas. If adequate margins can be achieved with limb salvage, the decision can then be based on **expected functional outcome.** The advantage of limb salvage versus amputation with regard to energy expenditure to ambulate, quality-of-life measures, and function with activities of daily living is controversial in the literature. Expected functional outcome should include the psychosocial and body-image values associated with limb salvage. These concerns should be balanced with improved task performance and lower concern for late mechanical injury associated with amputation and fitting of prosthetic limbs.

I. Technical considerations—Skin flaps should be of full thickness and avoid dissection between tissue planes. Periosteal stripping should be sufficient to allow for bone transection; this minimizes regenerative bone overgrowth. Wounds should not be sutured under tension. Muscles are best secured directly to bone at resting tension (myodesis) rather than to antagonist muscle (myoplasty). Stable residual limb muscle mass can improve function by reducing atrophy and providing a stable soft tissue envelope over the end of the bone. All transected nerves form neuromata. The nerve end should come to lie deep in a soft tissue envelope, away from potential pressure areas. Crushing the nerve may contribute to postoperative phantom or limb pain. Rigid dressings (postoperative) help reduce swelling, decrease pain, and protect the stump from trauma. Early prosthetic fitting is done within 5 to 21 days after surgery in selected patients.

J. Complications

1. Pain—**Phantom limb sensation,** the feeling that all or part of the amputated limb is present, occurs in almost all adults who have undergone amputation. It usually decreases with time. **Phantom pain** is a burning, painful sensation in the part having undergone amputation. It is diminished by prosthetic use, physical therapy, compression, and transcutaneous nerve stimulation. A common cause of residual pain is **complex regional pain syndrome** (reflex sympathetic dystrophy) or causalgia. Amputation should not be performed for this condition. **Localized stump pain** is often related to bony or soft tissue problems. **Referred pain to the limb** occurs in a frequent number of cases.
2. Edema—Postoperative edema occurs after amputation. It may impede wound healing and place significant tension on the tissues. Rigid dressings and soft compression help reduce the problem. Swelling occurring after stump maturation is usually caused by poor socket fit, medical problems, or trauma. Persistence of chronic swelling may lead to **verrucous hyperplasia,** a wartlike overgrowth of skin with pigmentation and serous discharge. It should be treated by a total-contact cast, which is changed regularly to accommodate the reduced edema.
3. Joint contractures—These complications are usually noted as hip and knee flexion contractures, which can be produced at the time of surgery by anchoring the respective muscles to the joints in a flexed position. They can be avoided by ensuring correct positioning of the amputated limb.

4. Wound failure to heal—This outcome occurs most often in diabetic and vascular disease patients. If the wound is not amenable to local care, wedge excision of soft tissue and bone, with closure and without tension, is the preferred treatment.

K. Upper limb amputations (Fig. 10–8)
  1. Wrist disarticulation
     a. Advantages—Wrist disarticulation has two advantages over transradial amputation: (1) preservation of more forearm rotation because of preservation of the distal radioulnar joint and (2) improved prosthetic suspension because of the flare of the distal radius. Effective function can be obtained at this level of amputation. Forearm rotation and strength are directly related to the length of the transradial (below-elbow) residual limb.
     b. Disadvantages—Wrist disarticulation provides challenges to the prosthetist that may outweigh its benefits. Cosmetically, the prosthetic limb is longer than the contralateral limb, and if myoelectric components are used, the motor and battery cannot be hidden within the prosthetic shank.
  2. Transradial amputation or elbow disarticulation—Patients with complete brachial plexus injury and a nonfunctioning hand and forearm may be best treated by a transradial amputation or elbow disarticulation, which can be fitted with a prosthesis. The optimum length of the residual limb is at the junction of the middle and distal thirds of the forearm, where the soft tissue envelope can be repaired by myodesis and the components of a myoelectric prosthesis can be hidden within the prosthetic shank. Because the patient can maintain function at this level prosthetically only by being able to open and close the terminal device, retention of the elbow joint is essential. The length and shape of elbow disarticulation provides improved suspension and lever-arm capacity. To enhance suspension and reduce the need for shoulder harnessing, a 45-60–degree distal humeral osteotomy is performed. Gangrene of the upper limb, when it is not due to Raynaud or Buerger disease, represents end-stage disease, especially in the diabetic patient. These patients experience a high mortality rate and do not survive beyond 24 months. Localized amputations are unlikely to heal. When surgery becomes necessary, amputation should be performed at the transradial level to achieve wound healing during the final months of the patient's life.

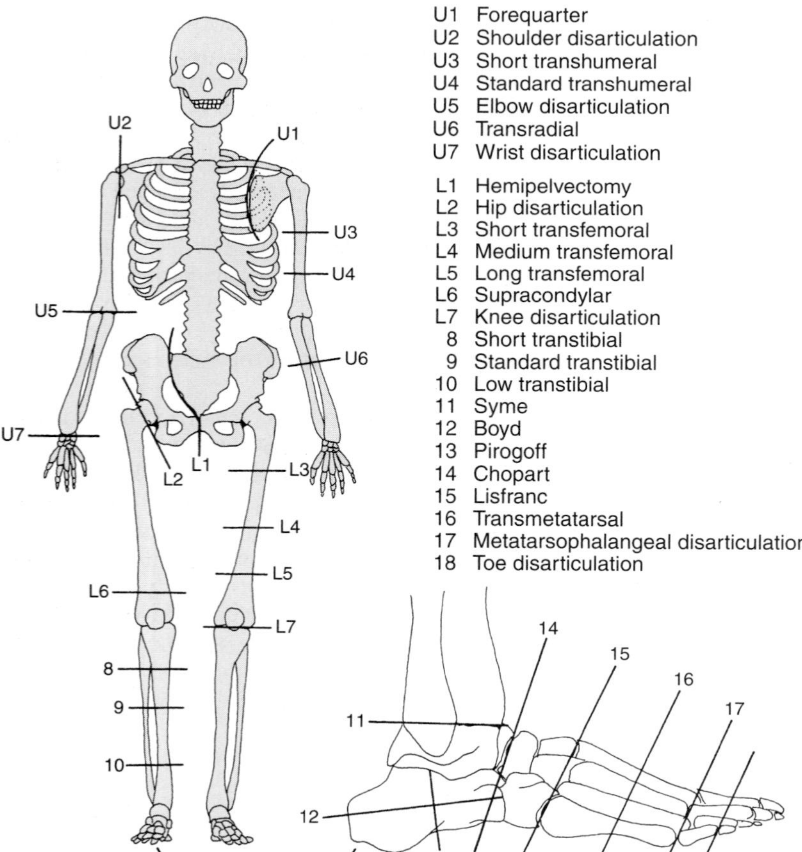

FIGURE 10–8 Composite illustration of common amputation levels.

L. Lower limb amputations (see Fig. 10–8)
1. Toe and ray amputation—Patients with ischemia generally ambulate with a propulsive gait pattern, so they suffer little disability from toe amputation. Traumatic amputees lose some stability after toe amputation in the late-stance phase. The great toe should be amputated distal to the insertion of the flexor hallucis brevis. Isolated second-toe amputation should be performed just distal to the proximal phalanx metaphyseal flare, leaving it to act as a buttress and prevent late hallux valgus. Patients who undergo single outer (first or fifth) ray resections function well in standard shoes. Resection of more than one ray leaves a narrow forefoot that is difficult to fit in shoes and often results in a late equinus deformity. Central ray resections are complicated by prolonged wound healing and rarely outperform midfoot amputation.
2. Transmetatarsal and Lisfranc tarsal-metatarsal amputation—There is little functional difference between these two. The long plantar flap acts as a myocutaneous flap and is preferred to fish-mouth dorsal-plantar flaps. Transmetatarsal amputation should be performed through the proximal metaphyses to prevent late plantar pressure ulcers under the residual bone ends. Percutaneous Achilles tendon lengthening should be performed with transmetatarsal and Lisfranc amputations to prevent the late development of equinus or equinovarus. Late varus can be corrected with the transfer of the tibialis anterior tendon to the neck of the talus. Some authors have reported reasonable functional outcomes with hindfoot amputation (i.e., Chopart or Boyd), but most experts recommend avoiding these levels if possible in diabetic and vascular disease patients. Although children have been reported to function reasonably well, adults retain an inadequate lever arm and are prone to experience fixed equinus of the heel if Achilles tendon lengthening and tibialis anterior tendon transfer are not performed.
3. Ankle disarticulation (Syme amputation)—This amputation allows direct load transfer and is rarely complicated by late residual limb ulcers or tissue breakdown. It provides a stable gait pattern that rarely requires prosthetic gait training after surgery. Surgery should be performed in one stage, even in ischemic limbs with insensate heel pads. A patent posterior tibial artery is necessary to ensure healing. The malleoli and metaphyseal flares should be removed from the tibia and fibula, but the remaining tibial articular surface should be retained to provide a resilient residual limb. The heel pad should be secured to the tibia either anteriorly through drill holes or posteriorly by securing the Achilles tendon.
4. Transtibial (below-knee) amputation—A long posterior myocutaneous flap is the preferred method of creating a soft tissue envelope. The optimum bone length is at least 12 cm below the knee joint or longer if adequate gastrocnemius or soleus muscle can be used to construct a durable soft tissue envelope. Posterior muscle should be secured to the beveled anterior tibia by myodesis. Rigid dressings are preferred during the early postoperative period, and early prosthetic fitting may be started 5-21 days after surgery if the residual limb is capable of transferring load and the patient has a satisfactory physical reserve.
5. Knee disarticulation (through-knee amputation)—The current technique uses a long posterior flap, with gastrocnemius muscle as end-padding. The alternative is to use sagittal skin flaps and cover the end of the femur with gastrocnemius muscle to act as a soft tissue envelope end-pad. The patella tendon is sutured to the cruciate ligaments in the notch, leaving the patella on the anterior femur. This level is generally used in the nonwalker who can support wound healing at the transtibial or distal level. Knee disarticulation is muscle balanced and provides an excellent weight-bearing platform for sitting and a lever arm for bed to chair transfer. When this amputation is performed in a potential walker, it provides a residual limb for direct bed to chair transfer (end-bearing).
6. Transfemoral (above-knee) amputation—This amputation increases the energy cost for walking. Transfemoral amputees with peripheral vascular disease are unlikely to become good walkers, so salvaging the limb at the knee disarticulation (transtibial level) is critical to maintaining functional walking independence. With greater femoral length, the lever arm, suspension, and limb advancement are optimized. The optimum transfemoral bone length is 12 cm above the knee joint to accommodate the prosthetic knee. Adductor myodesis is important for maintaining femoral adduction during the stance phase in order to allow optimum prosthetic function (Fig. 10–9). The major deforming force is toward abduction and flexion. Adductor myodesis at normal muscle tension eliminates the problem of adductor roll in the groin. Transecting the adductor magnus results in a loss of 70% of the adductor pull (Fig. 10–10). Rigid dressings are difficult to apply and maintain at this level. Elastic compression dressings are used and may be suspended about the opposite iliac crest.
7. Hip disarticulation—This is infrequently performed, and only an occasional few of these amputees become meaningful prosthesis users because of the high energy requirements for walking. Post-trauma or tumor patients occasionally use the prosthesis for limited activity. These patients sit in their prostheses and must use the torso in order to achieve momentum for "throwing" the limb forward to advance it.

III. Prostheses

A. Upper limb
1. Upper limb biomechanics—The shoulder provides the center of the radius of the functional sphere of the upper limb. The elbow acts as the caliper to position the hand at a workable

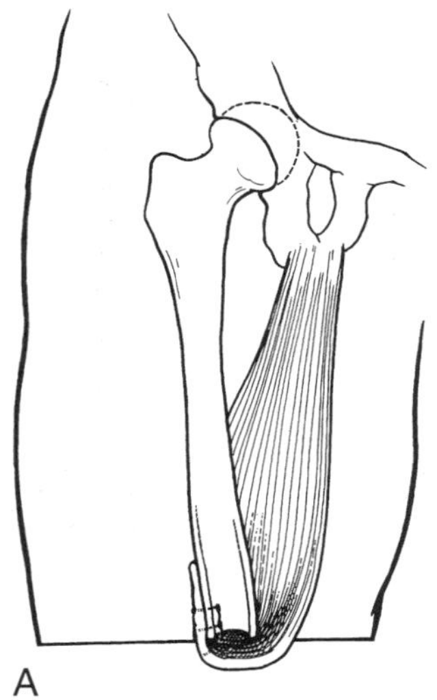

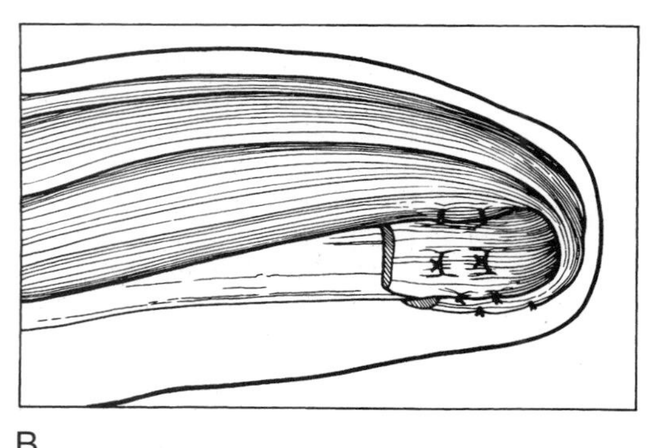

FIGURE 10–9 **A**, Diagram showing attachment of the adductor magnus to the lateral part of the femur. **B**, Diagram depicting attachment of the quadriceps over the adductor magnus. (From Gottschalk F: Transfemoral amputation. In Bowker J, Michael J, eds: Atlas of Limb Prosthetics, pp 479-486. St. Louis, Mosby-Year Book, 1992.)

distance from that center in order to perform its tasks. In a normal arm, tasks performed with the use of multiple joint segments usually occur simultaneously, whereas upper limb prostheses perform these same tasks sequentially; thus, joint- and residual-limb-length salvage is directly correlated with functional outcome. Motion at the retained joints is essential to maximize that function. Residual limb length is important for suspending the prosthetic socket and providing the lever arm necessary to "drive" the prosthesis through space.

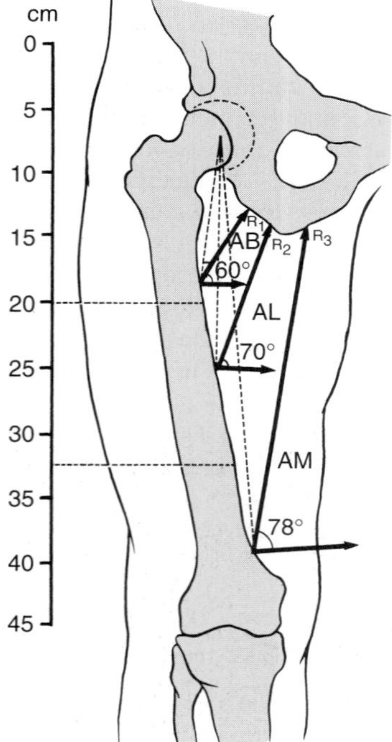

FIGURE 10–10 Diagram of moment arms of the three adductor muscles. Loss of the distal attachment of the adductor magnus (AM) will result in a loss of 70% of the adductor pull. AB, adductor brevis; AL, adductor longus. (From Gottschalk FA, Kourosh S, Stills M, et al: Does socket configuration influence the position of the femur in above-knee amputation? J Prosthet Orthot 2:94-102, 1989.)

2. Benefits of limb salvage—Limb salvage is more important for the upper limb, where sensation is critical to function. An insensate prosthesis provides less function than a partially sensate, partially functional salvaged limb.
3. Timing of prosthetic fitting—Prosthetic fitting should be done as soon as possible after amputation, even before complete wound healing has occurred. For transradial amputation, the outcomes for prosthetic limb use vary from 70-85% when prosthetic fitting occurs within 30 days of amputation, in contrast with less than 30% when the fitting starts late.
4. Types of prostheses for different levels of amputation
   a. **Midlength transradial amputation**—Myoelectric prostheses provide good cosmesis and are used for sedentary work. They can be used in any position, including overhead activity, and are the most successful in the midlength transradial amputee, for whom only the terminal device needs to be activated. Body-powered prostheses are used for heavy labor. The terminal device is activated by shoulder flexion and abduction. The optimum mechanical efficiency of figure-8 harnesses requires that the harness ring be at the spinous process of C7 and slightly to the nonamputated side.
   b. **Elbow disarticulation and transhumeral (above-elbow) amputations**—When the residual forearm is so short that it precludes an adequate lever arm for driving the prosthesis through space, **supracondylar suspension (Munster socket)** and **step-up hinges** can be used to augment function. Elbow disarticulation and transhumeral (above-elbow) amputations require two motions to develop prehension, making these levels of amputation significantly less

efficient and the prosthesis heavier than they are for amputation at the transradial level. Elbow flexion and extension are controlled by shoulder extension and depression. Amputations at these levels provide minimum function because the patient must sequentially control two joints and a terminal device. The best function with the least weight at the lowest cost is provided by hybrid prosthetic systems in which myoelectric, traditional body-powered, and body-driven switch components are combined.

c. **Proximal transhumeral and shoulder disarticulation amputations**—When the lever-arm capacity of the humerus is lost in proximal transhumeral or shoulder disarticulation amputations, limited function can be achieved with a manual universal shoulder joint positioned with the opposite hand and combined with lightweight hybrid prosthetic components.

B. Lower limb

1. Prosthetic feet—Several designs are available and divided into five classes.
   a. **Single-axis foot**—The single-axis foot is based on an ankle hinge that provides dorsiflexion and plantar flexion. The disadvantages of the single-axis foot include poor durability and cosmesis.
   b. **Solid-ankle, cushioned-heel (SACH) foot**—This has been the standard for decades and was appropriate for general use in low-demand patients. It may lead to overload problems on the nonamputated foot, and its use is being discontinued.
   c. **Dynamic-response foot**—The selection of the correct dynamic prosthetic foot requires information about the patient's height, weight, activity level, access for maintenance, cosmesis, and funding. The dynamic-response feet, including the Seattle foot, Carbon Copy II/III, and Flex Foot, allow amputees to undertake most normal activities (Fig. 10–11). Dynamic-response feet may be grouped into articulated feet and nonarticulated feet.
      (1) **Articulated dynamic-response foot**—These allow inversion/eversion and rotation of the foot and are useful for activities on uneven surfaces. They may absorb loads and decrease shear forces to the residual limb. Most dynamic-response feet have a **flexible keel** and are the standard for general use (Fig. 10–12). The keel deforms under load, becoming a spring and allowing dorsiflexion and thereby decreasing the loading on the normal side and providing a springlike response for push-off. Posterior projection of the keel provides a response at heel-strike for smooth transition through the stance phase.

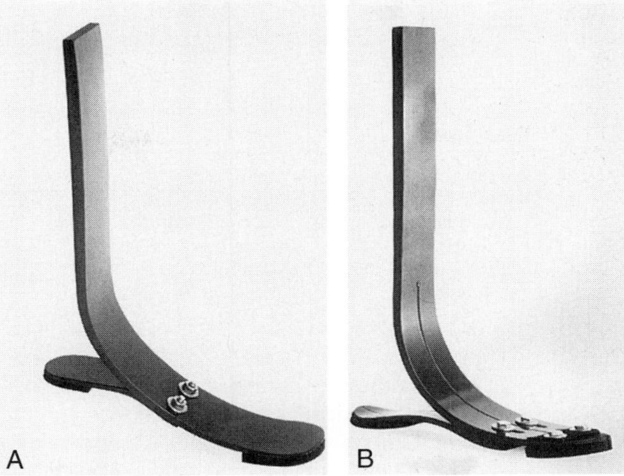

FIGURE 10–11 **A**, Flex Foot with carbon-fiber leaf and posterior projection of the keel for heel-strike. **B**, Flex Foot with split-toe configuration and spring-leaf design. (Courtesy of Flex Foot, Inc, Aliso Viejo, CA.)

A sagittal split allows for moderate inversion or eversion.
      (2) **Nonarticulated dynamic-response foot**—These can have short or long keels. Shortened keels are not as responsive and are indicated for the moderate-activity ambulator, whereas long keels are for very-high-demand activities. Separate prosthetic feet for running and lower-demand activities may be indicated.
2. Prosthetic shanks—These shanks provide the structural link between or among prosthetic components. Two varieties exist: **endoskeletal,** with a soft exterior and load-bearing tubing inside (the most common), and **exoskeletal,** with a hard load-bearing exterior shell. **Rotator units** are sometimes added for patients involved in twisting activities (e.g., golf) or for sitting.
3. Prosthetic knees (Table 10–4)—These prostheses are used in transfemoral and knee disarticulation and are chosen based on patient needs. Prosthetic knees provide controlled knee motion

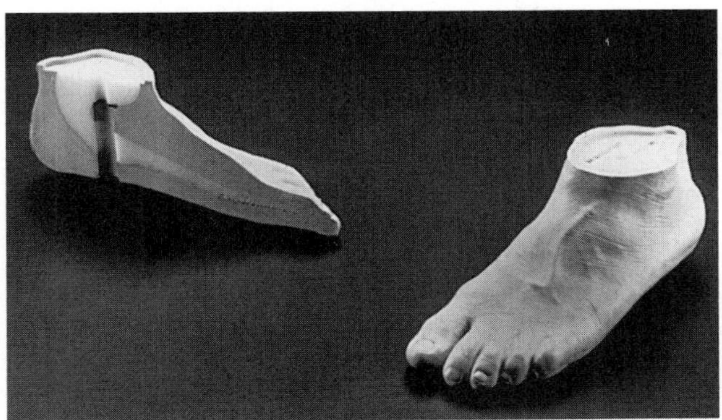
FIGURE 10–12 Cosmetic appearance of a dynamic-response foot (Seattle foot) and cross section showing internal configuration. (Courtesy of MIND, Seattle, WA.)

TABLE 10-4 CHARACTERISTICS OF VARIOUS PROSTHETIC KNEES

Knee Type	Characteristics		
	Action	*Advantages*	*Disadvantages*
Constant-friction	Limits flexion	Durable, long resistance	Decreased stability
Variable- friction	Varies with flexion	Variable cadence	Durability poor
Stance-control	Friction brake	Stability during stance	Durability poor, difficult on stairs
Polycentric	Instant center moves	Stable, increased flexion	Durability poor, heavy
Manual locking	Must unlock to sit	Maximum stability	Abnormal gait
Fluid-control	Deceleration in swing	Variable cadence	Weight, cost

in the prosthesis. **Alignment stability** (the position of the prosthetic knee in relation to the patient's line of weight bearing) is important to the design and fitting of prosthetic knees. Placing the knee center of rotation posterior to the line of weight bearing allows control in the stance phase but makes flexion difficult. Alternatively, with the knee center of rotation anterior to the line of weight bearing, flexion is made easier but at the expense of control. Only in the **polycentric knee** is there the possibility of both options by having a variable center of rotation. Six basic types of knees are available.

a. **Polycentric (four-bar linkage) knee**—This prosthesis has a moving instant center of rotation that provides for different stability characteristics during the gait cycle and may allow increased flexion for sitting. It is recommended for patients with transfemoral amputations, those with knee disarticulations, and bilateral amputees (Fig. 10–13).
b. **Stance-phase control (weight-activated [safety]) knee**—This knee functions like a constant-friction knee during the swing phase but "freezes" by application of high-friction housing when weight is applied to the limb. Its use is reserved primarily for older patients, those with very proximal amputations, or those walking on uneven terrain.
c. **Fluid-control (hydraulic and pneumatic) knee**—This knee allows adjustment of cadence response by changing resistance to knee flexion via a piston mechanism. The design prevents excessive flexion and is extended earlier in the gait cycle, allowing a more fluid gait. The knee is best used in active patients who prefer greater utility and variability at the expense of more weight.
d. **Constant-friction knee**—This knee prosthesis is essentially a hinge that is designed to dampen knee swing via a screw or rubber pad that applies friction to the knee bolt. It is a knee designed for general utility and may be used on uneven terrain. It is the most common knee used in childhood prostheses. Its major disadvantages are that it allows only single-speed walking and relies solely on alignment for stance-phase stability and is therefore not recommended for older, weaker patients.
e. **Variable-friction (cadence control) knee**—This device allows resistance to knee flexion to increase as the knee extends by employing a number of staggered friction pads. This knee allows walking at different speeds but is neither durable nor available in endoskeletal systems.
f. **Manual locking knee**—This knee consists of a constant-friction knee hinge with a positive lock in extension that can be unlocked to allow functioning similar to that of a constant-friction knee. The knee is often left locked in extension for more stability. It has limited indications and is used

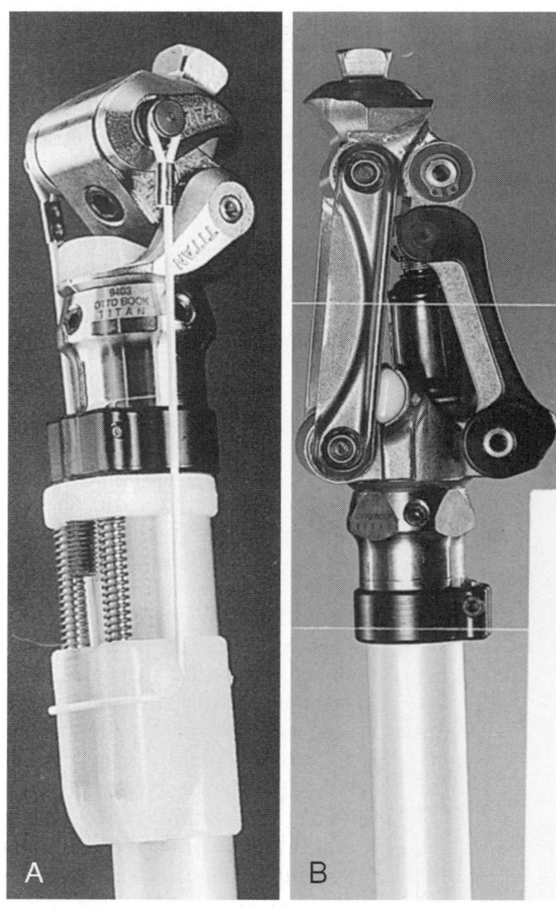

FIGURE 10–13 **A**, Stance-phase control unit for transfemoral prosthesis. **B**, Modular endoskeletal four-bar knee with hydraulic swing-phase control unit. (Courtesy of Otto Bock Orthopaedic Industries, Minneapolis.)

primarily in weak, unstable patients; those just learning to use prostheses; and blind amputees.

4. Suspension systems—Suspension is provided in modern lower extremity prostheses primarily through **socket design** and **suspension sleeves.** Straps and belts are usually used for supplementation.
   a. Sockets—**Sockets** are prosthetic components designed to provide comfortable functional control and even pressure distribution on the amputated stump. Sockets can be hard (rigid or unlined) or soft (lined with a resilient material and/or flexible shell). In general, the suction-and-socket contour is the primary suspension modality used. The suction socket provides an airtight seal via a pressure differential between the socket and atmosphere. Total-contact support of the residual limb surface prevents edema formation. In total-contact support, different areas have different loads.
      (1) Transfemoral sockets—**Quadrilateral sockets,** in which the posterior brim provides a shelf for the ischial tuberosity, have been the classic suspension system. However, the design made it difficult to keep the femur in adduction. **Narrow mediolateral (ischial containment) sockets** distribute the proximal and medial concentrations of forces more evenly as well as enhance rotational control of the socket (Fig. 10–14).

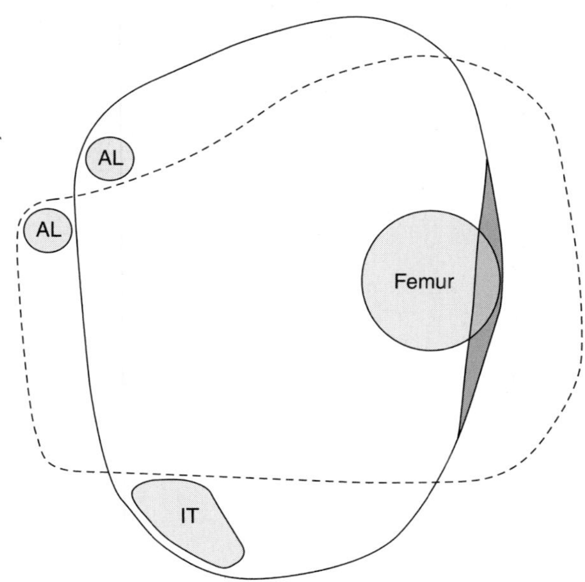

FIGURE 10–14 Comparison of transfemoral sockets. Note the inclusion of the ischial tuberosity (IT) and the narrow mediolateral design of newer contoured, adducted, trochanteric-controlled alignment method (CAT-CAM) socket shown by the solid line. AL, adductor longus. (Adapted from Sabolich J: Contoured adducted trochanteric controlled alignment method. Clin Prosthet Orthop 9:13-17, 1985.)

The ischium and ramus are contained within the socket of these more anatomic, comfortable, and functional designs. Socket design for transfemoral prosthesis allows for 10 degrees of adduction of the femur (to stretch the gluteus medius, allowing adequate strength for midstance stability) and 5 degrees of flexion (to stretch the gluteus maximus, allowing greater hip extension).
      (2) Transtibial sockets—Weight bearing by the patella tendon loads all areas of the residual limb that are weight tolerant (i.e., patella tendon, medial tibial flare, anterior compartment, gastrocnemius muscle, and fibular shaft). Weight-intolerant areas include the tibial crest and tubercle, distal fibula and fibular head, peroneal nerve, and hamstring tendons. The **patella tendon–bearing supracondylar/suprapatellar socket** has proximal extensions over the distal femoral condyles and patella. Total-surface weight bearing is different from total contact weight bearing. With total-surface weight bearing, pressure is distributed more equally across the entire surface of the transtibial residual limb, and the interface liner material in the socket is important. Urethane liners cope with multidirectional forces by easy material distortion and recovery to the original shape. Another liner is made of mineral oil gel with reinforcing fabric. These liners provide good shock-absorbing abilities and reduce skin problems. The anterior wedge shape of the socket helps control rotation of the socket on the limb.
      (3) Supracondylar suspension—This is recommended when the residual limb is less than 5 cm long. The socket is designed to increase the surface area for pressure distribution by raising the medial and lateral socket brim. A wedge may be used in the soft liner.
      (4) Supracondylar-suprapatellar suspension—This system encloses the patella in the socket and has a bar proximal to the patella. This design also provides mediolateral stability, and no additional cuffs or straps are required. Corset-type prostheses can lead to verrucous hyperplasia and thigh atrophy but reduce socket loads, control the direction of swing, and provide some additional weight support.
   b. Prosthetic sleeves—Prosthetic sleeves use friction and negative pressure for suspension. The sleeves fit snugly to the upper third of the tibial prosthesis and are made from

neoprene, latex, silicone, or thermoplastic elastomers.

(1) Transtibial suspension—**Gel-liner suspension systems with a locking pin** constitute the preferred method of suspension. Liners are made from silicone, urethane, or thermoplastic elastomer. The sleeve rolls onto the stump, and the locking pin is then locked into the socket (Fig. 10–15). The liners provide suspension through suction and friction and act as the socket interface. Prosthetic socks worn over the liner accommodate volume fluctuation. This suspension allows unrestricted knee flexion and minimal pistoning.

(2) Transfemoral suspension—Vacuum (suction) suspension is frequently used. It relies on surface tension, negative pressure, and muscle contraction. A one-way expulsion valve helps maintain negative pressure, and no belts or straps are required. Stable body weight is required for this intimate fit. Roll-on silicone or thermoplastic liners may be used with or without locking pins. The all-elastic suspension belt, which is made of neoprene, fastens around the waist and spreads over a larger surface area (Fig. 10–16). It is an excellent auxiliary suspension. Silesian belts are used to prevent socket rotation in limbs with redundant tissue. Such belts also prevent the socket from slipping off when suction sockets are fitted to short transfemoral stumps and the patient sits.

5. Common prosthetic problems (Table 10–5)
   a. Transtibial prostheses—**Pistoning during the swing phase** of gait is usually caused by an ineffective suspension system. **Pistoning in the stance phase** is due to a poor socket fit or volume changes in the stump (may require a change in thickness of the stump sock). **Alignment problems** are common (see Table 10–5). **Pressure-related pain or redness** should be corrected, with relief of the prosthesis in the affected area. Other problems may be **related to the foot**: Too soft a heel results in excessive knee extension, whereas too hard a heel causes knee flexion and lateral rotation of the toes.
   b. Transfemoral prostheses—Excessive prosthetic length and weak hip abductors or flexors can lead to circumduction, vaulting, and lateral trunk bending. Hip flexion

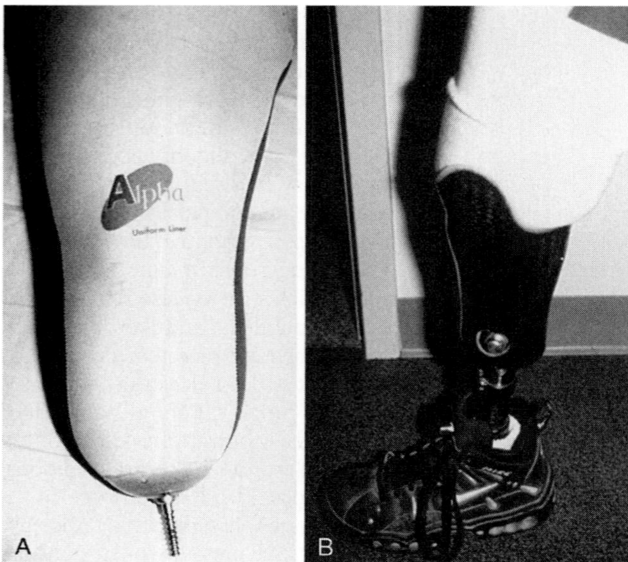

FIGURE 10–15 **A**, Gel liner suspension with locking pin. **B**, Transtibial prosthesis with liner locked in place.

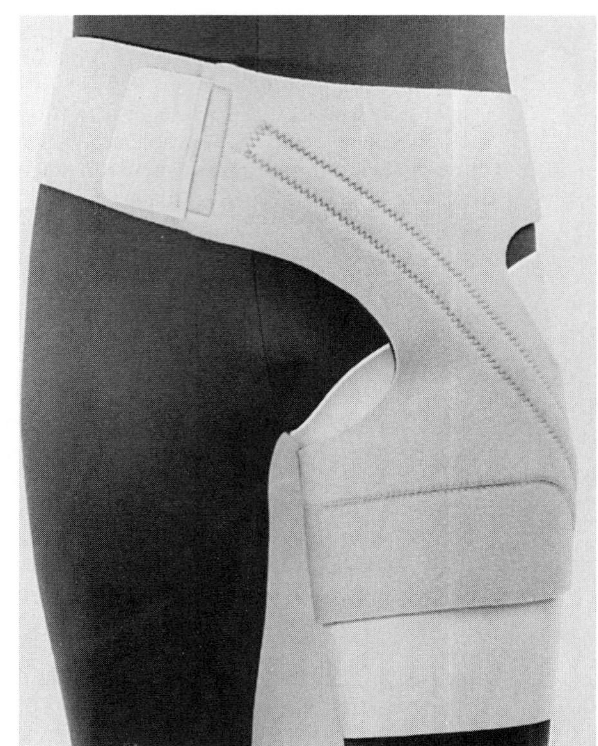

FIGURE 10–16 Total-elastic suspension belt for suspending a transfemoral socket. (Courtesy of Syncor Manufacturers, Green Bay, WI.)

TABLE 10-5 PROSTHETIC FOOT GAIT ABNORMALITIES

Foot Position	Gait Abnormality
Inset	Varus strain, pain (proximomedial, distolateral), circumduction
Outset	Valgus strain, pain (proximolateral, distomedial), broad-based gait
Forward placement	Increased knee extension (patellar pain) but stable
Posterior placement	Increased knee flexion/instability
Dorsiflexed foot	Increased patellar pressure
Plantar-flexed foot	Drop-off, patellar pressure

TABLE 10-6 TRANSFEMORAL PROSTHETIC GAIT ABNORMALITIES

Gait Abnormality	Prosthetic Problem
Lateral trunk bending	Short prosthesis, weak abductors, poor fit
Abducted gait	Poor socket fit medially
Circumducted gait	Prosthesis too long, excess knee friction
Vaulted gait	Prosthesis too long, poor suspension
Foot rotation at heel-strike	Heel too stiff, loose socket
Short stance phase	Painful stump, knee too loose
Knee instability	Knee too anterior, foot too stiff
Mediolateral whip	Excessive knee rotation, tight socket
Terminal snap	Quadriceps weakness, insecure patient
Foot slap, knee hyperextension	Heel too soft
Knee flexion	Heel too hard
Excessive lordosis	Hip flexion contracture, socket problems

contractures and insufficient anterior socket support can lead to excessive lumbar lordosis (compensatory). Inadequate prosthetic knee flexion can lead to a terminal knee snap. A medial whip (heel-in, heel-out) can be caused by a varus knee, excessive external rotation of the knee axis, or muscle weakness. A lateral whip (heel-out, heel-in) is caused by the opposite (valgus knee, internal rotation at knee, or muscle weakness). Table 10–6 summarizes common transfemoral prosthetic gait problems.

c. Stair climbing—In general, amputees ascend stairs by leading with the normal limb and descend by leading with the prosthetic limb ("the good goes up and the bad comes down").

IV. Orthoses

A. Introduction—The primary function of an orthosis is control of the motion of certain body segments. Orthoses are used to protect long bones or unstable joints, support flexible deformities, and occasionally substitute for a functional task. They may be static, dynamic, or a combination of these. With few exceptions, orthoses are not indicated for correction of fixed deformities or for spastic deformities that cannot be easily controlled manually. Orthoses are named according to the joints they control and the method used to obtain/maintain that control (e.g., a short leg, below-the-knee brace is an **ankle-foot orthosis** (AFO).

B. Shoes—Specific shoes can be used by themselves or in conjunction with foot orthoses. **Extra-depth shoes** with a high toe box designed to dissipate local pressures over bony prominences are recommended for diabetic patients. The plantar surface of an insensate foot is protected by use of a **pressure-dissipating material.** A paralytic or flexible foot deformity can be controlled with more rigid orthoses. **SACH heels** absorb the shock of initial loading and lessen the transmission of force to the midfoot as the foot passes through the stance phase. A **rocker sole** can lessen the bending forces on an arthritic or stiff midfoot during midstance, as the foot changes from accepting the weight-bearing load to pushing off. It is useful in treating metatarsalgia, hallux rigidus, and other forefoot problems. For the rocker sole to be effective, it must be rigid. Medial heel out-flaring is used to treat severe flatfoot of most causes. A foot orthosis is also necessary.

C. Foot orthoses—Most foot orthoses are used to align and support the foot; prevent, correct, or accommodate foot deformities; and improve foot function. Three main types of foot orthosis are used: **rigid, semirigid,** and **soft.** Rigid foot orthoses limit joint motion and stabilize flexible deformities. Semirigid orthoses have hinges and allow dorsiflexion and/or plantar flexion of the ankle. Soft orthoses have the best shock-absorbing ability and are used to accommodate fixed deformities of the feet, especially neuropathic, dysvascular, and ulcerative disorders.

D. AFO—The most commonly prescribed lower limb orthosis (AFO) is used to control the ankle joint. It may be fabricated with metal bars attached to the shoe or thermoplastic elastomer. The orthosis may be rigid, preventing ankle motion, or it can allow free or spring-assisted motion in either plane. After hindfoot fusions, the primary orthotic goals are absorption of the ground reaction forces, protection of the fusion sites, and protection of the midfoot. The thermoplastic foot section achieves mediolateral control with high trimlines. When subtalar motion is present, an articulating AFO permits motion by a mechanical ankle joint design. The primary factors in the selection of an orthotic joint include range of motion, durability, adjustability, and the biomechanical effect on the knee joint. A posterior leaf-spring AFO provides ankle instability in stance phase.

E. Knee-ankle-foot orthosis (KAFO)—This orthosis extends from the upper thigh to the foot. It is generally used to control an unstable or paralyzed knee joint. It provides mediolateral stability with the prescribed amounts of flexion or extension control. A subset of KAFOs are designated KOs **(knee orthoses)**. KOs can be made of elastic for the treatment of patellar pathology or of metal and plastic for the treatment of an unstable anterior cruciate ligament.

F. Hip-knee-ankle-foot orthosis (HKAFO)—This orthosis provides hip and pelvic stability but is rarely used by the adult paraplegic because of the cumbersome nature of the orthosis and the magnitude of effort in achieving minimum gains. Experimentally, it is being used in conjunction with implanted electrodes and the computerized functional stimulation of paraplegics. In children with upper-level lumbar myelomeningocele, the reciprocating gait orthoses are modified HKAFOs that can be used for standing and simulated walking.

G. Elbow orthoses—Hinged-elbow orthoses provide minimum stability in the treatment of ligament instability. Dynamic spring-loaded orthoses have been successfully used in the treatment of flexion and extension contractures.

H. Wrist-hand orthoses (WHOs)—The most common use of wrist and hand orthoses today is for postoperative care after injury or reconstructive surgery. These devices are static or dynamic. The opponens splint is successful in prepositioning the thumb but impairs tactile sensation. Wrist-driven hand orthoses are used in lower cervical quadriplegics. They may be body powered by tenodesis action or motor driven. Weight and cumbersomeness are the major limiting factors.

I. Fracture braces—Fracture bracing remains a valuable treatment option for isolated fractures of the tibia and fibula. Prefabricated fracture orthoses can be used in simple foot and ankle fractures, ankle sprains, and simple hand injuries.

J. Pediatric orthoses—Many dynamic orthoses are used by children to control motion without total immobilization. The Pavlik harness has become the mainstay for early treatment of developmental dislocation of the hip. Several dynamic orthoses have been used for containment in Perthes disease.

K. Spine orthoses

1. Cervical spine—Numerous orthoses are used to immobilize the cervical spine. Effective immobilization ranges from the various types of collars, to posted orthoses that gain purchase about the shoulders and under the chin, to the halo vest, which achieves the most stability by the nature of its fixation into the skull.
2. Thoracolumbar spine—Orthoses used to mechanically stabilize the back, thus reducing back pain, rely on increasing body cavity pressure. Three-point orthoses achieve their control by the length of their lever arm and the subsequent limitation of motion.

V. Surgery for Stroke and Closed Head Injury

A. Introduction—The orthopaedic surgeon can play a role in the early management of adult-acquired spasticity secondary to stroke or closed brain injury when the spasticity interferes with the rehabilitation program.

1. Nonsurgical treatment—Interventional modalities may include orthotic prescription, serial casting, and motor point nerve blocks with short-acting (bupivacaine HCl) or long-acting (phenol 6% in glycerol or Botox) agents. Splinting a joint (e.g., the ankle) in the neutral position is not sufficient to prevent the development of a contracture (e.g., an equinus contracture). When functional joint ranging is insufficient to control the deformity, intervention is often indicated. Local anesthetic injection to the posterior tibial nerve or sciatic nerve before casting relieves pain and allows for maximum correction of the deformity. Open nerve blocks may be warranted to avoid injecting mixed nerves with large sensory contributions.
2. Prerequisites for surgical treatment—Surgical intervention in adult-acquired spasticity should be delayed until the patient achieves maximum spontaneous motor recovery (6 months for stroke and 12-18 months for traumatic brain injury). When patients reach a plateau in functional progress or the deformity impedes further progress, intervention may be considered. Invasive procedures in this population should be an adjunct to a standard functional rehabilitation program, not an alternative. When surgery is considered as a method of improving function, patients should be screened for cognitive deficits, motivation, and body image awareness. Patients should not be confused and must have adequate short-term memory and the capacity for new learning. In addition to specific cognitive strengths, motivation is necessary for patients to use functional gains and participate in their rehabilitation program. Body image awareness is essential in order for surgical intervention to become meaningful and potentially beneficial. Patients who lack the awareness of a limb or its position in space should undergo therapy directed toward improving these deficits before undergoing surgical intervention.

B. Lower limb—Balance is the best predictor of a patient's ability to ambulate after acquired brain injury. The mainstay of treatment for the dynamic ankle equinus component of this gait deviation is to achieve ankle stability in the neutral position during initial floor contact (i.e., initial contact and stance) as well as floor clearance during the swing phase. An adjustable AFO with ankle dorsiflexion and a plantar flexion stop at the neutral position is often used during the recovery period, followed by a rigid AFO once the patient has reached a plateau in recovery. When the dynamic equinus overcomes the holding power of the orthosis and patients "walk out" of the brace, motor-balancing surgery is indicated. The equinus deformity is treated by percutaneous tendo Achillis lengthening. The dynamic varus-producing force in adults is the result of out-of-phase tibialis anterior muscle activity during the stance phase. This dynamic varus deformity is corrected by either split or complete lateral transfer of the tibialis anterior muscle.

C. Upper limb—There is a paucity of literature dealing with acquired spasticity in the upper limb. Invasive intervention can be considered for functional and nonfunctional goals.

1. Nonfunctional goals—Surgical release of static contracture is generally performed to complement nursing care or hygiene when the fixed contracture and/or spastic component results in skin maceration or breakdown.
2. Functional goals—One functional use of **static contracture release** is to improve upper extremity "tracking" (i.e., arm swing) during walking. Most upper extremity surgery performed in this patient population has the goal of increasing **prehensile hand function.** The goal may be simply to **improve placement,** enabling use of the hand as a "paperweight," or to achieve improved **fine motor control.** In patients with prehensile potential, surgery may allow the "one-handed" patient to be "two-handed" by increasing involved hand function from no

function to assistive or from assistive to independent.

a. Screening—When the goal of surgery is to improve function, patients must first be screened for **cognitive capacity, motivation, and body image awareness.** Patients must have the cognitive skills and learning capability to participate in their therapy after surgery and to functionally make use of their newly acquired skills at the completion of their rehabilitation program. If they are not motivated, they will not participate in the prolonged effort necessary to achieve meaningful functional improvement. Patients with poor stereognosis or neglect (i.e., poor body image awareness) find that the involved hand "drifts" in space and is not "available" for use if they have not been carefully trained in visual compensation techniques.

b. Grading—Once it has been determined that the patient has the potential to make functional upper extremity gains with surgery, he or she is graded on the basis of hand placement, proprioception and sensibility, and voluntary motor control. Dynamic electromyography is used when delineation of phasic motor activity is essential.

c. Methods—By means of fractional musculotendinous or step-cut methods, muscle unit lengthening of the agonist-deforming muscle units is combined with motor-balancing tendon transfers of the antagonists to achieve muscle balance and improved prehensile hand function.

VI. Spinal Cord Injury

A. Functional level—The functional level in a patient with spinal cord injury is determined by the most distal intact functional dermatome (sensory level) and the most distal motor level at which most of the muscles of that level function at least at a "fair" motor grade.

B. Mobility—The level at which spinal cord injury occurs determines mobility (Table 10–7). C4 and higher levels require high back and head support. At C5, mouth-driven accessories can control a motorized wheelchair. Various body-powered or motor-driven orthoses, such as a ratchet wrist-hand orthosis, can assist functional prehension. Manual wheelchairs and the use of a flexor hinge wrist-hand orthosis can be operated at C6 levels. Transfers are dependent at C4, assisted at C5, and independent at C6.

C. Activities of daily living—Patients at the C6 level can groom and dress themselves. Patients at the C7 level can cut meat. Bowel and bladder function can be controlled via rectal stimulation and intermittent catheterization.

D. Psychosocial factors—Men may be impotent but can often achieve a reflex erection.

E. Autonomic dysreflexia—This potentially catastrophic hypertensive event can occur with injuries above T5. It is usually caused by an obstructed urinary catheter or fecal impaction.

F. Surgery—Spinal fusion is frequently used to expedite rehabilitation and prevent the late development of pain or deformity at the fracture level. Anterior and/or posterior fusion with internal fixation should be performed soon after injury in order to facilitate early rehabilitation. Spasticity and contracture can produce hygiene problems or the development of pressure ulcers. Percutaneous (open) motor nerve blocks with phenol can be used to treat these deformities. When the deformity is a static contracture, muscle release or disarticulation may improve sitting or transfer potential. Tendon transfers can be used in the upper limb to eliminate the need for an

TABLE 10-7 TREATMENT OF SPINAL CORD INJURY BY FUNCTIONAL LEVEL

Functional Level	Working	Not Working	Treatment/Mobility
Above C4	—	Diaphragm, upper extremity muscles	Respirator dependent
C4	Diaphragm/trapezius	Upper extremity muscles	Wheelchair chin/puff
C5	Elbow flexors	Below elbow	Electric wheelchair, rachet
C6	Wrist extensors	Elbow extensors	Wheelchair, flexor hinge
C7	Elbow extensor	Grasp	Wheelchair, independent
C8	Finger flexors to middle finger		
T1	Intrinsic muscles	Abdominals/lower extremity muscles	Wheelchair, independent
T2-T12	Upper extremity muscles, abdominals	Lower extremity muscles	Wheelchair, HKAFO (nonfunctional ambulation)
L1	Upper extremity muscles, abdominals, quadriceps	Lower extremity muscles	KAFO; minimum ambulation
L2	Iliopsoas	Knee/ankle	KAFO, household ambulation
L3	Quadriceps	Ankle	AFO, community ambulation
L4	Tibialis anterior	Toe, plantar flexors	AFO, community ambulation
L5	EHL, EDL	Plantar flexors	AFO, independent
S1	Gastrocnemius/soleus	Bowel/bladder	± Metatarsal bar

AFO, ankle-foot orthosis; EDL, extensor digitorum longus; EHL, extensor hallucis longus; HKAFO, hip-knee-ankle-foot orthosis; KAFO, knee-ankle-foot orthosis; ±, with or without.

orthosis or allow the patient to achieve function with an orthosis.

VII. Postpolio Syndrome

A. Cause—Polio is a viral disease affecting the anterior horn cells of the spinal cord. Postpolio syndrome is not a reactivation of the polio virus. It is an aging phenomenon by which more nerve cells become inactive. The syndrome occurs after middle age. These patients use a high proportion of their capacity for normal activities of daily living. With aging and the drop-off of muscle units, they no longer have the reserves to perform their daily activities.

B. Treatment—Treatment comprises prescribed limited exercise combined with periods of rest, so muscles are maintained but not overtaxed. Standard polio surgeries, combining contracture release, arthrodesis, and tendon transfer, are indicated when the deformity overcomes functional capacity. The use of lightweight orthoses is important in helping patients to remain functionally independent.

Selected Bibliography

GAIT

Inman VT, Ralston H, Todd F: Human Walking. Baltimore, Williams & Wilkins, 1981.

Perry J: Gait Analysis: Normal and Pathological Function. New York, Slack [McGraw-Hill], 1992.

Ounpuu S: The biomechanics of running: A kinematic and kinetic analysis. Instr Course Lect 39:305, 1990.

AMPUTATIONS AND PROSTHESES

Smith D, Bowker J, Michael J, eds: Atlas of Amputations and Limb Deficiencies. Rosemont, IL, American Academy of Orthopaedic Surgeons, 2004.

Pinzur M, Gold J, Schwartz D, et al: Energy demands for walking in dysvascular amputees as related to the level of amputation. Orthopaedics 15:1033, 1992.

Waters RL, Perry J, Antonelli D, et al: Energy cost of walking of amputees: The influence of level of amputation. J Bone Joint Surg [Am] 58:42, 1976.

Wyss C, Harrington R, Burgess E, Matsen F: Transcutaneous oxygen tension as a predictor of success after an amputation. J Bone Joint Surg [Am] 70:203, 1988.

Gottschalk F, ed: Symposium on amputation. Clin Orthop 361:2, 1999.

Day H: The Proposed International Terminology for the Classification of Congenital Limb Deficiencies—The Recommendations of a Working Group of ISPO. London, Spastics International Medical Publications, Heinemann Medical Books [Philadelphia, JB Lippincott, 1975].

Bernd L, Blasius K, Lukoschek M, et al: The autologous stump plasty: Treatment for bony overgrowth in juvenile amputees. J Bone Joint Surg [Br] 73:203, 1991.

Gottschalk F: Traumatic amputations. In Bucholz RW, Heckman JD, eds: Fractures in Adults, pp 391–414. Philadelphia, Lippincott Williams & Wilkins, 2001.

Gottschalk F, Fisher D: Complications of amputation. In Conenwett JL, Gloviczki P, Johnston KW, et al, eds: Rutherford Vascular Surgery, pp 2213–2248. Philadelphia, WB Saunders, 2000.

Lagaard S, McElfresh E, Premer R: Gangrene of the upper extremity in diabetic patients. J Bone Joint Surg [Am] 71:257, 1989.

Gottschalk F, Kourosh S, Stills M, et al: Does socket configuration influence the position of the femur in above-knee amputation? J Prosthet Orthot 2:94, 1989.

ORTHOSES

Goldberg B, Hsu J, eds: Atlas of Orthoses and Assistive Devices, AAOS, 3rd ed. St. Louis, Mosby–Year Book, 1997.

STROKE AND CLOSED HEAD INJURY

Braun R: Stroke and brain injury. In Green D, ed: Operative Hand Surgery, pp 227–254. New York, Churchill Livingstone, 1988.

Pinzur M, Sherman R, Dimonte-Levine P, et al: Adult-onset hemiplegia: Changes in gait after muscle-balancing procedures to correct the equinus deformity. J Bone Joint Surg [Am] 68:1249, 1986.

CHAPTER 11

Trauma*

James P. Stannard, David A. Volgas, William M. Ricci, Daniel J. Sucato, Todd A. Milbrandt, and Matthew R. Craig

CONTENTS

SECTION 1 Care of the Multiply Injured Patient

Most orthopaedic surgeons, regardless of their subspecialty, will encounter trauma patients because trauma care is the foundation of orthopaedic practice in the United States. Therefore, an appreciation of the scope and treatment options for a wide variety of injuries is necessary.

I. Principles of Trauma Care

A. Trauma team—The orthopaedic surgeon is a member of the trauma team in all major teaching hospitals, reflecting the importance of fracture care for the management of the multiply injured patient. Fractures cause bleeding and pain and may lead to significant complications if they are not treated correctly from the initial presentation. As a member of the trauma team, the orthopaedic surgeon should be familiar with the overall management of the trauma patient. In the hectic environment of a trauma room, there must be a single "captain of the ship." This should be determined in advance. In most major trauma centers a trauma surgeon will assume that role, but in many smaller hospitals the ER physician may be that person. On rare occasions the orthopaedic surgeon may fulfill that role, especially in combat hospitals. Regardless of his or her role, the orthopaedic surgeon should communicate with the trauma team members and view his or her role as a part of an effort to maximize the patient's care. The orthopaedic surgeon should direct care in the management of fractures and their possible influence on the patient's outcome.

B. Primary assessment—Assessment begins with the primary survey, which seeks to identify any life-threatening injuries. A rapid assessment of the **a**irway, **b**reathing, and **c**irculation (ABC) is performed. The airway is often managed by intubation, especially in patients experiencing a great deal of pain or obtundation. The initial survey should include placement of

*The Appendix at the end of the book contains the pediatric and adult trauma tables.

TABLE 11-1 CLASSIFICATION AND TREATMENT OF HEMORRHAGIC SHOCK

	Parameters				
Class	*Blood Volume Loss (%)*	*Heart Rate*	*Blood Pressure*	*Urine Output*	**Treatment**
I	Up to 15%	< 100 bpm	Normal	> 30 mL/hr	Fluid replacement
II	15-30%	> 100 bpm	Decreased	20-30 mL/hr	Fluid replacement
III	30-40%	> 120 bpm	Decreased	5-15 mL/hr	Fluid and blood replacement
IV	> 40% (emergently life threatening)	> 140 bpm	Decreased	Negligible	Fluid and blood replacement

bpm, beats per minute.

From Browner BD, on behalf of the American College of Surgeons Committee on Trauma: Advanced Trauma Life Support: Skeletal Trauma: Basic Science, Management, and Reconstruction, 3rd ed, © 2003. Chicago, American College of Surgeons, 2001.

intravenous lines and treatment of any life-threatening injuries that are encountered. Aggressive fluid resuscitation should begin immediately in most cases. Hemodynamic instability may result from internal injury or fractures and is the most important consideration for the orthopaedic surgeon. Once the airway and breathing are controlled, circulation remains the biggest threat to life (Table 11–1).

C. Radiologic workup—A rapid radiologic workup that includes at a minimum anteroposterior (AP) chest, AP pelvis, and lateral cervical spine views is standard. Care should be taken not to focus on obvious radiographic findings such as an open-book pelvic injury and miss other important findings, such as a widened mediastinum. Pelvic fractures can be life-threatening. The orthopaedic surgeon may be called on to stabilize pelvic fractures in the ER and should be prepared to place a pelvic binder or sheet. Pelvic bleeding that does not respond rapidly to pelvic compression with a sheet or binder should be evaluated by angiography and embolization, if indicated.

D. Trauma scoring systems—Numerous scoring systems seek to quantify the injury that a patient sustained (Table 11–2 through 11–4). While some may yield prognostic value, none are perfect. Therefore, a thorough workup is needed to identify all injuries and prioritize their management. Although it may be desirable to repair all fractures on the day of admission, it may be inherently dangerous to do so because of hemodynamic instability and the added trauma that surgery creates. The **systemic inflammatory response syndrome** (SIRS) is a generalized response to trauma characterized by an increase in cytokines, complement, and many hormones. These changes are seen in varying degrees after trauma, and there is probably a genetic predisposition to an intense form of these changes. Patients are considered to have SIRS if they have 2 or more of the following criteria:

Heart rate greater than 90 beats per minute

White blood cell count (WBC) less than 4/mm^3 or greater than 10/mm^3

Respiration greater than 20, with $Paco_2$ less than 32 mm

Temperature less than 36°C or greater than 38°C

SIRS is associated with disseminated intravascular coagulopathy (DIC), acute respiratory distress syndrome (ARDS), renal failure, shock, and multisystem organ failure.

E. Damage-control orthopaedics—Principles of damage control have been applied to orthopaedic surgery and are now widely accepted. **Damage-control orthopaedics** (DCO) involves staging the definitive care of the patient to avoid adding to the overall trauma that the patient has undergone. Trauma is associated with a surge in inflammatory mediators, which peak 2 to 5 days after trauma. After the initial burst of cytokines and other mediators, leukocytes are "primed" and can be activated easily with further trauma, such as surgery. This may lead to multisystem organ failure or ARDS. Therefore, to minimize the additional trauma that is added with surgery, traumatologists will often treat only potentially life-threatening injuries during this acute inflammatory window. In the polytrauma patient or one with significant chest trauma, only emergent and urgent conditions should be treated. Compartment syndrome, fractures associated with vascular injury, unreduced dislocations, long bone fractures, open fractures, or unstable spine fractures should be stabilized acutely.

TABLE 11-2 GLASGOW COMA SCALE*

Response to Assessment	**Score**
Best Motor Response	
Obeys commands	6
Localizes pain	5
Normal withdrawal (flexion)	4
Abnormal withdrawal (flexion)—decorticate	3
Extension—decerebrate	2
None (flaccid)	1
Verbal Response	
Oriented	5
Confused conversation	4
Inappropriate words	3
Incomprehensible sounds	2
None	1
Eye Opening	
Spontaneous	4
To speech	3
To pain	2
None	1

**To calculate a Glasgow Coma Scale score, add the score for Eye Opening with the scores for Best Motor Response and Verbal Response. The best possible score is 15, and the worst possible score is 3.*

TABLE 11-3 ABBREVIATED INJURY SCORE

Examples of Abbreviated Injury Score	Score
Head	
Crush of head or brain	6
Brainstem contusion	5
Epidural hematoma (small)	4
Face	
Optic nerve laceration	2
External carotid laceration (major)	3
Le Fort III fracture	3
Neck	
Crushed larynx	5
Pharynx hematoma	3
Thyroid gland contusion	1
Thorax	
Open chest wound	4
Aorta, intimal tear	4
Esophageal contusion	2
Myocardial contusion	3
Pulmonary contusion (bilateral)	4
Two or three rib fractures	2
Abdominal and Pelvic Contents	
Bladder perforation	4
Colon transaction	4
Liver laceration with > 20% blood loss	3
Retroperitoneal hematoma	3
Splenic laceration—major	4
Spine	
Incomplete brachial plexus	2
Complete spinal cord, C4 or below	5
Herniated disc with radiculopathy	3
Vertebral body compression > 20%	3
Upper Extremity	
Amputation	3
Elbow crush	3
Shoulder dislocation	2
Open forearm fracture	3
Lower Extremity	
Amputation	
Below knee	3
Above knee	4
Hip dislocation	2
Knee dislocation	2
Femoral shaft fracture	3
Open pelvic fracture	3
External	
Hypothermia 31-30°C	3
Electrical injury with myonecrosis	3
Second- to third-degree burns—20-29% of body surface area	3

From Browner BD, et al, eds: Skeletal Trauma, 3rd ed, p 135. Philadelphia, WB Saunders, 2003.

TABLE 11-4 VARIABLES FOR THE MANGLED EXTREMITY SEVERITY SCORE

Component	Points
Skeletal and Soft Tissue Injury	
Low energy (stab, simple fracture, "civilian" gunshot wound)	1
Medium energy (open or multiplex fractures, dislocation)	2
High energy (close-range shotgun or "military" gunshot wound, crush injury)	3
Very high energy (same as above, plus gross contamination, soft tissue avulsion)	4
Limb Ischemia (score is doubled for ischemia > 6 hr***)***	
Pulse reduced or absent but perfusion normal	1
Pulseless, paresthesias, diminished capillary refill	2
Cool, paralyzed, insensate (numb)	3
Shock	
Systolic blood pressure always < 90 mm Hg	0
Transient hypotension	1
Persistent hypotension	2
Age (yr)	
< 30	0
30-50	1
> 50	2

From Johansen K, Daines M, Howey T, et al: Objective criteria accurately predict amputation following lower extremity trauma. J Trauma 30:568, 1990.

This may often be accomplished with an external fixator or splint. The definitive treatment of pelvic and acetabular fractures is usually delayed for 7-10 days in polytrauma patients to allow consolidation of the pelvic hematoma and resolution of the acute inflammatory response. Femur fractures may be converted from an external fixator to an intramedullary (IM) nail within 3 weeks, whereas tibia fractures should be converted within 7-10 days. If longer periods of time are necessary, a staged removal of the external fixator and subsequent nailing several days later are recommended.

II. Care of Injuries to Specific Tissues

A. Soft tissue injuries

1. Vascular injury—May be due to penetrating or blunt trauma.
   a. Diagnosis—The orthopaedic surgeon should recognize the injury and refer to a vascular surgery specialist or a microsurgeon, as indicated. Vascular injury can be present when pulses are palpable, and a change in pulse or a difference from the contralateral side may be the only harbinger of a serious vascular injury. If pulses are not equal to the uninjured side, a workup is indicated. Vascular compromise may develop over the course of hours in the case of knee dislocations and must be recognized promptly.
   b. Treatment—Reduction of fractures will often restore vascularity in the case of long bone fractures.
2. Compartment syndrome
   a. Diagnosis—One of the most frequently missed complications of trauma. It results when intracompartmental pressure exceeds capillary pressure, thus preventing exchange of waste

and nutrients across vessel walls. Unless it is treated within 4-6 hours, permanent injury will ensue. The diagnosis is clinical or made using a pressure monitor. Clinical hallmarks are pain out of proportion to the injury and pain with passive stretching of the muscle. Intracompartmental pressure measurement is abnormal if pressure is within 30 mm of the diastolic pressure *or* greater than 30 mm of the absolute pressure (the criteria are debated).

b. Treatment—Treatment is emergent decompression via fasciotomy.

c. Sequelae—Sequelae are common and include claw toes and contractures in the hand.

3. Nerve injury
   a. Cause—Caused when intracompartmental pressure exceeds capillary pressure, thus preventing exchange of nutrients across vessel walls. The most common form is nerve palsy (neurapraxia) caused by stretching of the nerve, which will recover over time (1 mm/day).
   b. Treatment
      (1) Nerve laceration (neurotmesis)—May be treated by repair or grafting. The results are variable according to the specific nerve injured and the degree of injury to the nerve.
      (2) Disruption of the nerve axon with an intact epineurium (axonotmesis)—May be treated initially by observation.
4. Bites
   a. Snake bites
      (1) Tend to occur in certain regions of the United States. Envenomation occurs in only 25% of cases. Venom may be neurotoxic (coral snakes) or hemotoxic (rattlesnake, cottonmouth).
      (2) Treatment and complications—Treatment is symptomatic and expectant—antivenom in a monitored setting, débridement of necrotic tissue, and fasciotomy. Antivenom is available for all endemic snakes, but there is a high incidence of anaphylaxis or serum sickness associated with its use. Complications can include severe local tissue necrosis, compartment syndrome, coagulopathies, and arrhythmias.
   b. Human and animal bites
      (1) Pathogens—Despite the association of certain bites with specific bacteria, *Staphylococcus* and *Streptococcus* remain the most prevalent pathogens. Other pathogens:
         Cat bites—*Pasteurella*
         Dog bites—*Eikenella*
         Human bites—Variable, including *Eikenella*
      (2) Treatment—A broad-spectrum antibiotic is commonly given, although regional variations are also common.
5. Thermal injury
   a. Hypothermia
      (1) Cause—Injury is caused by ice crystals forming outside the cell(s).
      (2) Treatment—Rapid rewarming and attention to arrhythmias are the current treatments. Amputation may be necessary.
   b. Burns—Generally treated by burn surgeons, but extremity burns may be treated by orthopaedic surgeons. Débridement of deep dermal burns and skin grafting are the hallmarks of treatment after early, aggressive fluid resuscitation. Antibiotic prophylaxis and tetanus are routine.
6. Electrical injury—May cause bone necrosis and massive soft tissue necrosis. The extent of tissue injury may not be apparent for days after injury because the skin may not be broken despite significant injury underneath. Treatment is similar to burns; débridement followed by reconstruction with amputation, a flap, or a skin graft is required.
7. Chemical burns—The first rule is to avoid contamination from other people and further damage to the victim. Dilution with copious irrigation is the initial treatment. After initial irrigation, the degree of necrosis is assessed, with débridement of necrotic tissue. Hydrofluoric acid is extremely toxic, causing profound hypocalcemia and cardiac death with little exposure; calcium gluconate may be used to treat skin exposure.
8. High-pressure injury (water, paint, grease)—Hand injuries are the most common. There may be extensive damage to underlying soft tissues despite a small entrance wound. Wide débridement of necrotic tissue and foreign material is required.

B. Joint injuries—Joint injuries may be caused by penetrating or blunt trauma.

1. Dislocations—These orthopaedic emergencies should be reduced as soon as possible to avoid injury to the nerve and vessels and the articular cartilage; general anesthesia may be needed. Neurovascular status should be assessed and documented both before and after reduction.
2. Open joint injuries
   a. Antibiotics—Penetrating trauma such as gunshot wounds may be treated with oral antibiotics if there is no debris in the joint; however, foreign matter is often carried into the joint as it is penetrated, even in "clean" gunshot wounds.
   b. Reverse arthrocentesis (injecting saline into the joint and observing the injured area for signs of extravasation)—This may miss a small puncture wound.
3. Fractures involving the joints—Must be reduced as anatomically as possible in order to reduce unequal wear.

C. Fractures

1. Open fractures
   a. Classification—The Gustillo and Anderson grading system is widely used (Table 11–5). There is considerable interobserver variability, and the grade may change with time.
      Grade I—No periosteal stripping, minimum soft tissue damage, small skin wound (1 cm)

TABLE 11-5 CLASSIFICATION OF OPEN FRACTURES

Fracture Type	Description
I	Skin opening of 1 cm or less, quite clean. Most likely from inside to outside. Minimum muscle contusion. Simple transverse or short oblique fractures.
II	Laceration more than 1 cm long, with extensive soft tissue damage, flaps, or avulsion. Minimum to moderate crushing component. Simple transverse or short oblique fractures with minimum comminution.
III	Extensive soft tissue damage, including muscles, skin, and neurovascular structures. Often a high-velocity injury with severe crushing component.
IIIA	Extensive soft tissue laceration, adequate bone coverage. Segmental fractures, gunshot injuries.
IIIB	Extensive soft tissue injury, with periosteal stripping and bone exposure. Usually associated with massive contamination.
IIIC	Vascular injury requiring repair

From Gustilo RB, Mendoza RM, Williams DN: Problems in the management of type III (severe) open fractures: A new classification of type III open fractures. J Trauma 24:742, 1984.

Grade II—Little periosteal stripping, moderate muscle damage, skin wound (1-10 cm)
Grade IIIA—Contaminated wound (high-energy gunshot wound, farm injury, shotgun) or extensive periosteal stripping with large skin wound (> 10 cm)
Grade IIIB—Same as IIIA, but will require flap coverage
Grade IIIC—same as IIIA, but with vascular injury that requires repair

b. Treatment
   (1) Débridement—Initial treatment should consist of local wound débridement that is adequate to clean the wound and débridement of all necrotic tissue.
   (2) Antibiotics—Usually started immediately. Antibiotic bead pouch with methylmethacrylate, tobramycin, and/or vancomycin may be used to temporize dirty wounds.
      (a) Grades I and II—First-generation cephalosporin (cephazolin) for 24 hours
      (b) Grade III—Cephalosporin and aminoglycoside for 72 hours after last incision and drainage
      (c) Heavily contaminated wounds and farm wounds—Cephalosporin, aminoglycosides, and high-dose penicillin
   (3) Stabilization of bony injuries—Will decrease further damage to soft tissue
   (4) Early coverage (< 5 days is the goal)
      (a) Gastrocnemius flap—For proximal third tibial fractures
      (b) Soleus flap—For middle third tibial fractures
      (c) Fasciocutaneous flap or free-tissue transfer—For distal third fractures
   (5) Negative-pressure therapy is commonly used to treat wounds.

2. Stabilization with external fixation
   a. Immediate treatment—Most fractures should be reduced and splinted promptly to avoid further soft tissue damage. External fixation may be used to treat grossly contaminated wounds and fractures that will require time for the soft tissues to heal before definitive fixation.
   b. Definitive treatment—External fixation may be used definitively for periarticular fractures, articular fractures that cannot be reconstructed, and segmental fractures.
3. Perioperative complications
   a. **Thromboembolic disease** (TED)—The incidence is very high in pelvic, spine, hip, and lower extremity fractures. Pulmonary embolus develops in as many as 5% of those who have **deep venous thrombosis** (DVT).
      (1) Diagnosis—Diagnosis of a DVT is by Doppler ultrasound, magnetic resonance venography, or D-dimer titers
      (2) Treatment—All patients with these injuries should receive some form of TED prophylaxis (mechanical or pharmacologic). The risks of pharmacologic prophylaxis include prolonged bleeding from surgical or traumatic wounds or a cerebral bleed.
   b. Fat embolus syndrome—Associated with reaming of long bones, but can occur with any long bone fracture. Hypoxia, a petechial rash on the chest, and tachycardia are the hallmarks. Treatment is supportive.
   c. ARDS—Patients with chest trauma and multiple fractures are at high risk. It is unclear whether reamed nailing of long bone fractures causes it directly, but may be implicated in the "second hit" phenomenon. Treatment is supportive (O_2, ventilator).
4. Fracture complications
   a. Delayed union—Defined as no progression of healing over serial radiographs. Treatment may include bone grafting and external bone stimulation.
   b. Nonunion
      (1) Classification (Fig. 11–1)
      (2) New treatments—Many new treatments, but scanty literature to support any one over the others
         (a) Calcium sulfate—Short resorption time
         (b) Calcium phosphate—Very long resorption time
         (c) BMP—Expensive, indicated in acute tibia and distal radius fractures, and possibly useful in nonunions
         (d) Platelet-derived growth factors—Seek to add osteoinductive factors to an osteoconductive matrix (cancellous bone, calcium)
      (3) Traditional treatment
         (a) Identify infection and treat appropriately

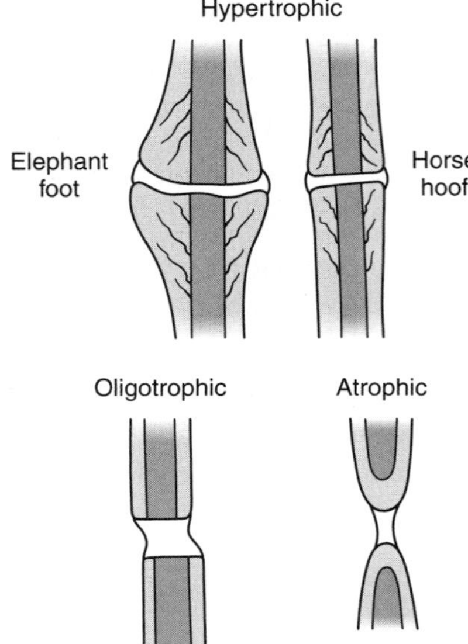

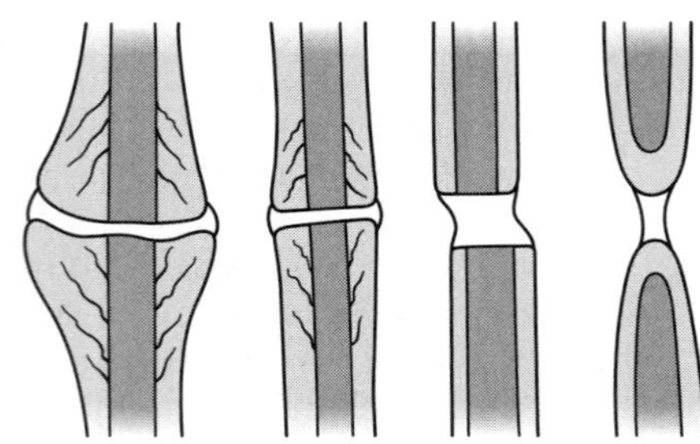

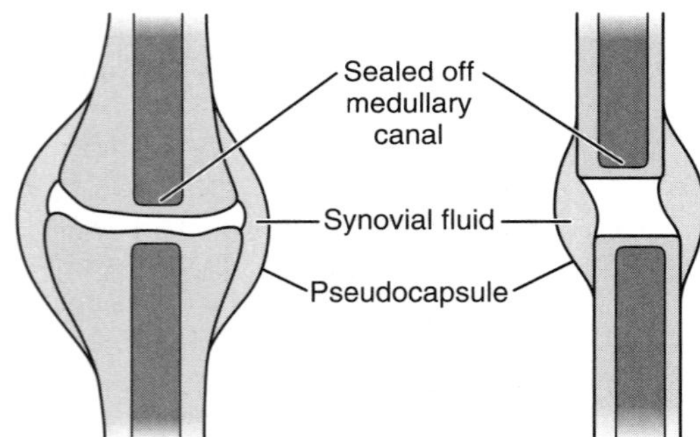

Synovial Pseudarthrosis

Sealed off medullary canal

Synovial fluid

Pseudocapsule

FIGURE 11–1 Classification of nonunions. (From Browner BD, et al, eds: Skeletal Trauma, 3rd ed, p 532. Philadelphia, WB Saunders, 2003.)

(b) Correct any deformity

(c) Provide stability (for hypertrophic nonunions)

(d) Preserve native biology

c. Segmental bone loss—Treatment includes treatment with bone graft and cage (similar to spine); interposition free tissue transfer (free-fibula transfer); bone transport (Ilizarov or Taylor spatial frame); and amputation.

d. **Heterotopic ossification** (HO)

(1) Diagnosis—Common in head-injured patients and in hip, elbow, and shoulder fractures. Any fracture associated with extensive muscle damage is subject to HO.

(2) Prophylaxis—Indomethacin 25 mg PO t.i.d. or indomethacin (sustained release) 75 mg PO q.d. for 6 weeks may be effective in preventing heterotopic bone formation.

(3) Treatment—Treatment is early, active **range of motion** (ROM) for the elbow and shoulder. Acetabular surgery usually requires postoperative radiation therapy (600-700 cGy).

e. Osteomyelitis

(1) Diagnosis

(a) Definitive diagnosis—By bone biopsy

(b) Other tests—May be used in combination with physical examination (draining wound, pain) to confirm the diagnosis.

(i) **Magnetic resonance imaging** (MRI)—95% sensitive and 90% specific

(ii) **Technetium 99m** (^{99m}Tc) study —85% sensitive and 80% specific

(iii) Indium study—95% sensitive and 85-90% specific

(2) Treatment—Based on grade and host type (Cierny/Mader)

(a) Grade

Grade I—**Intramedullary** (IM) nail removal and reaming

Grade II—Superficial; involves cortex; often seen in diabetic wounds; curettage

Grade III—Localized; involves cortical lesion, with extension into medullary canal; requires wide excision, bone grafting, and perhaps stabilization

TABLE 11-6 CLASSIFICATION OF CLOSED FRACTURES WITH SOFT TISSUE DAMAGE

Fracture Type	Description
0	Minimum soft tissue damage. Indirect violence. Simple fracture patterns. Example: torsion fracture of the tibia in skiers.
I	Superficial abrasion or contusion caused by pressure from within. Mild to moderately severe fracture configuration. Example: pronation fracture-dislocation of the ankle joint with soft tissue lesion over the medial malleolus.
II	Deep, contaminated abrasion associated with localized skin or muscle contusion. Impending compartment syndrome. Severe fracture configuration. Example: Segmental "bumper" fracture of the tibia
III	Extensive skin contusion or crush injury. Underlying muscle damage may be severe. Subcutaneous avulsion. Decompensated compartment syndrome. Associated major vascular injury. Severe or comminuted fracture configuration.

From Tscherne H, Oestern HJ: Die Klassifizierung des Weichteilschadens bei offenen und geschlossenen Frakturen. Unfallheilkunde 85:111–115, 1982. © Springer-Verlag.

Grade IV—Diffuse; involves spread through cortex and along medullary canal; wide sequestrectomy, muscle flap, bone graft, and stabilization

(b) Host

A—Normal, healthy patient

B—Locally compromised (vasculopathic)

C—Not considered a medical candidate for surgery; may require suppressive antibiotics

f. Fractures caused by gunshot wounds

(1) High-energy gunshot and shotgun wounds—These are considered grade III open fractures because they are often associated with considerable soft tissue injury (Table 11–6). They require extensive surgical débridement of necrotic tissue and require surgical stabilization of the fracture.

(2) Low-energy gunshot wounds—Can be treated as a closed fracture, but should get single-dose, first-generation cephalosporin.

(3) Bullets that pass through colon—Will contaminate any fracture caused by the bullet after perforation (pelvis, spine).

SECTION 2 Upper Extremity

I. Shoulder Injuries (Tables 11–7 and 11–8)

A. Sternoclavicular dislocation—"Serendipity" view or **computed tomographic** (CT) scan reveals dislocation of the sternoclavicular joint.

1. Anterior dislocation—Treated by closed reduction
2. Posterior dislocation—May cause dysphagia or difficulty breathing and sensation of fullness in the throat. Treated by closed reduction with a towel clip in the operating room. A thoracic surgeon should be on standby.
3. Chronic dislocation—Treated by resection of the medial clavicle, with preservation and reconstruction of costoclavicular ligaments.

B. Clavicle fracture (Fig. 11–2)

1. Classification—Classified by thirds (medial, middle, distal)
2. Diagnosis—**Coracoclavicular** (CC) and **acromioclavicular** (AC) ligaments may be ruptured.
3. Treatment
   a. Nonoperative treatment—Generally treated nonoperatively in a sling, but there is evidence for operative plate fixation of markedly displaced fractures.
   b. Operative treatment—Some authors recommend operative treatment of distal fractures that extend into the AC joint, while others recommend a late Mumford procedure.
   c. Fixation—Some authors recommend fixation when a clavicle fracture is associated with a displaced glenoid neck fracture, whereas others do not consider it necessary.

C. AC dislocation

1. Classification—Classified by extent of involvement of the ligamentous support and direction and magnitude of displacement (Fig. 11–3)
   Type I—Sprain of AC joint
   Type II—Rupture of AC ligaments and sprain of CC ligaments
   Type III—Rupture of both AC and CC ligaments
   Type IV—The clavicle is buttonholed through the trapezius posteriorly
   Type V—The trapezius and deltoid are detached
   Type VI—The clavicle is translocated beneath the coracoid
2. Treatment
   a. Types I and II—Always treated with brief immobilization in a sling.
   b. Type III—May be treated nonoperatively, but many would advocate early operative treatment in patients who are heavy laborers and throwers. The Weaver-Dunn procedure is the treatment of choice.
   c. Types IV-VI—Usually treated operatively.

D. Scapula fracture—Associated with pulmonary contusion and pneumothorax. Scapula body fractures are generally treated in a sling for 7-10 days and then early ROM.

E. Glenoid fracture

1. Nonoperative treatment—Used for nondisplaced fractures.
2. Operative treatment—Indicated for fractures that are displaced more than 2 mm. The approach is usually through a posterior portal, although the Nevaiser portal may be used to place a superoinferior screw in the glenoid.

F. Glenoid neck fracture

1. Nonoperative treatment—Many authors advocate nonoperative treatment in almost all cases.
2. Operative treatment—Many authors advocate reduction and plating through a posterior approach for the patient whose glenoid neck and humeral head are translocated anterior to the proximal fragment or are medially displaced.

G. Scapulothoracic dissociation—The result of significant trauma to the chest wall, lung, and heart. It is often associated with brachial plexus or vascular injury. Treatment is with immobilization in a sling.

H. Closed forequarter amputation—An uncommon injury, but associated with very high incidence of injury to the neurovascular structures. It may be associated with avulsion of brachial plexus roots and brachial or subclavian artery and may be life-threatening. Prompt repair of vascular injuries is required. Chronic flail arm and pain are the rule.

TABLE 11-7 ADULT SHOULDER DISLOCATIONS/LIGAMENTOUS INJURIES

Injury	Eponym/Other Name	Classification	Treatment	Complications
Anterior (glenohumeral [GH]) dislocation (most common))		Subcoracoid > subglenoid (also subclavicular and intrathoracic)	Must get axillary view of GH joint; reduce, immobilize (young patient, 4 wk; old patient, 2 wk); passive > active (Rockwood 7)	Axillary nerve neuropraxia, axillary artery injury, cuff injury (>40 yr old), recurrence (85% in <20 yr old), bone injury (head [Hill-Sachs], greater tuberosity, glenoid)
Recurrent/multidirectional		Anterior dislocation/subluxation atraumatic	Prolonged rehabilitation (rotator cuff strengthening); if failure, consider surgery (inferior capsular shift)	Look for generalized laxity; AMBRI
			Bankart repair: Anterior capsule → anterior rim	Late instability
			Staple capsulorrhaphy: Capsule → glenoid	Late degenerative joint disease (DJD), migration
			Putti-Platt repair: Subscapularis imbrication	Late DJD, ↓ external rotation (ER)
			Magnuson-Stack repair: Subscapularis → lesser tuberosity	Late DJD, ↓ER
			Bone block: Crest graft, anterior	↓range of motion, migration
			Bristow repair: Coracoid transfer	Nonunion, ↓ER, migration
			Capsular shift: Redundant capsule, advanced	Minimum procedure of choice with MDI
Posterior dislocation		Subacromial (seizures and shocks) (most common)	Reduce, immobilize for 3-6 wk; rotator cuff strengthening; operate if recurrent (glenoid osteotomy, bone block, posterior capsular shift)	Lesser tuberosity fracture, late recognition (may require advancement of lesser tuberosity into defect or total shoulder arthroplasty [place in less retroversion]); avoid by checking axial view
Inferior GH	Luxatio erecta		Reduce and immobilize; rotator cuff strengthening, rehabilitation	Neurovascular injury can resolve after reduction; axillary artery thrombosis; watch for rotator cuff tear
Acromioclavicular (AC) injury		I—AC sprain	7-10 days rest/immobilization, sling	Joint stiffness, deformity, CC ligament and soft tissue calcification, AC DJD, associated fractures, distal clavicle osteolysis
		II—AC tear, coracoclavicular (CC) sprain	Sling for 2 wk, rehabilitation, late-excision arthroplasty if required	
		III—AC tear, CC tear	Conservative vs. repair (athletes, laborers); Weaver-Dunn	
		IV—Clavicle through trapezius posteriorly	Reduce and repair	
		V—Clavicle 100-300% elevated; trapezius, deltoid detached	Reduce and repair (Weaver-Dunn)	
		VI—Clavicle inferior to coracoid	Reduce and repair	
Sternoclavicular injury			Evaluate with "serendipity" view or computed tomography	Bump (cosmetic), DJD, mediastinal impingement (dysphagia, throat fullness), hardware migration (with operative treatment)
		Anterior dislocation	Closed reduction with traction	
		Posterior dislocation	Closed reduction with towel clip or open; thoracic surgeon on standby	
		Chronic dislocation	Medial clavicle resection or ligament reconstruction (thoracic surgeon on standby)	
		Spontaneous atraumatic subluxation	Nonoperative	

*AMBRI, **a**traumatic, **m**ultidirectional, **b**ilateral, treated by **r**ehabilitation **i**nstability; MDI, multidirectional instability.*

TABLE 11-8 ADULT SHOULDER FRACTURES

Injury	Eponym	Classification	Treatment	Complications
Proximal humerus fracture		Neer (parts >5 mm or 45-degree displacement)		Missed dislocation, adhesive capsulitis (moist heat, gentle range of motion), malunion (reconstruction or total shoulder arthroplasty [TSA] required), avascular necrosis (AVN) (TSA required), nonunion (surgical neck, tuberosity fractures: ORIF), disrupted rotator cuff
		One-part (most common); impaction of the humeral neck	Sling for comfort, early motion; isometrics initially, advancing to progressive resistance	
		Two-part; displacement of the greater tuberosity >5 mm	Closed reduction unless articular segment (open reduction with internal fixation [ORIF]), shaft (impacted and angulated: traction, Velpeau; unimpacted: closed reduction, closed reduction with percutaneous pinning [CRPP] or ORIF), greater tuberosity (repair cuff), tuberosity with block to internal rotation (ORIF)	
		Three-part; displacement of the greater and lesser tuberosities >5 mm	ORIF in younger; prosthesis in older; repair of rotator cuff	
		Four-part; head splitting	Same as three-part; nonoperative in elderly/diabetic/ impacted four-part valgus pattern	
Proximal humerus fracture-dislocation		Anterior (greater tuberosity displacement)	Closed reduction; if >1 cm after reduction, open repair	As above, with the addition of axillary nerve or plexus injury, myositis ossificans (wait >1 yr to excise heterotopic bone)
		Posterior (lesser tuberosity displacement)	Closed reduction, ORIF if three-part; treatment for fracture as above	
Impression/ impaction of humeral head	Hill-Sachs	Stable (<20% articular surface)	Closed treatment	AVN, degenerative joint disease (DJD) (TSA)
		Unstable (20-50%)	Transfer of lesser tuberosity → defect (McLaughlin)	
		Unstable (>45%)	Prosthesis vs. rotational osteotomy	
Scapula fracture		Zdravkovic and Damholt		Associated injuries (clavicle, rib, pulmonary contusion, pneumothorax), axillary artery injury, plexus palsy, pressure symptoms, vascular and plexus injuries
		I—Body	Most treated nonoperatively	
		II—Coracoid and acromion	Associated injury common; ORIF of large, displaced fragments	
		III—Neck and glenoid	ORIF of large, unstable fractures (glenoid with displaced clavicle fracture)	
Clavicle fracture		Middle one third (most common)	Nonoperative: sling, figure 8 brace ORIF: displacement, ipsilateral displaced glenoid neck fracture	Vascular injury/pneumothorax, ligament injury (CC or AC), skin necrosis, malunion (osteotomy for young, active patient); nonunion (ORIF and bone graft), nerve injury (rare); muscle fatigue/ weakness, DJD (if articular)
		Distal one third (Neer)		
		I—Minimum interligamentous displacement (coracoclavicular [CC], acromioclavicular [AC])	Nonoperative; sling for comfort	
		II—Fracture medial to CC ligaments	Nonoperative if nondisplaced; consider ORIF for displaced fracture	
		IIA—Both ligaments attached to distal fragment	ORIF	
		IIB—Conoid torn, trapezoid attached to distal fragment	ORIF	
		III—AC joint	Closed treatment; late-excision arthroplasty if required	
		Proximal one third	Closed treatment	
Glenoid fracture		Ideberg		Nonoperative treatment if nondisplaced
		I—Anterior avulsion fracture	>25% of surface: ORIF if head is subluxated with major fragment; posterior approach	
		II—Transverse/obliquefracture,inferiorglenoidfree		
		III—Upper one third of glenoid and coracoid		
		IV—Horizontal glenoid through body		
		V—Combination of II-IV		
Scapulothoracic dissociation		(Seen on scapular lateral or chest radiograph)	Closed reduction, sling immobilization	Vascular and brachial plexus injuries, associated clavicle fracture

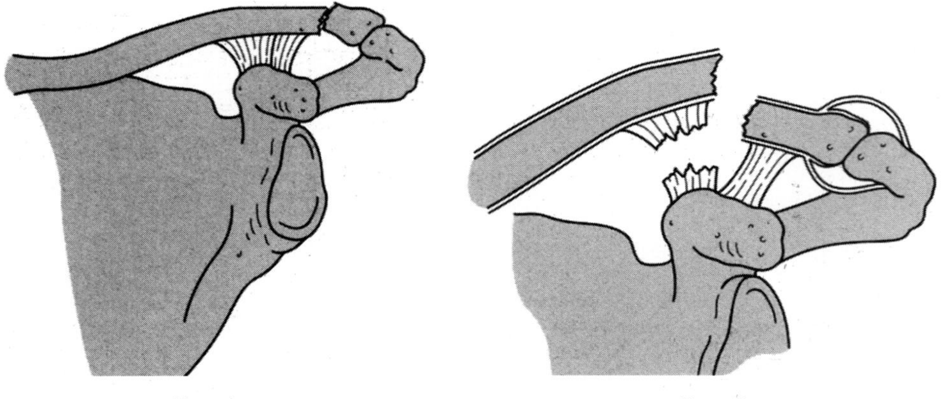

FIGURE 11–2 When the distal end of the clavicle is fractured, the ligaments may either remain intact and maintain apposition of the fracture fragments (Type I) or rupture, allowing wide displacement of the fragments (Type II). (Redrawn from Rockwood CA, Green DP, eds: Fractures, vol 1, 4th ed. Philadelphia, JB Lippincott, 1996.)

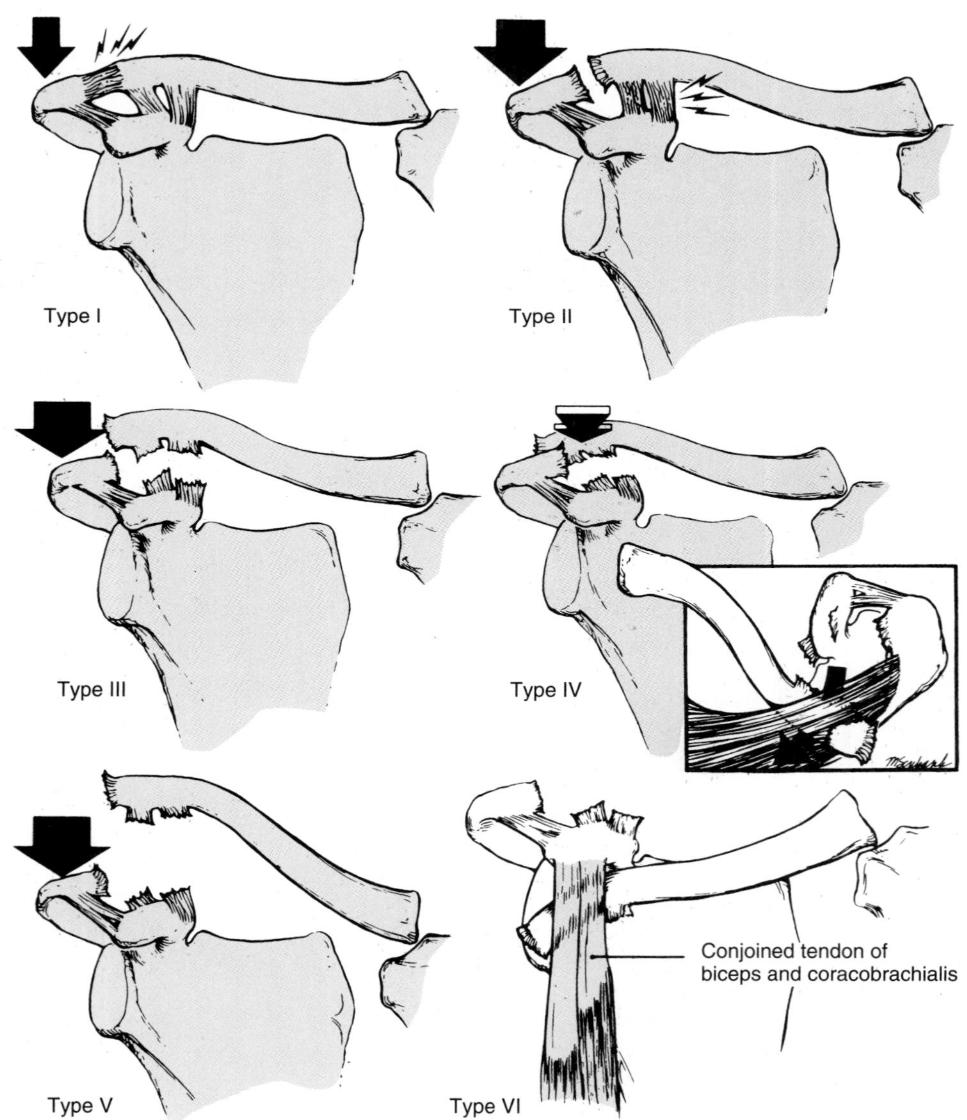

FIGURE 11–3 Classification of acromioclavicular injuries. (From Neer CS, Rockwood CA: Fractures dislocations of the shoulder. In Rockwood CA, Green DP, eds: Fractures in Adults, 2nd ed, p 871. Philadelphia, JB Lippincott, 1984. Reprinted by permission.)

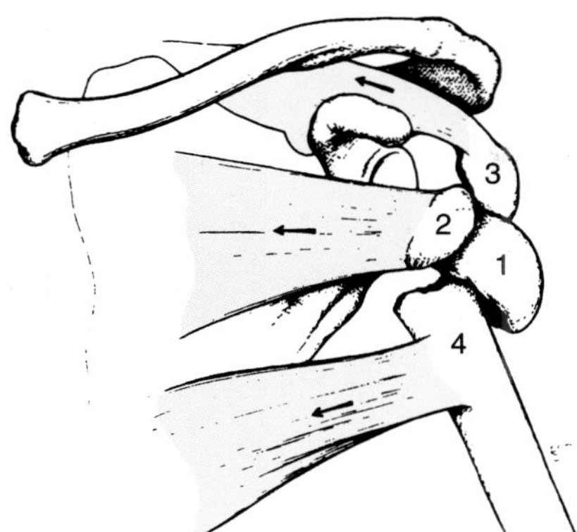

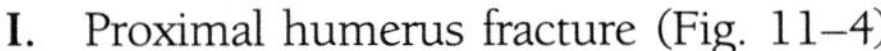

FIGURE 11–4 Proximal humeral fracture. There are four parts: 1, head; 2, lesser tuberosity; 3, greater tuberosity; and 4, humeral shaft. (From Neer CS, Rockwood CA: Fractures and dislocations of the shoulder. In Rockwood, CA, and Green, DP, eds: Fractures in Adults, 2nd ed, p 696. Philadelphia, JB Lippincott, 1984.)

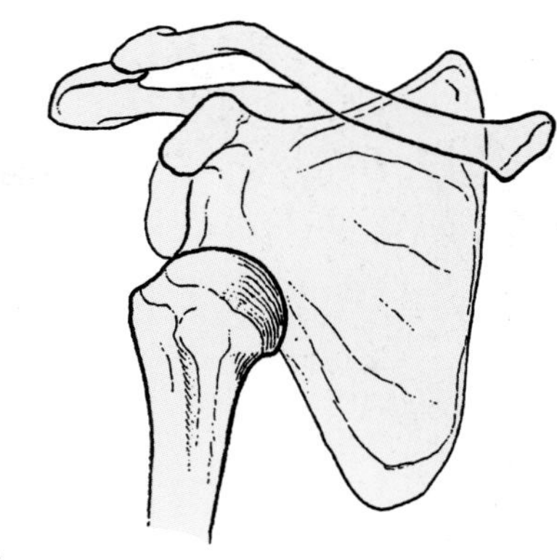

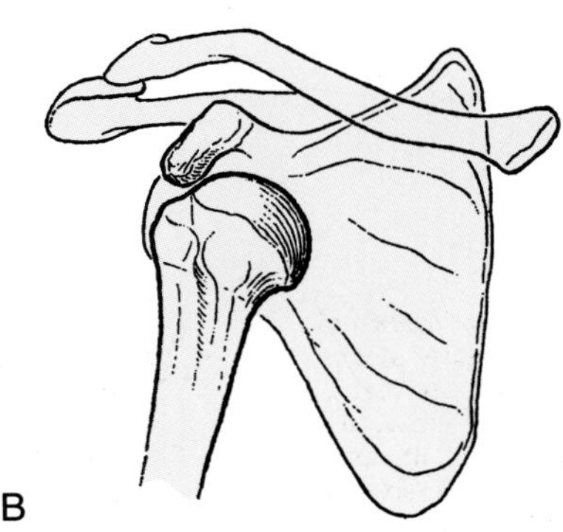

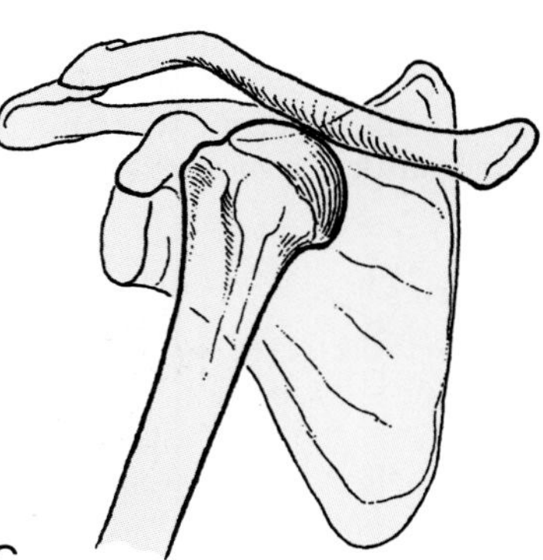

FIGURE 11–5 Anterior shoulder dislocation. **A**, Subglenoid. **B**, Subcoracoid. **C**, Subclavicular. (From Connolly JF, ed: DePalma's The Management of Fractures and Dislocations: An Atlas, 3rd ed, p 617. Philadelphia, WB Saunders, 1981.)

I. Proximal humerus fracture (Fig. 11–4)
1. Neer classification ("part" is defined as displacement of more than 5 mm or angulation of less than 45 degrees)
   a. One-part—Impaction of the humeral neck
   b. Two-part—Displacement of the greater tuberosity of more than 5 mm; associated with rotator cuff tear
   c. Three-part—Displacement of the greater and lesser tuberosities
   d. Four-part—"Head splitting"
2. Treatment
   a. One-part—Sling for comfort and early mobilization
   b. Two-part—Repair of the displaced tuberosity with sutures or tension band wiring; surgical neck fractures can normally be managed nonoperatively
   c. Three-part—**Open reduction with internal fixation** (ORIF) for young patients, with repair of the rotator cuff; hemiarthroplasty for older patients, with repair of the rotator cuff
   d. Four-part—Same as three-part

J. Shoulder dislocation
1. Anterior or anteroinferior (Fig. 11–5)
   a. Diagnosis
      (1) Apprehension sign
      (2) The axillary view is diagnostic
      (3) Usually traumatic and unilateral
      (4) Usually painful
   b. Treatment
      (1) Sling for 2 weeks in the elderly and 4 weeks in the young; followed by rotator cuff strengthening
      (2) Consider operative treatment in cases of recurrence or rotator cuff tear.
      (3) High recurrence rate in young patients
      (4) High incidence of rotator cuff injury in older patients
2. Multidirectional
   a. Diagnosis
      (1) Often bilateral
      (2) Often atraumatic, not painful
      (3) Examination of the shoulder reveals subluxation posteriorly as well as anteriorly and inferiorly
      (4) Generalized ligamentous laxity
   b. Treatment
      (1) Rotator cuff strengthening
      (2) Inferior capsular shift is indicated if instability is refractory to nonoperative treatment.
3. Posterior (Fig. 11–6)
   a. Diagnosis
      (1) Associated with seizures and electrical shock
      (2) Often missed but easily seen on axillary view

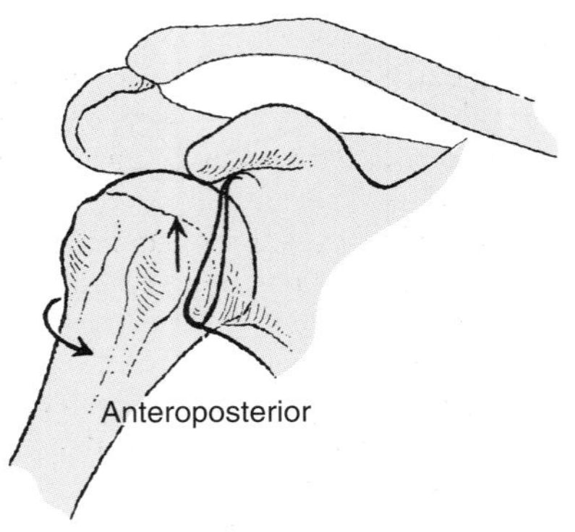

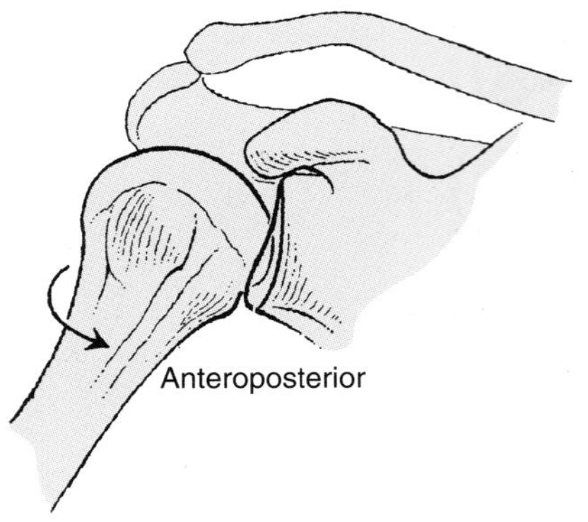

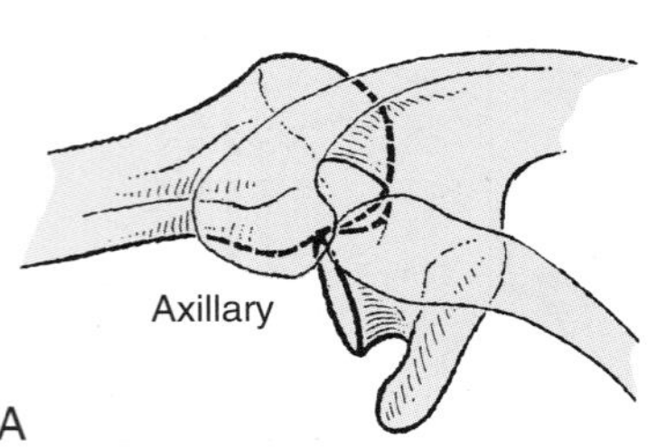

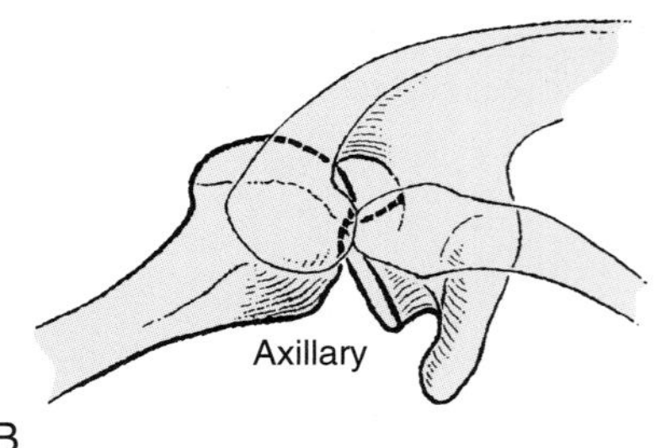

FIGURE 11–6 Posterior shoulder dislocation. **A**, Subacromial. **B**, Subcoracoid. (From Connolly JF, ed: DePalma's The Management of Fractures and Dislocations: An Atlas, 3rd ed, p 633. Philadelphia, WB Saunders, 1981.)

(3) May have fracture of lesser tuberosity or reverse Hill-Sachs lesion

b. Treatment
   (1) Immobilization for 3-6 weeks
   (2) Rotator cuff strengthening
   (3) Possible open bone grafting of humeral head defect and repair of posterior labral tear

II. Humeral Injuries

A. Shaft fracture (Table 11–9)
  1. Classification—By location and fracture pattern
  2. Treatment
     a. Nonoperative treatment—Functional brace if there is less than 20 degrees of anterior angulation, less than 30 degrees of valgus/varus angulation, or less than 3 cm of shortening
     b. Operative treatment—ORIF (probably the gold standard) or IM nail (possibly better for segmental or shaft/proximal humerus combination as well as pathologic fracture) if there is open fracture, floating elbow, polytrauma, or pathologic fracture
  3. Complications
     a. Radial nerve palsy (5-10%)—The vast majority (up to 92%) resolve with observation for 3-4 months. The exception is an open fracture, which has a higher likelihood of transection. The appropriate treatment of secondary nerve palsies is controversial.
     b. Nonunion—Treat with compression plate with bone graft if atrophic.
     c. Shoulder pain—Some papers report a high incidence of shoulder pain, whereas others do not.

B. Supracondylar fracture—Rare injury in adults
  1. Classification
     a. Anatomic location—High, low, abduction, and adduction (Fig. 11–7)

TABLE 11-9 ADULT HUMERAL SHAFT FRACTURES

Injury	Eponym	Classification	Treatment	Complications
Humeral shaft fracture	Holstein-Lewis (distal one third)	Based on location/ fracture pattern	Nonoperative: coaptation splint or cast brace if <20-degree anterior angulation, <30-degree varus/valgus, <3-cm shortening Operative: consider open reduction (with) internal fixation (ORIF) (compression plate) vs. intramedullary (IM) nail Indications: pathologic fracture, open fracture, floating elbow Relative indications: segmental fracture, distal spiral with nerve injury (Holstein-Lewis), obesity, thoracic trauma, polytrauma	Nonunion (treat with compression plate and bone graft), malunion, radial nerve injury (5-10% incidence; observe unless open fracture or persisting for 3-4 months), vascular injury; shoulder pain (IM nail)

b. AO/OTA distal humerus classification
Type A—Extra-articular
Type B—Intra-articular, single column
Type C—Intra-articular, with both columns fractured and no portion of the joint contiguous with the shaft

2. Treatment—ORIF
3. Complications—Neurovascular injury, nonunion, malunion, and loss of motion (contracture, fibrosis, bony block)

C. Distal single-column (condyle) fracture

1. Classification
   a. Classified as Milch types I and II lateral condyle fractures (more common) and types I and II medial condyle fractures. In type I lateral condyle fractures the lateral trochlear ridge is intact, and in type II lateral condyle fractures there is a fracture through lateral trochlear ridge (Fig. 11–8).
   b. AO/OTA distal humerus classification (see above)
2. Treatment—Type I nondisplaced: immobilize in supination (lateral condyle fracture) or pronation (medial condyle fracture); otherwise, closed reduction with percutaneous pinning (CRPP) or ORIF
3. Complications—Cubitus valgus (lateral) or cubitus varus (medial), ulnar nerve injury, and **degenerative joint disease** (DJD)

D. Distal two-column fracture

1. Presentation—Five major articular fragments are identified: capitellum/lateral trochlea, lateral epicondyle, posterolateral epicondyle, posterior trochlea, and medial trochlea/epicondyle (Fig. 11–9)
2. Classification
   a. Jupiter classification (Fig. 11–10)
      High T—Proximal or at level of olecranon fossa
      Low T (common)—Transverse component just proximal to the trochlea

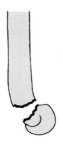

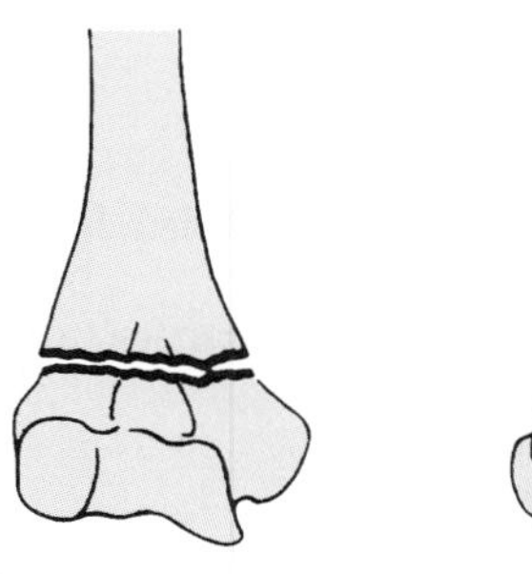
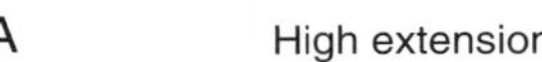
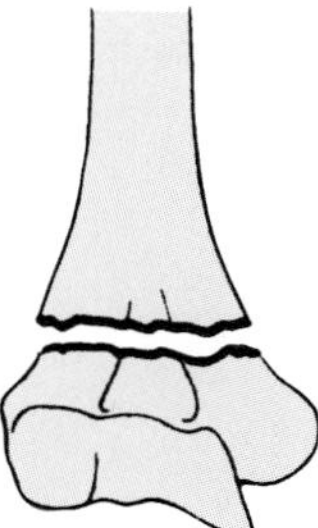
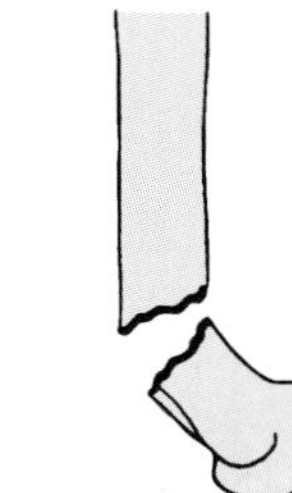
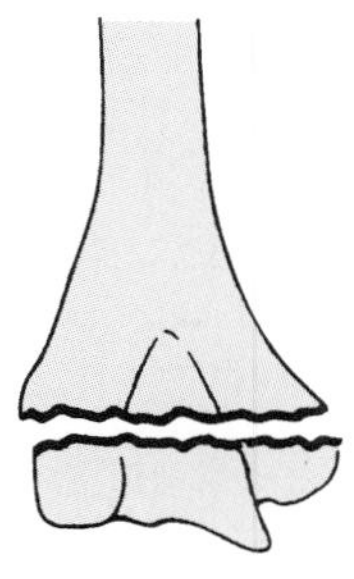
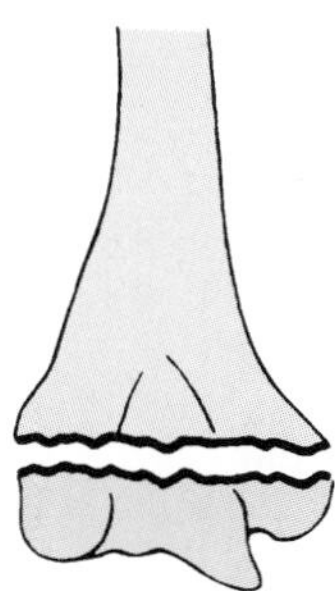
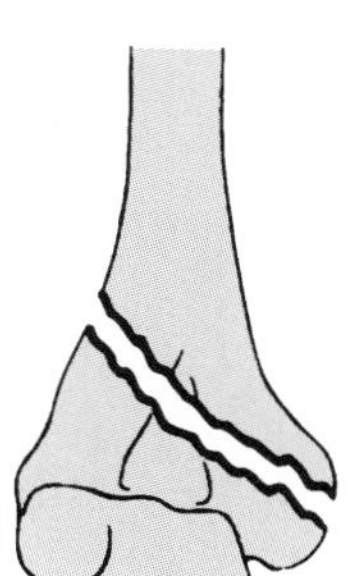
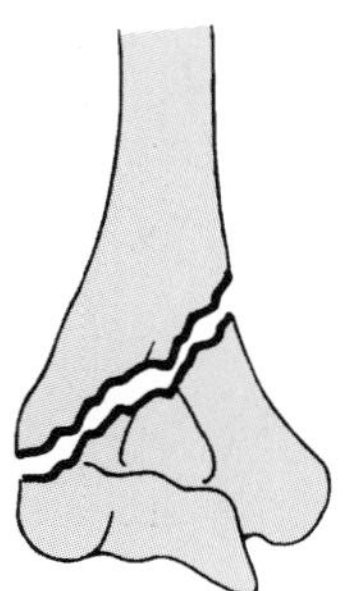

FIGURE 11–7 Transcolumn fractures. These fractures occur in four basic patterns: high, low, abduction, and adduction. The high and low fractures can be further subdivided into extension and flexion patterns. Transcolumn fractures are uncommon compared with other fractures of the distal humerus. (From Browner BD, et al, eds: Skeletal Trauma, 2nd ed, p 1515. Philadelphia, WB Saunders, 1998.)

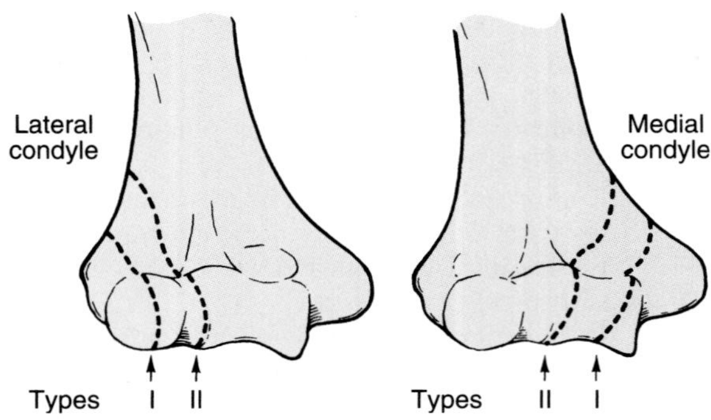

FIGURE 11–8 Humeral condyle fractures. (From Gelman MI: Radiology of Orthopedic Procedures: Problems and Complications, vol 24, p 56. Philadelphia, WB Saunders, 1984. Reprinted by permission.)

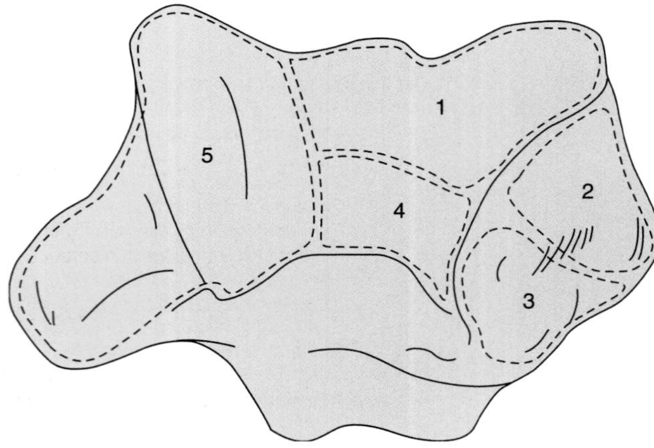

FIGURE 11–9 Schematic representation of the articular surface of the distal humerus showing the constituent parts of the articular fracture. 1, Capitellum and lateral portion of the trochlea. 2, Lateral epicondyle. 3, Lateral epicondyle, posterior metaphyseal portion. 4, Posterior aspect of the trochlea. 5, Medial aspect of the trochlea and medial epicondyle. (From Tornetta P III, Baumgaertner M: Orthopaedic Knowledge Update: Trauma 3, p 183. Rosemont, IL, American Academy of Orthopaedic Surgeons, 2005.)

Y—Oblique portion through both columns with distal vertical fracture

H—Trochlea is free fragment (**avascular necrosis** [AVN])

Medial lambda—Proximal fracture exits medially

Lateral lambda—Proximal fracture exits laterally

Multiplane—T type with additional fracture in coronal plane

b. AO/OTA distal humerus classification (see above)

3. Treatment
   a. ORIF using a posterior approach—Used with olecranon osteotomy or triceps split/peel (final muscle strength similar with both). In an open fracture, use ORIF by means of a triceps split through the defect, producing better results than osteotomy. Low-T fractures are more difficult and frequently require reoperation (almost 50%) for stiffness, but they can have good results.
   b. "Bag-of-bones" technique—Reasonable for demented patients and those who have severe medical comorbidities that prevent surgical treatment.
   c. Total elbow arthroplasty—Useful for patients over 65 years of age.
4. Complications—Stiffness, HO (4%), infection, and ulnar nerve injury (treat with anterior transposition)

E. Capitellum fracture
1. Classification
   a. Bryan and Morrey (Fig. 11–11)
      Type I—Hahn-Steinthal; complete fracture of capitellum
      Type II—Kocher-Lorenz; shear fracture of articular cartilage
      Type III—Comminuted
   b. McKee modification
      Type IV—Coronal shear fracture including capitellum and trochlea (Fig. 11–12)
2. Treatment
   a. Type I—If nondisplaced, splint 2-3 weeks and then allow motion; if displaced more than 2 mm, use ORIF.

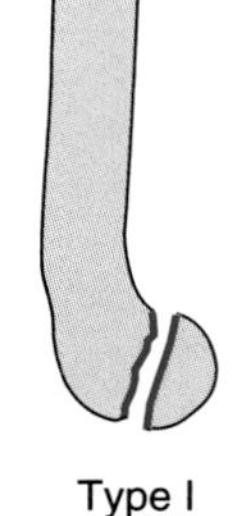

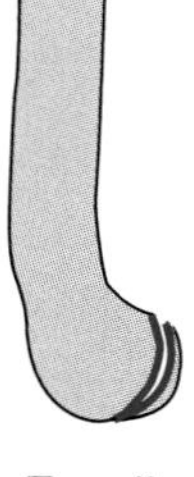

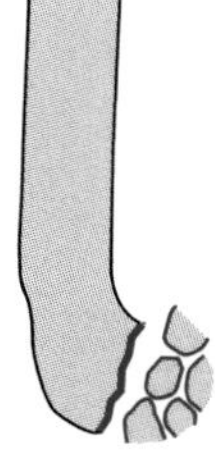

FIGURE 11–11 Fractures of the capitellum can be divided into type I, complete capitellum fracture; type II, the more superficial lesion of Kocher-Lorenz; and type III, comminuted capitellar fracture. (From Browner BD, et al, eds: Skeletal Trauma, 2nd ed, p 1511. Philadelphia, WB Saunders, 1998.)

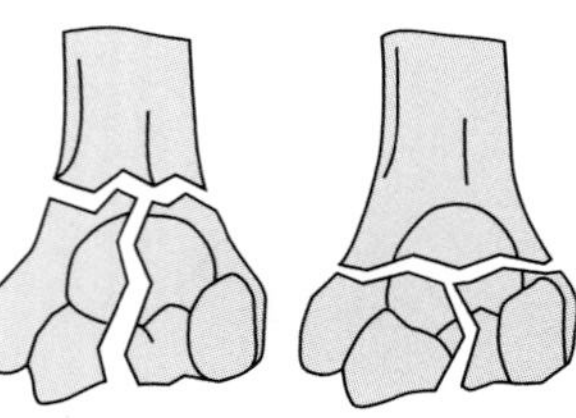
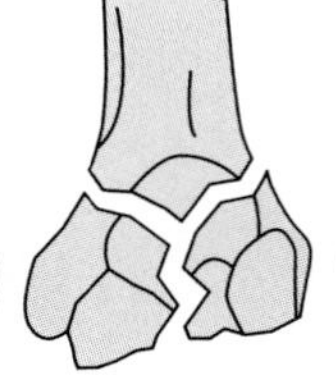
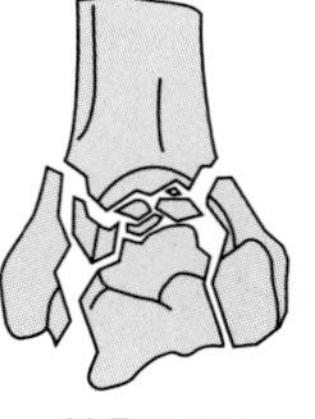
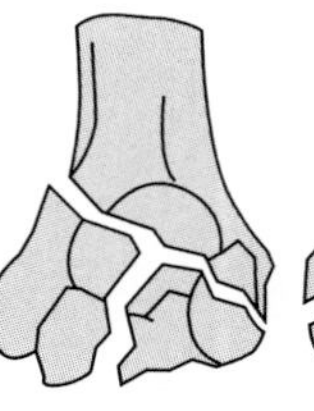
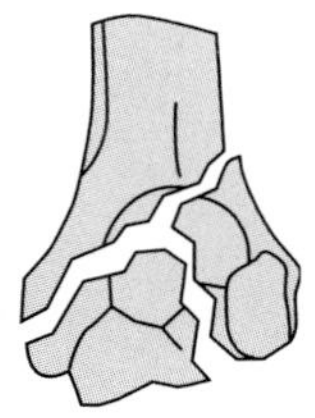

FIGURE 11–10 Jupiter classification of two-column distal humerus fractures. (From Jupiter J: Skeletal Trauma, vol 2, pp 1159-1163. Philadelphia, WB Saunders, 1992. Reprinted by permission.)

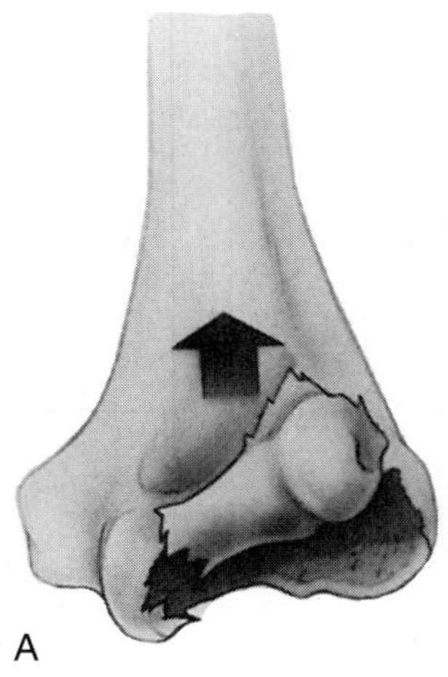
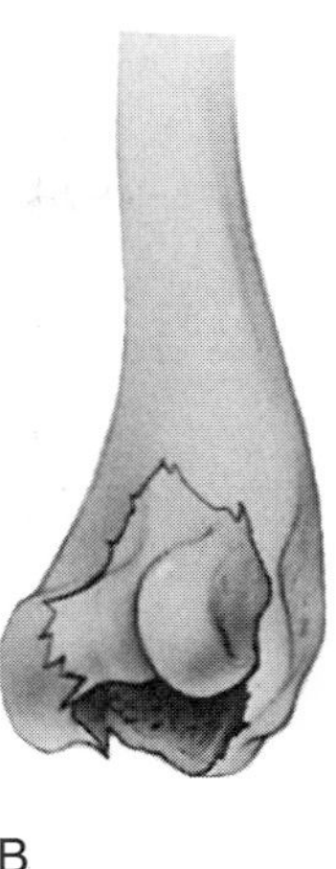

FIGURE 11–12 Coronal shear fracture of the distal humerus. **A**, Diagram showing separation and proximal migration rotation *(arrow)* of the distal fragment, which includes most of the anterior joint surface. **B**, Oblique view. (From Browner BD, et al, eds: Skeletal Trauma, 2nd ed, p 1512. Philadelphia, WB Saunders, 1998.)

b. Type II—If nondisplaced, splint 2-3 weeks and then allow motion; if displaced, excise fragments.
c. Type III—If displaced, excise fragments
d. Type IV—ORIF

3. Complications—Nonunion (1-11% with ORIF), olecranon osteotomy nonunion, ulnar nerve injury, HO (4% with ORIF), and AVN of capitellum.

III. Elbow Injuries (Table 11–10)

A. Olecranon fracture

1. Classification—Colton (Fig. 11–13)
   Type I—Avulsion
   Types IIA-D—Oblique fractures with increasing complexity
   Type III—Fracture-dislocation
   Type IV—Atypical, high-energy, comminuted fractures
2. Treatment
   a. Less than 1-2 mm displaced—Splint at 60-90 degrees for 7-10 days, followed by gentle active ROM exercises.
   b. Tension band—Use stainless steel wire or braided cable, not braided suture material. Migration of K-wires and prominent or painful hardware occurs in 71%.
   c. IM screw fixation—It is inadequate by itself, but a properly placed 7.3-mm partially threaded screw with tension band wiring works well.
   d. Plate fixation (dorsal or tension side)—The preferred technique for oblique fractures that extend distal to the coronoid process; more stable than tension band wiring.
   e. Excision—Used for nonreconstructable proximal olecranon fractures in low-demand patients. Reattach close to the articular surface. Avoid resecting more than 50% of the olecranon.
3. Complications—Decreased ROM, DJD, nonunion, ulnar nerve neurapraxia, and instability.

B. Coronoid fracture

1. Classification—Regan and Morrey (Fig. 11–14)
   Type I—Fracture of the tip of the coronoid process
   Type II—Fracture of 50% or less of coronoid
   Type III—Fracture of more than 50%
2. Treatment
   a. Type I—Associated with episodes of elbow instability. If instability persists, apply cerclage wire or No. 5 suture through drill holes; if instability does not persist, no operation.
   b. Types II and III—ORIF helps restore elbow stability. Must confirm stability before nonoperative treatment begins.
3. Complications—Instability (particularly medial) and DJD

C. Radial head fracture

1. Classification (Fig. 11–15)
   Type I—Nondisplaced
   Type II—Partial articulation with displacement
   Type III—Comminuted fractures involving the entire head of the radius
   Type IV—Fractures associated with ligamentous injury or other associated fractures
2. Treatment
   a. Type I—Splint for no more than 7 days, and then allow motion.
   b. Type II—Treatment is nonsurgical, with analgesics and active range of motion as symptoms resolve, if the elbow is stable and there is no block to motion with good reduction. Otherwise, use ORIF. Surgery provides better results (90-100% good or excellent).
   c. Type III—Replace the radial head, usually with a metal implant. ORIF if less than 3 pieces. Excise only in elderly patients with low functional demands.
   d. Type IV—Requires surgical repair. Must use either ORIF or metallic radial head replacement. Do not excise without adding radial head implant.
3. Complications—Loss of motion, posterior interosseous nerve (PIN) injury, radial shortening if Essex-Lopresti injury, and synovitis if a Silastic radial head implant is used.

D. Dislocation

1. Classification (Fig. 11–16)
   a. 80% are posterolateral; the rest are posterior, anterior, medial, lateral, or divergent
   b. Simple (no associated fracture) or complex (fracture)
2. Treatment
   a. Simple—Brief immobilization (1 week) for most and then allow motion. Long-term results are good.
   b. Complex—Surgical treatment is indicated. Anterior or divergent dislocations are usually high-energy injuries with a much higher incidence of open wounds, neurovascular injury, fracture, and recurrent instability.

TABLE 11-10 ADULT ELBOW FRACTURE-DISLOCATIONS

Injury	Eponym	Classification	Treatment	Complications
Supracondylar fracture		AO/OTA classification of distal humerus Type A—Extra-articular Type B—Intra-articular single column Type C—Intra-articular with both columns fractured and no portion of the joint contiguous with the shaft	Displaced: open reduction with internal fixation (ORIF) (double plating)	Neurovascular injury, nonunion, malunion, contracture, pain, decreased range of motion (ROM) (fibrosis, bony block)
Bicolumn fracture		Jupiter I—High T-pattern (at level of olecranon fossa) II—Low T-pattern (proximal to trochlea) III—Y-pattern (through both columns, distal vertical fracture) IV—H pattern (trochlea is free fragment) V—Medial lambda pattern (proximal fracture exits medially) VI—Lateral lambda pattern (proximal fracture exits laterally) VII—Multiplane: T-type with additional fracture in coronal plane	Nondisplaced: immobilize for 2 wk, then gentle motion Displaced: ORIF (posterior approach, olecranon osteotomy or triceps split/peel): fix condyles first, then epitrochlear ridge to humeral metaphysis) Arthroplasty (total elbow arthroplasty [TEA]) in elderly (consider >65 yr old) "Bag of bones" technique for demented patients or those medically unfit for surgery	Stiffness, heterotopic ossification, infection, ulnar neuropathy (treat with anterior transposition), avascular necrosis (AVN)
Transcondylar fracture	Kocher	Intra-articular (fragment posterior to humerus)	ORIF	↓ROM
	Posadas	Intra-articular (fragment anterior to humerus)	ORIF	
Capitellar fracture		Bryan and Morrey		Nonunion (1-11% with ORIF), olecranon osteotomy nonunion, ulnar nerve injury, heterotopic ossification (4% with ORIF), AVN of capitellum
	Hahn-Steinthal	I—Complete fracture of capitellum, large trochlear piece	Nondisplaced: splint for 2-3 wk, then motion; displaced >2 mm: ORIF	
	Kocher-Lorenz	II—Minimum subchondral bone (shear fracture of articular cartilage)	Nondisplaced: splint for 2-3 wk, then motion; displaced: excise displaced fragment	
		III—Comminuted fracture	Excise if displaced and unsalvageable	
		IV (McKee modification)—Coronal shear fracture, including capitellum and trochlea	ORIF	
Condylar fracture		Milch (lateral ≫ medial) I—Lateral trochlear ridge intact II—Fracture through lateral trochlear ridge	Nondisplaced: immobilize in supination (lateral condyle), pronation (medial condyle) Displaced: closed reduction with percutaneous pinning (CRPP) vs. ORIF ORIF	Cubitus valgus (lateral), cubitus varus (medial), ulnar nerve neuropraxia, degenerative joint disease (DJD)

Trochlear fracture	Laugier	Rare	Nondisplaced: splint for 3 wk; ORIF if displaced	
Epicondylar fracture	Granger	Medial ≫ lateral	Manipulation, immobilization for 10-14 days	Painful, unsightly fragment or ulnar nerve symptoms—late excision
Coronoid fracture		Regan and Morrey		Instability (medial) and DJD
		Type I—Fracture of the tip	Early motion if stable; ORIF with cerclage wire or suture if unstable	
		Type II—Fracture of <50% of coronoid	ORIF	
		Type III—Fracture of >50% of coronoid	ORIF	
Olecranon fracture		Colton (modified) Type I—Avulsion Type II (A-D)—Oblique fractures with increasing complexity Type III—Fracture-dislocations Type IV—Atypical high-energy, multifragmented fractures	Minimally displaced (<1-2 mm): splint at 69-90 degrees for 7-10 days, then motion Minimally displaced (<1-2 mm): splint at 69-90 degrees for 7-10 days, then motion Displaced: ORIF Tension band: use stainless steel wire or braided cable; migration of wire/prominent hardware in 71% Intramedullary 7.3-mm screw and tension band Plate fixation for oblique and comminuted fractures Excision for unreconstructible proximal olecranon fractures; reattach close to articular surface; avoid >50% resection	↓ROM, DJD, nonunion, ulnar nerve neuropraxia, instability (with removal of >80% of olecranon), symptomatic hardware/need for hardware removal
Radial head fracture		Mason (and Johnston)		Loss of motion, posterior interosseous nerve (PIN) injury; intraosseous membrane rupture; distal radioulnar joint disruption; Essex-Lopresti (distal radioulnar joint disruption); synovitis if Silastic radial head implant
		I—Nondisplaced	Nonoperative; splint for 7 days, then early motion with or without aspiration	
		II—Partially articular with displacement	If elbow stable and no block to motion: splint and early motion; otherwise, ORIF vs. arthroplasty	
		III—Comminuted fractures involving the entire head of the radius	Arthroplasty; ORIF if < three pieces, good bone quality; excise in elderly, low functional demands	
		IV—Fractures associated with ligamentous injury (elbow dislocation) or other associated fractures	Reduce dislocation and then address fracture surgically (arthroplasty for stability)	
Dislocation (pure ligamentous)		Posterolateral (most common), posterior, anterior, medial, lateral, divergent; simple (no fracture) or complex (fracture)	Closed reduction; check ROM/stability; splint for 2-7 days and then gentle, active ROM; open reduction unstable/interposed soft tissue ORIF complex (fracture) dislocations	Irreducibility, median and ulnar nerve injury, brachial artery injury, flexion contracture, heterotopic ossification, fractures (medial epicondyle, radial head, coronoid)

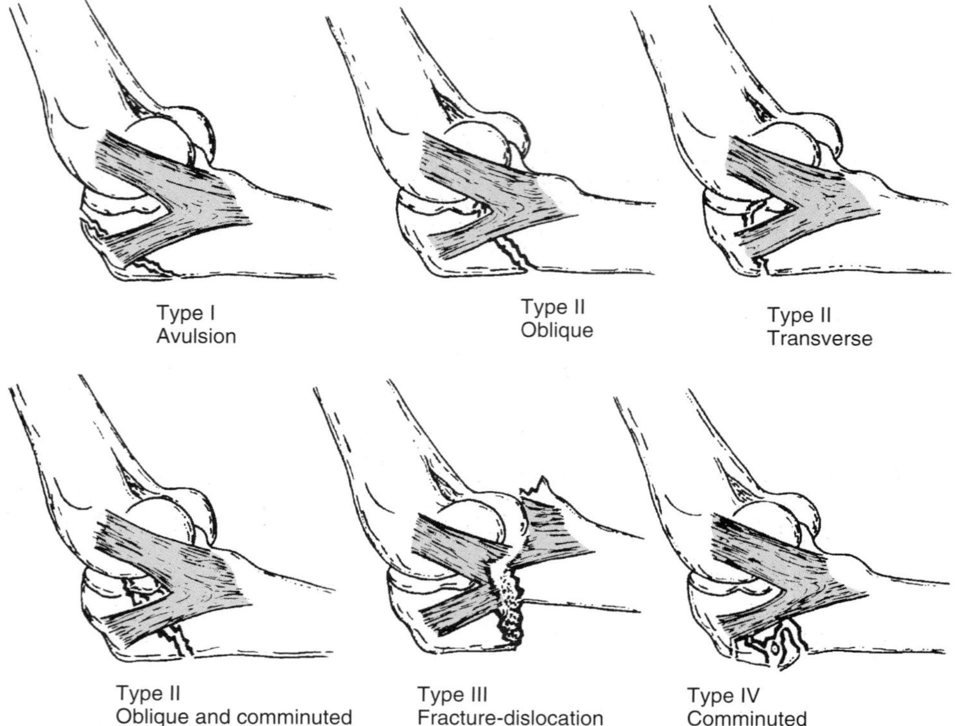

FIGURE 11–13 Colton classification of olecranon fractures. (From Browner BD, et al, eds: Skeletal Trauma, 2nd ed, p 1469. Philadelphia, WB Saunders, 1998.)

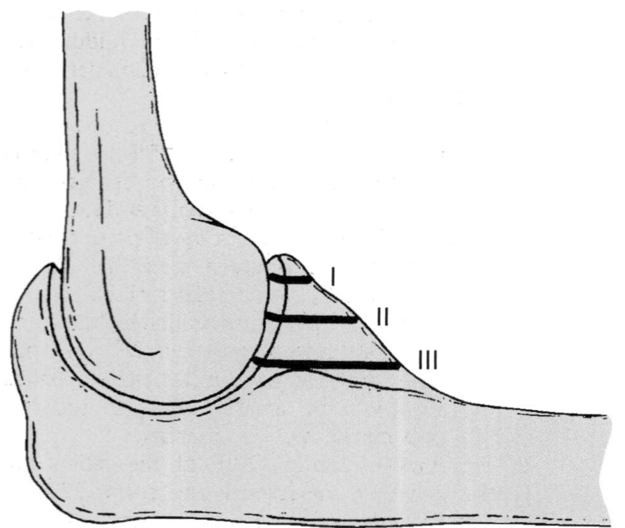

FIGURE 11–14 The coronoid fracture has been classified into three types by Regan and Morrey. (From Browner BD, et al, eds: Skeletal Trauma, 2nd ed, p 1480. Philadelphia, WB Saunders, 1998.)

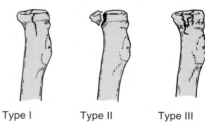

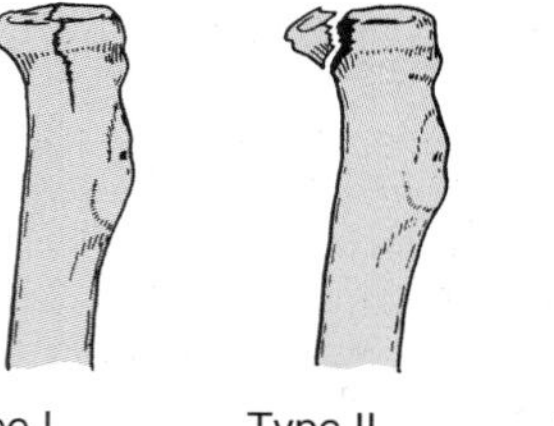

FIGURE 11–15 Classification of radial head fractures. (From Gelman MI: Radiology of Orthopedic Procedures: Problems and Complications, vol 24, p 59. Philadelphia, WB Saunders, 1984. Reprinted by permission.)

3. Complications—Radial head and neck fractures (50-60%), epicondyle fractures (10%), coronoid fractures (10%), median or ulnar nerve injury, brachial artery injury, flexion contracture, and HO.

IV. Forearm Fractures (Table 11–11)

A. Monteggia fractures

1. Diagnosis/classification

a. Bado classification (Fig. 11–17)

Type 1 (60%)—Anterior radial head dislocation and apex anterior proximal third ulna fracture

Type 2 (15%)—Posterior radial head dislocation and apex posterior proximal third ulna fracture

Type 3—Lateral radial head dislocation and proximal ulnar metaphyseal fracture

Type 4—Anterior radial head dislocation and proximal third radius and ulna fractures

b. Interosseous membrane evaluation is important with Monteggia and Monteggia-equivalent (fracture of radial head rather than dislocation) injuries.

(1) Physical examination—Considered abnormal if greater than 3-mm instability is noted when the radius pulled proximally, indicating injury. If injury is

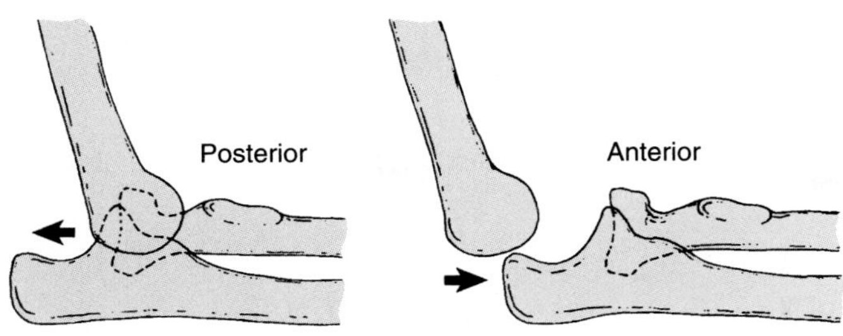

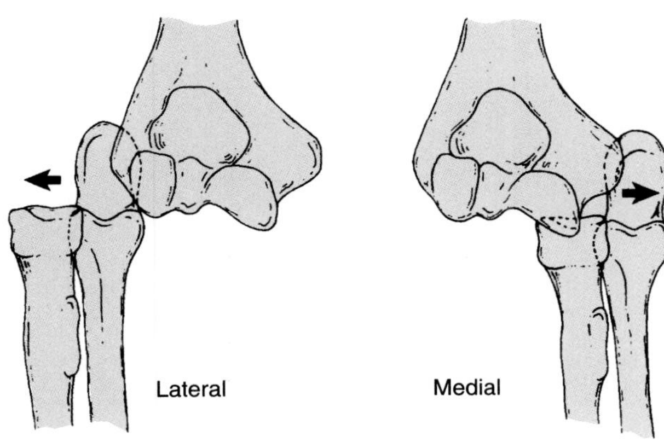

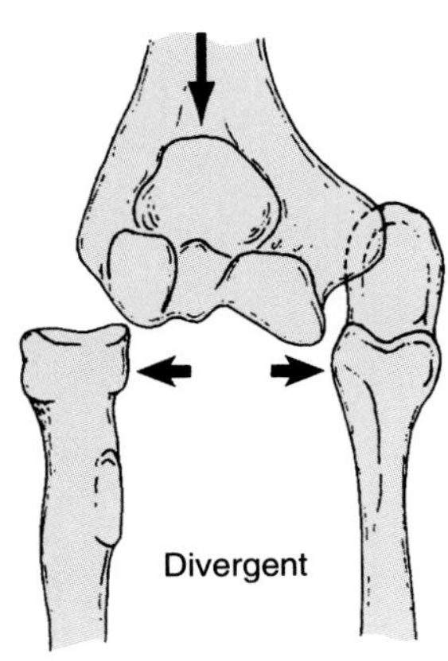

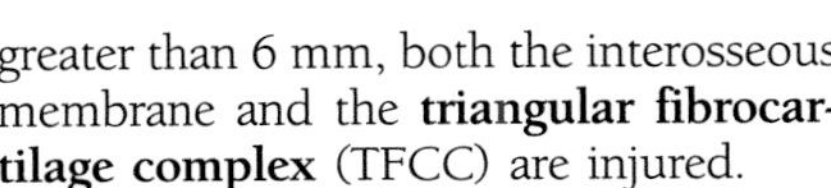

FIGURE 11–16 An elbow dislocation is defined by the direction of the forearm bones. (From Browner BD, et al, eds: Skeletal Trauma, 2nd ed, p 1475. Philadelphia, WB Saunders, 1998.)

greater than 6 mm, both the interosseous membrane and the **triangular fibrocartilage complex** (TFCC) are injured.

(2) Confirm diagnosis with MRI or ultrasound.

2. Treatment—All Monteggia fractures in adults should be treated with ORIF. The radial head will normally reduce and be stable. If not, the most common cause is a nonanatomic reduction of the ulna. If the ulna is anatomic and the radial head does not reduce, an open reduction with a separate approach is required.
3. Complications—The complication rate is higher for Monteggia-equivalent and Bado type II injuries. Common problems include PIN injury (usually resolves spontaneously), redislocation/subluxation, synostosis, and loss of motion.

B. Both-bone forearm fractures

1. Classification—Displaced versus nondisplaced
2. Treatment—ORIF in adults
3. Complications—Malunion, nonunion, vascular injury, PIN injury, synostosis, and refracture after plate removal

C. Ulna "nightstick" fractures

1. Classification—Stable (traditional definition is < 50% displacement) versus unstable (newer literature suggests that 25-50% displacement or 10-15 degrees angulation is unstable)
2. Treatment
   a. Distal two thirds, less than 50% displaced, and less than 10 degrees angulation—Long-arm cast (LAC) to functional fracture brace with good interosseous mold
   b. Proximal third, over 50% displaced, or over 10 degrees angulation—ORIF
3. Complications—Malunion/nonunion

D. Distal third radius fracture with radioulnar dislocation (Galeazzi)

1. Diagnosis/classification—Fracture of the radius (usually at the junction of the middle and distal thirds), with distal radioulnar joint (DRUJ) instability.
   a. DRUJ instability
      (1) DRUJ is unstable in 55% of patients when the radial fracture is less than 7.5 cm from the articular surface.
      (2) DRUJ is unstable in 6% of patients when the radial fracture is more than 7.5 cm away from the articular surface.
      (3) Signs of DRUJ instability include ulnar styloid fracture, widened DRUJ on posteroanterior view, dislocation on lateral view, and greater than or equal to 5 mm of radial shortening.
2. Treatment—Perform ORIF of the radius and then supinate the forearm and assess DRUJ. If it is unstable, reduce and pin in supination.
3. Complications—Malunion/nonunion and DRUJ subluxation

V. Wrist Fractures (Table 11–12)

A. Distal radius fractures

1. Classification
   a. Frykman classification—Types I-VIII (Fig. 11–18)

      Types II, IV, VI, and VIII—Include the ulnar styloid
      Type I—Extra-articular
      Type III—Enters radiocarpal joint
      Type V—Enters radioulnar joint
      Type VII—Enters both joints

TABLE 11-11 ADULT RADIAL AND ULNAR SHAFT FRACTURES AND DISLOCATIONS

Injury	Eponym/ Other Name	Classification	Treatment	Complications
Radius and ulna fractures	"Both-bone"	Degree of displacement	Open reduction with internal fixation (ORIF) with six-hole dynamic compression plate (DCP); external fixation for type III open fracture, bone graft if >one-third (shaft) comminution	Malunion/nonunion, vascular injury, percutaneous interosseous nerve (PIN) injury, compartment syndrome, synostosis, infection, refracture (after plate removal)
Ulna fracture	Nightstick	Nondisplaced	Distal two thirds, <50% displaced, <10-degree angulation: long-arm cast (LAC) to functional brace with good interosseous mold	Malunion, nonunion
		Displaced	Proximal one third, >50% displaced, >10-degree angulation: ORIF; look for wrist/elbow injury	
Proximal ulna and radial head fracture	Monteggia	Bado		PIN injury (usually spontaneously resolves), redislocation/subluxation (inadequate reduction), synostosis, loss of motion
		Type I (60%)—radial head dislocation, anterior and apex anterior proximal one-third ulna fracture	ORIF of ulna (DCP), closed-reduction head, immobilize; if radial head irreducible, ulna fracture reduction may be nonanatomic	
		Type II (15)%—radial head dislocation, posterior and apex posterior proximal one-third ulna shaft fracture	ORIF of ulna (DCP), closed reduction head, immobilize at 70 degrees	
		Type III—radial head dislocation, lateral and proximal ulnar metaphyseal fracture	ORIF of ulna (DCP), closed reduction head, immobilize	
		Type IV—radial head dislocatiion, anterior fracture and forearm fracture of both bones	ORIF of radius and ulna, closed reduction head, immobilize	
Proximal radius fracture		Nondisplaced	LAC in supination, close follow-up	
		Displaced	Proximal one fifth: closed; one fifth–two thirds: ORIF	
Distal radius (distal one third) and radioulnar dislocation	Galeazzi/ Piedmont	Supination/pronation (signs of instability: ulnar styloid fracture, widened distal radioulnar joint on posteroanterior view, dislocation on lateral view, ≥5-mm radial shortening)	ORIF of radius (volar), closed reduction with or without percutaneous pinning to radioulnar joint (in supination) if unstable	Angulation, distal subluxation, malunion, nonunion; displaced by gravity, pronator quadratus, brachioradialis

b. Melone classification (Fig. 11–19—Describes radiocarpal joint fragments
   - Radial styloid
   - Shaft
   - Lunate facet
     - Palmar
     - Dorsal

   Types I-IV represent increasingly comminuted fractures of the aforementioned four anatomic regions and their parts. Type V is an extremely comminuted, unstable fracture without large, identifiable facet fragments).
c. Fernandez classification (Fig. 11–20) based on the mechanism of injury and designed to guide treatment decision making.
   - Type I—Bending fractures
   - Type II—Articular shear fractures
   - Type III—Compression fractures
   - Type IV—Fractures-dislocations
   - Type V—Combined mechanisms

2. Treatment—Based on the Fernandez classification
   a. Type I—Usually an extra-articular metaphyseal fracture. Comminution determines stability. The volarly displaced radial fracture is much more unstable. Conservative treatment with reduction and casting if stable. CRPP versus external fixation if unstable.
   b. Type II—Shearing injury of the joint surface (volar or dorsal lip or radial styloid). Usually unstable, and carpal subluxation frequently occurs. Treatment is with ORIF.
   c. Type III—Articular compression (die-punch) injuries follow the patterns described by Melone. Conservative treatment if

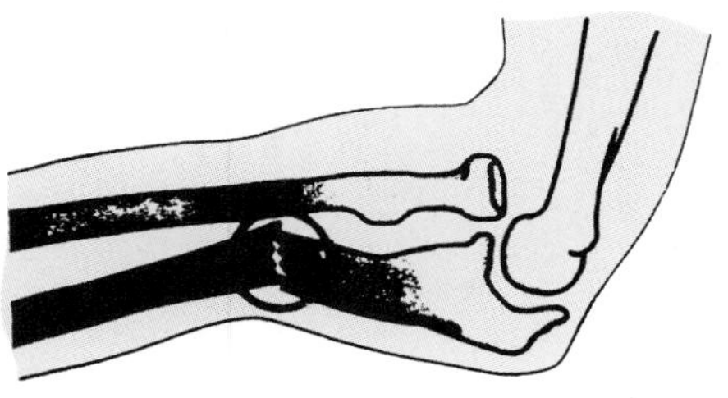
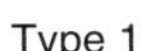

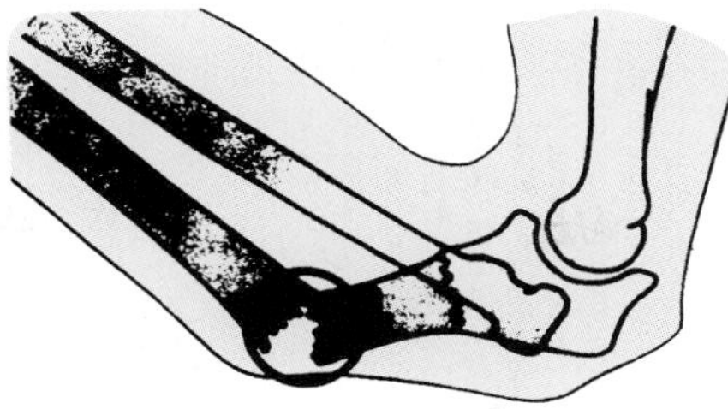

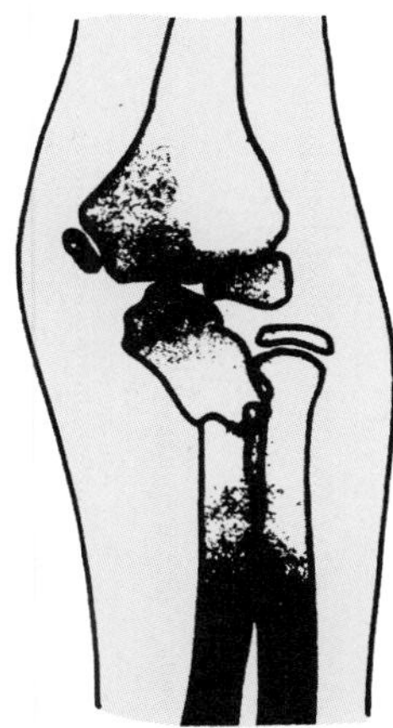

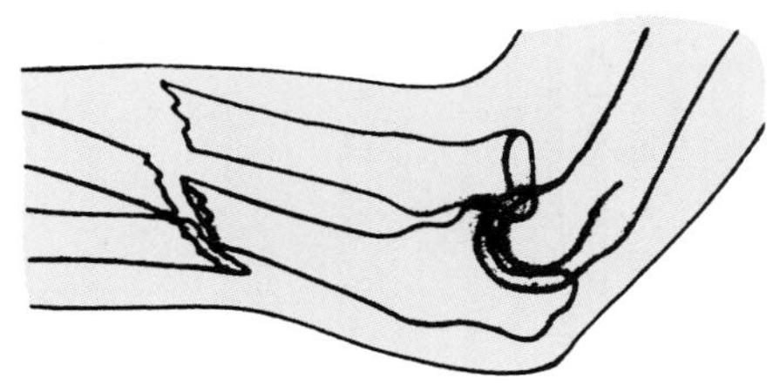

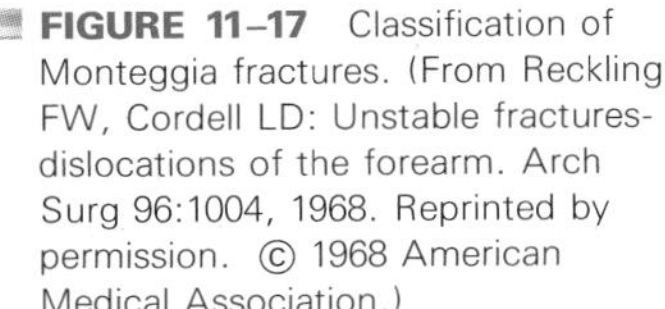

FIGURE 11–17 Classification of Monteggia fractures. (From Reckling FW, Cordell LD: Unstable fractures-dislocations of the forearm. Arch Surg 96:1004, 1968. Reprinted by permission. © 1968 American Medical Association.)

nondisplaced. ORIF with disimpaction of the articular surface if displaced.

d. Type IV—Rare and follows high-energy trauma. These are avulsion fractures with radiocarpal fracture dislocations. Surgical repair of the avulsed styloid usually restores stability. Treat with closed or, more frequently, open reduction, pin or screw fixation, or tension wiring.

e. Type V—Combination fractures of types I-IV after high-energy trauma. These are very severe and unstable fractures. There are always associated injuries. Treatment is open, with combined methods.

3. Outcomes—Restoration of anatomic alignment is the best predictor of a good outcome. The loss of radial length and volar tilt is the most important, and radial inclination is less important. Articular step-offs of more than 1-2 mm also predict poor outcome.

4. Complications—Loss of reduction, malunion/nonunion, median nerve neuropathy, weakness, tendon adhesion, instability, extensor pollicis longus (EPL) rupture, dorsal intercalated segment instability (DISI), and Volkmann ischemic contracture.

B. Dorsal rim radius fractures—Dorsal Barton (Fig. 11–21)
1. Classification—Fernandez type II
2. Treatment—ORIF with dorsal approach in the vast majority.
3. Complications—The same as the complications for distal radius fracture.

C. Radial styloid fractures—Chauffeur fracture (Fig. 11–22)
1. Diagnosis/classification—Frequently high-energy trauma in young adults. Fernandez type II is associated with perilunate injuries.
2. Treatment—CRPP or ORIF with screws. Immobilize in ulnar deviation.
3. Complications—The same as the complications for distal radius fracture.

D. Volar rim radius fractures—Volar Barton fracture (Fig. 11–23)
1. Classification—Fernandez type II
2. Treatment—Usually with ORIF by means of the volar approach. Closed reduction (rarely).
3. Complications—The same as the complications for distal radius fracture.

E. DRUJ injuries
1. Diagnosis/classification—Fracture of the base of the ulnar styloid, associated with TFCC tear.
2. Treatment—Closed or open reduction to achieve anatomic ulnar styloid reduction; immobilize in supination.
3. Complications—Osteochondral fracture, ulnar nerve compression, instability, arthrosis, weak grip, and decreased forearm rotation.

VI. Carpal Injuries (see Table 11–12)

A. Scaphoid fracture
1. Classification—Based on anatomic location (Fig. 11–24)
   Neck
   Waist

TABLE 11-12 ADULT WRIST AND CARPAL FRACTURES

Injury	Eponym	Classification	Treatment	Complications
Distal radius fracture	Colles (dorsal displacement)	Frykman (I- VIII; even number = ulnar styloid fracture I—Extra-articular III—Intra-articular radiocarpal joint fracture V—Intra-articular radioulnar joint fracture VII—Displaced intra-articular radiocarpal and radioulnar joint fractures	Distract, manipulate, splint 15 degrees palmar flexion and ulnar deviation, external fixation, and/or open reduction (with) internal fixation (ORIF) if comminuted/unstable; external fixation for severe comminution, ORIF for large fragments with a >15-degree dorsal tilt; >1-2–mm articular displacement; bone graft comminuted fractures	Loss of reduction, nonunion, malunion, median neuropathy/carpal tunnel syndrome, weakness, tendon adhesion/rupture, instability, extensor pollicis longus rupture, dorsal intercalated segment instability (DISI) >15 degrees (extension), ulnar side pain (shortening), complex regional pain syndrome (CRPS), Volkmann ischemic contracture
	Smith (volar displacement)	Intra- vs. extra-articular	Distract, manipulate, splint in supination, flexion; CRPP vs. ORIF (volar approach)	Missed diagnosis, similar to Colles fracture
Dorsal rim of radius fracture	Dorsal Barton	Fernandez type II	Majority: ORIF with dorsal approach	Similar to Colles fracture
Radial styloid fracture	Chauffeur	Fernandez type II	Reduction, CRPP, cannulated screw or plate; immobilize in ulnar deviation	Similar to Colles fracture; rule out associated perilunate injury (ORIF)
Volar rim of radius fracture	Volar Barton	Fernandez type II	Majority: ORIF with volar buttress plate	Similar to Colles fracture
Distal radioulnar joint dissociation		Based on ulna displacement; fracture of base of ulnar styloid associated with TFCC tear	Dorsal—reduction, full supination, long-arm cast (LAC) for 6 wk Volar—reduction (may require open reduction), LAC for 6 wk in pronation	Osteochondral fracture, triangular fibrocartilage complex (TFCC) injury, ulnar nerve compression, instability, arthrosis, weak grip, decreased forearm rotation
Scaphoid fracture		Based on anatomic location (neck, waist, body, proximal pole)	Evaluate with anteroposterior, lateral, navicular, and clenched-fist views; plain radiographs; magnetic resonance imaging (MRI) for occult fracture; CT to characterize fracture, evaluate nonunion nondisplaced: thumb spica, (LAC for proximal and mid-body, short-arm cast [SAC] for distal pole) ORIF if displaced, unstable, proximal pole, nonunion	Nonunion (computed tomographic [CT] evaluation; bone graft), instability, refracture, nerve injury, CRPS, degenerative joint disease (DJD), pain, missed fracture (MRI best for diagnosis of occult injury)
Triquetrum fracture		Dorsal shear (most common) vs. body (rare)	SAC for 4 wk; ORIF if displaced body fracture	
Pisiform fracture		Uncommon (1-3% of all carpal fractures)	SAC in flexion/ulnar deviation for 6 wk	Nonunion (treat with excision); associated with distal radius, hamate, triquetrum fractures
Trapezium fracture		Body, trapezial ridge	Nonoperative: SAC with molded abduction of first ray; ORIF of intra-articular displaced-body fractures	Body: associated carpometacarpal (CMC) dislocation or Bennett fracture; trapezial ridge fracture: chronic pain (treat with excision)

Capitate fracture		Rare	Closed treatment if nondisplaced, ORIF if displaced	Associated with perilunate dislocations, scaphoid fractures, and CMC fracture-dislocations; osteonecrosis; nonunion (treat with fusion of capitate, scaphoid, and lunate)
Perilunate instability/ dislocation (with or without scaphoid fracture)		Mayfield I—Scapholunate dissociation II—Lunocapitate disruption III—Lunotriquetral disruption IV—Lunate dislocation	Early (6-8 wk)—open (dorsal) ligament repair and ORIF scaphoid fracture (if present) Late—triscaphoid fusion, proximal row carpectomy, or wrist fusion	Rotatory instability of scaphoid, median nerve palsy, late flexor rupture
Rotatory scapholunate dissociation	Terry Thomas sign	>3-mm scapholunate interval on anteroposterior vs. contralateral wrist view; scapholunate angle >60 degrees, scaphoid ring sign	Closed reduction, immobilization; ORIF if scaphoid fracture displaced; open repair of ligaments (volar and dorsal, capsulodesis)	Late DJD (advanced collapse of scapholunate)
Lunate fracture		Based on fracture location (volar pole most common)	ORIF for displaced fracture; nonoperative for nondisplaced injury	Disorganization, disintegration; distinguish from Kienböck
Hamate fracture		Based on location and size of fragment—body or hook	Body: closed treatment if nondisplaced; CRPP or ORIF if displaced or unstable Hook: closed treatment if acute, excise if chronic and symptomatic	Missed on plain films (CT view required); body: associated with fourth and fifth CMC fracture-dislocation; hook: ulnar nerve symptoms, flexor tendon problems
Carpal instability		DISI (most common)—dorsal intercalated segment instability, scapholunate angle >70 degrees Volar intercalated segment instability (VISI), scapholunate angle <35 degrees Axial injury	Closed reduction of acute injuries followed by early repair; open scapholunate reconstruction for failed/late reduction/scapholunate advanced collapse (SLAC) for wrist; ORIF axial injuries	DISI, VISI: DJD, stiffness, treatment for chronic instability controversial; axial: usually high energy with soft tissue injury, nerve/vascular/muscle injury

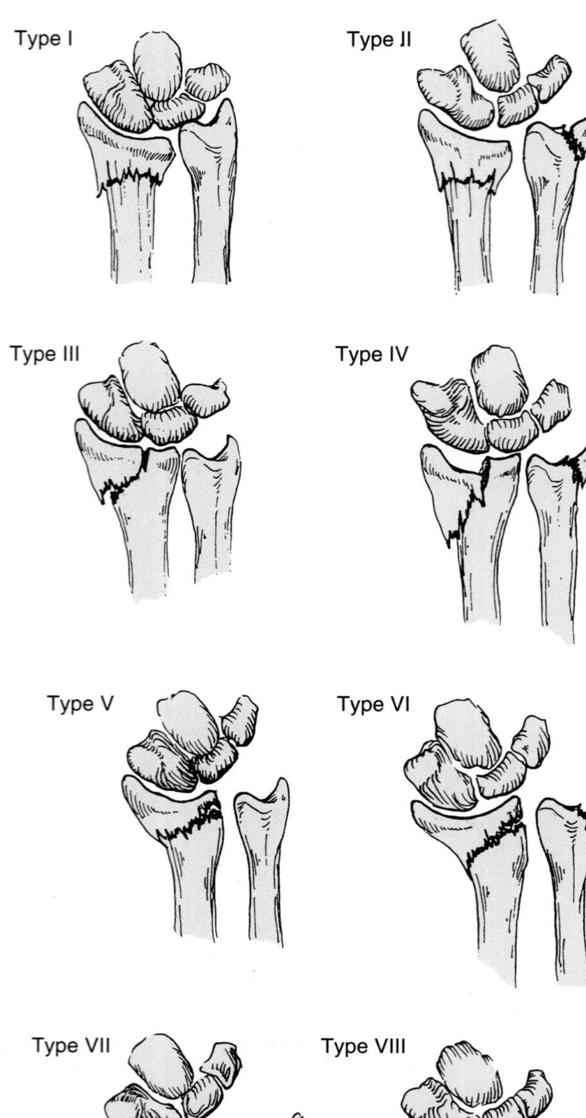

FIGURE 11–18 The Frykman classification of distal radius fractures. Note even numbers with ulnar styloid involvement. (From Kozin SH, Berlet AC: Handbook of Common Orthopaedic Fractures, pp 17, 19. West Chester, PA, Medical Surveillance, 1989.)

Body
Proximal pole

2. Diagnosis
   a. Radiographs—Anteroposterior, lateral, navicular, and clenched-fist views
   b. MRI scan—To rule out occult fracture
   c. CT scan with sagittal and coronal reconstructions—Characterizes fracture and evaluates union
3. Treatment
   a. General principles
      (1) Short arm–thumb spica immobilization until definitive diagnosis and treatment plan are made.
      (2) Rule out occult fracture in those with a high index of suspicion and negative plain radiographs.
      (3) Stable fixation and immobilization
   b. Nonoperative treatment
      (1) Nondisplaced distal fracture—Short arm–thumb spica cast for 8-12 weeks.
      (2) Nondisplaced proximal and midbody fractures—Long arm–thumb spica cast for 6 weeks, followed by short arm–thumb spica cast until union.
   c. Operative treatment
      (1) Indications—Operative treatment is used for displaced fractures, unstable fractures, proximal pole fractures, and delayed diagnosis.
      (2) ORIF—Percutaneous screw fixation under arthroscopic assistance using headless variable-pitch screws
4. Complications—Complications include nonunion (treat with Russe bone graft), instability, refracture, nerve injury, DJD, pain, and missed fracture (bone scan or MRI helpful).

B. Lunate fracture
1. Diagnosis/classification—The mechanism of injury is direct trauma. The classification is based on fracture location, with fracture of the volar pole being most common. Lunate fracture must be distinguished from Kienböck disease.
2. Treatment
   a. Nonoperative treatment—Used for nondisplaced fractures.
   b. Operative treatment—ORIF is used for displaced fractures.
3. Complications—Complications are disorganization and disintegration of the lunate.

C. Triquetrum fracture
1. Diagnosis/classification
   a. Dorsal shear injury—Very common; the third most common carpal fracture after scaphoid and lunate.
   b. Body fracture (rare)
2. Treatment
   a. Nonoperative treatment
      (1) Dorsal shear injury—Closed treatment for 4-6 weeks; excision of fragment if symptoms continue.
      (2) Body fracture—Closed treatment if nondisplaced.
   b. Operative treatment—ORIF for displaced body fracture.
3. Complications—Usually asymptomatic.

D. Pisiform fracture
1. Diagnosis/classification
   a. Uncommon—1-3% of all carpal fractures
   b. 50% with distal radius, hamate, or triquetrum fracture
2. Treatment—Short-arm cast (SAC) with 30 degrees of wrist flexion and ulnar deviation for 6 weeks

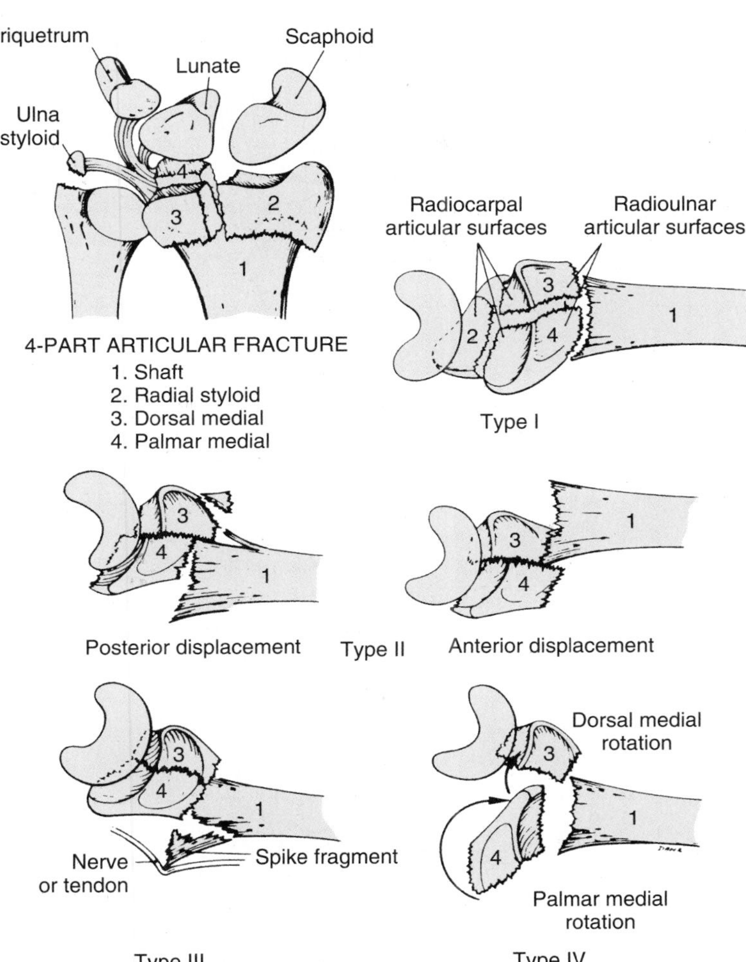

FIGURE 11–19 The Melone classification of distal radius fractures. (From Melone CP Jr: Open treatment for displaced articular fractures of the distal radius. Clin Orthop 202:104, 1986. Reprinted by permission.)

3. Complications—Nonunion (treat with excision)

E. Trapezium fracture
   1. Classification
      a. Body fracture
      b. Trapezial ridge fracture
         (1) Base of ridge
         (2) Tip of ridge
   2. Treatment
      a. Nonoperative treatment
         (1) Trapezial ridge I—Attempted closed treatment and early excision for nonunion common
         (2) Trapezial ridge II—Closed treatment for 6 weeks (molded abduction of first ray)
      b. Operative treatment—For body fractures, treatment is ORIF for intra-articular displaced fracture
   3. Complications
      a. Body—Associated carpometacarpal (CMC) dislocation or Bennett fracture
      b. Trapezial ridge I fracture—Chronic pain (requires excision)

F. Capitate fracture
   1. Evaluation—Rarely occurs in isolation
   2. Treatment—Treatment is with ORIF
   3. Complications
      a. Associated with perilunate dislocations, scaphoid fracture, and CMC fracture/dislocation
      b. Osteonecrosis
      c. Nonunion (may be treated by fusion of the capitate, scaphoid, and lunate)

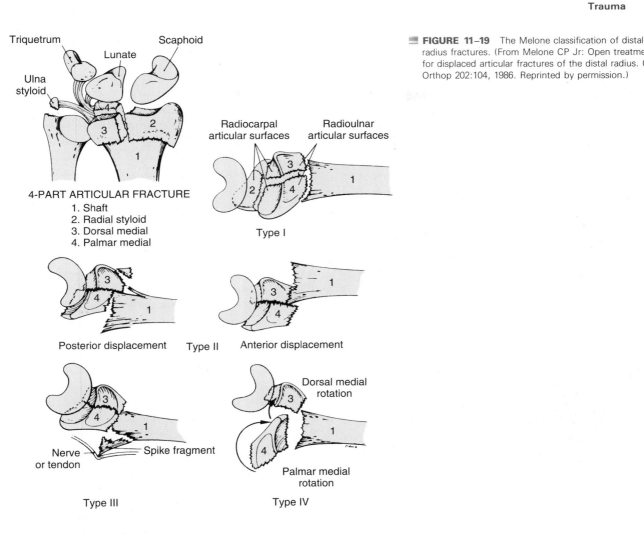

G. Hamate fracture
   1. Diagnosis/classification
      a. Body fracture—Uncommon
      b. Hook-of-hamate fracture—Common in golf, baseball, and racquet sports
   2. Treatment
      a. Nonoperative treatment
         (1) Body fracture—Closed treatment for nondisplaced fracture
         (2) Hook-of-hamate fracture—Closed treatment for 6 weeks if acute
      b. Operative treatment
         (1) Body fracture—CRPP or ORIF if displaced or unstable
         (2) Hook-of-hamate fracture—Excision or (rarely) ORIF
   3. Complications
      a. Body fracture—Associated with fourth and fifth CMC fracture-dislocation
      b. Hook-of-hamate fracture—Ulnar nerve and flexor tendon symptoms or attritional rupture

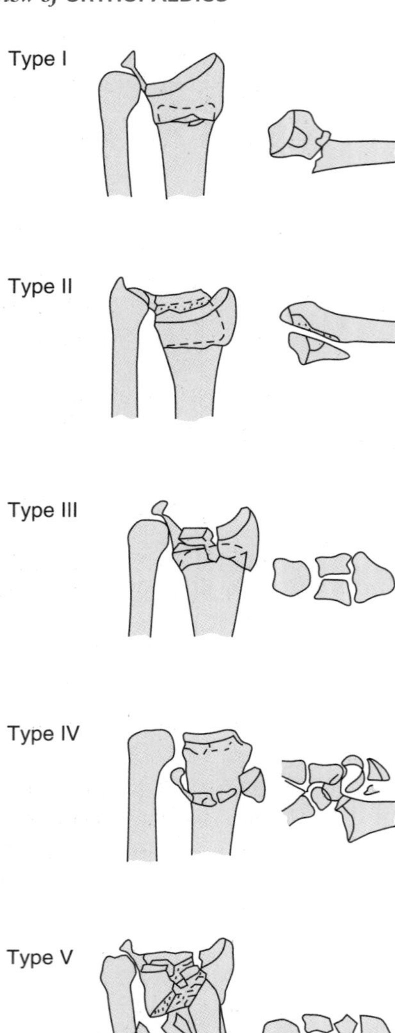

FIGURE 11–20 The Fernandez classification of distal radius fractures (fracture types in adults based on the mechanism of injury). (From Tornetta P III, Baumgaertner M: Orthopaedic Knowledge Update: Trauma 3, p 206. Rosemont, IL, American Academy of Orthopaedic Surgeons, 2005.)

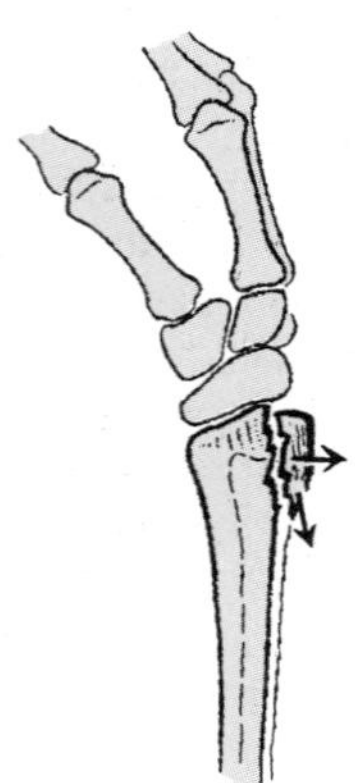

FIGURE 11–21 The Barton fracture (dorsal). (From Connolly JF, ed: DePalma's The Management of Fractures and Dislocations: An Atlas, 3rd ed, p 1032. Philadelphia, WB Saunders, 1981. Reprinted by permission.)

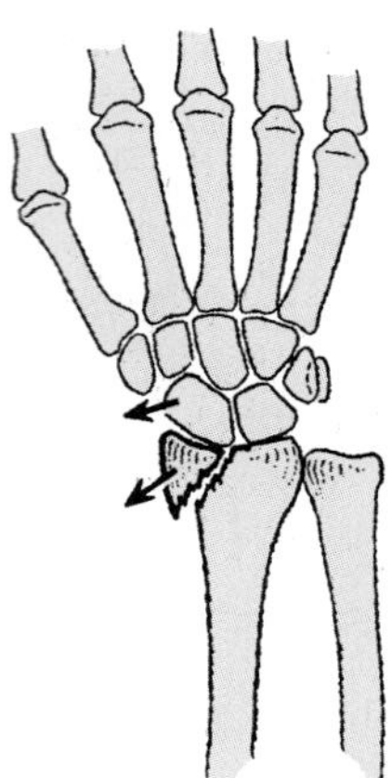

FIGURE 11–22 Radial styloid fractures. (From Connolly JF, ed: DePalma's The Management of Fractures and Dislocations: An Atlas, 3rd ed, p 1033. Philadelphia, WB Saunders, 1981. Reprinted by permission.)

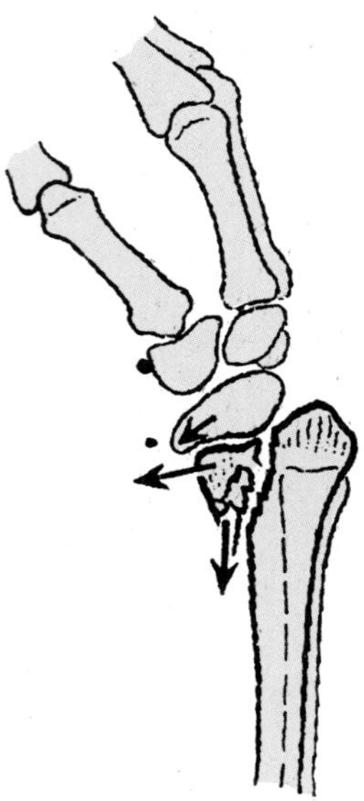

FIGURE 11–23 The Barton fracture (volar). (From Connolly JF, ed: DePalma's The Management of Fractures and Dislocations: An Atlas, 3rd ed, p 1028. Philadelphia, WB Saunders, 1981. Reprinted by permission.)

H. Perilunate instability
1. Mayfield classification (Fig. 11–25)
   a. **Scapholunate** (SL) dissociation
   b. Lunocapitate disruption
   c. Lunotriquetral disruption
   d. Lunate dislocation
2. Operative treatment
   a. Early (6-8 weeks)—Open (dorsally); ligament repair and ORIF scaphoid fracture (if present)
   b. Late—Triscaphoid fusion, proximal row carpectomy, or wrist fusion
3. Complications—These include rotatory instability of the scaphoid, median nerve palsy, and late flexor rupture.

I. SL dissociation
1. Diagnosis

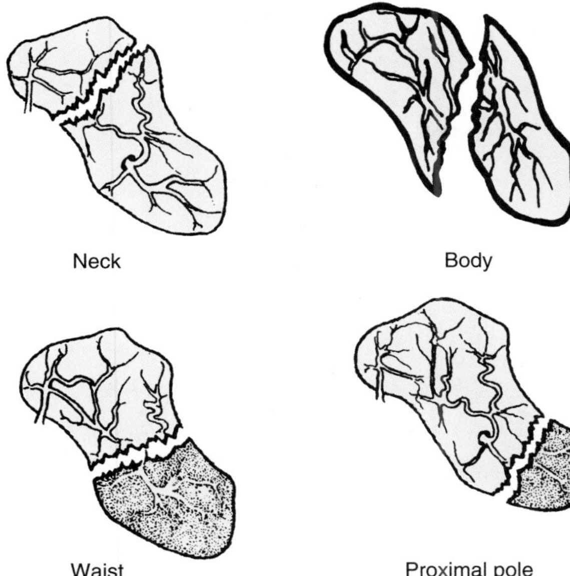

FIGURE 11–24 Classification of scaphoid fractures. Note progressive risk of avascular necrosis with proximal transverse fractures. (From Weissman BN, Sledge CB: Orthopedic Radiology, p 1060. Philadelphia, WB Saunders, 1986. Reprinted by permission.)

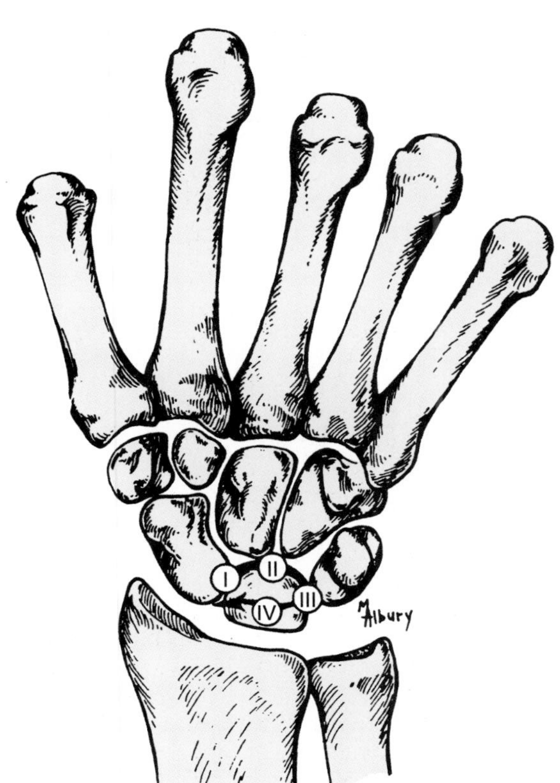

FIGURE 11–25 Perilunar stages of instability. I, Scapholunate. II, Capitolunate. III, Triquetrolunate. IV, Dorsal radiocarpal (leading to lunate dislocation). (From Mayfield JK: Mechanism of carpal injuries. Clin Orthop 149:50, 1980. Reprinted by permission.)

a. Terry Thomas sign
   (1) SL angle greater than 60 degrees
   (2) Scaphoid ring sign
b. A 3-mm or larger SL gap versus the opposite side

2. Treatment
   a. Nonoperative treatment—Closed treatment if minor
   b. Operative treatment—For early treatment (< 3 weeks), open reduction of scaphoid and lunate, with ligament repair and pinning.
3. Complications—Widening of SL is common. Another complication is late DJD.

J. Carpal instability
1. Diagnosis
   a. DISI—The most common (SL angle > 70 degrees)
   b. **Volar intercalated segmental instability** (VISI) (volar SI angle < 35 degrees)
   c. Axial injury
2. Treatment—Treatment is operative
   a. DISI and VISI—Open reduction and ligament repair
   b. Axial injury—ORIF
3. Complications
   a. DISI and VISI—DJD and stiffness; treatment for chronic instability is controversial
   b. Axial injury—Usually of high energy, with skin and soft tissue, neurovascular (ulnar nerve the most common), and intrinsic muscle injuries

VII. Hand Injuries (Tables 11–13 and 11–14)

A. Hamatometacarpal fracture-dislocation
1. Cain classification
   IA—Ligamentous injury
   IB—Dorsal hamate fracture (most common)
   II—Comminuted dorsal hamate fracture
   III—Coronal hamate fracture
2. Treatment
   a. IA—Stable, cast; unstable, CRPP
   b. IB—Stable, cast; unstable, ORIF
   c. II—ORIF to restore dorsal buttress
   d. III—ORIF to restore congruent joint surface

B. First CMC dislocation
1. Evaluation—Rare injury without associated fracture
2. Treatment—CRPP with traction/pronation
3. Complication—Chronic instability

C. First metacarpal fracture
1. Classification (Fig. 11–26)
   a. Bennett fracture—Volar ulnar lip fracture
   b. Rolando fracture—Comminuted intra-articular fracture
   c. Extra-articular fracture—This can be transverse or oblique.
2. Treatment
   a. Bennett fracture
      (1) CRPP if the volar-ulnar fragment is too small for screw fixation and anatomic reduction is achieved

TABLE 11-13 ADULT HAND DISLOCATIONS

Injury	Eponym/ Other Name	Classification	Treatment	Complications
Distal interphalangeal dislocation		Dorsal dislocation (most common)	Closed reduction; immobilize for 2 wk, then range of motion; late diagnosis or irreducible: open reduction (with) internal fixation (ORIF)	Extensor lag—treated with 8-wk course of splinting, similar to a mallet finger
		Collateral ligament injury	Sprain: buddy tape for 3-6 wk Tear: repair radial collateral of index, ring, middle finger; ulnar collateral of small (dominant hand)	
Proximal interphalangeal dislocation		Dorsal dislocation (most common) (volar plate disruption)		
		I—Hyperextension, volar plate avulsion	Buddy tape or extension block splint for 4 days, then motion	Stiffness, contractures (treat with volar plate arthroplasty)
		II—Dislocation, major ligamentous injury	Extension block splint	
		III—Proximal dislocation (middle phalanx fracture)	If >4-mm displacement, reduce; ORIF if irreducible	
	Boutonniere	Volar dislocation (central slip injury)	Closed reduction; splint in full extension for 6 wk if congruous	Late recognition: therapy to restore motion, ORIF or volar plate arthroplasty
		Rotatory	ORIF if irreducible or incongruous	
		Dorsal fracture-dislocation	Extension block splint if congruous; if unstable, ORIF or volar plate arthroplasty	
Thumb metacarpophalangeal (MCP) dislocation	Gamekeeper/skier thumb	Ulnar collateral ligament injury (most common)	Sprain: does not open >35 degrees with stress; treat with thumb spica cast for 4 wk Complete rupture: open repair (interposition of adductor aponeurosis—Stener lesion)	Unrecognized Stener lesion, chronic pain, instability, degenerative joint disease
		Radial collateral ligament injury (rare)	Splint vs. repair if complete rupture and symptomatic	
		Dorsal (simple or complex [interposition of volar plate])	Simple: splint; complex: open	
MCP dislocation		Collateral ligament injury (index finger most common)	Reduce with traction/volar–directed force to proximal phalanx; splint in 50-degree MCP flexion for 3 wk, then buddy tape for 3 additional wk Open if irreducible, >2-mm displacement of associated fracture fragments, or 20% of joint	Late recognition—injection, splinting, operation (rare)
		Dorsal dislocation (most common)		
		Simple	Closed reduction, immobilization for 7-10 days	Failure to recognize complex dislocation
		Complex	Soft tissue volar plate interposition (pucker, sesamoid in joint, and parallelism of metacarpal and P1 (phalanx) require ORIF and volar plate arthroplasty)	Stiffness, contractures, neurovascular injury (open)
		Volar dislocation	Rare, requires ORIF	
Carpometacarpal (CMC) dislocation			Closed reduction with percutaneous pinning (CRPP); ORIF—fourth CMC dislocations and open dislocations	
Thumb CMC dislocation		Rare injury without associated fracture	CRPP with traction/pronation; immobilize for 6-10 wk	Chronic instability
Hamate/metacarpal fracture-dislocation		Cain		Delay in diagnosis (pronation oblique films required)
		IA—Ligamentous injury	Reduce—If stable, cast; if unstable, CRPP	
		IB—Dorsal hamate fracture (most common)	Reduce—If stable, cast; if unstable, ORIF	
		II—Comminuted dorsal hamate fracture	ORIF, restore dorsal buttress	
		III—Coronal hamate fracture	ORIF, restore congruent joint	

TABLE 11-14 ADULT HAND FRACTURES

Injury	Eponym	Classification	Treatment	Complications
Distal phalanx (P3) fracture		Longitudinal, comminuted, transverse, crush (frequent)	Splint distal interphalangeal (DIP) for 3-4 wk; evacuate hematoma and repair nail bed with fine absorbable suture	Nail bed injury
Extensor digitorum communis avulsion	Mallet finger	Watson-Jones Extensor tendon stretch: >15-30–degree extensor lag Extensor tendon rupture: 30-60–degree extensor lag Bony mallet	Volar/stack splint for 6-8 wk full time, then 4 wk at night only; closed reduction with percutaneous pinning (CRPP)/open reduction with internal fixation (ORIF) if >50% of articular surface; volar subluxation of P3 or occupation prevents splinting	Dorsal skin necrosis, deformity, nail bed injury (with ORIF), subluxation, extensor lag, nail bed deformity, pin tract infections, osteomyelitis, hot-cold intolerance, hypersensitivity
Flexor digitorum profundus (FDP) avulsion	Jersey finger	Leddy and Packer		Can lead to lumbrical and finger (late), missed diagnosis (therapy or fuse DIP late); quadregia if FDP advanced >1 cm during repair
		I—Tendon in palm	Repair within 7-10 days (vincula disruption)	
		II—Tendon at level of Proximal interphalangeal (PIP) (held by A3 pulley)	Repair within 6 wk	
		III—Tendon at level of A4 pulley	ORIF of large, bony fragment with K-wires; keep A4 pulley intact with repair	
		IV—Bony fragment at P3 base	Early fixation of bony fragments and tendon	
Proximal (P1) and middle (P2) phalanges fracture		Extra-articular base (stable)	Buddy tape	Decreased range of motion (ROM) (flexor tendon adhesions), contractures, malunion/malrotation (may require osteotomy), lateral deviation, volar angulation (osteotomy), nonunion, tendon adherence
		Extra-articular base (unstable)	Reduce and immobilize (CRPP/ORIF if irreducible; external fixation for comminuted fractures, soft tissue injuries)	
		Intra-articular nondisplaced	Buddy tape, early ROM, close follow-up	
		Intra-articular condylar	Reduction, CRPP, or ORIF; restore articular surface if >1-mm displacement	
		Intra-articular P1 base	Small/nondisplaced—buddy tape Large/displaced—ORIF	
	Boutonniere	Intra-articular P2 base	Splint PIP (extension) for 6 wk; ORIF if large, bony fragment	
Metacarpal (MC) fracture		Head (transverse, oblique, spiral, comminuted)	ORIF for large piece, external fixation with early motion of comminuted fractures	Soft tissue injury (look for fight bite!), malunion (rotation); prominent MC head in palm (affects grip); loss of reduction (no volar buttress); nonunion, contracture of intrinsic muscles; claw deformity with extrinsic tendon imbalance
	Boxer	Neck—fourth and fifth MCs	40-70–degree angulation OK; reduce with Jahss maneuver, splint; operative if rotational deformity, extensor lag, multiple fracture, irreducible	
		Neck—second and third MCs	Usually requires CRPP to adjacent MC or ORIF	
		Shaft—transverse	Closed reduction, immobilize, or CRPP; accept 20-30–degree angulation in IV and V, 10-degree angulation in II and III; ORIF if irreducible	
		Shaft—oblique	ORIF if >5-mm shortening or rotated	
		Shaft—comminuted	Nondisplaced: splint; displaced: CRPP to adjacent MC or ORIF	
Thumb (first) MC base fracture	Bennett	I—Intra-articular volar ulnar lip	Attempt CRPP to trapezium; ORIF if irreducible	Displaced by abductor pollicis longus
	Rolando	II—Intra-articular "Y" (volar and dorsal)	Large fragments: ORIF; comminuted: external fixation or early motion	Degenerative joint disease
		III—Extra-articular (transverse or oblique)	Closed reduction, splint for 4 wk; CRPP if angulation >30 degrees	
Small (fifth) MC base fracture	"Baby Bennett"	Base fracture (epibasal, two-part, three-part, comminuted)	Evaluate with semipronated, semisupinated, distraction views; CRPP to adjacent MC or ORIF	Watch carpometacarpal fracture-dislocation, painful arthritis, fragment displaced by extensor carpi ulnaris

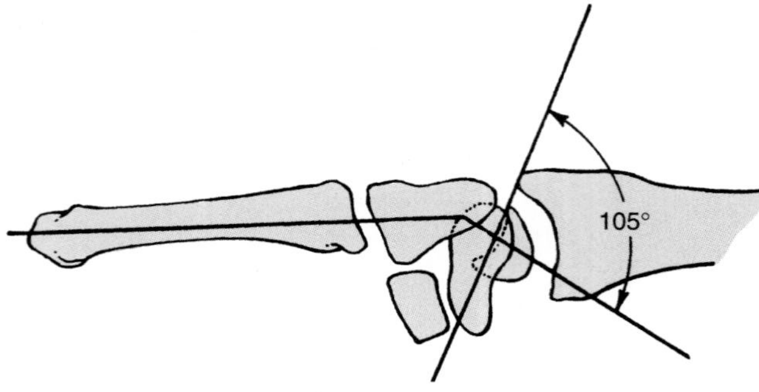

FIGURE 11–26 Dorsal intercalary segmental instability (DISI). Note scapholunate angle > 70 degrees, consistent with a DISI pattern. (From Connolly JF, ed: DePalma's The Management of Fractures and Dislocations: An Atlas, 3rd ed, p 1085. Philadelphia, WB Saunders, 1981. Reprinted by permission.)

(2) ORIF if there is a large fragment and/or the fracture is irreducible

b. Rolando fracture—ORIF with 2-mm T-plate or blade plate if there are larger fragments, K-wires for smaller fragments, and spanning external fixator for very severe comminution

c. Extra-articular—Spica cast for 4 weeks and CRPP if there is greater than 30 degrees angulation

D. First metacarpophalangeal (MCP) joint injury/dislocation

1. Diagnosis/classification
   a. Ulnar collateral ligament injury (gamekeeper's thumb)—The most common injury.
      (1) Sprain (joint opens < 35-45 degrees) or complete tear.
      (2) Stener lesion—Interposition of adductor aponeurosis.
   b. Radial collateral ligament injury (rare)
   c. Dorsal—Simple or complex (interposition of the volar plate) (Fig. 11–27)
2. Treatment
   a. Gamekeeper's thumb
      (1) Sprain—Thumb spica cast for 4-6 weeks.

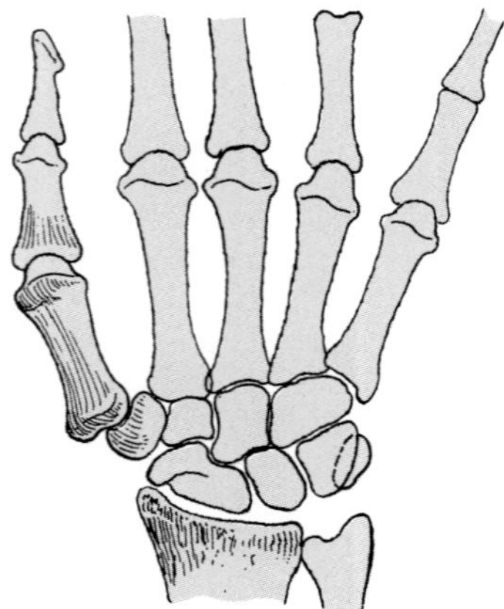

FIGURE 11–27 Subluxation/dislocation of the thumb carpometacarpal joint. (From Connolly JF, ed: DePalma's The Management of Fractures and Dislocations: An Atlas, 3rd ed, p 1165. Philadelphia, WB Saunders, 1981. Reprinted by permission.)

      (2) Stener lesion—Open-repair aponeurosis.
   b. Radial collateral ligament injury—Splint; late reconstruction only if necessary.
   c. Dorsal—For a simple dislocation, splint for 3 weeks; for a complex dislocation, perform open repair.
3. Complications—Unrecognized injury or Stener lesion, leading to chronic instability and pain.

E. Finger MCP dislocation

1. Diagnosis/classification—Index is finger most often affected; characteristic skin puckering in the palm at the level of injury
   a. Collateral ligament injury—Uncommon aponeurosis
   b. Dorsal—By far the most common (simple or complex)
   c. Volar (rare)
2. Treatment—Reduce with volar force to the dorsal base of the proximal phalanx. May be irreducible; do not make multiple forceful attempts at reduction.
   a. Collateral ligament injury—Splint in 50 degrees MCP flexion for 3 weeks and then buddy tape for 3 more weeks. Use ORIF if there is an avulsion fragment with greater than 2-mm displacement or greater than 20% articular involvement.
   b. Dorsal—For a simple dislocation, splint for 7-10 days and then buddy tape. For a complex dislocation, perform open reduction (irreducible).
   c. Volar—Open reduction
3. Complications—Loss of motion (can be severely disabling)

F. Proximal interphalangeal (PIP) dislocation

1. Diagnosis/classification
   a. Dorsal—The most common dislocation. Avulsion of the volar plate occurs first, followed by a rent between the accessory and proper collateral ligaments. It can be further classified as stable or unstable as determined by maintenance of reduction. A fracture-dislocation of greater than 40% of the middle phalangeal joint surface will yield an unstable fracture-dislocation.
   b. Lateral
   c. Volar
2. Treatment—Reduce with volar force to the dorsal base of the proximal phalanx. May be irreducible; do not make multiple forceful attempts at reduction.
   a. Dorsal dislocation—Reduce with digital block anesthesia, longitudinal traction, and dorsal pressure applied to the proximal phalangeal head. Confirm concentric reduction and then apply dorsal block (about 30 degrees) splinting for 4 days, followed by vigorous joint motion to avoid stiffness.
   b. Dorsal fracture-dislocation—Similar reduction and stability test in extension. If stable, apply dorsal block splinting, excluding the last 45 degrees of extension; apply

30-degree block after 5-7 days; and buddy tape a week later. Unstable fracture-dislocation requires surgical fixation.

c. Volar or lateral dislocation—Closed reduction; ORIF if irreducible or incongruous. Try to reduce volar dislocation with MCP and PIP in flexion to avoid irreducible dislocation. Open treatment can be with pinning, external fixation, or open screw fixation.

3. Complications—Loss of motion (can be severely disabling)
   a. Dorsal dislocations are at significant risk for permanent stiffness and contractures (treat with volar plate arthroplasty).
   b. Central slip avulsion or marginal fracture avulsion—Look for these conditions with volar dislocations, leading to boutonniere deformity. Treat with acute ORIF repair of central slip.

G. Distal interphalangeal (DIP) dislocation
1. Diagnosis/classification
   a. Dorsal—The most common dislocation
   b. Collateral ligament injury
2. Treatment—Reduce with volar force to the dorsal base of the proximal phalanx. May be irreducible; do not make multiple forceful attempts at reduction.
   a. Dorsal—If the dislocation is acute, use closed reduction and splint for 1-2 weeks. If it is chronic or irreducible, use open reduction.
   b. Collateral ligament injury—For a sprain, buddy tape for 3-6 weeks. For a tear, perform open repair.
3. Complications—Extensor lag, which is treated with 8-week course of splinting, similar to a mallet finger.

H. Small metacarpal (MC) base fractures
1. Diagnosis—Reverse or baby Bennett fracture. Radiographic diagnosis can be difficult. Confirm the diagnosis with direct examination and special radiographs (semi pronated, semi supinated, or distraction films).
2. Classification
   Epibasal
   Two-part
   Three-part
   Comminuted
3. Treatment—Controversial, whether nonsurgical management or ORIF. If surgical treatment is elected, use CRPP and cast for 6 weeks or ORIF.
4. Complications—Painful arthritis and displacement by extensor carpi ulnaris (ECU).

I. MC shaft fracture
1. Classification (descriptive)
   Transverse
   Oblique
   Spiral
   Comminuted
2. Treatment
   a. Transverse—Reduce and immobilize or use percutaneous pinning (PCP). Accept 10 degrees for the index and long fingers and 20-30 degrees for the ring and small fingers. Use ORIF if fracture is irreducible.
   b. Oblique and spiral—CRPP or ORIF if fracture is unstable and/or displaced.
   c. Comminuted—For a nondisplaced fracture, splint. For a displaced fracture, pin to adjacent MC (preferred) or ORIF.

J. MC neck fracture
1. Diagnosis/classification—Common injury from flexed MC head striking an unyielding object. A fracture of the fifth MC neck is called a boxer fracture.
2. Treatment
   a. Nonoperative treatment—Reduce with the Jahss maneuver (flexed MCP joint with dorsally directed force through MC head and proximal phalanx). It is critical to assess rotational deformity. Splint in MCP flexion and PIP extension for 2-3 weeks, and then free the PIP joint and start motion. MCP motion begins after 4-5 weeks.
   b. Operative treatment—Usually percutaneous pinning. Indications are rotational deformity despite closed reduction, extension lag due to excessive MC head flexion, multiple fractures, or excessive displacement (> 50-60° for the ring and small fingers and > 15-20° for the index and long fingers).
3. Complications—Claw deformity with extrinsic tendon imbalance; prominent MC head in palm (may impair grip), loss of reduction; nonunion; and intrinsic contracture

K. MC head fracture
1. Diagnosis—Check carefully; these are frequently open fractures.
2. Classification (descriptive)
   Vertical
   Horizontal
   Oblique
   Comminuted
3. Treatment—ORIF for large fragments and external fixation with early motion if fracture is comminuted

L. Proximal and middle phalanx fracture
1. Diagnosis/classification
   a. Transverse, oblique, spiral, or comminuted for diaphyseal fracture
   b. Other anatomic locations—Extra-articular base, neck, and condylar region
   c. Intra-articular base—Three types of fractures
      (1) Collateral ligament avulsion
      (2) Compression
      (3) Vertical shear
   d. Diaphyseal
   e. Neck
   f. Condylar
2. Treatment
   a. Extra-articular base fracture—The Eaton-Belsky technique of transarticular pinning is popular for the proximal phalanx (Fig. 11–28).

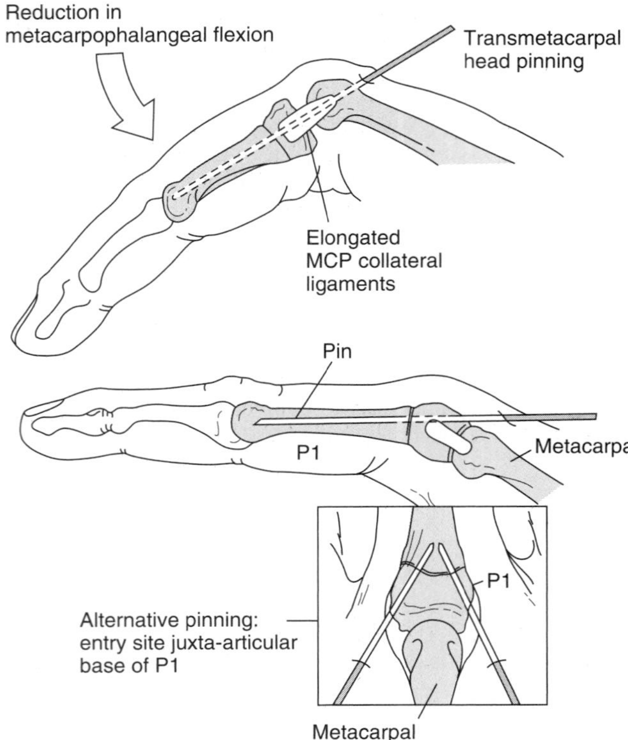

FIGURE 11–28 Intramedullary (Eaton-Belsky) pinning of proximal phalangeal base fractures. MCP, metacarpophalangeal. (From Stannard J, Schmidt A, Kregor P: Surgical Treatment of Orthopaedic Trauma. New York, Thieme Medical Publishers, 2007, Fig. 18-5.)

b. Collateral ligament avulsion—Tension band or ORIF if it is displaced or unstable and buddy tape if nondisplaced
c. Compression fracture of intra-articular base—ORIF with bone graft if needed
d. Vertical shear—ORIF or CRPP
e. Diaphyseal fracture—Buddy tape if fracture is stable and CRPP or ORIF if unstable. No difference in recovery rate, pain score, alignment, motion, or grip strength in a trial between ORIF with screws and CRPP.
f. Neck—CRPP
g. Condylar—Nondisplaced; digital splint for 7-10 days. Displaced ORIF.

3. Complications—Flexor tendon adhesions, flexion contracture, malunion or nonunion, malrotation, volar angulation (watch with proximal phalanx fractures; the middle phalanx may angulate toward either the volar or dorsal apex), and lateral deviation

M. Distal phalanx fracture

1. Diagnosis/classification
   a. Descriptive—Longitudinal, comminuted, and transverse
   b. Frequently crush injuries
2. Treatment
   a. Associated nail bed injuries may require surgery and are open fractures. Irrigate/débride, reduce, and splint with a digital splint and with the DIP extended and PIP free.
   b. Repair nail bed sterile matrix

N. EDL avulsion (mallet finger)

1. Classification—Watson-Jones classification
   a. Extensor tendon stretch—15-30 degrees extensor lag
   b. Extensor tendon torn—30-60 degrees extensor lag
   c. Extensor tendon avulsion with bone flaking
   d. Extensor tendon avulsion fragment—bony mallet
2. Treatment
   a. Vast majority treated closed with splinting. The first three classifications are treated with extensor splint for 6-8 weeks, followed by 3-4 weeks of night splinting.
   b. CRPP if occupation prevents splinting.
   c. Volar subluxation of distal phalanx (absolute indication) or greater than 50% of the

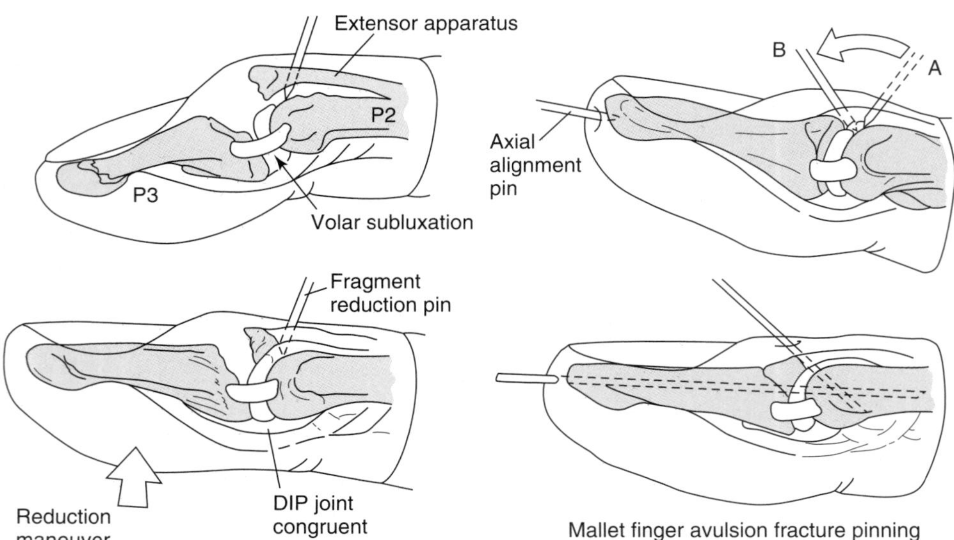

FIGURE 11–29 Technique of reduction and stabilization of a displaced mallet fracture with volar subluxation. The dorsal pin "levers" the avulsion fragment attached to the terminal tendon into place. The body of the phalanx is reduced and secured with a transarticular pin. DIP, distal interphalangeal joint. (From Stannard J, Schmidt A, Kregor P: Surgical Treatment of Orthopaedic Trauma. New York, Thieme Medical Publishers, 2007, Fig. 18-5.)

articular surface involved (relative indication at best). CRPP with extension block pinning (Fig. 11–29) or ORIF.

3. Complications—Dorsal skin necrosis, extensor lag, permanent nail deformities, pin tract infections, and osteomyelitis reported in up to 41% of surgically treated patients.

O. **Flexor digitorum longus** (FDL) avulsion (Jersey finger)

1. Classification—Leddy and Packer
   - Type I—Nonbony avulsion retracting into the palm
   - Type II—Avulsion, with small fragment retracting to PIP joint (held by A3 pulley)
   - Type III—Large-fragment avulsion to A4 pulley (just proximal to the DIP joint) (less common)
2. Treatment—All three types should be treated surgically.
   - Type I—Repair as acutely as possible (7-10 days maximum) due to complete disruption of vincula/blood supply
   - Type II—Repair by 6 weeks at the latest (easiest in first 7-10 days)
   - Type III—ORIF on large, bony fragment with K-wires
3. Complications—Missed diagnosis leads to lumbrical-plus finger requiring therapy or DIP arthrodesis (late); bony avulsion can have tendon avulsion separate from fragment, requiring fixation within 7-10 days.

SECTION 3 Lower Extremity and Pelvis

I. Pelvic and Acetabular Injuries

A. Pelvic ring injuries (Table 11–15)

1. Diagnosis
   a. Mechanism of injury
      (1) Often of high energy
      (2) Associated injuries common
      (3) Nonpelvic sources of bleeding must be ruled out.
      (4) Mortality usually related to nonpelvic injuries
   b. Radiographs
      (1) Anteroposterior pelvis
      (2) Inlet—Evaluate anteroposterior displacement of sacroiliac joint and rotational deformity
      (3) Outlet—Evaluate vertical displacement of sacroiliac joint
   c. CT scan—Particularly useful to evaluate posterior pelvic injury patterns
2. Classification
   a. Young-Burgess (Fig. 11–30)—Based on injury mechanism
      (1) Lateral compression (LC)
      (2) Anteroposterior compression (APC)
      (3) Vertical shear (VS)
      (4) Combined mechanism (CM)
   b. Tile—Based on fracture stability
      (1) Stable
         (a) Avulsion fractures
         (b) Iliac wing fractures
         (c) Transverse sacral fractures
      (2) Partially stable—Rotationally unstable and vertically stable
         (a) Anterior pelvic disruption alone
         (b) Anterior pelvic and anterior sacroiliac ligament disruption (intact posterior sacroiliac ligaments)
      (3) Unstable
         (a) Disruption of anterior pelvis (symphysis or rami fractures)
         (b) Complete posterior disruption (anterior and posterior SI ligaments or sacral or posterior ilium fracture)
3. Treatment
   a. General principles
      (1) Emergent treatment—To control hemorrhage and provisionally stabilize the pelvic ring
         (a) Volume resuscitation
         (b) Angiographic embolization
         (c) Pelvic binder
         (d) External fixation
         (e) Skeletal traction—For vertically unstable patterns
         (f) Pelvic C clamp
   b. Nonoperative treatment
      (1) Indicated for stable fracture patterns
      (2) Weight bearing as tolerated (WBAT) for isolated anterior injuries
      (3) Protected weight bearing for ipsilateral anterior and posterior ring injuries
   c. Operative treatment
      (1) Indications
         (a) Symphysis diastasis greater than 2.5 cm
         (b) Anterior and posterior SI ligament disruption
         (c) Vertical instability of posterior hemipelvis
         (d) Sacral fracture, with displacement greater than 1 cm
      (2) Anterior injuries
         (a) ORIF with plate fixation

TABLE 11-15 ADULT PELVIC FRACTURES

Injury	Eponym	Classification	Treatment	Complications
Pelvic fracture			Emergent management (advanced trauma life support, resuscitation, embolization of bleeding arteries if necessary, binder/external fixation/traction/pelvic C-clamp based on injury pattern)	
		Young and Burgess		Posterior skin slough, life-threatening hemorrhage, gastrointestinal injury, genitourinary injury (bladder, urethrea, impotency), neurologic injury, nonunion, post-traumatic degenerative joint disease, pain, deep venous thrombosis, pulmonary embolism, loss of reduction, sepsis, thrombophlebitis, malunion (leg-length discrepancy, sitting problems), vascular injuries (including aortic rupture), SI pain; APC-III highest rate of associated injury
		Lateral compression (LC)		
		I (most common)—Transverse rami fracture and sacral compression fracture	Protected weight bearing (WB), pain control	
		II—Rami fracture and posterior iliac wing fracture	Protected WB or delayed open reduction with internal fixation (ORIF)	
		III—Symphysis or rami and anterior and posterior sacroiliac (SI) ligament torn	Based on contralateral injury (ORIF of unstable injuries)	
		Anteroposterior compression (APC)		
		I—Symphysis (<2 cm) or rami (vertical) and anterior SI ligament stretched	Bed rest, early mobilization, pain control	
		II—Symphysis or rami and anterior SI ligament torn	Acute external fixation/anterior ORIF if concurrent laparotomy	
		III—Symphysis or rami and anterior and posterior SI ligament torn	Acute external fixation/anterior ORIF if concurrent laparotomy; posterior SI ORIF	
	Malgaigne	Vertical shear—Anterior and posterior vertical displacement	Acute external fixation/anterior ORIF if concurrent laparotomy; posterior SI ORIF (SI screws, anterior SI plate, posterior transiliac sacral bars, spinal-pelvic fixation)	
		Combined mechanical—Combination of other injuries	Based on injuries; ORIF if posterior SI displaced	
Sacral fracture		Denis—Fracture location relative to foramen		
		Stable, nondisplaced	Nonoperative (weight bearing as tolerated if fracture incomplete, toe-touch weight bearing for complete fracture)	Neurologic (highest with zone II fractures), chronic low-back pain, malunion
		Unstable, displaced (>1 cm)	Percutaneous SI screws, posterior ORIF, transiliac sacral bars, open foraminal decompression for neuron injury with zone II fractures	

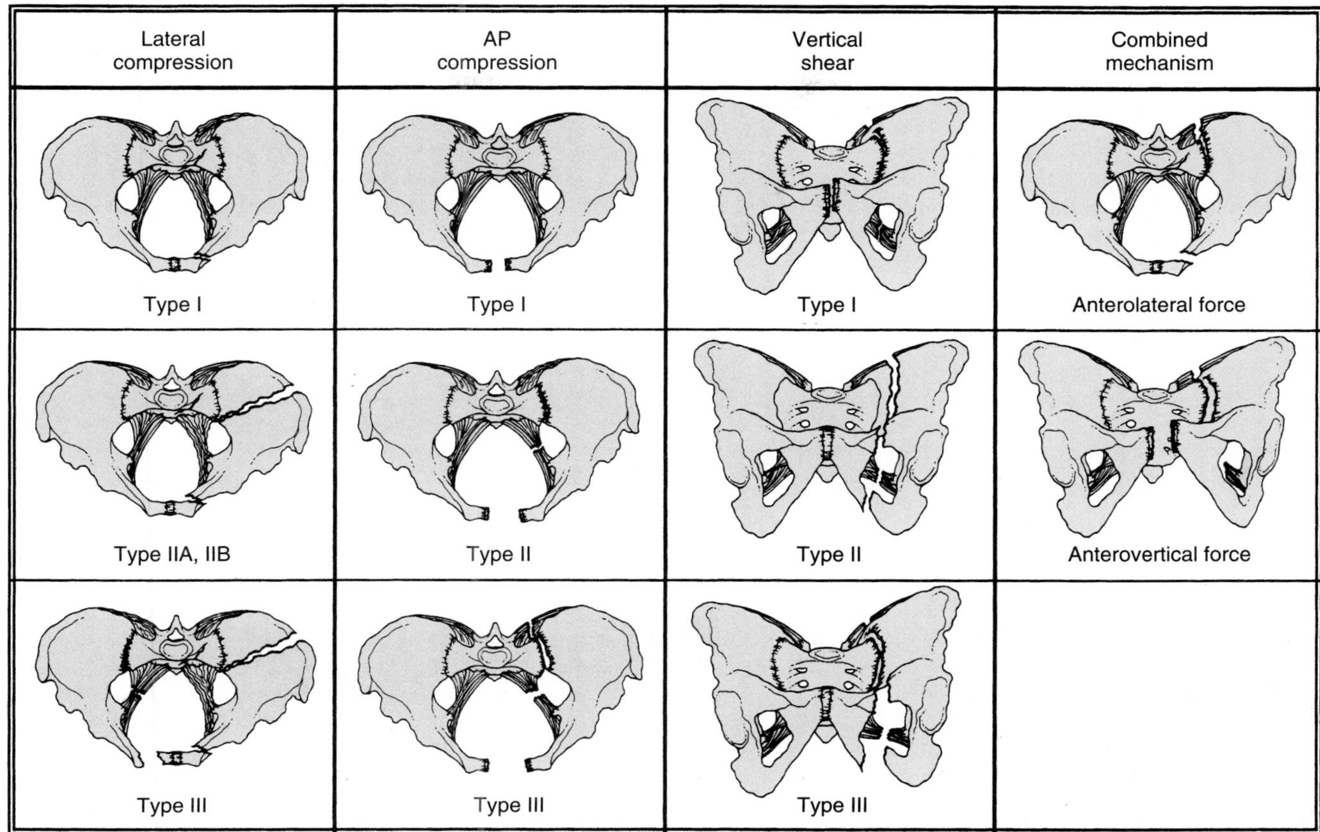

FIGURE 11–30 The modified Young-Burgess classification system. AP, anteroposterior. (From Tornetta P III, Baumgaertner M: Orthopaedic Knowledge Update: Trauma 3. Rosemont, IL, American Academy of Orthopaedic Surgeons, 2005.)

(b) External fixation via pins through anterior-inferior iliac spine

(3) Posterior injuries

(a) Percutaneous iliosacral screw fixation

(b) Anterior plate fixation across the SI joint

(c) Posterior transiliac sacral bars

(d) Spinal-pelvic fixation considered for vertically unstable patterns

4. Complications
   a. Severe, life-threatening hemorrhage (highest risk with APC2, APC3, and LC3 patterns)
   b. Neurologic injury
   c. Urogenital injury/dysfunction
   d. Malunion
   e. Nonunion
   f. DVT and/or pulmonary embolus (PE)—Should rule out DVT prior to definitive operative treatment
   g. Infection—Open fracture and associated contaminated laparotomy
   h. Death—The highest risk is open fracture, LC3, APC2, and APC3 patterns

B. Sacral fractures

1. Diagnosis
   a. Mechanism of injury—High energy
   b. Radiographs—Anteroposterior pelvis, inlet, outlet, and lateral views
   c. CT scans (usually required)
2. Classification—Denis classification (Fig. 11–31) based on fracture location relative to foramen (zones I, II, and III)
3. Treatment
   a. Nonoperative treatment

(1) Indicated for stable and minimally displaced fractures

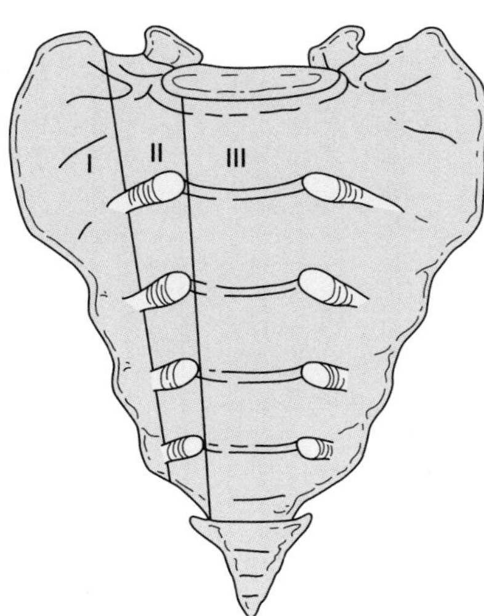

FIGURE 11–31 The Denis classification of sacral fractures. (From Browner BD, et al, eds: Skeletal Trauma, p 820. Philadelphia, WB Saunders, 1992.)

(2) WBAT for incomplete fractures in which the ilium is contiguous with the intact sacrum (e.g., anterior impaction fractures from LC compression mechanism or isolated sacral ala fractures)
(3) Touch-toe weight bearing (TTWB) for complete fractures

b. Operative treatment
(1) Indicated for displaced fractures (> 1 cm)
(2) Percutaneous iliosacral screws
(3) Posterior plating
(4) Transiliac sacral bars
(5) Open foraminal decompression considered for neurologic injury associated with zone II fracture

4. Complications
a. Neurologic injury
(1) Highest incidence with displaced zone II fractures
(2) L2 nerve root usually involved with zone II fractures
(3) Cauda equina syndrome can be associated with zone III injuries

b. Chronic low-back pain
c. Malunion

C. Acetabular fractures (Table 11–16)
1. Diagnosis
a. Mechanism of injury
(1) Young high-energy patients
(2) Pattern of injury dependent on position of hip and direction of impact
(3) Flexed hip with axial load (dashboard injury mechanism) the most common injury

b. Plain radiographs
(1) Anteroposterior pelvis—Six cardinal lines (Fig. 11–32)

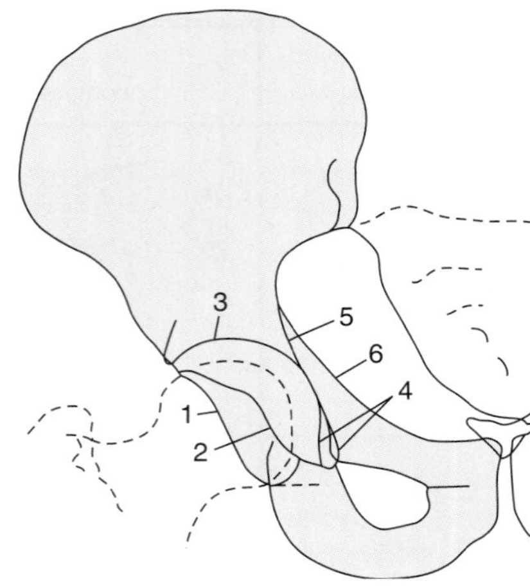

FIGURE 11–32 Six cardinal radiographic lines of the acetabulum. 1, Posterior wall. 2, Anterior wall. 3, Roof. 4, Teardrop. 5, Ilioischial line. 6, Iliopectineal line. (From Tornetta P III, Baumgaertner M: Orthopaedic Knowledge Update: Trauma 3, p 264. Rosemont, IL, American Academy of Orthopaedic Surgeons, 2005.)

TABLE 11-16 ADULT ACETABULAR FRACTURES

Injury	Classification	Treatment	Complications
Acetabular fracture	Letournel—based on involvement of acetabular columns and wall Simple types Anterior wall (AW) Anterior column (AC) Posterior wall (PW)—most common simple type Posterior column (PC) Transverse—involves both AC and PC Associated types PC/PW Transverse/PW—most common associated type AC/posterior hemitransverse (ACPHT)—least common type T-type—transverse with vertical limb through ischium Both columns (BCs)—dissociation of acetabular dome from axial skeleton. "Spur sign" seen on obturator oblique view	Nonoperative: <1-mm step-off and <2-mm gap; roof arc angle >45 degrees on anteroposterior, inlet, and outlet views—computed tomographic correlate is fracture >10 mm from dome apex; PW fractures without instability (<20% of PW); associated fractures of BCs with secondary congruence; severe comminution in elderly in whom total hip arthroplasty is planned after fracture healing Relative contraindications to surgery: morbid obesity, physiologically elderly/nonambulatory, contaminated wound, delay to operation >4 wk, presence of deep venous thrombosis with contraindication for filter Operative: displaced fracture, incongruous or unstable joint, intra-articular bone fragments, irreducible fracture-dislocation ***Surgical approaches:*** Kocher-Langenbeck (posterior approach) indicated for PW, PC, transverse, transverse/PW (when PW requires fixation), PC/PW, T-type Ilioinguinal (anterior approach) indicated for AW, AC, ACPHT, BCs Extensile approaches considered for fractures >3 wk old and complex associated fractures Combined anterior and posterior approaches Extended iliofemoral Triradiate Posterior with trochanteric osteotomy	Nerve injury (sciatic 16-33%, femoral, superior gluteal), vascular injury (inferior gluteal artery), heterotopic ossification (3-69%—consider radiation therapy or Indocin), avascular necrosis (with posterior injury), chondrolysis, post-traumatic degenerative joint disease, soft tissue degloving (Morel-Lavalle lesion), osteonecrosis (damage to medial femoral circumflex artery), malreduction (delay to surgery), bleeding (shorter time to surgery)

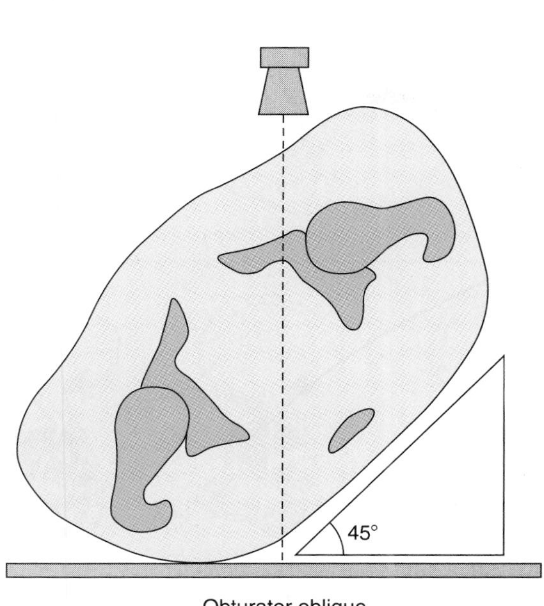

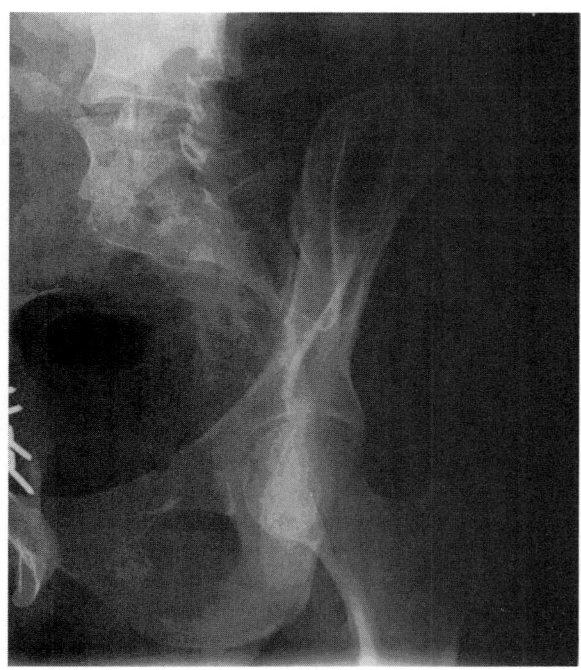

FIGURE 11–33 **A**, Obturator oblique view of the pelvis obtained with the patient tilted 45 degrees, with the unaffected hip down and adjacent to the x-ray cassette. The x-ray beam was centered over the affected hip. (From Tornetta P III, Baumgaertner M: Orthopaedic Knowledge Update: Trauma 3, p 263. Rosemont, IL, American Academy of Orthopaedic Surgeons, 2005.) **B**, Obturator oblique radiograph profiles the anterior column and the posterior wall of the acetabulum.

(2) Obturator oblique—Profiles anterior column and posterior wall (Fig. 11–33)

(3) Iliac oblique—Profiles posterior column and anterior wall (Fig. 11–34)

c. CT scan

(1) Thin-cut (1-2 mm) axial

(2) Three-dimensional (3D) reconstruction, with femur subtracted

2. Classification—Letournel classification (Fig. 11–35) based on involvement of acetabular columns and walls

a. Simple types

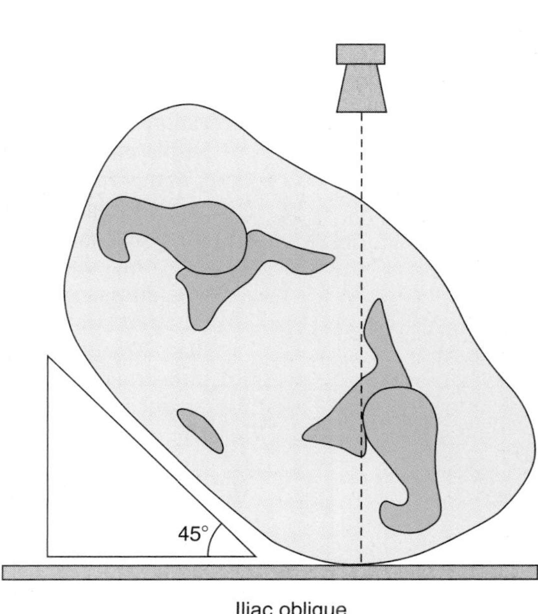

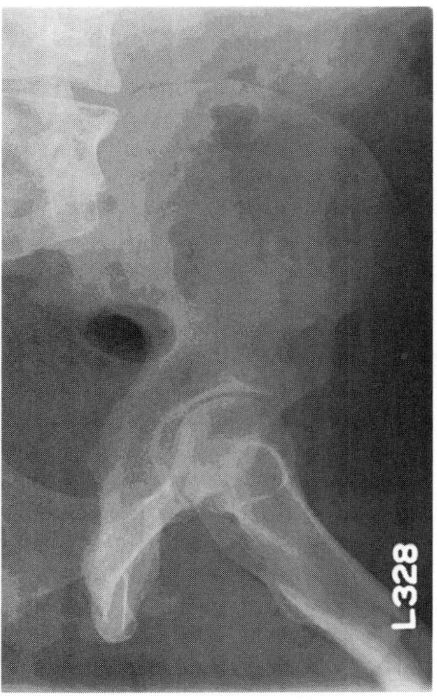

FIGURE 11–34 **A**, Iliac oblique view of the pelvis obtained with the patient tilted 45 degrees, with the affected hip down and adjacent to the x-ray cassette. The x-ray beam was centered over the affected hip. (From Tornetta P III, Baumgaertner M: Orthopaedic Knowledge Update: Trauma 3, p 263. Rosemont, IL, American Academy of Orthopaedic Surgeons, 2005.) **B**, Iliac oblique radiograph profiles the posterior column and the anterior wall of the acetabulum.

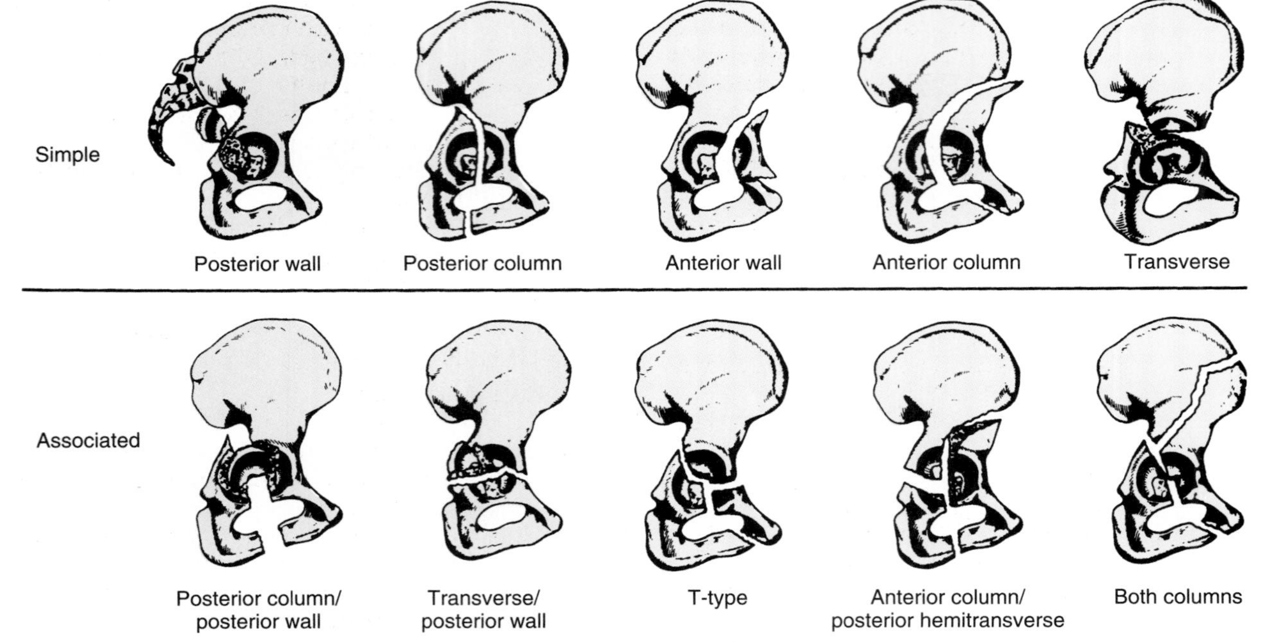

FIGURE 11–35 The Letournel classification of acetabular fractures. (From Tornetta P III, Baumgaertner M: Orthopaedic Knowledge Update: Trauma 3, p 370. Rosemont, IL, American Academy of Orthopaedic Surgeons, 2005.)

(1) Posterior wall (PW)—The most common simple type
(2) Posterior column (PC)
(3) Anterior wall (AW)
(4) Anterior column (AC)
(5) Transverse—Involves both the anterior and posterior columns (but without criteria for "AC" and "PC" types)

b. Associated types
(1) Posterior column/posterior wall (PC/PW)
(2) Transverse/posterior wall (TPW)—The most common associated type
(3) T-type—Transverse and vertical limbs through ischium
(4) Anterior column/posterior hemitransverse (ACPHT) (least common type)
(5) Both columns—Dissociation of acetabular dome from axial skeletal. "Spur sign" seen on obturator oblique view.

3. Treatment
a. General principles
(1) Restore articular congruity and hip stability
(2) Avoid injury to blood supply to femoral head
(3) DVT screening and prophylaxis

b. Nonoperative treatment
(1) Indications
(a) Nondisplaced or minimally displaced fracture (< 1-mm step and < 2-mm gap)
(b) Roof arc angle greater than 45 degrees on anteroposterior, inlet, and outlet views—The CT correlate is a fracture greater than 10 mm from the dome apex.
(c) Posterior wall fracture without instability (< 20% of posterior wall)
(d) Fracture of both columns, with secondary congruence
(e) Severe comminution in the elderly in whom **total hip replacement** (THR) is planned after fracture healing
(2) Protected weight bearing for approximately 6 weeks
(3) Femoral traction for 2-3 weeks, followed by TTWB for 3-4 weeks

c. Operative treatment
(1) Indications
(a) Displacement with a greater than 1-mm step or greater than 2-mm gap associated with the roof is an angle less than 45 degrees on any view or documented instability with stress examination.
(b) Posterior wall fracture of greater than 20% or hip instability
(c) Intra-articular bone fragments
(d) Irreducible fracture-dislocation
(2) Relative contraindications to surgery
(a) Morbid obesity
(b) Physiologically elderly and nonambulatory
(c) Presence of DVT, with contraindication to inferior vena cava (IVC) filter
(d) Contaminated wound compromising surgical approach
(e) Delay to operation more than 4 weeks
(3) Surgical approaches

(a) Kocher-Langenbeck (posterior approach) procedure indicated for PW, PC, transverse, transverse/PW (when PW requires fixation), PC/PW, and T-type
(b) Ilioinguinal (anterior approach) procedure indicated for AW, AC, ACPHT, and both columns
(c) Extensile approaches considered for fractures over 3 weeks old and complex associated fractures
   i. Combined anterior and posterior approaches
   ii. Extended iliofemoral procedure
   iii. Triradiate
   iv. Posterior and trochanteric osteotomy

4. Complications
   a. Soft tissue degloving (Morel-Lavalle lesion) associated with higher infection rates
   b. DVT—Preoperative screening and IVC filter when is DVT present. Postoperative screening and anticoagulation if DVT is present
   c. PE—Treatment similar to that for DVT indicated above
   d. HO associated with extended approaches > Kocher-Langenbeck > anterior approach, prophylaxis with indomethacin, or **radiation therapy** (XRT) of 600 cGy within 48 hours of surgery
   e. Neurologic injury—Sciatic nerve injury associated with posterior dislocations. Intraoperative monitoring is not associated with reduced iatrogenic nerve injury. Hip extension and knee flexion reduce tension on sciatic nerve. Iatrogenic injury to lateral femoral cutaneous nerve with anterior approach.
   f. Osteonecrosis—The highest incidence with posterior fractures, especially fracture-dislocations. Iatrogenic damage to medial femoral circumflex artery.
   g. Post-traumatic DJD—The highest in patterns with PW involvement
   h. Malreduction—Associated with greater delay due to surgery
   i. Bleeding—Associated with shorter time to surgery
   j. Functional deficit—Especially abductor weakness (posterior more than anterior approach)

II. Femoral and Hip Injuries (Tables 11–17 and 11–18)

A. Hip dislocations
1. Diagnosis
   a. Mechanism of injury—Axial load. The position of the hip determines the direction of dislocation.
   b. Plain radiographs—Anteroposterior and lateral views of the hip. Anteroposterior pelvis and Judet views after reduction to evaluate associated acetabular fractures.
   c. CT scan—Performed after reduction to evaluate associated acetabular and/or femoral head fracture and loose bodies in joint.
2. Classification—Based on direction of dislocation and presence or absence of associated acetabular or femoral head fracture.
   a. Posterior dislocation—The most common; associated with posterior wall acetabular fracture and anterior femoral head fracture. Leg flexed, adducted, and internally rotated at hip.
   b. Anterior dislocation—Uncommon; leg extended, abducted, and externally rotated at hip.
3. Treatment
   a. Emergent, closed reduction.
   b. Emergent, open reduction if irreducible after closed reduction.

TABLE 11-17 ADULT HIP DISLOCATIONS

Injury	Classification	Treatment	Complications
Hip dislocation	Direction: posterior (most common), anterior, obturator; associated fractures (acetabular, femoral head)	Emergent, closed reduction (open if irreducible); computed tomography/plain films (Judet views) after reduction; traction/abduction pillow (depends on stability); weight bearing as tolerated if hip stable	Associated with increased-energy trauma and often associated with other injuries; femoral artery/nerve injuries (anterior dislocation), sciatic nerve injury (up to 20%; peroneal division most common), osteonecrosis (up to 15%), post-traumatic arthritis, recurrent dislocation (rare), post-traumatic degenerative joint disease (especially with retained fragments); instability (with >30-40% fracture of posterior wall); unrecognized femoral neck fracture

TABLE 11-18 ADULT—HIP FRACTURES

Injury	Classification	Treatment	Complications
Femoral head fracture	Pipkin—based on location of fracture relative to fovea and associated fractures of acetabulum or femoral neck	Restore articular congruity (open reduction [with] internal fixation [ORIF] when >1-mm step-off), restore hip stability, remove loose bodies, treat associated fractures, avoid injury to femoral head blood supply	Osteonecrosis (up to 15%), post-traumatic arthritis, sciatic nerve injury (up to 20%), recurrent dislocation (rare); Pipkin III highest rate of avascular necrosis
	Type I—Fracture below fovea	Nonoperative if small fragment, congruent joint, protected weight bearing (WB); ORIF with anterior approach (headless countersunk screws)	
	Type II—Fracture above fovea	Nonoperative if stable, nondisplaced fragment, protected WB; ORIF with anterior approach (headless countersunk screws)	
	Type III—Associated femoral neck fracture	ORIF of femoral neck and head; arthroplasty if older patient	
	Type IV—Associated acetabular fracture	ORIF of acetabulum and head via posterior approach; arthroplasty if older patient	
Femoral neck fracture	Garden (low energy in elderly) I—Incomplete/valgus impaction (stable) II—Complete, nondisplaced (stable) III—Complete, partially displaced (unstable) IV—Complete, totally displaced (unstable)	Based on orientation of trabecular lines and displacement Medical optimization; closed reduction with percutaneous pinning (CRPP) with 3 screws or sliding compression hip screw with derotation screw; prosthesis for elderly (>70 yr old physiologically), sick, pathologic fracture, Parkinson, rheumatoid arthritis, Dilantin therapy with displaced fractures (Garden III or IV); results of unipolar vs. bipolar prosthesis similar; consider total hip arthroplasty for more active patients, acetabular degenerative joint disease (higher dislocation rate than hemiarthroplasty)	Osteonecrosis (10-40%; injury to medial femoral circumflex), nonunion (10-30% of displaced fractures), infection, malunion (accept <15 degrees valgus and 10 degrees anteroposterior displacement); infection, pulmonary embolism, mortality (≈30% at 1 year; increases with advancing age, medical problems, males); cardiopulmonary decompensation with cemented stems
	Pauwels (high energy in the young)	Based on orientation of fracture line; increased vertical orientation associated with less stability; ORIF with sliding hip screw (fixed-angle device) for vertically oriented fracture lines	

Intertrochanteric fracture	Number of fracture fragments, ability to resist compressive loads when fixed Two-part: stable with little risk of collapse Three-part: intermediate stability Four-part and comminuted: least stable	Nonoperative treatment with nondisplaced fractures in compliant patients, those with high operative risk ORIF with sliding compression hip screw and side plate most reliable; lag screw in center-center position (TAD <25 mm); intramedullary (IM) nail for unstable, reverse oblique, subtrochanteric fractures; calcar-replacing arthroplasty for patients with severe osteopenia, comminution	Excessive collapse (limb shortening, medialization of shaft, sliding hip screw ≫ IM device), prominent hardware; nail cutout (TAD >25 mm); loss of fixation (increased with superolateral screws); joint penetration (screw ideally placed center-center and deep); mortality, infection
Greater trochanteric fracture	Amount of displacement	ORIF if >1 cm displacement in young patient	
Lesser trochanteric fracture	Amount of displacement	ORIF if >2 cm displacement in young athlete	Consider pathologic fracture
Subtrochanteric fracture	Russell-Taylor—based on involvement of lesser trochanter and piriformis fossa	Restore limb length, alignment, rotation; indirect reduction (open or percutaneous if necessary); avoid piriformis entry when fossa involved; fixed-angle device (95-degree blade plate) for proximal comminution	Apex anterior and varus most common deformity; nonunion (minimized with IM nail), infection (increased with soft tissue dissection)
	IA—Fracture below lesser trochanter	IM nail, standard proximal interlock	
	IB—Fracture involves lesser trochanter; greater trochanter intact	IM nail, reconstructed interlock	
	IIA—Greater trochanter involved, lesser trochanter intact	IM nail, standard proximal interlock	
	IIB—Greater and lesser trochanters involved	ORIF with fixed-angle device (95-degree blade plate) vs. IM nail, reconstructed interlock	

TAD, tip to apex distance.

c. Evaluate stability after reduction.
d. Traction and/or hip abduction pillow for unstable injuries pending definitive management of associated injuries (e.g., acetabular fracture).
e. Postreduction radiographs (anteroposterior pelvis and Judet views) and CT scan to rule out associated acetabular fracture, femoral head fracture, and intra-articular loose bodies.
f. WBAT (if hip is stable and without associated injuries)

4. Complications
   a. Osteonecrosis (up to 15%)
   b. Post-traumatic arthritis—More common when associated with PW acetabular fracture.
   c. Sciatic nerve injury (up to 20%)—Peroneal nerve division usually the most affected.
   d. Recurrent dislocation (rare)

B. Femoral head fractures
1. Diagnosis
   a. Plain radiographs—Anteroposterior and lateral views of hip
   b. CT scan—To evaluate location and size of fragment and rule out associated acetabular fracture.
2. Classification—Pipkin classification (Fig. 11–36) based on location of fracture relative to fovea and presence or absence of associated fractures of the acetabulum or femoral neck
   Type I—Fracture below fovea
   Type II—Fracture above fovea
   Type III—Associated femoral neck fracture
   Type IV—Associated acetabular fracture

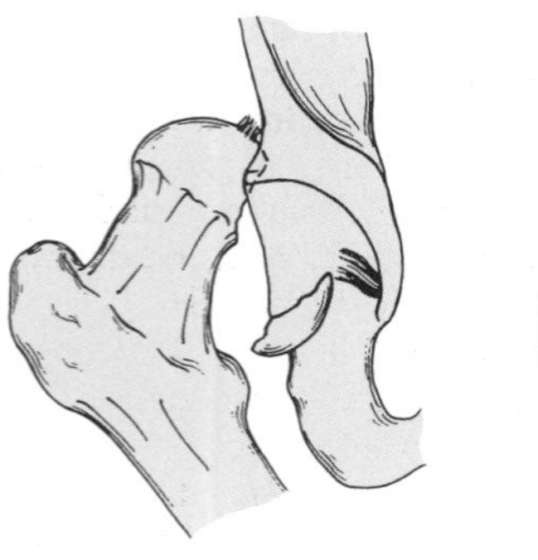

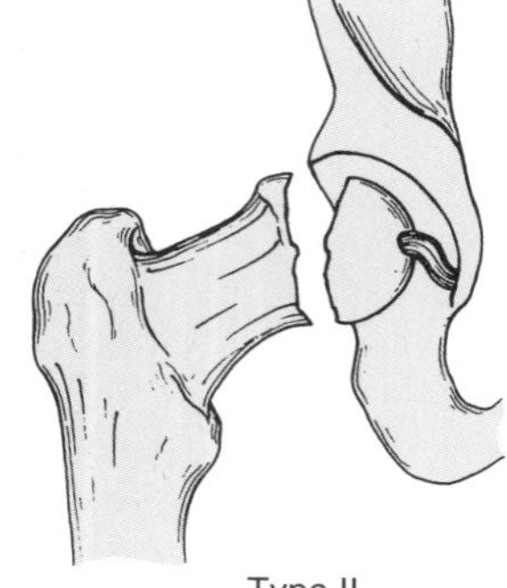

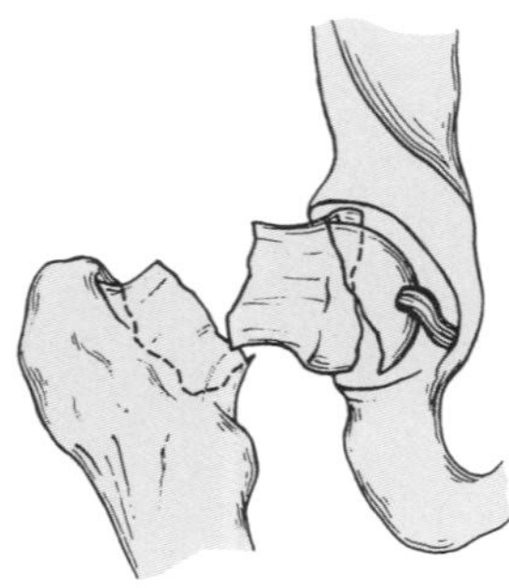

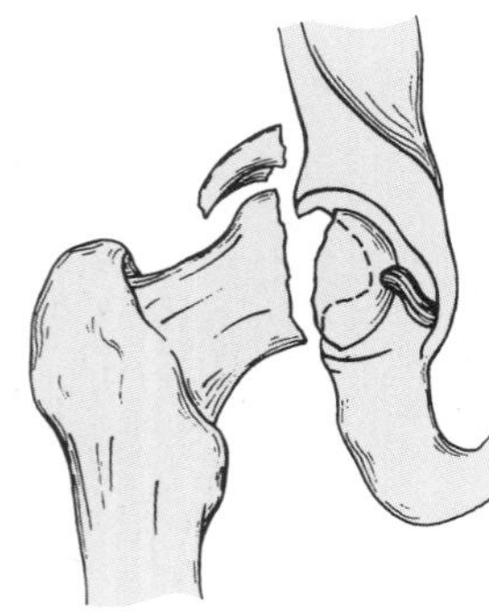

FIGURE 11–36 The Pipkin classification of femoral neck fractures. (From Tornetta P III, Baumgaertner M: Orthopaedic Knowledge Update: Trauma 3, p 370. Rosemont, IL, American Academy of Orthopaedic Surgeons, 2005.)

3. Treatment
   a. General principles
      (1) Restore articular congruity of weight-bearing portion of head and hip stability.
      (2) Remove associated loose bodies.
      (3) Treat associated acetabular fracture.
      (4) Avoid injury to structures involved in blood supply to femoral head.
   b. Nonoperative treatment
      (1) Indications
         (a) Pipkin type I—Small fragment and congruent joint or nondisplaced larger fragment
         (b) Pipkin type II—Nondisplaced; frequent (weekly) radiographs for 3-4 weeks to rule out secondary displacement
      (2) Protected weight bearing for 4-6 weeks
   c. Operative treatment
      (1) Indications
         (a) Greater than 1-mm step-off (except small Pipkin type I)
         (b) Associated loose bodies in joint
         (c) Associated neck or acetabular fracture requiring surgical management
      (2) Fixation with headless countersunk lag screws
         (a) Anterior approach for Pipkin types I and II without associated operative PW fracture
         (b) Posterior approach for Pipkin type IV
      (3) Hip arthroplasty for older patient
4. Complications
   a. Same as those for hip dislocation
   b. The highest rate of AVN for Pipkin type III injuries

C. Femoral neck fractures
1. Diagnosis
   a. Mechanism of injury
      (1) Low energy (fall from standing height) in elderly—Associated with osteoporosis
      (2) High energy in young patients—Associated with vertical fracture orientation
   b. Plain radiographs
      (1) Anteroposterior and lateral views of hip
      (2) Anteroposterior and lateral views of femur
      (3) Anteroposterior pelvis
   c. MRI or bone scan to rule out occult fracture
2. Classification
   a. Garden classification (Fig. 11–37) based on orientation of trabecular lines and displacement
      (1) Garden types I and II considered stable
      (2) Garden types III and IV considered unstable
   b. Pauwels classification (Fig. 11–38) based on orientation of fracture line
      (1) Increased vertical orientation associated with more shear force and reduced inherent stability
      (2) Nonunion and AVN associated with vertical patterns (Pauwels type III)

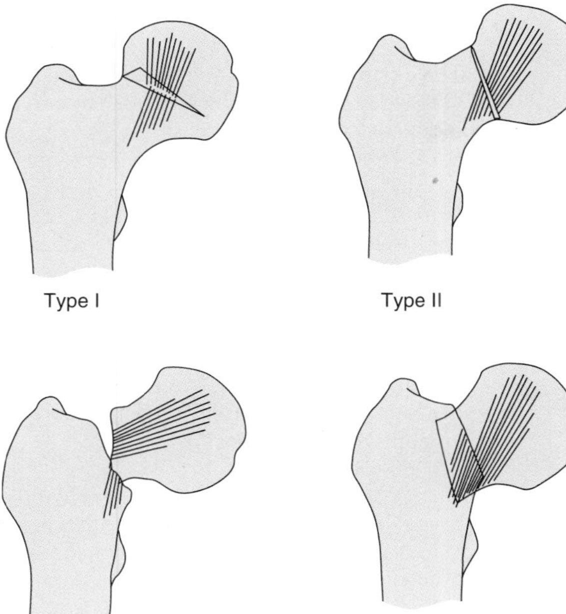

FIGURE 11–37 Schematic representation of the Garden classification of femoral neck fractures. Type I is an incomplete, impacted fracture in valgus malalignment (generally stable). Type II is a nondisplaced fracture. Type III is an incompletely displaced fracture in varus malalignment. Type IV is a completely displaced fracture, with no engagement of the two fragments. The compression trabeculae in the femoral head line up with the trabeculae on the acetabular side. Displacement is generally more evident on the lateral view in type IV. For prognostic purposes, these groupings can be lumped into nondisplaced/impacted (types I and II) and displaced (types III and IV) because the risks of nonunion and aseptic necrosis are similar within these grouped types. (From Tornetta P III, Baumgaertner M: Orthopaedic Knowledge Update: Trauma 3, p 370. Rosemont, IL, American Academy of Orthopaedic Surgeons, 2005.)

3. Treatment
    a. General principles
        (1) Preoperative medical optimization
        (2) Stable fixation and early mobilization
    b. Nonoperative treatment
        (1) Indications
            (a) Nondisplaced fractures in patients able to comply with weight-bearing restrictions
            (b) Displaced fractures in patients with extremely limited functional demands and/or those with high risk for surgery
        (2) TTWB for 6-8 weeks
    c. Operative treatment
        (1) Indications
            (a) Displaced fractures
            (b) Most nondisplaced fractures
        (2) Internal fixation
            (a) Indicated for Garden types I and III fractures in young patients, occult fractures, and displaced fractures in young patients
            (b) Three parallel screws for Garden types I and II and occult fractures
                i. Inverted V pattern
                ii. Screws distal to lesser trochanter associated with increased risk of peri-implant subtrochanteric fracture
                iii. Consider fourth screw when posterior comminution exists
            (c) Sliding hip screw (fixed-angle device) plus derotation screw indicated for basal cervical fractures and vertically oriented fractures
            (d) Anatomic reduction associated with the best results for displaced fractures in young patients
                i. Open reduction often required
                ii. Anatomic reduction more critical than reduced time to fixation
            (e) Decompression of intracapsular hematoma thought to reduce risk of AVN (not proven and controversial)
            (f) Internal fixation associated with decreased perioperative morbidity and an increased need for secondary procedures relative to arthroplasty
        (3) Hemiarthroplasty
            (a) Indicated for elderly patients with displaced fractures
            (b) Lower risk of dislocation than in total hip arthroplasty (THA), especially in patients unable to comply with dislocation precautions (e.g., dementia, Parkinson disease)

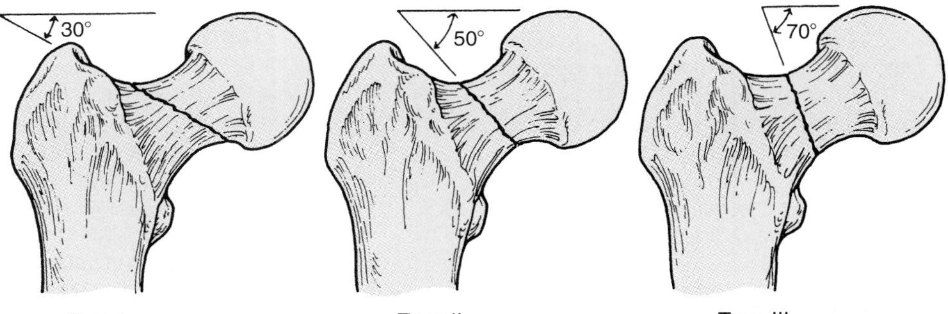

FIGURE 11–38 The Pauwels classification of femoral neck fractures. With progression from type I to type III, there are increasing shear forces placed across the fracture site. (From Evarts CM, ed: Surgery of the Musculoskeletal System, 2nd ed, p 2556. New York, Churchill Livingstone, 1990.)

(c) The cemented femoral component yields better results than those for the uncemented component in patients with "stove pipe"–type canals.
(d) The cemented femoral component has a higher risk of cardiopulmonary decompensation than that associated with the noncemented component, especially in patients with significant preexisting cardiopulmonary disease.
(e) The results of unipolar and bipolar prostheses are similar.
(4) THA
(a) Indicated for elderly patients with displaced fractures
(b) Preferred to hemiarthroplasty for patients with preexisting hip arthropathy (osteoarthritis and rheumatoid arthritis)
(c) Better functional results than those associated with hemiarthroplasty in active patients
(d) Higher dislocation rate than hemiarthroplasty

4. Complications
a. Osteonecrosis—Occurs in 10-40%; associated with injury to femoral head blood supply, the main contribution being the terminal branch of the medial femoral circumflex artery
(1) Higher risk with greater initial displacement
(2) Higher risk with poor or deficient reduction
(3) Decompression of intracapsular hematoma may reduce risk (controversial)
(4) Reduced time to reduction may reduce risk (controversial)
b. Nonunion—Occurs in 10-30% of displaced fractures
(1) Higher risk with malreduction
(2) Treatment options include conversion to hip arthroplasty (worse results than those associated with primary arthroplasty) and valgus osteotomy.
c. Infection
d. Mortality—One-year mortality in elderly patients approximately 30%

D. Intertrochanteric fractures
1. Diagnosis
a. Mechanism of injury—Fall from standing height
b. Risk factors include osteoporosis, prior hip fracture, and risk of falls
c. More common than femoral neck fracture in patients with preexisting hip arthritis
d. Plain radiographs
(1) Anteroposterior and lateral views of hip
(2) Anteroposterior and lateral views of femur
(3) Anteroposterior pelvis
e. MRI or bone scan to rule out occult fracture
2. Classification—Based on the number of fracture fragments and ability to resist compression loads once they are reduced and fixed.
a. Two-part fractures—Usually stable, with little risk of excessive collapse
b. Three-part fractures—Intermediate stability
(1) Size and location of lesser trochanteric fragment determine stability.
(2) Large posterior medial fragments are less stable.
c. Four-part and severely comminuted fractures are the least stable. They have the highest risk for excessive collapse, varus collapse, and nonunion.
3. Treatment
a. General principles
(1) Stable fixation to allow early weight bearing
(2) Minimize potential for implant failure.
b. Nonoperative treatment
(1) Indications
(a) Nondisplaced fractures in patients able to comply with non–weight-bearing restrictions
(b) Displaced fractures in nonambulatory individuals or those with prohibitive operative risk
(2) Management with TTWB for 6-8 weeks
c. Operative treatment
(1) Indications
(a) Displaced fractures
(b) Most nondisplaced fractures
(2) Internal fixation indicated for the vast majority of intertrochanteric fractures.
(a) Sliding hip screw device
i. Indicated for most intertrochanteric fractures except reverse oblique and subtrochanteric fractures
ii. High union rate
iii. Associated with moderate amount of collapse, resulting limb shortening, and medialization when used for unstable fractures. More collapse than that seen with IM implants.
iv. Lower peri-implant fracture rate than that seen with IM implants
v. Lag screw placed in center—Center position with tip–apex distance (TAD) of less than 25 mm associated with the lowest screw failure rate
vi. Two-hole side place sufficient for stable fractures
(b) IM nail
i. Indicated for most intertrochanteric fractures
ii. Reduced collapse relative to sliding hip screw plate devices due to IM buttress effect of nail
iii. Short nails indicated for standard obliquity fractures, with distal interlocking optional
iv. Long nails indicated for standard obliquity, reverse obliquity, and subtrochanteric fractures. Risk of distal anterior perforation due to

mismatch of anterior bow between femur and nail.

v. Higher peri-implant fracture rate than that associated with sliding hip screw plate devices

vi. Multiple screws into head fragment may provide improved rotational control (advantage controversial)

vii. Single lag screw design should aim center—Center in head with less than 25 mm TAD

(c) 95-degree fixed-angle plate device—Indicated for reverse obliquity, comminuted fracture, and nonunion repair

(3) Arthroplasty

(a) Indicated for severely comminuted fractures

(b) Still requires union of greater trochanter to shaft

(c) Calcar-replacing design often required

4. Complications

a. Excessive collapse—Stable fixation to allow early weight bearing

1. Results in limb shortening and medialization of shaft

2. Reduced abductor moment arm may cause functional deficit.

3. Associated with displacement of lesser trochanter

4. More collapse associated with sliding hip screw device than that associated with IM implant

5. May result in painful, prominent hardware

b. Implant failure/cutout—Associated with TAD (Fig. 11–39) greater than 25 mm

c. Peri-implant fracture

(1) More common with nails than plates

(2) Low risk with current nail designs

(a) Smaller distal interlocking screws further from tip of nail than earlier designs

(b) Reduced trochanteric bend compared with earlier designs

d. Infection

e. Mortality

E. Subtrochanteric fractures

1. Diagnosis

a. Mechanism of injury—Higher energy than intertrochanteric fractures

b. Plain radiographs

(1) Anteroposterior and lateral views of hip

(2) Anteroposterior and lateral views of femur

2. Classification—Russell-Taylor classification (Fig. 11–40) based on involvement of lesser trochanter and piriformis fossa

Type IA—Fracture below lesser trochanter

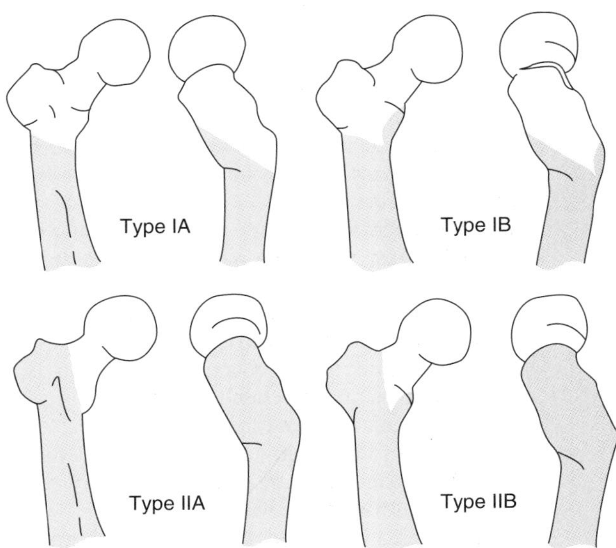

FIGURE 11–40 Russell-Taylor classification of subtrochanteric fractures. (From Russell TA, Taylor JC: Subtrochanteric fractures of the femur. In Browner BD, et al, eds: Skeletal Trauma, p 1491. Philadelphia, WB Saunders, 1992.)

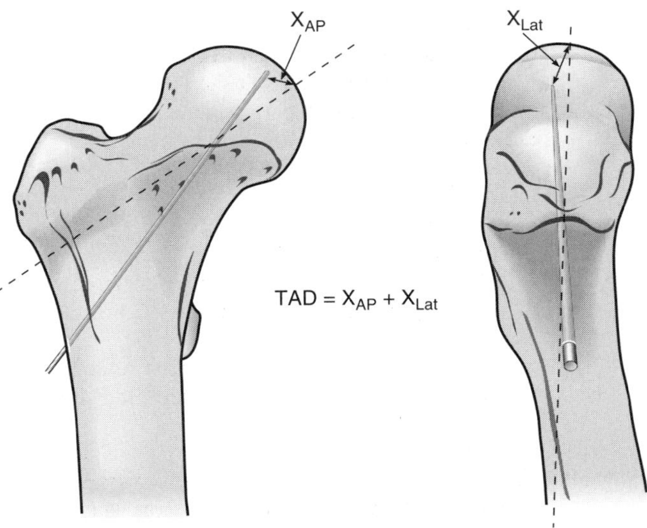

FIGURE 11–39 Tip-apex distance (TAD) should be < 25 mm. (Redrawn from Orthopaedic Knowledge Update: Trauma 2, p 127. Rosemont, IL, American Academy of Orthopaedic Surgeons, 2000.)

Type IB—Fracture involves lesser trochanter. Greater trochanter intact
Type IIA—Greater trochanter involved. Lesser trochanter intact
Type IIB—Greater and lesser trochanter involved

3. Treatment
   a. General principles
      (1) Restore limb length alignment and rotation.
      (2) Indirect reduction techniques obviate the need for bone grafting in acute fractures.
   b. Nonoperative treatment is rarely indicated.
   c. Operative treatment—Implant must withstand high medial compressive loads and high lateral tensile loads.
      (1) Indications—The most subtrochanteric fracture
      (2) IM fixation
         (a) Indirect reduction preserves biologic environment.
         (b) Standard proximal interlocking for fractures with intact lesser trochanter
         (c) Reconstruction interlocking for fractures with involvement of lesser trochanter
         (d) Piriformis entry nail is a contraindication for fractures involving piriformis fossa.
         (e) Apex anterior and varus angles are the most common deformities.
         (f) Open or percutaneous reduction indicated when closed reduction inadequate
      (3) Fixed-angle plate fixation
         (a) Indicated for fractures with proximal comminution and nonunion
         (b) 95-degree devices
         (c) 135-degree devices contraindicated
         (d) Must avoid soft tissue stripping
         (e) Acute bone grafting usually not required when biologic plating techniques are used
4. Complications
   a. Nonunion—Minimized with IM nailing and biologic plating
   b. Malalignment—Varus and apex anterior angulation with IM nailing. Consider adjunctive reduction aids and percutaneous reduction.
   c. Infection—Associated with increased soft tissue dissection

F. Femoral shaft fractures (Table 11–19)

1. Diagnosis
   a. Mechanism of injury—Often associated with high-energy mechanisms
   b. Associated fractures and other injuries are common.
   c. Associated neck fractures are uncommon (< 10%); when present, they are often missed (up to 50%).
   d. Plain radiographs
      (1) Anteroposterior and lateral views of femur
      (2) Anteroposterior and cross-table lateral hip to rule out femoral neck fracture
   e. CT scan to rule out occult femoral neck fracture
      (1) If the scan is obtained for abdominal or pelvic evaluation, it should be reviewed.
      (2) Consider dedicated, thin-cut CT.
2. Classification—Winquist-Hansen classification (Fig. 11–41) based on degree of comminution and amount of cortical continuity
   Type 0—No comminution
   Type I—Comminution less than 25%
   Type II—Comminution 25-50%
   Type III—Comminution greater than 50%
   Type IV—Comminution 100%
3. Treatment
   a. General principles
      (1) Restore limb length, alignment, and rotation.
      (2) Early stabilization reduces systemic complications associated with multiply injured patients.
   b. Nonoperative treatment (rarely indicated)
      (1) Long-leg cast for nondisplaced distal shaft fracture
      (2) Pillow splint for nonambulatory individuals
   c. Operative treatment—Indicated for most fractures
      (1) IM nail
         (a) Indicated for most femoral shaft fractures
         (b) High union rates (> 95%)
         (c) More hip problems with antegrade than retrograde insertion; problems include pain and weakness.
         (d) More knee problems retrograde than antegrade insertion; problems include pain and chondral injury to patella if nail left proud
         (e) Piriformis and trochanteric starting points indicated when they are used with approximately designed nails
            i. Piriformis entry contraindicated when fracture extends to piriformis fossa
            ii. Anterior starting point in piriformis fossa associated with increased hoop stress and risk of iatrogenic comminution
            iii. Anterior trochanteric starting point with minimal hoop stress
            iv. Trochanteric starting point risks medial comminution of shaft due to off-axis starting point and varus if straight (no trochanteric bend) nail used
         (f) Static interlocking for most fractures
         (g) Reamed nailing for most fractures
            i. Higher union rates than unreamed nails
            ii. Unreamed nails associated with decreased fat embolization; clinical relevance unclear
            iii. Appropriate reaming technique includes sharp reamers, slow

TABLE 11-19 ADULT FEMORAL SHAFT FRACTURES

Injury	Eponym/ Other Name	Classification	Treatment	Complications
Femoral fracture (2.0 cm below lesser trochanter to 8 cm from knee joint)		Winquist—based on degree of comminution and amount of cortical continuity I—Transverse, comminution <25% of circumference (e.g., butterfly fragment) II—Comminution 25-50% of circumference III—>50% comminution (unstable) IV—Extensive (100%) comminution, no cortical contact, unstable V—Segmental bone loss (unstable)	Most often high-energy mechanism; early stabilization as patient status permits; most fractures are treated by closed intramedullary (IM) nail; statically locked, reamed nail for most fractures; antegrade (piriformis or trochanter) or retrograde; obesity a relative indication for trochanteric entry nail; multitrauma patients temporized with external fixation (damage control), converted to IM nail later; plate fixation for neck/shaft fractures, periprosthetic treatment (lower union, higher infection, longer time to weight bearing)	Infection (<5% closed fractures), nonunion (<5% closed fractures; treat with exchange nail vs. ORIF/ICBG), delayed union (exchange nail vs. dynamization), malalignment (malrotation, limb length discrepancy), hip pain/weakness (antegrade nail), knee pain (retrograde nail), pudendal nerve injury (excessive traction through post), missed knee ligament injury, knee stiffness (especially with distal external fixation), refracture, failure of fixation, deep venous thrombosis, pulmonary embolism, acute respiratory distress syndrome (ARDS)
Femoral neck and shaft fractures		Garden or Pauwels/Winquist (2.5-5.0% of femoral shaft fractures, BUT ≈30% are missed)	Neck takes priority; 135-degree fixed-angle device vs. parallel screws for neck, retrograde nail vs. plate for shaft; reconstructed nail for nondisplaced neck or intertrochanteric and shaft fractures	Infection, delayed union, nonunion, loss of fixation, avascular necrosis
Periprosthetic femur fracture		Vancouver	Stable prosthesis—lateral plate vs. lateral plate and allograft strut Unstable prosthesis—revision arthroplasty with uncemented long stem and lateral plate Allograft struts for bone loss	
Femoral and tibial shaft fractures	"Floating knee"		Retrograde nail for femur, antegrade nail for tibia	Multiple other injuries, fat emboli syndrome, ARDS

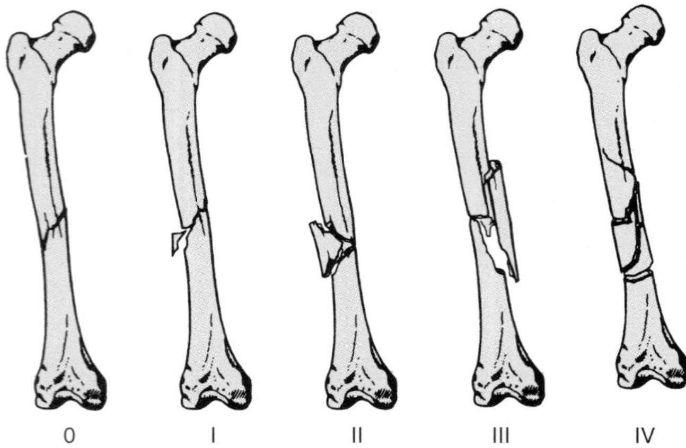

FIGURE 11–41 The Winquist-Hansen classification of femoral shaft fractures. (Note: type V [not shown] has segmental bone loss.) (From Johnson KD: Femur: Trauma. In Tornetta P III, Baumgaertner M: Orthopaedic Knowledge Update: Trauma 3, p 514. Rosemont, IL, American Academy of Orthopaedic Surgeons, 1990.)

advancement, less heat generation, and less embolization

iv. Minimum cortical reaming preferred

v. Nail diameter 1-2 mm smaller than largest reamer

(h) Multitrauma patients may benefit from delayed nailing with immediate provisional external fixation (damage control principles). Benefits include reduced blood loss, reduced hypothermia, and reduced inflammatory mediator release.

(2) External fixation
- (a) Indicated for provisional fixation
  - i. Application of damage control principles
  - ii. Severe contamination requiring repeated access to medullary canal
  - iii. Vascular injury
- (b) Safely converted to IM nail in absence of pin tract infection up to at least 3 weeks

(3) Plate fixation
- (a) Indicated for periprosthetic fractures
- (b) Indicated for neck shaft fractures
- (c) Reduced union rate, higher infection and implant failure rates, and longer time to weight bearing than IM nail

4. Complications
   - a. Infection—Less than 5% of closed fractures
   - b. Nonunion—Less than 5% of closed fractures. Exchange nailing less successful than repair with plate and screws in bone grafting.
   - c. Delayed union—Less than 5% of closed fractures. Dynamization is less successful than exchange nailing.
   - d. Malalignment
     - (1) Proximal fracture more often malaligned with retrograde than antegrade nailing
     - (2) Distal fractures more often malaligned with antegrade than retrograde nailing
     - (3) Malrotation difficult to diagnose, especially with comminuted fractures
       - (a) Compare to the contralateral limb before leaving operating room
       - (b) Supine nailing has a higher incidence of internal rotation.
       - (c) Lateral nailing has a higher incidence of external rotation.
     - (4) Length discrepancy is associated with comminuted fractures.
   - e. Hip pain/weakness is associated with antegrade nailing.
   - f. Knee pain is associated with retrograde nailing.
   - g. Patellar chondral injury is associated with retrograde nailing, with nail left protruding into the knee joint.
   - h. Pudendal nerve injury is associated with excessive traction.
   - i. HO is associated with antegrade nailing (rarely clinically relevant).
5. Special circumstances
   - a. Obese patients
     - (1) High complication rates with piriformis nailing
     - (2) Relative indication for retrograde nailing
   - b. Ipsilateral femoral neck and shaft fractures
     - (1) Uncommon (< 10%), but when present, missed in up to 30% of cases
     - (2) Neck component the highest priority
       - (a) Neck often vertical
       - (b) 135-degree fixed-angle plate or parallel screws preferred for neck
       - (c) Retrograde nail or plate fixation for shaft
       - (d) Reconstruction nail for nondisplaced neck fractures or associated intertrochanteric and shaft fractures
   - c. Multiply injured patient—Consider damage control principles.
   - d. Periprosthetic fracture
     - (1) Stable prosthesis—A lateral plate with the use of biologic plating techniques yields results similar to those obtained with a lateral plate and an allograft strut.
     - (2) Unstable prosthesis—Revision arthroplasty with uncemented long stem + lateral plate
     - (3) Allograft struts indicated for bone loss

G. Supracondylar and intracondylar fractures

1. Diagnosis
   - a. Mechanism of injury—High energy in young patients and low energy in older patients
   - b. Plain radiographs
     - (1) Anteroposterior and lateral views of femur
     - (2) Anteroposterior and lateral views of knee
   - c. CT scan—Usually not required; helpful for comminuted intra-articular fractures
2. Classification—OTA classification (Fig. 11–42) based on the degree of comminution and articular involvement

   33-A—Extra-articular
   33-B—Partial articular (unicondylar)
   33-C—Intra-articular

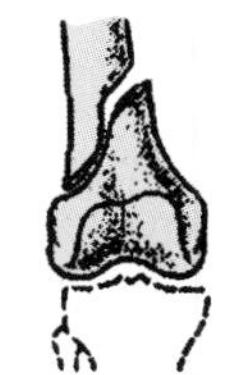

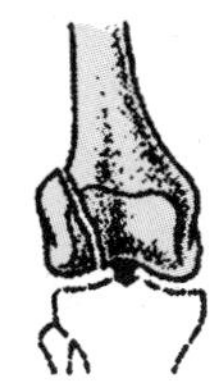

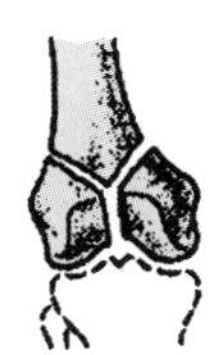

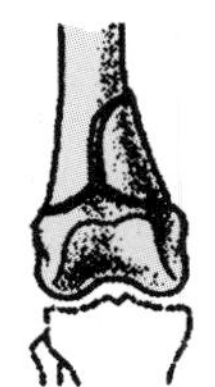

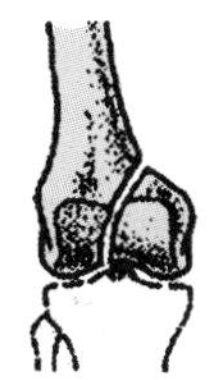

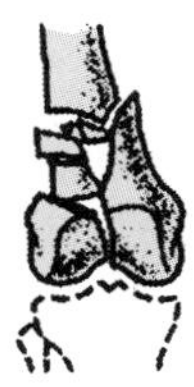

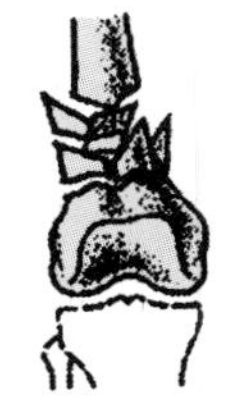

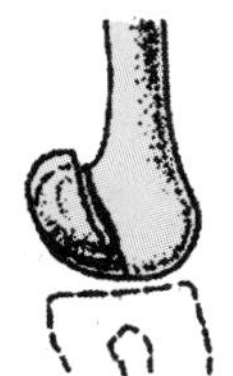

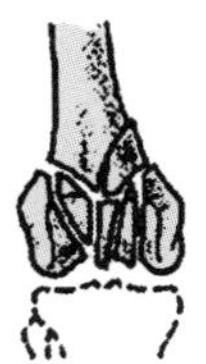

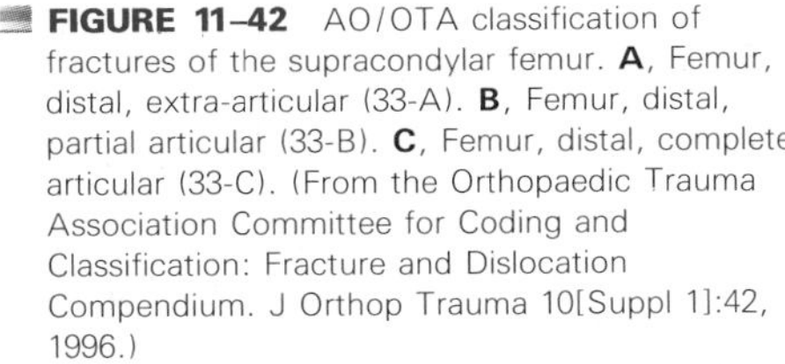

FIGURE 11–42 AO/OTA classification of fractures of the supracondylar femur. **A**, Femur, distal, extra-articular (33-A). **B**, Femur, distal, partial articular (33-B). **C**, Femur, distal, complete articular (33-C). (From the Orthopaedic Trauma Association Committee for Coding and Classification: Fracture and Dislocation Compendium. J Orthop Trauma 10[Suppl 1]:42, 1996.)

3. Treatment
   a. General principles
      (1) Restore articular congruity.
      (2) Rigid stabilization of articular fracture
      (3) Indirect reduction of metaphyseal component to preserve vascularity to fracture fragments
      (4) Stable (not necessarily rigid) fixation of articular block to shaft
      (5) Early knee ROM
   b. Nonoperative treatment—Indicated for nondisplaced fractures
      (1) Brace or knee immobilized
      (2) Full-time bracing for 6-8 weeks
      (3) Closed-chain ROM at 3-4 weeks
   c. Operative treatment—Indicated for most displaced fractures
      (1) Plate fixation—Indicated for most fractures
         (a) Fixed-angle plates required when metaphyseal comminution exists
            i. Traditional 95-degree devices limited by number and location of distal fixation
            ii. Locked plates offer multiple fixed-angle points of fixation in distal fragment in multiple planes.
            iii. Non–fixed-angle plates prone to varus collapse, especially in metaphyseal comminution
         (b) High union rates (> 80%) with indirect reduction technique without bone graft
         (c) Lateral approach—Indirect reduction of metaphyseal fracture and arthrotomy with direct reduction of articular component
            i. Sagittal intra-articular split the most common
            ii. Condyles are malrotated in sagittal plane with respect to each other
            iii. Coronal (Hoffa) fractures require interfragmentary lag screws and condylar plate that spans fracture (locked plate preferred).
      (2) Retrograde IM nail
         (a) Indicated for extra-articular fractures and simple intra-articular fractures
         (b) Reduced stability compared with plate fixation for osteoporotic fractures, especially those with wide metaphyseal flares
            i. Blocking screws can help provide reduction and improved stability.
            ii. Fixed-angle, distal interlocking screws may provide improved stability.
         (c) Long nails that cross the femoral isthmus are preferred to short "supracondylar" nails.

(3) Arthroplasty
(a) Indicated when associated with preexisting joint arthropathy and select cases when stable internal fixation not achievable
(b) Usually requires distal femoral replacement prosthesis
(c) Reduced longevity compared with internal fixation
(d) Allows immediate weight bearing

4. Complications
a. Nonunion—Associated with soft tissue stripping in metaphyseal region
b. Malalignment
(1) Valgus malreduction the most common
(2) Malalignment more common with IM nails
c. Loss of fixation
(1) Varus collapse the most common
(a) Plate fixation associated with toggle of distal non–fixed-angle screws used for comminuted metaphyseal fractures
(b) IM nail fixation
(2) Proximal (diaphyseal) screw failure associated with short plates and nonlocked diaphyseal fixation—Plate fixation is associated with toggle of distal non–fixed-angle screws used for comminuted metaphyseal fractures.
d. Infection—Associated with diabetic patients, especially those with active foot ulcers
e. Knee pain/stiffness
f. Painful hardware—Avoid prominent medial screws.

5. Special circumstances—Periprosthetic fractures
a. Good results with locked plates
b. Retrograde nails require a sufficiently large intercondylar box.

III. Knee Injuries (Table 11–20)

A. Dislocation
1. Diagnosis/classification
a. Direction—Anterior (30-40%), posterior (30-40%), medial, lateral, and rotatory (posterolateral the most common) (Fig. 11–43)
b. Schenck anatomic classification of knee dislocation (KD)
KD I—Dislocation with either anterior cruciate ligament (ACL) or posterior cruciate ligament (PCL) intact
KD II—Torn ACL/PCL
KD III—Torn ACL/PCL and either posterolateral corner (PLC) or posteromedial corner (PMC)
KD IV—Torn ACL/PCL/PLC/PMC
KD V—Fracture-dislocation
c. More than 50% present reduced (easily missed diagnosis)
d. Vascular injury in 5-15% in recent studies. Selective arteriography with the use of a physical examination rather than an immediate arteriogram is now the standard of care. The most common finding in patients with vascular injury is a diminished or absent pedal pulse.
e. Significant soft tissue injuries

2. Treatment
a. Emergent reduction if patient did not present reduced
b. Revascularize within 6 hours if there is significant arterial injury.
c. Care for soft tissue injuries (open-knee dislocations)
d. Ligament repair or reconstruction
(1) Reconstruction with allograft becoming the most common
(2) Acute reconstruction may be better than chronic
(3) Early motion rehabilitation
(4) Possible role for hinged external fixator

3. Complications
a. Vascular injury—The highest with KD IV; an **ankle-brachial index** (ABI) of greater than 0.9 is associated with an intact artery
b. Neurologic injury—Peroneal nerve injury common (about 25%), but up to 50% recover at least partially. May benefit from neurolysis.
c. Stiffness/arthrofibrosis—The most common complication (38%)
d. Ligamentous laxity also very common (37%)

B. Patella fractures
1. Diagnosis/classification
a. Descriptive—Transverse, vertical (rarely requires surgical treatment), comminuted, proximal or distal (30%) pole, and nondisplaced (Fig. 11–44).
b. An inability to extend the knee or do a straight-leg raise demonstrates an incompetent extensor mechanism.
c. Displaced fracture is 3 mm fragment separation or 2 mm step-off.
2. Treatment—Preserve patella whenever possible (i.e., avoid patellectomy).
a. Nonoperative treatment—Nondisplaced with intact extensor mechanism, hinged knee brace in extension, and progress in flexion after 2-3 weeks
b. Tension band wiring—22%, with early motion displaced 2 mm or more during early postoperative period. Catastrophic failure with unprotected weight bearing. May use cannulated screws with tension band wire.
c. Partial patellectomy—Useful with extra-articular distal pole fractures. Also used with severely comminuted fractures; preserve the largest pieces and reattach patella ligament (Fig. 11–45).
3. Complications—Symptomatic hardware (very common), loss of reduction (22%), nonunion (< 5%), infection, and arthrofibrosis/stiffness

C. Patella dislocations
1. Diagnosis—Frequently involves young adults or adolescents, usually laterally, and involves injury to the medial patellofemoral ligament.

TABLE 11-20 ADULT KNEE FRACTURES AND DISLOCATIONS

Injury	Eponym	Classification	Treatment	Complications
Supracondylar fracture	"Hoffa" fracture (33-B3)	AO/OTA—degree of comminution and articular involvement 33-A—Extra-articular 33-B—Partially articular (unicondylar) 33-C—Intra-articular	Restore articular congruity, rigid stabilization of articular fracture, preserve vascularity, stable fixation of joint to shaft, early range of motion (ROM) Nonoperative: Brace or knee immobilizer, Non–weight bearing for 6-8 wk, closed-chain ROM at 3-4 wk Plate fixation: most fractures; fixed-angle plate for metaphyseal comminution (nonfixed: varus collapse) Retrograde intramedullary (IM) nail: extra-articular or simple intra-articular fractures, long nail preferred Arthroplasty when fixation not achievable, arthropathy present	Nonunion (soft tissue stripping of metaphyseal region), malalignment (valgus malreduction most common, nails ≫ plates), loss of fixation (varus collapse), infection, knee stiffness, degenerative joint disease (DJD), unstable fixation, deep venous thrombosis (DVT), fracture fragments from missed coronal plane ("Hoffa fracture"), prominent hardware
Periprosthetic fracture			Locked plate vs. retrograde nail (need size of intercondylar box in total knee arthroplasty for nail to fit)	
Patella fracture		Nondisplaced, transverse, proximal or distal (30%) pole, comminuted, vertical (nonoperative)	Nonoperative: nondisplaced (<2 mm) with intact extensor mechanism; hinged knee brace in extension, progress in flexion after 2-3 wk Open reduction (with) internal fixation (ORIF) (tension band wiring, screws) if patient cannot actively extend knee (extensor mechanism rupture) or there is a >2-mm separation or incongruent articular surface (>2-mm step-off); excise fragments that are extremely comminuted; avoid patellectomy	Symptomatic hardware, loss of reduction, nonunion (<5%), infection, arthrofibrosis/stiffness, quadriceps weakness, infection, DJD, extensor lag
Patella dislocation		Acute, recurrent, subluxation, habitual, usually lateral	Immobilize, controlled motion for 6 wk; arthroscopy for displaced or osteochondral fracture; recurrent: lateral release, medial plication (repair/reconstruct MPFL); bony transplant if abnormal Q angle. Avoid surgery in those with habitual dislocation.	Redislocation

Continued

TABLE 11-20 ADULT KNEE FRACTURES AND DISLOCATIONS—cont'd

Injury	Eponym	Classification	Treatment	Complications
Knee dislocation		Anterior (30-40%), posterior (30-40%), lateral, medial, rotatory (anteromedial, anterolateral, posteromedial, posterolateral) Schenck anatomic classification: KD I—Dislocation with anterior cruciate ligament (ACL) or posterior cruciate ligament (PCL) intact KD II—Torn ACL/PCL KD III—Torn ACL/PCL and either posterolateral corner (PLC) or posteromedial corner (PMC) KD IV—Torn ACL/PCL/PLC/PMC KD V—Fracture-dislocation	May present spontaneously reduced—easily missed; reduce dislocations emergently; open reduction if needed (posterolateral rotation); arteriogram based on physical exam findings (absent/asymmetrical pulses); repair vascular injuries (5-15%); ligament repair (within 2-3 wk) or reconstruction, allograft vs. autograft, early motion	Vascular injury (5-15%, highest with KD-IV; ankle-brachial index >0.9 associated with intact artery); neurologic injury (tibial/peroneal nerve), stiffness/arthrofibrosis (most common complication), ligamentous laxity
Quadriceps rupture		Generally older than 40 and metabolic disorders (CRF, RA, steroid use), M ≫ F	Incomplete rupture: nonoperative management Complete: repair through osseous drill holes or suture anchors; repair acutely: >2 wk or ≤5-cm retraction	Strength deficit; stiffness, inability to resume preinjury athletic/recreational activity; bilateral ruptures (identify underlying medical problem, repair both); DVT; chronic ruptures (allograft reconstruction, quadriceps tendon lengthening)
Patella tendon rupture		Younger than 40, overload of extensor mechanism; increased risk with metabolic disorders (rheumatoid arthritis, diabetes mellitus, infection)	Direct repair with nonabsorbable suture and locking (Krackow) stitch through drill holes; can protect repair with cerclage	Missed diagnosis (high-riding patella seen on radiographs), stiffness, extensor weakness

MPFL, medial patellofemoral ligament.

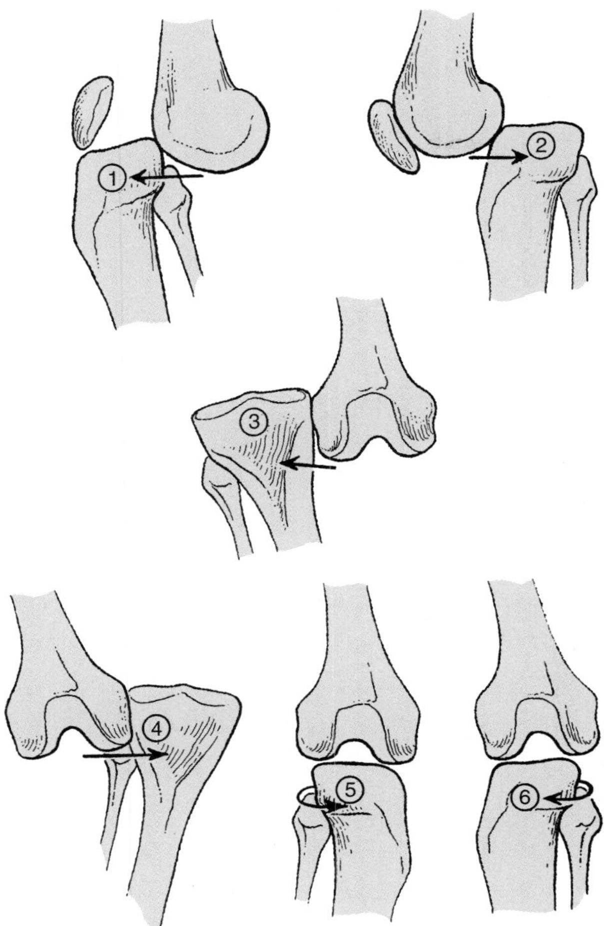

FIGURE 11–43 Dislocations of the knee. 1, Anterior. 2, Posterior. 3, Lateral. 4, Medial. 5, Anteromedial. 6, Anterolateral. (From Connolly JF, ed: DePalma's The Management of Fractures and Dislocations: An Atlas, 3rd ed, p 1621. Philadelphia, WB Saunders, 1981.)

2. Treatment—Immobilize with controlled motion for 6 weeks.
3. Complications—Redislocation

D. Patella ligament rupture
1. Diagnosis/classification—Patients younger than 40 with overload of extensor mechanism during athletic activity. Increased risk with metabolic disorders, rheumatologic disease, renal failure, corticosteroid injection, patellar tendinitis, and infection. A frequently missed diagnosis.
2. Treatment—Direct primary repair with a nonabsorbable suture and locking (Krakow) stitch through patellar drill holes. Can supplement

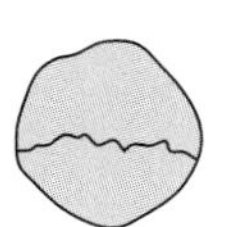

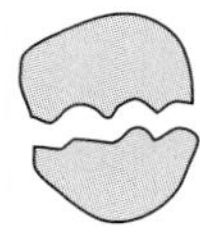

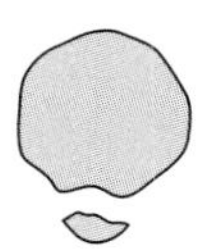

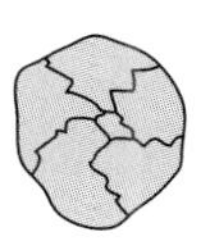

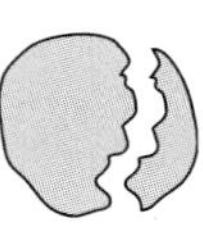

FIGURE 11–44 Types of patellar fractures. (From Weissman BN, Sledge CB: Orthopedic Radiology, p 553. Philadelphia, WB Saunders, 1986.)

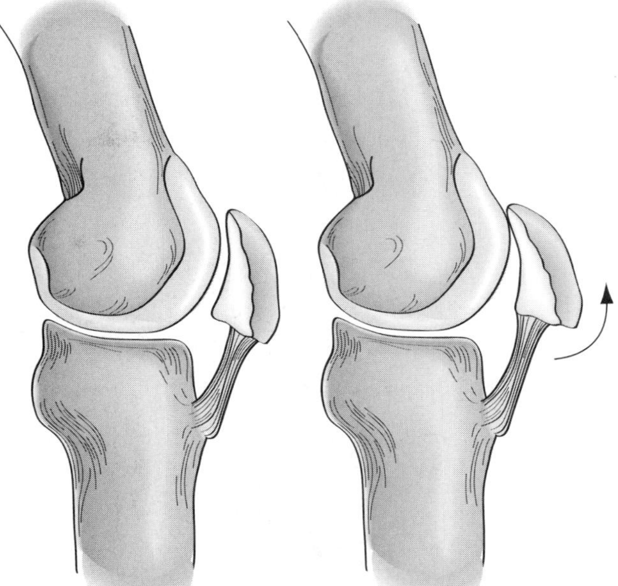

FIGURE 11–45 Anterior reattachment of the patellar ligament, which is recommended to prevent tilting of the patella superiorly. (Redrawn with permission from Marder RA, et al: Effects of partial patellectomy and reattachment of the patellar tendon on patellofemoral contact areas and pressures. J Bone Joint Surg [Am] 75:35-45, 1993.)

with semitendinosus graft and/or cerclage wire to protect repair.
3. Complications—Stiffness and extensor weakness

E. Quadriceps tendon rupture
1. Diagnosis—Patients may be younger than 40, but this condition most commonly occurs in older patients with medical problems. 20-33% associated with renal failure, diabetes, rheumatoid arthritis, hyperparathyroidism, connective tissue disorders, steroid use, and intra-articular injections. Males are affected more often (up to 8:1). The nondominant limb is affected two times more than the dominant limb.
2. Treatment
   a. Incomplete rupture—Nonoperative management; warn of risk for future rupture
   b. Acute unilateral rupture—Repair through osseous drill holes or suture anchors. Repair acutely; ruptures more than 2 weeks old may be retracted 5 cm.
   c. Bilateral ruptures—Identify the underlying medical problem; otherwise, treat the same as a unilateral rupture. Requires non–weight bearing (NWB), DVT, and prophylaxis.
   d. Chronic tendon ruptures—Less successful than the acute ones. May require Co-divilla procedure or quadriceps tendon lengthening.
3. Complications—Strength deficit (33-50% of patients), stiffness, and the inability to resume prior level of athletic/recreational activity (50%)

IV. Tibial Injuries (Table 11–21)

A. Plateau fracture
1. Diagnosis/classification

TABLE 11-21 ADULT TIBIA FRACTURES AND DISLOCATIONS

Injury	Eponym/ Other Name	Classification	Treatment	Complications
Tibial plateau fracture		Schatzker classification I—Split II—Split depression III—Pure depression IV—Medial plateau split V—Bicondylar with intact metaphysis VI—Bicondylar with metaphyseal/diaphyseal dissociation AO/OTA classification 41-A—Extra-articular fracture 41-B—Partial articular fracture (Schatzker I–IV) 41-C—Complete articular/bicondylar (Schatzker V and VI)	Magnetic resonance imaging can change treatment or classification in most cases (soft tissue injury); medial cruciate ligament > anterior cruciate ligament (ACL); lateral > bicondylar > medial (think dislocation with medial); spanning external fixation for high-energy injuries (soft tissue stabilization) Nonoperative: stable knees (<10 degrees varus/valgus in full extension, <3 mm articular step-off); cast brace, early range of motion (ROM), delayed weight bearing for 4-6 wk Open reduction with external fixation (ORIF) if articular step-off >3 mm, condylar widening >5 mm, knee unstable, medial and bicondylar; plate fixation (locked vs nonlocked, single vs. dual [posteromedial] incision) vs. external fixation (bicondylar or severe soft tissue injury, wires >15 mm from joint)	Degenerative joint disease (DJD), infection (surgical approach most important factor), malunion (varus collapse with non-op or conventional plates/bicondylar fracture), ligament instability, peroneal nerve injury, compartment syndrome, stiffness, loss of reduction, avascular necrosis
Tibial spine fracture		I—Anterior tilt II—Complete anterior tilt III—No contact A—No rotation B—Rotated	I/II/IIIA closed reduction, long-leg cast (LLC) for 6 wk if knee can be brought into full extension; IIIB and all irreducible types require open reduction	Block to motion (arthroscopic loose-body removal), ACL laxity
Tibial tubercle fracture			ORIF with screw or staple	Loss of fixation, quadriceps weakness
Subcondylar tibial fracture		Stable	Cast immobilization	Arterial injury, decreased ROM
		Displaced	ORIF with buttress plate	
Tibial stress fracture		Upper one third (recruits)	Modify activity for 6-10 wk	Progression to complete fracture
Tibial shaft fracture		AO/OTA classification 42-A—Simple, two parts 42-B—Butterfly comminution 42-C—Comminuted; no direct contact between proximal and distal fragments Gustillo and Anderson—open fracture grade Grade I—No periosteal stripping, <1-cm wound Grade II—No periosteal stripping, >1-cm wound Grade IIIA—Periosteal stripping, no flap required Grade IIIB—Periosteal stripping, flap required Grade IIIC—Periosteal stripping, flap required, vascular injury requiring repair	Most respond to closed reduction, LLC, wedge as needed, PTB at 6-8 wk; intramedullary (IM) nail for transverse oblique fracture of mid–one third or segmental and also for vascular injury, bilateral injury, pathologic fractures, severe ligamentous injuries to knee (statically locked IM nail); open fractures: unreamed nail up to and including some IIIB injuries, early flap coverage, delayed bone grafting. Consider early amputation in grade IIIC injuries, posterior tibial nerve injury, warm ischemia >6 hr, and severe ipsilateral foot injury (unreconstructible limb).	Delayed union (>20 wk; increased with greater initial displacement and middle-third fractures; treatment includes fibulectomy and posterolateral bone graft), nonunion (posterolateral bone graft or reamed IM nail), infection (flap/graft or amputation), malunion (varus/valgus, shortening [accept <5 degrees varus/valgus, <10 degrees anteroposterior angulation]), vascular injuries (upper one fourth of anterior tibial artery), compartment syndrome, peroneal nerve injury, CRPS
Tibial plafond fracture	Pilon	Ruedi and Allgöwer I—Minimally displaced II—Incongruous III—Comminuted	LLC and non–weight bearing ORIF if displaced and ankle involved; consider minimally invasive small-pin external fixation techniques	DJD (may require late fusion), infection, varus/valgus angulation, skin slough
Fibular shaft fracture		Mid to lower one third (athletes)	Cast only if needed for pain relief	Missed syndesmotic injury
Proximal fibula fracture			Open if unstable	Injury to biceps, peroneal nerve
Proximal tibia-fibula dislocation		Anterior (most common), posterior, superior	Reduce (90 degrees flexion), ORIF fails with recurrence	
Chondral/osteochondral fracture		Endogenous vs. exogenous	Arthroscopic evaluation of locked, acute condylar defects; remove small fragments (pin large fragments)	DJD

CRPS, complex regional pain syndrome; PTB, patella tendon–bearing cast.

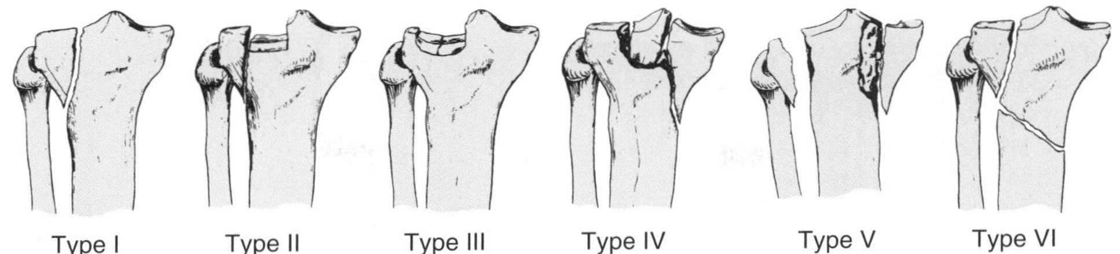

FIGURE 11–46 Diagram of the Schatzker classification of tibial plateau fractures. Type I, cleavage of wedge fracture of the lateral tibial plateau. Type II, lateral split/depression fracture. Type III, pure central depression. Type IV, fracture of the medial condyle (may involve tibial spine). Type V, bicondylar fracture. Type VI, metaphyseal/diaphyseal dissociation. (From Schatzker J, McBroom R, Bruce D: The tibial plateau fracture: The Toronto experience, 1968-1975. Clin Orthop 138:94-104, 1979.)

a. Schatzker classification (Fig. 11–46)
   Type I—Split
   Type II—Split depression
   Type III—Pure depression
   Type IV—Medial tibial plateau
   Type V—Bicondylar with intact metaphysis
   Type VI—Bicondylar with metaphyseal/diaphyseal dissociation

b. AO/OTA classification (Fig. 11–47)
   41-A—Extra-articular fracture
   41-B—Partial articular fracture (Schatzker I-IV)
   41-C—Complete articular/bicondylar (Schatzker V and VI)

c. MRI changes treatment or classification in most cases. Soft tissue injury is demonstrated (50-90% incidence). Medial collateral ligament (MCL) > ACL; meniscus tears in over 50% of cases.

d. Lateral > bicondylar > medial (think *dislocation* with medial)

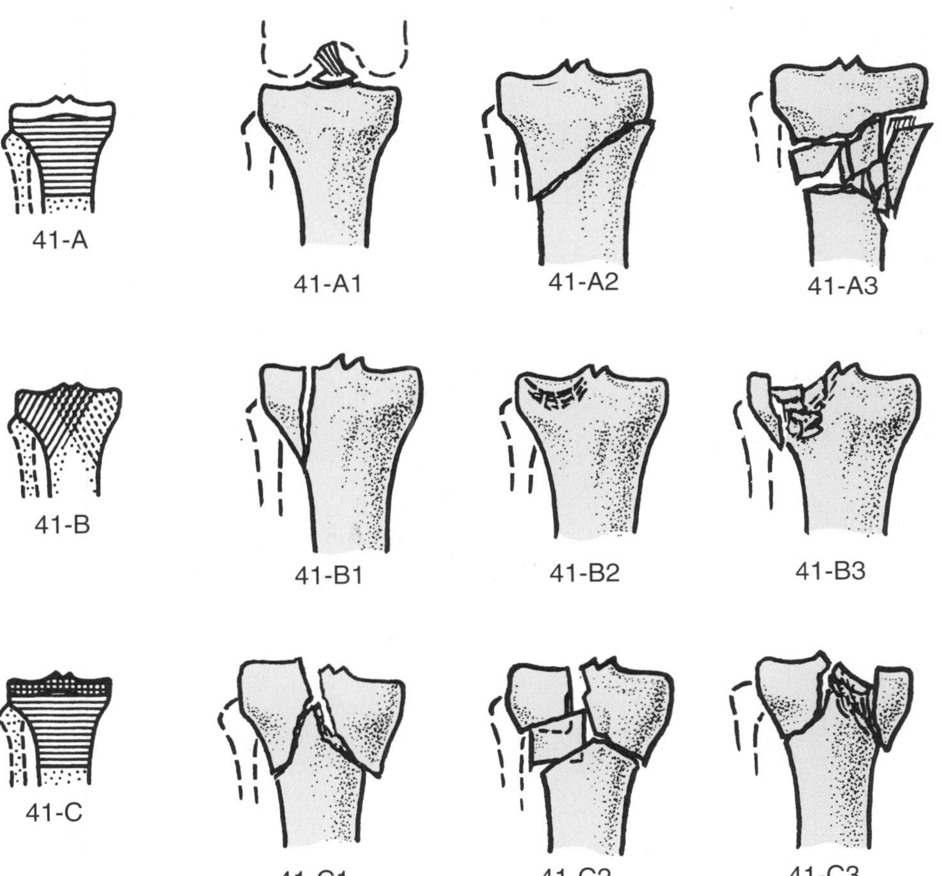

FIGURE 11–47 AO/OTA universal classification system for fractures of the tibial plateau (see text). (From Müller ME, et al, eds: The Comprehensive Classification of Fractures of Long Bones. Berlin, Springer-Verlag, 1990.)

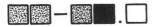

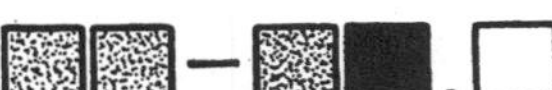

2. Treatment
   a. Nonoperative treatment—Indicated in stable knees (< 10 degrees coronal plane instability with the knee in full extension) with less than 3 mm articular step-off. Cast brace, early ROM, and delayed weight bearing for at least 4-6 weeks.
   b. Operative treatment—Indicated with articular step-off greater than 3 mm, condylar widening greater than 5 mm, instability of the knee, and all medial and bicondylar plateau fractures.
      (1) ORIF—Plate fixation with early motion. Percutaneous locked plating for poor-quality bone in bicondylar fractures. No stripping. Separate posteromedial incision if second plate is needed.
      (2) External fixation—Hybrid or Ilizarov useful for bicondylar fractures with severe soft tissue injuries. Keep small wires at least 15 mm from the joint to avoid septic joint.
      (3) Spanning external fixators—Used temporarily with selected high-energy injuries. Controversial with regard to when or if these devices should be used.
3. Complications—**Degenerative joint disease** (DJD), infection (surgical approach the most important factor), malunion (varus collapse with nonoperative or conventional plates in severe bicondylar fractures), ligament instability (left untreated, has an adverse impact on outcome), peroneal nerve injury, and compartment syndrome

B. Shaft fractures
1. Diagnosis
   a. Mechanism of injury
      (1) Low energy
         (a) Spiral oblique fracture
         (b) Tibia and fibula at same level
         (c) Closed fracture with minor soft tissue trauma
      (2) High energy
         (a) Comminuted fracture
         (b) Tibia and fibula at same level
         (c) Transverse fracture pattern
         (d) Diastasis between tibia and fibula
         (e) Segmental fracture
         (f) Open fracture or closed with significant soft tissue trauma
   b. The most common long bone fracture
   c. Often associated with soft tissue injuries
      (1) Soft tissue management critical to outcome
      (2) Open fractures often require repeated incision and drainage.
         (a) Number of instances of débridement, type of irrigation, and pressure of irrigant controversial
         (b) Sharp débridement of nonvariable soft tissue and bone the most important aspect of incision and drainage
   d. Plain radiographs
      (1) Anteroposterior and lateral tibia views must include knee and ankle.
      (2) Dedicated knee and ankle radiographs for intra-articular extension
2. Classification
   a. OTA classification (Fig. 11–48)—Based on comminution
      42-A—Simple (two parts)
      42-B—Butterfly comminution
      42-C—Comminuted; no direct contact between proximal and distal fragments
   b. Open fracture grade (Gustillo and Anderson)—Based on degree of periosteal stripping and requirement for soft tissue coverage
      Grade I—No periosteal stripping, less than 1-cm wound
      Grade II—No periosteal stripping, greater than 1-cm wound
      Grade IIIA—Periosteal stripping, no flap required
      Grade IIIB—Periosteal stripping, flap required
      Grade IIIC—Periosteal stripping and vascular injury requiring repair
   c. Grade of closed-fracture soft tissue injury—Tscherne classification
      Grade 0—Injuries from indirect forces, with negligible soft tissue injury
      Grade I—Superficial contusion/abrasion, simple fracture
      Grade II—Deep abrasion, muscle/skin contusion; direct trauma, and impending compartment syndrome
      Grade III—Excessive skin contusion; crushed skin or destruction of muscle, subcutaneous degloving, acute compartment syndrome, and rupture of a major blood vessel or nerve
3. Treatment
   a. General principles
      (1) Degree of shortening and translation seen on injury radiographs can be expected to be present on union with nonoperative management.
      (2) Angular and rotational alignment well controlled with cast
      (3) Timely and thorough soft tissue management critical to outcome
      (4) Restore limb length, alignment, and rotation.
      (5) Stable fixation
      (6) Early ROM of knee and ankle
   b. Nonoperative treatment
      (1) Indications
         (a) Low-energy fractures
         (b) Shortening less than 1-2 cm
         (c) Cortical apposition greater than 50%
         (d) Angulation maintained with cast
            i. Varus—Valgus less than 5 degrees
            ii. Flexion—Extension less than 10 degrees

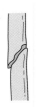

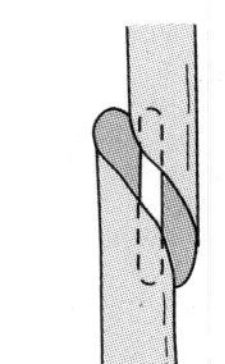
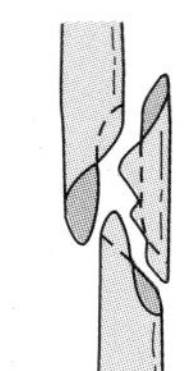
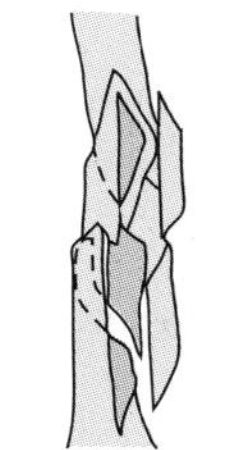
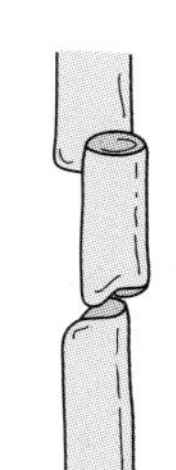
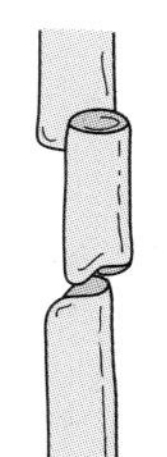
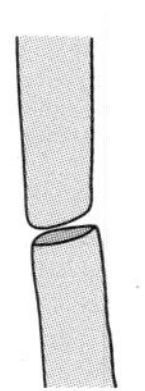
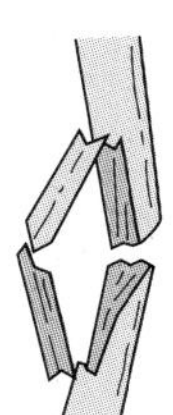
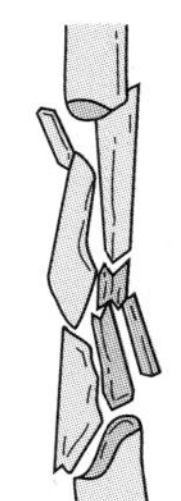
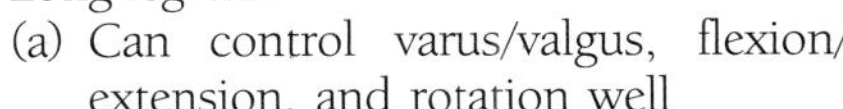

FIGURE 11–48 AO/OTA classification of fractures of the tibial shaft. **A**, Tibia/fibula, diaphyseal, simple (42-A). **B**, Tibia/fibula, diaphyseal, wedge (42-B). **C**, Tibia/fibula, diaphyseal, complex (42-C). (From the Orthopaedic Trauma Association Committee for Coding and Classification. Fracture and Dislocation Compendium. J Orthop Trauma 10[Suppl 1]: 52, 1996.)

- (2) Long-leg cast
  - (a) Can control varus/valgus, flexion/extension, and rotation well
  - (b) Shortening and cortical apposition seen on injury radiograph are equivalent to shortening at union.
  - (c) Convert to functional brace at 4-6 weeks
  - (d) Non–weight bearing for 4-6 weeks

c. Operative treatment
- (1) Indications
  - (a) Open fractures
  - (b) Criteria for nonoperative management not met
  - (c) Soft tissue injury not amenable to cast
  - (d) Ipsilateral femoral fracture
  - (e) Morbid obesity
- (2) IM nailing
  - (a) Reduced time of immobilization compared with cast management
  - (b) Earlier weight bearing than that achieved with cast
  - (c) Union rate greater than 80% for closed injuries
  - (d) Reamed nailing associated with higher union rates than those achieved with nonreamed nailing
    - i. Reamed nailing safe for open fractures
    - ii. Severity of soft tissue injury more prognostic than reaming status
  - (e) Static interlocking indicated for stable and unstable fractures
  - (f) Dynamic interlocking indicated only for stable fracture (Winquist I or II)
  - (g) Avoidance of proximal fractures associated with valgus and apex anterior angulation achieved by the following
    - i. Blocking screws
    - ii. Provisional unicortical plates
  - (h) Gaps at fracture site associated with nonunion
- (3) External fixation
  - (a) Temporary during application of damage control principles
  - (b) Temporary or definitive for highly contaminated fractures
  - (c) Higher incidence of malalignment than IM nails

(d) Circular frames indicated for very proximal and distal shaft fractures and when these fractures are associated with severe soft tissue injury

(4) Plate fixation

(a) For extreme proximal and distal shaft fractures

(b) Higher infection risk than that for IM nailing in open fractures

4. Complications
   a. Nonunion
      (1) Dynamization if axially stable
      (2) Reamed-exchange nailing
      (3) Bone graft for bone defects
   b. Malunion—The most common with proximal third fractures, which are avoided/treated with blocking screws and a proper starting point and insertion angle (critical)
   c. Infection—Risk increases with increased severity of soft tissue injury.
   d. Compartment syndrome
      (1) Diagnosed by compartment pressure within 30 mm Hg of diastolic blood pressure
      (2) Emergent fasciotomy indicated
      (3) Can occur with open fractures
   e. Anterior knee pain—Occurs in more than 30% of IM nailing cases; resolves with removal of nail in 50% of cases.
5. Ipsilateral femoral shaft and tibial shaft fractures (“floating knee”)—Treated by retrograde femoral nailing and antegrade tibial nailing.

C. Tibial plafond fractures

1. Classification
   a. Reudi-Allgöwer (Fig. 11–49)
      Type I—A nondisplaced fracture
      Type II—Displacement of the articular surface
      Type III—Comminution of the articular surface
   b. AO/OTA (Fig. 11–50)
      43-A—Extra-articular
      43-B—Partially articular
      43-C—Completely articular
2. Treatment
   a. Nonoperative treatment—Nonoperative management is indicated only if the patient is too ill or has significant risk of skin problems (diabetes and vascular disease).
   b. Operative treatment
      (1) Limited internal fixation with external fixation
         (a) Proponents cite a decreased infection rate, soft tissue breakdown, and stiffness, even when ORIF is used.
         (b) With a hybrid fixator, thin wires may be placed within the joint capsule.
         (c) Thin wires may often be placed within the zone of injury.
         (d) Anatomic articular reconstruction may not be possible, especially when there is central depression.

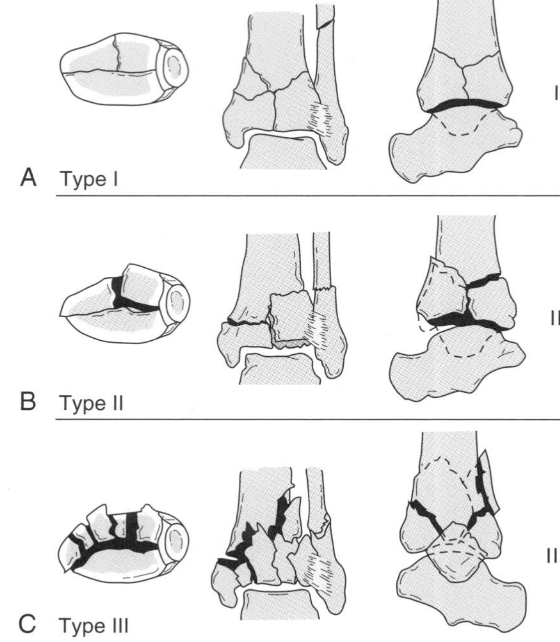

FIGURE 11–49 The Reudi-Allgöwer classification of tibial plafond fractures. (**A** Reproduced with permission from Ruedi TP, Allgöwer M: Fractures of the lower end of the tibia into the ankle joint: Results of 9 years after open reduction. Injury 5:130, 1973. **B** Reproduced with permission from Muller ME, ed: The Comprehensive Classification of Fractures of Long Bones. Berlin, Springer-Verlag, 1990. **C** From Anglen JD: Orthopaedic Knowledge Update: Trauma 2, p 192. Rosemont, IL, American Academy of Orthopaedic Surgeons, 2000.)

      (2) Primary temporizing external fixation with delayed ORIF
         (a) Proponents advocate anatomic restoration of the joint despite a higher risk of wound problems and infection.
         (b) Typically ORIF of the fibula to maintain length and external fixation across the ankle; delay definitive ORIF of tibia until soft tissue swelling has subsided
         (c) May be necessary for fractures with significant joint depression or displacement
         (d) Hardware may become prominent and require later removal.
3. Complications
   a. Wound dehiscence 9-30%—Recommend waiting until soft tissue edema has subsided before ORIF (1-2 weeks)
   b. Infection 5-15%—May occur with either method of treatment
   c. Malunion
   d. Nonunion—Especially in metaphysis and more common with hybrid fixation
   e. Post-traumatic arthritis
   f. Chondrolysis

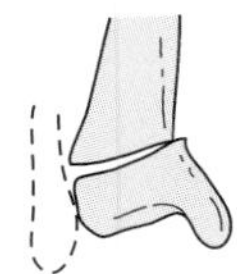

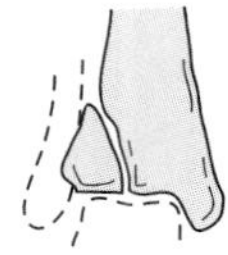

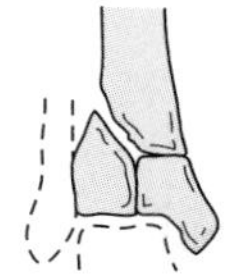

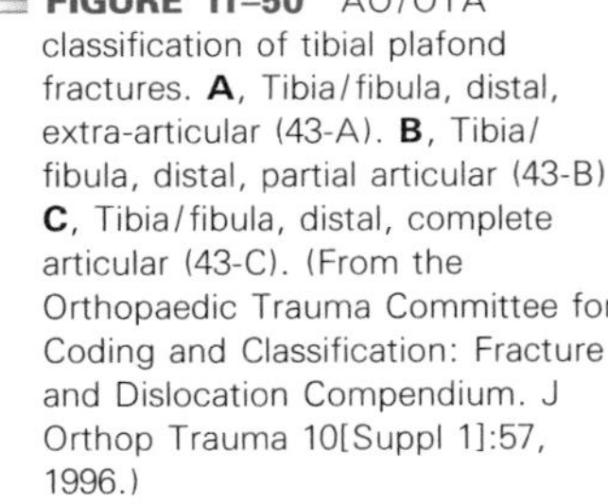

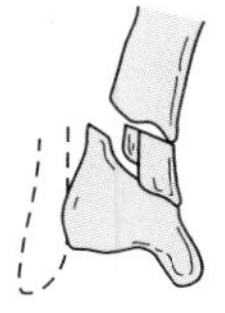

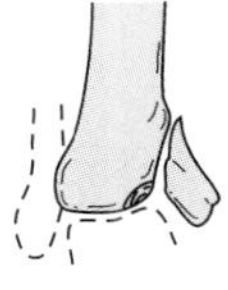

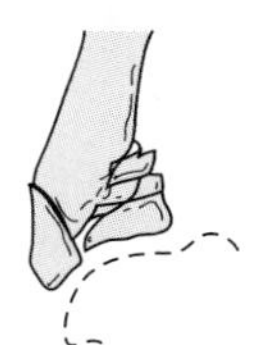

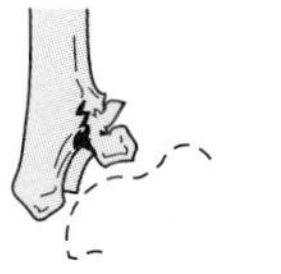

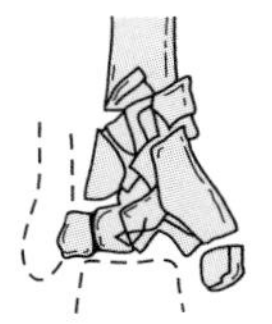

FIGURE 11–50 AO/OTA classification of tibial plafond fractures. **A**, Tibia/fibula, distal, extra-articular (43-A). **B**, Tibia/fibula, distal, partial articular (43-B). **C**, Tibia/fibula, distal, complete articular (43-C). (From the Orthopaedic Trauma Committee for Coding and Classification: Fracture and Dislocation Compendium. J Orthop Trauma 10[Suppl 1]:57, 1996.)

V. Ankle and Foot Injuries (Tables 11–22 and 11–23)

A. Ankle fractures
   1. Diagnosis
      a. Mechanism of injury—Rotation
      b. Associated syndesmotic instability must be ruled out.
      c. Associated deltoid ligament incompetence must be ruled out.
   2. Classification
      a. Lauge-Hansen (Box 11–1)—Based on the foot's position (first word of classification) and motion (talus) relative to the leg (second word of classification)
         (1) Supination-adduction
            (a) Stage I—Transverse fracture of lateral malleolus at or below the level of the anterior talofibular ligament or a tear of the lateral collateral ligament structures, with the anterior talofibular ligament disrupted most often and frequently the calcaneofibular ligament also being torn
            (b) Stage II—Oblique fracture of the medial malleolus
         (2) Supination—External (eversion) rotation (the most common)
            (a) Stage I—Rupture of the anterior inferior tibiofibular ligament
            (b) Stage II—Oblique fracture or spiral fracture of the lateral malleolus
            (c) Stage III—Rupture of the post–tibiofibular ligament or fracture of the posterior malleolus of the tibia
            (d) Stage IV—Transverse (sometimes oblique) fracture of the medial malleolus
         (3) Pronation-abduction
            (a) Stage I—Rupture of the deltoid ligament or transverse fracture of the medial malleolus
            (b) Stage II—Rupture of the anterior and posterior inferior tibiotalofibular ligaments or bony avulsion
            (c) Stage III—Oblique fracture of the fibula at the level of the syndesmosis
         (4) Pronation-eversion
            (a) Stage I—Rupture of the deltoid ligament or transverse fracture of the medial malleolus
            (b) Stage II—Rupture of the anterior inferior tibiotalofibular ligaments or bony avulsion
            (c) Stage III—Spiral/oblique fracture of the fibula above the level of the syndesmosis
            (d) Stage IV—Rupture of the posterior inferior tibiofibular ligament or fracture of the posterior malleolus
         (5) Pronation-dorsiflexion
            (a) Stage I—Fracture of the medial malleolus
            (b) Stage II—Fracture of the anterior lip of the tibia
            (c) Stage III—Fracture of the supramalleolar aspect of the fibula
            (d) Stage IV—Rupture of the posterior inferior tibiofibular ligament or fracture of the posterior malleolus

TABLE 11-22 ADULT TRAUMA, LOWER EXTREMITY—ANKLE FRACTURES AND DISLOCATIONS

Injury	Eponym	Classification	Treatment	Complications
Ankle fracture		Lauge-Hansen (position of foot—motion of foot relative to leg) Supination-adduction 1—Transverse lateral malleolus fracture 2—Oblique medial malleolus fracture Supination–external rotation 1—AITFL 2—Spiral fracture of lateral malleolus 3—Posteromedial fracture or PITFL injury 4—Transverse/oblique medial malleolus fracture/deltoid injury Pronation-abduction 1—Transverse medial malleolus fracture/deltoid injury 2—Anterior and posterior ITFL/posterior malleolus 3—Oblique lateral malleolus (supramalleolar) fracture Pronation–external rotation 1—Medial malleolus fracture/deltoid ligament injury 2—AITFL/intraosseous ligament 3—High fibular fracture 4—Posterior malleolus fracture Pronation-dorsiflexion 1—Medial malleolus fracture 2—Fracture of anterior lip of tibia 3—Supramalleolar fibular fracture 4—Posteromedial fracture or PITFL injury	Rotational injury; rule out syndesmotic injury and deltoid ligament incompetence Anatomic restoration of ankle mortise; 1-mm talar shift = 42% decrease in tibiotalar contact area; isolated lateral malleolus fractures with intact deltoid ligament can be treated with short-leg walking boot; isolated medial malleolus fractures Open reduction (with) internal fixation (ORIF): displaced bimalleolar/trimalleolar ankle fractures, displaced lateral malleolus with deltoid rupture, displaced medial malleolus, syndesmotic disruption, posterior malleolus >25% ORIF fibula: lateral buttress plate with or without interfragment screw vs. posterolateral plate (peroneal irritation) ORIF medial malleolus: lag screws or tension band, buttress plate for vertical shear fractures ORIF posterior malleolus: anteroposterior/posteroanterior lag screws, buttress plate	Wound complications (diabetics), deep infection (diabetics), stiffness, post-traumatic arthrosis, nonunion, malunion Diabetic complications: skin breakdown, loss of reduction, up to 30% amputation rate; augment fixation with transarticular screws/pins or syndesmotic fixation
High tibia fracture	Maisonneuve	Danis-Weber (AO/OTA; position of fibular fracture) 44-A—At or below the syndesmosis 44-B—Obliquely up from joint 44-C—High fibula fracture	In general, treatment of AO/OTA type A fractures is closed; treatment of AO types B and C is ORIF. Assess syndesmosis stability.	

AITFL, anterior inferior talofibular ligament; ITFL, inferior talofibular ligament; PITFL, posterior inferior talofibular ligament.

TABLE 11-23 ADULT TRAUMA, LOWER EXTREMITY—FOOT FRACTURES AND DISLOCATIONS

Injury	Eponym/Other Name	Classification	Treatment	Complications
Talar neck fracture	Aviator astragalus	Hawkins and Canale I—Nondisplaced II—Displaced and subtalar dislocation/subluxation III—Displaced and talar body dislocation IV—With talar body and head dislocation (pantalar dislocation)	Nonoperative: nondisplaced fracture, poor soft tissue; short-leg cast (SLC), non–weight bearing (NWB) for 8-12 wk (high shear stresses) Open reduction (with) internal fixation (ORIF): obtain and maintain anatomic reduction	Avascular necrosis (AVN) (especially types III/IV [Hawkins sign indicates a good prognosis]); delayed/nonunion, malunion, post-traumatic arthrosis, skin necrosis
Talar body fracture		Rare	Usually requires ORIF with or without medial malleolus osteotomy for exposure	AVN, malunion, degenerative joint disease (DJD)
Talar head fracture		Rare	Nondisplaced—splint/ice/elevation	Talonavicular DJD
Talar process fracture		Lateral process ≫ medial	SLC for 6 wk; excise if comminuted, symptomatic ORIF if large and displaced	Medial malleolus fracture (26%); rule out os trigonum (50%)
	Shepherd	Posterior process	SLC for 3-6 wk, excise symptomatic nonunions	
Subtalar dislocation		Calcaneus medial displacement (most common)	Reduce, immobilization 4 wk, open reduction if irreducibly closed	Posterior tibial tendon entrapment
Total talar dislocation		Talar and Chopart injury	Open reduction, late fusion	AVN
Calcancal fracture (most common)		Extra-articular (anterior process, tuberosity, medial process, sustentaculum talus, body)	Principles of treatment: avoid wound complications, restore articular congruity, restore height and width; computed tomographic scan helpful	Wound complications in up to 20% of cases; diabetics and smokers at increased risk; subtalar arthritis (need for fusion), peroneal tendon subluxation, neuroma, chronic pain (heel widening, nerve entrapment), DJD, malunion, associated fractures (spine, lower extremity), heel skin slough, compartment syndrome
		Intra-articular (nondisplaced, tongue, joint depression, comminuted), (Böhler angle and crucial angle of Gissane)	Nonoperative for nondisplaced and extra-articular fractures and high-risk patients (smokers, diabetics); walking boot/cast, NWB for 8-10 wk, early range of motion, edema control	
		Sanders classification Type I—Nondisplaced fracture Type II—Two-part fracture Type III—Three-part fracture with central depression Type IV—Comminuted fracture of four or more parts	ORIF: lateral approach after soft tissue subsides, articular reduction, internal fixation with or without bone graft (controversial)	
Navicular fracture		Anatomic location (body, tuberosity, avulsion), mechanism of energy (high vs. low energy) Compressed medial column	ORIF: displaced intra-articular and tuberosity fractures; stress fractures—SLC, NWB for 6 wk; avulsion fracture: treat as symptomatic sprain	Osteonecrosis (ORIF nonunion), associated with midfoot fractures
Cuboid fracture	Nutcracker	Compressed calcaneus and metatarsals (lateral column)	ORIF with bone graft or external fixation to 5th metatarsal to maintain length of lateral column SLC, NWB for 6-8 wk	Nonunion, malunion, chronic pain, stiffness
Tarsometatarsal fracture-dislocation	Lisfranc (Lisfranc ligament from base of second metatarsal [MT] to medial cuneiform)	High (forced dorsiflexion) vs. low (dorsiflexion/twisting) energy Homolateral—all five digits in same direction Partial (isolated)—first or second MT displaced Divergent—displacement in sagittal and coronal planes	Anatomic reduction of all affected joints; avoid soft tissue complications Nonoperative management for low-grade sprains, no subluxation ORIF for displaced fracture-dislocation vs. closed reduction with or without percutaneous pinning; ORIF of MT disruptions with screws is successful; consider primary arthrodesis for pure ligamentous disruptions	Chronic pain or disability (arthrodesis preferred); post-traumatic arthritis; delay in diagnosis (medial border of second MT base must align with medial border of middle cuneiform); compartment syndrome; broken implants—removal not required

Continued

TABLE 11-23 ADULT TRAUMA, LOWER EXTREMITY—FOOT FRACTURES AND DISLOCATIONS—cont'd

Injury	Eponym/Other Name	Classification	Treatment	Complications
Metatarsal fracture		Shaft	Majority treated nonoperatively; closed reduction with percutaneous pinning (CRPP) if needed; short-leg walking cast (SLWC) for 4 wk	Post-traumatic DJD, nonunion (most common with Jones fracture; ORIF, bone graft)
	March	Second MT stress fracture (most common)	Symptomatic; SLWC if late	
		Head	Reduction (traction and manipulation), cast; CRPP vs. ORIF if needed (avoid plantar prominent MT head)	
	Pseudo-Jones	Base avulsion (fifth MT)	SLWC for 2-3 wk, late removal of fragments if needed	
	Jones	Fifth MT base transverse fracture (differentiate from metadiaphyseal stress fracture)	6-8 wk NWB, SLC vs. percutaneous screw for faster recovery (return to play)	
Metatarsophalangeal (MTP) dislocation		Direction of dislocation (dorsal, first MTP most common)	Reduce promptly, immobilize (consider CRPP)	Post-traumatic arthrosis
Phalangeal fractures		Crush, associated nail bed injury	Majority treated nonoperatively; buddy tape for comfort, weight bearing as tolerated; ORIF of intra-articular fracture of hallux (great toe)	Post-traumatic arthrosis

Box 11–1 The Lauge-Hansen Classification

SUPINATION-ADDUCTION

- Stage 1: Transverse fracture of the lateral malleolus at or below the level of the anterior talofibular ligament or a tear of the structures of the lateral collateral ligament, with the anterior talofibular ligament most often disrupted. The calcaneofibular ligament is also frequently torn.
- Stage 2: Oblique fracture of the medial malleolus.

SUPINATION-EXTERNAL (EVERSION) ROTATION*

- Stage 1: Rupture of the anterior inferior tibiofibular ligament
- Stage 2: Oblique fracture or spiral fracture of the lateral malleolus
- Stage 3: Rupture of the post-tibiofibular ligament or fracture of the posterior malleolus of the tibia
- Stage 4: Transverse (sometimes oblique) fracture of the tibial malleolus

PRONATION-ABDUCTION†

- Stage 1: Rupture of the deltoid ligament or transverse fracture of the medial malleolus
- Stage 2: Rupture of the anterior and posterior inferior tibiotalofibular ligaments or bony avulsion
- Stage 3: Oblique fracture of the fibula at the level of the syndesmosis

PRONATION-EVERSION

- Stage 1: Rupture of the deltoid ligament or transverse fracture of the medial malleolus
- Stage 2: Rupture of the anterior inferior tibiotalofibular ligaments or bony avulsion
- Stage 3: Spiral/oblique fracture of the fibula above the level of the syndesmosis
- Stage 4: Rupture of the posterior inferior tibiofibular ligament or fracture of the posterior malleolus

PRONATION-DORSIFLEXION

- Stage 1: Fracture of the medial malleolus
- Stage 2: Fracture of the anterior lip of the tibia
- Stage 3: Fracture of the supramalleolar aspect of the fibula
- Stage 4: Rupture of the posterior inferior tibiofibular ligament or fracture of the posterior malleolus

*40% to 70% of all ankle fractures
†Less than 5% of ankle fractures

b. Danis-Weber and OTA classifications—Based primarily on the location of the fibular fracture (Fig. 11–51)
   44-A—Fibular fracture infrasyndesmotic
   44-B—Fibular fracture trans-syndesmotic
   44-C—Fibular fracture suprasyndesmotic

3. Treatment
   a. General principles
      (1) Anatomic reduction of ankle mortise required
      (2) One millimeter of lateral talar shift is equivalent to 42% decreased tibiotalar contact area
      (3) Confirm syndesmotic stability after operative fixation
   b. Nonoperative treatment
      (1) Indications
         (a) Isolated lateral malleolus fractures with intact deltoid ligament
         (b) Isolated medial malleolus fractures—Tip avulsion (nondisplaced or minimally displaced)
         (c) Nondisplaced bimalleolar fractures
      (2) Short-leg weight-bearing cast or walker boot for 6 weeks
   c. Operative treatment
      (1) Indications
         (a) Displaced bimalleolar and trimalleolar fractures
         (b) Displaced lateral malleolar fractures, with incompetent deltoid ligament
         (c) Displaced medial malleolus fractures
         (d) Syndesmotic disruption
         (e) Posterior malleolar fractures greater than 25%
      (2) ORIF
         (a) Fibular fixation
            i. Lateral plate with anteroposterior lag screw (for spiral/oblique patterns)
            ii. Posterior lateral plate—More stable than the lateral plate but more soft tissue irritation (peroneal tendon)
         (b) Medial malleolar fixation
            i. Medial lag screws or tension band for transverse fractures
            ii. Medial buttress plate for vertical fractures
         (c) Posterior malleolus
            i. Anteroposterior lag screws
            ii. Posterior buttress plate
         (d) Cast or walker boot for 6 weeks
4. Complications
   a. Wound complications, especially with diabetics
   b. Deep infection, especially in diabetics
   c. Stiffness (common)
   d. Post-traumatic arthrosis—Associated with persistent mortise instability or malreduction
5. Special circumstances
   a. Diabetic patients
      (1) High rate of complications with both nonoperative and operative management
         (a) Worse in patients with neuropathy
         (b) Skin breakdown, loss of reduction, and nonunion with cast treatment
         (c) Wound complications, deep infection, loss of reduction, and hardware failure with operative management
         (d) Up to 30% amputation rate
      (2) Augment fixation with transarticular screws or pins or with syndesmotic fixation.
   b. Open fractures
      (1) Emergent incision and drainage
      (2) Immediate ORIF
      (3) Results similar to closed fractures
   c. Syndesmotic instability

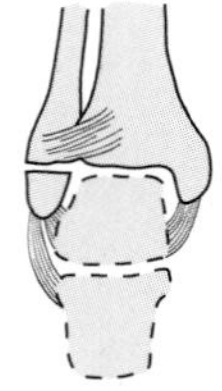

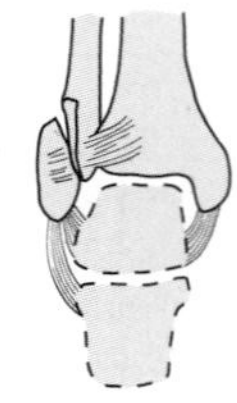

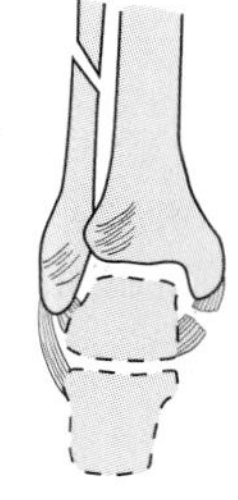

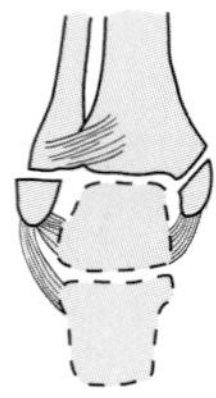

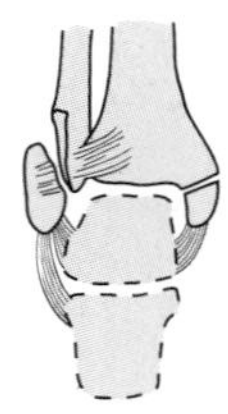

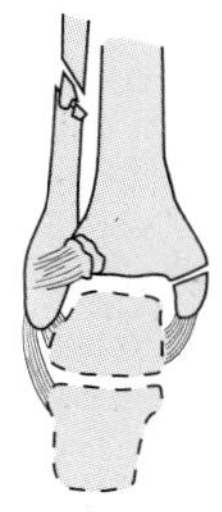

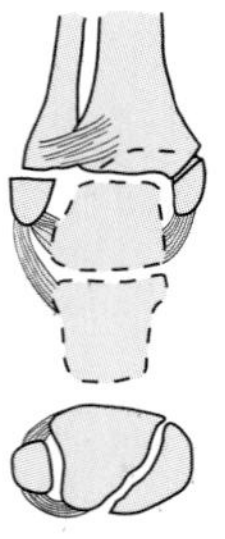

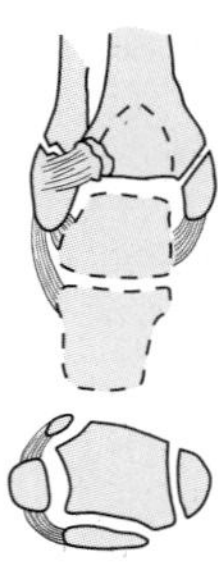

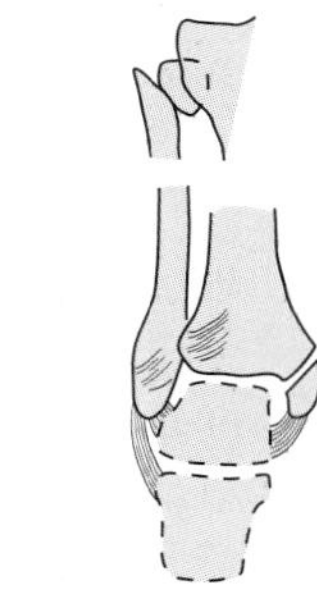

FIGURE 11–51 AO/OTA classification of ankle fractures. **A**, Tibia/fibula, malleolar, infrasyndesmotic lesions (44-A). **B**, Tibia/fibula, malleolar, trans-syndesmotic fibula fracture (44-B). **C**, Tibia/fibula, malleolar, suprasyndesmotic (44-C). (Redrawn from the Committee for Coding and Classification: Fracture and dislocation compendium. J Orthop Trauma 10[Suppl 1]:62, 1996.)

(1) Common with fibula fractures more than 6 cm above the ankle joint
(2) Uncommon after fixation of low fibula fractures—Test stability after fixation.
(3) The reduction of joints of the tibia-fibula should be compared with uninjured side on true lateral view.
(4) Malreduction associated with poor functional results
(5) Fixation with two 3.5-mm position screws (not lag screws)
(6) Non–weight bearing for 6-8 weeks
(7) Screw removal after 3 months optional

B. Talus fractures

1. Diagnosis
   a. Mechanism of injury—Usually high-energy injuries; forced dorsiflexion with axial load
   b. Neck fractures the most common
   c. Associated dislocation surgical emergency due to skin tenting and neurovascular stretch injury
2. Classification—Hawkins classification (Fig. 11–52) based on displacement and associated dislocation
   Type I—Nondisplaced
   Type II—Displaced, with subtalar dislocation
   Type III—Displaced, with talar body dislocation (subtalar and tibiotalar dislocations)
   Type IV—Displaced, with talar body and head dislocation (plantar dislocation)
3. Treatment
   a. General principles—Avoid secondary displacement, provide proper foot alignment, and avoid AVN.
   b. Nonoperative treatment—Indicated for nondisplaced fractures is use of a short-leg cast (SLC) with non–weight bearing for

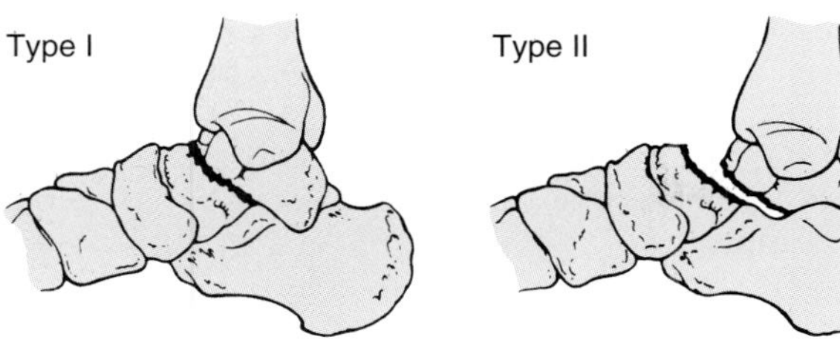

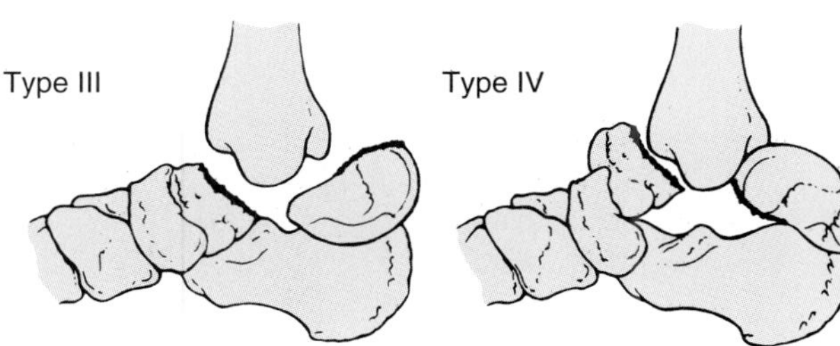

FIGURE 11–52 The Hawkins classification of talar neck fractures. (From Sangeorzan BJ, Hansen ST: Ankle and foot: Trauma. In Orthopaedic Knowledge Update 3, p 616. Rosemont, IL, American Academy of Orthopaedic Surgeons, 1990. Reprinted by permission.)

10-12 weeks; high shear stress requires prolonged immobilization and non–weight bearing.

c. Operative treatment
   (1) Indicated for displacement fractures
   (2) Associated dislocations often require open reduction.
   (3) Dual-incision approach recommended to assure anatomic reduction
   (4) Posterior-to-anterior or anterior-to-posterior screws
   (5) Non–weight bearing for 10-12 weeks

4. Complications
   a. AVN—Increased risk with increased initial displacement and associated dislocation
   b. Nonunion
   c. Post-traumatic arthritis or tibiotalar and subtalar joints
   d. Malunion
5. Special circumstances
   a. Talar body fractures— Unusual; treated with ORIF with or without medial malleolar osteotomy for exposure
   b. Talar process fractures
      (1) Lateral more common than medial
      (2) Often misdiagnosed as ankle sprain
      (3) Treat with SLC and subsequent protected weight bearing for 6 weeks
   c. Open fracture with extruded fragment—Preserve extruded fragment when it is articular and large

C. Calcaneus fractures
   1. Diagnosis
      a. Mechanism of injury—Axial load
      b. Significant soft tissue injury often associated with fracture
      c. Typical deformity—Heel shortened, widened, and in varus; forced dorsiflexion with axial load
   2. Classification—Sanders classification (Fig. 11–53) based on location and comminution of posterior facet on coronal CT scan
   3. Treatment
      a. General principles
         (1) Avoid wound complications
         (2) Restore articular congruity
         (3) Restore normal calcaneal width and height
         (4) Maximum functional recovery may take longer than 12 months.
      b. Nonoperative treatment
         (1) Indicated for nondisplaced fractures, extra-articular fractures, and those at high risk for operative complications (diabetics and smokers)
         (2) Cast or walker boot, non–weight bearing for 8-10 weeks, early ROM, and compression stocking to control swelling
      c. Operative treatment
         (1) Indicated for displaced intra-articular fractures
         (2) Extensile lateral approach associated with up to 20% wound complications
         (3) Low-profile implants
         (4) Percutaneous reduction and screw fixation

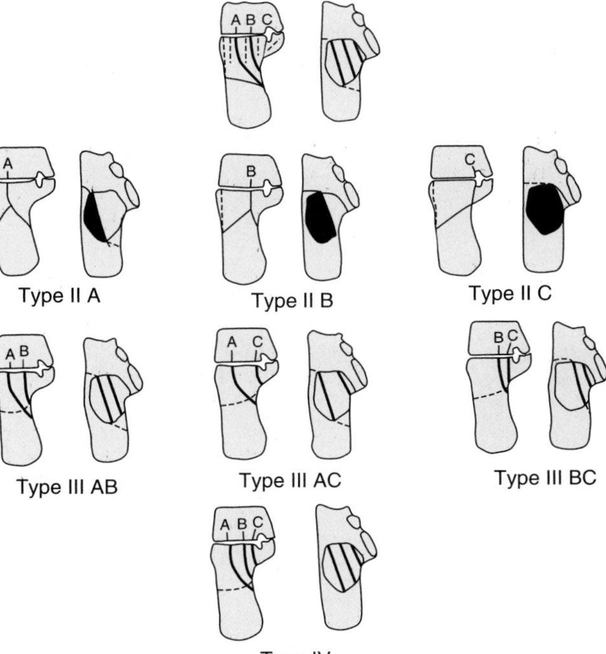

FIGURE 11–53 The Sanders classification of calcaneus fractures based on a coronal CT scan. Roman numerals describe the numbers of fracture fragments of the posterior facet. Letters describe the locations of the primary fracture line through the posterior facet. Type A, lateral. Type B, central. Type C, medial. (Reproduced with permission from Benirschke SK, Sangeorzan BS: Extensive intra-articular fractures of the foot: surgical management of calcaneal fractures. Clin Orthop 292:128-134, 1993.)

(5) Delay surgery until soft tissue envelope shows wrinkling (7-14 days).

4. Complications
   a. Wound complications in up to 20% of cases (increased in diabetics and smokers)
      (1) Local wound care and oral antibiotics usually sufficient
      (2) Implant removal usually not required
   b. Subtalar arthritis
   c. Peroneal impingement with nonoperative treatment from lateral wall blowout
   d. Poor functional outcome in patients over age 50, obese patients, manual laborers, and those receiving workers' compensation
   e. Compartment syndrome
5. Special circumstances—Open fractures
   a. Usually a medial open wound
   b. Poorer results than those associated with closed fractures
   c. Associated with severe comminution

D. Navicular fractures

1. Diagnosis/classification
   a. High-energy fractures usually via compression of medial column (nutcracker)
   b. Low-energy injuries—Avulsions
      (1) Dorsal avulsion of joint capsule
      (2) Tuberosity fracture—Avulsion of posterior tibial tendon
   c. Stress fracture
2. Treatment
   a. Displaced intra-articular fractures—ORIF
   b. Avulsion fractures—Protocol for symptomatic sprains
   c. Stress fracture—SLC with non–weight bearing for 6 weeks

E. Cuboid fractures

1. Diagnosis—Compression of lateral column
2. Treatment
   a. Restore column length—ORIF or external fixation spanning from the calcaneus to the fifth metatarsal.
   b. SLC with non–weight bearing for 6-8 weeks

F. Tarsometatarsal fractures-dislocations (**Lisfranc injury**)

1. Diagnosis
   a. Mechanism of injury
      (1) High energy—Forced dorsiflexion
      (2) Low energy—Dorsiflexion/twisting
   b. High index of suspicion for subtle injury when it is associated with midfoot swelling and/or tenderness
      (1) Stress view (standing)
      (2) Comparison view of noninjured foot
   c. Lisfranc ligament—Base of second metatarsal to medial cuneiform
   d. Plain radiographs
      (1) Anteroposterior—Medial midfoot evaluation
      (2) Oblique—Lateral midfoot evaluation
      (3) Lateral—Dorsal displacement
2. Classification—Based on the direction of dislocation (Fig. 11–54)
   Homolateral
   Partial (isolated)
   Divergent
3. Treatment
   a. General principles
      (1) Anatomic reduction of all affected joints
      (2) Avoid soft tissue complications.
      (3) Immediate reduction of widely dislocated joints—Minor subluxation acceptable
      (4) Definitive management after recovery of soft tissues
      (5) Provisional K-wire fixation for grossly unstable joints

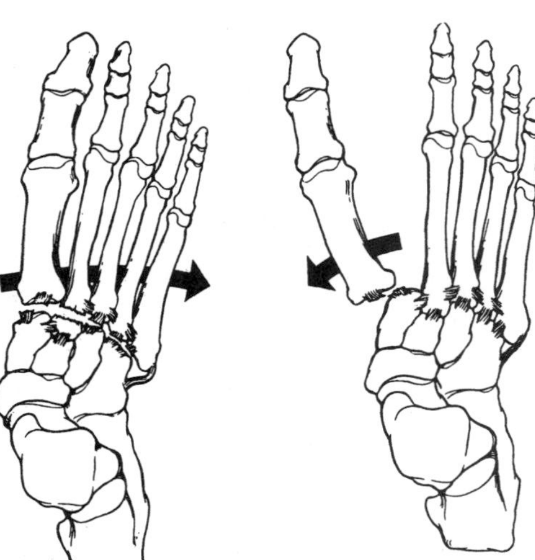
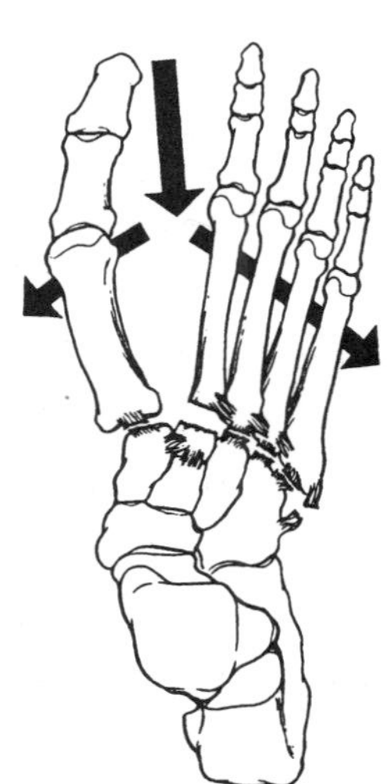

FIGURE 11–54 Classification of midfoot tarsometatarsal injuries.

b. Nonoperative treatment—Indicated for low-grade sprains with no subluxation
c. Operative treatment
(1) Indicated for displacement
(2) Screw fixation of affected medial joints
(3) Screw or K-wire fixation of lateral joints
(4) Non–weight bearing for 6-8 weeks; no removal of implants before 12 weeks
4. Complications
a. Long-term pain and/or disability—Maximum recovery longer than 12 months
b. Post-traumatic arthritis
c. Fractured implants—Removal not required

G. Metatarsal fractures
1. Diagnosis/classification
a. Rule out associated Lisfranc injury.
b. Distinguished midshaft, distal, and base fifth metatarsal fractures
c. **Jones fracture** at metaphyseal diaphyseal junction of fifth metatarsal
(1) Vascular watershed area
(2) Relatively high healing complication rate with weight-bearing protocols
(3) Requires prolonged non–weight bearing
d. Pseudo–Jones fracture—More proximal than Jones; avulsion of peroneus brevis tendon
(1) Healing much more reliable than true Jones fracture
(2) Weight-bearing protocol acceptable
2. Treatment
a. Shaft fractures usually treated nonoperatively
b. Avoid prominent metatarsal heads.
c. Jones fracture—SLC with non–weight bearing for 6-8 weeks or percutaneous screw fixation for faster recovery
d. Pinning for widely displaced shaft fractures or distal fractures
3. Complications
a. Nonunion—The most common complication with Jones fracture; treated by screw fixation with or without bone grafting

H. Metatarsophalangeal joint dislocation
1. Classification
a. First metatarsophalangeal (the most common dislocation)
b. Dorsal
2. Treatment—Closed reduction, a hard shoe, and WBAT

I. Phalangeal fractures
1. Diagnosis
a. The Cruch mechanism
b. Associated nail injury
2. Treatment
a. Nonoperative for most
b. Buddy taping for comfort
c. WBAT
d. Operative for intra-articular fractures of the great toe

SECTION 4 Spine

I. Upper Cervical Spine Injuries

A. General concepts—The first goal of treatment is stabilization. Traction should not be used in distraction injuries. Distraction injuries tend to be more unstable than compression injuries. Neurogenic shock is rare, characterized by massive vasodilation causing the loss of autonomic tone. Treatment is with vasopressors. The role of steroids is unclear.
1. If they are given within 3 hours, administer for 24 hours.
2. If they are given within 3-8 hours, administer for 48 hours.
3. A bolus of 30 mg/kg over 15 minutes, with a maintenance infusion of 5.4 mg/kg per hour

B. ASIA (American Spinal Injury Association) classification (Table 11–24)

C. Clinical syndromes
1. **Brown-Séquard syndrome**
a. Motor function is disrupted on the side of injury, while pain and temperature are affected on the contralateral side.
b. Ninety percent of patients will recover the ability to walk.
2. **Central cord syndrome**
a. The upper extremity is affected more than the lower extremity.
b. The prognosis is good for the recovery of ambulation, but the patient is less likely to recover upper extremity function.
3. Anterior cord syndrome
a. Motor response, pain reception, and temperature reception are not functioning; vibration sensation, proprioception, and deep pressure sensation are intact.
b. The prognosis is poor.

D. Occipitocervical dissociation
1. The Power ratio* of both columns to OA is less than 1.
2. The odontoid tip lines up with the basion.
3. The distance between the odontoid and basion is 4-5 mm in adults and up to 10 mm in children.
4. Classification—Harborview classification
Stage I—MRI evidence of injury to ligamentous stabilizers, alignment within 2 mm of normal, and distraction of 2 mm or less on manual traction radiograph

*The Power ratio $\left(\frac{\text{basion–posterior arch}}{\text{opsithion–anterior arch}}\right) > 1.0$ indicates instability of the atlantoaxial junction.

TABLE 11-24 ADULT SPINE TRAUMA

Level	Injury Type	Classification	Common Name	Mechanism of Injury	Risk of Neurologic Injury	Treatment	Indication for Surgery	Important Points
Occipitocervical dislocation	I	Traynelis et al	Anterior	Anterior translation	Very high	Occipitocervical fusion	Surgery indicated	Very unstable; rarely survive injury
	II		Distraction	Pure distraction	Very high	Occipitocervical fusion	Surgery indicated	Very unstable; rarely survive injury
	III		Posterior	Posterior translation	Very high	Occipitocervical fusion	Surgery indicated	Very unstable; rarely survive injury
Occipital condyle fracture	I	Anderson-Montesano	Impacted condyle fracture	Compression of skull	Low	Collar	Usually not required	Alar ligament and tectorial membrane usually intact
	II		Occipital condyle and basilar skull fracture	Compression of skull	Low	Collar	Usually not required	Alar ligament and tectorial membrane usually intact
	III		Avulsion fracture of alar ligament	Distraction of skull	Moderate to high	Collar, halo, or surgery, depending on stability	More than 1 mm of displacement	Potential for ligament disruption
C1 ring fracture	Posterior arch fracture		Lamina fracture	Hyperextension	Low	Immobilization	Not indicated	Hyperextension
	Two- and three-part fractures		Lateral mass fracture	Lateral compression	Low	Immobilization	Not indicated	
	Four-part fracture		Jefferson fracture	Axial compression	Low	Immobilization, sometimes traction	Optional for widely displaced lateral masses	>7-mm offset of lateral mass indicates transverse ligament rupture
C2 fracture	Traumatic spondylolisthesis	Levine	Hangman fracture					
	I or IA		IA called atypical hangman	Hyperextension	Low	Collar		Prove stable with supervised flexion–extension radiographs
	II or IIA			Hyperextension with secondary flexion	Low to moderate	Immobilization; avoid traction with IIA	Osteosynthesis optional	Type II, use traction; type IIA, avoid traction
	III		Bilateral facet dislocation	Hyperextension with secondary flexion/ distraction	High	Surgical reduction of facet dislocation and C2-C3 fusion	Surgery required to reduce facets	Open reduction of facets required
	Odontoid fracture							
	I	Anderson-D'Alonzo	Avulsion fracture	Hyperextension of distraction	Low	Collar	None	Watch for associated occipitocervical instability
	II		Fracture at junction of odontoid and body	Multiple mechanisms	Moderate	Halo vs. internal fixation	Unstable fracture or nonunion	Most common; high rate of nonunion
	III		Fracture into C2 body	Multiple mechanisms	Moderate	Halo vest immobilization	Displacement, instability	Usually stable

C2 body fracture				Similar to subaxial cervical spine	Low			
Transverse ligament disruption			C1-C2 instability	Severe flexion	Moderate to high	C1-C2 fusion	ADI >3-5 mm	Often associated with dizziness, syncope, respiratory problems, and blurred vision
C1-C2 rotatory subluxation	I	Fielding-Hawkins	Rotatory fixation	Rotational trauma	Low	Immobilization/ traction/surgery	Indicated for chronic cases with fixed deformity and spasm or instability	Many causes; infection and trauma most common
	II		Rotatory fixation with 3-5 mm of anterior displacement	Rotational trauma	Moderate	Immobilization/ traction/surgery	Indicated for chronic cases with fixed deformity and spasm or instability	
	III		Rotatory fixation with >5 mm anterior displacement	Rotational trauma	Moderate	Immobilization/ traction/surgery	Indicated for chronic cases with fixed deformity and spasm or instability	
	IV		Rotatory fixation with posterior displacement	Rotational trauma	Moderate to high	Immobilization/ traction/surgery	Indicated for chronic cases with fixed deformity and spasm or instability	
Subaxial cervical spine		Allen-Ferguson		Mechanisms implied by name	Depends on stage of injury	Depends on stage of injury		
	Compressive flexion			Compression and flexion	Low to high		Instability or neurologic deficit with cord compression	
	Distractive flexion			Distraction and flexion	Low to high		Instability or neurologic deficit with cord compression	
	Axial compression			Axial compression	Low to high		Instability or neurologic deficit with cord compression	
	Compressive extension			Compression and extension	Low to high		Instability or neurologic deficit with cord compression	
	Distractive extension			Distraction and extension	Low to high		Instability or neurologic deficit with cord compression	
	Lateral flexion			Lateral bending	Low to moderate		Instability or neurologic deficit with cord compression	
	Compression		Compression	Flexion	Low	Collar		Watch for signs of posterior ligament disruption.

Continued

TABLE 11-24 ADULT SPINE TRAUMA—cont'd

Level	Injury Type	Classification	Common Name	Mechanism of Injury	Risk of Neurologic Injury	Treatment	Indication for Surgery	Important Points
Subaxial cervical spine (cont'd)	Burst		Burst	Axial compression	Moderate to high	Halo vs. anterior decompression/ fusion	Cord compression	Anterior decompression specifically indicated in cases of incomplete cord injury
			Flexion teardrop	Compression and flexion	High	Halo vs. anterior decompression/ fusion	Cord compression	Very unstable
			Facet dislocation	Flexion and distraction	High	Reduction of facet, fusion	Bilateral facet dislocation	Possible disc herniation; consider MRI prior to reduction
	Posterior element fracture		Spinous process	Extension (sometimes flexion or rotation)	Low	Collar	Floating lateral mass	Most are stable
Thoracolumbar spine	Compression	Denis		Flexion and axial loading		Bracing	Greater than 50% anterior collapse or widening of spinous process	Osteoporotic compression fracture requires workup and treatment of underlying condition; watch for ileus.
	Burst			Axial loading				
	Stable					Bracing	Progressive deformity or neurologic compromise	Watch for any signs of posterior ligament rupture vs. MRI; watch for ileus.
	Unstable					Surgery	>30 degrees kyphosis; incomplete cord injury with cord compromise	Cord decompression required if neurologic deficit present
	Seatbelt injury		Chance fracture (bony injury)	Distraction and flexion		Surgery for posterior ligament ruptures, bracing for postoperative treatment	>17% kyphosis with bony injury, posterior ligament injury	High rate of associated intra-abdominal injury
	Fracture-dislocation			Rotation and shear		Surgical alignment, fusion, instrumentation	All require surgery	Long segmental posterior construct

ADI, atlanto–dens interval; MRI, magnetic resonance imaging.

Stage II—Same as Stage 1, except distraction of less than 2 mm on a manual-traction radiograph

Stage III—Distraction of more than 2 mm on static radiographs

5. Treatment
   a. Operative treatment indications—Stage II or III injuries or any injury with associated neurologic deficit
6. Operative procedure—Occipitocervical fusion

E. Occipital fracture

1. Classification—Anderson-Montesano classification

   Type I—Comminuted impaction fracture of occiput; generally stable

   Type II—Shear or compression fracture extending into the base of the skull; variably stable

   Type III—Avulsion injuries that have a transverse fracture component; generally unstable
2. Treatment
   a. Operative treatment—Indicated with evidence of instability or neurologic deficit
   b. Stable vs. unstable injuries—A cervical collar for stable injuries and surgical stabilization for unstable injuries

F. C1 fracture

1. Classification—Levine and Edwards classification
   a. Posterior arch fractures—Hyperextension
   b. Lateral mass fractures—Axial load with lateral bend
   c. Isolated anterior arch fractures—Hyperextension
   d. Burst fractures (Jefferson)—Axial load
2. Treatment—Operative treatment
   a. Indications
      (1) Combined lateral mass displacement of 7 mm (8.1 mm with standard x-ray magnification) indicates transverse ligament rupture.
      (2) ADI of greater than 3 mm indicates that the transverse ligament is damaged and ADI of greater than 5 mm indicates that both the transverse and alar ligaments are damaged.
      (3) Residual displacement after halo of more than 7 mm or ADI of more than 3 mm
   b. A halo for 6-12 weeks for fractures with an intact transverse ligament
   c. Posterior spinal fusion (C1-C2 or occiput-C2) if the transverse ligament is incompetent

G. Atlantoaxial instability

1. Fielding and Hawkins classification

   Type I—Rotationally unstable but transverse alar ligament (TAL) intact. The odontoid is the pivot point.

   Type II—Rotationally unstable, with TAL incompetence; one facet acts as the pivot.

   Type III—Both facets subluxed anteriorly, more than 5 mm ADI

   Type IV—Both facets subluxed posteriorly

   Type V—Frank dislocation
2. Treatment—Operative treatment
   a. Indications
      (1) Chronic deformity
      (2) Less than 2-mm distraction
      (3) Types IB and IC
      (4) Failure of immobilization
   b. A halo for 3 months—Types IIA and IIB
   c. C1-C2 posterior fusion—Include the occiput if the instability is associated with occipitocervical dislocation.

H. Odontoid fracture

1. Classification—Anderson-D'Alonso classification

   Type I—Avulsion of the alar ligaments from the tip

   Type II—Fracture at the base of the odontoid

   Type IIA—Comminuted fracture of the base of the odontoid

   Type III—Fractures that extend into the body of C2
2. Treatment—Operative treatment
   a. Indications—Types II and IIA fractures are generally considered operative because of the high rate of nonunion.
   b. Immobilization in rigid cervical orthosis for type I
   c. Posterior C1-C2 fusion for type II
   d. An anterior screw may be used in type II fractures unless body habitus, fracture geometry, or other injuries preclude it. This procedure is associated with a higher failure rate than posterior fusion, but it does preserve atlantoaxial motion.
   e. Halo vest for type III—Consider operative treatment if initial displacement is greater than 5 mm.

I. C2 fracture (traumatic spondylolisthesis of the axis)

1. Classification—Levine classification

   Type I—Minimally displaced fracture of the pars 2 degrees to hyperextension and axial loading

   Type IA—Same as type I except fracture lines are asymmetrical

   Type II—Displaced fractures (> 3 mm) of the pars, with subsequent flexion after hyperextension and axial loading

   Type IIa—Flexion without displacement; BE CAREFUL not to mistake this for a type I fracture, which represents total disc avulsion

   Type III—Bilateral pars fracture with bilateral facet dislocations (rare)
2. Treatment
   a. Indications
      (1) Operative treatment for type II fractures with more than 3-5–mm displacement
      (2) Operative treatment for type III fractures
   b. Type I—Rigid cervical orthosis
   c. Type IIA—Halo vest or surgery (no traction!)
   d. Type III—Generally operative, usually C2-C3 fusion
3. Complications—Vascular injury; vertebral artery injury is rare but increasingly diagnosed by magnetic resonance angiogram (MRA)

II. Lower Cervical Spine Injuries

A. Classification—Allen-Ferguson classification based on mechanism; described as the position of the head and neck at the time of injury (flexion/extension) and the mode of failure (distraction/compression)
   Compressive flexion
   Vertical compression
   Distractive flexion
   Compressive extension
   Distractive extension
   Lateral flexion

B. Stability
   1. White and Punjabi—Point system based on anatomic, radiographic, and neurologic criteria; less than 5 points is equivalent to instability.
   2. Several patterns are inherently unstable.
      a. "Teardrop" fractures, which result from compressive flexion injury, contrast with the small avulsion-type teardrop injury, which may be treated with immobilization.
      b. Flexion-type injuries tend to be more unstable than extension injuries.
      c. Any fracture associated with neurologic injury is assumed to be unstable.
      d. Facet dislocations
      e. Fractures with significant initial displacement

C. Treatment
   1. Fractures that are primarily bony without ligamentous injury are usually treated with immobilization.
   2. Posterior ligamentous injury is usually treated with surgical stabilization.

III. Thoracic Spine Injuries

A. Classification—Magerl classification
   Type A—Compression fractures caused by axial loading
   Type B—Distraction injuries with ligamentous (B1) or osseoligamentous (B2) injury posteriorly
   Type C—Multidirectional injuries, often fracture dislocations; very unstable with very high likelihood of neurologic injury

B. Treatment
   1. Most burst fractures and compression fractures can be treated with an orthosis for 12 weeks and a shorter period of time for less severe fractures.
   2. Flexion-distraction injuries with a bony avulsion posteriorly (type B2) can be treated with an orthosis.
   3. Types B1 and C injuries usually require surgical stabilization.
   4. Some compression fractures with more than 50% anterior collapse may also require stabilization.

IV. Thoracolumbar and Lumbar Spine Injuries

A. Classification—Denis classification
   1. Columns
      a. The anterior column is equivalent to the anterior one third of the body and annulus and the anterior longitudinal ligament (ALL).
      b. The middle column is equivalent to the posterior two thirds of the body and annulus and the posterior longitudinal ligament (PLL).
      c. The posterior column is equivalent to the spinous process, lamina, pedicles, transverse process, and ligamentum flavum; interspinous ligament; supraspinous ligament; and facets.
   2. Compression fractures involve only the anterior column.
   3. Burst fractures involve the middle and anterior and often the posterior columns.
   4. Flexion-distraction injuries involve failure of the posterior and middle columns in tension.
   5. Fracture-dislocations involve the failure of all three columns.

B. Associated injuries
   1. Adynamic ileus is common.
   2. Calcaneus fractures are associated in approximately 10% of cases.

C. Treatment
   1. Most compression fractures can be managed in an orthosis unless kyphosis is greater than 30 degrees.
   2. Burst fractures may be treated in an orthosis if kyphosis is less than 20 degrees, there is no neurologic deficit, canal compromise is less than 50%, and there is less than a 50% loss of anterior body height; otherwise, they are operative.
   3. Flexion-distraction and fracture-dislocations are routinely treated with surgical stabilization.

SECTION 5 Pediatric Trauma

I. Introduction

A. Several features of fractures and dislocations in children are not found in adults (Tables 11–25 through 11–36; Figs. 11–55 through 11–80). Children's bones are more ductile than adults' bones, and bowing is thus unique to children. The terms **greenstick** and **torus** imply a partial fracture with some part of the bone intact. The periosteum in children is much thicker and often remains intact on the concave (compression) side, allowing for less displacement and better reduction of fractures. Children's fractures heal more quickly and with less immobilization than adults' fractures. Contractures are also less likely. However, because bones are actively growing in pediatric fractures, malunion and growth plate injuries are important concerns. Remodeling is more thorough; thus, displacement and angulation that would not be

TABLE 11-25 SALTER-HARRIS CLASSIFICATION OF PHYSEAL INJURIES

Type	Description	Prognosis
I	Transverse fractures through the physis	Excellent
II	Fractures through the physis, with metaphyseal fragment	Excellent
III	Fractures through the physis and epiphysis	Good but with the potential for intra-articular deformity; may require ORIF
IV	Fractures through the epiphysis, physis, and metaphysis	Good but unstable; fragment requires ORIF
V	Crush injury to the physis	Poor, with growth arrest
VI	Injury to the perichondrial ring	Good; may cause angular deformities

ORIF, open reduction with internal fixation.

acceptable in an adult are often acceptable in children. The exception to this rule is an intra-articular fracture, in which the same axioms apply.

II. Child Abuse

A. Introduction—One must always be alert for the "battered child." All states now require physicians to report suspected child abuse. Suspicion should be raised when fractures are seen in children less than 3 years old (the most common age group for sustaining abuse), with multiple healing bruises, skin marks, burns, unreasonable histories, and signs of neglect, among other indications.

B. Fracture location—The most common locations of fractures in children of abuse are the humerus, tibia, and femur, in that order. If suspicion is high, skeletal surveys are appropriate in children with delayed development and in some metaphyseal and spiral fractures. Diaphyseal fractures are also common in abuse cases (four times as likely as metaphyseal fractures). Skeletal surveys are not as helpful in children over 5 years old. Instead, a bone scan may be done as an alternative or adjunctive study. Nonorthopaedic injuries found in abuse include head injuries, burns, and blunt abdominal visceral injuries.

C. Treatment—In addition to normal fracture care, early involvement of social workers and pediatricians is essential. If the abuse is missed, there is a greater than 33% chance of further abuse and a 5-10% chance of death in affected children.

TABLE 11-26 PEDIATRIC HAND AND WRIST TRAUMA

Injury	Eponym/Other Name	Classification	Treatment	Complications
Phalanx fracture (see Fig. 11–56)	(Watch for mallet equivalent)	Based on phalanx and SH classification	Closed reduction for most; ORIF if condylar, SH III/IV >25 degrees if <10 yr old, >10 degrees if >10 yr old; dynamic traction for pilon equivalents	Residual deformities, tendon imbalance, nail deformities
Metacarpal fracture (see Fig. 11–57)		Based on location	Reduce; ORIF if irreducible	Avascular necrosis of metacarpal head
Thumb MC fracture (see Fig. 11–58)	Type D = Bennett equivalent	Type A—metaphyseal Type B—SH II (medial) Type C—SH II (lateral) Type D—SH III	Closed reduction except for type D, which requires ORIF	
IP dislocation			Closed reduction and splint; ORIF if unable to obtain or maintain a congruous reduction	
MCP dislocation			Attempt closed reduction; ORIF if irreducible	
CMC dislocation			Reduce with finger traps; CRPP with K-wire to carpus and adjacent MC	
Distal radius fracture		SH fractures I-V	CRPP types III and IV	Deformity, loss of reduction, infection with open fracture, Volkmann contracture, growth arrest, malunion, refracture, TFCC tears, carpal tunnel syndrome
	Torus	Tension side intact	SAC for 3 wk	
	Greenstick	Tension side with plastic deformation	Reduce if angulation >10 degrees	
	Complete	Both cortices disrupted	Reduce and place in LAC	

CMC, carpometacarpal; CRPP, closed reduction with percutaneous pinning; LAC, long-arm cast; MC, metacarpal; MCP, metacarpophalangeal joint; ORIF, open reduction with internal fixation; SAC, short-arm cast; SH, Salter-Harris; TFCC, triangular fibrocartilage complex.

TABLE 11-27 PEDIATRIC RADIAL AND ULNAR SHAFT TRAUMA

Injury	Eponym/Other Name	Classification	Treatment	Complications
Radius and ulna fractures	"Both-bone"	Greenstick, compression, complete	Correct rotation, with pronation/supination and <10 degrees angulation: LAC 3-4 wk if <10 yr old; bayonet apposition OK if growth remains	Refracture, limb ischemia, malunion (especially in <10 yr old with inadequate reduction), nerve injury, synostosis
Plastic deformation		Based on bones involved (ulna >radius)	Reduction with pressure as a fulcrum, the most deformed bone first; must reduce >20 degrees in 4 yr old, less in older children	Persistence of deformity
Ulna fracture and radial head dislocation (see Fig. 11–59)	Monteggia	Type I—Ulna angulation and radial head anterior (extension)	Reduce (traction flexion); LAC, 100 degrees flexion in supination	Late diagnosis (reconstruct annular ligament), decreased ROM Missed wrist injury, nonunion, persistent radial head dislocation, periarticular ossification
		Type II—Ulna angulation and radial head posterior (flexion)	Reduce (traction extension); LAC in some extension	
		Type III—Ulna anterior angulation, radial head lateral (adduction)	Reduce (extension); LAC, 90 degrees flexion in supination	
		Type IV—Ulna and proximal (one third) radius fracture (both anterior angulation)	Reduce (supinate); may require ORIF	
Radial head dislocation (anterior)	Monteggia equivalent		Supination and pressure on radial head; LAC, 100 degrees flexion in supination	Synostosis, PIN injury, loss of reduction
Ulna and radial neck fractures	Check for Monteggia equivalent		Reduce (traction, pressure on radial head, varus stress); LAC, 90 degrees flexion	
Ulna and proximal radius fractures	Check for Monteggia equivalent		Reduce (traction supination); LAC, 90 degrees in supination	
Radius fracture and distal radioulnar dislocation	Galeazzi		Reduce (traction supination if ulna dorsal, pronation if ulna volar); ORIF if >12 yr old or reduction fails	Malunion, nerve injury (AIN), RU subluxation, loss of radial bow

AIN, anterior interosseous nerve; LAC, long-arm cast; ORIF, open reduction with internal fixation; PIN, posterior interosseous nerve; ROM, range of motion; RU, radioulnar.

III. Physeal Fractures

A. Introduction—Fracture of the physis, or growth plate, is more likely than injury to attached ligaments; thus, assume that there is a fracture of the physis until evidence proves otherwise.

B. Characteristics—Although physeal fractures are classically thought to be through the zone of provisional calcification (within the zone of hypertrophy) of the growth plate, the fracture can be through many different layers. The blood supply of the epiphysis is tenuous, and injuries can disrupt small physeal vessels supplying the growth center. This can lead to many complications associated with these injuries (e.g., limb length discrepancies, malunion, bony bars). The most common physeal injuries occur in the distal radius, followed by the distal tibia.

C. Classification—The **Salter-Harris** (SH) classification modified by Rang is the gold standard for physeal injuries (see Fig. 11–55; see Table 11–8).

D. Treatment and results—Gentle reduction should be attempted initially for SH I and II fractures, sometimes using conscious sedation protocols. With reduction and immobilization, these fractures will do well without a significant amount of growth arrest (except in the distal femur). SH III and IV fractures are intra-articular by definition and usually require ORIF. Follow-up radiographs are required for all physeal injuries. Remodeling is also common in pediatric fractures (up to 20 degrees). This depends on the location and age of the patient. Table 11–8 to 11–19 detail the tolerance for each fracture during childhood. Harris-Park growth arrest lines (transverse radiodense lines) may be the only evidence of a physeal injury on follow-up radiographs.

E. Partial growth arrest—Physeal bars or bridges result from growth plate injuries that arrest a part of the physis and leave the uninjured physis to grow normally. This results in angular growth and deformity. Physeal bridge resection with interposition of a fat graft or artificial material is reserved for patients with over 2 cm of growth remaining and less than 50% physeal involvement. Treatment of smaller peripheral bars in young patients have the highest success rate. MRI and CT scans can help define the location and amount of physeal closure. Arrest involving more than 50% of the physis should be treated with ipsilateral completion of the arrest and contralateral epiphysiodesis or ipsilateral limb lengthening.

TABLE 11-28 PEDIATRIC ELBOW TRAUMA

Injury	Eponym/Other Name	Classification	Treatment	Complications
Supracondylar fracture (6-8 yr old) (see Fig. 11–60)		I—Extension (98%), nondisplaced	Immobilize 3 wk Minimally displaced (<2 mm), splint	Nerve injury (AIN and radial), vascular injury (1%), decreased ROM; if pulse present but then lost, explore; if-pulse present but then lost, explore; if no pulse present but pink hand, watch; if no pulse present and cold, explore.
		II—Displaced (posterior cortex intact)	Reduce; cast vs. CRPP (must re-create Baumann angle) (see Fig. 11–61)	
		III—Displaced (posterior periosteal hinge intact)	Reduce; CRPP versus open pinning	
		IV—Displaced (posterior periosteal hinge disrupted)	Reduce; CRPP versus open pinning	
		Flexion (distal fragment anterior)	Reduce; CRPP versus ORIF	HO, cubitus varus (5-10%), ipsilateral fractures Nerve injury (ulnar), malunion (decreased extension)
Lateral condyle fracture (6 yr old) (see Fig. 11–62)		Milch I—SH IV Milch II—SH II into trochlea	Minimally displaced (<2 mm), splint; displaced, ORIF with pins or cannulated screws	Overgrowth/spur "fishtail" deformity, nonunion, cubitus valgus, AVN, ulnar nerve palsy
Medial condyle fracture (9-14 yr old)		Nondisplaced— <10 mm displacement		Cubitus varus, AVN
		Displaced— >10 mm displacement	Minimally displaced, splint Displaced, ORIF	
Entire distal humeral physis fracture (<7 yr old) (see Fig. 11–63)		A—Infant (SH I) B—7 mo–3 yr old (SH I) C—3-7 yr old (SH II)	Closed reduction, LAC; displaced, CRPP	Child abuse, common late diagnosis, cubitus varus
Medial epicondylar apophysis fracture (11 yr old) (see Fig. 11–64)	Little Leaguer's elbow	I—Acute injuries		Highly associated with elbow dislocation (50%), valgus instability, loss of extension
		A—Nondisplaced	Immobilize 1 wk	
		B—Minimally displaced	Immobilize 1 wk	
		C—Significantly displaced (may be dislocated)	ORIF for valgus instability; otherwise, early ROM	
		D—Entrapment of fragment in joint	Manipulative extraction, ORIF (especially with ulnar nerve entrapment)	
		E—Fracture through epicondylar apophysis	Immobilization vs. ORIF	
		II—Chronic tension stress injury	Change in throwing activities	
T condylar fracture		Based on fracture	ORIF with cannulated screws	Decreased ROM
Radial head and neck fractures (<4 yr old) (see Fig. 11–65)		A—SH I or II physeal fracture B—SH IV fracture C—Transmetaphyseal fracture D and E—With elbow dislocation	Immobilize if <60 degrees in pronation/supination; ORIF if markedly displaced or >60 degrees primarily	Decreased ROM, radial head overgrowth, neck notching, AVN, synostosis, nonunion
Proximal olecranon physis fracture (rare)		I—Physeal-metaphyseal border (younger children) II—Physis with large metaphyseal fragment (older children)		
Olecranon metaphysis fracture		A—Flexion	If undisplaced (<3 mm), immobilize 3 wk; ORIF if defect	Rare: delay/nonunion
		B—Extension	Reduction in extension	
		C—Shear	Immobilize in hyperflexion	ORIF if periosteal tear
Elbow dislocation (11-20 yr old)		Based on direction of dislocation	Reduction and cast for <2 wk	Watch for associated fractures and nerve injuries (ulnar >median), HO, recurrent dislocation.
Radial head subluxation (15 mo-3 yr old)	Nursemaid's elbow	Stretching of annular ligaments	Reduce (supination/flexion)	

AIN, anterior interosseous nerve; AVN, avascular necrosis; CRPP, closed reduction/percutaneous pinning; HO, heterotopic ossification; LAC, long-arm cast; ORIF, open reduction with internal fixation; ROM, range of motion; SH, Salter-Harris.

TABLE 11-29 PEDIATRIC SHOULDER TRAUMA

Injury	Classification	Treatment	Complications
Humeral shaft fracture	Neonate	Small splint or splint to side	Compartment syndrome, radial nerve palsy, rotational palsy
	<3 yr old	Collar and cuff OK	
	3-12 yr old	Sarmiento brace	
	>12 yr old	Sarmiento brace	
Proximal humeral physis fracture	SH (I most common in <5 yr old)	Sling if minimally displaced, gentle manipulation for displaced fractures, CRPP vs. ORIF for <50% apposition, >45 degrees angulation	
Proximal humeral metaphysis fracture (common)	Based on location	Sling	
Midshaft clavicle fracture	≤2 yr old	Supportive sling if symptomatic	Rare: malunion or nonunion, neurovascular compromise
	>2 yr old	Figure 8 brace vs. sling	
Medial clavicle fracture	Usually SH I or II physeal separations	Sling for 1 wk	
Lateral clavicle fracture	I—Nondisplaced; intact AC and CC ligaments	Sling vs. figure 8 brace	
	IIA—Clavicle displaced superiorly; fracture medial to CC ligament	Type II may need ORIF	
	IIB—Clavicle displaced superiorly; conoid ligaments tear		
AC joint injury	Same as adult	Same as adult	Watch for coracoid fracture
SC joint injury	Anterior and posterior	Same as adult	
Clavicle dislocation (rare)	Anterior and posterior	ORIF with repair of periosteal tube	
Scapula fracture	Anterior and posterior	Same as adult	
Glenohumeral dislocation	Anterior and posterior	Initial immobilization followed by rehabilitation; reconstruction for recurrent instability	Recent research shows >60% chance of redislocation when patient is <21 yr old

AC, acromioclavicular; CC, coracoclavicular; ORIF, open reduction with internal fixation; CRPP, closed reduction with percutaneous pinning; SC, sternoclavicular; SH, Salter-Harris.

TABLE 11-30 PEDIATRIC SPINE TRAUMA

Injury	Eponym/ Other Name	Classification	Treatment	Complications
Occiput-C1 dissociations			Reduced with traction; craniovertebral fusion later	Often fatal
C1-C2 dissociations		Traumatic ligament disruption	Reduce in extension, immobilize with halo for 8-12 wk	Vertebral artery is at risk with surgery
	Grisel syndrome	Ligament laxity from local inflammation	Traction; immobilize for 6-8 wk	
	Rotatory subluxation	I—Without C1 shift II—<5 mm C1 anterior shift III—>5 mm C1 anterior shift IV—Posterior shift Odontoid physeal or os odontoideum	Traction; if no improvement, then open reduction and fusion	
C2-C3 dislocation		True vs. pseudo (more likely)		
Cervical facet dislocation			Same as in adults	
Thoracic and lumbar fractures		Same as in adults	Same as in adults	
Spondylosis		Stress fracture of pars (likely at L5-S1)	Acute: immobilize in brace; otherwise, surgical treatment; fusion for refractory cases	
Spinal cord injury without radiographic abnormality (SCIWORA)		Spinal cord injury without radiographic abnormality	Evaluation with magnetic resonance imaging and supportive treatment	Scoliosis (especially <8 yr old)

TABLE 11-31 PEDIATRIC PELVIC TRAUMA

Injury	Eponym	Classification (Key and Cornwell)	Treatment	Complications
Pelvic fracture				In general, less than adults because of remodeling
		I—Ring intact (see Figs. 11–67 and 11–68)		
		Avulsions (ASIS, AIIS, IT)	BR flexed hip for 2 wk; guarded WB for 4 wk	Loss of reduction, delayed union
		Pubis/ischium	BR 3-7 days; limited WB for 4 wk	DJD, malunion, organ injury
	Duverney	Iliac wing	BR with leg abducted; progress to full WB	Sacral nerve injury
		Sacrum/coccyx	BR 3-6 wk, if severe (sacral)	
		II—Single break in ring (see Fig. 11–69)		
		Ipsilateral rami	BR 2-4 wk; non-WB	
		Symphysis pubis	BR with sling or spica	
		SI joint (rare)	BR with progressive WB	
		III—Double break in ring (see Fig. 11–69)		
	Straddle	Bilateral pubic rami	BR with flexed hip 2-4 wk	Often unstable, with associated injuries
	Malgaigne	Anterior and posterior ring with migration	Skeletal traction; external fixator for 3-6 wk	
		IV—Acetabular fractures		
		Small fragment with dislocation	BR followed by progressive ambulation	
		Linear: Nondisplaced	Treat associated pelvic fracture	
		Linear: Hip unstable	Skeletal traction; ORIF if incongruous	
		Central	Lateral traction for reduction; ORIF if severe	HO, especially if severe

AIIS, anterior inferior iliac spine; ASIS, anterior superior iliac spine; BR, bed rest; DJD, degenerative joint disease; HO, heterotopic ossification; IT, ischial tuberosity; ORIF, open reduction with internal fixation; SI, sacroiliac; WB, weight bearing.

TABLE 11-32 PEDIATRIC HIP TRAUMA

Injury	Classification	Treatment	Complications
Hip fracture (see Fig. 11–70)	Delbet		
	IA—Transepiphyseal with dislocation	Closed reduction or ORIF with pin	AVN close to 100%
	IB—Transepiphyseal without dislocation	CRPP with spica	AVN in up to 60%
	II—Transcervical	CRPP with spica	Coxa vara (25%): treat with subtrochanteric valgus osteotomy
	IIIA—Cervical trochanteric (displaced)	CRPP with spica	Nonunion (6%)
	IIIB—Cervical trochanteric (nondisplaced)	Spica cast in abduction	Growth arrest
	IV—Intertrochanteric	Spica cast; ORIF if unstable	May cross physis if it creates greater fracture stability
Femoral neck stress fracture	Devas		
	Superior transverse	CRPP (otherwise is displaced)	Displacement causes more problems; varus deformities
	Inferior (compressive)	NWB	
Traumatic dislocation	Posterior or anterior	Closed reduction; open if joint incongruous	AVN (10%), recurrent dislocation, HO, DJD

AVN, avascular necrosis; CRPP, closed reduction/percutaneous pinning; DJD, degenerative joint disease; HO, heterotopic ossification; NWB, non–weight bearing; ORIF, open reduction with internal fixation.

TABLE 11-33 PEDIATRIC FEMORAL SHAFT TRAUMA

Injury	Classification	Treatment	Complications
Femur fracture (including subtrochanteric fractures)	≤6 yr old	Spica cast; may need short period of traction if shortened >2 cm and followed by spica casting	LLD: Angular deformity (avoid >10 degrees frontal and >10 degrees sagittal malalignment)
	6-13 yr old	Current trend to use flexible titanium nails, with possible additional immobilization, but may also use external fixation (higher refracture rate), plate (need to remove, causes large scar formation), or traction (rare)	Rotational deformity (>10 degrees); expect 0.9 cm overgrowth in <10 yr old
	≥14 yr old	IM nail (trochanteric entry)	AVN reported with IM nails in children with growth remaining

AVN, avascular necrosis; IM, intramedullary; LLD, leg length discrepancy.

TABLE 11-34 PEDIATRIC KNEE TRAUMA

Injury	Eponym/Other Name	Classification	Treatment	Complications
Distal femoral epiphysis fracture (see Figs. 11–71 to 11–73)	"Wagon wheel"	SH I-IV (II most common)	Closed reduction: LLC; CRPP in SH III or IV; open if soft tissue interposition or displaced III and IV	Popliteal artery or peroneal nerve injury, recurrent displacement; growth plate injuries because of undulating physis
Proximal tibial epiphysis fracture		SH I-IV (II most common)	Nondisplaced: LLC in 30° of flexion; displaced: CRPP	Popliteal artery injury, growth plate injury
Floating knee		Letts		Infection, nonunion, malunion, injuries
		A—Both fractures diaphyseal	ORIF in one, closed reduction in the other	
		B—One fracture diaphyseal and one metaphyseal	ORIF of diaphyseal and closed reduction of metaphyseal	
		C—One fracture diaphyseal and one epiphyseal	CRPP of epiphyseal and ORIF of diaphyseal	
		D—One fracture open and one closed	Débride/external fixation, open and closed reductions of closed fracture	
		E—Both fractures open	Débride/external fixation of both	
Tibial tubercle avulsion fracture (14-16 yr old in jumping sport) (see Fig. 11–75)		Odgen		
		1—Small distal piece fractured	If minimally displaced with extension, then cast; otherwise, ORIF	Genu recurvatum, decreased ROM, laxity
		2—Fracture at junction of primary and secondary ossification centers		
		3—Fracture through one epiphysis (SH III)		
Tibial spine fracture (most common hemarthrosis in preadolescent) (see Fig. 11–75)		Meyers and McKeever		
		I—Incomplete/ nondisplaced	Attempt closed reduction in extension for all; if it remains displaced, then may use arthroscope and ACL guide to fix with suture	Meniscal entrapment
		II—Hinged (posterior rim intact)		
		III—Completely displaced		
Patella fracture		Nondisplaced	Aspiration and cast vs. brace in 5 degrees of flexion	Patella alta, extensor lag, infection
		Displaced (>2 mm)	ORIF with tension band	
	Sleeve fracture (see Fig. 11–76)	Avulsion of the distal pole and articular cartilage	ORIF with tension band	
Femorotibial dislocation		Same as in adults	Same as in adults: Arteriogram	Popliteal artery injury
Patella dislocation		Same as in adults	Closed-reduction cast for 3 wk; consider fixing MPFL; open if fragment	Predisposition: Down syndrome, arthrogryposis

ACL, anterior cruciate ligament; CRPP, closed reduction/percutaneous pinning; LLC, long-leg cast; MPFL, medial patellofemoral ligament; ORIF, open reduction with internal fixation; ROM, range of motion; SH, Salter-Harris.

TABLE 11-35 PEDIATRIC TIBIAL SHAFT TRAUMA

Injury	Eponym/ Other Name	Classification	Treatment	Complications
Tibia-fibula fracture	Greenstick	Incomplete	LLC in slight flexion for 6-8 wk unless >10 degrees AP or >5 degrees varus/ valgus; then must do manipulation	Angular deformity (valgus)
		Complete	Closed reduction and cast	LLD (may see overgrowth with <10 yr old), malrotation, vascular injury
Tibial spiral fracture	Toddler	Spiral fracture in <6 yr old	LLC for 3-4 wk	
Bike spoke injury		Soft tissue disruption	Admit and observe	Compartment syndrome; need for soft tissue coverage
Proximal tibial metaphysis fracture (see Fig. 11–77)	Cozen	Greenstick in 3-6 yr old (complete in older children)	LLC in varus for 6 wk	Genu valgum, arterial injury, physeal injury

AP, anteroposterior; LLC, long-leg cast; LLD, leg length discrepancy.

TABLE 11-36 PEDIATRIC ANKLE AND FOOT TRAUMA

Injury	Eponym/Other Name	Classification	Treatment	Complications
Ankle fracture		SH and Dias-Tachdjian (see Fig. 11–78)	If SH I or II injury, treat with SLWC; if SH III or IV injury, treat with CRPP vs. ORIF	Angular deformity, bony bridge (poor prognosis with distal tibia), LLD, DJD, rotational deformity, AVN
	Juvenile Tillaux (see Fig. 11–79)	SH III of lateral tibial physis (because distal-medial tibial physis is closed in this age group)	May use LLC if <2 mm displacement; if greater, treat with ORIF and visualization of joint line	
	Wagstaff	SH III of distal fibular physis	Closed reduction and cast; ORIF if necessary	
	Triplane (see Fig. 11–80)	Complex SH IV, with components in all three planes	ORIF if >2 mm articular step-off (fixation achieved parallel to physis in metaphysis and epiphysis)	Must use CT to delineate fracture
Talus fracture		Same as in adults	Closed reduction and cast unless >5 mm or 5 degrees of displacement	AVN
Calcaneus fracture	Essex-Lopresti	Same as in adults	Same as in adults	
Tarsometatarsal fracture		Fracture of base of second metatarsal and cuboid fracture	Closed reduction vs. CRPP if unstable	
Base of the fifth metatarsal fracture	Jones/pseudo-Jones	Same as in adults	Same as in adults	Nonunion

AVN, avascular necrosis; CRPP, closed reduction/percutaneous pinning; CT, computed tomography; DJD, degenerative joint disease; LLC, long-leg cast; LLD, leg length discrepancy; ORIF, open reduction with internal fixation; SH, Salter-Harris; SLWC, short-leg walking cast.

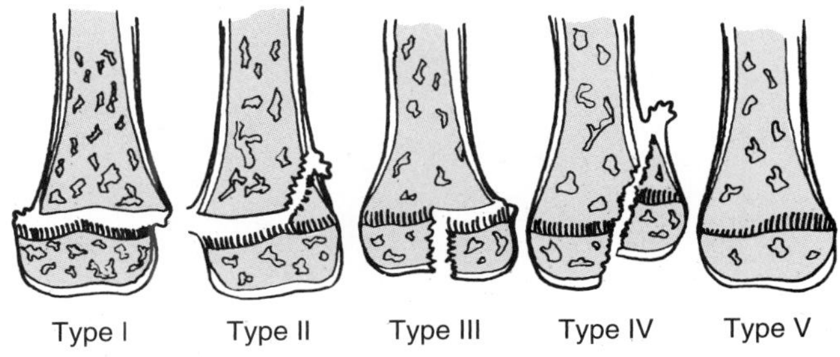

FIGURE 11–55 The Salter-Harris classification of injuries to the physis. (From Bora FW: The Pediatric Upper Extremity, p 154. Philadelphia, WB Saunders, 1986.)

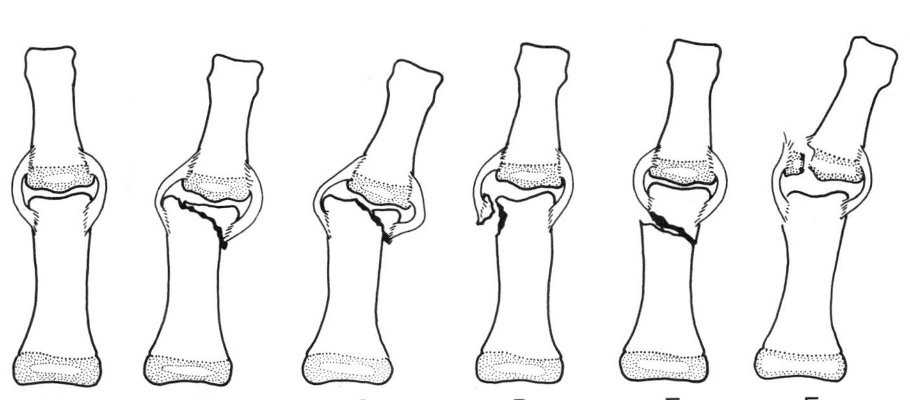

FIGURE 11–56 Pediatric interphalangeal finger fractures. **A**, Normal. **B**, Unicondylar. **C**, Partially condylar. **D**, Lateral avulsion. **E**, Bicondylar. **F**, Salter-Harris III. (From Ogden JA: Skeletal Injury in the Child, 2nd ed, p 530. Philadelphia, WB Saunders, 1990.)

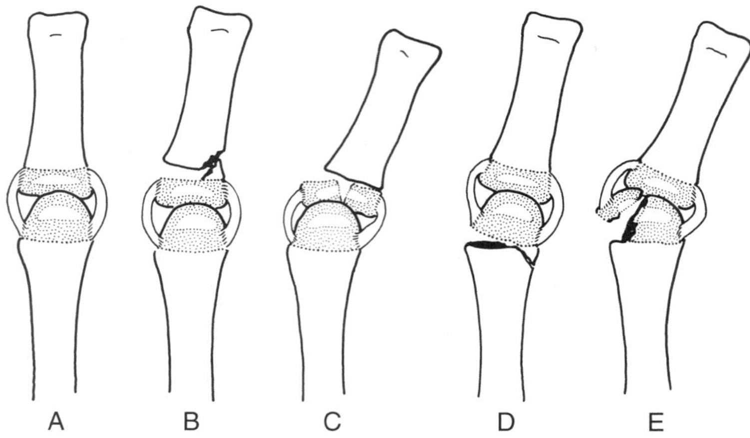

FIGURE 11–57 Pediatric metacarpophalangeal (MCP) fractures. **A**, Normal. **B**, Salter-Harris (SH) II proximal phalanx. **C**, SH III proximal phalanx. **D**, SH II metacarpal. **E**, SH III metacarpal. (From Ogden JA: Skeletal Injury in the Child, 2nd ed, p 530. Philadelphia, WB Saunders, 1990.)

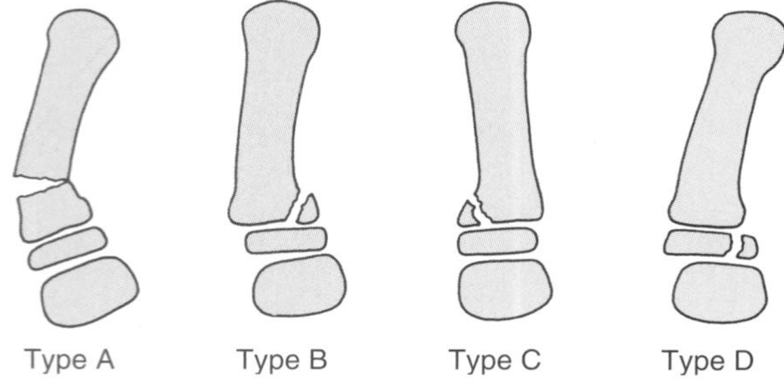

FIGURE 11–58 Classification of pediatric thumb metacarpal fractures. Type A, metaphyseal. Type B, Salter-Harris (SH) II medial. Type C, SH II lateral. Type D, SH III. (From O'Brien ET: Fractures of the hand and wrist region. In Rockwood CA Jr, Wilkins KE, King RE, eds: Fractures in Children, 2nd ed, p 257. Philadelphia, JB Lippincott, 1984.)

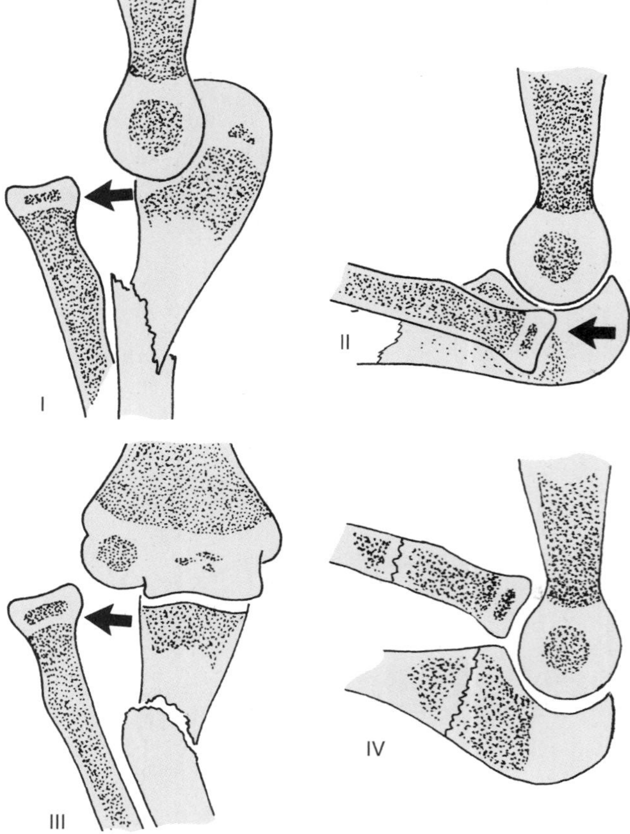

FIGURE 11–59 The pediatric Monteggia fractures. Type I, Anterior. Type II, Posterior. Type III, Lateral. Type IV, BB fracture. (I-III from Ogden JA: Skeletal Injury in the Child, 2nd ed, pp 480-481. Philadelphia, WB Saunders, 1990.)

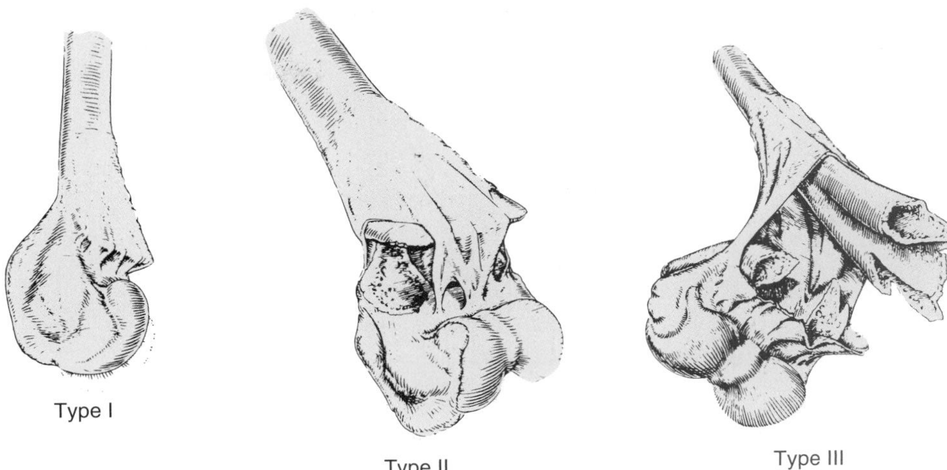

FIGURE 11–60 Supracondylar fractures. (From Abraham E, et al: Experimental hyperextension supracondylar fractures in monkeys. Clin Orthop 171:313-314, 1982.)

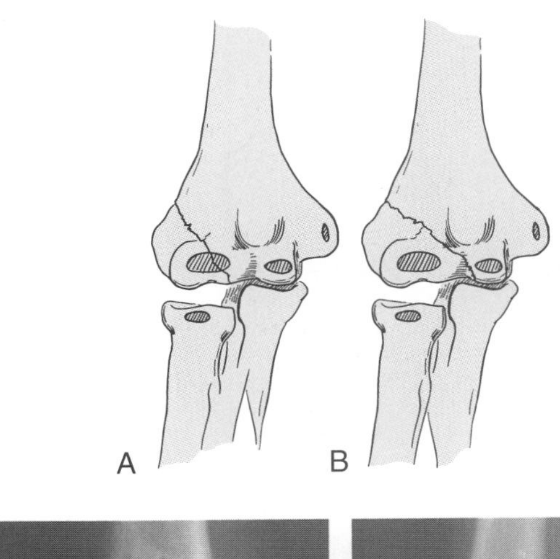

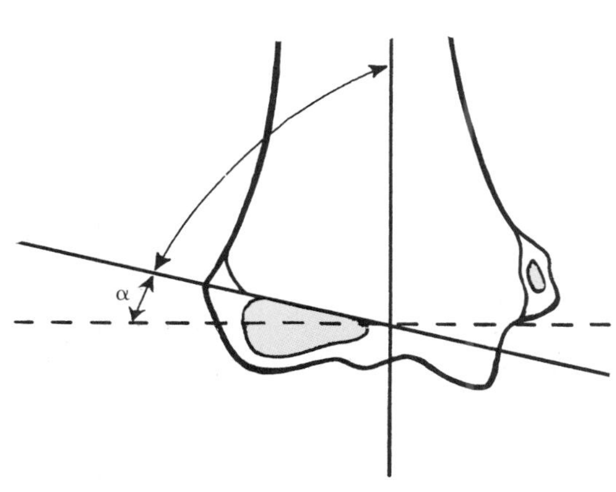

FIGURE 11–61 The Baumann angle is created by the intersection of a line drawn down the proximal margin of the capitellar ossification center and a line drawn perpendicular to the long axis of the humeral shaft. (From Herring JA: Tachdjian's Pediatric Orthopaedics, 4th ed, p 2459. Philadelphia, WB Saunders, 2008.)

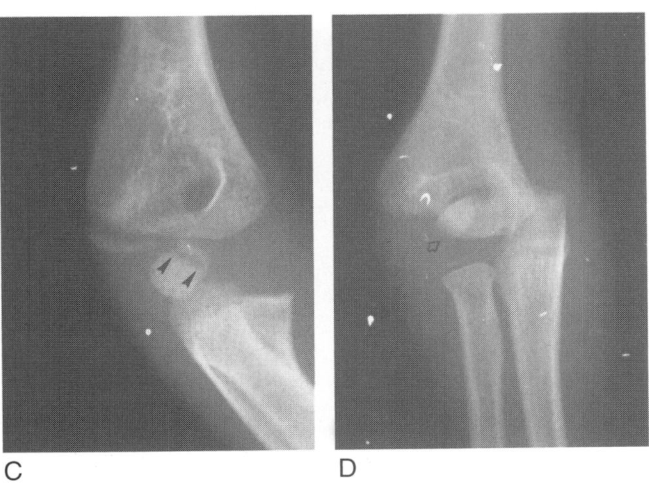

FIGURE 11–62 The Milch classification of lateral condyle fractures. **A** and **C**, Type I—The fracture extends through the secondary ossification center of the capitellum *(arrowheads)*. **B** and **D**, Type II—The fracture crosses the epiphysis and enters the joint medial to the trochlear groove. The capitellar articular surface is subtly rotated *(arrowhead)*. (From Herring JA: Tachdjian's Pediatric Orthopaedics, 4th ed, p 2489. Philadelphia, WB Saunders, 2008.)

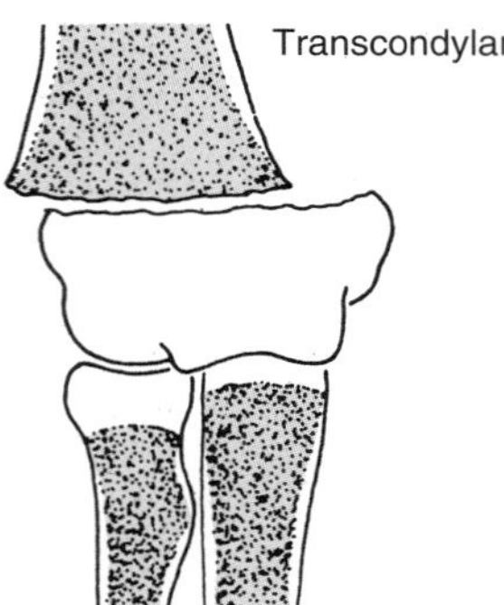

FIGURE 11–63 Transcondylar fracture. (From Ogden JA: Skeletal Injury in the Child, 2nd ed, p 388. Philadelphia, WB Saunders, 1990.)

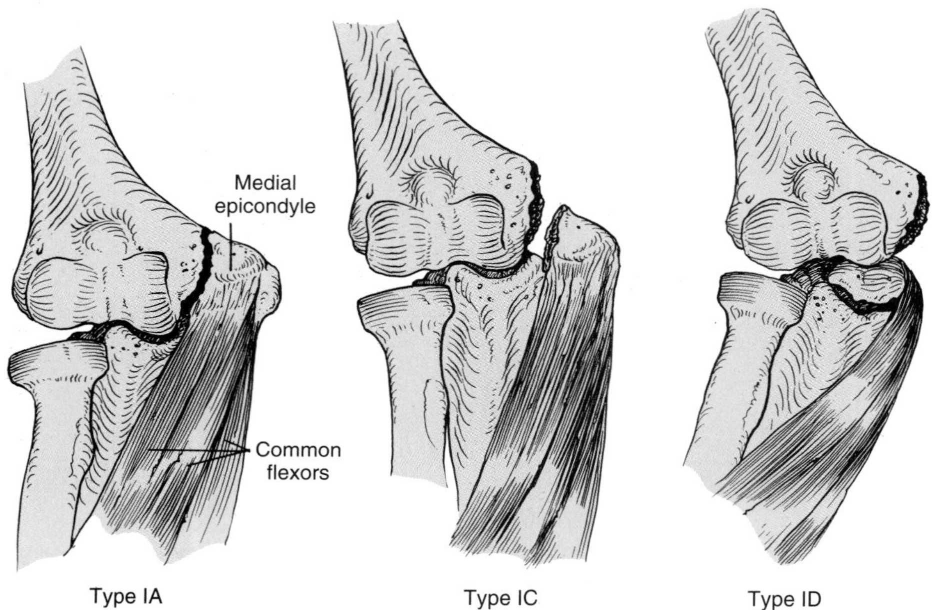

FIGURE 11–64 Medial epicondyle fractures. Type IA, Undisplaced. Type IC, Displaced. Type ID, Entrapped. (From Tachdjian MO: Pediatric Orthopaedics, 2nd ed, p 3122. Philadelphia, WB Saunders, 1990.)

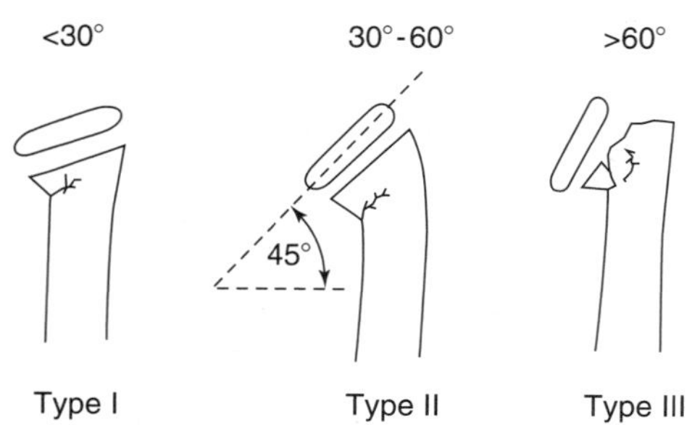

FIGURE 11–65 Radial head fractures. (From Tachdjian MO: Pediatric Orthopaedics, 2nd ed, p 3140. Philadelphia, WB Saunders, 1990.)

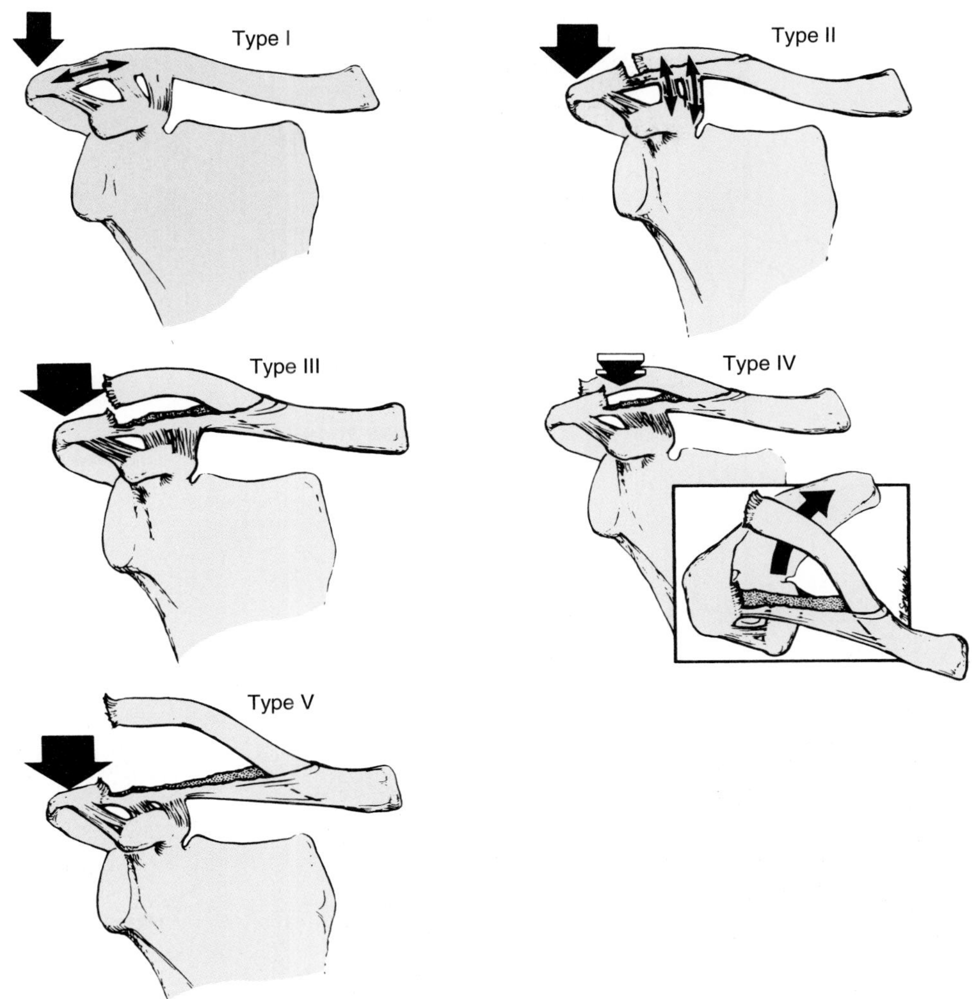

FIGURE 11–66 Classification of pediatric acromioclavicular injuries. (From Rockwood CA Jr, Wilkins KE, King RE, eds: Fractures in Children, 2nd ed, p 636. Philadelphia, JB Lippincott, 1984.)

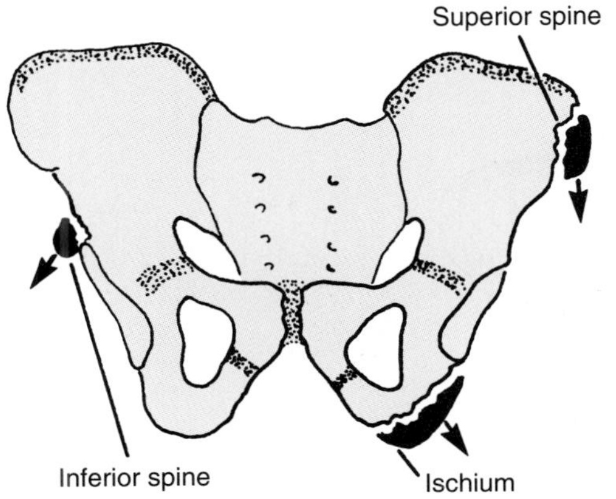

FIGURE 11–67 Avulsion fractures of the pelvis. Superior spine, sartorius avulsion; inferior spine, rectus avulsion; ischium, hamstring avulsion. (From Ogden JA: Skeletal Injury in the Child, 2nd ed, p 635. Philadelphia, WB Saunders, 1990.)

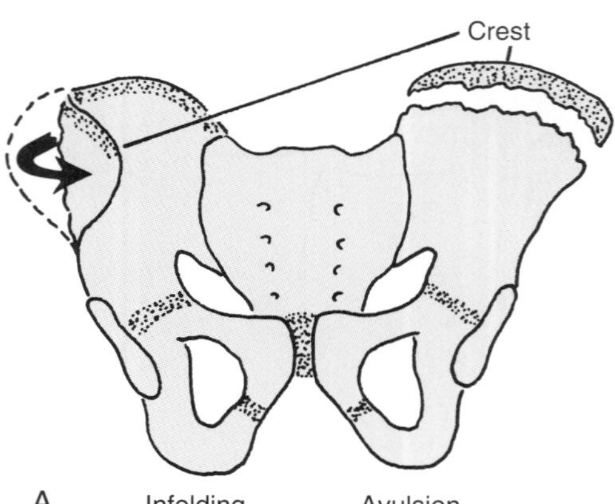

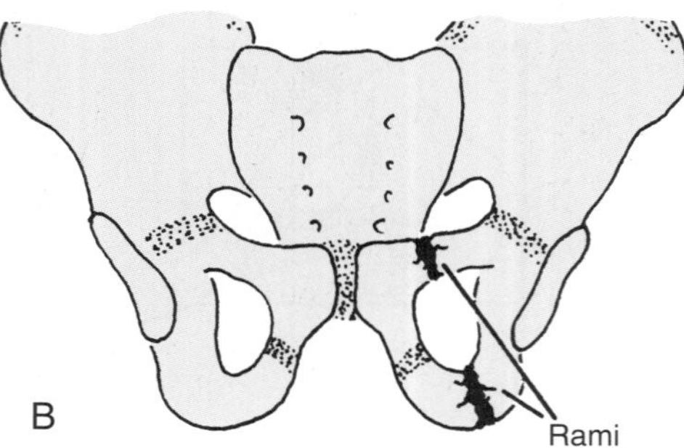

FIGURE 11–68 Stable pelvic fractures. **A,** Examples of infolding and crest avulsion. **B,** Unilateral nondisplaced superior/inferior public rami fractures. (From Ogden JA: Skeletal Injury in the Child, 2nd ed, p 634. Philadelphia, WB Saunders, 1990.)

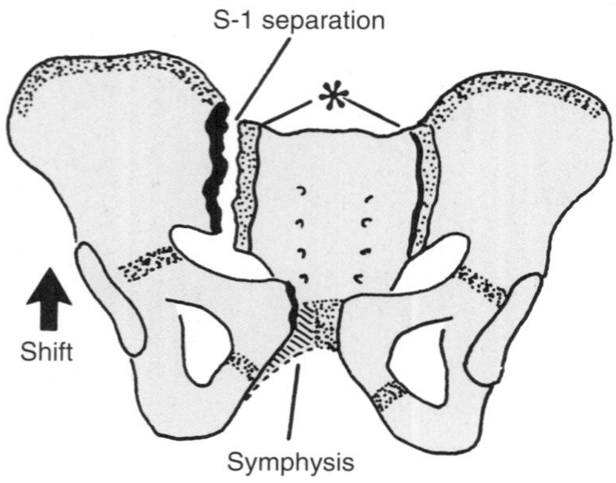

FIGURE 11–69 Unstable pelvic fractures. (From Ogden JA: Skeletal Injury in the Child, 2nd ed, p 388. Philadelphia, WB Saunders, 1990.)

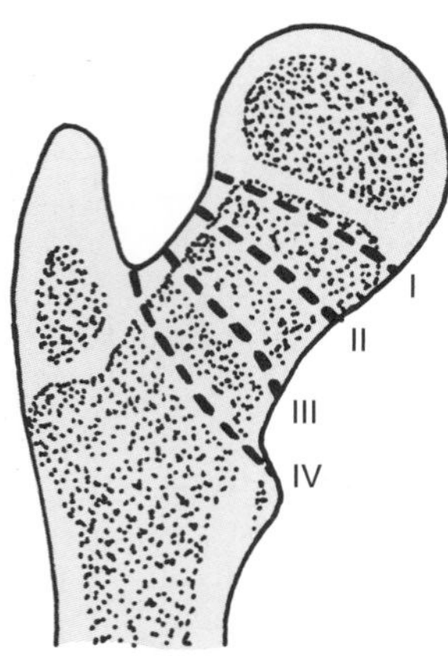

FIGURE 11–70 Femoral neck fractures in children. I, Transepiphyseal. II, Transcervical. III, Cervical-trochanteric. IV, Intertrochanteric. (From Ogden JA: Skeletal Injury in the Child, 2nd ed, p 689. Philadelphia, WB Saunders, 1990.)

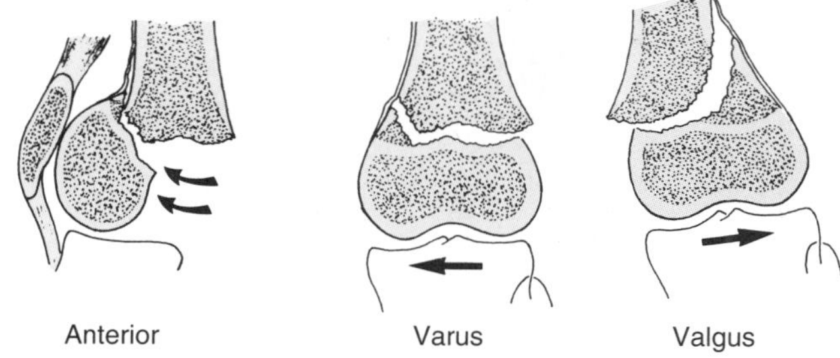

FIGURE 11–71 Distal femoral physeal fractures. (From Ogden JA: Skeletal Injury in the Child, 2nd ed, p 725. Philadelphia, WB Saunders, 1990.)

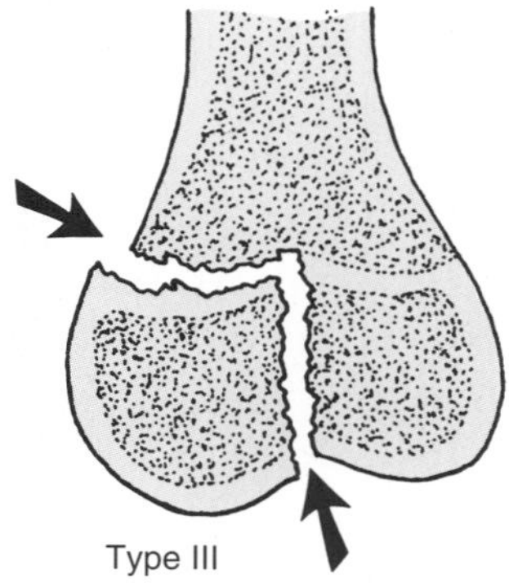

FIGURE 11–72 Distal femoral Salter-Harris type III fracture. (From Ogden JA: Skeletal Injury in the Child, 2nd ed, p 727. Philadelphia, WB Saunders, 1990.)

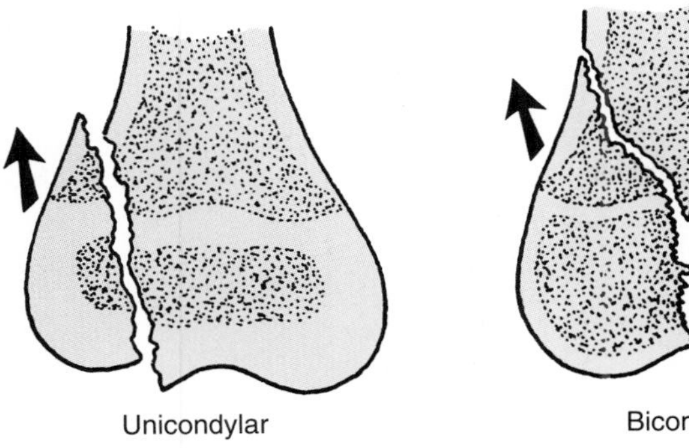

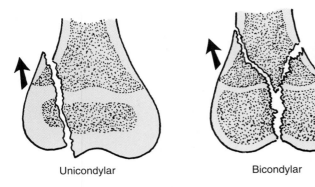

FIGURE 11–73 Salter-Harris types III and IV fractures of the distal femur. (From Ogden JA: Skeletal Injury in the Child, 2nd ed, p 689. Philadelphia, WB Saunders, 1990.)

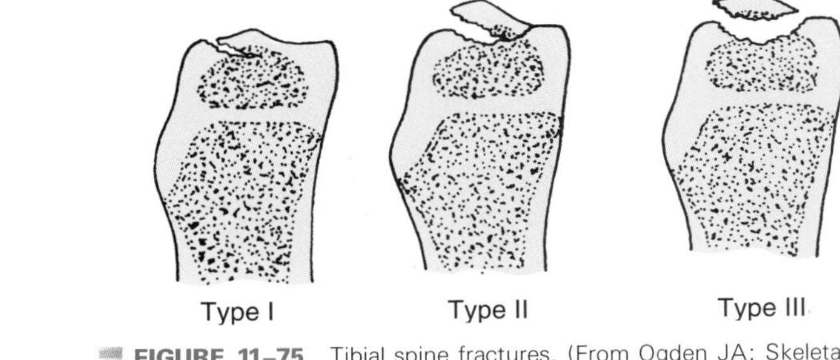

FIGURE 11–75 Tibial spine fractures. (From Ogden JA: Skeletal Injury in the Child, 2nd ed, p 689. Philadelphia, WB Saunders, 1990.)

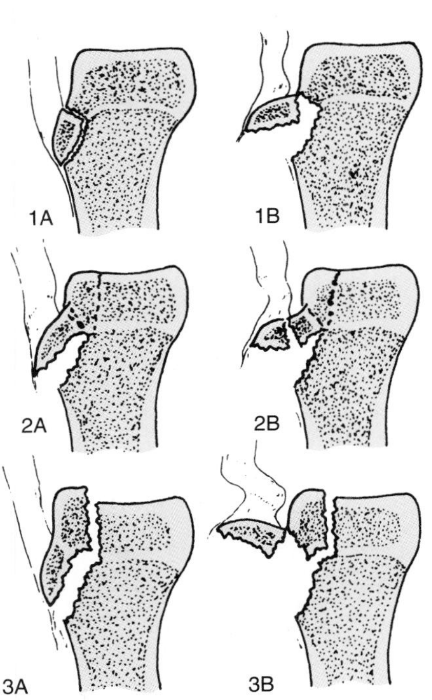

FIGURE 11–74 Fractures of the tibial tubercle. (From Ogden JA: Skeletal Injury in the Child, 2nd ed, p 808. Philadelphia, WB Saunders, 1990.)

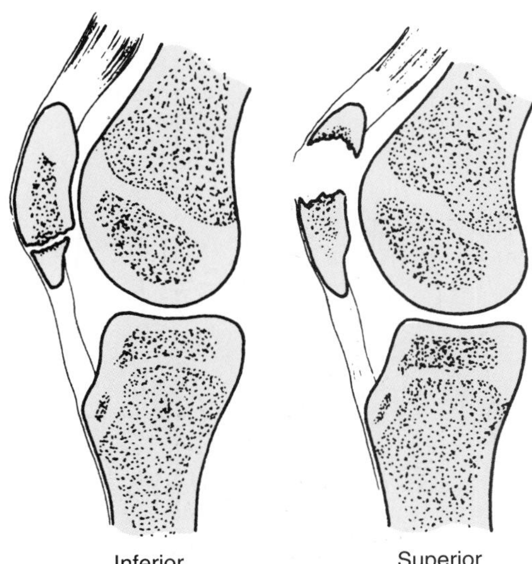

FIGURE 11–76 Patellar sleeve fractures. (From Ogden JA: Skeletal Injury in the Child, 2nd ed, p 762. Philadelphia, WB Saunders, 1990.)

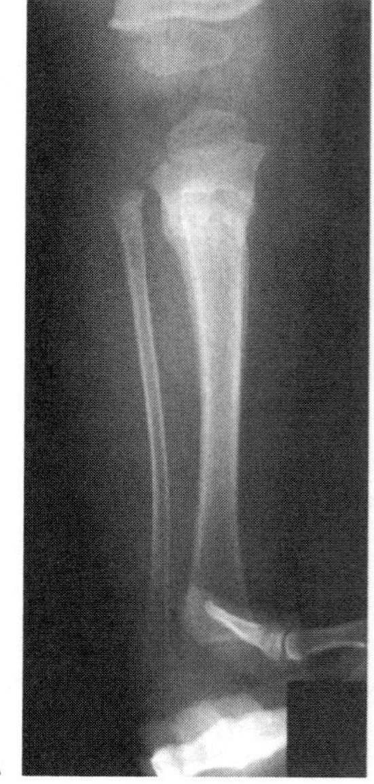

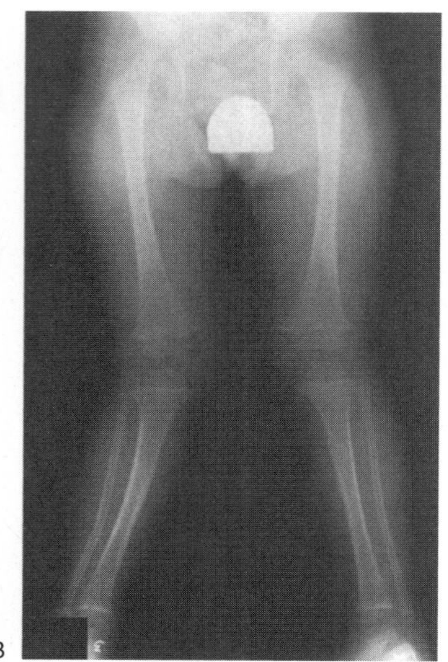

FIGURE 11–77 Valgus deformity after a proximal metaphyseal tibial fracture in a 3-year-old boy. **A**, Radiograph showing healing at 4 weeks. **B**, There was obvious valgus deformity of the injured leg 1 year later. (From Herring JA: Tachdjian's Pediatric Orthopaedics, 4th ed, p 2713. Philadelphia, WB Saunders, 2008.)

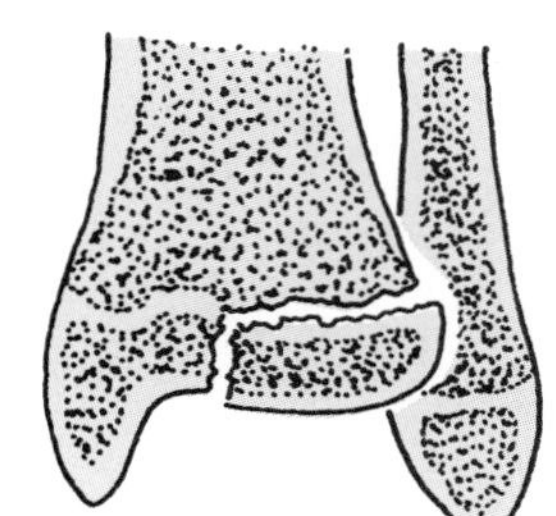
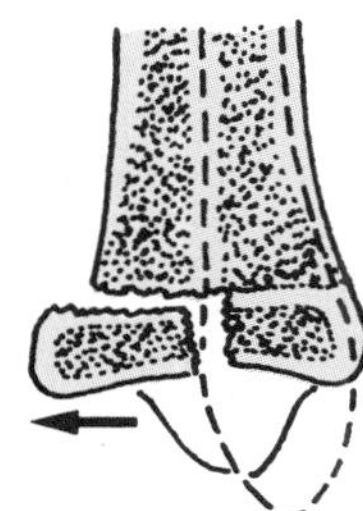
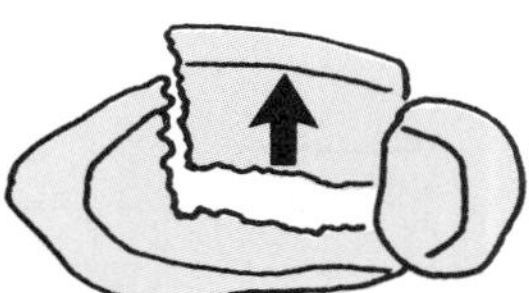

FIGURE 11–79 Juvenile Tillaux fracture. (From Ogden JA: Skeletal Injury in the Child, 2nd ed, p 838. Philadelphia, WB Saunders, 1990.)

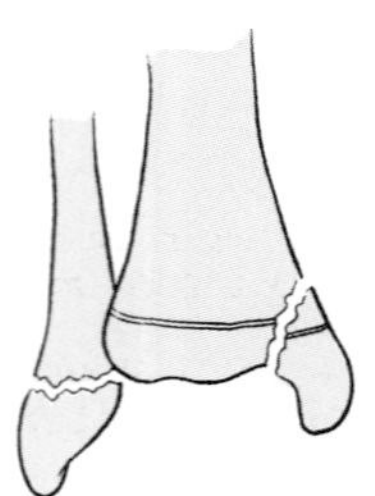

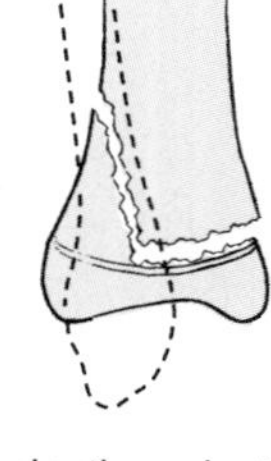

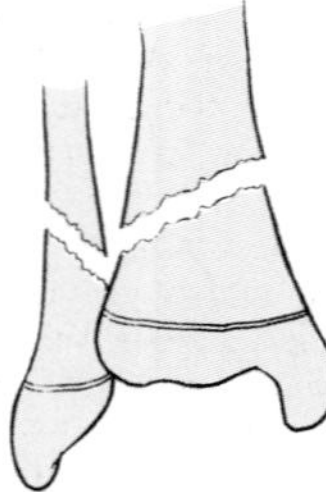

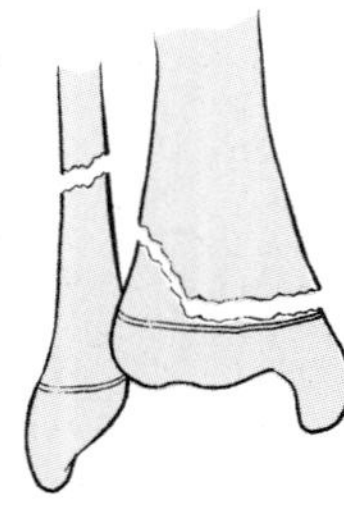

FIGURE 11–78 The Dias-Tachdjian modification of the Lauge-Hansen classification of ankle fractures in children. (From Herring JA: Tachdjian's Pediatric Orthopaedics, 3rd ed, p 2393. Philadelphia, WB Saunders, 2002.)

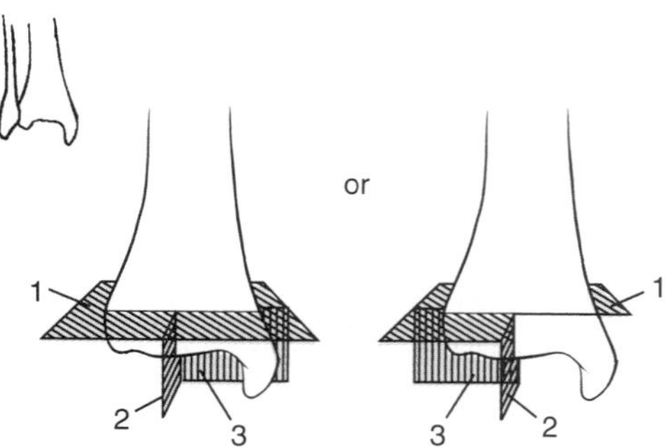

FIGURE 11–80 The triplane fracture pattern. Note the fracture pattern in three planes: axial (1), sagittal (2), and frontal (3). (From Herring JA: Tachdjian's Pediatric Orthopaedics, 4th ed, p 2751. Philadelphia, WB Saunders, 2008.)

Selected Bibliography

MULTIPLY INJURED PATIENTS

Keel M, Trentz O: Pathophysiology of polytrauma. Injury 36:691–709, 2005.

Nowotarski PJ, Turen CH, Brumback RJ, Scarboro JM: Conversion of external fixation to intramedullary nailing for fractures of the shaft of the femur in multiply injured patients. J Bone Joint Surg [Am] 82:781–788, 2000.

Pape HC, Grimme K, Van Griensven M, et al: Impact of intramedullary instrumentation versus damage control for femoral fractures on immunoinflammatory parameters: Prospective randomized analysis by the EPOFF Study Group. J Trauma 55:7–13, 2003.

Pape HC, Hildebrand F, Pertschy S, et al: Changes in the management of femoral shaft fractures in polytrauma patients: From early total care to damage control orthopedic surgery. J Trauma 53:452–461, discussion 461–462, 2002.

Roberts CS, Pape HC, Jones AL, et al: Damage control orthopaedics: Evolving concepts in the treatment of patients who have sustained orthopaedic trauma. Instr Course Lect 54:447–462, 2005.

Strecker W, Gebhard F, Rager J, et al: Early biochemical characterization of soft-tissue trauma and fracture trauma. J Trauma 47:358–364, 1999.

SOFT TISSUE INJURY

Harris IA, Kadir A, Donald G: Continuous compartment pressure monitoring for tibia fractures: Does it influence outcome? J Trauma 60:1330–1335, discussion 1335, 2006.

Hogan CJ, Ruland RT: High-pressure injection injuries to the upper extremity: A review of the literature. J Orthop Trauma 20:503–511, 2006.

Marko P, Layon AJ, Caruso L, et al: Burn injuries. Curr Opin Anaesthesiol 16:183–191, 2003.

Spies C, Trohman RG: Narrative review: Electrocution and life-threatening electrical injuries. Ann Intern Med 145:531–537, 2006.

Spiller HA, Bosse GM: Prospective study of morbidity associated with snakebite envenomation. J Toxicol Clin Toxicol 41:125–130, 2003.

Weisz RD, Egol KA, Koval KJ: Soft-tissue principles for orthopaedic surgeons. Bull Hosp Joint Dis 60:150–154, 2001.

White J: Snake venoms and coagulopathy. Toxicon 45:951–967, 2005.

FRACTURE MANAGEMENT

Calhoun JH, Manring MM: Adult osteomyelitis. Infect Dis Clin North Am 19:765–786, 2005.

Giannoudis PV, Tzioupis C, Pape HC: Fat embolism: The reaming controversy. Injury 37(Suppl. 4):S50–S58, 2006.

Habashi NM, Andrews PL, Scalea TM: Therapeutic aspects of fat embolism syndrome. Injury 37(Suppl. 4):S68–S73, 2006.

Hildebrand F, Giannoudis P, van Griensven M, et al: Secondary effects of femoral instrumentation on pulmonary physiology in a standardised sheep model: What is the effect of lung contusion and reaming? Injury 36:544–555, 2005.

Hoff WS, Hoey BA, Wainwright GA, et al: Early experience with retrievable inferior vena cava filters in high-risk trauma patients. J Am Coll Surg 199:869–874, 2004.

Kelsey LJ, Fry DM, VanderKolk WE: Thrombosis risk in the trauma patient: Prevention and treatment. Hematol Oncol Clin North Am 14:417–430, 2000.

Morgan SJ, Jeray KJ, Phieffer LS, et al: Attitudes of orthopaedic trauma surgeons regarding current controversies in the management of pelvic and acetabular fractures. J Orthop Trauma 15:526–532, 2001.

Ochsner PE, Hailemariam S: Histology of osteosynthesis associated bone infection. Injury 37(Suppl. 2):S49–S58, 2006.

Pape HC, Hildebrand F, Pertschy S, et al: Changes in the management of femoral shaft fractures in polytrauma patients: From early total care to damage control orthopedic surgery. J Trauma 53:452–461, discussion 461–462, 2002.

Volgas DA, Stannard JP, Alonso JE: Current orthopaedic treatment of ballistic injuries. Injury 36:380–386, 2005.

Wang J, Li F, Calhoun JH, Mader JT: The role and effectiveness of adjunctive hyperbaric oxygen therapy in the management of musculoskeletal disorders. J Postgrad Med 48:226–231, 2002.

Wolf JM, DiGiovanni CW: A survey of orthopedic surgeons regarding DVT prophylaxis in foot and ankle trauma surgery. Orthopedics 27:504–508, 2004.

SHOULDER

Collinge C, Devinney S, Herscovici D, et al: Anterior-inferior plate fixation of middle-third fractures and nonunions of the clavicle. J Orthop Trauma 20:680–686, 2006.

Court-Brown CM, Caesar B: Epidemiology of adult fractures: A review. Injury 37:691–697, 2006.

Edwards SG, Whittle AP, Wood GW II: Nonoperative treatment of ipsilateral fractures of the scapula and clavicle. J Bone Joint Surg [Am] 82:774–780, 2000.

Estrada LS, Alonso J, Rue LW III: A continuum between scapulothoracic dissociation and traumatic forequarter amputation: A review of the literature. Am Surg 67:868–872, 2001.

Gove N, Ebraheim NA, Glass E: Posterior sternoclavicular dislocations: A review of management and complications. Am J Orthop 35:132–136, 2006.

Jadobsen BW, Johannsen HV, Suder P, Sojbjerg JO: Primary repair versus conservative treatment of first-time traumatic anterior dislocation of the shoulder: A randomized study with 10-year follow-up. Arthroscopy 23:118–123, 2007.

Lenters TR, Wolf FM, Leopold SS, et al: Arthroscopic compared with open repairs for recurrent anterior shoulder instability: A systematic review and meta-analysis of the literature. J Bone Joint Surg [Am] 89:244–254, 2007.

Schandelmaier P, Blauth M, Schneider C, Krettek C: Fractures of the glenoid treated by operation: A 5- to 23-year follow-up of 22 cases. J Bone Joint Surg [Br] 84:173–177, 2002.

Zelle BA, Pape HC, Gerich TG, et al: Functional outcome following scapulothoracic dissociation. J Bone Joint Surg [Am] 86:2–8, 2004.

Zlowodzki M, Bhandari M, Zelle BA, et al: Treatment of scapula fractures: Systematic review of 520 fractures in 22 case series. J Orthop Trauma 20:230–233, 2006.

PROXIMAL HUMERUS FRACTURE

Nho SJ, Brophy RH, Barker JU, et al: Innovations in the management of displaced proximal humerus fractures. J Am Acta Orthop Surg 15: 12–26, 2007.

Robinson CM, Page RS, Hill RM, et al: Primary hemiarthroplasty for treatment of proximal humeral fractures. J Bone Joint Surg [Am] 85:1215–1223, 2003.

HUMERUS

Chapman JR, Henley MB, Agel J, Benca PJ: Randomized prospective study of humeral shaft fracture fixation: Intramedullary nails versus plates. J Orthop Trauma 14:162–166, 2000.

Lin J: Treatment of humeral shaft fractures with humeral locked nail and comparison with plate fixation. J Trauma 44:859–864, 1998.

McCormack RG, Brien D, Buckley RE, et al: Fixation of fractures of the shaft of the humerus by dynamic compression plate or intramedullary nail. J Bone Joint Surg [Br] 82:336–339, 2000.

McKee MD, Wilson TL, Winston L, et al: Functional outcome following surgical treatment of intra-articular distal humeral fractures through a posterior approach. J Bone Joint Surg [Am] 82:1701–1707, 2000.

McKee MD, Kim J, Kebaish K, et al: Functional outcome after open supracondylar fractures of the humerus. J Bone Joint Surg [Br] 82:646–651, 2000.

Ring D, Jupiter JB, Gulotta L: Articular fractures of the distal part of the humerus. J Bone Joint Surg [Am] 85:232–238, 2003.

ELBOW

Harrell RM, Tong J, Weinhold PS, Dahners LE: Comparison of the mechanical properties of different tension band materials and suture techniques. J Orthop Trauma 17:119–122, 2003.

Josefsson PO, Johnell O, Gentz CF: Long-term sequelae of simple dislocation of the elbow. J Bone Joint Surg [Am] 66:927–930, 1984.

Khalfayan EE, Culp RW, Alexander AH: Mason type II radial head fractures: Operative versus nonoperative treatment. J Orthop Trauma 6:283–289, 1992.

King GJ, Zarzour ZD, Rath DA, et al: Metallic radial head arthroplasty improves valgus stability of the elbow. Clin Orthop 368:114–125, 1999.

Moro JK, Werier J, MacDermid JC, et al: Arthroplasty with a metal radial head for unreconstructible fractures of the radial head. J Bone Joint Surg [Am] 83:1201–1211, 2001.

Mullett JH, Shannon F, Noel J, et al: K-wire position in tension band wiring of the olecranon: A comparison of two techniques. Injury 31:427–431, 2000.

Ring D, Quintero J, Jupiter JB: Open reduction and internal fixation of fractures of the radial head. J Bone Joint Surg [Am] 84:1811–1815, 2002.

Romero JM, Miran A, Jensen CH: Complications and reoperation rate after tension-band wiring of olecranon fractures. J Orthop Sci 5:318–320, 2000.

Smith GR, Hotchkiss RN: Radial head and neck fractures: Anatomic guidelines for proper placement of internal fixation. J Shoulder Elbow Surg 5:113–117, 1996.

FOREARM

Fester EW, Murray PM, Sanders TG, et al: The efficacy of magnetic resonance imaging and ultrasound in detecting disruptions of the forearm interosseous membrane: A cadaver study. J Hand Surg [Am] 27:418–424, 2002.

Rettig ME, Raskin KB: Galeazzi fracture-dislocation: A new treatment-oriented classification. J Hand Surg [Am] 26:228–235, 2001.

Ring D, Jupiter JB, Simpson NS: Monteggia fractures in adults. J Bone Joint Surg [Am] 80:1733–1744, 1998.

Smith AM, Urbanosky LR, Castle JA, et al: Radius pull test: Predictor of longitudinal forearm instability. J Bone Joint Surg [Am] 84:1970–1976, 2002.

HAND AND WRIST

Amadio PC, Beckenbaugh RD, Bishop AT, et al: Fractures of the hand and wrist. In Jupiter JB, ed: Flynn's Hand Surgery, pp 122–185. Baltimore, Williams & Wilkins, 1991.

Dorsay TA, Major NM, Helms CA: Cost effectiveness of immediate MR imaging versus traditional follow-up for revealing radiographically occult scaphoid fractures. AJR Am J Roentgenol 177:1257–1263, 2001.

Fernandez DL, Palmer AK: Fractures of the distal radius. In Green DP, Hotchkiss RN, Pederson WC, eds: Green's Operative Hand Surgery, 4th ed, p 940. New York, Churchill Livingstone, 1999.

Galanakis I, Aligizakis A, Katonis P, et al: Treatment of closed unstable metacarpal fractures using percutaneous transverse fixation with Kirschner wires. J Trauma 55:509–513, 2003.

Gellman H, Caputo RJ, Carter V, et al: Comparison of short and long thumb spica casts for non-displaced fractures of the carpal scaphoid. J Bone Joint Surg [Am] 71:354–357, 1989.

Hambidge JE, Desai VV, Schranz PJ, et al: Acute fractures of the scaphoid: Treatment by cast immobilization with the wrist in flexion or extension?. J Bone Joint Surg [Br] 81:91–92, 1999.

Herzberg G, Comtet JJ, Linscheid RL, et al: Perilunate dislocations and fracture-dislocations: A multicenter study. J Hand Surg [Am] 18:768–779, 1993.

Hornbach EE, Cohen MS: Closed reduction and percutaneous pinning of fractures of the proximal phalanx. J Hand Surg [Br] 26:45–49, 2001.

Horton TC, Hatton M, Davis TR: A prospective randomized controlled study of fixation of long oblique and spiral shaft fractures of the proximal phalanx: Closed reduction and percutaneous Kirschner wiring versus open reduction and lag screw fixation. J Hand Surg [Br] 28:5–9, 2003.

King HJ, Shin SJ, Kang ES: Complications of operative treatment for mallet fractures of the distal phalanx. J Hand Surg [Br] 26:28–31, 2001.

Leddy JP, Packer JW: Avulsion of the profundus tendon insertion in athletes. J Hand Surg [Am] 2:66–69, 1977.

Papaloizos MY, Le Moine P, Prues-Latour V, et al: Proximal fractures of the fifth metacarpal: A retrospective analysis of 25 operated cases. J Hand Surg [Br] 25:253–257, 2000.

Pegoli L, Toh S, Arai K, et al: The Ishiguro extension block technique for the treatment of mallet finger fracture: Indications and clinical results. J Hand Surg [Br] 28:15–17, 2003.

Saxena P, McDonald R, Gull S, Hyder N: Diagnostic scanning for suspected scaphoid fractures: An economic evaluation based on cost-minimisation models. Injury 34:503–511, 2003.

Simic PM, Weiland AJ: Fractures of the distal aspect of the radius: Changes in treatment over the past two decades. Instr Course Lect 52:185–195, 2003.

Slade JF III, Gutow AP, Geissler WB: Percutaneous internal fixation of scaphoid fractures via an arthroscopically assisted dorsal approach. J Bone Joint Surg [Am] 84(Suppl. 2):21–36, 2002.

Slade JF III, Geissler WB, Gutow AP, Merrell GA: Percutaneous internal fixation of selected scaphoid nonunions with an arthroscopically assisted dorsal approach. J Bone Joint Surg [Am] 85(Suppl. 4):20–32, 2003.

Tetik C, Gudemez E: Modification of the extension block Kirschner wire technique for mallet fractures. Clin Orthop 404:284–290, 2002.

Trumble TE, Schmitt SR, Vedder NB: Factors affecting functional outcome of displaced intra-articular distal radius fractures. J Hand Surg [Am] 19:325–340, 1994.

CARPAL

Adolfsson L, Lindau T, Arner M: Acutrak screw fixation versus cast immobilization for undisplaced scaphoid waist fractures. J Hand Surg [Br] 26:192–195, 2001.

Bone CD, Shin AY, McBride MT, Dao KD: Percutaneous screw fixation or cast immobilization for nondisplaced scaphoid fractures. J Bone Joint Surg [Am] 83:483–488, 2001.

Brydie A, Raby N: Early MRI in the management of clinical scaphoid fracture. Br J Radiol 76:296–300, 2003.

Dorsay TA, Major NM, Helms CA: Cost-effectiveness of immediate MR imaging versus traditional follow-up for revealing radiographically occult scaphoid fractures. AJR Am J Roentgenol 177:1257–1263, 2001.

Herzberg G, Comtet JJ, Linscheid RL, et al: Perilunate dislocations and fracture-dislocations: A multicenter study. J Hand Surg [Am] 18:768–779, 1993.

Herzberg G, Forissier D: Acute dorsal trans-scaphoid perilunate fracture-dislocations: Medium-term results. J Hand Surg [Br] 27:498–502, 2002.

Hildebrand KA, Ross DC, Patterson SD, et al: Dorsal perilunate dislocations and fracture-dislocations: Questionnaire, clinical, and radiographic evaluation. J Hand Surg [Am] 25:1069–1079, 2000.

McAdams TR, Spisak S, Beaulieu CF, Ladd AL: The effect of pronation and supination on the minimally displaced scaphoid fracture. Clin Orthop 411:255–259, 2003.

Melone CP Jr, Murphy MS, Raskin KB: Perilunate injuries: Repair by dual dorsal and volar approaches. Hand Clin 16:439–448, 2000.

Parvizi J, Wayman J, Kelly P, Moran CG: Combining the clinical signs improves diagnosis of scaphoid fractures: A prospective study with follow-up. J Hand Surg [Br] 23:324–327, 1998.

Rettig ME, Kozin SH, Cooney WP: Open reduction and internal fixation of acute displaced scaphoid waist fractures. J Hand Surg [Am] 26:271–276, 2001.

Saeden B, Tornkvist H, Ponzer S, Hoglund M: Fracture of the carpal scaphoid: A prospective, randomized 12-year follow-up comparing operative and conservative treatment. J Bone Joint Surg [Br] 83:230–234, 2001.

Slade JF III, Gutow AP, Geissler WB: Percutaneous internal fixation of scaphoid fractures via an arthroscopically assisted dorsal approach. J Bone Joint Surg [Am] 84(Suppl. 2):21–36, 2002.

Slade JF III, Geissler WB, Gutow AP, Merrell GA: Percutaneous internal fixation of selected scaphoid nonunions with an arthroscopically assisted dorsal approach. J Bone Joint Surg [Am] 85(Suppl. 4):20–32, 2003.

Soejima O, Iida H, Naito M: Transscaphoid-transtriquetral perilunate fracture dislocation: Report of a case and review of the literature. Arch Orthop Trauma Surg 123:305–307, 2003.

Trumble TE: Management of scaphoid nonunions. J Am Acad Orthop Surg 11:380–391, 2003.

PELVIS/SACRUM

Barei DP, Bellabarba C, Mills WJ, Routt ML Jr: Percutaneous management of unstable pelvic ring disruptions. Injury 32(Suppl. 1):SA33–SA44, 2001.

Bellabarba C, Ricci WM, Bolhofner BR: Distraction external fixation in lateral compression pelvic fractures. J Orthop Trauma 14:475–482, 2000.

Blackmore CC, Jurkovich GJ, Linnau KF, et al: Assessment of volume of hemorrhage and outcome from pelvic fracture. Arch Surg 138: 504–508, 2003.

Bottlang M, Simpson T, Sigg J, et al: Noninvasive reduction of open-book pelvic fractures by circumferential compression. J Orthop Trauma 16:367–373, 2002.

Connor GS, McGwin G Jr, MacLennan PA, et al: Early versus delayed fixation of pelvic ring fractures. Am Surg 69:1019–1023, 2003.

Cook RE, Keating JF, Gillespie I: The role of angiography in the management of haemorrhage from major fractures of the pelvis. J Bone Joint Surg [Br] 84:178–182, 2002.

Copeland CE, Bosse MJ, McCarthy ML, et al: Effect of trauma and pelvic function on female genitourinary, sexual, and reproductive function. J Orthop Trauma 11:73–81, 1997.

Duane TM, Tan BB, Golay D, et al: Blunt trauma and the role of routine pelvic radiographs: A prospective analysis. J Trauma 53:463–468, 2002.

Eastridge BJ, Starr A, Minei JP, O'Keefe GE: The importance of fracture pattern in guiding therapeutic decision-making in patients with hemorrhagic shock and pelvic ring disruptions. J Trauma 53:446–451, 2002.

Griffin DR, Starr AJ, Reinert CM, et al: Vertically unstable pelvic fractures fixed with percutaneous iliosacral screws: Does posterior injury pattern predict fixation failure?. J Orthop Trauma 17:399–405, 2003.

Grimm MR, Vrahas MS, Thomas KA: Pressure-volume characteristics of the intact and disrupted pelvic retroperitoneum. J Trauma 44:454–459, 1998.

Kabak S, Halici M, Tuncel M, et al: Functional outcome of open reduction and internal fixation for completely unstable pelvic ring fractures (type C): A report of 40 cases. J Orthop Trauma 17:555–562, 2003.

Mayher BE, Guyton JL, Gingrich JR: Impact of urethral injury management on the treatment and outcome of concurrent pelvic fractures. Urology 57:439–442, 2001.

McCormick JP, Morgan SJ, Smith WR: Clinical effectiveness of the physical examination in diagnosis of posterior pelvic ring injuries. J Orthop Trauma 17:257–261, 2003.

Miller PR, Moore PS, Mansell E, et al: External fixation or arteriogram in bleeding pelvic fracture: Initial therapy guided by markers of arterial hemorrhage. J Trauma 54:437–443, 2003.

Nork SE, Jones CB, Harding SP, et al: Percutaneous stabilization of U-shaped sacral fractures using iliosacral screws: Technique and early results. J Orthop Trauma 15:238–246, 2001.

Routt ML, Simonian PT, Mills WJ: Iliosacral screw fixation: Early complications of the percutaneous technique. J Orthop Trauma 11:584–589, 1997.

Routt ML, Nork SE, Mills WJ: Treatment of complex fractures: High-energy pelvic ring disruptions. Orthop Clin North Am 33:59–72, 2002.

Starr AJ, Griffin DR, Reinert CM, et al: Pelvic ring disruptions: Prediction of associated injuries, transfusion requirement, pelvic arteriography, complications, and mortality. J Orthop Trauma 16:553–561, 2002.

Velmahos GC, Toutouzas KG, Vassiliu P, et al: A prospective study on the safety and efficacy of angiographic embolization for pelvic and visceral injuries. J Trauma 53:303–308, 2002.

ACETABULUM

Borrelli J Jr, Goldfarb C, Catalano L, Evanoff BA: Assessment of articular fragment displacement in acetabular fractures: A comparison of computerized tomography and plain radiographs. J Orthop Trauma 16:449–456, 2002.

Borrelli J Jr, Goldfarb C, Ricci W, et al: Functional outcome after isolated acetabular fractures. J Orthop Trauma 16:73–81, 2002.

Borrelli J, Ungacta F, and Kantor J: Intraneural sciatic nerve pressures relative to the position of the hip and knee. In Final Program of the 14th Annual Meeting of the Orthopaedic Trauma Association, Vancouver, BC, Canada, October 8-10, 1998. Available at http://www.hwbf.org/ota/am/ota98/otapa/OTA98106.htm. Accessed April 27, 2005.

Carmack DB, Moed BR, McCarroll K, Freccero D: Accuracy of detecting screw penetration of the acetabulum with intraoperative fluoroscopy and computed tomography. J Bone Joint Surg [Am] 83:1370–1375, 2001.

Haidukewych GJ, Scaduto J, Herscovici D Jr, et al: Iatrogenic nerve injury in acetabular fracture surgery: A comparison of monitored and unmonitored procedures. J Orthop Trauma 16:297–301, 2002.

Kloen P, Siebenrock KA, Ganz R: Modification of the ilioinguinal approach. J Orthop Trauma 16:586–593, 2002.

Letournel E, Judet R, eds: Fractures of the Acetabulum, 2nd ed. Berlin, Springer-Verlag, 1993.

Levine RG, Renard R, Behrens FF, Tornetta P III: Biomechanical consequences of secondary congruence after both-column acetabular fracture. J Orthop Trauma 16:87–91, 2002.

Malkani AL, Voor MJ, Rennirt G, et al: Increased peak contact stress after incongruent reduction of transverse acetabular fractures: A cadaveric model. J Trauma 51:704–709, 2001.

Mears DC, Velyvis JH: Acute total hip arthroplasty for selected displaced acetabular fractures: Two to twelve-year results. J Bone Joint Surg [Am] 84:1–9, 2002.

Moed BR, Carr SEW, Watson JT: Results of operative treatment of fractures of the posterior wall of the acetabulum. J Bone Joint Surg [Am] 84:752–758, 2002.

Moed BR, Carr SE, Gruson KI, et al: Computed tomographic assessment of fractures of the posterior wall of the acetabulum after operative treatment. J Bone Joint Surg [Am] 85:512–522, 2003.

Moed BR, Yu PH, Gruson KI: Functional outcomes of acetabular fractures. J Bone Joint Surg [Am] 85:1879–1883, 2003.

Moore KD, Goss K, Anglen JO: Indomethacin versus radiation therapy for prophylaxis against heterotopic ossification in acetabular fractures: A randomized, prospective study. J Bone Joint Surg [Br] 80:259–263, 1998.

Olson SA, Matta JM: The computerized tomography subchondral arc: A new method of assessing acetabular articular continuity after fracture (a preliminary report). J Orthop Trauma 7:402–413, 1993.

Rice J, Kaliszer M, Dolan M, et al: Comparison between clinical and radiologic outcome measures after reconstruction of acetabular fractures. J Orthop Truama 16:82–86, 2002.

Starr AJ, Watson JT, Reinert CM, et al: Complications following the "T extensile" approach: A modified extensile approach for acetabular fracture surgery—report of forty-three patients. J Orthop Trauma 16:535–542, 2002.

Tornetta P III: Nonoperative management of acetabular fractures: The use of dynamic stress views. J Bone Joint Surg [Br] 81:67–70, 1999.

Tornetta P III: Displaced acetabular fractures: Indications for operative and nonoperative management. J Am Acad Orthop Surg 9:18–28, 2001.

FEMUR

Adams CI, Robinson CM, Court-Brown CM, McQueen MM: Prospective randomized controlled trial of an intramedullary nail versus dynamic screw and plate for intertrochanteric fractures of the femur. J Orthop Trauma 15:394–400, 2001.

Bartonicek J: Pauwels' classification of femoral neck fractures: Correct interpretation of the original. J Orthop Trauma 15:358–360, 2001.

Baumgaertner MR, Curtin SL, Lindskog DM, Keggi JM: The value of the tip-apex distance in predicting failure of fixation of peritrochanteric fractures of the hip. J Bone Joint Surg [Am] 77:1058–1064, 1995.

Bolhofner BR, Carmen B, Clifford P: The results of open reduction and internal fixation of distal femur fractures using a biologic (indirect) reduction technique. J Orthop Trauma 10:372–377, 1996.

Brumback RJ, Toal TR Jr, Murphy-Zane MS, et al: Immediate weight-bearing after treatment of a comminuted fracture of the femoral shaft with a statically locked intramedullary nail. J Bone Joint Surg [Am] 81:1538–1544, 1999.

Haidukewych GJ, Israel TA, Berry DJ: Reverse obliquity fractures of the intertrochanteric region of the femur. J Bone Joint Surg [Am] 83:643–650, 2001.

Hak DJ, Lee SS, Goulet JA: Success of exchange reamed intramedullary nailing for femoral shaft non-union or delayed union. J Orthop Trauma 14:178–182, 2000.

Kauffman JI, Simon JA, Kummer FJ, et al: Internal fixation of femoral neck fractures with posterior comminution: A biomechanical study. J Orthop Trauma 13:155–159, 1999.

Kregor PJ, Stannard JA, Zlowodski M, Cole PA: Treatment of distal femur fractures using the less invasive stabilization system: Surgical experience and early clinical results in 103 fractures. J Orthop Trauma 18:509–520, 2004.

Morgan E, Ostrum RF, DiCicco J, et al: Effects of retrograde femoral intramedullary nailing on the patellofemoral articulation. J Orthop Trauma 13:13–16, 1999.

Nowotarski PJ, Turen CH, Brumback RJ, Scarboro JM: Conversion of external fixation to intramedullary nailing for fractures of the shaft of the femur in multiply injured patients. J Bone Joint Surg [Am] 82:781–788, 2000.

Ostrum RF, Agarwal A, Lakatos R, Poka A: Prospective comparison of retrograde and antegrade femoral intramedullary nailing. J Orthop Trauma 14:496–501, 2000.

Pape HC, Hildebrand F, Pertschy S, et al: Changes in the management of femoral shaft fractures in poly-trauma patients: From early total care to damage control orthopedic surgery. J Trauma 53:452–462, 2002.

Ricci WM, Bellabarba C, Evanoff B, et al: Retrograde versus antegrade nailing of femoral shaft fractures. J Orthop Trauma 15:161–169, 2001.

Ricci WM, Devinney S, Haidukewych G, et al: Trochanteric nail insertion for the treatment of femoral shaft fractures. J Orthop Trauma 19:511–517, 2005.

Ricci WM, Loftus T, Cox C, Borrelli J: Locked plates combined with minimally invasive insertion technique for the treatment of periprosthetic supracondylar femur fractures above a total knee arthroplasty. J Orthop Trauma 20:190–196, 2006.

Ricci WM, Schwappach J, Tucker M, et al: Trochanteric versus piriformis entry portal for the treatment of femoral shaft fractures. J Orthop Trauma 20:663–667, 2006.

Ricci WM, Bellabarba C, Lewis R, et al: Angular malalignment after intramedullary nailing of femoral shaft fractures. J Orthop Trauma 15:90–95, 2001.

Ricci WM, Bolhofner BR, Loftus T, et al: Indirect reduction and plate fixation, without grafting, for periprosthetic femoral shaft fractures about a stable intramedullary implant. J Bone Joint Surg 87:2240–2245, 2005.

Rizzo PF, Gould ES, Lyden JP, Asnis SE: Diagnosis of occult fracture about the hip: Magnetic resonance imaging compared with bone-scanning. J Bone Joint Surg [Am] 75:395–401, 1993.

Russell T, Taylor J: Subtrochanteric fractures of the femur. In Browner B, Jupiter J, Levine A, Trafton P, eds: Skeletal Trauma, pp 1883–1926. Philadelphia, WB Saunders, 1992.

Sadowski C, Lubbeke A, Saudan M, et al: Treatment of reverse oblique and transverse intertrochanteric fractures with use of an intramedullary nail or a 95-degree screw-plate. J Bone Joint Surg [Am] 84A:372–381, 2002.

Scalea TM, Boswell SA, Scott JD, et al: External fixation as a bridge to intramedullary nailing for patients with multiple injuries and femur fractures: Damage control orthopedics. J Trauma 48:613–621, 2000.

Stannard JP, Harris HW, Volgas DA, Alonso JE: Functional outcome of patients with femoral head fractures associated with hip dislocations. Clin Orthop 377:44–56, 2000.

Swiontkowski MF, Thorpe M, Seiler JG, Hansen ST: Operative management of displaced femoral head fractures: Case-matched comparison of anterior versus posterior approaches for Pipkin I and Pipkin II fractures. J Orthop Trauma 6:437–442, 1992.

Tornetta P III, Tiburzi D: Antegrade or retrograde reamed femoral nailing: A prospective, randomized trial. J Bone Joint Surg [Br] 82:652–654, 2000.

Tornetta P III, Tiburzi D: Reamed versus non-reamed anterograde femoral nailing. J Orthop Trauma 14:15–19, 2000.

Watson JT, Moed BR: Ipsilateral femoral neck and shaft fractures. Clin Orthop 399:78–86, 2002.

Weight M, Collinge C: Early results of the less invasive stabilization system for mechanically unstable fractures of the distal femur (AO/OTA types A2, A3, C2, and C3). J Orthop Trauma 18:503–508, 2004.

Weresh MJ, Hakanson R, Stover MD, et al: Failure of exchange reamed intramedullary nails for ununited femoral shaft fractures. J Orthop Trauma 14:335–338, 2000.

Wolinsky PR, Banit D, Parker RE, et al: Reamed intramedullary femoral nailing after induction of an "ARDS-like" state in sheep: Effect on clinically applicable markers of pulmonary function. J Orthop Trauma 12:169–175, 1998.

Yoon TR, Rowe SM, Chung JY, et al: Clinical and radiographic outcome of femoral head fractures: 30 patients followed for 3-10 years. Acta Orthop Scand 72:348–353, 2001.

KNEE

Goitz RJ, Tomaino MM: Management of peroneal nerve injuries associated with knee dislocation. Am J Orthop 32:14–16, 2003.

Ilan DI, Tejwani N, Keschner M, Leibman M: Quadriceps tendon rupture. J Am Acad Orthop Surg 11:192–200, 2003.

Konrath GA, Chen D, Lock T, et al: Outcomes following repair of quadriceps tendon ruptures. J Orthop Trauma 12:273–279, 1998.

Mills WJ, Barei DP, McNair P: The value of the ankle brachial index for diagnosing arterial injury after knee dislocation: A prospective study. J Trauma 56:1261–1265, 2004.

Miranda FE, Dennis JW, Veldenz HC, et al: Confirmation of the safety and accuracy of physical examination in the evaluation of knee dislocation for injury of the popliteal artery: A prospective study. J Trauma 52:247–251, 2002.

Noyes FR, Barber-Westin SD: Reconstruction of the anterior and posterior cruciate ligaments after knee dislocation: Use of early protected postoperative motion to decrease arthrofibrosis. Am J Sports Med 25:769–778, 1997.

O'Shea K, Kenny P, Donovan J, et al: Outcomes following quadriceps tendon ruptures. Injury 33:257–260, 2002.

Richards DP, Barber FA: Repair of quadriceps tendon ruptures using suture anchors. Arthroscopy 18:556–559, 2002.

Schenck RC Jr: The dislocated knee. Instr Course Lect 43:127–136, 1994.

Siwek CW, Rao JP: Ruptures of the extensor mechanism of the knee joint. J Bone Joint Surg [Am] 63:932–937, 1981.

Smith ST, Cramer KE, Karges DE, et al: Early complications in the operative treatment of patella fractures. J Orthop Trauma 11:183–187, 1997.

Stannard JP, Wilson TC, Sheils TM, et al: Heterotopic ossification associated with knee dislocation. Arthroscopy 18:835–839, 2002.

Stannard JP, Sheils TM, McGwin G, et al: Use of a hinged external knee fixator after surgery for knee dislocation. Arthroscopy 19:626–631, 2003.

Stannard JP, Sheils TM, Lopez-Ben RR, et al: Vascular injuries in knee dislocations: The role of physical examination in determining the need for arteriography. J Bone Joint Surg [Am] 86:910–915, 2004.

Stannard JP, Schenck RJ Jr.: Knee dislocations and ligamentous injuries. In Stannard JP, Schmidt AH, Kregor PJ, eds: Surgical Treatment of Orthopaedic Trauma. New York, Thieme Medical Publishers, 2007.

Treiman GS, Yellin AE, Weaver FA, et al: Examination of the patient with knee dislocation: The case for selective arteriography. Arch Surg 127:1056–1063, 1992.

TIBIA

Holt MD, Williams LA, Dent CM: MRI in the management of tibial plateau fractures. Injury 26:595–599, 1995.

Kumar A, Whittle AP: Treatment of complex (Shatzker type VI) fractures of the tibial plateau with circular wire external fixation: Retrospective case review. J Orthop Trauma 14:339–344, 2000.

Mils WJ, Nork SE: Open reduction and internal fixation of high-energy tibial plateau fractures. Orthop Clin North Am 33:177–198, 2002.

Shepherd I, Abdollahi K, Lee J, Vangsness CT Jr.: The prevalence of soft tissue injuries in nonoperative tibial plateau fractures as determined by magnetic resonance imaging. J Orthop Trauma 16:628–631, 2002.

Stannard JP, Wilson TC, Volgas DA, Alonso JE: The less invasive stabilization system in the treatment of complex fractures of the tibial plateau: Short term results. J Orthop Trauma 18:552–558, 2004.

Stannard JP, Martin SL: In Stannard JP, Schmidt AH, Kregor PJ, eds: Tibial Plateau Fractures in Surgical Treatment of Orthopaedic Trauma. New York, Thieme Medical Publishers, 2007.

Watson JT, Coufal C: Treatment of complex lateral plateau fractures using Ilizarov techniques. Clin Orthop Relat Res 353:97–106, 1998.

Yacoubian SC, Nevins RT, Sallis JG, et al: Impact of MRI on treatment plan and fracture classification of tibial plateau fractures. J Orthop Trauma 16:632–637, 2002.

TIBIAL SHAFT

Bhandari M, Guyatt GH, Tornetta P III, et al: Current practice in the intramedullary nailing of tibial shaft fractures: An international survey. J Trauma 53:725–732, 2002.

Bhandari M, Guyatt GH, Tong D, et al: Reamed versus non-reamed intramedullary nailing of lower extremity long bone fractures: A systemic overview and meta-analysis. J Orthop Trauma 14:2–9, 2000.

Court-Brown CM, Keating JF, Christie J, McQueen MM: Exchange intramedullary nailing: Its use in aseptic tibial nonunion. J Bone Joint Surg [Br] 77:407–411, 1995.

Court-Brown CM, Gustilo T, Shaw AD: Knee pain after intramedullary tibial nailing: Its incidence, etiology, and outcome. J Orthop Trauma 11:103–105, 1997.

Finkemeier CG, Schmidt AH, Kyle RF, et al: A prospective, randomized study of intramedullary nails inserted with and without reaming for the treatment of open and closed fractures of the tibial shaft. J Orthop Trauma 14:187–193, 2000.

Fischer MD, Gustilo RB, Varecka TF: The timing of flap coverage, bone-grafting, and intramedullary nailing in patients who have a fracture of the tibial shaft with extensive soft-tissue injury. J Bone Joint Surg [Am] 73:1316–1322, 1991.

Freedman EL, Johnson EE: Radiographic analysis of tibial fracture malalignment following intramedullary nailing. Clin Orthop 315:25–33, 1995.

Gopal S, Majumder S, Batchelor AG, et al: Fix and flap: The radical orthopaedic and plastic treatment of severe open fractures of the tibia. J Bone Joint Surg [Br] 82:959–966, 2000.

Gregory P, DiCicco J, Karpik K, et al: Ipsilateral fractures of the femur and tibia: Treatment with retrograde femoral nailing and unreamed tibial nailing. J Orthop Trauma 10:309–316, 1996.

Henley MB, Chapman JR, Agel J, et al: Treatment of Type II, IIIA, and IIIB open fractures of the tibial shaft: A prospective comparison of unreamed

interlocking intramedullary nails and half-pin external fixators. J Orthop Trauma 12:1–7, 1998.
Keating JF, O'Brien PJ, Blachut PA, et al: Locking intramedullary nailing with and without reaming for open fractures of the tibial shaft: A prospective, randomized study. J Bone Joint Surg [Am] 79:334–341, 1997.
Krettek C, Miclau T, Schandelmaier P, et al: The mechanical effect of blocking screws ("Poller screws") in stabilizing tibia fractures with short proximal or distal fragments after insertion of small-diameter intramedullary nails. J Orthop Trauma 13:550–553, 1999.
Milner SA, Davis TR, Muir KR, et al: Long-term outcome after tibial shaft fracture: Is malunion important? J Bone Joint Surg [Am] 84:971–980, 2002.
Ricci WM, O'Boyle M, Borrelli J, et al: Fractures of the proximal third of the tibial shaft treated with intramedullary nails and blocking screws. J Orthop Trauma 15:264–270, 2001.
Schmidt AH, Finkemeier CG, Tornetta P: Treatment of closed tibial fracture. Instr Course Lect 52:607–622, 2003.
Tornetta P, Collins E: Semiextended position of intramedullary nailing of the proximal tibia. Clin Orthop 328:185–189, 1996.

TIBIAL PLAFOND

Blauth M, Bastian L, Krettek C, et al: Surgical options for the treatment of severe tibial pilon fractures: A study of three techniques. J Orthop Trauma 15:153–160, 2001.
Bone L, Stegemann P, McNamara K, Seibel R: External fixation of severely comminuted and open tibial pilon fractures. Clin Orthop Relat Res 292:101–107, 1993.
Borrelli J Jr, Catalano L: Open reduction and internal fixation of pilon fractures. J Orthop Trauma 13:573–582, 1999.
Borrelli J Jr, Ellis E: Pilon fractures: Assessment and treatment. Orthop Clin North Am 33x:231–245, 2002.
Chen SH, Wu PH, Lee YS: Long-term results of pilon fractures. Arch Orthop Trauma Surg 127:55–60, 2007.

DISTAL TIBIA FRACTURES

Borrelli J Jr, Ellis E: Pilon fractures: Assessment and treatment. Orthop Clin North Am 33x:231–245, 2002.
Chen SH, Wu PH, Lee YS: Long-term results of pilon fractures. Arch Orthop Trauma Surg 127:55–60, 2007.
Pollak AN, McCarthy ML, Bess RS, et al: Outcomes after treatment of high-energy tibial plafond fractures. J Bone Joint Surg [Am] 85:1893–1900, 2003.
Sirkin M, Sanders R, DiPasquale T, Herscovici D Jr: A staged protocol for soft tissue management in the treatment of complex pilon fractures. J Orthop Trauma 18(8 Suppl):S32–S38, 2004.
Topliss CJ, Jackson M, Atkins RM: Anatomy of pilon fractures of the distal tibia. J Bone Joint Surg [Br] 87:692–697, 2005.

ANKLE

Ebraheim NA, Elgafy H, Padanilam T: Syndesmotic disruption in low fibular fractures associated with deltoid ligament injury. Clin Orthop 409:260–267, 2003.
Egol KA, Dolan R, Koval KJ: Functional outcome of surgery for fractures of the ankle: A prospective, randomized comparison of management in a cast or a functional brace. J Bone Joint Surg [Br] 82:246–249, 2000.
Egol KA, Sheikhazadeh A, Mogatederi S, et al: Lower-extremity function for driving an automobile after operative treatment of ankle fracture. J Bone Joint Surg [Am] 85:1185–1189, 2003.
Lamontagne J, Blachut PA, Broekhuyse HM, et al: Surgical treatment of a displaced lateral malleolus fracture: The antiglide technique versus lateral plate fixation. J Orthop Trauma 16:498–502, 2002.
Lehtonen H, Jarvinen TL, Honkonen S, et al: Use of a cast compared with a functional ankle brace after operative treatment of an ankle fracture: A prospective, randomized study. J Bone Joint Surg [Am] 85:205–211, 2003.
McConnell T, Creevy W, Tornetta P III: Stress examination of supination external rotation-type fibular fractures. J Bone Joint Surg [Am] 86:2171–2178, 2004.
Obremskey WT, Dirschl DR, Crowther JD, et al: Change over time of SF-36 functional outcomes for operatively treated unstable ankle fractures. J Orthop Trauma 16:30–33, 2002.
Tornetta P III, Spoo JE, Reynolds FA, Lee C: Over-tightening of the ankle syndesmosis: Is it really possible? J Bone Joint Surg [Am] 83:489–492, 2001.

FOOT

Abidi N, Dhawan S, Gruen G, et al: Wound-healing risk factors after open reduction and internal fixation of calcaneal fractures. Foot Ankle Int 19:856–861, 1998.
Borrelli J Jr, Lashgari C: Vascularity of the lateral calcaneal flap: A cadaveric injection study. J Orthop Trauma 13:73–77, 1999.
Buckley R, Tough S, McCormack R, et al: Operative compared with non-operative treatment of displaced intra-articular calcaneal fractures: A prospective, randomized, controlled multicenter trial. J Bone Joint Surg [Am] 84:1733–1744, 2002.
Csizy M, Buckley R, Tough S, et al: Displaced intra-articular calcaneal fractures: Variables predicting late subtalar fusion. J Orthop Trauma 17:106–112, 2003.
Fleuriau Chateau PB, Brokaw DS, Jelen BA, et al: Plate fixation of talar neck fractures: Preliminary review of a new technique in twenty-three patients. J Orthop Trauma 16:213–219, 2002.
Kuo RS, Tejwani NC, Digiovanni CW, et al: Outcome after open reduction and internal fixation of Lisfranc joint injuries. J Bone Joint Surg [Am] 82:1609–1618, 2000.
Loucks C, Buckley R: Bohler's angle: Correlation with outcome in displaced intra-articular calcaneal fractures. J Orthop Trauma 13:554–558, 1999.
Pajenda G, Vecsei V, Reddy B, Heinz T: Treatment of talar neck fractures: Clinical results of 50 patients. J Foot Ankle Surg 39:365–375, 2000.
Peicha G, Labovitz J, Seibert FJ, et al: The anatomy of the joint as a risk factor for Lisfranc dislocation and fracture dislocation: An anatomical and radiological case control study. J Bone Joint Surg [Br] 84:981–985, 2002.
Philbin T, Rosenberg G, Sterra JJ: Complications of missed or untreated Lisfranc injuries. Foot Ankle Clin 8:61–71, 2003.
Sanders R: Displaced intra-articular fractures of the calcaneus. J Bone Joint Surg [Am] 82:225–250, 2000.
Smith JW, Arnoczky SP, Hersh A: The intraosseous blood supply of the fifth metatarsal: Implications for proximal fracture healing. Foot Ankle 13:143–152, 1992.
Tornetta P III: Percutaneous treatment of calcaneal fractures. Clin Orthop 375:91–96, 2000.
Vallier HA, Nork SE, Benirschke SK, Sangeorzan BJ: Surgical treatment of talar body fractures. J Bone Joint Surg [Am] 85:1716–1724, 2003.
Weber M, Lochner A: Reconstruction of the cuboid in compression fractures: Short to midterm results in 12 patients. Foot Ankle Int 23:1008–1013, 2002.
Ziran BH, Abidi NA, Scheel MJ: Medial malleolar osteotomy for exposure of complex talar body fractures. J Orthop Trauma 15:513–518, 2001.

UPPER CERVICAL SPINE

Askins V, Eismont FJ: Efficacy of five cervical orthoses in restricting cervical motion: A comparison study. Spine 22:1193–1198, 1997.
Borm W, Kast E, Richter HP, Mohr K: Anterior screw fixation in type II odontoid fractures: Is there a difference in outcome between age groups? Neurosurgery 52:1089–1092, discussion 1092–1094, 2003.
Eismont FJ, Arena MJ, Green BA: Extrusion of an intervertebral disc associated with traumatic subluxation or dislocation of cervical facets: Case report. J Bone Joint Surg [Am] 73:1555–1560, 1991.
Eismont FJ, Currier BL, McGuire RA Jr: Cervical spine and spinal cord injuries: Recognition and treatment. Instr Course Lect 53:341–358, 2004.
Fielding JW, Cochran GB, Lawsing JF III, Hohl M: Tears of the transverse ligament of the atlas: A clinical and biomechanical study. J Bone Joint Surg [Am] 56:1683–1691, 1974.
Govender S, Grootboom M: Fractures of the dens—the results of non-rigid immobilization. Injury 19:165–167, 1988.
Greene KA, Dickman CA, Marciano FF, et al: Acute axis fractures: Analysis of management and outcome in 340 consecutive cases. Spine 22:1843–1852, 1997.
Guiot B, Fessler RG: Complex atlantoaxial fractures. J Neurosurg 91(2 Suppl):139–143, 1999.
Levine AM, Edwards CC: Fractures of the atlas. J Bone Joint Surg [Am] 73:680–691, 1991.

Levine AM, Edwards CC: Traumatic lesions of the occipitoatlantoaxial complex. Clin Orthop Relat Res 239:53–68, 1989.

LOWER CERVICAL SPINE

Allen BL Jr, Ferguson RL, Lehmann TR, O'Brien RP: A mechanistic classification of closed, indirect fractures and dislocations of the lower cervical spine. Spine 7:1–27, 1982.
Andreshak JL, Dekutoski MB: Management of unilateral facet dislocations: A review of the literature. Orthopedics 20:917–926, 1997.
Torg JS, Pavlov H, O'Neill MJ, et al: The axial load teardrop fracture: A biomechanical, clinical and roentgenographic analysis. Am J Sports Med 19:355–364, 1991.
Torg JS, Thibault L, Sennett B, Pavlov H: The Nicolas Andry Award: The pathomechanics and pathophysiology of cervical spinal cord injury. Clin Orthop Relat Res 321:259–269, 1995.

PHYSEAL INJURY (PEDIATRIC)

Ogden JA: The evaluation and treatment of partial physeal arrest. J Bone Joint Surg [Am] 69:1297–1302, 1987.
Salter RB, Harris WR: Injuries involving the epiphyseal plate. J Bone Joint Surg [Am] 45:587–622, 1963.

WRIST AND HAND (PEDIATRIC)

Campbell RM Jr: Operative treatment of fractures and dislocations of the hand and wrist region in children. Orthop Clin North Am 21:217–243, 1990.
Dicke TE, Nunley JA: Distal forearm fractures in children: Complications and surgical indications. Orthop Clin North Am 24:333–340, 1993.
Light TR: Carpal injuries in children. Hand Clin 16:513–522, 2000.
Noonan KJ, Price CT: Forearm and distal radius fractures in children. J Am Acad Orthop Surg 6:146–156, 1998.
Torre BA: Epiphyseal injuries in the small joints of the hand. Hand Clin 4:113–121, 1988.

RADIAL AND ULNAR SHAFT (PEDIATRIC)

Flynn JM: Pediatric forearm fractures: Decision making, surgical techniques, and complications. AAOS Instr Course Lect 51:355–360, 2002.
Goodwin RC, Kuivila TE: Pediatric elbow and forearm fractures requiring surgical treatment. Hand Clin 18:135–148, 2002.
Ring D, Jupiter JB, Waters PM: Monteggia fractures in children and adults. J Am Acad Orthop Surg 6:215–224, 1998.
Ring D, Waters PM, Hotchkiss RN, Kasser JR: Pediatric floating elbow. J Pediatr Orthop 21:456–459, 2001.

ELBOW (PEDIATRIC)

Bast SC, Hoffer MM, Aval S: Nonoperative treatment for minimally and nondisplaced lateral humeral condyle fractures in children. J Pediatr Orthop 18:448–450, 1998.
Dias JJ, Johnson GV, Hoskinson J, Sulaiman K: Management of severely displaced medial epicondyle fractures. J Orthop Trauma 1:59–62, 1987.
Finnbogason T, Karlsson G, Lindberg L, Mortensson W: Nondisplaced and minimally displaced fractures of the lateral humeral condyle in children: A prospective radiographic investigation of fracture stability. J Pediatr Orthop 15:422–425, 1995.
Lins RE, Simovitch RW, Waters PM: Pediatric elbow trauma. Orthop Clin North Am 30:119–132, 1999.
Shimada K, Masada K, Tada K, Yamamoto T: Osteosynthesis for the treatment of non-union of the lateral humeral condyle in children. J Bone Joint Surg [Am] 79:234–240, 1997.
Skaggs DL, Hale JM, Bassett J, et al: Operative treatment of supracondylar fractures of the humerus in children: The consequences of pin placement. J Bone Joint Surg [Am] 83:735–740, 2001.
Sponseller PD: Problem elbow fractures in children. Hand Clin 10:495–505, 1994.

SPINE (PEDIATRIC)

Akbarnia BA: Pediatric spine fractures. Orthop Clin North Am 30:521–536, 1999.
Bosch PP, Vogt MT, Ward WT: Pediatric spinal cord injury without radiographic abnormality (SCIWORA): The absence of occult instability and lack of indication for bracing. Spine 27:2788–2800, 2002.
Sun PP, Poffenbarger GJ, Durham S, Zimmerman RA: Spectrum of occipitoatlantoaxial injury in young children. J Neurosurg 93(Suppl. 1):28–39, 2000.

PELVIS (PEDIATRIC)

Grisoni N, Conner S, Marsh E, et al: Pelvic fractures in a pediatric level I trauma center. J Orthop Trauma 16:458–463, 2002.
Tolo VT: Orthopaedic treatment of fractures of the long bones and pelvis in children who have multiple injuries. AAOS Instr Course Lect 49: 415–423, 2000.

HIP (PEDIATRIC)

Bagatur AE, Zorer G: Complications associated with surgically treated hip fractures in children. J Pediatr Orthop 11(Part B):219–228, 2002.
Canale ST: Fractures of the hip in children and adolescents. Orthop Clin North Am 21:341–352, 1990.
Davison BL, Weinstein SL: Hip fractures in children: A long-term follow-up study. J Pediatr Orthop 12:355–358, 1992.
Hughes LO, Beaty JH: Fractures of the head and neck of the femur in children. J Bone Joint Surg [Am] 76:283–292, 1994.
Spiegel PG, Mast JW: Internal and external fixation of fractures in children. Orthop Clin North Am 11:405–421, 1980.
Thompson GH, Bachner EJ, Ballock RT: Salter-Harris type II fractures of the capital femoral epiphysis. J Orthop Trauma 14:510–514, 2000.

FEMUR (PEDIATRIC)

Buckley SL: Current trends in the treatment of femoral shaft fractures in children and adolescents. Clin Orthop 338:60–73, 1997.
Sponseller PD: Surgical management of pediatric femoral fractures. AAOS Instr Course Lect 51:361–365, 2002.

KNEE (PEDIATRIC)

Beaty JH, Kumar A: Fractures about the knee in children. J Bone Joint Surg [Am] 76:1870–1880, 1994.
Davies EM, McLaren MI: Type III tibial spine avulsions treated with arthroscopic Acutrak screw reattachment. Clin Orthop 388:205–208, 2001.
Hallam PJ, Fazal MA, Ashwood N, et al: An alternative to fixation of displaced fractures of the anterior intercondylar eminence in children. J Bone Joint Surg [Br] 84:579–582, 2002.
Qidwai SA: Intramedullary Kirschner wiring for tibia fractures in children. J Pediatr Orthop 21:294–297, 2001.
Roberts JM: Operative treatment of fractures about the knee. Orthop Clin North Am 21:365–379, 1990.
Zionts LE: Fractures around the knee in children. J Am Acad Orthop Surg 10:345–355, 2002.

TIBIA (PEDIATRIC)

D'Souza LG, Hynes DE, McManus F, et al: The bicycle spoke injury: an avoidable accident? Foot Ankle Int 17(3):170–173, 1996.
Letts M, Vincent N, Gouw G: The "floating knee" in children. J Bone Joint Surg [Br] 68:442–446, 1986.
Müller I, Muschol M, Mann M, Hassenpflug J: Results of proximal metaphyseal fractures in children. Arch Orthop Trauma Surg 122:331–333, 2002.
Yue JJ, Churchill RS, Cooperman DR, et al: The floating knee in the pediatric patient: Nonoperative versus operative stabilization. Clin Orthop Relat Res 376:124–136, 2000.

FOOT AND ANKLE (PEDIATRIC)

Buoncristiani AM, Manos RE, Mills WJ: Plantar-flexion tarsometatarsal joint injuries in children. J Pediatr Orthop 21:324–327, 2001.
Crawford AH: Ankle fractures in children. AAOS Instr Course Lect 44: 317–324, 1995.
Kling TF Jr: Operative treatment of ankle fractures in children. Orthop Clin North Am 21:381–392, 1990.
Trott AW: Fractures of the foot in children. Orthop Clin North Am 7: 677–686, 1976.

CHAPTER 12

Principles of Practice and Statistics

S. Raymond Golish AND Marc M. DeHart

CONTENTS

SECTION 1 Principles of Practice

The practice of orthopaedic surgery involves complex relationships among the ethics of patient care, the business of orthopaedics, and the law. The duty of the orthopaedic surgeon to provide ethical care is the principal consideration; however, the management of potential conflicts of interest among the areas of ethical patient care, business goals, and legal considerations is also of paramount importance. Careful attention to business and legal issues can allow the practicing orthopaedic surgeon greater freedom and ability to provide ethical patient care. Principles of professionalism are also important tools in the effective practice of modern orthopaedic surgery. With the help of other organizations, the **American Academy of Orthopaedic Surgeons** (AAOS) has developed several documents regarding the principles of ethics in the practice of orthopaedic surgery. These documents include *Code of Ethics for Orthopaedic Surgeons* (2004), *Principles of Medical Ethics in Orthopaedic Surgery* (2002), *Medical Professionalism in the New Millennium: A Physician Charter* (2002), *Standards of Professionalism* (2005), and most recently *A Guide to the Ethical Practice of Orthopaedic Surgery* (2006). While many of the documents are aspirational, the principles outlined in *Standards of Professionalism* serve as the mandatory minimal level of acceptable conduct for orthopaedic surgeons, and nonadherance to these principles can result in the loss of membership. Violations of these standards may serve as grounds for formal complaints to and action by the

Academy, as outlined in the AAOS Bylaws. Violations are determined by the Professional Compliance Program of the AAOS and can be reported to the National Practitioner Data Bank, State Medical Licensing Boards, and the **American Board of Orthopaedic Surgery** (ABOS).

I. Principles of Ethics and Professionalism

A. Introduction—Ethics is the discipline dealing with the principles or moral values that govern relationships between and among individuals and defines what the orthopaedic surgeon ought to do.

B. Key elements of the AAOS Code of Medical Ethics and Professionalism (1988)—These include the following principles of conduct.

1. The physician–patient relationship is the "central focus of all ethical concerns." The relationship is based on trust but also has a contractual basis. Medical contracts and medical confidentiality are discussed in Section 3, Ethics and Medicolegal Issues.
2. The personal conduct of the orthopaedic surgeon should emphasize the patient's best interests through truth, honesty, and the provision of "competent and compassionate care." The surgeon must obey the law and maintain professional dignity and discipline.
3. Conflicts of interest are possible in the complex relationships existing among ethical patient care, the business of orthopaedics, and medicolegal concerns. Relationships with industry and ownership of medical facilities are the most common areas of conflict and are best managed with full disclosure. The other six sections of the code address important issues such as maintaining competence; relationships with orthopaedic surgeons, nurses, and allied health professionals; relationship to the public; general principles of care; research and academic responsibilities; and community responsibility.

C. Medical professionalism in the new millennium—A physician charter

1. The AAOS adopted the charter that was crafted by physicians throughout the industrialized world who were concerned about changes in health care delivery systems that threaten the values of professionalism. Three fundamental principles of professionalism define the basis of medicine's contract with society:
   a. The primacy of patient welfare—Serve the patient's interest
   b. Autonomy—Respect a patient's informed choices
   c. Social justice—Fair distribution of health care resources
2. The charter also defines a set of 10 professional responsibilities that apply to physicians: maintain commitments to professional competence, honesty with patients, patient confidentiality, appropriate relations, improving the quality of care, improving access to care, just distribution of finite resources, scientific knowledge, managing conflicts of interest, and professional responsibilities.

D. Standards of professionalism—These standards represent the mandatory minimum levels of acceptable conduct for orthopaedic surgeons. Violations of them may serve as grounds for formal complaints to and action by the Academy, as outlined in the AAOS Bylaws. Violations are determined by the Professional Compliance Program of the AAOS and can be reported to the National Practitioner Data Bank, State Medical Licensing Boards, and the ABOS. The current Standards (2006) include the following principles and practice.

1. Providing musculoskeletal services to patients
   a. Be aware that responsibility to the patient is paramount
   b. Provide needed and appropriate care
   c. Advocate for the most appropriate care
   d. Safeguard patient confidentiality and privacy
   e. Maintain appropriate relations with patients
   f. Respect a patient's request for additional opinions
   g. Present medical facts and obtain informed consent
   h. Pursue lifelong scientific and medical learning
   i. Provide services and use techniques only for which he or she is qualified by personal education, training, or experience
   j. If impaired by substance abuse, seek professional care and limit/cease practice as directed
   k. If impaired by mental/physical disability, seek professional care and limit/cease practice as directed
2. Professional relationships
   a. Be aware that responsibility to the patient is paramount
   b. Maintain fairness, respect, and confidentiality with other professionals
   c. Act in a professional manner with other professionals
   d. Work collaboratively to reduce medical errors, increase patient safety, and improve outcomes
   e. Facilitate and cooperate in transferring patient care
3. Orthopaedic expert witness testimony
   a. Do not testify falsely
   b. Provide impartial opinions
   c. Evaluate care by standards of time, place, situation
   d. Do not condemn standard care or condone substandard care
   e. Explain any opinion that varies from standard
   f. Seek and review all pertinent records
   g. Have knowledge and experience and respond accurately to questions
   h. Testify only when having relevant experience/knowledge
   i. State basis of testimony: experience and/or scientific evidence
   j. Have a current unrestricted license
   k. Have current board certification in orthopaedic surgery (i.e., ABOS)
   l. Have an active practice/familiarity with present practices
   m. Do not misrepresent your credentials
   n. Fees should not be contingent on outcome
   o. Expect reasonable compensation

4. Research and academic responsibilities
   a. Responsibility to patient is paramount
   b. Informed consent is required
   c. Honor withdrawal request
   d. Seek peer review and follow regulations
   e. Be truthful with patients and colleagues
   f. Report fraudulent or deceptive research
   g. Claim credit only if substantial contributions made
   h. Give credit when presenting others' ideas
   i. Expose fraud and deception
   j. Warrant contributions to publications
   k. Disclose duplicate publications
   l. Credit contributors
   m. Acknowledge funding sources or consulting agreements

II. Child, Elder, and Spousal Abuse

A. Violence—Each year intentional violence claims 20,000 lives, is responsible for more than 300,000 hospitalizations, and causes millions of injuries. It is estimated that 1.4 million children in the United States suffer some form of maltreatment each year. As many as 2000 children die each year from abuse.

B. Child abuse—The U.S. Child Abuse Prevention and Treatment Act of 1974 requires orthopaedic surgeons to report all suspected cases of child abuse to local authorities. Failure to report suspected child abuse might result in state disciplinary actions.
   1. Child protective services and social workers should be alerted, and the events and home circumstances should be investigated.
   2. These statutes provide immunity for physicians when reporting such cases provided that they act in good faith, even if the information is protected by the physician–patient privilege.

C. Elder abuse—Elder abuse has been estimated to affect 2 million older Americans each year. A 1989 Congressional study indicated that 1 of every 25 Americans over age 65 suffers some serious form of abuse, neglect, or exploitation. Many states have provided legislation to protect physicians who report elderly abuse from liability.

D. Spousal abuse—The reporting of suspected spousal abuse is not required, and there is a corresponding absence of legal protection for physicians. A physician may encourage a patient to seek self-protection. If the physician believes that an individual is truly incapable of self-protection, a court order may be obtained to permit reporting.

III. Diversity in Orthopaedics

A. Importance of diversity—Our understanding of the value of diversity in race, gender, creed, and sexual orientation is increasing in all areas of life. It is essential to be sensitive to diversity issues with respect to colleagues in orthopaedic surgery and medicine, allied medical professionals, and patients. Other aspects of diversity and nondiscrimination are also important, such as obesity, psychiatric disease, income class, physical disability, and the status of **human immunodeficiency virus** (HIV). Several important lines of research have addressed diversity and discrimination in medicine. The factors involved in these issues are complex, but this research has raised our awareness of the importance of diversity in modern medical practice.

B. Treatment decisions—The AAOS Code of Medical Ethics states that treatment decisions should not be made due to "race, color, gender, sexual orientation, religion, or national origin or on any basis that would constitute illegal discrimination."

C. Sensitivity to diversity issues—Sensitivity to diversity issues is an increasingly important aspect of professionalism. Each practitioner must examine the attitudes, preconceptions, and emotions exhibited in the workplace in this dimension. One must be aware of how speech and behaviors might be perceived by others of different backgrounds. It is possible for the actions of someone with good intentions to be interpreted as threatening or derogatory by others of different backgrounds.

IV. Sexual Misconduct

A. Introduction—Avoiding sexual misconduct is an important aspect of diversity awareness in relationships with patients, coworkers, staff, and colleagues. Sexual relationships, even if consensual, between individuals in a professional supervisor/trainee relationship create the potential for sexual exploitation and the loss of objectivity. In the workplace, some general guidelines have been broadly instituted as a policy for responding to instances of sexual misconduct.

B. Sexual harassment in employment
   1. Quid pro quo—Harassment is directly linked to employment or advancement.
   2. Hostile environment harassment—Verbal or physical conduct (e.g., gestures, innuendo, humor, pictures) of a sexual nature or general hostility due to gender that promotes a hostile environment in the workplace. Actual sexual advances are not necessary to create a hostile work environment.
   3. "Reasonable woman" test—The adopted standard for offensive behavior is the "reasonable woman" test. If a reasonable woman would have found the behavior objectionable, then harassment may have occurred.
   4. Individuals in medical training programs are considered employees of the school that is training them. This status allows them to pursue harassment claims under the Civil Rights Act.

C. Sexual misconduct in the patient care setting—Sexual misconduct with patients is a form of exploitation. Such misconduct is unethical and may represent malpractice or even criminal acts of assault. Courts have maintained that a patient is unable to give meaningful consent to sexual or romantic advances. Physicians are encouraged to report instances of sexual misconduct by their colleagues. Many states have laws prohibiting physicians from pursuing relationships with current or former patients. The physician–patient relationship must be terminated before pursuing any romantic interest. Even then, it may still be unethical if the physician exploits certain confidences, trust, or emotions learned while serving as the patient's physician.

V. The Impaired Physician

A surgeon (resident, fellow, or attending) who discovers chemical impairment, dependence, or incompetence in a colleague or supervisor has the responsibility to ensure that the problem is identified and treated. Mechanisms exist for the proper identification and treatment of the impaired physician. Misconduct can be reported to state and local agencies. One must be sure to act in good faith with reasonable evidence when reporting such incidences. If a patient is at risk for immediate harm or injury by an impaired physician, one should assert authority and relieve the physician of the patient care and then address the problem with the senior hospital staff as soon as possible.

VI. Orthopaedic Education

A. Maintenance of competence—The practicing orthopaedic surgeon should strive to continually improve. These efforts should extend beyond the effort devoted to clinical care during the course of practice. Although a surgeon's daily practice and caseload represent an invaluable self-teaching opportunity, formal education beyond one's practice is essential.
   1. AAOS Code of Medical Ethics—States that orthopaedic surgeons should undertake "continuing medical educational activities." Countless courses on a variety of topics offer formal **continuing medical education** (CME) credits. Accrual of these credits is one way of demonstrating vigorous and ongoing self-education.
   2. ABOS—Requires CME coursework for recertification. An average of 40 hours of CME credit per year is recommended. Some state medical boards may require more hours.

B. Residency and Guidelines of the **American Council on Graduate Medical Education** (ACGME)
   1. Work hour restrictions—The ACGME has significantly changed the nature of resident education in recent years. The momentum for work hour restrictions resulted from high-profile medical malpractice cases and from a variety of academic studies regarding impaired performance with long duty hours. Significant work hour restrictions have affected resident education. Residency programs must comply with restrictions and document compliance. Failure to comply can result in probation or suspension of residency accreditation.
   2. **Duty hours**—Defined as clinical (patient care), academic, and administrative work, including time on call. Duty hours must be limited to 80 hours per week averaged over a 4-week period. However, in addition to the 80-hour week, other restrictions apply. Residents must have 1 day in seven off, averaged over a 4-week period. A "day" is defined as a continuous 24-hour period free from duties. There must be a 10-hour time period off-duty between daily clinical duties or after being on call. This last restriction has been difficult to comply with in some situations. An in-house call must be confined to no more than 1 in 3 days, no more than 24 hours of continuous duty, no new patients after 24 hours, and a maximum of 6 additional hours for transfer of patient care.

C. **Core competencies**—The ACGME has defined core competencies for all resident education.
   1. Patient care skills should be acquired, including the provision of "compassionate, appropriate, and effective" care.
   2. Medical knowledge must be assimilated, including information regarding "established and evolving biomedical, clinical, and cognate sciences, as well as the application of this knowledge to patient care."
   3. Practice-based learning includes improving patient care with investigation and the appraisal of scientific evidence.
   4. Interpersonal and communication skills facilitate effective and compassionate exchange of information with patients, families, and health professionals.
   5. Professionalism consists of handling responsibilities while adhering to ethical principles and considering diversity issues in patient care and social services.
   6. System-based practice is aided by an awareness of the larger context of medical decisions at the levels of the social, economic, and information systems.

VII. Research

A. Introduction—Clinical and basic research provides a tremendous opportunity for improvement of the diagnosis and treatment of orthopaedic disease.

B. Ethical research—Research is considered "ethical" when the primary goal is to improve methods of detection or treatment of illness. It should be designed to produce useful, reproducible information and should not be redundant or serve to further individuals or institutions financially or professionally.
   1. Results should be reported honestly, accurately, and in a timely fashion. Misrepresentation or falsifying data is unethical.
   2. Withholding critical information to protect financial interests may create an ethical conflict and jeopardize patient care.
   3. Sponsorship by industry has represented a potential conflict of interest or bias; however, significant developments have been made possible by their involvement, and this form of cooperative effort is gaining acceptance. Specific ethical problems arise with this type of research funding.

C. Informed consent—Human research subjects must provide voluntary, informed consent before participating in any research protocol. Their medical care must not be contingent on their participation, and they must be allowed to withdraw from the study at any time without penalty. Each subject must be able to demonstrate understanding of the information and the ability to make a responsible decision. The decision must be voluntary and not the result of undue pressure or influence. Voluntary, informed consent includes the following requirements.

1. An explanation of the proposed procedure
2. The likely effects and risks of the procedure
3. An explanation of the possible side effects in language easily understood by the patient
4. Methods and conditions of participation

D. Animal use in research

1. The AAOS states that the humane use of animals in research is justified in order to enhance the quality of life of both humans and animals.
2. The use of animals is ethical only when no suitable alternatives are available.
3. Protocols should be designed to minimize the number of animals used. The animals must be used in a manner that avoids abuse and maintains all appropriate animal care standards.
4. The approval of the Animal Care and Use Committee is mandatory, as is following all the applicable regulations and standards.

E. Responsibilities of the **principal investigator** (PI) and coauthors

1. The PI remains responsible for all aspects of the research project, even when duties have been delegated to others.
2. The PI is also responsible for accurately representing the efforts of individuals or agencies involved in the research and citing contributions from other researchers or publications.
3. The coauthors must have made a significant contribution to the design of, collection of data for, and formation of the research project.
4. Each coauthor should sign an affidavit stating that he or she has reviewed the manuscript and agrees with all the results and conclusions presented therein before publication.
5. Resident research should be conducted under the supervision of an attending surgeon. However, the attending surgeon must contribute to the work in actual fact or in a consultative capacity.
6. Scientific publications create information that affects other research and the direct care of patients. If an error in scientific method or failure to replicate results is found, the PI is responsible for accurately reporting this.

F. World Medical Association Declaration of Helsinki (October 2000)— This document was written by the World Medical Association to provide ethical guidance for medical research. It is based on the duty of a physician to "promote and safeguard the health of the people."

VIII. Impairment, Disability, and Handicap

A. Impairment

1. Definition—**Impairments** are conditions that interfere with an individual's activities of daily living. They are characterized by the loss of use or derangement of any body part, system, or function. Impairments are determined by the physician based on the objective results of a physical examination. An impaired individual is not necessarily disabled. For example, a surgeon who loses a hand will be disabled in terms of the ability to operate; however, the surgeon may be fully capable of being the chief of a hospital medical staff and may not be at all disabled with respect to that occupation.
2. **Permanent impairment**—An impairment is permanent when it has become static or well-stabilized with or without medical treatment and is not likely to remit despite maximum medical treatment.

B. Disability

1. Definition—**Disability** is an alteration of an individual's capacity to meet personal, social, or occupational demands or statutory or regulatory requirements because of impairment. Disability may be thought of as the gap between what a person can do and what she or he needs or wants to do. To meet the definition of disability, an individual's impairment or combination of impairments must be of such severity that she or he is not only unable to do the work previously done but also cannot perform any other kind of substantial gainful work, considering the individual's age, education, and work experience.
2. **Permanent disability**—A disability is permanent when it has become static or well-established and is not likely to change despite continuing use of medical or rehabilitative measures.
3. Provisions of the **Americans with Disabilities Act** (ADA)—This legislation, which became effective on July 22, 1992, applies to organizations in the private sector that employ 25 or more employees.
   a. **Accommodation** refers to modifications of a job or workplace that enable a disabled employee to meet the same job demands and conditions as those required of any other employee in the same or similar job.
   b. Under the ADA, the identification of an individual as having a disability does not depend on the results of a medical examination.
   c. An individual may be identified as having a disability if there is a record of an impairment that has substantially limited one or more major life activities.
4. Morbidity associated with disability
   a. Feelings of displacement, depression, and suicide increase as the disability becomes protracted.
   b. There is a higher incidence of drug and alcohol abuse, family disruption, and divorce among disabled workers.

c. Return to employment must be the goal of treatment.

C. Handicap—A **handicap** is related to, but different from, the concepts of disability and impairment. Under federal law, an individual is handicapped if she or he has an impairment that substantially limits one or more of the activities of daily living, has a record of such an impairment, or is regarded as having such an impairment.

SECTION 2 Ethics and the Business of Orthopaedics

I. Conflict of Interest

A. Maintain focus on patient care—Orthopaedic surgery involves complex financial relationships among payers, hospitals, surgeons, other physicians, implant and device manufacturers, attorneys, and the government. Patient care is pre-eminent when conflicts of interest arise in the business of orthopaedics.

B. Disclosure—**Disclosure** is a primary tool for managing potential conflicts of interest in patient care. It may be important in several forums, but disclosure of potential conflicts to patients by physicians is mandatory for maintaining trust. The AAOS Code of Medical Ethics states: "If the orthopaedic surgeon has a financial or ownership interest in a durable medical goods provider, imaging center, surgery center, or other health care facility where the orthopaedic surgeon's financial interest is not immediately obvious, the orthopaedic surgeon must disclose this interest to the patient." Disclosure is important with respect to intellectual property, royalties, and devices as well.

II. Global Services

Physicians have the opportunity to bill for services rendered at a variety of times and venues. However, some services are considered part of a whole and cannot be billed separately. The AAOS Code of Medical Ethics states: "It is unethical for orthopaedic surgeons to bill individually for services that are properly considered a part of the "global service" package where defined, i.e., services that are a necessary part of the surgical procedure." For example, one does not bill separately for office visits scheduled for routine postsurgical follow-up for a period of 90 days. In a similar manner, it is often not possible to bill for certain surgical codes separately when one code is considered a component of a larger procedure. The unethical billing of separate codes has sometimes been called "unbundling." Unbundling can cause significant ethical and legal ramifications in some circumstances.

III. Referrals and Ownership of Medical Services

A. Introduction—There are significant legal and ethical restrictions on patterns of referral among physicians and ownership of medical services. These restrictions and their exceptions are crucial to the day-to-day business of many physicians, including orthopaedic surgeons.

B. Stark laws—Federal legislation was passed in 1995 enacting the **Stark laws**, which continue to be reinterpreted and modified. These laws apply to those physicians serving Medicare and Medicaid patients who refer such patients for medical services called **designated health services** (DHS). In practice, DHS includes most diagnostic and therapeutic services relevant to orthopaedic surgery. In general, the Stark laws prohibit the referral of Medicare and Medicaid patients for DHS to entities in which the referring physician or immediate family member have a financial relationship. Violations may result in a $15,000 civil penalty per claim.

C. Exceptions—In principle, the Stark laws are very broad, prohibiting orthopaedic surgeons from expanding their business interests to include medical services over which they have referral influence. However, the statute has been interpreted to have numerous exceptions. While it is beyond our scope to cover all the nuances of this complex matter, the exception for "in-house ancillary services" has been a matter of special importance and debate. In this exception, orthopaedic surgery groups have been allowed to refer patients for x-rays, MRIs, physical therapy, and outpatient surgical facilities that are within their own practice. While there is potential for abuse, in-house ancillary services constitute an important source of income for some groups, can provide an important service and convenience for the patient, and may offer economic efficiency.

IV. Relationship with Industry

A. Conflict of interest—Medicine and industry work together in improving the treatment of patients. This relationship is even more pronounced in orthopaedics because of the required implants, materials, and techniques. The Code of Medical Ethics and Professionalism for Orthopaedic Surgeons states: "The practice of medicine inherently presents potential conflicts of interest. When a conflict of interest arises, it must be resolved in the best interest of the patient." The physician's role is to use his or her expertise to select the best possible orthopaedic hardware, medication, or treatment for a particular patient's needs. Decisions should be based on the following criteria.

1. Clinical trials in the published medical literature
2. The clinician's expertise
3. The clinician's perspective of the patient's preference

4. Monetary issues, which should enter into the decision process in the realm of cost-effectiveness
   a. Monetary considerations may include limitations of the patient's resources or needs.
   b. There is no role in this decision for consideration of factors that benefit the physician. This is particularly true for financial compensation.

B. Consulting and intellectual property—The practice of individual orthopaedic surgeons' consulting for orthopaedic device and implant manufacturers has come under extreme scrutiny and has generated State Department subpoenas of five large pieces of orthopaedic equipment. Orthopaedic leaders have increased the intensity of the debate about the relationship with industry. This relationship has been described as comprising four types:

Type I is a surgeon possessing intellectual property rights.

Type II is a consulting agreement based on specific expertise.

Type III is a surgeon who is compensated for product promotional activities.

Type IV is a surgeon who is provided benefits in exchange for product use.

There seems little doubt that interactions characteristic of types I and II can be useful for the improvement of patient care. While some type III activities are considered ethical, all type IV activities are ethical violations.

1. Consultation and compensation—Compensation may potentially affect a physician's decision making concerning the choice of particular hardware, medication, or treatment. In this circumstance, the physician must disclose to the patient that she or he receives this financial compensation. Compensation for consulting and speaking engagements must follow the principle of reasonable compensation for demonstrable work that leverages a consultant's unique expertise. Similar to financial interests, any items of money, including royalties received from a manufacturer, must be disclosed to the patient. It is unethical to receive any payment (excluding royalties) from the manufacturer for the use of its product. It is unethical for the physician to agree to exclusively use a product for which the physician receives royalties.
2. Intellectual property—The nature of medical practice builds on innovations and ideas, and to claim exclusive rights to a procedure denies all former individual contributions. The additional fallout from such patents would limit medical education, increase the cost of delivered services, and jeopardize the quality of patient care. The AAOS states that procedure patents are unethical.

C. Industry and educational support

1. Educational support from industry should benefit the patient by providing background information regarding therapy and management without attempting to directly influence treatment decisions.
2. Social functions not associated with an educational element or cash gifts should not be offered to or accepted by orthopaedic surgeons.
3. **Continuing medical education** (CME) subsidies that support educational programs (CME credits provided) are acceptable when they improve patient care. Educational subsidies should not be applied to personal expenses (travel, lodging) for attendees. Any subsidy should be paid directly to the conference sponsor. The faculty at CME courses may accept reasonable honoraria and reimbursement for travel, lodging, and meal expenses.
4. Educational events not tied to CME credits are acceptable at the discretion of the orthopaedic surgeon. There is potential for conflict of interest in these circumstances, and the surgeon must use sound ethical judgment when evaluating and considering such offers.
5. Scholarships to allow residents or fellows to attend CME courses are permitted. Selection for those attending must be made by the resident or fellows program director.

V. Second Opinions

A. Introduction—The definition of specific relationships between physicians and their responsibilities to colleagues and patients can help prevent inappropriate actions. Clear and direct communication between the parties involved can eliminate most problems.

B. **Consultation** implies that the treating physician retains care for the patient but is requesting additional diagnostic or treatment expertise from the consultant. It is unethical for the consulting physician to solicit the care of a patient or make slanderous accusations about the referring physician.

C. **Referral** implies that the treating physician desires to share the care of the patient for a specific service. This request may be temporary or permanent and should be made clear at the outset by the physicians involved.

D. **Transfer by the treating physician** implies complete transfer of care to the accepting physician. All transfers must be made with the consent of the patient.

E. **Second opinions secured** by third-party payers before authorizing procedures are usually governed by contractual agreements. The physician must be aware of provisions in the contract regarding the assumption of care.

VI. Truth in Advertising

A. Principles

1. Federal and state antitrust laws protect truthful advertising.
2. Truthful advertising must not contain any overtly false claim or imply a false claim that would affect a reasonably prudent person. It should include only claims that can be substantiated by the physician and not omit any fact that would influence a reasonably prudent person.

3. Claims should be representative of expected results for the average patient.
4. Care should be exercised when using terms such as "safe and effective" because the layperson equates these terms with no risk and a guarantee of a good result.
5. The advertising of a physician's qualifications should reflect the amount of formal training and degree of expertise and competence.

VII. Insurance and Reimbursement

A. **Centers for Medicare and Medicaid Services** (CMSs)—CMSs are the federal agencies that administer public health programs in the United States. Public health care programs were initiated as part of the Social Security movement in 1965 and have become perhaps the most important economic entities in modern health care.

1. Programs—**Medicare** is a federal health care insurance system for individuals over age 65. **Medicaid** is a federally funded but state-administered health care insurance system for certain low-income and other individuals. Medicare is the larger of the two entities. Medicare covers a very large range of health care services, including all aspects of clinical medicine, some aspects of nursing care, and many advanced technologies. Coverage decisions are made on the basis of medical evidence, government bureaucracy, and politics. The most recent major change has been the addition in 2003 of a prescription drug benefit called Medicare, Part D.
2. Economic impact—The Medicare program is one of the most significant aspects of the federal budget and costs hundreds of billions of dollars annually. The cost of Medicare in 2005 was approximately 2.7% of the United States **gross domestic product** (GDP) and is expected to rise relative to the GDP. Medicare is in a financial crisis because 75-year projections indicate that the program will be underfunded by tens of trillions of dollars based on current trends. Most orthopaedic surgeons accept Medicare insurance. The **Medicare Payment Advisory Commission** (MedPAC) reported in 2006 that 87% of Medicare patients had no or only a minor problem getting an appointment.
3. Reimbursement trends—Concern regarding Medicare reimbursement is growing. Reimbursements for orthopaedic surgical services have steadily declined. Some years there has been no decrease in payments, but the overall trend has been downward, especially for common services such as total joint arthroplasty. More decreases are projected. Some physicians have expressed concern that senior citizens will not be able to receive care based on negative Medicare reimbursement trends. At present, approximately 3% of the practices open to private patients are totally closed to Medicare patients. This proportion may increase, but closure to Medicare patients is unlikely to be effective for most practices because Medicare is the largest payer. Many private insurance plans closely follow Medicare reimbursement decisions and attempt to reimburse for similar services at similar rates.

B. Insurance and reimbursement tools

1. **Relative value units** (RVUs)—Physicians are reimbursed for patient care under a system of relative value units. RVUs are assigned to patient care activities in the clinic, operating room, emergency room, or interventional suite. The RVU for a patient care activity is a combination of the work (time, intensity, effort—about 50% of value), practice expense (overhead, staffing—about 45%), and professional liability insurance (regional malpractice costs—5%). The RVU calculation for thousands of codes and procedures is complex; both government and physician groups are represented in determining updates. Recently, there have been broad measures to increase the RVUs for clinical as opposed to operative work in an effort to encourage conservative care.
2. **Diagnosis-related groups** (DRGs)—DRGs constitute an administrative tool that was developed for Medicare use in the 1980s to assess health care costs and reimbursement for inpatients at an acute care hospital. A DRG is a set of medical conditions (based on a principal diagnosis) that require similar resources for treatment. Reimbursement decisions for hospitals are made by the DRG. Historically, the most important group for orthopaedic surgeons was DRG 209, which included total knee and total hip arthroplasty as well as several less common lower extremity procedures. Although DRG 209 was recently divided into two groups for primary and revision work, the history of the 209 code is telling. The importance of DRG 209 to hospitals, orthopaedic surgeons, and implant manufacturers is hard to overestimate. DRG 209 has routinely been one of the top 10 DRGs since the 1990s. Excluding childbirth, it is the most common major surgical DRG. Concern has been growing about reimbursement for common DRGs. Some reports show that hospitals on average register a loss for many if not all of the 10 most common DRGs. Several potential explanations have been offered, including the rising cost of medical equipment and supplies, the rising cost of nursing and support personnel, and decreasing DRG reimbursement.
3. Gainsharing—The rising cost of implants has been cited as a major issue for orthopaedic surgeons and hospitals alike. The cost of implants has increased, while DRG reimbursement to the hospital has decreased. Whereas the implant is purchased by the hospital with part of the DRG reimbursement, the professional fees of the surgeon are not reimbursed from the DRG. Because the surgeon usually chooses the implant, this has been identified by some as a profound conflict

of interest between the surgeon and hospital. Several schemes have been studied to try to control costs; these are often called **gainsharing** plans. Concerns about the ethics and legality of gainsharing have proliferated. There are powerful stakeholders, including implant manufacturers and hospitals.

4. Pay for performance—An important trend in reimbursement and quality assurance is the adoption of **pay-for-performance** (or P4P) measures by CMS and private insurers. The goal of pay for performance is to ensure that important elements of quality care are standardized for hospitals, orthopaedic surgeons, and managed care organizations. Many pay-for-performance measures have been discussed for orthopaedics. The universal use of systemic anticoagulation postoperatively, the administration of prophylactics antibiotics preoperatively, timely cessation of prophylactic antibiotics postoperatively, and medical management of osteoporosis after osteoporotic fracture treatment have received attention. Various methods have been considered as financial incentives for pay-for-performance measures. It is possible that Medicare payments will ultimately be lowered for organizations and individuals who do not adhere to pay-for-performance guidelines.

C. Emergency room call—Response to an emergency room (ER) call is an increasingly important issue in orthopaedics. Numerous factors have been cited as contributing to a decreasing desire among surgeons to cover an emergency room call, including lifestyle issues and the work attitudes of younger surgeons. However, there is also an important economic component because some orthopaedists increasingly see the emergency room call as a source of underinsured patients who may have difficult pathology. A night call may also interfere with a productive elective schedule during the day. Incentive plans have been tried by some hospitals to increase call participation; some orthopaedic groups have also recruited surgeons specifically for trauma coverage. The Orthopaedic Trauma Association (OTA) has a policy statement suggesting that some trauma patients may be outside the purview of the general orthopaedist. However, many cases found in the emergency room are in the realm of general orthopaedics. Coverage will need to be maintained for many of these patients at many hospitals. There are also significant legal issues involved ER coverage, which are discussed in the subsection on the **Emergency Medical Treatment and Active Labor Act** (EMTALA).

SECTION 3 Ethics and Medicolegal Issues

I. Informed Consent

A. Introduction—Informed consent is a legal doctrine closely associated with the right to autonomy. It requires a physician to obtain permission for treatment to be rendered, an operation to be performed, and many diagnostic procedures. Informed consent is a process, not simply a form or document. It represents an exchange of information between the surgeon and patient (or legal representative) that results in the selection of and agreement to undergo a specific form of treatment. Without proper consent, the surgeon may be guilty of an assault, battery, or trespass against the patient. Most litigation results from unexpected consequences of a procedure. Properly informed patients will be aware of and have decided to accept both the benefits and risks. Consent must be obtained by the attending surgeon. The attending surgeon should explain in layperson's terms the following information.

   The patient's diagnosis and the nature of the condition or illness necessitating intervention
   The nature and purpose of the proposed treatment/procedural plan
   The risk and complications of the treatment or procedure
   All options or alternatives (including no treatment), with their associated risks/complications
   The probability of success (no guarantee of success should be expressed or implied)

B. Decision-making capacity
   1. A patient must be able to understand the clinical circumstances and indications for a procedure.
   2. A patient must be able to understand the alternative approaches to the procedure.
   3. A patient must be able to weigh the alternative approaches and be able and willing to express in an understandable fashion his or her choices.
   4. The level of capacity required of a patient is related to the risks of a procedure and the risk-benefit ratio.
   5. In circumstances in which a patient lacks the ability to make decisions, informed consent may be obtained by a legal guardian or, in situations deemed medically necessary, by a physician.
   6. Special informed-consent rules apply to emergencies and minors.
      a. A medical emergency concerns an unconscious or incapacitated person with a life- or limb-threatening condition who requires immediate medical attention. Treatment can proceed without informed consent. The surgeon must ensure that a description of the patient's medical condition at the time of the emergency is documented in the record, specifically addressing the reason for the emergent condition and why treatment needed to be rendered.
      b. Consent rules for minors vary greatly from state to state. The surgeon must be aware of the

rules that apply locally. Generally, consent for treatment of minors is obtained from the parent or guardian for all but emergency conditions.

C. Documentation of informed consent

A long form (i.e., a detailed form that includes all the specific details of elements noted in the previous discussion)

A short form (may not contain all the specific details; simply states that the risks/benefits have been explained)

A detailed note in the patient's record. A short or long form is usually combined with the note, creating so-called double consent.

D. Standards of disclosure—The degree of disclosure varies among the states, and the courts have developed two standards that may be applied.

1. Professional or reasonable physician standard—This standard is used by most states. It is based on what is customary practice in a specific medical community for surgeons to divulge to their patients.
2. Patient viewpoint standard—This standard is based on the level of information a reasonable person would want to know in a similar circumstance. The courts have shown some preference for this standard in recent years.

II. Physician–Patient Contract

A. Introduction—The AAOS Code of Medical Ethics states: "The physician–patient relationship has a contractual basis and is based on confidentiality, trust, and honesty. Both the patient and the orthopaedic surgeon are free to enter or discontinue the relationship within any existing constraints of a contract with a third party. An orthopaedic surgeon has an obligation to render care only for those conditions that he or she is competent to treat." Within those general guidelines, there a numerous principles, restrictions, and subtleties. Only an experienced attorney can provide advice in this domain, but a few general principles are outlined here.

B. Initiating the physician–patient contract

1. Clearly, a contract may be initiated when a physician actually sees a patient in an office visit or hospital consultation that results in a plan of treatment. Even if initial consultation results in a plan for follow-up as needed or follow-up with another provider, the relationship is ongoing unless certain terms are met, which are outlined below. The relationship may be exclusive to a single operation and appropriate aftercare, with no implication that further unrelated orthopaedic care will be provided.
2. Orthopaedic surgeons do have an obligation to adhere to a "standard of care," although this concept is hard to define precisely. A standard of care is set by what a reasonable orthopaedic surgeon might do under similar circumstances. It is not ethical or legal to offer a perceived undesirable patient substandard care (e.g., nonoperative treatment of a fracture that is typically considered operative) in the hope that the patient will go away. The standard of care is often considered to be regional or local in nature, but several legal cases have been decided on the notion of a national standard of care. This is a complex concept that is often determined on a case-by-case basis.

C. Terminating the physician–patient contract—Once a relationship has been established, it is expected that the relationship will continue except under certain circumstances. The following principles apply.

1. Physicians must always provide emergent treatment to patients.
2. For patients with whom an unsolvable conflict occurs or for those who can no longer pay for services, the physician may sever the physician–patient relationship as long as an alternative source of care can be identified. When an alternative source cannot be identified, caution must be exercised. Even for nonemergent care, there is debate over whether an orthopaedist may terminate care due to an inability to pay.
3. Identifying an alternative source of care is best accomplished in writing and should provide the patient with ample time to establish care with the new provider. This situation also applies if an orthopaedic surgeon withdraws from a managed care contract or no longer accepts an insurance plan.
4. Medical records should be forwarded to the accepting physician, including a medical history and a summary of the treatment rendered. The date of shipping and receipt of records should be documented.
5. A physician is not required to provide therapy that is found to be ethically inappropriate or medically ineffective. Initiation and termination of the physician–patient relationship in the setting of the emergency room are governed by EMTALA and discussed in a separate subsection.

D. Abandonment

1. Wrongful termination of the physician–patient relationship consists of four basic elements.
   a. There must be an established physician–patient relationship.
   b. The patient must have a reasonable expectation that care will be provided.
   c. The patient must have a medical need that requires medical attention, the absence of which will result in harm or injury.
   d. Causation must be established. The failure to provide care must produce injury or harm.
2. Abandonment may take many forms.
   a. It may be alleged that the patient's follow-up is inadequate to recognize common complications.
   b. It could be failure to provide an appointment to an established patient, even if the patient has not paid previous bills, has missed other appointments, has been noncompliant, or has sought interim care from another provider.
   c. There may be a premature discharge from an inpatient setting.

d. If illness, personal conflict, or vacation prevents the physician from attending to patient care, immediate notice must be issued to allow the patient the opportunity to seek care elsewhere.

e. If a patient does not appear for important follow-up appointments, a certified letter should be sent instructing him or her to follow up.

E. Scope of practice—The AAOS Code of Medical Ethics states: "An orthopaedic surgeon should practice only within the scope of his or her personal education, training, and experience." In general, an orthopaedic surgeon may decline to treat a patient with pathology that is outside the scope of his or her practice. However, the restrictions regarding terminating the relationship still apply. Contractual obligations may also be important, especially in the managed care setting, in which an orthopaedic surgeon manages general musculoskeletal care. The AAOS Code of Medical Ethics states: "If an orthopaedic surgeon contracts to provide comprehensive musculoskeletal care, then he or she has the obligation to ensure that appropriate care is provided in areas outside of his or her personal expertise."

III. Medical Liability

A. Crisis and reform—Although the principles of medical liability remain constant, the modern landscape of medical liability is undergoing rapid evolution and reassessment. It is widely felt that there is an ongoing crisis in medical liability that threatens the well-being of patients and physicians alike.

B. Elements of malpractice litigation

1. **Malpractice**—Negligence by a health care provider that results in injury to a patient. A **malpractice suit** is a civil action filed by a patient alleging that a physician's negligence resulted in an injury for which the patient desires compensation. The requirement of the law is proof by a preponderance of the evidence.

   a. **Negligence** is the result of failure to exercise the degree of diligence and care that a reasonable and prudent person would exercise under the same or similar conditions.

   b. **Medical negligence** comprises four elements: duty, breach of duty, causation, and damages.

   (1) **Duty** begins when the surgeon offers to treat the patient and the patient accepts the offer. The duty of the physician is to provide care equal to the same standard of care ordinarily executed by surgeons in the same medical specialty.

   (a) The standard of care is not uniform and is usually established by local expert opinion.

   (b) Residents and fellows are held to the same standard of care as that for board-certified orthopaedists.

   (2) **Breach of duty** occurs when action or failure to act deviates from the standard of care. This may be an **act of commission** (doing what one should not have done) or an **act of omission** (failing to do what one should have done).

   (3) **Causation** is present when it is demonstrated that failure to meet the standard of care was the direct cause of the patient's injuries.

   (4) **Damages** are monies awarded as compensation for injuries sustained as the result of medical negligence.

   (a) **Special damages** are actual expenses, such as medical/rehabilitative expenses and lost wages.

   (b) **General damages**, or noneconomic losses, are awards for pain and suffering, disfigurement, and other causes.

   (c) **Punitive/exemplary damages** serve as a penalty for blatant disregard or incompetence. These are seldom awarded in medical malpractice cases.

   (d) The ***ad quod damnum*** **clause** is the portion of a plaintiff's complaint that specifies the amount of money sought for damages in a suit. Some states do not allow this clause to be included as part of a lawsuit.

2. The **comparative negligence doctrine** awards damages based on the percentage of responsibility for the result by each party.

3. **Contributory negligence** bars the recovery of damages if there was negligence on the part of the plaintiff.

4. **Modified comparative fault** bars the recovery of damages if the plaintiff's percentage of negligence exceeds 50%.

C. Bad faith action—Sometimes a claim is filed and an action pursued regardless of the lack of reasonable grounds for filing the claim. In these circumstances, the physician may countersue for damages.

D. Expert testimony

1. Purpose—Expert testimony is used to determine the standard of care and whether a breach of conduct has occurred. An orthopaedic treating physician has an ethical and legal responsibility to provide accurate and truthful testimony at a patient's request.

2. Requirements to testify—According to the AAOS guidelines for expert testimony, a testifying physician must meet the following requirements:

   Have a current, valid, and unrestricted license to practice medicine in the applicable state

   Have satisfactorily completed the educational requirements of the American Board of Orthopaedic Surgery or a recognized specialty board

   Have experience, education, and/or demonstrated competence in the subject of the case

   Be familiar with clinical practice and applicable standards of care in orthopaedic surgery at the time of the incident

Be fully aware of all the pertinent facts and history of the case at the time of the incident

3. Validity of testimony—The expert should ensure that the testimony is nonpartisan, scientifically correct, and clinically accurate. The expert should testify only to the facts and be prepared to provide documentation for the basis of testimony (personal experience, clinical references, and currently accepted orthopaedic opinion).
4. Compensation—It is unethical to accept compensation based on the outcome of the litigation; however, reasonable compensation commensurate with time and expertise is acceptable.

E. *Res ipsa loquitur*—Certain cases do not require expert testimony. This is the legal doctrine of *res ipsa loquitur* ("the thing speaks for itself"). Examples of this principle are the wrong site of surgery, surgical equipment inadvertently left in the patient, and failure of a physician to attend to a persistently complaining patient in distress.

F. Statute of limitations—A plaintiff must file a malpractice suit within the statute of limitations.
1. The statute of limitations is generally 2 years. However, the time limit varies by state.
2. The statute of limitations for minors may also vary by state; it is generally 2 years from the time of the incident or until the individual's 18th birthday.

G. Discovery
1. Discovery is the process by which both parties find out about each other's cases and is a period of information gathering.
2. Discovery is formed by several techniques of gathering facts.
   a. Interrogatories—Written questions answered in writing under oath.
   b. Deposition—Pretrial oral testimony given under oath.
   c. Production request—Producing documents regarding a claim.
   d. Request for admission—Admitting or denying factual statements under oath.

IV. Malpractice Insurance

A. Two basic types of malpractice insurance: occurrence and claims made.
1. **Occurrence coverage** covers the insured for all claims resulting from action during the period of employment covered by the policy, regardless of when the claim is filed. It continues to cover the physician for occurrences during a specific period even after the physician has ceased working at that particular job/location.
2. **Claims-made coverage** insures the physician during a particular period of employment covered by the policy. Claims filed after the expiration of the policy (usually when the physician leaves a particular job/employer) are not covered even if the events occurred during the period of coverage.

B. Other malpractice coverage
1. **Tail coverage** is a separate policy that covers the physician for all claims made for actions occurring during the period of coverage; this essentially constitutes an occurrence policy.
2. **Prior-act coverage** protects the insured from potential claims resulting from events for which claims have yet to be filed.
3. ***Locum tenens* coverage** provides extended insurance coverage to a physician who temporarily replaces the policyholder.
4. **Slot coverage** covers duties encountered while practicing in a specific position through which several physicians may rotate.

C. Policies may have specific restrictions or exclusions.
1. Some policies cover only direct patient care.
2. Activities such as peer review, quality assurance, and utilization review may be covered by the insurance policy or a health care contract.
3. Nearly all policies for residents/fellows have an exclusion for moonlighting. The residents and fellows must either ensure that the institution where they are moonlighting provides coverage or purchase professional liability insurance on their own behalf.
4. The **hold harmless clause** is a contractual statement that attempts to shift liability from the employer to the physician. Insurance carriers do not generally cover this contractual obligation.

D. Surcharging or experience rating—Insurance plans may assess points against a physician based on the number of claims filed and dollar amounts awarded on behalf of the insured.

E. The **Good Samaritan Act**—This act grants immunity for actions performed in good faith by persons at the scene of an emergency. Immunity is not given if the act constitutes gross, willful, or wanton neglect. This does not extend to care given in expectation of payment by persons who routinely render care in an emergency room or by the patient's admitting, attending, or treating physician.

F. The AAOS recommends that a resident or fellow make a point of obtaining evidence of insurance for each year of residency and saving this evidence in personal files.

V. Liability Status of Residents and Fellows

A. Introduction—The status of residents and fellows as licensed physicians who are functioning as employees while they are in a training/educational program creates a special relationship between them and their patients and supervisors.

B. Disclosure to patients—Failure to inform a patient of residency/fellow status may result in claims of fraud, deceit, misrepresentation, assault, battery, and lack of informed consent.

C. Levels of responsibility
1. Residents and fellows are responsible for their own actions.
2. Supervisors may be held accountable for the actions of the residents and fellows. This is known as **vicarious liability**.
3. ***Respondeat superior*** ("Let the master answer")—This doctrine is also known as "borrowed

servant'' or the ''captain of the ship.'' An agency relationship is established by the fact that the resident has been authorized to act for or represent the supervising physician. As an agent for the supervisor, all acts of the relationship are considered to be under the direction of the supervisor. This relationship is independent of the specific employer of the trainee.

4. Residents and fellows are held to the same standard of care as a fully trained, practicing orthopaedist, regardless of their level of training. Residents should not attempt to perform procedures that are beyond their level of training. Appropriate consultation with their supervisors is imperative in any situation. The lack of appropriate consultation puts the resident at risk of acting independent of the supervisor.

D. The AAOS recommends that residents and fellows retain permanent documentation regarding the resolution of any adverse decision in which they may be named. Adverse decisions will be reported to the National Practitioner Data Bank and the resulting information made available to all health care facilities, as will any pending litigation. Documentation regarding the individual cases and information on the resolution of adverse decisions will be necessary when the individual seeks privileges at any health care facility.

VI. Emergency Medical Treatment and Active Labor Act (EMTALA)

A. Elements

1. EMTALA is a set of laws from 1986 and updated in 2003 that govern how hospitals treat and transfer patients presenting with unstable medical conditions. This is sometimes called an ''anti-dumping'' law. In general, hospitals must treat a patient in order to ''stabilize'' an unstable medical condition regardless of the ability to pay.
2. EMTALA applies to hospitals that provide emergency services to Medicare and Medicaid patients. The regulations apply to all patients at such hospitals, not just Medicare patients. In practice, it applies to nearly all hospitals except some specialty and military hospitals. Any patient who comes to the emergency room requesting treatment must receive a screening exam to identify a possible emergency condition. A patient in whom an emergency condition exists must receive treatment until the condition is ''stabilized'' or until transfer or discharge is unlikely to result in deterioration of the condition. Once stabilized, a patient may be transferred if the benefits of transfer outweigh the risks (documented) and the receiving institution accepts the transfer. Records must accompany the transfer.

B. On-call and follow-up care

1. In general, EMTALA places responsibility on the hospital itself. However, important restrictions apply to physicians. An ''on-call'' physician who fails to respond to an emergency medical condition is in violation of these laws. An orthopaedic surgeon who affirms that an unstable patient is stable and authorizes his or her transfer is also in violation. Even a physician who accepts a transfer by telephone may have established a relationship and thus be liable under some circumstances.
2. A more common scenario involves follow-up care, but the law is unclear. An orthopaedist who is on call for the emergency room and either sees the patient or formulates a plan of care without seeing the patient has established a relationship. This does not constitute a clear obligation to provide follow-up care under EMTALA once the patient has been stabilized. However, it may be interpreted in different ways, and the orthopaedist may have some obligation for ongoing care regardless of the patient's ability to pay.
3. There is no law forcing orthopaedists to be on call. Hospitals have a federally mandated responsibility to provide care to emergency patients. Orthopaedists in every community have a responsibility to ensure that emergency patients receive appropriate and timely musculoskeletal care. The AAOS position statement concerning on-call responsibilities notes that hospitals are obligated to assume a portion of the growing costs of providing emergency care. Many effective strategies are emerging, with hospitals providing stipends or other reimbursements to orthopaedic surgeons to help defray the extra expenses of on-call services.

C. Medical records—The medical record is a complex document with several important purposes in addition to its critical role in patient care. Whether it is used in legal proceedings or not, the medical record is a legal document. The record should be treated as if it is being constantly reviewed by parties with differing perspectives and objectives. Communication must be complete and clear. The following statements cover several legal and practical aspects of the medical record.

1. Medical records represent the best defense in a malpractice lawsuit.
   a. Medical records must be maintained for 7 years after the last date of treatment.
   b. Medical records are confidential and cannot be reproduced or discussed with parties not involved in treating the patient without the patient's written approval.
2. Accurate and complete medical records protect both the patient and physician from errors and misinterpretations. Records should be
   - Well-documented, detailing the history, observations, reasons for the treatment provided, and patient noncompliance
   - Legible and clear
   - Accurate and should properly identify the patient
   - A logical sequence of the events and factors affecting treatment decisions
   - An outline of the treatment plan, including the risks, benefits, and alternatives
   - Free from editorial comments or casual criticism of the patient or other health care providers

3. Medical records should never be altered.
   a. All corrections should be made by amendments. These amendments should accurately reflect the reason for correction and be placed after the last entry.
   b. An errant entry should be lined through so that it remains legible. The reason for the correction, the date, the time, and the physician's initials must be included.
   c. Removing or obscuring an entry shatters credibility and is indefensible.
   d. Attempts to supplement or clarify entries after notification of a lawsuit constitute tampering.
4. On notification of a lawsuit, the medical records should be secured, inventoried, and copied. Copies of the medical record must be made available to the patient or the attorney in a reasonable amount of time. The medical record must not be withheld as ransom for outstanding bills.
5. **Health Insurance Portability and Accountability Act** (HIPAA)—This legislation describes the federal security and privacy laws that regulate the disclosure of a patient's personal medical records. Practices must develop specific policies on the use of private patient information. Patients must sign notices describing the policies for practices to release the private information. In addition, patients would have to sign a specific authorization form before a covered entity could release their medical information to a life insurer, a bank, a marketing firm, or another outside business for purposes not related to their health care.

SECTION 4 Probability and Statistics

As a consumer of medical research, the orthopaedic surgeon needs to have a firm grasp of statistical concepts. The ability to discern superior from inferior research allows the surgeon to make sound clinical decisions. Probability theory is a mathematical construct that underlies the practical use of statistics. Concepts and terms are often used interchangeably between probability and statistics. We discuss the fundamental concepts of probability and statistics in turn.

I. Probability Distributions

A. Introduction—A **probability distribution** is a mathematical object that allows one to answer any meaningful question about the likelihood and probability of a given scientific problem. There are many distributions, but only a few are very useful.

B. **Random variables** are described by probability distributions. These variables represent the quantities involved in a scientific problem. Random variables can be continuous numbers (e.g., 100.0) such as leg length or angle of radial inclination. They can be categorical or discrete, such as fracture versus no fracture or male versus female. Some categorical random variables result from cutoff values of continuous random variables (e.g., leg-length discrepancy >2 cm or radial inclination > 11 degrees).

C. Types of probability distribution
   1. Normal (Gaussian) distribution
      a. The most important continuous distribution is the **normal distribution** (Fig. 12–1). The normal distribution is determined by two quantities, the **mean** and **standard deviation** (SD). The mean is a measure of central tendency. Changing the mean shifts the entire curve along the x-axis, whereas changing the SD changes the width of the curve along the x-axis. The normal distribution is unimodal, bell shaped, and symmetrical at a horizontal line equal to the mean value. Virtually all observations in a normal distribution occur within mean ±3 SD, 95% within mean ±2 SD, and 66% within mean ±1 SD.
      b. In real-world research, there are important reasons for assuming that the distributions of many continuous variables are normal. One can also test statistically whether a distribution is normal. In summary, one will usually assume a continuous distribution is normal unless there are warning signs that indicate otherwise, which are discussed below. Statistics that assume a normal distribution are called **parametric statistics** and include the most common statistics, such as the t-test, mean, and SD. Statistics for continuous variables that do not assume a normal distribution are called **nonparametric statistics**; there are nonparametric versions of most parametric statistics, which are discussed below.
   2. 2 × 2 tables as distributions—The most important categorical distribution is the 2 × 2 table. This familiar distribution is usually used in orthopaedic surgery to compare a diagnosis with a diagnostic test, resulting in sensitivities and specificities that are discussed in detail below. In practice, a 2 × 2 table is a statistic because the boxes are filled in with real data. However, in theory, a table is also a probability distribution under certain circumstances. We devote an entire subsection to the analysis of the 2 × 2 table. However, it is useful to think of the table as a probability distribution because it makes concepts such as sensitivity/specificity, positive/negative predictive value, the p-value, and power much clearer.

II. Statistics

A. Populations and samples—A **population** is a collection of all possible measurements that could be used to address a hypothesis. A **sample** is a subset of a population that is analyzed with statistics because it is

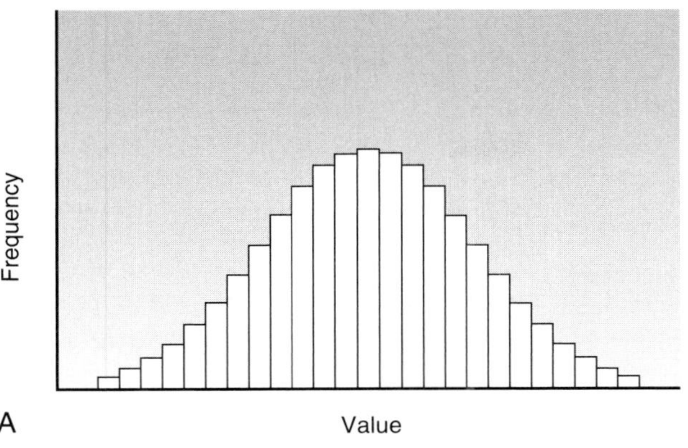

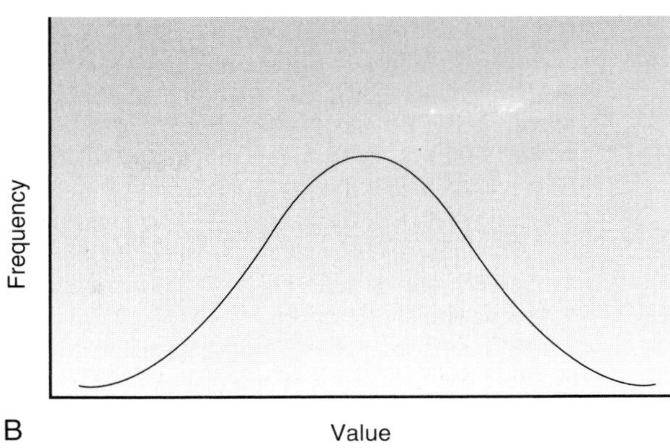

FIGURE 12–1 Normal (Gaussian) distribution. **A**, Probability distribution of actual data plotted as a histogram with very narrow ranges. **B**, The idealized way this is represented in textbooks, articles, and tests. (From Jekel JF, Elmore JG, Katz DL: Epidemiology, Biostatistics, and Preventive Medicine. Philadelphia, WB Saunders, 1996.)

usually not possible to study the whole population. **Criteria of inclusion and exclusion** define the sample and the population to which the study applies. **Statistical inference** is the process of drawing conclusions about the population from analysis of the sample. Ideally, the sample is a random subset of the population, so any member of the population is equally likely to be represented. To the extent that the sample is not random, the inferences will be biased. Several different types of bias are discussed below.

B. Inference, hypothesis testing, and decision analysis—In **statistical inference**, the goal is to estimate a population quantity from a sample. A **point estimate** is a single number that provides the best estimate in some sense. A **confidence interval** is a range of values that represents an interval in which the value is likely to lie (e.g., with 95% confidence). Inference is one large branch of statistics. In **hypothesis testing**, the goal is to reach a statistical judgment on whether a given question is true (e.g., "Is the treatment effective?"). In **decision analysis**, the goal is to combine the results of inference and hypothesis testing with information about outcomes to determine an optimum treatment.

C. Clinical research studies—Clinical research studies are addressed in detail later. In **observational studies**, the management of clinical patients as it currently exists is the object of study. In **experimental studies**, the management of patients is altered in order to conduct an experiment. By far the most important experimental study is the **randomized controlled trial** (RCT), in which a single variable (e.g., a treatment) is randomly assigned. The goal is to assess the effect of the treatment on some outcome variables. Variables other than the treatment may also affect the outcome. These other factors in the design are often called **confounding variables** because they may influence the conclusions if not properly addressed. In experimental studies, randomization controls for confounding variables.

D. Bias—**Bias** is a flaw in impartiality that alters the manner in which measurement, analysis, or assessment is recorded, conducted, or interpreted. Randomization controls the bias that would otherwise be introduced by confounding variables, but other types of bias exist. **Blinding** controls bias that arises when orthopaedic surgeons have information about study subjects that may compromise their impartiality, however subconsciously or subtly it may occur. Meticulous attention to the study protocol is also important in minimizing bias. **Selection bias** is introduced by a nonrandom selection of a sample from a given population. **Observational or informational bias** occurs when a measurement/outcome is affected by the characteristics of the study group itself. There are numerous potential sources of bias that are given special names. The most important issue is to understand that potential biases exist and to research ways to minimize or assess their effects.

E. Clinical instruments (Fig. 12–2)—**Clinical instruments** are outcome variables that are designed by experts to assess function, pain, or other clinically important judgments. They usually have multiple components involving multiple-choice questions, scales, or ratings completed by the patient or clinician. In a diagnostic study, **intraobserver variability** may occur between successive observations by the

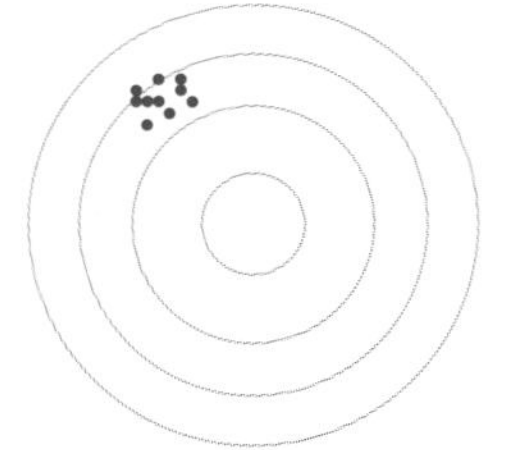

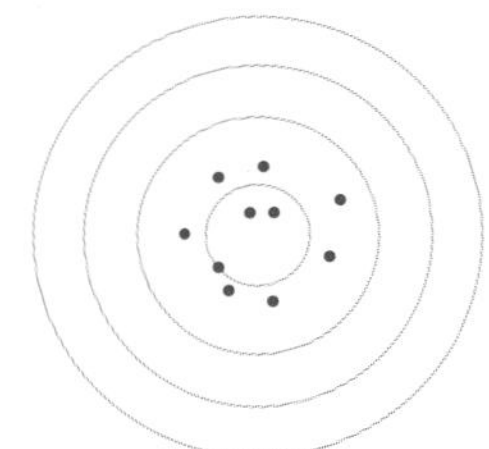

Precision (high)	Accuracy (high)
Reliability (high)	Validity (high)
Variability (low)	Bias (low)

A B

FIGURE 12–2 Measurements of instrument properties.

same surgeon. **Interobserver variability** occurs between observations by different surgeons.

1. An instrument is **valid** if it produces an average measure of the outcome of interest, such as the familiar WOMAC (Western Ontario and McMaster University) score for lower extremity function. Validity in clinical instruments is an example of the general notion of accuracy in statistics.
2. An instrument is **reliable** if it produces similar scores in similar situations.
3. A measure is **accurate** if it produces an average estimate of the quantity of interest. A measure that is not accurate is biased.
4. A measure is **precise** if it produces very similar outcomes under similar circumstances. A measure that is not precise has high variability.

F. Dependency, correlation, and causation—Probability and statistics in general are concerned with dependency and correlation. **Dependency** occurs when two or more variables are known to affect each other without any indication of which one is the cause and which the effect. **Correlation** is the term given to two dependent continuous variables. Probability and statistics usually do not involve judgments about **causation**, with one important exception. RCTs can prove causation directly by isolating the randomized variable from the web of dependencies and correlations. There are sophisticated methods for attempting to prove causation without RCTs, but they are beyond our scope.

III. 2 × 2 Table Analysis

A. Tests for disease—The concept of a 2 × 2 table as a statistical comparison of two categorical random variables was introduced earlier. Here we define the concepts of table analysis, which are familiar to most orthopaedic surgeons. However, we approach them in a systematic way so that the many relationships among the concepts are more apparent. Figure 12–3 demonstrates the quantities graphically. The cells of the table are often filled with counts when the data are initially gathered. **Counts** are the numbers of patients in each situation (e.g., 15 patients with a positive test who also have disease). Because the properties of a table are **probabilities** (or frequencies), the table must be normalized by dividing each cell by the total number of patients.

1. Basic 2 × 2 table—The basic 2 × 2 table is shown in Figure 12–3A. It is important to construct the table the same way each time. Label the columns +/− for **disease** (D). Then label the rows +/− for the **test** (T). Label the cells of the table a, b, c, and d as you would read, left to right and top to bottom. Some authors like to label the cells as a = **true positive** (TP), b = **false positive** (FP), c = **false negative** (FN), and d = **true negative** (TN). However, this notation is cumbersome and can be distracting. Once the patterns are clear, the T/F and P/N notation is easy to re-create if desired.
2. Sensitivity—**Sensitivity** is the probability of a positive test, given the presence of disease. It is a property of the test itself and is computed from columns (see Fig. 12–3B).

$$\text{sensitivity} = a/(a + c)$$

3. Specificity—**Specificity** is the probability of a negative test, given the absence of disease. It is a property of the test itself and is computed from columns (see Fig. 12–3C).

$$\text{specificity} = d/(b + d)$$

4. Positive predictive value—**Positive predictive value** is the probability of disease, given a positive test. It is a property of the test's interacting with the prevalence of disease in the community (see below). It is computed from rows (see Fig. 12–3D).

$$\text{positive predictive value} = a/(a + b)$$

5. Negative predictive value—**Negative predictive value** is the probability of health, given a negative test. It is a property of the test's interacting with the prevalence of health in the community (see below). It is computed from rows (see Fig. 12–3E).

$$\text{negative predictive value} = d/(c + d)$$

6. Accuracy—The **accuracy of a test** is the probability of a correct test result. It is a property of the test's interacting with the prevalence of disease and health in the community (see below). Accuracy is computed from both rows and columns (see Fig. 12–3F).

$$\text{accuracy} = (a + d)/(a + b + c + d)$$

7. Prevalence of disease—The **prevalence of disease** is the probability of disease in the community, given no test information. Prevalence is computed from both rows and columns (see Fig. 12–3G).

$$\text{prevalence of disease} = (a + c)/(a + b + c + d)$$

8. Prevalence of health—The **prevalence of health** is the probability of health in the community, given no test information. Prevalence is computed from both rows and columns (see Fig. 12–3H).

$$\text{prevalence of health} = (b + d)/(a + b + c + d)$$

9. False-positive rate—The **false-positive rate** is the probability of a positive test, given the absence of disease. It is computed from columns (see Fig. 12–3I).

$$\text{false-positive rate} = b/(b + d)$$

10. False-negative rate—The **false-negative rate** is the probability of a negative test, given the presence of disease. It is computed from columns (see Fig. 12–3J).

$$\text{false-negative rate} = c/(a + c)$$

B. Relationships—Four numbers uniquely define a 2 × 2 table. We have listed seven different summary

- Draw the table
- Write "Disease" on top
- Letter left to right and top to bottom
- You are asked for **probabilities**

A

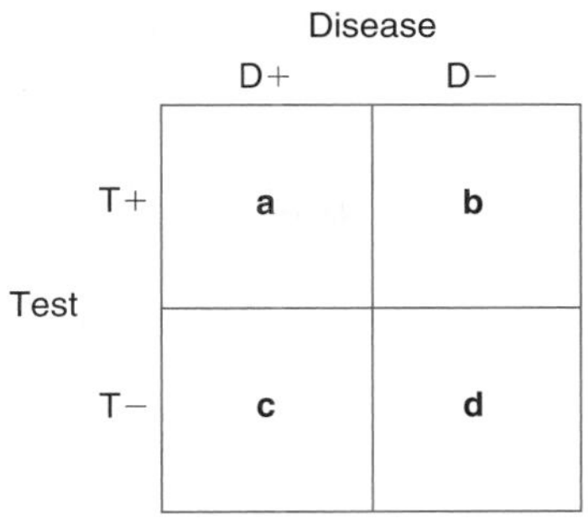

	Disease D+	Disease D−
Test T+	**a**	**b**
Test T−	**c**	**d**

- Accuracy
- (a + d)/(a + b + c + d)
- Correct test results irrespective of positive/negative results

B

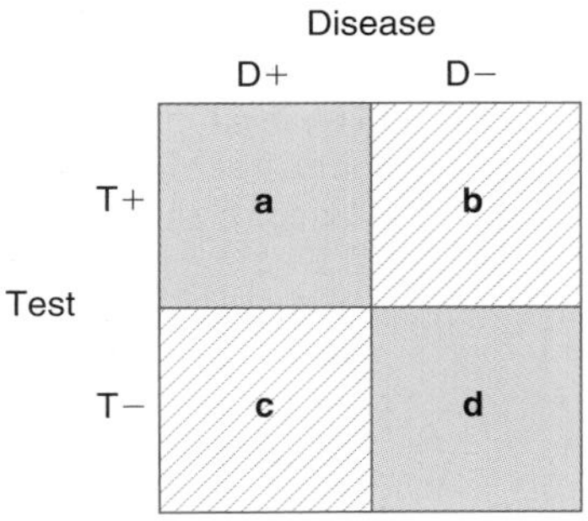

	Disease D+	Disease D−
Test T+	**a**	**b**
Test T−	**c**	**d**

- Sensitivity
- a/(a + c)
- Probability of a positive test, given the presence of disease

C

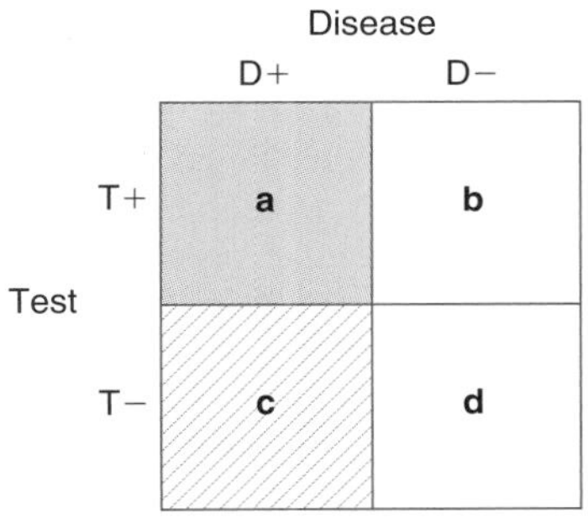

	Disease D+	Disease D−
Test T+	**a**	**b**
Test T−	**c**	**d**

- Specificity
- d/(b + d)
- Probability of a negative test, given the absence of disease

D

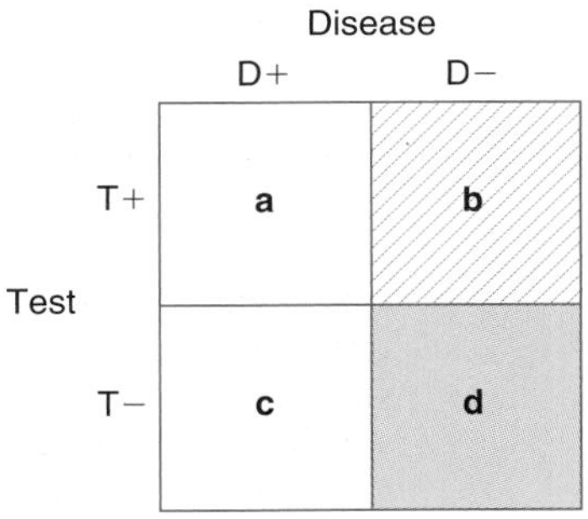

	Disease D+	Disease D−
Test T+	**a**	**b**
Test T−	**c**	**d**

- Positive predictive value
- a/(a + b)
- Probability of disease, given a positive test

E

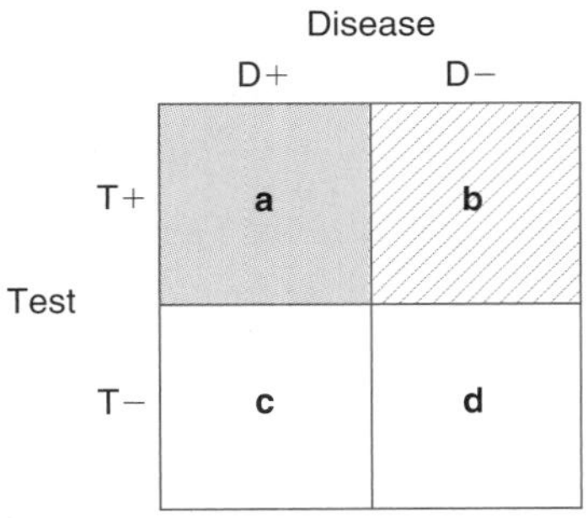

	Disease D+	Disease D−
Test T+	**a**	**b**
Test T−	**c**	**d**

- Negative predictive value
- d/(c + d)
- Probability of health, given a negative test

F

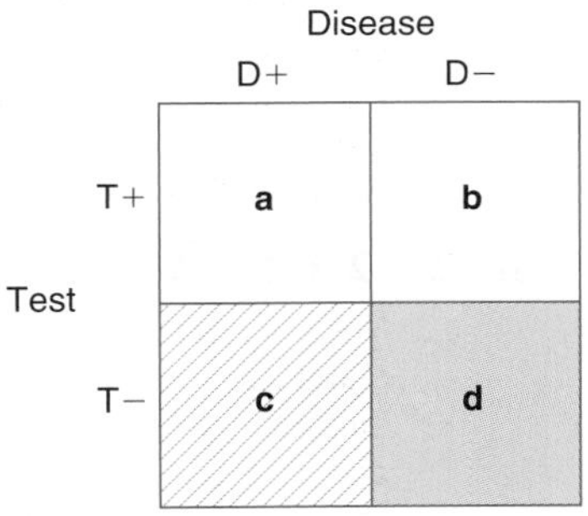

	Disease D+	Disease D−
Test T+	**a**	**b**
Test T−	**c**	**d**

- Prevalence of disease
- (a + c)/(a + b + c + d)
- Probability of disease, given no test information

G

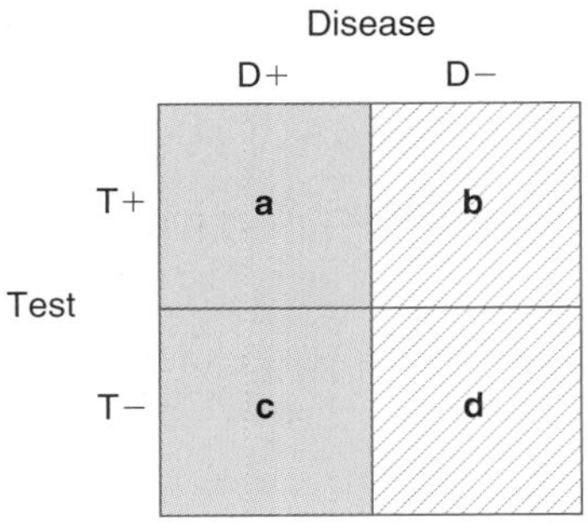

	Disease D+	Disease D−
Test T+	**a**	**b**
Test T−	**c**	**d**

- Prevalence of health
- (b + d)/(a + b + c + d)
- Probability of health, given no test information

H

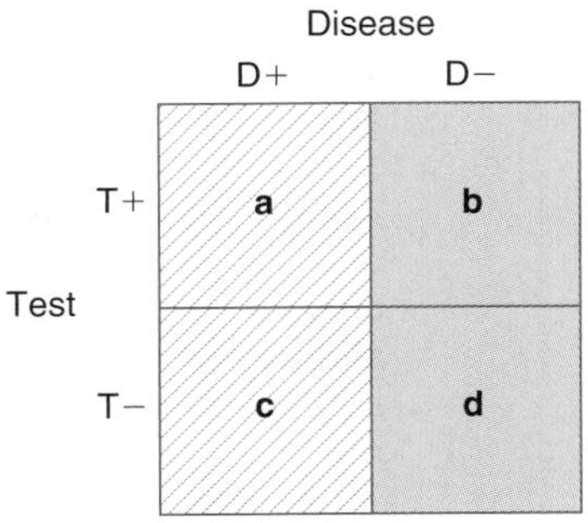

	Disease D+	Disease D−
Test T+	**a**	**b**
Test T−	**c**	**d**

- False-positive rate
- b/(b + d)
- Probability of a positive test, given the absence of disease

I

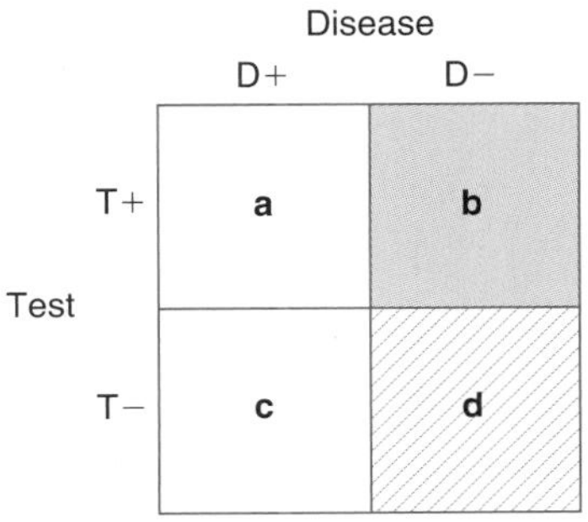

	Disease D+	Disease D−
Test T+	**a**	**b**
Test T−	**c**	**d**

- False-negative rate
- c/(a + c)
- Probability of a negative test, given the presence of disease

J

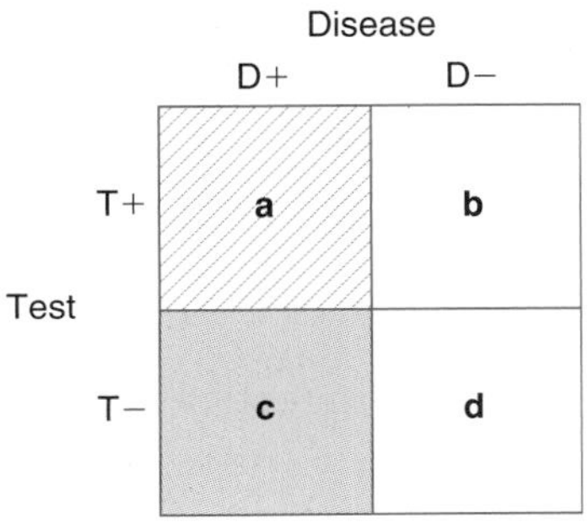

	Disease D+	Disease D−
Test T+	**a**	**b**
Test T−	**c**	**d**

FIGURE 12–3 Examples of 2 × 2 tables.

measures of a table as tests for disease; therefore, there must be relationships among these quantities. These relationships are called **constraints**, and they should accord with your intuition of the relationships and their clinical meanings.

$$\text{false-positive rate} = 1 - \text{sensitivity}$$

$$\text{false-negative rate} = 1 - \text{specificity}$$

$$\text{positive predictive value} \propto \text{prevalence of disease} \times \text{sensitivity}$$

$$\text{negative predictive value} \propto \text{prevalence of health} \times \text{specificity}$$

The two relationships among the predictive values, prevalences, sensitivities, and specificities are fundamental. They are a form of the **Bayes theorem**, a basic result in probability theory.

C. Screening and confirmation with diagnostic tests—Different types of tests are used for screening and confirmation of a diagnosis.

1. **Screening** involves testing a large number of individuals, presuming that there is a low prevalence of disease in the population and many healthy individuals. Sensitive tests are used for screening because they have a low false-negative rate. They are unlikely to miss an affected individual. A sensitive test increases the positive predictive value in the presence of a low prevalence of disease.
2. **Confirmation** of a diagnosis involves testing a smaller number of individuals, presuming that there is a high prevalence of disease in the population and many affected individuals. Specific tests are used for confirmation because they are unlikely to result in false treatment of a healthy individual. A specific test increases the negative predictive value in the presence of a low prevalence of health.

D. Tests with continuous variables

1. Cutoff value of a test—The analysis of 2 × 2 tables is presented for categorical variables. But many of these variables result from a cutoff value applied to a continuous variable. A **cutoff value** is a number above or below which a laboratory result is considered significant (e.g., serum potassium > 5.5). There are important issues involved in both choosing the cutoff value and designing the test itself so that a useful cutoff value may be chosen. In brief, choosing a cutoff value involves trading sensitivity for specificity.
2. Receiver operating characteristic (ROC) curves—The **ROC curve** is a graphical representation of the tradeoffs involved in designing a diagnostic test with a cutoff value. A typical ROC curve is a plot of sensitivity (on the y-axis) versus 1 − specificity (or false-positive rate) on the x-axis. Before a cutoff value is chosen, the test itself must be designed. An ideal ROC curve rises quickly to the upper left corner of the graph and then continues to rise slowly. A poor ROC curve rises more slowly to a point short of the upper left corner of the graph and then continues to rise (Fig. 12–4). The overall shape of a test is determined by physical law, biochemical properties, or the financial resources used in the design or manufacturing of the test. Once the overall ROC curve is fixed, the surgeon or experimenter decides how to use the test by choosing a cutoff value. Different cutoff values result in a balanced test, or a test that is optimized for use in screening or confirmation (Fig. 12–5).

IV. Hypothesis Testing

A. Null and alternative hypotheses

1. The nature of scientific inquiry—The basic nature of scientific inquiry with the use of statistics revolves around the null hypothesis and collecting data regarding it. The **null hypothesis** (H_0) is the hypothesis to be tested; often there is no difference between two sets of data or between or among subsets of a data set. The **alternative hypothesis** is just the opposite of the null hypothesis. One important point is that data are gathered to comment on the null hypothesis. This hypothesis is never truly proven, but data can cast doubt on it. The null hypothesis is finally accepted when a preponderance of data have failed to cast doubt on it.

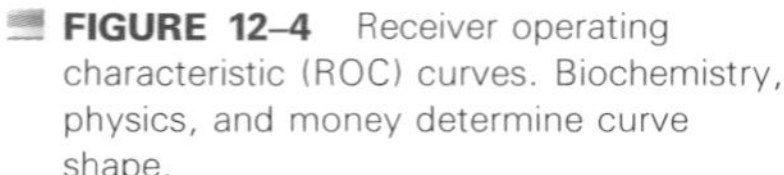
FIGURE 12–4 Receiver operating characteristic (ROC) curves. Biochemistry, physics, and money determine curve shape.

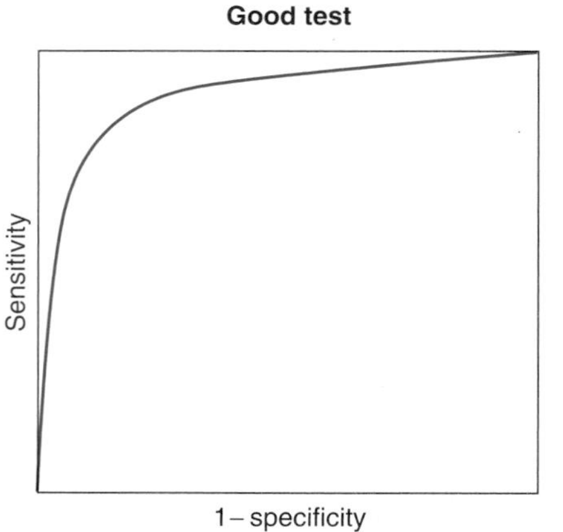

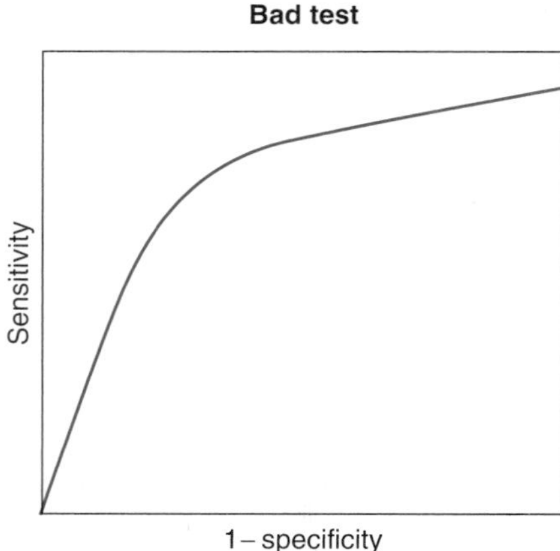

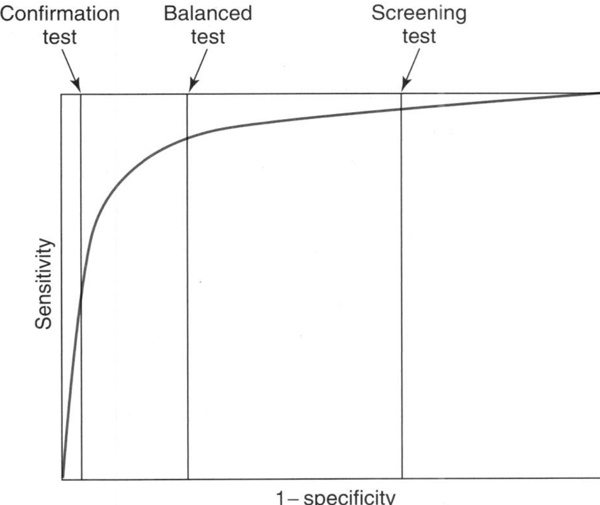

FIGURE 12–5 Receiver operating characteristic (ROC) curves. The surgeon, experimenter, and manufacturer determine the cutoff values.

2. Probability of data, given the null hypothesis—It is useful to consider the probability of the data, given the null hypothesis. Figure 12–6A is a schematic of an idealized probability distribution for the probability of the data, given the null hypothesis. The **p-value** can be calculated for a statistic; it is the probability that the data arose by chance, supposing that the null hypothesis is true. As such, a small p-value casts doubt that the null hypothesis is true. In the schematic (Fig. 12–6B), the p-value is the area under the tails of the probability distribution for the data, given the null hypothesis. The process of accepting or rejecting the null hypothesis involves choosing a cutoff for the p-value. In practice, $p < 0.05$ is usually termed a **significant difference** (Fig. 12–6C), and the experimenter rejects the null hypothesis. In practice, $p > 0.05$ is usually termed **no significant difference**, and the experimenter accepts the null hypothesis. This process constitutes the core procedure of hypothesis testing. The various tradeoffs and characteristic values are discussed below in greater detail.

B. Type I error rate (α)—By setting a cutoff for the p-value as above, the experimenter is choosing the allowable rate of false-positive errors. By setting the cutoff for the p-value at 0.05, the experimenter is saying that it is acceptable to detect a false-positive difference that occurs by pure chance 5% of the time in an attempt to detect true negative differences. A **type I error** is a **false-positive difference**.

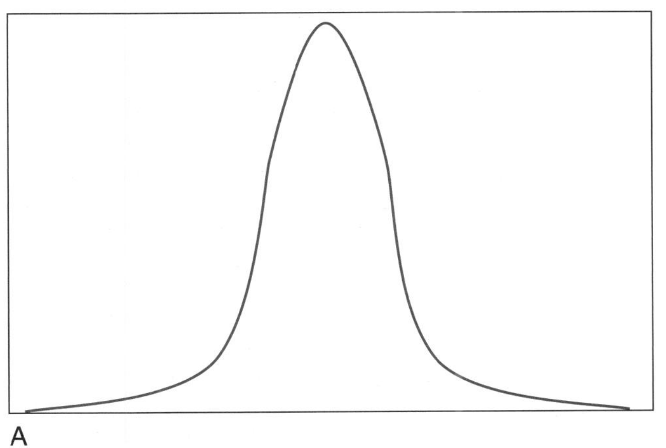

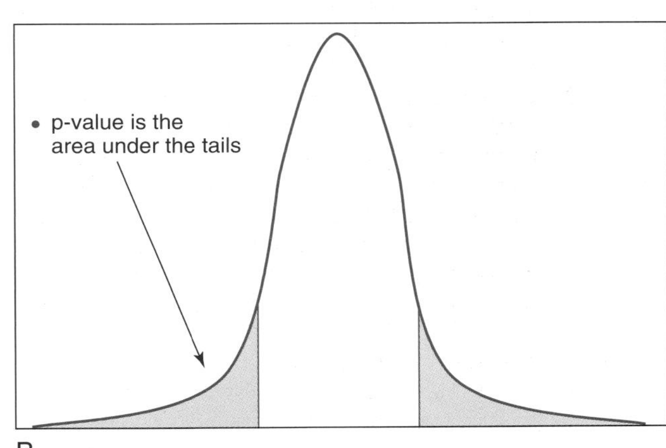

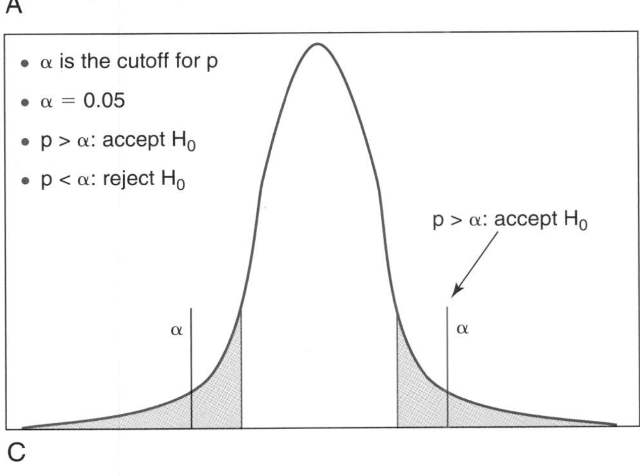

FIGURE 12–6 **A**, Schematic of an idealized probability distribution for the data, given the null hypothesis. **B**, The p-value is the area under the tails of the probability distribution for the data, given the null hypothesis. **C**, The process of accepting or rejecting the null hypothesis involves choosing a cutoff for the p-value. In practice, $p < 0.05$ is usually termed a significant difference.

This outcome corresponds to detecting a difference when in fact there is no difference or rejecting the null hypothesis when one should accept it. The type I error rate is the false-positive rate, sometimes called alpha (α), and it is the cutoff for the p-value chosen by the experimenter.

C. Type II error rate (β)—Choosing the type I error rate is familiar to most readers. The type II error rate is equally important; however, it is possible to do an entire study and be ignorant of the type II error rate inherent in the study design, although it is ill-advised. A **type II error** is a **false-negative difference**. This outcome corresponds to detecting no difference when in fact there is a difference or accepting the null hypothesis when one should reject it. The type II error rate can be calculated given the type I error rate and the sample size (for most experiments). The conventional value for the type II error rate is 0.2. By setting the type II error rate at 0.2, the experimenter is saying that it is acceptable to conclude a false-negative difference that occurs by pure chance 20% of the time in an attempt to detect true-negative differences. The type II error rate is the false-negative rate, sometimes called beta (ß), and it is chosen by the experimenter. The power is $1-\beta$, or the probability of detecting a true-positive difference. The experimenter chooses the false-negative rate or **power** (usually 80%).

D. Experimental design
   1. There is an intimate relationship among the type I error rate, type II error rate (or power), and sample size. Ideally, wouldn't we like to have the type I error rate be very low and the power very high? One must trade the type I error rate and power for a fixed sample size. The experimenter can decrease type I errors and increase power simultaneously only by increasing the sample size. Increasing the sample size costs time and money and increases the study complexity, and it also may entail patient morbidity. So the tradeoffs must be managed carefully in designing an experiment.
   2. ***A priori* power analysis** is the preferred method for experimental design. In a priori power analysis, the type I error rate is chosen (e.g., 0.05), the power is chosen (e.g., 80%), and then the sample size needed to achieve the desired power is calculated. The experiment is executed with the needed number of samples. Exactly how the calculations are performed is beyond our scope, but they are well-defined for many statistics. To perform the calculations, one must have an estimate of the effect size, which is the expected size of the difference between the null and alternative hypotheses, an idea that can be made mathematically precise.
   3. ***Post-hoc* power analysis** refers to how many experiments are performed in practice. In post hoc power analysis, the type I error rate is chosen and then a number of samples are chosen that are reasonable to do. The experimenter asks, "How many patients are in my series?" or "How much funding do I have?" and obtains the number of samples that is practical under this constraint. From the type I error rate and number of samples, the power is calculated. If the number of samples is too small, the power to detect true-positive differences will be small and the type II error rate will be large. A negative result will be less meaningful.
   4. Implications—The asymmetry between type I and type II errors and the prevalence of post hoc power analysis have several implications for orthopaedic science. Literature reviews have been performed claiming that many negative results are from underpowered studies; these results may be false-negatives. Many studies omit even post hoc power analysis. In such reports, not only may the study be underpowered but also an estimate of the effect is not even offered. Finally, the type I error rate is often set at 0.05, whereas the type II error rate is often set at 0.20 even in well-designed studies. Are type I errors worse? Is it worse to pollute the scientific literature with a claim of an effect where none exists? Or is it worse to claim that there is no effect with a beneficial therapy? These are difficult questions. Designing good experiments takes experience and resources.

V. Statistics and Tests

A. Introduction—There are numerous statistics and statistical tests for various situations and distributions. Here we cover some general principles of statistics and several of the most commonly used and tested statistical procedures.

B. Descriptive statistics—These are used to summarize data in a few numbers, such as the mean and SD. Often the goal of statistics is **inference**, to learn something about the properties of the population from the sample. The mean and SD are also used for inference, because these statistics are estimates of the population mean and SD if the distribution is normal. Statistics are also useful for hypothesis testing, as described above. A common pattern is to perform inference and hypothesis testing in sequence. We might calculate the correlation coefficient between two variables and then test the hypothesis that the correlation is significant. Statistics are also used for decision analysis, which is discussed briefly.

C. Review of statistics—Statistics are relevant to either **continuous** or **categorical distributions**. Parametric statistics are relevant to **normal (bell-curve) distributions**, and nonparametric statistics apply when the distribution is not normal or unknown. Most statistical procedures apply when all of the variables are assumed to be dependent, although it is occasionally possible to control one or more variables experimentally (the **independent variables**) and measure the other variables (the **dependent variables**). The most common statistics compare two variables. However, sophisticated procedures exist for analyzing the relationships among many variables simultaneously. These procedures are discussed briefly. Some of them exist for comparing matched samples, samples that correspond value by value rather than just as a whole group. Statistics such as the median and mean are measures of **central tendency or location**: they give a single summary measure. Statistics such as the SD and range are measures of **variability or spread**: they give a summary measure of the width of a sample.

D. One-variable and descriptive statistics
   1. The **mean** is the average of a group of numbers. The **median** is the number that divides the sample into two groups: half above and half below. The **mode** is the most common single number in a sample. The **SD** is the square root of the average squared deviation from the mean. The **variance** is the SD squared. The **interquartile range** is the relationship among the minimum, median, and maximum.
   2. A **histogram** is a graphical representation of all the numbers in a sample divided into bins (see Fig. 12–1). The histogram can be considered an estimate of the probability distribution function.

E. Two-variable statistics
   1. Comparing means—**Comparing means** involves comparing continuous with categorical variables. Not all the tests involve means per se, but the general term is a useful indicator of the procedure. Figure 12–7 is a schematic of the comparison of means, and Figure 12–8 summarizes the tests. The **t-test** (also called student's t-test) compares the mean of a sample with a single fixed value. The **two-sample t-test** compares the means of two samples. The t-test can be paired. **Analysis of variance** (ANOVA) compares one dependent variable among three or more groups. It can be modified to compare multiple dependent variables among three or more groups (**multiple analysis of variance** [MANOVA]). MANOVA compares multiple dependent variables among three or more groups. There are nonparametric methods for most of these approaches; the nonparametric statistics measure the responses to questions occasionally asked on examinations in addition to being useful in practice. The method of **discriminant analysis** is related to ANOVA and is useful for predicting groups.

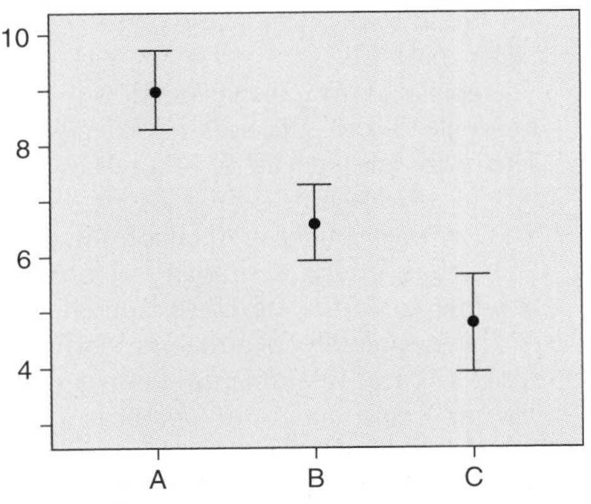

FIGURE 12–7 Schematic of the comparison of means.

	Normal	Nonparametric
Two categories	t-test	Wilcoxon rank sum Mann-Whitney U
Two categories (paired)	Paired t-test	Wilcoxon signed rank
Three or more categories	ANOVA	Kruskal-Wallis
Three or more categories (paired)	ANOVA	Friedman

FIGURE 12–8 Summary of comparison test results. ANOVA, analysis of variance.

The method of analysis of covariance (ANCOVA) is a variant of ANOVA that allows one to control for continuous confounding variables (e.g., age).

   2. Linear regression
      a. Comparing two continuous variables is given the general name of **linear regression**. Figure 12–9 is a schematic of the procedure, and Figure 12–10 is a summary of the tests. By far the most common situation involves just two variables. The **Pearson correlation coefficient** compares two groups of numbers so that +1 is a perfect correlation (straight line agreement), 0 is uncorrelated (independent in a normal distribution), and −1 is a perfect negative correlation (high values of one predict low values of the other). Another measure is the **R-squared** (R^2) (or the coefficient of determination). R^2 is the correlation coefficient squared and denotes the proportion of one variable that is "explained" by another. One tests the significance of a correlation coefficient with a t-test. The null hypothesis shows that there is no correlation. (This illustrates that one statistical test can be used for many different purposes.) Note that the correlation coefficient tests only for a linear correlation. Two variables can be

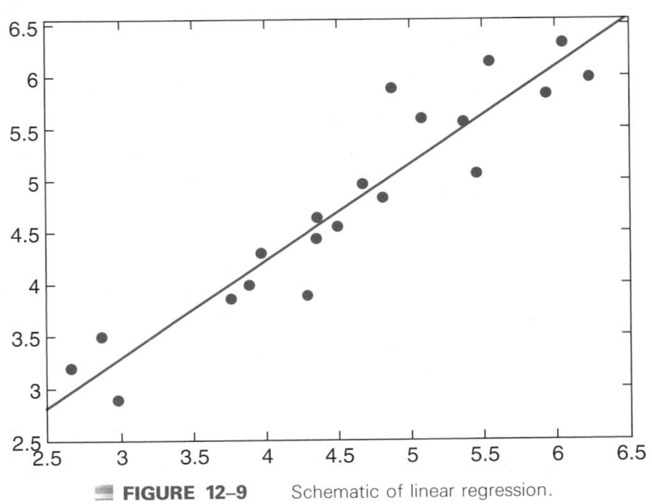

FIGURE 12–9 Schematic of linear regression.

	Normal	Nonparametric
Two variables	Pearson correlation	Spearman correlation
Three or more variables	Linear regression	Nonparametric regression

FIGURE 12–10 Summary of the results of linear regression.

closely related (e.g., one is simply the square of the other) but poorly linearly correlated.

b. Strictly speaking, the correlation coefficient is a parametric statistic most applicable to normal distributions. The **Spearman correlation** (or rank correlation) is a nonparametric measure of correlation.

c. The case of two variables is a highly simplified one of the general process of linear regression for any number of variables. The analysis of linear relationships is a broad field with a variety of methods, some quite sophisticated. Options also exist for the nonparametric analysis of linear relationships among several continuous variables. The calculation of partial correlations among several variables is part of linear regression as well.

3. Logistic regression

a. The prediction of a categorical variable from a continuous variable is termed **logistic regression**. A basic approach involves an S-shaped function that approximates a cutoff value between two groups. Figure 12–11 is a schematic of the procedure. More generally, logistic regression methods may predict a categorical variable from many continuous or categorical variables simultaneously. This general class of approaches also includes related methods such as generalized regression, probit, and logit models. Despite technical distinctions, logistic regression is the most widely used term.

b. One of the most important aspects of logistic regression is the idea of **model building**, which is the selection or elimination of predictor variables in a systematic way, with the use of both statistical criteria and expert opinion for variable selection. Model building is applicable to many multivariate statistical approaches; many orthopaedic surgeons first encounter this process in logistic regression. In general, variables are either sequentially added or sequentially removed based on whether the model's ability to predict the data improves with a predictor variable. This is an important procedure in many practical clinical studies.

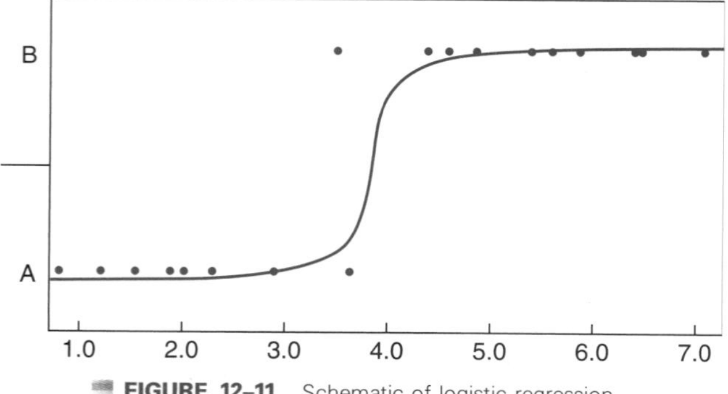

FIGURE 12–11 Schematic of logistic regression.

4. Table analysis

a. We have already considered the analysis of 2×2 tables in terms of various measures (e.g., sensitivity, specificity). We now consider hypothesis testing in tables. By far the most common approach is the **chi-squared** (χ^2) statistic, which can be used for 2×2 tables or tables with more categories per variable (e.g., 3×3) table. The χ^2 statistic tests the null hypothesis that the cells of the table are random and that there are no dependencies among the cell counts. In the situation in which there are relatively few total cases (the sum of all cells less approximately 50), the **Fisher exact test** is a useful substitute for χ^2.

b. Occasionally, there is a need to analyze the relationships among many categorical variables. There are advanced methods such as **log-linear analysis** and **Bayes networks** for such problems, the details of which are beyond our scope. However, these methods highlight an important aspect of model building in general: the question of **covariate selection** and how to control for **confounding**. In a prior section, we discussed the use of randomization to control for confounding. However, it is sometimes necessary to estimate the effect of a treatment by using observational data (e.g., retrospective data) alone, without any randomization. In these cases, it is necessary to control for confounders that can affect the outcome so that the effect of the treatment on the outcome can be isolated. There are folklore and conventional practice about how to select the variables that must be controlled for. Also, there are advanced theoretical studies of this question. It is accepted that one should control for variables that affect both the treatment and the outcome, and one should not control for variables that are affected by the treatment. The details may be found in the references.

F. Decision analysis

1. The goal of clinical management is to make appropriate decisions. Although knowledge such as the sensitivity and specificity of a test is helpful, this type of information is only a start.

2. The key component of **decision analysis** is some knowledge of the desirability of outcomes. It is possible to formulate basic numerical measures of the desirability of outcomes on a numerical scale. Clinical instruments, discussed previously, are important tools in this process. But the questions here are complex. How can one assign a value to life and death, quality of life, mobility, freedom from pain, and range of motion? Despite the

difficulties, serious efforts seek to tackle these problems. Decision analysis is an indispensable tool in debates on public health and medical policy. When billions of dollars and the lives of many people are at stake, it is essential to have quantitative information, however imperfect or crude.

3. **Decision trees** are statistical tools to make decisions based on outcome measures. In a decision tree, the experiment simply enumerates every possible test, decision, and outcome in a management scenario and formulates them as a clinical algorithm. Once this challenging process is complete, it is relatively simple to calculate the optimum strategy, or at least the time/money/morbidity tradeoffs in alternative strategies. Clearly, some clinical scenarios are much more amenable to an algorithmic approach than others because some scenarios involve rare, distinct, or complex management decisions. However, the approach can help guide policy decisions. It is used at the highest levels of the government and corporate insurance industries.
4. Because management decisions involve tradeoffs in time/money/life and quality of life, a scale has been developed to assess **quality-adjusted life-years** (QALYs). QALYs are used by the CMSs to assess the cost-effectiveness of therapies. One tentative guideline is that tests or therapies that cost less than $50,000 per QALY are cost-effective.

VI. Clinical Study Types

A. Introduction—There are numerous distinct types of clinical research studies. We will not attempt to survey them all but rather to identify the major types and the conceptual distinctions among them. Each type has advantages and disadvantages. Many orthopaedic surgeons are more focused on clinical research than laboratory research, so we focus on that.

B. Experimental versus observational studies (Fig. 12–12)—A critical distinction exists between experimental and observational studies. In experimental studies, the management of patients is altered in order to conduct an experiment. In observational studies, the management of clinical patients as it currently exists is the object of study. Observational studies may be further divided into prospective and retrospective studies; in general, prospective is preferred. But this distinction is not as overarching as the difference between experiments and observations, which require different analytic tools and admit different types of conclusions.

1. Experimental studies
   a. Randomized controlled trial—By far the most important experimental study is the RCT, in which a single variable is randomly assigned; this may be called the **independent variable** and is usually a treatment. Each different treatment is called an **arm** of the study. The **outcome variables** are clinical, radiographic, or functional measures of the success of management. Randomization severs the dependence of outcome variables on other factors in the study (e.g., gender, age, fracture severity), thus helping to isolate the effect of the treatment on outcomes. These other factors in the design are often called **confounding variables**, because they may also influence the outcome variables if they are not properly addressed. RCTs have the advantage of the powerful effect of randomization to control for confounding and bias and isolate the effect of the treatment on the outcomes. The disadvantages are cost, complexity, and the ethical considerations involved in randomly assigning treatments.
   b. Several modifications of RCTs are important.
      (1) **Crossover studies**—These involve switching patients between different arms of the study. For example, one arm may receive physical therapy for 4 weeks and another arm medical therapy for 4 weeks. Then the patients switch therapies for another 4 weeks. Such patients may act as their own controls and increase the power of the

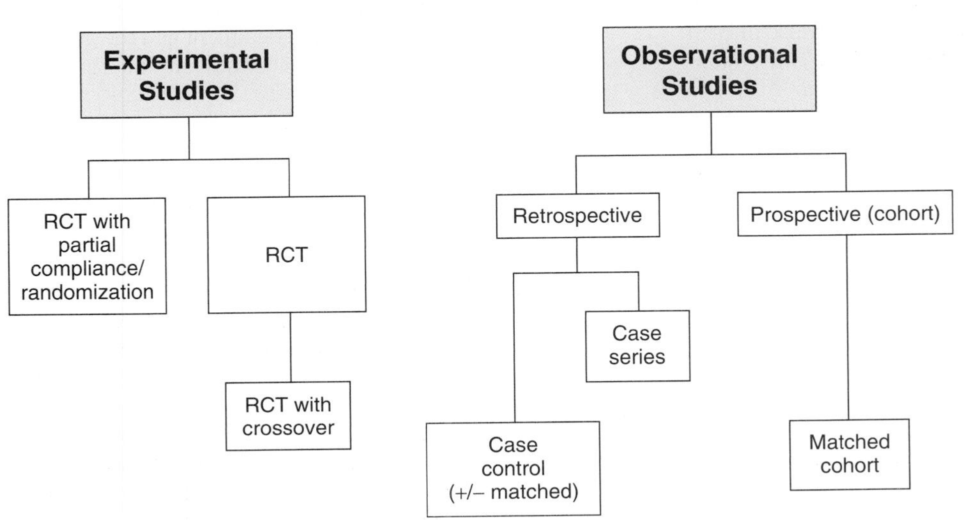

FIGURE 12–12 Summary of experimental versus observational study types. RCT, randomized controlled trial.

study. If patients wait a period of time between therapies, receiving no therapy, this is a **washout period** in which the effect of the first therapy is allowed to wear off.

(2) Partial compliance—Many RCTs involve imperfect compliance with the study protocol by patients who find the protocol difficult to adhere to. If this effect is large, special analytic methods are needed to increase confidence in the results.

2. Observational studies—Observational studies may be divided into prospective and retrospective studies.
   a. A **prospective observational study** is usually called a cohort study. In a **cohort study**, a group of patients is identified to receive a specific treatment and then treated, and their results are followed serially over time.
      (1) The essential feature of a cohort is its prospective nature. First, the study design is considered, and a priori power analysis is performed to determine the necessary sample size. The study is announced publicly (in a sense) by institutional review boards for human subjects. Then, the treatment is administered. The outcomes of interest are followed at well-defined intervals. All data are gathered up to a minimum interval (e.g., 2 years of follow-up) for analysis.
      (2) In practice, all cohort studies involve a **control group**, which consists of patients who have the same diagnosis but different treatment, such as a gold-standard treatment or conservative management. Ideally, the control group is defined prospectively as well and follows an identical clinical protocol, except for the treatment. It is possible to use a **historical control group** by identifying control patients from their medical records. In some cohort studies, **matching** is used to identify control patients. In matching, patients who have similar demographic or clinical variables, such as gender, age, and comorbidity, are compared. Matching is a way of controlling for confounding variables in observational studies.
      (3) Prospective studies have the advantage of being a well-defined and principled type of observational study, but there is no randomization in the choice of treatment between the cohort and control groups. All the potential biases and confounders exist in this type of study.
   b. Retrospective observational study
      (1) The most common type of **retrospective observational study** is a **case series**, which presents information from multiple patients with a similar disease or condition. The data usually come from a review of charts, looking back in time to what occurred with each patient. One advantage of case series is that they can generate speculative associations, which can be further tested by other study types. The major drawback is a lack of any control group with which to compare results. Statistical associations may be sought within the series patients, but exploratory statistics are very relevant here.
      (2) An improvement on case series is the **case-control study**, a case series with a historical control group with which comparisons can be made. Because many case-control studies have relatively small numbers of patients, it is useful to choose control patients matched by gender, age, pathology, and/or other experimental variables.

C. Other study types—Numerous other study types exist. Epidemiologists use **cross-sectional studies**, a study of a population segment at one point in time, to determine disease prevalence or the proportion of a sample with a disease under study. **Longitudinal studies** follow a population segment over time to determine incidence, or the rate of the new occurrences of a disease per unit of time.

D. 2 × 2 tables for epidemiology
   1. The analysis of 2 × 2 tables for analyzing diagnostic tests is presented earlier. 2 × 2 tables are also useful for epidemiologic studies relating outcome to exposure. In the table shown in Figure 12–3A, outcome (O) replaces disease (D), and exposure (E) replaces test (T).
   2. Two useful summary measures are important in this type of 2 × 2 table.
      a. When the table is from an RCT (or cohort study),

$$\text{relative risk} = (a \times [c + d])/(c \times [a + b])$$

A relative risk of >1 is a warning sign. The 95% confidence intervals for the relative risk are calculated, so both confidence values of >1 signal a significant risk.

      b. For case-control studies,

$$\text{odds ratio} = (a \times d)/(c \times b)$$

An odds ratio of > 1 works the same as the relative risk ratio, as described above. In a rare condition, it can be shown that the odds ratio approximates the relative risk. The relative risk reduction, absolute risk reduction, and number needed to treat are related measures used in interventional studies.

Selected Bibliography

American Academy of Orthopaedic Surgeons: Principles of medical ethics and professionalism in orthopaedic surgery (rev. May 2002). Accessed November 2006 from http://www.aaos.org/about/papers/ethics/prin.asp.

American Academy of Orthopaedic Surgeons: Code of Ethics and Professionalism for Orthopaedic Surgeons (rev. Dec. 2004). Accessed November 2006 from http://www.aaos.org/about/papers/ethics/code.asp.

American Academy of Orthopaedic Surgeons: Guide to the ethical practice of orthopaedic surgery (2006). Accessed November 2006 from http://www.aaos.org/about/papers/ethics.asp.

American Academy of Orthopaedic Surgeons: AAOS Position Statement: On-call coverage and emergency care services in orthopaedics (Sept. 2006), Document No. 1172. Accessed November 2006 from http://www.aaos.org/about/papers/position/1172.asp.

Ayanian JZ, Cleary PD, Weissman JS, Epstein AM: The effect of patients' preferences on racial differences in access to renal transplantation. N Engl J Med 341:1661–1669, 1999.

Bosse MJ, Henley MB, Bray T, Vrahas MS: An AOA critical issue. Access to emergent musculoskeletal care: Resuscitating orthopaedic emergency-department coverage. J Bone Joint Surg [Am] 88:1385–1394, 2006.

Feder BJ: Subpoenas seek data on orthopedics makers' ties to surgeons. *NY Times,* March 31, 2005.

Grace SL, Abbey SE, Shnek ZM, et al: Cardiac rehabilitation II: Referral and participation. Gen Hosp Psychiatry 24:127–134, 2002.

Healy WL: Gainsharing: A primer for orthopaedic surgeons. J Bone Joint Surg [Am] 88:1880–1887, 2006.

Jacobs JJ, Galante JO, Mirza SK, Zdeblick T: Relationships with industry: Critical for new technology or an unnecessary evil? J Bone Joint Surg [Am] 88:1650–1663, 2006.

Oppel R: Bush enters fray over malpractice, *NY Times,* January 17, 2003.

Project of the ABIM Foundation, ACP-ASIM Foundation, and European Federation of Internal Medicine: "Medical professionalism in the new millennium: A physician charter" (2002). Accessed November 2006 from http//www.aaos.org/about/papers/ethics/profess.asp.

U.S. Department of Health and Human Services: Fact sheet: Protecting the privacy of patients' health information (April 2003). Accessed November 2006 from http//www.hhs.gov/news/facts/privacy.html.

Pay-for-performance: What surgeons, hospitals and stakeholders need to know. Orthop Today 26:84, 2006.

Senate fails to pass two medical liability reform bills. Orthop Today 26:58–60, 2006. http//www.aaos.org/about/papers/ethics.asp.

What does dropping out as a Medicare provider mean? Orthop Today 26:62, 2006.

INDEX

Note: Page numbers followed by the letter b refer to boxed material; those followed by the letters f refer to figures, and t to tables.

B

C

D

E

F

G

H

I

J

K

N

O

Q

R

S

T

Appendix

ADULT UPPER EXTREMITY—ELBOW FRACTURE-DISLOCATIONS

Injury	Eponym	Classification	Treatment	Complications
Supracondylar fracture		AO/OTA classification of distal humerus Type A—Extra-articular Type B—Intra-articular single column Type C—Intra-articular with both columns fractured and no portion of the joint contiguous with the shaft	Displaced: open reduction with internal fixation (ORIF) (double plating)	Neurovascular injury, nonunion, malunion, contracture, pain, decreased range of motion (ROM) (fibrosis, bony block)
Bicolumn fracture		Jupiter I—High T-pattern (at level of olecranon fossa) II—Low T-pattern (proximal to trochlea) III—Y-pattern (through both columns, distal vertical fracture) IV—H pattern (trochlea is free fragment) V—Medial lambda pattern (proximal fracture exits medially) VI—Lateral lambda pattern (proximal fracture exits laterally) VII—Multiplane: T-type with additional fracture in coronal plane	Nondisplaced: immobilize for 2 wk, then gentle motion Displaced: ORIF (posterior approach, olecranon osteotomy or triceps split/peel): fix condyles first, then epitrochlear ridge to humeral metaphysis) Arthroplasty (total elbow arthroplasty [TEA]) in elderly (consider >65 yr old) "Bag of bones" technique for demented patients or those medically unfit for surgery	Stiffness, heterotopic ossification, infection, ulnar neuropathy (treat with anterior transposition), avascular necrosis (AVN)
Transcondylar fracture	Kocher Posadas	Intra-articular (fragment posterior to humerus) Intra-articular (fragment anterior to humerus)	ORIF ORIF	↓ROM
Capitellar fracture	 Hahn-Steinthal Kocher-Lorenz	Bryan and Morrey I—Complete fracture of capitellum, large trochlear piece II—Minimum subchondral bone (shear fracture of articular cartilage) III—Comminuted fracture IV (McKee modification)—Coronal shear fracture, including capitellum and trochlea	 Nondisplaced: splint for 2-3 wk, then motion; displaced >2 mm: ORIF Nondisplaced: splint for 2-3 wk, then motion; displaced: excise displaced fragment Excise if displaced and unsalvageable ORIF	Nonunion (1-11% with ORIF), olecranon osteotomy nonunion, ulnar nerve injury, heterotopic ossification (4% with ORIF), AVN of capitellum
Condylar fracture		Milch (lateral ≫ medial) I—Lateral trochlear ridge intact II—Fracture through lateral trochlear ridge	Nondisplaced: immobilize in supination (lateral condyle), pronation (medial condyle) Displaced: closed reduction with percutaneous pinning (CRPP) vs. ORIF ORIF	Cubitus valgus (lateral), cubitus varus (medial), ulnar nerve neuropraxia, degenerative joint disease (DJD)
Trochlear fracture	Laugier	Rare	Nondisplaced: splint for 3 wk; ORIF if displaced	

ADULT UPPER EXTREMITY—ELBOW FRACTURE-DISLOCATIONS—cont'd

Injury	Eponym	Classification	Treatment	Complications
Epicondylar fracture	Granger	Medial ≫ lateral	Manipulation, immobilization for 10-14 days	Painful, unsightly fragment or ulnar nerve symptoms—late excision
Coronoid fracture		Regan and Morrey		Instability (medial) and DJD
		Type I—Fracture of the tip	Early motion if stable; ORIF with cerclage wire or suture if unstable	
		Type II—Fracture of <50% of coronoid	ORIF	
		Type III—Fracture of >50% of coronoid	ORIF	
Olecranon fracture		Colton (modified)	Minimally displaced (<1-2 mm): splint at 69-90 degrees for 7-10 days, then motion	↓ROM, DJD, nonunion, ulnar nerve neuropraxia, instability (with removal of >80% of olecranon), symptomatic hardware/need for hardware removal
		Type I—Avulsion	Minimally displaced (<1-2 mm): splint at 69-90 degrees for 7-10 days, then motion	
		Type II (A-D)—Oblique fractures with increasing complexity	Displaced: ORIF	
		Type III—Fractures-dislocations	Tension band: use stainless steel wire or braided cable; migration of wire/prominent hardware in 71%	
		Type IV—Atypical high-energy, multifragmented fractures	Intramedullary 7.3-mm screw and tension band	
			Plate fixation for oblique and comminuted fractures	
			Excision for unreconstructible proximal olecranon fractures; reattach close to articular surface; avoid >50% resection	
Radial head fracture		Mason (and Johnston)		Loss of motion, posterior interosseous nerve (PIN) injury; intraosseous membrane rupture; distal radioulnar joint disruption; Essex-Lopresti (distal radioulnar joint disruption); synovitis if Silastic radial head implant
		I—Nondisplaced	Nonoperative; splint for 7 days, then early motion with or without aspiration	
		II—Partially articular with displacement	If elbow stable and no block to motion: splint and early motion; otherwise, ORIF vs. arthroplasty	
		III—Comminuted fractures involving the entire head of the radius	Arthroplasty; ORIF if < three pieces, good bone quality; excise in elderly, low functional demands	
		IV—Fractures associated with ligamentous injury (elbow dislocation) or other associated fractures	Reduce dislocation and then address fracture surgically (arthroplasty for stability)	
Dislocation (pure ligamentous)		Posterolateral (most common), posterior, anterior, medial, lateral, divergent; simple (no fracture) or complex (fracture)	Closed reduction; check ROM/stability; splint for 2-7 days and then gentle, active ROM; open reduction unstable/interposed soft tissue ORIF complex (fracture) dislocations	Irreducibility, median and ulnar nerve injury, brachial artery injury, flexion contracture, heterotopic ossification, fractures (medial epicondyle, radial head, coronoid)

ADULT UPPER EXTREMITY—HAND DISLOCATIONS

Injury	Eponym/ Other Name	Classification	Treatment	Complications
Distal interphalangeal dislocation		Dorsal dislocation (most common)	Closed reduction; immobilize for 2 wk, then range of motion; late diagnosis or irreducible: open reduction (with) internal fixation (ORIF)	Extensor lag—treated with 8-wk course of splinting, similar to a mallet finger
		Collateral ligament injury	Sprain: buddy tape for 3-6 wk Tear: repair radial collateral of index, ring, middle finger; ulnar collateral of small (dominant hand)	
Proximal interphalangeal dislocation		Dorsal dislocation (most common) (volar plate disruption)		
		I—Hyperextension, volar plate avulsion	Buddy tape or extension block splint for 4 days, then motion	Stiffness, contractures (treat with volar plate arthroplasty)
		II—Dislocation, major ligamentous injury	Extension block splint	
		III—Proximal dislocation (middle phalanx fracture)	If >4-mm displacement, reduce; ORIF if irreducible	
	Boutonniere	Volar dislocation (central slip injury)	Closed reduction; splint in full extension for 6 wk if congruous	Late recognition: therapy to restore motion, ORIF or volar plate arthroplasty
		Rotatory	ORIF if irreducible or incongruous	
		Dorsal fracture-dislocation	Extension block splint if congruous; if unstable, ORIF or volar plate arthroplasty	
Thumb metacarpophalangeal (MCP) dislocation	Gamekeeper/skier thumb	Ulnar collateral ligament injury (most common)	Sprain: does not open >35 degrees with stress; treat with thumb spica cast for 4 wk Complete rupture: open repair (interposition of adductor aponeurosis—Stener lesion)	Unrecognized Stener lesion, chronic pain, instability, degenerative joint disease
		Radial collateral ligament injury (rare)	Splint vs. repair if complete rupture and symptomatic	
		Dorsal (simple or complex [interposition of volar plate])	Simple: splint; complex: open	
MCP dislocation		Collateral ligament injury (index finger most common)	Reduce with traction/volar–directed force to proximal phalanx; splint in 50-degree MCP flexion for 3 wk, then buddy tape for 3 additional wk Open if irreducible, >2-mm displacement of associated fracture fragments, or 20% of joint	Late recognition—injection, splinting, operation (rare)
		Dorsal dislocation (most common)		
		Simple	Closed reduction, immobilization for 7-10 days	Failure to recognize complex dislocation
		Complex	Soft tissue volar plate interposition (pucker, sesamoid in joint, and parallelism of metacarpal and P1 (phalanx) require ORIF and volar plate arthroplasty)	Stiffness, contractures, neurovascular injury (open)
		Volar dislocation	Rare, requires ORIF	
Carpometacarpal (CMC) dislocation			Closed reduction with percutaneous pinning (CRPP); ORIF—fourth CMC dislocations and open dislocations	
Thumb CMC dislocation		Rare injury without associated fracture	CRPP with traction/pronation; immobilize for 6-10 wk	Chronic instability
Hamate/metacarpal fracture-dislocation		Cain		Delay in diagnosis (pronation oblique films required)
		IA—Ligamentous injury	Reduce—If stable, cast; if unstable, CRPP	
		IB—Dorsal hamate fracture (most common)	Reduce—If stable, cast; if unstable, ORIF	
		II—Comminuted dorsal hamate fracture	ORIF, restore dorsal buttress	
		III—Coronal hamate fracture	ORIF, restore congruent joint	

ADULT UPPER EXTREMITY—HAND FRACTURES

Injury	Eponym	Classification	Treatment	Complications
Distal fracture phalanx (P3)		Longitudinal, comminuted, transverse, crush (frequent)	Splint distal interphalangeal (DIP) for 3-4 wk; evacuate hematoma and repair nail bed with fine absorbable suture	Nail bed injury
Extensor digitorum communis avulsion	Mallet finger	Watson-Jones Extensor tendon stretch: >15-30–degree extensor lag Extensor tendon rupture: 30-60–degree extensor lag Bony mallet	Volar/stack splint for 6-8 wk full time, then 4 wk at night only; closed reduction with percutaneous pinning (CRPP)/open reduction with internal fixation (ORIF) if >50% of articular surface; volar subluxation of P3 or occupation prevents splinting	Dorsal skin necrosis, deformity, nail bed injury (with ORIF), subluxation, extensor lag, nail bed deformity, pin tract infections, osteomyelitis, hot-cold intolerance, hypersensitivity
Flexor digitorum profundus (FDP) avulsion	Jersey finger	Leddy and Packer		Can lead to lumbrical and finger (late), missed diagnosis (therapy or fuse DIP late); quadregia if FDP advanced >1 cm during repair
		I—Tendon in palm	Repair within 7-10 days (vincula disruption)	
		II—Tendon at level of Proximal interphalangeal (PIP) (held by A3 pulley)	Repair within 6 wk	
		III—Tendon at level of A4 pulley	ORIF of large, bony fragment with K-wires; keep A4 pulley intact with repair	
		IV—Bony fragment at P3 base	Early fixation of bony fragments and tendon	
Proximal (P1) and middle (P2) phalanges fracture		Extra-articular base (stable)	Buddy tape	Decreased range of motion (ROM) (flexor tendon adhesions), contractures, malunion/malrotation (may require osteotomy), lateral deviation, volar angulation (osteotomy), nonunion, tendon adherence
		Extra-articular base (unstable)	Reduce and immobilize (CRPP/ORIF if irreducible; external fixation for comminuted fractures, soft tissue injuries)	
		Intra-articular nondisplaced	Buddy tape, early ROM, close follow-up	
		Intra-articular condylar	Reduction, CRPP, or ORIF; restore articular surface if >1-mm displacement	
		Intra-articular P1 base	Small/nondisplaced—buddy tape Large/displaced—ORIF	
	Boutonniere	Intra-articular P2 base	Splint PIP (extension) for 6 wk; ORIF if large, bony fragment	
Metacarpal (MC) fracture		Head (transverse, oblique, spiral, comminuted)	ORIF for large piece, external fixation with early motion of comminuted fractures	Soft tissue injury (look for fight bite!), malunion (rotation); prominent MC head in palm (affects grip); loss of reduction (no volar buttress); nonunion, contracture of intrinsic muscles; claw deformity with extrinsic tendon imbalance
	Boxer	Neck—fourth and fifth MCs	40-70–degree angulation OK; reduce with Jahss maneuver, splint; operative if rotational deformity, extensor lag, multiple fracture, irreducible	
		Neck—second and third MCs	Usually requires CRPP to adjacent MC or ORIF	
		Shaft—transverse	Closed reduction, immobilize, or CRPP; accept 20-30–degree angulation in IV and V, 10-degree angulation in II and III; ORIF if irreducible	
		Shaft—oblique	ORIF if >5-mm shortening or rotated	
		Shaft—comminuted	Nondisplaced: splint; displaced: CRPP to adjacent MC or ORIF	
Thumb fracture (first) MC base fracture	Bennett	I—Intra-articular volar ulnar lip	Attempt CRPP to trapezium; ORIF if irreducible	Displaced by abductor pollicis longus
	Rolando	II—Intra-articular "Y" (volar and dorsal)	Large fragments: ORIF; comminuted: external fixation or early motion	Degenerative joint disease
		III—Extra-articular (transverse or oblique)	Closed reduction, splint for 4 wk; CRPP if angulation >30 degrees	
Small (fifth) MC base fracture	"Baby Bennett"	Base fracture (epibasal, two-part, three-part, comminuted)	Evaluate with semipronated, semisupinated, distraction views; CRPP to adjacent MC or ORIF	Watch carpometacarpal fracture-dislocation, painful arthritis, fragment displaced by extensor carpi ulnaris

ADULT UPPER EXTREMITY—HUMERAL SHAFT FRACTURES

Injury	Eponym	Classification	Treatment	Complications
Humeral shaft fracture	Holstein-Lewis (distal one third)	Based on location/ fracture pattern	Nonoperative: coaptation splint or cast brace if <20-degree anterior angulation, <30-degree varus/valgus, <3-cm shortening Operative: consider open reduction (with) internal fixation (ORIF) (compression plate) vs. intramedullary (IM) nail Indications: pathologic fracture, open fracture, floating elbow Relative indications: segmental fracture, distal spiral with nerve injury (Holstein-Lewis), obesity, thoracic trauma, polytrauma	Nonunion (treat with compression plate and bone graft), malunion, radial nerve injury (5-10% incidence; observe unless open fracture or persisting for 3-4 months), vascular injury; shoulder pain (IM nail)

ADULT UPPER EXTREMITY—RADIAL AND ULNAR SHAFT FRACTURES AND DISLOCATIONS

Injury	Eponym/ Other Name	Classification	Treatment	Complications
Radius and ulna fractures	"Both-bone"	Degree of displacement	Open reduction with internal fixation (ORIF) with six-hole dynamic compression plate (DCP); external fixation for type III open fracture, bone graft if >one-third (shaft) comminution	Malunion/nonunion, vascular injury, percutaneous interosseous nerve (PIN) injury, compartment syndrome, synostosis, infection, refracture (after plate removal)
Ulna fracture	Nightstick	Nondisplaced	Distal two thirds, <50% displaced, <10-degree angulation: long-arm cast (LAC) to functional brace with good interosseous mold	Malunion, nonunion
		Displaced	Proximal one third, >50% displaced, >10-degree angulation: ORIF; look for wrist/elbow injury	
Proximal ulna and radial head fractures	Monteggia	Bado Type I (60%)—radial head dislocation, anterior and apex anterior proximal one-third ulna fracture	ORIF of ulna (DCP), closed-reduction head, immobilize; if radial head irreducible, ulna fracture reduction may be nonanatomic	PIN injury (usually spontaneously resolves), redislocation/subluxation (inadequate reduction), synostosis, loss of motion
		Type II (15)%—radial head dislocation, posterior and apex posterior proximal one-third ulna shaft fracture	ORIF of ulna (DCP), closed reduction head, immobilize at 70 degrees	
		Type III—radial head dislocation, lateral and proximal ulnar metaphyseal fracture	ORIF of ulna (DCP), closed reduction head, immobilize	
		Type IV—radial head dislocatiion, anterior fracture and forearm fracture of both bones	ORIF of radius and ulna, closed reduction head, immobilize	
Proximal radius fracture		Nondisplaced	LAC in supination, close follow-up	
		Displaced	Proximal one fifth: closed; one fifth–two thirds: ORIF	
Distal radius (distal one third) and radioulnar dislocation	Galeazzi/ Piedmont	Supination/pronation (signs of instability: ulnar styloid fracture, widened distal radioulnar joint on posteroanterior view, dislocation on lateral view, ≥5-mm radial shortening)	ORIF of radius (volar), closed reduction with or without percutaneous pinning to radioulnar joint (in supination) if unstable	Angulation, distal subluxation, malunion, nonunion; displaced by gravity, pronator quadratus, brachioradialis

ADULT UPPER EXTREMITY—SHOULDER DISLOCATIONS/LIGAMENTOUS INJURIES

Injury	Eponym/Other Name	Classification	Treatment	Complications
Anterior (glenohumeral [GH]) dislocation (most common))		Subcoracoid > subglenoid (also subclavicular and intrathoracic)	Must get axillary view of GH joint; reduce, immobilize (young patient, 4 wk; old patient, 2 wk); passive > active (Rockwood 7)	Axillary nerve neuropraxia, axillary artery injury, cuff injury (>40 yr old), recurrence (85% in <20 yr old), bone injury (head [Hill-Sachs], greater tuberosity, glenoid)
Recurrent/multidirectional		Anterior dislocation/subluxation atraumatic	Prolonged rehabilitation (rotator cuff strengthening); if failure, consider surgery (inferior capsular shift)	Look for generalized laxity; AMBRI
			Bankart repair: Anterior capsule → anterior rim	Late instability
			Staple capsulorrhaphy: Capsule → glenoid	Late degenerative joint disease (DJD), migration
			Putti-Platt repair: Subscapularis imbrication	Late DJD, ↓ external rotation (ER)
			Magnuson-Stack repair: Subscapularis → lesser tuberosity	Late DJD, ↓ER
			Bone block: Crest graft, anterior	↓range of motion, migration
			Bristow repair: Coracoid transfer	Nonunion, ↓ER, migration
			Capsular shift: Redundant capsule, advanced	Minimum procedure of choice with MDI
Posterior dislocation		Subacromial (seizures and shocks) (most common)	Reduce, immobilize for 3-6 wk; rotator cuff strengthening; operate if recurrent (glenoid osteotomy, bone block, posterior capsular shift)	Lesser tuberosity fracture, late recognition (may require advancement of lesser tuberosity into defect or total shoulder arthroplasty [place in less retroversion]); avoid by checking axial view
Inferior GH	Luxatio erecta		Reduce and immobilize; rotator cuff strengthening, rehabilitation	Neurovascular injury can resolve after reduction; axillary artery thrombosis; watch for rotator cuff tear
Acromioclavicular (AC) injury		I—AC sprain	7-10 days rest/immobilization, sling	Joint stiffness, deformity, CC ligament and soft tissue calcification, AC DJD, associated fractures, distal clavicle osteolysis
		II—AC tear, coracoclavicular (CC) sprain	Sling for 2 wk, rehabilitation, late-excision arthroplasty if required	
		III—AC tear, CC tear	Conservative vs. repair (athletes, laborers); Weaver-Dunn	
		IV—Clavicle through trapezius posteriorly	Reduce and repair	
		V—Clavicle 100-300% elevated; trapezius, deltoid detached	Reduce and repair (Weaver-Dunn)	
		VI—Clavicle inferior to coracoid	Reduce and repair	
Sternoclavicular injury			Evaluate with "serendipity" view or computed tomography	Bump (cosmetic), DJD, mediastinal impingement (dysphagia, throat fullness), hardware migration (with operative treatment)
		Anterior dislocation	Closed reduction with traction	
		Posterior dislocation	Closed reduction with towel clip or open; thoracic surgeon on standby	
		Chronic dislocation	Medial clavicle resection or ligament reconstruction (thoracic surgeon on standby)	
		Spontaneous atraumatic subluxation	Nonoperative	

*AMBRI, **a**traumatic, **m**ultidirectional, **b**ilateral, treated by **r**ehabilitation **i**nstability; MDI, multidirectional instability.*

ADULT UPPER EXTREMITY—SHOULDER FRACTURES

Injury	Eponym	Classification	Treatment	Complications
Proximal humerus fracture		Neer (parts >5 mm or 45-degree displacement)		Missed dislocation, adhesive capsulitis (moist heat, gentle range of motion), malunion (reconstruction or total shoulder arthroplasty [TSA] required), avascular necrosis (AVN) (TSA required), nonunion (surgical neck, tuberosity fractures: ORIF), disrupted rotator cuff
		One-part (most common); impaction of the humeral neck	Sling for comfort, early motion; isometrics initially, advancing to progressive resistance	
		Two-part; displacement of the greater tuberosity >5 mm	Closed reduction unless articular segment (open reduction with internal fixation [ORIF]), shaft (impacted and angulated: traction, Velpeau; unimpacted: closed reduction, closed reduction with percutaneous pinning [CRPP] or ORIF), greater tuberosity (repair cuff), tuberosity with block to internal rotation (ORIF)	
		Three-part; displacement of the greater and lesser tuberosities >5 mm	ORIF in younger, prosthesis in older; repair of rotator cuff	
		Four-part; head splitting	Same as three-part; nonoperative in elderly/diabetic/impacted four-part valgus pattern	
Proximal humerus fracture-dislocation		Anterior (greater tuberosity displacement)	Closed reduction; if >1 cm after reduction, open repair	As above, with the addition of axillary nerve or plexus injury, myositis ossificans (wait >1 yr to excise heterotopic bone)
		Posterior (lesser tuberosity displacement)	Closed reduction, ORIF if three-part; treatment for fracture as above	
Impression/impaction of humeral head	Hill-Sachs	Stable (<20% articular surface)	Closed treatment	AVN, degenerative joint disease (DJD) (TSA)
		Unstable (20-50%)	Transfer of lesser tuberosity → defect (McLaughlin)	
		Unstable (>45%)	Prosthesis vs. rotational osteotomy	
Scapula fracture		Zdravkovic and Damholt		Associated injuries (clavicle, rib, pulmonary contusion, pneumothorax), axillary artery injury, plexus palsy, pressure symptoms, vascular and plexus injuries
		I—Body	Most treated nonoperatively	
		II—Coracoid and acromion	Associated injury common; ORIF of large, displaced fragments	
		III—Neck and glenoid	ORIF of large, unstable fractures (glenoid with displaced clavicle fracture)	
Clavicle fracture		Middle one third (most common)	Nonoperative: sling, figure 8 brace ORIF: displacement, ipsilateral displaced glenoid neck fracture	Vascular injury/pneumothorax, ligament injury (CC or AC), skin necrosis, malunion (osteotomy for young, active patient); nonunion (ORIF and bone graft), nerve injury (rare); muscle fatigue/weakness, DJD (if articular)
		Distal one third (Neer)		
		I—Minimum interligamentous displacement (coracoclavicular [CC], acromioclavicular [AC])	Nonoperative; sling for comfort	
		II—Fracture medial to CC ligaments	Nonoperative if nondisplaced; consider ORIF for displaced fracture	
		IIA—Both ligaments attached to distal fragment	ORIF	
		IIB—Conoid torn, trapezoid attached to distal fragment	ORIF	
		III—AC joint	Closed treatment; late-excision arthroplasty if required	
		Proximal one third	Closed treatment	
Glenoid fracture		Ideberg		Nonoperative treatment if nondisplaced
		I—Anterior avulsion fracture	>25% of surface: ORIF if head is subluxated with major fragment; posterior approach	
		II—Transverse/obliquefracture;inferiorglenoidfree		
		III—Upper one third of glenoid and coracoid		
		IV—Horizontal glenoid through body		
		V—Combination of II-IV		
Scapulothoracic dissociation		(Seen on scapular lateral or chest radiograph)	Closed reduction, sling immobilization	Vascular and brachial plexus injuries, associated clavicle fracture

ADULT UPPER EXTREMITY—WRIST AND CARPAL FRACTURES

Injury	Eponym	Classification	Treatment	Complications
Distal radius fracture	Colles (dorsal displacement)	Frykman (I- VIII; even number = ulnar styloid fracture I—Extra-articular III—Intra-articular radiocarpal joint fracture V—Intra-articular radioulnar joint fracture VII—Displaced intra-articular radiocarpal and radioulnar joint fractures	Distract, manipulate, splint 15 degrees palmar flexion and ulnar deviation, external fixation, and/or open reduction (with) internal fixation (ORIF) if comminuted/unstable; external fixation for severe comminution, ORIF for large fragments with a >15-degree dorsal tilt; >1-2–mm articular displacement; bone graft comminuted fractures	Loss of reduction, nonunion, malunion, median neuropathy/carpal tunnel syndrome, weakness, tendon adhesion/rupture, instability, extensor pollicis longus rupture, dorsal intercalated segment instability (DISI) >15 degrees (extension), ulnar side pain (shortening), complex regional pain syndrome (CRPS), Volkmann ischemic contracture
	Smith (volar displacement)	Intra- vs. extra-articular	Distract, manipulate, splint in supination, flexion; CRPP vs. ORIF (volar approach)	Missed diagnosis, similar to Colles fracture
Dorsal rim of radius fracture	Dorsal Barton	Fernandez type II	Majority: ORIF with dorsal approach	Similar to Colles fracture
Radial styloid fracture	Chauffeur	Fernandez type II	Reduction, CRPP, cannulated screw or plate; immobilize in ulnar deviation	Similar to Colles fracture; rule out associated perilunate injury (ORIF)
Volar rim of radius fracture	Volar Barton	Fernandez type II	Majority: ORIF with volar buttress plate	Similar to Colles fracture
Distal radioulnar joint dissociation		Based on ulna displacement; fracture of base of ulnar styloid associated with TFCC tear	Dorsal—reduction, full supination, long-arm cast (LAC) for 6 wk Volar—reduction (may require open reduction), LAC for 6 wk in pronation	Osteochondral fracture, triangular fibrocartilage complex (TFCC) injury, ulnar nerve compression, instability, arthrosis, weak grip, decreased forearm rotation
Scaphoid fracture		Based on anatomic location (neck, waist, body, proximal pole)	Evaluate with anteroposterior, lateral, navicular, and clenched-fist views; plain radiographs; magnetic resonance imaging (MRI) for occult fracture; CT to characterize fracture, evaluate nonunion nondisplaced: thumb spica, (LAC for proximal and mid-body, short-arm cast [SAC] for distal pole) ORIF if displaced, unstable, proximal pole, nonunion	Nonunion (computed tomographic [CT] evaluation; bone graft), instability, refracture, nerve injury, CRPS, degenerative joint disease (DJD), pain, missed fracture (MRI best for diagnosis of occult injury)
Triquetrum fracture		Dorsal shear (most common) vs. body (rare)	SAC for 4 wk; ORIF if displaced body fracture	
Pisiform fracture		Uncommon (1-3% of all carpal fractures)	SAC in flexion/ulnar deviation for 6 wk	Nonunion (treat with excision); associated with distal radius, hamate, triquetrum fractures
Trapezium fracture		Body, trapezial ridge	Nonoperative: SAC with molded abduction of first ray; ORIF of intra-articular displaced-body fractures	Body: associated carpometacarpal (CMC) dislocation or Bennett fracture; trapezial ridge fracture: chronic pain (treat with excision)
Capitate fracture		Rare	Closed treatment if nondisplaced, ORIF if displaced	Associated with perilunate dislocations, scaphoid fractures, and CMC fracture-dislocations; osteonecrosis; nonunion (treat with fusion of capitate, scaphoid, and lunate)

Continued

ADULT UPPER EXTREMITY—WRIST AND CARPAL FRACTURES—cont'd

Injury	Eponym	Classification	Treatment	Complications
Perilunate instability/ dislocation (with or without scaphoid fracture)		Mayfield I—Scapholunate dissociation II—Lunocapitate disruption III—Lunotriquetral disruption IV—Lunate dislocation	Early (6-8 wk)—open (dorsal) ligament repair and ORIF scaphoid fracture (if present) Late—triscaphoid fusion, proximal row carpectomy, or wrist fusion	Rotatory instability of scaphoid, median nerve palsy, late flexor rupture
Rotatory scapholunate dissociation	Terry Thomas sign	>3-mm scapholunate interval on anteroposterior vs. contralateral wrist view; scapholunate angle >60 degrees, scaphoid ring sign	Closed reduction, immobilization; ORIF if scaphoid fracture displaced; open repair of ligaments (volar and dorsal, capsulodesis)	Late DJD (advanced collapse of scapholunate)
Lunate fracture		Based on fracture location (volar pole most common)	ORIF for displaced fracture; nonoperative for nondisplaced injury	Disorganization, disintegration; distinguish from Kienböck
Hamate fracture		Based on location and size of fragment—body or hook	Body: closed treatment if nondisplaced; CRPP or ORIF if displaced or unstable Hook: closed treatment if acute, excise if chronic and symptomatic	Missed on plain films (CT view required); body: associated with fourth and fifth CMC fracture-dislocation; hook: ulnar nerve symptoms, flexor tendon problems
Carpal instability		DISI (most common)—dorsal intercalated segment instability, scapholunate angle >70 degrees Volar intercalated segment instability (VISI), scapholunate angle <35 degrees Axial injury	Closed reduction of acute injuries followed by early repair; open scapholunate reconstruction for failed/late reduction/scapholunate advanced collapse (SLAC) for wrist; ORIF axial injuries	DISI, VISI: DJD, stiffness, treatment for chronic instability controversial; axial: usually high energy with soft tissue injury, nerve/vascular/muscle injury

ADULT SPINE TRAUMA

Level	Injury Type	Classification	Common Name	Mechanism of Injury	Risk of Neurologic Injury	Treatment	Indication for Surgery	Important Points
Occipitocervical dislocation	I	Traynelis et al	Anterior	Anterior translation	Very high	Occipitocervical fusion	Surgery indicated	Very unstable; rarely survive injury
	II		Distraction	Pure distraction	Very high	Occipitocervical fusion	Surgery indicated	Very unstable; rarely survive injury
	III		Posterior	Posterior translation	Very high	Occipitocervical fusion	Surgery indicated	Very unstable; rarely survive injury
Occipital condyle fracture	I	Anderson-Montesano	Impacted condyle fracture	Compression of skull	Low	Collar	Usually not required	Alar ligament and tectorial membrane usually intact
	II		Occipital condyle and basilar skull fracture	Compression of skull	Low	Collar	Usually not required	Alar ligament and tectorial membrane usually intact
	III		Avulsion fracture of alar ligament	Distraction of skull	Moderate to high	Collar, halo, or surgery, depending on stability	More than 1 mm of displacement	Potential for ligament disruption
C1 ring fracture	Posterior arch fracture		Lamina fracture	Hyperextension	Low	Immobilization	Not indicated	Hyperextension
	Two- and three-part fractures		Lateral mass fracture	Lateral compression	Low	Immobilization	Not indicated	
	Four-part fracture		Jefferson fracture	Axial compression	Low	Immobilization, sometimes traction	Optional for widely displaced lateral masses	>7-mm offset of lateral mass indicates transverse ligament rupture
C2 fracture	Traumatic spondylolisthesis	Levine	Hangman fracture					
	I or IA		IA called atypical hangman	Hyperextension	Low	Collar		Prove stable with supervised flexion–extension radiographs
	II or IIA			Hyperextension with secondary flexion	Low to moderate	Immobilization; avoid traction with IIA	Osteosynthesis optional	Type II, use traction; type IIA, avoid traction
	III		Bilateral facet dislocation	Hyperextension with secondary flexion/distraction	High	Surgical reduction of facet dislocation and C2-C3 fusion	Surgery required to reduce facets	Open reduction of facets required
	Odontoid fracture I	Anderson-D'Alonzo	Avulsion fracture	Hyperextension of distraction	Low	Collar	None	Watch for associated occipitocervical instability
	II		Fracture at junction of odontoid and body	Multiple mechanisms	Moderate	Halo vs. internal fixation	Unstable fracture or nonunion	Most common; high rate of nonunion
	III		Fracture into C2 body	Multiple mechanisms	Moderate	Halo vest immobilization	Displacement, instability	Usually stable

Continued

ADULT SPINE TRAUMA—cont'd

Level	Injury Type	Classification	Common Name	Mechanism of Injury	Risk of Neurologic Injury	Treatment	Indication for Surgery	Important Points
C2 body fracture				Similar to subaxial cervical spine	Low			
Transverse ligament disruption			C1-C2 instability	Severe flexion	Moderate to high	C1-C2 fusion	ADI >3-5 mm	Often associated with dizziness, syncope, respiratory problems, and blurred vision
C1-C2 rotatory subluxation	I	Fielding-Hawkins	Rotatory fixation	Rotational trauma	Low	Immobilization/ traction/surgery	Indicated for chronic cases with fixed deformity and spasm or instability	Many causes; infection and trauma most common
	II		Rotatory fixation with 3-5 mm of anterior displacement	Rotational trauma	Moderate	Immobilization/ traction/surgery	Indicated for chronic cases with fixed deformity and spasm or instability	
	III		Rotatory fixation with >5 mm anterior displacement	Rotational trauma	Moderate	Immobilization/ traction/surgery	Indicated for chronic cases with fixed deformity and spasm or instability	
	IV		Rotatory fixation with posterior displacement	Rotational trauma	Moderate to high	Immobilization/ traction/surgery	Indicated for chronic cases with fixed deformity and spasm or instability	
Subaxial cervical spine		Allen-Ferguson		Mechanisms implied by name	Depends on stage of injury	Depends on stage of injury		
	Compressive flexion			Compression and flexion	Low to high		Instability or neurologic deficit with cord compression	
	Distractive flexion			Distraction and flexion	Low to high		Instability or neurologic deficit with cord compression	
	Axial compression			Axial compression	Low to high		Instability or neurologic deficit with cord compression	
	Compressive extension			Compression and extension	Low to high		Instability or neurologic deficit with cord compression	
	Distractive extension			Distraction and extension	Low to high		Instability or neurologic deficit with cord compression	

Subaxial cervical spine (cont'd)	Lateral flexion			Lateral bending	Low to moderate		Instability or neurologic deficit with cord compression	
	Compression		Compression	Flexion	Low	Collar		Watch for signs of posterior ligament disruption.
	Burst		Burst	Axial compression	Moderate to high	Halo vs. anterior decompression/ fusion	Cord compression	Anterior decompression specifically indicated in cases of incomplete cord injury
			Flexion teardrop	Compression and flexion	High	Halo vs. anterior decompression/ fusion	Cord compression	Very unstable
			Facet dislocation	Flexion and distraction	High	Reduction of facet, fusion	Bilateral facet dislocation	Possible disc herniation; consider MRI prior to reduction
	Posterior element fracture		Spinous process	Extension (sometimes flexion or rotation)	Low	Collar	Floating lateral mass	Most are stable
Thoracolumbar spine	Compression	Denis		Flexion and axial loading		Bracing	Greater than 50% anterior collapse or widening of spinous process	Osteoporotic compression fracture requires workup and treatment of underlying condition; watch for ileus.
	Burst			Axial loading				
	Stable					Bracing	Progressive deformity or neurologic compromise	Watch for any signs of posterior ligament rupture vs. MRI; watch for ileus.
	Unstable					Surgery	>30 degrees kyphosis; incomplete cord injury with cord compromise	Cord decompression required if neurologic deficit present
	Seatbelt injury		Chance fracture (bony injury)	Distraction and flexion		Surgery for posterior ligament ruptures, bracing for postoperative treatment	>17% kyphosis with bony injury, posterior ligament injury	High rate of associated intra-abdominal injury
	Fracture-dislocation			Rotation and shear		Surgical alignment, fusion, instrumentation	All require surgery	Long segmental posterior construct

ADI, atlanto–dens interval; MRI, magnetic resonance imaging.

ADULT LOWER EXTREMITY—ACETABULAR FRACTURES

Injury	Classification	Treatment	Complications
Acetabular fracture	Letournel—based on involvement of acetabular columns and wall Simple types Anterior wall (AW) Anterior column (AC) Posterior wall (PW)—most common simple type Posterior column (PC) Transverse—involves both AC and PC Associated types PC/PW Transverse/PW—most common associated type AC/posterior hemitransverse (ACPHT)—least common type T-type—transverse with vertical limb through ischium Both columns (BCs)—dissociation of acetabular dome from axial skeleton. "Spur sign" seen on obturator oblique view	Nonoperative: <1-mm step-off and <2-mm gap; roof arc angle >45 degrees on anteroposterior, inlet, and outlet views—computed tomographic correlate is fracture >10 mm from dome apex; PW fractures without instability (<20% of PW); associated fractures of BCs with secondary congruence; severe comminution in elderly in whom total hip arthroplasty is planned after fracture healing Relative contraindications to surgery: morbid obesity, physiologically elderly/nonambulatory, contaminated wound, delay to operation >4 wk, presence of deep venous thrombosis with contraindication for filter Operative: displaced fracture, incongruous or unstable joint, intra-articular bone fragments, irreducible fracture-dislocation ***Surgical approaches:*** Kocher-Langenbeck (posterior approach) indicated for PW, PC, transverse, transverse/PW (when PW requires fixation), PC/PW, T-type Ilioinguinal (anterior approach) indicated for AW, AC, ACPHT, BCs Extensile approaches considered for fractures >3 wk old and complex associated fractures Combined anterior and posterior approaches Extended iliofemoral Triradiate Posterior with trochanteric osteotomy	Nerve injury (sciatic 16-33%, femoral, superior gluteal), vascular injury (inferior gluteal artery), heterotopic ossification (3-69%—consider radiation therapy or Indocin), avascular necrosis (with posterior injury), chondrolysis, post-traumatic degenerative joint disease, soft tissue degloving (Morel-Lavalle lesion), osteonecrosis (damage to medial femoral circumflex artery), malreduction (delay to surgery), bleeding (shorter time to surgery)

ADULT LOWER EXTREMITY—ANKLE FRACTURES AND DISLOCATIONS

Injury	Eponym	Classification	Treatment	Complications
Ankle fracture		Lauge-Hansen (position of foot—motion of foot relative to leg) Supination-adduction 1—Transverse lateral malleolus fracture 2—Oblique medial malleolus fracture Supination–external rotation 1—AITFL 2—Spiral fracture of lateral malleolus 3—Posteromedial fracture or PITFL injury 4—Transverse/oblique medial malleolus fracture/ deltoid injury Pronation-abduction 1—Transverse medial malleolus fracture/deltoid injury 2—Anterior and posterior ITFL/posterior malleolus 3—Oblique lateral malleolus (supramalleolar) fracture Pronation–external rotation 1—Medial malleolus fracture/deltoid ligament injury 2—AITFL/intraosseous ligament 3—High fibular fracture 4—Posterior malleolus fracture Pronation-dorsiflexion 1—Medial malleolus fracture 2—Fracture of anterior lip of tibia 3—Supramalleolar fibular fracture 4—Posteromedial fracture or PITFL injury	Rotational injury; rule out syndesmotic injury and deltoid ligament incompetence Anatomic restoration of ankle mortise; 1-mm talar shift = 42% decrease in tibiotalar contact area; isolated lateral malleolus fractures with intact deltoid ligament can be treated with short-leg walking boot; isolated medial malleolus fractures Open reduction (with) internal fixation (ORIF): displaced bimalleolar/trimalleolar ankle fractures, displaced lateral malleolus with deltoid rupture, displaced medial malleolus, syndesmotic disruption, posterior malleolus >25% ORIF fibula: lateral buttress plate with or without interfragment screw vs. posterolateral plate (peroneal irritation) ORIF medial malleolus: lag screws or tension band, buttress plate for vertical shear fractures ORIF posterior malleolus: anteroposterior/ posteroanterior lag screws, buttress plate	Wound complications (diabetics), deep infection (diabetics), stiffness, post-traumatic arthrosis, nonunion, malunion Diabetic complications: skin breakdown, loss of reduction, up to 30% amputation rate; augment fixation with transarticular screws/ pins or syndesmotic fixation
High tibia fracture	Maisonneuve	Danis-Weber (AO/OTA; position of fibular fracture) 44-A—At or below the syndesmosis 44-B—Obliquely up from joint 44-C—High fibula fracture	In general, treatment of AO/OTA type A fractures is closed; treatment of AO types B and C is ORIF. Assess syndesmosis stability.	

AITFL, anterior inferior talofibular ligament; ITFL, inferior talofibular ligament; PITFL, posterior inferior talofibular ligament.

ADULT LOWER EXTREMITY—FEMORAL SHAFT FRACTURES

Injury	Eponym/Other Name	Classification	Treatment	Complications
Femoral fracture (2.0 cm below lesser trochanter to 8 cm from knee joint)		Winquist—based on degree of comminution and amount of cortical continuity I—Transverse, comminution <25% of circumference (e.g., butterfly fragment) II—Comminution 25-50% of circumference III—>50% comminution (unstable) IV—Extensive (100%) comminution, no cortical contact, unstable V—Segmental bone loss (unstable)	Most often high-energy mechanism; early stabilization as patient status permits; most fractures are treated by closed intramedullary (IM) nail; statically locked, reamed nail for most fractures; antegrade (piriformis or trochanter) or retrograde; obesity a relative indication for trochanteric entry nail; multitrauma patients temporized with external fixation (damage control), converted to IM nail later; plate fixation for neck/shaft fractures, periprosthetic treatment (lower union, higher infection, longer time to weight bearing)	Infection (<5% closed fractures), nonunion (<5% closed fractures; treat with exchange nail vs. ORIF/ICBG), delayed union (exchange nail vs. dynamization), malalignment (malrotation, limb length discrepancy), hip pain/weakness (antegrade nail), knee pain (retrograde nail), pudendal nerve injury (excessive traction through post), missed knee ligament injury, knee stiffness (especially with distal external fixation), refracture, failure of fixation, deep venous thrombosis, pulmonary embolism, acute respiratory distress syndrome (ARDS)
Femoral neck and shaft fractures		Garden or Pauwels/Winquist (2.5-5.0% of femoral shaft fractures, BUT ≈30% are missed)	Neck takes priority; 135-degree fixed-angle device vs. parallel screws for neck, retrograde nail vs. plate for shaft; reconstructed nail for nondisplaced neck or intertrochanteric and shaft fractures	Infection, delayed union, nonunion, loss of fixation, avascular necrosis
Periprosthetic femur fracture		Vancouver	Stable prosthesis—lateral plate vs. lateral plate and allograft strut Unstable prosthesis—revision arthroplasty with uncemented long stem and lateral plate Allograft struts for bone loss	
Femoral and tibial shaft fractures	"Floating knee"		Retrograde nail for femur, antegrade nail for tibia	Multiple other injuries, fat emboli syndrome, ARDS

ADULT LOWER EXTREMITY—FOOT FRACTURES AND DISLOCATIONS

Injury	Eponym/ Other Name	Classification	Treatment	Complications
Talar neck fracture	Aviator astragalus	Hawkins and Canale I—Nondisplaced II—Displaced and subtalar dislocation/ subluxation III—Displaced and talar body dislocation IV—With talar body and head dislocation (pantalar dislocation)	Nonoperative: nondisplaced fracture, poor soft tissue; short-leg cast (SLC), non–weight bearing (NWB) for 8-12 wk (high shear stresses) Open reduction (with) internal fixation (ORIF): obtain and maintain anatomic reduction	Avascular necrosis (AVN) (especially types III/IV [Hawkins sign indicates a good prognosis]); delayed/nonunion, malunion, post-traumatic arthrosis, skin necrosis
Talar body fracture		Rare	Usually requires ORIF with or without medial malleolus osteotomy for exposure	AVN, malunion, degenerative joint disease (DJD)
Talar head fracture		Rare	Nondisplaced—splint/ice/elevation	Talonavicular DJD
Talar process fracture		Lateral process ≫ medial	SLC for 6 wk; excise if comminuted, symptomatic ORIF if large and displaced	Medial malleolus fracture (26%); rule out os trigonum (50%)
	Shepherd	Posterior process	SLC for 3-6 wk, excise symptomatic nonunions	
Subtalar dislocation		Calcaneus medial displacement (most common)	Reduce, immobilization 4 wk, open reduction if irreducibly closed	Posterior tibial tendon entrapment
Total talar dislocation		Talar and Chopart injury	Open reduction, late fusion	AVN
Calcaneal fracture (most common)		Extra-articular (anterior process, tuberosity, medial process, sustentaculum talus, body)	Principles of treatment: avoid wound complications, restore articular congruity, restore height and width; computed tomographic scan helpful	Wound complications in up to 20% of cases; diabetics and smokers at increased risk; subtalar arthritis (need for fusion), peroneal tendon subluxation, neuroma, chronic pain (heel widening, nerve entrapment), DJD, malunion, associated fractures (spine, lower extremity), heel skin slough, compartment syndrome
		Intra-articular (nondisplaced, tongue, joint depression, comminuted), (Böhler angle and crucial angle of Gissane)	Nonoperative for nondisplaced and extra-articular fractures and high-risk patients (smokers, diabetics); walking boot/cast, NWB for 8-10 wk, early range of motion, edema control	
		Sanders classification Type I—Nondisplaced fracture Type II—Two-part fracture Type III—Three-part fracture with central depression Type IV—Comminuted fracture of four or more parts	ORIF: lateral approach after soft tissue subsides, articular reduction, internal fixation with or without bone graft (controversial)	

Continued

ADULT LOWER EXTREMITY—FOOT FRACTURES AND DISLOCATIONS—cont'd

Injury	Eponym/ Other Name	Classification	Treatment	Complications
Navicular fracture		Anatomic location (body, tuberosity, avulsion), mechanism of energy (high vs. low energy) Compressed medial column	ORIF: displaced intra-articular and tuberosity fractures; stress fractures—SLC, NWB for 6 wk; avulsion fracture: treat as symptomatic sprain	Osteonecrosis (ORIF nonunion), associated with midfoot fractures
Cuboid fracture	Nutcracker	Compressed calcaneus and metatarsals (lateral column)	ORIF with bone graft or external fixation to 5th metatarsal to maintain length of lateral column SLC, NWB for 6-8 wk	Nonunion, malunion, chronic pain, stiffness
Tarsometatarsal fracture-dislocation	Lisfranc (Lisfranc ligament from base of second metatarsal [MT] to medial cuneiform)	High (forced dorsiflexion) vs. low (dorsiflexion/twisting) energy Homolateral—all five digits in same direction Partial (isolated)—first or second MT displaced Divergent—displacement in sagittal and coronal planes	Anatomic reduction of all affected joints; avoid soft tissue complications Nonoperative management for low-grade sprains, no subluxation ORIF for displaced fracture-dislocation vs. closed reduction with or without percutaneous pinning; ORIF of MT disruptions with screws is successful; consider primary arthrodesis for pure ligamentous disruptions	Chronic pain or disability (arthrodesis preferred); post-traumatic arthritis; delay in diagnosis (medial border of second MT base must align with medial border of middle cuneiform); compartment syndrome; broken implants—removal not required
Metatarsal fracture		Shaft	Majority treated nonoperatively; closed reduction with percutaneous pinning (CRPP) if needed; short-leg walking cast (SLWC) for 4 wk	Post-traumatic DJD, nonunion (most common with Jones fracture; ORIF, bone graft)
	March	Second MT stress fracture (most common)	Symptomatic; SLWC if late	
		Head	Reduction (traction and manipulation), cast; CRPP vs. ORIF if needed (avoid plantar prominent MT head)	
	Pseudo-Jones	Base avulsion (fifth MT)	SLWC for 2-3 wk, late removal of fragments if needed	
	Jones	Fifth MT base transverse fracture (differentiate from metadiaphyseal stress fracture)	6-8 wk NWB, SLC vs. percutaneous screw for faster recovery (return to play)	
Metatarsophalangeal (MTP) dislocation		Direction of dislocation (dorsal, first MTP most common)	Reduce promptly, immobilize (consider CRPP)	Post-traumatic arthrosis
Phalangeal fractures		Crush, associated nail bed injury	Majority treated nonoperatively; buddy tape for comfort, weight bearing as tolerated; ORIF of intra-articular fracture of hallux (great toe)	Post-traumatic arthrosis

ADULT LOWER EXTREMITY—HIP DISLOCATIONS

Injury	Classification	Treatment	Complications
Hip dislocation	Direction: posterior (most common), anterior, obturator; associated fractures (acetabular, femoral head)	Emergent, closed reduction (open if irreducible); computed tomography/plain films (Judet views) after reduction; traction/abduction pillow (depends on stability); weight bearing as tolerated if hip stable	Associated with increased-energy trauma and often associated with other injuries; femoral artery/nerve injuries (anterior dislocation), sciatic nerve injury (up to 20%; peroneal division most common), osteonecrosis (up to 15%), post-traumatic arthritis, recurrent dislocation (rare), post-traumatic degenerative joint disease (especially with retained fragments); instability (with >30-40% fracture of posterior wall); unrecognized femoral neck fracture

ADULT LOWER EXTREMITY—HIP FRACTURES

Injury	Classification	Treatment	Complications
Femoral head fracture	Pipkin—based on location of fracture relative to fovea and associated fractures of acetabulum or femoral neck	Restore articular congruity (open reduction [with] internal fixation [ORIF] when >1-mm step-off), restore hip stability, remove loose bodies, treat associated fractures, avoid injury to femoral head blood supply	Osteonecrosis (up to 15%), post-traumatic arthritis, sciatic nerve injury (up to 20%), recurrent dislocation (rare); Pipkin III highest rate of avascular necrosis
	Type I—Fracture below fovea	Nonoperative if small fragment, congruent joint, protected weight bearing (WB); ORIF with anterior approach (headless countersunk screws)	
	Type II—Fracture above fovea	Nonoperative if stable, nondisplaced fragment, protected WB; ORIF with anterior approach (headless countersunk screws)	
	Type III—Associated femoral neck fracture	ORIF of femoral neck and head; arthroplasty if older patient	
	Type IV—Associated acetabular fracture	ORIF of acetabulum and head via posterior approach; arthroplasty if older patient	
Femoral neck fracture	Garden (low energy in elderly)	Based on orientation of trabecular lines and displacement	
	I—Incomplete/valgus impaction (stable) II—Complete, nondisplaced (stable) III—Complete, partially displaced (unstable) IV—Complete, totally displaced (unstable)	Medical optimization; closed reduction with percutaneous pinning (CRPP) with 3 screws or sliding compression hip screw with derotation screw; prosthesis for elderly (>70 yr old physiologically), sick, pathologic fracture, Parkinson, rheumatoid arthritis, Dilantin therapy with displaced fractures (Garden III or IV); results of unipolar vs. bipolar prosthesis similar; consider total hip arthroplasty for more active patients, acetabular degenerative joint disease (higher dislocation rate than hemiarthroplasty)	Osteonecrosis (10-40%; injury to medial femoral circumflex), nonunion (10-30% of displaced fractures), infection, malunion (accept <15 degrees valgus and 10 degrees anteroposterior displacement); infection, pulmonary embolism, mortality (≈30% at 1 year; increases with advancing age, medical problems, males); cardiopulmonary decompensation with cemented stems
	Pauwels (high energy in the young)	Based on orientation of fracture line; increased vertical orientation associated with less stability; ORIF with sliding hip screw (fixed-angle device) for vertically oriented fracture lines	

ADULT LOWER EXTREMITY—HIP FRACTURES—cont'd

Injury	Classification	Treatment	Complications
Intertrochanteric fracture	Number of fracture fragments, ability to resist compressive loads when fixed Two-part: stable with little risk of collapse Three-part: intermediate stability Four-part and comminuted: least stable	Nonoperative treatment with nondisplaced fractures in compliant patients, those with high operative risk ORIF with sliding compression hip screw and side plate most reliable; lag screw in center-center position (TAD <25 mm); intramedullary (IM) nail for unstable, reverse oblique, subtrochanteric fractures; calcar-replacing arthroplasty for patients with severe osteopenia, comminution	Excessive collapse (limb shortening, medialization of shaft, sliding hip screw ≫ IM device), prominent hardware; nail cutout (TAD >25 mm); loss of fixation (increased with superolateral screws); joint penetration (screw ideally placed center-center and deep); mortality, infection
Greater trochanteric fracture	Amount of displacement	ORIF if >1 cm displacement in young patient	
Lesser trochanteric fracture	Amount of displacement	ORIF if >2 cm displacement in young athlete	Consider pathologic fracture
Subtrochanteric fracture	Russell-Taylor—based on involvement of lesser trochanter and piriformis fossa	Restore limb length, alignment, rotation; indirect reduction (open or percutaneous if necessary); avoid piriformis entry when fossa involved; fixed-angle device (95-degree blade plate) for proximal comminution	Apex anterior and varus most common deformity; nonunion (minimized with IM nail), infection (increased with soft tissue dissection)
	IA—Fracture below lesser trochanter	IM nail, standard proximal interlock	
	IB—Fracture involves lesser trochanter; greater trochanter intact	IM nail, reconstructed interlock	
	IIA—Greater trochanter involved, lesser trochanter intact	IM nail, standard proximal interlock	
	IIB—Greater and lesser trochanters involved	ORIF with fixed-angle device (95-degree blade plate) vs. IM nail, reconstructed interlock	

TAD, tip to apex distance.

ADULT LOWER EXTREMITY—KNEE FRACTURES AND DISLOCATIONS

Injury	Eponym	Classification	Treatment	Complications
Supracondylar fracture	"Hoffa" fracture (33-B3)	AO/OTA—degree of comminution and articular involvement 33-A—Extra-articular 33-B—Partially articular (unicondylar) 33-C—Intra-articular	Restore articular congruity, rigid stabilization of articular fracture, preserve vascularity, stable fixation of joint to shaft, early range of motion (ROM) Nonoperative: Brace or knee immobilizer, Non–weight bearing for 6-8 wk, closed-chain ROM at 3-4 wk Plate fixation: most fractures; fixed-angle plate for metaphyseal comminution (nonfixed: varus collapse) Retrograde intramedullary (IM) nail: extra-articular or simple intra-articular fractures, long nail preferred Arthroplasty when fixation not achievable, arthropathy present	Nonunion (soft tissue stripping of metaphyseal region), malalignment (valgus malreduction most common, nails ≫ plates), loss of fixation (varus collapse), infection, knee stiffness, degenerative joint disease (DJD), unstable fixation, deep venous thrombosis (DVT), fracture fragments from missed coronal plane ("Hoffa fracture"), prominent hardware
Periprosthetic fracture			Locked plate vs. retrograde nail (need size of intercondylar box in total knee arthroplasty for nail to fit)	
Patella fracture		Nondisplaced, transverse, proximal or distal (30%) pole, comminuted, vertical (nonoperative)	Nonoperative: nondisplaced (<2 mm) with intact extensor mechanism; hinged knee brace in extension, progress in flexion after 2-3 wk Open reduction (with) internal fixation (ORIF) (tension band wiring, screws) if patient cannot actively extend knee (extensor mechanism rupture) or there is a >2-mm separation or incongruent articular surface (>2-mm step-off); excise fragments that are extremely comminuted; avoid patellectomy	Symptomatic hardware, loss of reduction, nonunion (<5%), infection, arthrofibrosis/stiffness, quadriceps weakness, infection, DJD, extensor lag
Patella dislocation		Acute, recurrent, subluxation, habitual, usually lateral	Immobilize, controlled motion for 6 wk; arthroscopy for displaced or osteochondral fracture; recurrent: lateral release, medial plication (repair/reconstruct MPFL); bony transplant if abnormal Q angle. Avoid surgery in those with habitual dislocation.	Redislocation

ADULT LOWER EXTREMITY—KNEE FRACTURES AND DISLOCATIONS—cont'd

Injury	Eponym	Classification	Treatment	Complications
Knee dislocation		Anterior (30-40%), posterior (30-40%), lateral, medial, rotatory (anteromedial, anterolateral, posteromedial, posterolateral) Schenck anatomic classification: KD I—Dislocation with anterior cruciate ligament (ACL) or posterior cruciate ligament (PCL) intact KD II—Torn ACL/PCL KD III—Torn ACL/PCL and either posterolateral corner (PLC) or posteromedial corner (PMC) KD IV—Torn ACL/PCL/PLC/PMC KD V—Fracture-dislocation	May present spontaneously reduced—easily missed; reduce dislocations emergently; open reduction if needed (posterolateral rotation); arteriogram based on physical exam findings (absent/asymmetrical pulses); repair vascular injuries (5-15%); ligament repair (within 2-3 wk) or reconstruction, allograft vs. autograft, early motion	Vascular injury (5-15%, highest with KD-IV; ankle-brachial index >0.9 associated with intact artery); neurologic injury (tibial/peroneal nerve), stiffness/ arthrofibrosis (most common complication), ligamentous laxity
Quadriceps rupture		Generally older than 40 and metabolic disorders (CRF, RA, steroid use), M $\gg$ F	Incomplete rupture: nonoperative management Complete: repair through osseous drill holes or suture anchors; repair acutely: >2 wk or $\leq$5-cm retraction	Strength deficit; stiffness, inability to resume preinjury athletic/recreational activity; bilateral ruptures (identify underlying medical problem, repair both); DVT; chronic ruptures (allograft reconstruction, quadriceps tendon lengthening)
Patella tendon rupture		Younger than 40, overload of extensor mechanism; increased risk with metabolic disorders (rheumatoid arthritis, diabetes mellitus, infection)	Direct repair with nonabsorbable suture and locking (Krackow) stitch through drill holes; can protect repair with cerclage	Missed diagnosis (high-riding patella seen on radiographs), stiffness, extensor weakness

MPFL, medial patellofemoral ligament.

ADULT LOWER EXTREMITY—PELVIC FRACTURES

Injury	Eponym	Classification	Treatment	Complications
Pelvic fracture			Emergent management (advanced trauma life support, resuscitation, embolization of bleeding arteries if necessary, binder/external fixation/traction/pelvic C-clamp based on injury pattern)	
		Young and Burgess		Posterior skin slough, life-threatening hemorrhage, gastrointestinal injury, genitourinary injury (bladder, urethrea, impotency), neurologic injury, nonunion, post-traumatic degenerative joint disease, pain, deep venous thrombosis, pulmonary embolism, loss of reduction, sepsis, thrombophlebitis, malunion (leg-length discrepancy, sitting problems), vascular injuries (including aortic rupture), SI pain; APC-III highest rate of associated injury
		Lateral compression (LC)		
		I (most common)—Transverse rami fracture and sacral compression fracture	Protected weight bearing (WB), pain control	
		II—Rami fracture and posterior iliac wing fracture	Protected WB or delayed open reduction with internal fixation (ORIF)	
		III—Symphysis or rami and anterior and posterior sacroiliac (SI) ligament torn	Based on contralateral injury (ORIF of unstable injuries)	
		Anteroposterior compression (APC)		
		I—Symphysis (<2 cm) or rami (vertical) and anterior SI ligament stretched	Bed rest, early mobilization, pain control	
		II—Symphysis or rami and anterior SI ligament torn	Acute external fixation/anterior ORIF if concurrent laparotomy	
		III—Symphysis or rami and anterior and posterior SI ligament torn	Acute external fixation/anterior ORIF if concurrent laparotomy; posterior SI ORIF	
	Malgaigne	Vertical shear—Anterior and posterior vertical displacement	Acute external fixation/anterior ORIF if concurrent laparotomy; posterior SI ORIF (SI screws, anterior SI plate, posterior transiliac sacral bars, spinal-pelvic fixation)	
		Combined mechanical—Combination of other injuries	Based on injuries; ORIF if posterior SI displaced	
Sacral fracture		Denis—Fracture location relative to foramen		
		Stable, nondisplaced	Nonoperative (weight bearing as tolerated if fracture incomplete, toe-touch weight bearing for complete fracture)	Neurologic (highest with zone II fractures), chronic low-back pain, malunion
		Unstable, displaced (>1 cm)	Percutaneous SI screws, posterior ORIF, transiliac sacral bars, open foraminal decompression for neuron injury with zone II fractures	

ADULT LOWER EXTREMITY—TIBIA FRACTURES AND DISLOCATIONS

Injury	Eponym/ Other Name	Classification	Treatment	Complications
Tibial plateau fracture		Schatzker classification I—Split II—Split depression III—Pure depression IV—Medial plateau split V—Bicondylar with intact metaphysis VI—Bicondylar with metaphyseal/diaphyseal dissociation AO/OTA classification 41-A—Extra-articular fracture 41-B—Partial articular fracture (Shatzker I–IV) 41-C—Complete articular/bicondylar (Shatzker V and VI)	Magnetic resonance imaging can change treatment or classification in most cases (soft tissue injury); medial cruciate ligament > anterior cruciate ligament (ACL); lateral > bicondylar > medial (think dislocation with medial); spanning external fixation for high-energy injuries (soft tissue stabilization) Nonoperative: stable knees (<10 degrees varus/valgus in full extension, <3 mm articular step-off); cast brace, early range of motion (ROM), delayed weight bearing for 4-6 wk Open reduction with external fixation (ORIF) if articular step-off >3 mm, condylar widening >5 mm, knee unstable, medial and bicondylar; plate fixation (locked vs nonlocked, single vs. dual [posteromedial] incision) vs. external fixation (bicondylar or severe soft tissue injury, wires >15 mm from joint)	Degenerative joint disease (DJD), infection (surgical approach most important factor), malunion (varus collapse with non-op or conventional plates/bicondylar fracture), ligament instability, peroneal nerve injury, compartment syndrome, stiffness, loss of reduction, avascular necrosis
Tibial spine fracture		I—Anterior tilt II—Complete anterior tilt III—No contact A—No rotation B—Rotated	I/II/IIIA closed reduction, long-leg cast (LLC) for 6 wk if knee can be brought into full extension; IIIB and all irreducible types require open reduction	Block to motion (arthroscopic loose-body removal), ACL laxity
Tibial tubercle fracture			ORIF with screw or staple	Loss of fixation, quadriceps weakness
Subcondylar tibial fracture		Stable	Cast immobilization	Arterial injury, decreased ROM
		Displaced	ORIF with buttress plate	
Tibial stress fracture		Upper one third (recruits)	Modify activity for 6-10 wk	Progression to complete fracture
Tibial shaft fracture		AO/OTA classification 42-A—Simple, two parts 42-B—Butterfly comminution 42-C—Comminuted; no direct contact between proximal and distal fragments Gustillo and Anderson—open fracture grade Grade I—No periosteal stripping, <1-cm wound Grade II—No periosteal stripping, >1-cm wound Grade IIIA—Periosteal stripping, no flap required Grade IIIB—Periosteal stripping, flap required Grade IIIC—Periosteal stripping, flap required, vascular injury requiring repair	Most respond to closed reduction, LLC, wedge as needed, PTB at 6-8 wk; intramedullary (IM) nail for transverse oblique fracture of mid–one third or segmental and also for vascular injury, bilateral injury, pathologic fractures, severe ligamentous injuries to knee (statically locked IM nail); open fractures: unreamed nail up to and including some IIIB injuries, early flap coverage, delayed bone grafting. Consider early amputation in grade IIIC injuries, posterior tibial nerve injury, warm ischemia >6 hr, and severe ipsilateral foot injury (unreconstructible limb).	Delayed union (>20 wk; increased with greater initial displacement and middle-third fractures; treatment includes fibulectomy and posterolateral bone graft), nonunion (posterolateral bone graft or reamed IM nail), infection (flap/graft or amputation), malunion (varus/valgus, shortening [accept <5 degrees varus/valgus, <10 degrees anteroposterior angulation]), vascular injuries (upper one fourth of anterior tibial artery), compartment syndrome, peroneal nerve injury, CRPS
Tibial plafond fracture	Pilon	Ruedi and Allgöwer I—Minimally displaced II—Incongruous III—Comminuted	LLC and non–weight bearing ORIF if displaced and ankle involved; consider minimally invasive small-pin external fixation techniques	DJD (may require late fusion), infection, varus/valgus angulation, skin slough
Fibular shaft fracture		Mid to lower one third (athletes)	Cast only if needed for pain relief	Missed syndesmotic injury
Proximal fibula fracture			Open if unstable	Injury to biceps, peroneal nerve
Proximal tibia-fibula dislocation		Anterior (most common), posterior, superior	Reduce (90 degrees flexion), ORIF fails with recurrence	
Chondral/osteochondral fracture		Endogenous vs. exogenous	Arthroscopic evaluation of locked, acute condylar defects; remove small fragments (pin large fragments)	DJD

CRPS, complex regional pain syndrome; PTB, patella tendon–bearing cast.

PEDIATRIC UPPER EXTREMITY—ELBOW TRAUMA

Injury	Eponym/Other Name	Classification	Treatment	Complications
Supracondylar fracture (6-8 yr old)		I—Extension (98%), nondisplaced	Immobilize 3 wk Minimally displaced (<2 mm), splint	Nerve injury (AIN and radial), vascular injury (1%), decreased ROM; if pulse present but then lost, explore; if pulse present but then lost, explore; if no pulse present but pink hand, watch; if no pulse present and cold, explore.
		II—Displaced (posterior cortex intact)	Reduce; cast vs. CRPP (must re-create Baumann angle)	
		III—Displaced (posterior periosteal hinge intact)	Reduce; CRPP versus open pinning	
		IV—Displaced (posterior periosteal hinge disrupted)	Reduce; CRPP versus open pinning	HO, cubitus varus (5-10%), ipsilateral fractures
		Flexion (distal fragment anterior)	Reduce; CRPP versus ORIF	Nerve injury (ulnar), malunion (decreased extension)
Lateral condyle fracture (6 yr old)		Milch I—SH IV Milch II—SH II into trochlea	Minimally displaced (<2 mm), splint; displaced, ORIF with pins or cannulated screws	Overgrowth/spur "fishtail" deformity, nonunion, cubitus valgus, AVN, ulnar nerve palsy
Medial condyle fracture (9-14 yr old)		Nondisplaced— <10 mm displacement		Cubitus varus, AVN
		Displaced— >10 mm displacement	Minimally displaced, splint Displaced, ORIF	
Entire distal humeral physis fracture (<7 yr old)		A—Infant (SH I) B—7 mo–3 yr old (SH I) C—3-7 yr old (SH II)	Closed reduction, LAC; displaced, CRPP	Child abuse, common late diagnosis, cubitus varus
Medial epicondylar apophysis fracture (11 yr old)	Little Leaguer's elbow	I—Acute injuries		Highly associated with elbow dislocation (50%), valgus instability, loss of extension
		A—Nondisplaced	Immobilize 1 wk	
		B—Minimally displaced	Immobilize 1 wk	
		C—Significantly displaced (may be dislocated)	ORIF for valgus instability; otherwise, early ROM	
		D—Entrapment of fragment in joint	Manipulative extraction, ORIF (especially with ulnar nerve entrapment)	
		E—Fracture through epicondylar apophysis	Immobilization vs. ORIF	
		II—Chronic tension stress injury	Change in throwing activities	
T condylar fracture		Based on fracture	ORIF with cannulated screws	Decreased ROM
Radial head and neck fractures (<4 yr old)		A—SH I or II physeal fracture B—SH IV fracture C—Transmetaphyseal fracture D and E—With elbow dislocation	Immobilize if <60 degrees in pronation/supination; ORIF if markedly displaced or >60 degrees primarily	Decreased ROM, radial head overgrowth, neck notching, AVN, synostosis, nonunion
Proximal olecranon physis fracture (rare)		I—Physeal-metaphyseal border (younger children) II—Physis with large metaphyseal fragment (older children)		
Olecranon metaphysis fracture		A—Flexion	If undisplaced (<3 mm), immobilize 3 wk; ORIF if defect	Rare: delay/nonunion
		B—Extension	Reduction in extension	
		C—Shear	Immobilize in hyperflexion	ORIF if periosteal tear
Elbow dislocation (11-20 yr old)		Based on direction of dislocation	Reduction and cast for <2 wk	Watch for associated fractures and nerve injuries (ulnar >median), HO, recurrent dislocation.
Radial head subluxation (15 mo-3 yr old)	Nursemaid's elbow	Stretching of annular ligaments	Reduce (supination/flexion)	

AIN, anterior interosseous nerve; AVN, avascular necrosis; CRPP, closed reduction/percutaneous pinning; HO, heterotopic ossification; LAC, long-arm cast; ORIF, open reduction with internal fixation; ROM, range of motion; SH, Salter-Harris.

SALTER-HARRIS CLASSIFICATION OF PHYSEAL INJURIES

Type	Description	Prognosis
I	Transverse fractures through the physis	Excellent
II	Fractures through the physis, with metaphyseal fragment	Excellent
III	Fractures through the physis and epiphysis	Good but with the potential for intra-articular deformity; may require ORIF
IV	Fractures through the epiphysis, physis, and metaphysis	Good but unstable; fragment requires ORIF
V	Crush injury to the physis	Poor, with growth arrest
VI	Injury to the perichondrial ring	Good; may cause angular deformities

ORIF, open reduction with internal fixation.

PEDIATRIC UPPER EXTREMITY—HAND AND WRIST TRAUMA

Injury	Eponym/ Other Name	Classification	Treatment	Complications
Phalanx fracture	(Watch for mallet equivalent)	Based on phalanx and SH classification	Closed reduction for most; ORIF if condylar, SH III/IV >25 degrees if <10 yr old, >10 degrees if >10 yr old; dynamic traction for pilon equivalents	Residual deformities, tendon imbalance, nail deformities
Metacarpal fracture		Based on location	Reduce; ORIF if irreducible	Avascular necrosis of metacarpal head
Thumb MC fracture	Type D = Bennett equivalent	Type A—metaphyseal Type B—SH II (medial) Type C—SH II (lateral) Type D—SH III	Closed reduction except for type D, which requires ORIF	
IP dislocation			Closed reduction and splint; ORIF if unable to obtain or maintain a congruous reduction	
MCP dislocation			Attempt closed reduction; ORIF if irreducible	
CMC dislocation			Reduce with finger traps; CRPP with K-wire to carpus and adjacent MC	
Distal radius fracture		SH fractures I-V	CRPP types III and IV	Deformity, loss of reduction, infection with open fracture, Volkmann contracture, growth arrest, malunion, refracture, TFCC tears, carpal tunnel syndrome
	Torus	Tension side intact	SAC for 3 wk	
	Greenstick	Tension side with plastic deformation	Reduce if angulation >10 degrees	
	Complete	Both cortices disrupted	Reduce and place in LAC	

CMC, carpometacarpal; CRPP, closed reduction with percutaneous pinning; LAC, long-arm cast; MC, metacarpal; MCP, metacarpophalangeal joint; ORIF, open reduction with internal fixation; SAC, short-arm cast; SH, Salter-Harris; TFCC, triangular fibrocartilage complex.

PEDIATRIC UPPER EXTREMITY—RADIAL AND ULNAR SHAFT TRAUMA

Injury	Eponym/Other Name	Classification	Treatment	Complications
Radius and ulna fractures	"Both-bone"	Greenstick, compression, complete	Correct rotation, with pronation/supination and <10 degrees angulation: LAC 3-4 wk if <10 yr old; bayonet apposition OK if growth remains	Refracture, limb ischemia, malunion (especially in <10 yr old with inadequate reduction), nerve injury, synostosis
Plastic deformation		Based on bones involved (ulna >radius)	Reduction with pressure as a fulcrum, the most deformed bone first; must reduce >20 degrees in 4 yr old, less in older children	Persistence of deformity
Ulna fracture and radial head dislocation	Monteggia	Type I—Ulna angulation and radial head anterior (extension)	Reduce (traction flexion); LAC, 100 degrees flexion in supination	Late diagnosis (reconstruct annular ligament), decreased ROM
		Type II—Ulna angulation and radial head posterior (flexion)	Reduce (traction extension); LAC in some extension	Missed wrist injury, nonunion, persistent radial head dislocation, periarticular ossification
		Type III—Ulna anterior angulation, radial head lateral (adduction)	Reduce (extension); LAC, 90 degrees flexion in supination	
		Type IV—Ulna and proximal (one third) radius fracture (both anterior angulation)	Reduce (supinate); may require ORIF	
Radial head dislocation (anterior)	Monteggia equivalent		Supination and pressure on radial head; LAC, 100 degrees flexion in supination	Synostosis, PIN injury, loss of reduction
Ulna and radial neck fractures	Check for Monteggia equivalent		Reduce (traction, pressure on radial head, varus stress); LAC, 90 degrees flexion	
Ulna and proximal radius fractures	Check for Monteggia equivalent		Reduce (traction supination); LAC, 90 degrees in supination	
Radius fracture and distal radioulnar dislocation	Galeazzi		Reduce (traction supination if ulna dorsal, pronation if ulna volar); ORIF if >12 yr old or reduction fails	Malunion, nerve injury (AIN), RU subluxation, loss of radial bow

AIN, anterior interosseous nerve; LAC, long-arm cast; ORIF, open reduction with internal fixation; PIN, posterior interosseous nerve; ROM, range of motion; RU, radioulnar.

PEDIATRIC UPPER EXTREMITY—SHOULDER TRAUMA

Injury	Classification	Treatment	Complications
Humeral shaft fracture	Neonate	Small splint or splint to side	Compartment syndrome, radial nerve palsy, rotational palsy
	<3 yr old	Collar and cuff OK	
	3-12 yr old	Sarmiento brace	
	>12 yr old	Sarmiento brace	
Proximal humeral physis fracture	SH (I most common in <5 yr old)	Sling if minimally displaced, gentle manipulation for displaced fractures, CRPP vs. ORIF for <50% apposition, >45 degrees angulation	
Proximal humeral metaphysis fracture (common)	Based on location	Sling	
Midshaft clavicle fracture	≤2 yr old	Supportive sling if symptomatic	Rare: malunion or nonunion, neurovascular compromise
	>2 yr old	Figure 8 brace vs. sling	
Medial clavicle fracture	Usually SH I or II physeal separations	Sling for 1 wk	
Lateral clavicle fracture	I—Nondisplaced; intact AC and CC ligaments	Sling vs. figure 8 brace	
	IIA—Clavicle displaced superiorly; fracture medial to CC ligament	Type II may need ORIF	
	IIB—Clavicle displaced superiorly; conoid ligaments tear		
AC joint injury	Same as adult	Same as adult	Watch for coracoid fracture
SC joint injury	Anterior and posterior	Same as adult	
Clavicle dislocation (rare)	Anterior and posterior	ORIF with repair of periosteal tube	
Scapula fracture	Anterior and posterior	Same as adult	
Glenohumeral dislocation	Anterior and posterior	Initial immobilization followed by rehabilitation; reconstruction for recurrent instability	Recent research shows >60% chance of redislocation when patient is <21 yr old

AC, acromioclavicular; CC, coracoclavicular; ORIF, open reduction with internal fixation; CRPP, closed reduction with percutaneous pinning; SC, sternoclavicular; SH, Salter-Harris.

PEDIATRIC SPINE TRAUMA

Injury	Eponym/ Other Name	Classification	Treatment	Complications
Occiput-C1 dissociations			Reduced with traction; craniovertebral fusion later	Often fatal
C1-C2 dissociations		Traumatic ligament disruption	Reduce in extension, immobilize with halo for 8-12 wk	Vertebral artery is at risk with surgery
	Grisel syndrome	Ligament laxity from local inflammation	Traction; immobilize for 6-8 wk	
	Rotatory subluxation	I—Without C1 shift II—<5 mm C1 anterior shift III—>5 mm C1 anterior shift IV—Posterior shift Odontoid physeal or os odontoideum	Traction; if no improvement, then open reduction and fusion	
C2-C3 dislocation		True vs. pseudo (more likely)		
Cervical facet dislocation			Same as in adults	
Thoracic and lumbar fractures		Same as in adults	Same as in adults	
Spondylosis		Stress fracture of pars (likely at L5-S1)	Acute: immobilize in brace; otherwise, surgical treatment; fusion for refractory cases	
Spinal cord injury without radiographic abnormality (SCIWORA)		Spinal cord injury without radiographic abnormality	Evaluation with magnetic resonance imaging and supportive treatment	Scoliosis (especially <8 yr old)

PEDIATRIC LOWER EXTREMITY—ANKLE AND FOOT TRAUMA

Injury	Eponym/ Other Name	Classification	Treatment	Complications
Ankle fracture		SH and Dias-Tachdjian	If SH I or II injury, treat with SLWC; if SH III or IV injury, treat with CRPP vs. ORIF	Angular deformity, bony bridge (poor prognosis with distal tibia), LLD, DJD, rotational deformity, AVN
	Juvenile Tillaux	SH III of lateral tibial physis (because distal-medial tibial physis is closed in this age group)	May use LLC if <2 mm displacement; if greater, treat with ORIF and visualization of joint line	
	Wagstaff	SH III of distal fibular physis	Closed reduction and cast; ORIF if necessary	
	Triplane	Complex SH IV, with components in all three planes	ORIF if >2 mm articular step-off (fixation achieved parallel to physis in metaphysis and epiphysis)	Must use CT to delineate fracture
Talus fracture		Same as in adults	Closed reduction and cast unless >5 mm or 5 degrees of displacement	AVN
Calcaneus fracture	Essex-Lopresti	Same as in adults	Same as in adults	
Tarsometatarsal fracture		Fracture of base of second metatarsal and cuboid fracture	Closed reduction vs. CRPP if unstable	
Base of the fifth metatarsal fracture	Jones/pseudo-Jones	Same as in adults	Same as in adults	Nonunion

AVN, avascular necrosis; CRPP, closed reduction/percutaneous pinning; CT, computed tomography; DJD, degenerative joint disease; LLC, long-leg cast; LLD, leg length discrepancy; ORIF, open reduction with internal fixation; SH, Salter-Harris; SLWC, short-leg walking cast.

PEDIATRIC LOWER EXTREMITY—FEMORAL SHAFT TRAUMA

Injury	Classification	Treatment	Complications
Femur fracture (including subtrochanteric fractures)	≤6 yr old	Spica cast; may need short period of traction if shortened >2 cm and followed by spica casting	LLD: Angular deformity (avoid >10 degrees frontal and >10 degrees sagittal malalignment)
	6-13 yr old	Current trend to use flexible titanium nails, with possible additional immobilization, but may also use external fixation (higher refracture rate), plate (need to remove, causes large scar formation), or traction (rare)	Rotational deformity (>10 degrees); expect 0.9 cm overgrowth in <10 yr old
	≥14 yr old	IM nail (trochanteric entry)	AVN reported with IM nails in children with growth remaining

AVN, avascular necrosis; IM, intramedullary; LLD, leg length discrepancy.

PEDIATRIC LOWER EXTREMITY—HIP TRAUMA

Injury	Classification	Treatment	Complications
Hip fracture	Delbet		
	IA—Transepiphyseal with dislocation	Closed reduction or ORIF with pin	AVN close to 100%
	IB—Transepiphyseal without dislocation	CRPP with spica	AVN in up to 60%
	II—Transcervical	CRPP with spica	Coxa vara (25%): treat with subtrochanteric valgus osteotomy
	IIIA—Cervical trochanteric (displaced)	CRPP with spica	Nonunion (6%)
	IIIB—Cervical trochanteric (nondisplaced)	Spica cast in abduction	Growth arrest
	IV—Intertrochanteric	Spica cast; ORIF if unstable	May cross physis if it creates greater fracture stability
Femoral neck stress fracture	Devas		
	Superior transverse	CRPP (otherwise is displaced)	Displacement causes more problems; varus deformities
	Inferior (compressive)	NWB	
Traumatic dislocation	Posterior or anterior	Closed reduction; open if joint incongruous	AVN (10%), recurrent dislocation, HO, DJD

AVN, avascular necrosis; CRPP, closed reduction/percutaneous pinning; DJD, degenerative joint disease; HO, heterotopic ossification; NWB, non–weight bearing; ORIF, open reduction with internal fixation.

PEDIATRIC LOWER EXTREMITY—KNEE TRAUMA

Injury	Eponym/ Other Name	Classification	Treatment	Complications
Distal femoral epiphysis fracture	"Wagon wheel"	SH I-IV (II most common)	Closed reduction: LLC; CRPP in SH III or IV; open if soft tissue interposition or displaced III and IV	Popliteal artery or peroneal nerve injury, recurrent displacement; growth plate injuries because of undulating physis
Proximal tibial epiphysis fracture		SH I-IV (II most common)	Nondisplaced: LLC in 30° of flexion; displaced: CRPP	Popliteal artery injury, growth plate injury
Floating knee		Letts		Infection, nonunion, malunion, injuries
		A—Both fractures diaphyseal	ORIF in one, closed reduction in the other	
		B—One fracture diaphyseal and one metaphyseal	ORIF of diaphyseal and closed reduction of metaphyseal	
		C—One fracture diaphyseal and one epiphyseal	CRPP of epiphyseal and ORIF of diaphyseal	
		D—One fracture open and one closed	Débride/external fixation, open and closed reductions of closed fracture	
		E—Both fractures open	Débride/external fixation of both	
Tibial tubercle avulsion fracture (14-16 yr old in jumping sport)		Odgen		
		1—Small distal piece fractured	If minimally displaced with extension, then cast; otherwise, ORIF	Genu recurvatum, decreased ROM, laxity
		2—Fracture at junction of primary and secondary ossification centers		
		3—Fracture through one epiphysis (SH III)		
Tibial spine fracture (most common hemarthrosis in preadolescent)		Meyers and McKeever		
		I—Incomplete/ nondisplaced	Attempt closed reduction in extension for all; if it remains displaced, then may use arthroscope and ACL guide to fix with suture	Meniscal entrapment
		II—Hinged (posterior rim intact)		
		III—Completely displaced		
Patella fracture		Nondisplaced	Aspiration and cast vs. brace in 5 degrees of flexion	Patella alta, extensor lag, infection
		Displaced (>2 mm)	ORIF with tension band	
	Sleeve fracture	Avulsion of the distal pole and articular cartilage	ORIF with tension band	
Femorotibial dislocation		Same as in adults	Same as in adults: Arteriogram	Popliteal artery injury
Patella dislocation		Same as in adults	Closed-reduction cast for 3 wk; consider fixing MPFL; open if fragment	Predisposition: Down syndrome, arthrogryposis

ACL, anterior cruciate ligament; CRPP, closed reduction/percutaneous pinning; LLC, long-leg cast; MPFL, medial patellofemoral ligament; ORIF, open reduction with internal fixation; ROM, range of motion; SH, Salter-Harris.

PEDIATRIC LOWER EXTREMITY—PELVIC TRAUMA

Injury	Eponym	Classification (Key and Cornwell)	Treatment	Complications
Pelvic fracture				In general, less than adults because of remodeling
		I—Ring intact		
		Avulsions (ASIS, AIIS, IT)	BR flexed hip for 2 wk; guarded WB for 4 wk	Loss of reduction, delayed union
		Pubis/ischium	BR 3-7 days; limited WB for 4 wk	DJD, malunion, organ injury
	Duverney	Iliac wing	BR with leg abducted; progress to full WB	Sacral nerve injury
		Sacrum/coccyx	BR 3-6 wk, if severe (sacral)	
		II—Single break in ring		
		Ipsilateral rami	BR 2-4 wk; non-WB	
		Symphysis pubis	BR with sling or spica	
		SI joint (rare)	BR with progressive WB	
		III—Double break in ring		
	Straddle	Bilateral pubic rami	BR with flexed hip 2-4 wk	Often unstable, with associated injuries
	Malgaigne	Anterior and posterior ring with migration	Skeletal traction; external fixator for 3-6 wk	
		IV—Acetabular fractures		
		Small fragment with dislocation	BR followed by progressive ambulation	
		Linear: Nondisplaced	Treat associated pelvic fracture	
		Linear: Hip unstable	Skeletal traction; ORIF if incongruous	
		Central	Lateral traction for reduction; ORIF if severe	HO, especially if severe

AIIS, anterior inferior iliac spine; ASIS, anterior superior iliac spine; BR, bed rest; DJD, degenerative joint disease; HO, heterotopic ossification; IT, ischial tuberosity; ORIF, open reduction with internal fixation; SI, sacroiliac; WB, weight bearing.

PEDIATRIC LOWER EXTREMITY—TIBIAL SHAFT TRAUMA

Injury	Eponym/ Other Name	Classification	Treatment	Complications
Tibia-fibula fracture	Greenstick	Incomplete	LLC in slight flexion for 6-8 wk unless >10 degrees AP or >5 degrees varus/valgus; then must do manipulation	Angular deformity (valgus)
		Complete	Closed reduction and cast	LLD (may see overgrowth with <10 yr old), malrotation, vascular injury
Tibial spiral fracture	Toddler	Spiral fracture in <6 yr old	LLC for 3-4 wk	
Bike spoke injury		Soft tissue disruption	Admit and observe	Compartment syndrome; need for soft tissue coverage
Proximal tibial metaphysis fracture	Cozen	Greenstick in 3-6 yr old (complete in older children)	LLC in varus for 6 wk	Genu valgum, arterial injury, physeal injury

AP, anteroposterior; LLC, long-leg cast; LLD, leg length discrepancy.